Postgraduate Ophthalmology
An Exam Preparatory Manual

Postgraduate Ophthalmology
An Exam Preparatory Manual

Editors

Prafulla Kumar Maharana
MD DNB
Associate Professor
Department of Ophthalmology
Dr Rajendra Prasad Centre for Ophthalmic Sciences
All India Institute of Medical Sciences
New Delhi, India
Email: drpraful13@gmail.com

Ritu Nagpal
MD FLVPEI (Cornea)
Consultant
Eye7 Hospitals
New Delhi, India
Email: doc.ritunagpal@gmail.com

Pranita Sahay
MD (AIIMS, New Delhi) FRCOphth (London) FRCS (Glasgow) FICO (Cornea) FAICO (Refractive Surgery) DNB
Consultant
Department of Ophthalmology
(Cataract, Cornea and Refractive Surgery Services)
Centre for Sight Eye Hospital
New Delhi, India
Email: drpranitasahay@gmail.com

Namrata Sharma
MD FRCOphth FRCSEd
Professor
Department of Ophthalmology
(Cataract, Cornea and Refractive Surgery Services)
Dr Rajendra Prasad Centre for Ophthalmic Sciences
All India Institute of Medical Sciences
New Delhi, India
Email: namrata.sharma@gmail.com

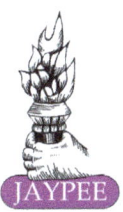

JAYPEE BROTHERS MEDICAL PUBLISHERS
The Health Sciences Publisher
New Delhi | London

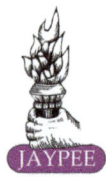 **Jaypee Brothers Medical Publishers (P) Ltd**

Headquarters
Jaypee Brothers Medical Publishers (P) Ltd
EMCA House, 23/23-B
Ansari Road, Daryaganj
New Delhi 110 002, India
Landline: +91-11-23272143, +91-11-23272703
+91-11-23282021, +91-11-23245672
Email: jaypee@jaypeebrothers.com

Corporate Office
Jaypee Brothers Medical Publishers (P) Ltd
4838/24, Ansari Road, Daryaganj
New Delhi 110 002, India
Phone: +91-11-43574357
Fax: +91-11-43574314
Email: jaypee@jaypeebrothers.com

Overseas Office
JP Medical Ltd
83 Victoria Street, London
SW1H 0HW (UK)
Phone: +44 20 3170 8910
Fax: +44 (0)20 3008 6180
Email: info@jpmedpub.com

Website: www.jaypeebrothers.com
Website: www.jaypeedigital.com

© 2023, Jaypee Brothers Medical Publishers

The views and opinions expressed in this book are solely those of the original contributor(s)/author(s) and do not necessarily represent those of editor(s) or publisher of the book.

All rights reserved. No part of this publication may be reproduced, stored or transmitted in any form or by any means, electronic, mechanical, photo copying, recording or otherwise, without the prior permission in writing of the publishers.

All brand names and product names used in this book are trade names, service marks, trademarks or registered trademarks of their respective owners. The publisher is not associated with any product or vendor mentioned in this book.

Medical knowledge and practice change constantly. This book is designed to provide accurate, authoritative information about the subject matter in question. However, readers are advised to check the most current information available on procedures included and check information from the manufacturer of each product to be administered, to verify the recommended dose, formula, method and duration of administration, adverse effects and contra indications. It is the responsibility of the practitioner to take all appropriate safety precautions. Neither the publisher nor the author(s)/editor(s) assume any liability for any injury and/or damage to persons or property arising from or related to use of material in this book.

This book is sold on the understanding that the publisher is not engaged in providing professional medical services. If such advice or services are required, the services of a competent medical professional should be sought.

Every effort has been made where necessary to contact holders of copyright to obtain permission to reproduce copyright material. If any have been inadvertently overlooked, the publisher will be pleased to make the necessary arrangements at the first opportunity.

Inquiries for bulk sales may be solicited at: jaypee@jaypeebrothers.com

Postgraduate Ophthalmology: An Exam Preparatory Manual

First Edition: **2023**

ISBN: 978-93-5465-494-7

Dedication

I would like to dedicate this book to the ophthalmology students across India who have given me tremendous love and respect for my previous books.

– **Prafulla Kumar Maharana**

I would like to dedicate this book to my Parents.

– **Ritu Nagpal**

I would like to dedicate this book to my Parents.

– **Pranita Sahay**

I would like to dedicate this book to my Parents.

– **Namrata Sharma**

Contributors

Aafreen Bari MD
Senior Resident
Dr Rajendra Prasad Centre for
Ophthalmic Sciences
All India Institute of Medical Sciences
New Delhi, India
Email: aafreen.aiims@gmail.com

Adarsh Shashni MD
Senior Resident
Dr Rajendra Prasad Centre for
Ophthalmic Sciences
All India Institute of Medical Sciences
New Delhi, India
Email: shashni009@gmail.com

Adit Gupta MD
Consultant
Mumbai Eye Plastic Surgery
Mumbai, Maharashtra, India
Email: draditgupta@yahoo.in

Aditi Dubey MS
Associate Professor
Gandhi Medical College
Bhopal, Madhya Pradesh, India
Email: Aditi.dubey1585@gmail.com

Akruti Desai MD
Associate Faculty
Shantilal Shanghvi Eye Institute
Mumbai, Maharashtra, India
Email: desai.akruti@gmail.com

Akshay Gopinathan Nair DNB
Consultant
Department of Ophthalmic Plastic
Surgery and Ocular Oncology Services
Advanced Eye Hospital and Institute
Navi Mumbai, Maharashtra, India
Email: akshaygn@gmail.com

Akshaya Balaji MD DNB
Senior Resident
Department of Cornea, Cataract and
Refractive Services
Dr Rajendra Prasad Centre for
Ophthalmic Sciences
All India Institute of Medical Sciences
New Delhi, India
Email: akshayabalajiv@gmail.com

Alisha Kishore MD
Assistant Professor
Government Medical College
and Hospital
Chandigarh, India
Email: alishakishore7@gmail.com

Ananya Parampalli Ravindra MD
Senior Resident
Department of Cornea, Cataract and
Refractive Services
Dr Rajendra Prasad Centre for
Ophthalmic Sciences
All India Institute of Medical Sciences
New Delhi, India
Email: ananyaherle96@gmail.com

Anasua G Kapoor MD
Head of Campus and Consultant
Department of Ophthalmic Plastic
Surgery and Ocular Oncology
LV Prasad Eye Institute
Vijayawada, Andhra Pradesh, India
Email: anasua21@yahoo.com

Anushka Agarwala MBBS
Junior Resident
Dr Rajendra Prasad Centre for
Ophthalmic Sciences
All India Institute of Medical Sciences
New Delhi, India
Email: anushka.agarwalla@gmail.com

Archita Singh MD FAICO FICO
Consultant
Department of Cornea, Cataract and
Refractive Surgery
ASG Eye Hospital
Indore, Madhya Pradesh, India
Email: architasingh88@gmail.com

Arpit Sharma MD
Fellow
Department Vitreoretinal Surgery
Aravind Eye Hospital, Madurai
Email: arpitpolistes@gmail.com

Ashi Morawala MD
Consultant
Pushpagiri Eye Hospital
Hyderabad, Telangana, India
Email: ashi.morawala@gmail.com

Athul S Puthalath MD DNB MNAMS FICO
Fellow
Department of Retina Vitreous Services
Aravind Eye Hospital
Madurai, Tamil Nadu, India
Email: asputhalath@gmail.com

Barkha Gupta
MD MCh (Cornea, Cataract and Refractive
Surgery) FICO
Consultant
Department of Cornea and
Refractive Services
Dr Agarwal Eye Institute
Chennai, Tamil Nadu, India
Email: barkha19gupta@gmail.com

Bhagabat Nayak MD FAICO
Associate Professor
All India Institute of Medical Sciences
Bhubaneswar, Odisha, India
Email: bhagabat80@gmail.com

Chirakshi Dhull MD
Senior Ophthalmologist
Eye Q Hospital
Rohtak, Haryana, India
Email: chirakshi@gmail.com

Deepali Singhal MD
Consultant Ophthalmology
Anil Eye Hospital
Dombivli, Maharashtra, India
Email: deepali.singhal88@gmail.com

Devesh Kumawat MD
Assistant Professor
Department of Ophthalmology
Dr Rajendra Prasad Centre for
Ophthalmic Sciences
All India Institute of Medical Sciences
New Delhi, India
Email: deveshkumawat21@gmail.com

Devjyoti Tripathy MD
Consultant
Department of Ophthalmic Plastic
Surgery and Ocular Oncology
LV Prasad Eye Institute
Bhubaneswar, Odisha, India
Email: drdtripathy@gmail.com

Dewang Angmo
MD DNB FRCS FICO MNAMS
Associate Professor
Department of Ophthalmology
Dr Rajendra Prasad Centre for
Ophthalmic Sciences
All India Institute of Medical Sciences
New Delhi, India
Email: dewang45@gmail.com

Dhwni Shahanand
DNB Fellowship in Cornea and Refractive Surgery
Cornea Consultant
Nethradhama
Bengaluru, Karnataka, India
Email: dhwanishahanand@gmail.com

Gazella Bruce Warjri MS
Consultant Ophthalmologist
LV Prasad Eye Institute
Hyderabad, Telangana, India
Email: gazellabr@gmail.com

Gitanjli Sood Sirkek MS
Consultant
Department of Vitreo-Retina
SM Eye Institute
Kangra, Himachal Pradesh, India
Email: gitz.sood@gmail.com

Gunjan Saluja
MD DNB FICO FAICO (Pediatric Ophthalmology and Strabismus)
Consultant Squint
Department of Oculoplasty and
Neuro-ophthalmology Services
Bhatia Netralaya
Bhilai, Chhattisgarh, India
Email: gunjansaluja2015@gmail.com

Harathy Selvan MD
Specialty Registrar
Sandwell and West Birmingham NHS Trust, UK
Email: sharathy2012@gmail.com

Jyoti Batra MD
Consultant
Department of Ophthalmic Plastic
Surgery and Ocular Oncology
ICARE Eye Hospital
Noida, Uttar Pradesh, India
Email: drjyotibatra@gmail.com

Kanchangouri Satpute DNB
Senior Resident
Dr Rajendra Prasad Centre for
Ophthalmic Sciences
All India Institute of Medical Sciences
New Delhi, India
Email: kanchangouri2014@gmail.com

Karthikeyan Mahalingam MD
Assistant Professor
Department of Ophthalmology
Dr Rajendra Prasad Centre for
Ophthalmic Sciences
All India Institute of Medical Sciences
New Delhi, India
Email: kalingachit@gmail.com

Kavya B Madhuri MD
Consultant
Department of Ophthalmic Plastic
Surgery and Ocular Oncology
LV Prasad Eye Institute
Vijayawada, Andhra Pradesh, India
Email: bejjanki.kavyamadhuri@gmail.com

Luci Kaweri MD
Consultant
Department of Cataract and
Refractive Services
Narayana Nethralaya
Bengaluru, Karnataka, India
Email: dr.lucikaweri@gmail.com

Mahesh Kumar MH MD
Head
Department of Vitreo-Retina
ASG Eye Hospital
Mysuru, Karnataka, India
Email: mayu.doc@gmail.com

Manasi Tripathi MD
Senior Resident
Dr Rajendra Prasad Centre for
Ophthalmic Sciences
All India Institute of Medical Sciences
New Delhi, India
Email: manasitripathirpc@gmail.com

Manpreet Singh MS
Associate Professor
Department of Ophthalmology
Advanced Eye Centre
Postgraduate Institute of Medical
Education and Research
Chandigarh, India
Email: drmanu83@gmail.com

Manthan Chaniyara MD
Assistant Professor
GMERS Medical College
Morbi, Gujarat, India
Email: dr.chaniyara@gmail.com

Mohamed Ibrahime Asif MD
Consultant
Department of Cornea, Cataract, and
Refractive Surgery
Eye7 Chaudhary Eye Centre
New Delhi, India
Email: mohamedasif1991@yahoo.co.in

Monika Kapoor MD
Consultant
Department of Vitreo-Retina
Nethradhama Super Speciality
Eye Hospital
Bengaluru, Karnataka, India

Nagesh BN MD
Managing Director
Senior Consultant
Department of Cornea, Cataract
and Refractive Surgery
Yashoda Nethralaya
Bengaluru, Karnataka, India
Email: drnageshbn@gmail.com

Namrata Bhuta MS
Fellow
Department of Cataract and
Refractive Surgery
Narayana Nethralaya
Bengaluru, Karnataka, India
Email: bhuta.namrata510@gmail.com

Namrata Sharma MD FRCOphth FRCSEd
Professor
Department of Ophthalmology
(Cataract, Cornea and Refractive
Surgery Services)
Dr Rajendra Prasad Centre for
Ophthalmic Sciences
All India Institute of Medical Sciences
New Delhi, India
Email: namrata.sharma@gmail.com

Nandini Bothra MD
Consultant
Department of Ophthalmic
Plastic Surgery
LV Prasad Eye Institute
Hyderabad, Telangana, India
Email: nan_bothra@yahoo.com

Navneet Sidhu MD
Senior Resident
Dr Rajendra Prasad Centre for
Ophthalmic Sciences
All India Institute of Medical Sciences
New Delhi, India
Email: navneet2408@yahoo.com

Neha Midha MD
Director
Avantika Eye Care and Glaucoma Services
New Delhi, India
Email: neha.midha1@gmail.com

Nikitha Ayyadurai MD
Department of Ophthalmology
Dr Rajendra Prasad Centre for
Ophthalmic Sciences
All India Institute of Medical Sciences
New Delhi, India

Niranjana Balasubramaniam MBBS
Fellow
Dr Rajendra Prasad Centre for
Ophthalmic Sciences
All India Institute of Medical Sciences
New Delhi, India

Nirav Raichura MD
Ophthalmic Plastic, Orbital and
Lacrimal Surgeon
Consultant and Director
Darshan Netralaya
Mumbai, Maharashtra, India
Email: niravdraichura@gmail.com

Nupur Goel MD
Consultant
Department of Anterior Segment
and Oculoplasty
ICARE Eye Hospital and PG Institute
Noida, Uttar Pradesh, India
Email: nupurgoel.ms@gmail.com

Oshin Bansal MD
Consultant
Ophthalmic Plastic Surgery
CL Gupta Eye Institute
Moradabad, Uttar Pradesh, India
Email: oshin.hp7@gmail.com

Payal Pandit MS
Fellow
Department of Cataract and
Refractive Surgery
Narayana Nethralaya
Bengaluru, Karnataka, India
Email: drpayalpandit@gmail.com

Prafulla Kumar Maharana MD DNB
Associate Professor
Department of Ophthalmology
Dr Rajendra Prasad Centre for
Ophthalmic Sciences
All India Institute of Medical Sciences
New Delhi, India
Email: drpraful13@gmail.com

Pranita Sahay
MD (AIIMS, New Delhi) FRCOphth (London)
FRCS (Glasgow) FICO (Cornea) FAICO
(Refractive Surgery) DNB
Consultant
Department of Ophthalmology
(Cataract, Cornea and Refractive
Surgery Services)
Centre for Sight Eye Hospital
New Delhi, India
Email: drpranitasahay@gmail.com

Prerana Tahiliani DNB
Department of Ophthalmology
Deenanath Mangeshkar Hospital
Pune, Maharashtra, India
Email: preranast@gmail.com

Priyanka Mishra MD
Senior Resident
Dr Rajendra Prasad Centre for
Ophthalmic Sciences
All India Institute of Medical Sciences
New Delhi, India
Email: priyankamishra16october@gmail.com

Priyanka Ramesh MD
Consultant Ophthalmologist
Ramesh Eye Clinic and Ophthalmic
Microsurgical Center
Glaucoma Squint and Paediatric
Ophthalmologist – The Eye Foundation—
Retina Institute of Karnataka
Bengaluru, Karnataka, India
Email: priya.ramesh91@gmail.com

Priyanka V Walvekar MD
Faculty
Narayana Nethralaya
Bengaluru, Karnataka, India
Email: priyanka.walvekar@gmail.com

Pulak Agrawal MD FICO
Director
JRM Multispecialty Hospital
Bikaner, Rajasthan, India
Email: pulak.mamc@gmail.com

Richa Dharap Wagh
MBBS DNB (Ophthalmology) FICO (UK)
FAICO (Oculoplasty) FLVPEI
Assistant Professor and
Oculoplasty Surgeon
Ophthalmology Department
Government Medical College
Nagpur, Maharashtra, India
Email: richa_dharap@hotmail.com

Ritika Mukhija MD FRCOphth
Fellow
Sussex Eye Hospital
Brighton, UK
Email: ritika190@gmail.com

Ritu Nagpal
MD FLVPEI (Cornea)
Consultant
Eye7 Hospitals
New Delhi, India
Email: doc.ritunagpal@gmail.com

Ritweez Sahu MD
Senior Resident
Vitreoretina, Uvea and ROP Services
Dr Rajendra Prasad Centre for
Ophthalmic Sciences
All India Institute of Medical Sciences
New Delhi, India
Email: ritweezsahu@yahoo.co.in

Roshmi Gupta MD
Head
Department of Ophthalmic Plastics
Orbital Surgery and Ocular Oncology
Narayana Nethralaya
Bengaluru, Karnataka, India
Email: roshmi.gupta@gmail.com

Samir Mahapatra MD
Consultant
Department of Ophthalmic Plastic
Surgery Services
LV Prasad Eye Institute
Bhubaneswar, Odisha, India
Email: samirmahapatra.eye@gmail.com

Sanjana M MD
Fellow
Department of Ophthalmic Plastic
Surgery Services
LV Prasad Eye Institute
Vijayawada, Andhra Pradesh, India
Email: sanjanalvp93@gmail.com

Saumya Yadav MD
Consultant Ophthalmologist
Ansari Hospital
New Delhi, India
Email: dr.sy17@gmail.com

Savari T Desai MD
Oculoplasty, Orbit, Ocular Oncology and
Facial Aesthetics Surgeon
Consultant
PD Hinduja National Hospital, Mumbai
Hinduja Healthcare Surgical, Mumbai
Breach Candy Hospital, Mumbai
Ex-Honorary Consultant
Tata Memorial Hospital
Mumbai, Maharashtra, India
Email: savaridesai@gmail.com

Shreyas Temkar MD
Senior Resident
Dr Rajendra Prasad Centre for
Ophthalmic Sciences
All India Institute of Medical Sciences
New Delhi, India
Email: shreyastemkar@gmail.com

Shruthi Gunda MD
Fellow
Department of Ocular Oncology and
Ophthalmic Plastic Surgery
LV Prasad Eye Institute
Vijayawada, Andhra Pradesh, India
Email: shruthi.gunda@gmail.com

Shweta Gupta MD
Consultant Oculoplastic Surgeon and
Ocular Oncologist
Sankara Eye Foundation
Indore, Madhya Pradesh, India
Email: shwetaguptapgi@gmail.com

Siddhi Goel MD
Consultant
Department of Ophthalmology
Asian Institute of Medical Sciences
Faridabad, Haryana, India
Email: siddhigoel91@gmail.com

Sohini Mandal MD
Senior Resident
Dr Rajendra Prasad Centre for
Ophthalmic Sciences
All India Institute of Medical Sciences
New Delhi, India
Email: sohinimandal59@gmail.com

Suryasnata Rath MD
Network Director Operations
and Consultant
Department of Ophthalmic Plastic
Surgery, Orbit and Ocular
Oncology Services
LV Prasad Eye Institute
Bhubaneswar, Odisha, India
Email: drsuryasnata@gmail.com

Swati Singh MS
Consultant
LV Prasad Eye Institute
Hyderabad, Telangana, India
Email: dr.swati888@yahoo.com

Tarjani Dave MD
Associate Director and Consultant
LV Prasad Eye Institute
Hyderabad, Telangana, India
Email: tvdeye@gmail.com

Tejaswini V MD
Consultant
Department of Vitreo-Retina and Cataract
Sankara Netra Chikitsalaya
Vijayawada, Andhra Pradesh, India
Email: teja217@gmail.com

Vaishali Rakheja MD FICO
Consultant
Department of Pediatric Ophthalmology
Glaucoma and Neuro-ophthalmology
Services
Grewal Eye Institute
Chandigarh, India
Email: vaishali.rakheja@gmail.com

Varshita H Vasanthapuram MD
Consultant
Department of Ophthalmic Plastic
Surgery
Narayana Nethralaya
Bengaluru, Karnataka, India
Email: vivavarsh@gmail.com

Vathsalya Vijay MD
Honorary Consultant Orbit and
Oculoplastic Surgeon
Department of Oral and
Maxillofacial Surgery
Goa Dental College and Hospital
Bambolim, Goa, India
Email: vathsramraj@gmail.com

Vatsala Nidhi MD
Cornea Fellow
Shroff's Charity Eye Hospital
New Delhi, India
Email: vatsalanidhi28393@gmail.com

Vijitha S Vempuluru MD
Consultant
Department of Ocular Oncology and
Ophthalmic Plastic Surgery
LV Prasad Eye Institute
Hyderabad, Telangana, India
Email: vijithavenus@gmail.com

Vineeta Pai
Fellowship in Cornea and External
Diseases (RGUHS)
Cornea Consultant
Nethradhama
Bengaluru, Karnataka, India
Email: paivineeta@gmail.com

Vishal Raval MD
Consultant
Operation Eyesight Universal Institute
for Eye Cancer
LV Prasad Eye Institute
Hyderabad, Telangana, India
Email: drvishalraval@gmail.com

Preface

Postgraduate ophthalmology examinations are tough and challenging. Previously we had the pleasure to come out with two books, *Ophthalmology Clinics I and II*, which were largely focused on practical examination of postgraduate ophthalmology students. The tremendous love and respect that we received from the students and ophthalmologists across the country prompted us to do something more to help the students pass the litmus test of postgraduate examinations with minimal stress.

Theory examination is the first part of any postgraduate ophthalmology examinations. The standard textbooks provide a comprehensive information on any particular topic. With every passing year the questions are becoming more focused on one aspect of a topic or the answer requires a compilation from more than one chapter. While reading the standard textbooks allow you to build your knowledge on any particular topic, it may not guide you about how to answer a particular question.

The aim of this book is to provide a "Question & Answer" type of description of individual topic. It will guide you how to attempt different types of questions such as essay type or short notes. We have compiled the questions from various postgraduate ophthalmology examinations across the country. We have attempted to answer individual questions in this book instead of writing a comprehensive description. However, the questions are numerous and it is beyond the scope of this book to answer every one of them. Thus, in the end we have provided a question bank that will help you to revise at the time of your exam preparation.

Lastly, we would like to emphasize here that, this book is not a replacement for standard textbooks. We would advise you people to read standard textbooks at least once and then refer to this book. If you keep our previous book *Ophthalmology Clinics for Postgraduates* side-by-side and read one topic, it will improve your knowledge many folds.

Prafulla Kumar Maharana
Ritu Nagpal
Pranita Sahay
Namrata Sharma

Acknowledgments

We would like to express our deep gratitude to Ms Nikita and Dr Deepali Singhal for helping us in compiling the questions from various ophthalmology examinations across the country.

Contents

CHAPTER 1	**OCULOPLASTY AND TUMORS**	1

- **1.1 Eyelid Anatomy** 1
  Oshin Bansal, Jyoti Batra

- **1.2 Eyelid Embryology and Congenital Eyelid Anomalies** 10
  Oshin Bansal, Jyoti Batra

- **1.3 Blepharitis** 14
  Oshin Bansal, Jyoti Batra

- **1.4 Blepharoptosis** 19
  Kavya B Madhuri, Devjyoti Tripathy

- **1.5 Entropion and Ectropion** 40
  Akruti Desai, Suryasnata Rath

- **1.6 Eyelid Reconstruction** 51
  Kavya B Madhuri, Anasua G Kapoor

- **1.7 Botulinum Toxin and Dermal Fillers in Ophthalmology** 60
  Akshay Gopinathan Nair, Swati Singh

- **1.8 Eyelid Retraction** 65
  Akruti Desai, Roshmi Gupta

- **1.9 Anomalies of Eyelid Position and Function** 70
  Vathsalya Vijay, Akruti Desai

- **1.10 Anatomy of Lacrimal System** 85
  Priyanka V Walvekar, Nandini Bothra

- **1.11 Congenital Disorders of the Lacrimal System** 90
  Priyanka V Walvekar, Nandini Bothra

- **1.12 Acquired Lacrimal Disorders** 96
  Richa Dharap Wagh, Swati Singh, Nandini Bothra

- **1.13 Evaluation of Epiphora** 108
  Nandini Bothra

- **1.14 Tumors of the Eyelids** 111
  Vijitha S Vempuluru, Shruthi Gunda, Anasua G Kapoor

- **1.15 Orbital Anatomy** 120
  Akruti Desai, Anasua G Kapoor

- **1.16 Orbital Fracture** 129
  Adit Gupta, Prerana Tahiliani, Manpreet Singh

- **1.17 Proptosis** 136
  Nirav Raichura, Savari T Desai

- **1.18 Thyroid Eye Disease** 150
  Varshita H Vasanthapuram, Kavya B Madhuri

1.19	**Orbital Cellulitis**	171
	Ashi Morawala, Anasua G Kapoor	
1.20	**Intraocular Tumor**	186
	Vijitha S Vempuluru, Vishal Raval, Anasua G Kapoor	
1.21	**Conjunctival Pigmented Tumors**	195
	Shweta Gupta, Anasua G Kapoor	
1.22	**Orbital Imaging**	202
	Samir Mahapatra, Sanjana M	
1.23	**Congenital Lesions of Orbit**	220
	Vijitha S Vempuluru, Anasua G Kapoor	
1.24	**Orbital Cysts and Tumors**	225
	Vijitha S Vempuluru, Anasua G Kapoor, Shruthi Gunda	
1.25	**Socket**	245
	Richa Dharap Wagh, Tarjani Dave	
1.26	**Conjunctival Epithelial Tumors and OSSN**	267
	Nupur Goel, Anasua G Kapoor	

CHAPTER 2 — NEURO-OPHTHALMOLOGY — 280

2.1	**Cranial Nerve Palsy**	280
	Gunjan Saluja	
2.2	**Ocular Myopathies**	289
	Gunjan Saluja	
2.3	**Anatomy and Physiology**	295
	Gunjan Saluja	
2.4	**Optic Nerve**	307
	Gunjan Saluja	
2.5	**Pupil**	335
	Gunjan Saluja	
2.6	**Chiasmal and Retrochiasmal Lesion**	342
	Gunjan Saluja	
2.7	**Miscellaneous**	347
	Gunjan Saluja	

CHAPTER 3 — STRABISMUS — 352

Priyanka Ramesh, Gunjan Saluja

CHAPTER 4 — SCLERA — 399

Aditi Dubey

CHAPTER 5 — RETINA — 405

5.1	**Common Retinal Disorders and Surgery**	405
	Mahesh Kumar MH, Navneet Sidhu, Monika Kapoor	
5.2	**Photoreceptors**	448
	Mahesh Kumar MH, Navneet Sidhu, Monika Kapoor	

	5.3	Vitreous Hemorrhage	450
		Mahesh Kumar MH, Monika Kapoor	
	5.4	Pars Plana Vitrectomy	453
		Mahesh Kumar MH, Monika Kapoor	
	5.5	Posteriorly Dislocated Nucleus	454
		Mahesh Kumar MH, Monika Kapoor	
	5.6	Photodynamic Therapy	455
		Mahesh Kumar MH, Monika Kapoor	
	5.7	Macular Function Tests in Opaque Media	456
		Mahesh Kumar MH, Monika Kapoor	

CHAPTER 6 UVEA 459

6.1 Uveitis 459
Gitanjli Sood Sirkek, Devesh Kumawat, Mahesh Kumar MH

CHAPTER 7 GLAUCOMA 522

7.1 Developmental Anomalies of the Angle 522
Dewang Angmo, Ritweez Sahu, Karthikeyan Mahalingam, Kanchangouri Satpute

7.2 Anterior Cleavage Syndromes 525
Dewang Angmo, Akshaya Balaji, Karthikeyan Mahalingam, Kanchangouri Satpute

7.3 Epidemiology of Glaucoma 528
Neha Midha, Dewang Angmo

7.4 Optic Nerve Head Damage and Visual Field Changes 529
Priyanka Mishra, Dewang Angmo

7.4.1 Short-wavelength Automated Perimetry 537
Dewang Angmo, Karthikeyan Mahalingam

7.5 Optical Coherence Tomography in Glaucoma 539
Bhagabat Nayak, Dewang Angmo

7.6 Juvenile Open-angle Glaucoma 541
Harathy Selvan, Dewang Angmo, Karthikeyan Mahalingam

7.7 Medical Management of Glaucoma 544
Vaishali Rakheja, Dewang Angmo

7.8 Laser Peripheral Iridotomy 549
Barkha Gupta, Dewang Angmo

7.9 Newer Antiglaucoma Medications 553
Aafreen Bari, Dewang Angmo

7.10 Advances in Management of Glaucoma 554
Dewang Angmo, Karthikeyan Mahalingam

7.11 Nonpenetrating Glaucoma Surgery 557
Neha Midha, Dewang Angmo

7.12 Selective Laser Trabeculoplasty 559
Barkha Gupta, Dewang Angmo

7.13 Bleb 560
Dewang Angmo, Niranjana Balasubramaniam, Karthikeyan Mahalingam

	7.14	**Complications of Glaucoma Surgery** 565
		Bhagabat Nayak, Dewang Angmo
	7.15	**Releasable Sutures in Trabeculectomy** 572
		Dewang Angmo, Vatsala Nidi, Karthikeyan Mahalingam
	7.16	**Classification of Secondary Glaucoma** 576
		Gazella Bruce Warjri, Dewang Angmo
	7.17	**Drug-induced Glaucoma** 580
		Gazella Bruce Warjri, Dewang Angmo
	7.18	**Lens-induced Glaucoma** 582
		Gazella Bruce Warjri, Dewang Angmo
	7.19	**Normal-tension Glaucoma** 585
		Neha Midha, Dewang Angmo
	7.20	**Refractory Glaucoma** 586
		Dewang Angmo, Nikitha Ayyadurai, Karthikeyan Mahalingam
	7.21	**Primary Congenital Glaucoma and its Associated Syndromes** 589
		Dewang Angmo, Karthikeyan Mahalingam
	7.22	**Surgical Management of Congenital Glaucoma** 591
		Dewang Angmo, Karthikeyan Mahalingam
	7.23	**Ocular Blood Flow and Glaucoma** 593
		Neha Midha, Dewang Angmo
	7.24	**Neuroprotective Agents** 594
		Aafreen Bari, Dewang Angmo
	7.25	**Advanced Glaucoma and Painful Blind Eye** 596
		Bhagabat Nayak, Dewang Angmo
CHAPTER 8		**CORNEA AND CONJUNCTIVA** — 600
	8.1	**Anatomy and Physiology of Cornea** 600
		Sohini Mondal, Ritu Nagpal
	8.2	**Acute Conjunctivitis** 613
		Siddhi Goel, Ritu Nagpal
	8.3	**Ophthalmia Neonatorum** 618
		Ritika Mukhija, Prafulla Kumar Maharana, Ritu Nagpal
	8.4	**Corneal Infection and Inflammatory Disorders** 622
		Deepali Singhal, Pranita Sahay, Ananya Parampalli Ravindra, Siddhi Goel, Ritika Mukhija, *Saumya Yadav, Alisha Kishore, Aafreen Bari, Ritu Nagpal*
	8.5	**Corneal Dystrophy** 671
		Sohini Mondal, Ritu Nagpal, Prafulla Kumar Maharana
	8.6	**Fuchs Endothelial Corneal Dystrophy** 688
		Ritu Nagpal, Prafulla Kumar Maharana, Siddhi Goel
	8.7	**Keratoconus** 693
		Prafulla Kumar Maharana, Pranita Sahay
	8.8	**Limbal Stem Cell Deficiency** 702
		Ritu Nagpal, Alisha Kishore, Prafulla Kumar Maharana
	8.9	**Corneal Transplantation** 706
		Aafreen Bari, Arpit Sharma, Ritu Nagpal

8.10	**Keratomalacia**	761
	Ritu Nagpal, Archita Singh, Prafulla Kumar Maharana	
8.11	**Shield Ulcer**	768
	Pranita Sahay	
8.12	**Toxic Anterior Segment Syndrome**..	772
	Pranita Sahay, Prafulla Kumar Maharana	
8.13	**Ectatic Disorders of the Cornea**	777
	Nagesh BN, Dhwni Shahanand, Vineeta Pai	

CHAPTER 9   CATARACT AND REFRACTIVE SURGERY   801

9.1.1	**Preoperative Laboratory Testing for Cataract Surgery**	801
	Archita Singh, Ritu Nagpal, Prafulla Kumar Maharana	
9.1.2	**Congenital Cataract**	806
	Chirakshi Dhull, Ritu Nagpal, Prafulla Kumar Maharana	
9.1.3	**Traumatic Cataract**	810
	Manthan Chaniyara	
9.1.4	**Nondilating Pupil**	813
	Chirakshi Dhull, Ritu Nagpal, Prafulla Kumar Maharana	
9.1.5	**Uveitis and Cataract Surgery**	817
	Tejaswini V, Ritu Nagpal	
9.1.6	**Ectopia Lentis**	821
	Pulak Agrawal, Manasi Tripathi	
9.2	**Refractive Surgery**	825
	Luci Kaweri, Namrata Bhuta, Payal Pandit	

CHAPTER 10   OCULAR TRAUMA   859

10.1	**Eyelid Trauma**	859
	Adarsh Shashni, Anushka Agarwala	
10.2	**Penetrating Ocular Trauma**	862
	Tejaswini V, Anushka Agarwala	
10.3	**Acute Chemical Injury**	868
	Mohamed Ibrahime Asif, Ritika Mukhija, Pranita Sahay	
10.4	**Blunt Ocular Trauma**	874
	Shreyas Temkar, Pranita Sahay	

CHAPTER 11   SYSTEMIC DISORDERS AND EYE   877

Athul S Puthalath, Devesh Kumawat, Pranita Sahay

QUESTION BANK   907

Deepali Singhal, Pranita Sahay

Anatomy and Physiology	907
Optics and Refraction..	910
Eyelids	912

Lacrimal Drainage System 913
Orbit 914
Conjunctiva 916
Cornea and External Diseases 916
Refractive Surgery 920
Sclera 921
Glaucoma 921
Lens 924
Uveitis 926
Retina 928
Vitreous 932
Ocular Tumors 932
Strabismus 933
Neuro-ophthalmology 935
Investigations 937
Ocular Trauma 938
Community Ophthalmology and Biostatistics 939
Ophthalmic Microbiology, Pharmacology, and Pathology 941
Recent Advances 942
Systemic Disorders and Eye, Drug Toxicity 942
Miscellaneous 943

Index *945*

CHAPTER 1

Oculoplasty and Tumors

1.1 Eyelid Anatomy

Oshin Bansal, Jyoti Batra

Q 1. Describe in detail eyelid anatomy and its applied aspects.

The eyelids help to keep the corneas moist and protect against injury and excessive light, regulating the amount of light reaching the retina.

Gross Anatomy

The upper eyelid extends over the orbital margin to the eyebrow above and the lower more smoothly into the cheek, where nasojugal and malar sulci may limit it.

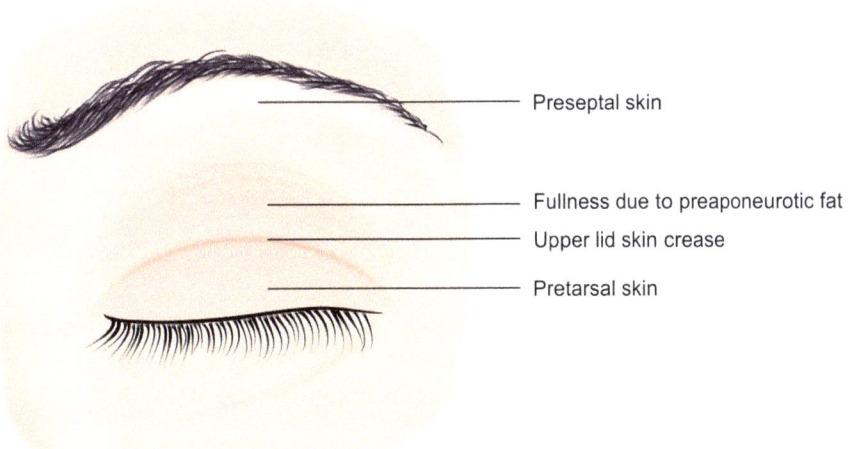

Lid Crease

- Upper/superior lid crease—situated 6–10 mm above the lash line. It is formed by the insertion of levator aponeurosis to orbicularis oculi. It divides the upper lid into:
  - Preseptal part above
  - Pretarsal part below
- Inferior lid crease—4–5 mm from the lash line. It is less evident in adults.
- The nasojugal fold medially and malar fold laterally separate the thin lower eyelid skin from the thicker skin of the cheek. At the nasojugal sulcus, a band of connective tissue passes between orbicularis oculi and levator labii superioris. The sulci mark the junctions between the loose palpebral and denser tissues in the cheek, hence limiting edema and demarcating adipose herniation.

Position of Lids

In primary position of gaze, the upper lid covers one sixth of the cornea and the lower lid just touches the cornea.

Canthi

The upper and the lower eyelids meet at medial and lateral canthi.
- Lateral canthus—located 5-7 mm from the lateral orbital margin—lies in contact with the eyeball.
- Medial canthus is separated from the globe by the tear lake (lacus lacrimalis). A yellowish conjunctival fold, the lacrimal caruncle, projects into the lacus, and lateral to it is the pink plica semilunaris.

Palpebral fissure height measured at the level of pupil is as follows:
- 8-10 mm in males
- 10-12 mm in females.

Lid Margins

Lid measures nearly 2 mm in width.

Lacrimal papilla—a small elevation on the medial aspect of lid-harboring lacrimal punctum—divides the lid into two parts:
1. Lacrimal portion medially known as *pars lacrimalis*—rounded and devoid of lashes
2. Ciliary portion laterally known as *pars ciliaris*—has rounded anterior border and sharp posterior border and intermarginal strip in between

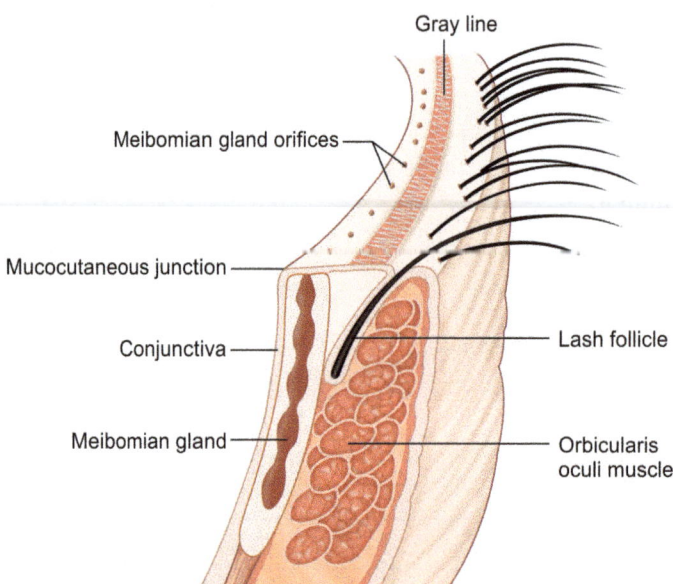

Important landmarks from posterior to anterior are as follows:
- Mucocutaneous junction represents the anterior limit of the marginal strip of tear fluid.
- Meibomian gland orifices
- Gray line—muscle of Riolan (pars ciliaris part of orbicularis oculi) lies deep to it, forms bloodless plane of dissection, and divides the intermarginal strip into anterior and posterior parts.

Structure of Eyelid

From anterior to posterior
1. Skin
2. Subcutaneous areolar tissue
3. Orbicularis oculi muscle   } Anterior lamella
4. Submuscular areolar tissue
5. Orbital septa
6. Eyelid retractors
7. Tarsal plate   } Posterior lamella
8. Conjunctiva

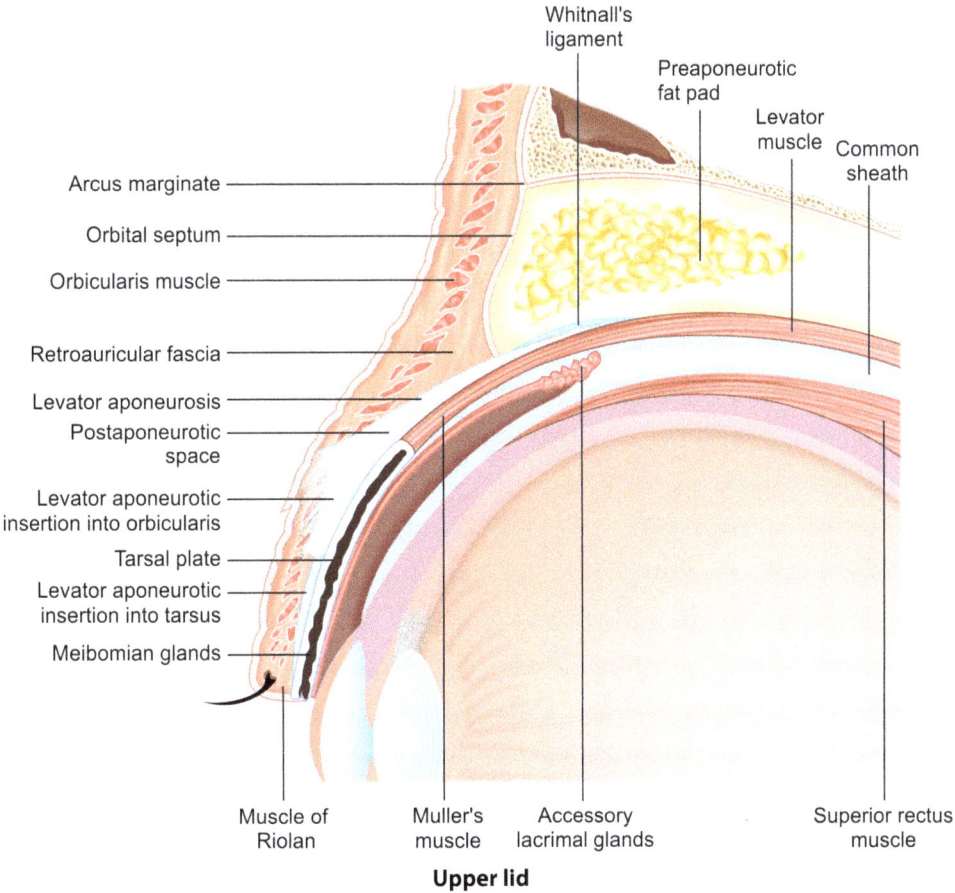

Upper lid

Skin
- Eyelid has the thinnest skin in the body and is loosely attached to orbicularis oculi muscle but more firmly attached to regions of canthal tendons. *These two properties provide more mobility to the lids.*
- Fine hairs are present.

Subcutaneous Areolar Tissue
- Loose areolar tissue with no fat—readily distended by blood or edema
- Absent at lid margins, skin folds, and medial and lateral angles.

Orbicularis Oculi Muscle
Orbicularis oculi muscle is divided into three parts:
1. Orbital—rests on orbital bone
    - *Origin:*
        - Medial canthal ligament
        - Frontal process of maxilla
        - Orbital process of frontal bone
    - Insertion—Its fibers run in an elliptical fashion and insert medially just below the point of origin. Few fibers insert into the dermis at the medial brow.
2. *Preseptal:*
    - Origin—single head in lower lid: medial canthal ligament.
        - *Two heads in upper lid:*
            - *Superficial head:* Common medial canthal ligament
            - *Deep head:* Superior limb of medial canthal tendon (MCT), which is fused to lacrimal sac fundus by layer of fibrovascular fascia
    - Insertion—lateral canthal tendon and lateral horizontal raphe

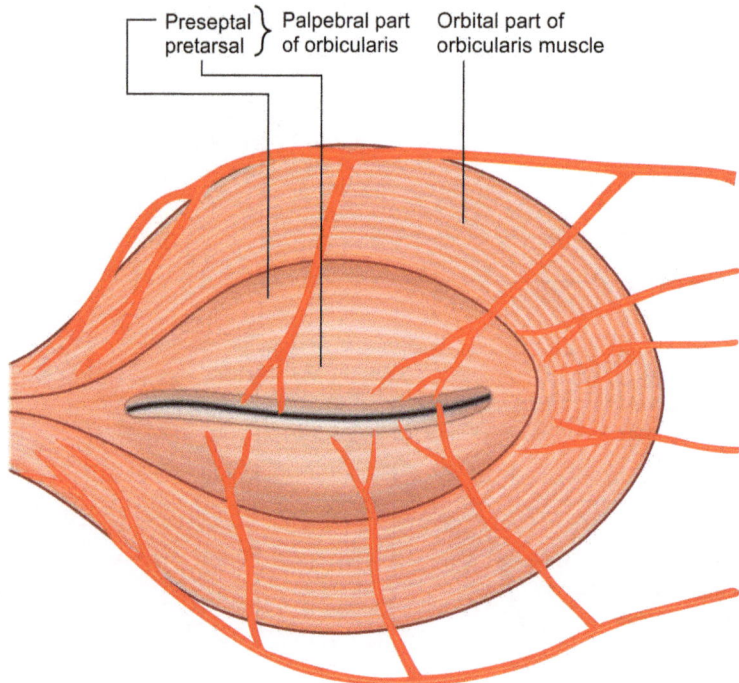

From its orientation, the preseptal orbicularis muscle appears to counteract opposing tone in the retractors of the eyelids, both levator aponeurosis in the upper lid and capsulopalpebral fascia (CPF) in the lower lid. Secondarily, its contraction pulls the lacrimal sac fascia laterally, thereby contributing to the lacrimal pump mechanism.

3. *Pretarsal:*
    - Origin:
        - MCT (superficial head)
        - Lacrimal fascia and posterior lacrimal crest (deep head)
    - Insertion—lateral canthal tendon and lateral horizontal raphe

Horner's muscle/pars lacrimalis is the part of pretarsal fibers, which arise from the lacrimal fascia and helps in the drainage of tears.

Muscle of Riolan/pars ciliaris—pretarsal orbicularis fibers that lie along the lid margin behind the ciliary follicles.
Nerve supply—facial nerve.

Applied Anatomy
- Palpebral part causes reflex/involuntary closure of the eyelid and orbital part causes voluntary lid closure.
- Dysfunction of orbicularis can be due to multiple etiologies:
    - Myokymia—benign involuntary spontaneous localized twitching of few superficial muscle bundles of orbicularis oculi
    - Benign essential blepharospasm—focal cranial dystonia of uncertain etiology. It typically affects older individuals and is characterized by involuntary contractions of the orbicularis, procerus, and corrugator muscles.
    - Hemifacial spasms—a unilateral condition seen in older individuals and characterized by tonic and clonic spasms of facial muscles in the distribution of the ipsilateral facial nerve. In most cases, it is caused by a vascular compression of the seventh nerve.
    - Bell's palsy—idiopathic, unilateral, paralysis of the seventh cranial nerve. It is characterized by weakness of the facial muscles on one side including orbicularis oculi resulting in lagophthalmos.

Orbital Septum
- It originates from the orbital rim at thickening called arcus marginale.
- Superior orbital septum fuses with levator aponeurosis 10 mm from the superior edge of the upper tarsal plate.
- Lower orbital septum fuses with the CPF and they together attach to the lower edge of the lower tarsal plate.

Applied Anatomy
- In older patients, and in younger individuals as a familial trait, the septum may be a flimsy, transparent film through which orbital fat pockets easily herniated causing eyelid fat bags.

- Following trauma to the eyelids, prolapse of orbital fat into the wound occurs with lacerations of the orbital septum. The septum should not be repaired, since this frequently causes shortening of this structure, with resultant lagophthalmos.

Tarsal Plates

- Dense fibrous tissues of 1.0–1.5 mm thickness that provide structural integrity to the eyelids
- Measure—29 mm horizontally
- Upper tarsus—10-11 mm in height
- Lower tarsus—4-5 mm in height
- Meibomian/tarsal glands are embedded in the substance of tarsal plate: approximately 25 in the upper lid and 20 in the lower lid.
- Lateral ends of the tarsal plates are attached to Whitnall's tubercle by lateral canthal tendon. Medial ends are attached by MCT to the anterior lacrimal crest and frontal process of maxilla.

Applied Anatomy

Obstruction of the meibomian gland ductules by lipid and cellular debris, or by abnormalities of keratinization, may result in lipogranulomatous inflammation and frank infection, presenting as hordeolum or chalazion.

Canthal Tendons

1. *Lateral canthal tendon:*
   Formed by:
   - Y-shaped fibrous thickening of orbital septum connecting the tarsal plates and lateral orbital tubercle (tubercle of Whitnall)
   - Common tendon formed by pretarsal orbicularis oculi
   - Lateral raphe formed by preseptal orbicularis oculi
2. *Medial canthal tendon:*
   - Fibrous component—Y-shaped band attaching the medial ends of tarsal plates to the frontal process of maxilla just anterior to the anterior lacrimal crest
   - Muscular component formed by the attachment of preseptal and pretarsal orbicularis oculi
   The MCT has superficial and deep parts.
   - The superficial part is attached to the anterior lacrimal crest—stronger— and gives support.
   - The posterior part is attached to the posterior lacrimal crest and facilitates lacrimal drainage.

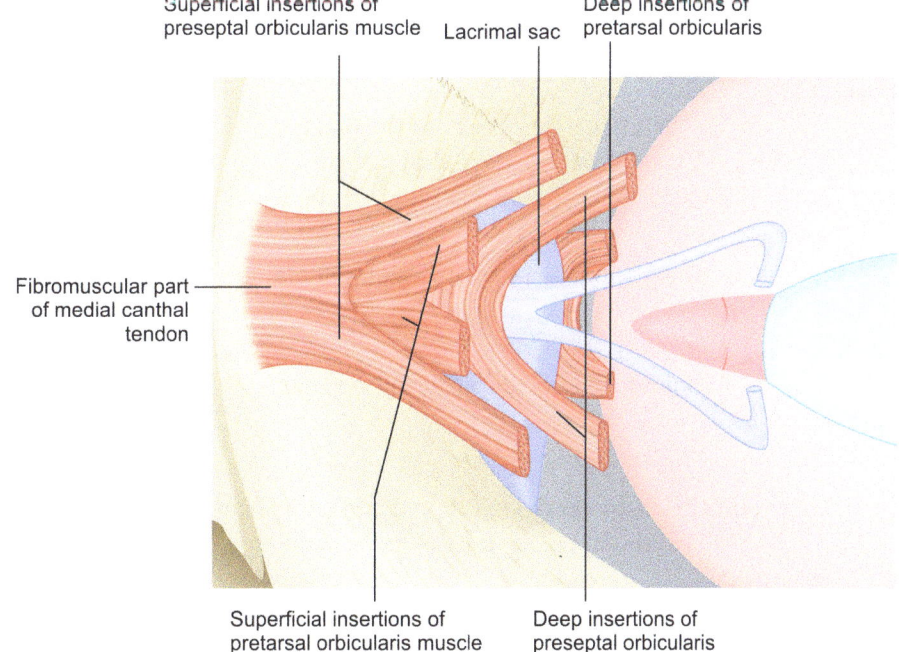

Levator Palpebrae Superioris

- Origin—from the orbital surface of the lesser wing of sphenoid, above the annulus of Zinn
- Has muscular part—about 40 mm and runs horizontally—above the superior rectus.
- The direction changes at the level of superior transverse ligament of Whitnall, which then continues vertically down as aponeurosis.
- Levator aponeurosis gets inserted to the superior two-thirds of the anterior surface of the upper tarsal plate.
- Medial horn of levator aponeurosis attaches to the posterior limb of MCT and posterior lacrimal crest.
- Lateral horn attaches to the lateral tubercle of Whitnall and fibers of capsulopalpebral fascia (CPF). The lateral horn divides the lacrimal gland into palpebral and orbital parts.
  Nerve supply—superior division of oculomotor nerve

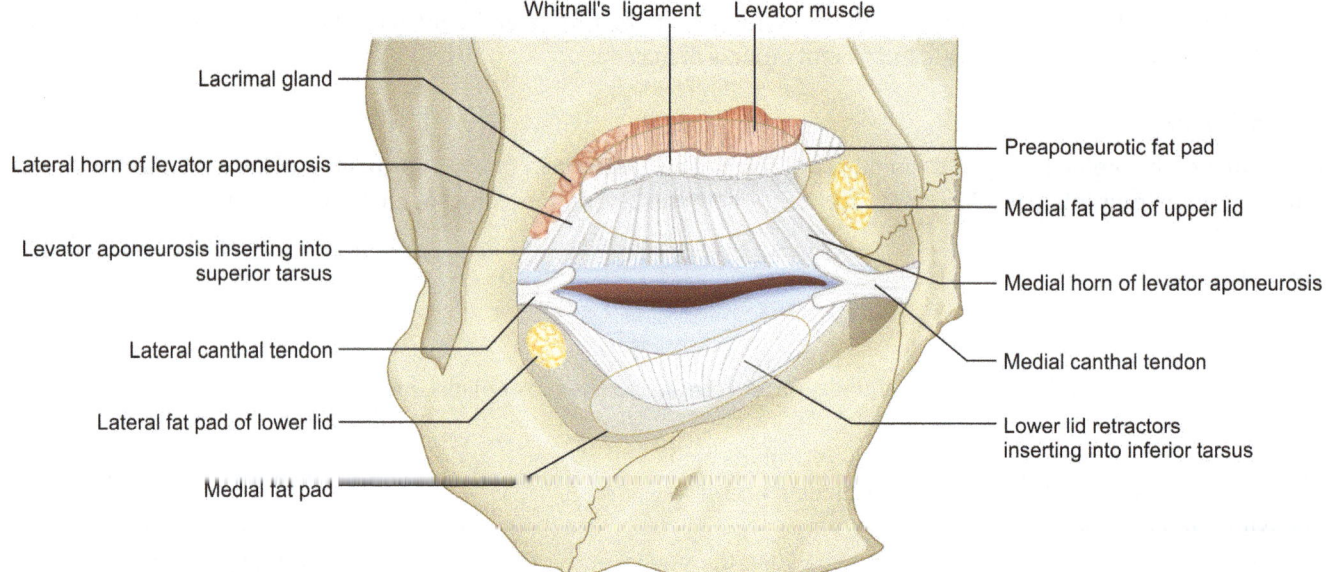

Muller's Muscle

- Origin—from levator palpebrae superioris (LPS) close to muscle–aponeurosis junction.
- Insertion—upper border of tarsal plate of the upper lid.
  Nerve supply—sympathetic nerves

Inferior Lid Retractors

1. *Capsulopalpebral fascia (CPF):*

   It originates as capsulopalpebral head
   from inferior rectus muscle
   ↓
   Divides into two—encircles inferior oblique
   ↓
   Joins together to form Lockwood ligament
   ↓
   Extends from Lockwood's ligament, sends strands to the inferior fornix, and inserts to the lower border of the inferior tarsal plate

2. Inferior tarsal muscle—analogous to Muller's muscle—poorly developed

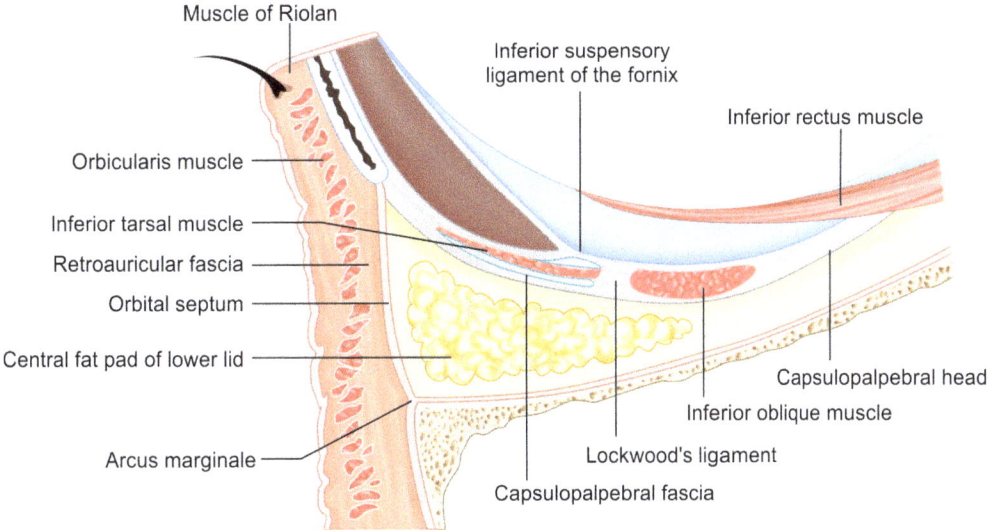

Applied Anatomy

- The most common causes of adult-acquired ptosis are involutional thinning and stretching of the levator aponeurosis.
- With horizontal eyelid lacerations, the presence of orbital fat suggests deep eyelid injury to the level of the orbit and should alert the clinician for the possibility of aponeurotic injury.
- Entropion and ectropion frequently result from involutional stretching of the CPF, horizontal laxity of the tarsus or canthal ligaments, or both.
- Disruption of sympathetic innervation to Muller's muscles, anywhere from its origin in the hypothalamus to its terminal postsynaptic branches in the eyelids, results in Horner's syndrome. This is characterized by the classic triad of ptosis, miosis, and ipsilateral anhidrosis of the face.

Glands of Eyelid

- Lacrimal gland—palpebral part
- Accessory lacrimal gland
  - Krause
  - Wolfring
- Meibomian gland
- Zeis gland
- Moll gland
- Goblet cells—in conjunctiva, plica, caruncle.

 2. Describe the lymphatic drainage of eyelids and its applied aspects.

The lymphatic channels form pretarsal and post-tarsal plexuses, connected by cross-channels.

Pretarsal plexus	Post-tarsal plexus
Have many valves	No valves
Drains skin and its appendages	Drains the conjunctiva and tarsal glands

Both groups drain as follows:
1. *Upper lid:*
   - Lateral two-thirds—preauricular and parotid lymph nodes (LNs)
   - Medial one third—submandibular, submental, and anterior cervical LN
2. *Lower lid:*
   - Lateral one third—preauricular and parotid LNs
   - Medial two-thirds—submandibular and submental anterior cervical LN.

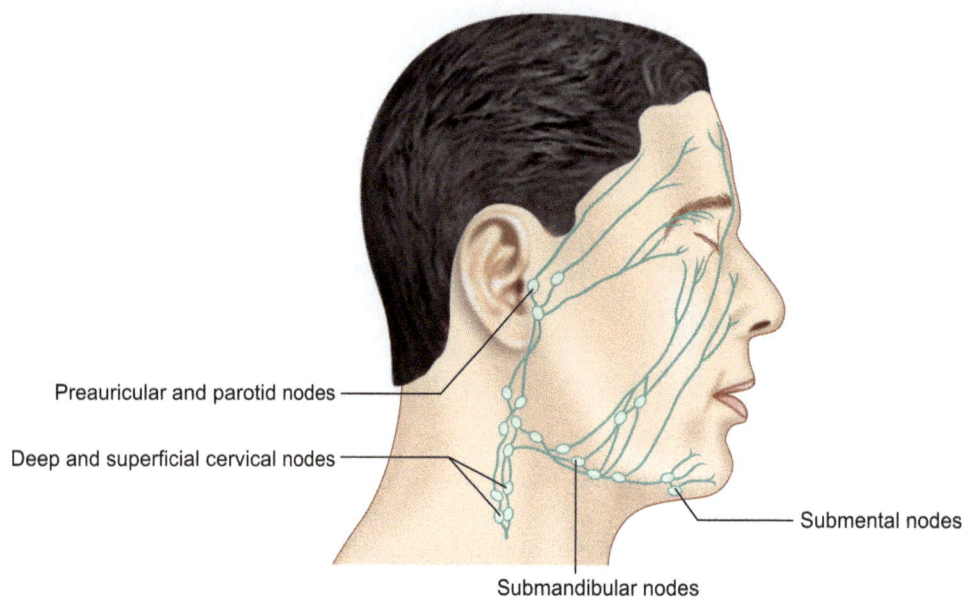

Applied Anatomy

- Extensive excision of subcutaneous eyelid tissues or deep incisions in the inferolateral eyelid area may result in persistent lymphedema due to the disruption of these vessels.
- Regional metastases of eyelid tumors are rare for basal cell and squamous cell carcinoma, but may occur more commonly with sebaceous cell carcinoma.
- The orbitomalar retaining ligament along the inferior orbital rim is the principal suspensory structure for the infraorbital soft tissues, but it also separates the lymphatic drainage fields of the lid from those of the cheek. This explains why significant lower eyelid edema is often seen to stop at the orbital rim.

 3. Describe the vascular supply to eyelids. What are the clinical applications of the same?

Eyelid has extensive vascularity, promotes healing, and defends against infection.

Arterial supply is through two main sources:
1. Internal carotid artery (ICA)—ophthalmic artery and its branches
   - Supraorbital—supplies levator, superior rectus, and superior oblique muscles
   - Lacrimal—through lateral palpebral artery
   - Dorsal nasal artery—through medial palpebral artery
2. *External carotid artery (ECA):*
   - Facial artery → angular artery (terminal branch)
   - Internal maxillary artery → gives infraorbital artery in pterygopalatine fossa; supplies the cheek, lower eyelid, and conjunctiva
   - Superficial temporal artery—terminal branch of the ECA
     - *Branches and area supplied:*
       - Frontal artery—frontalis, orbicularis muscles
       - Zygomatic artery—lateral portion of the lids
       - Transverse facial artery—lateral portion of the lower lids and cheek

Oculoplasty and Tumors

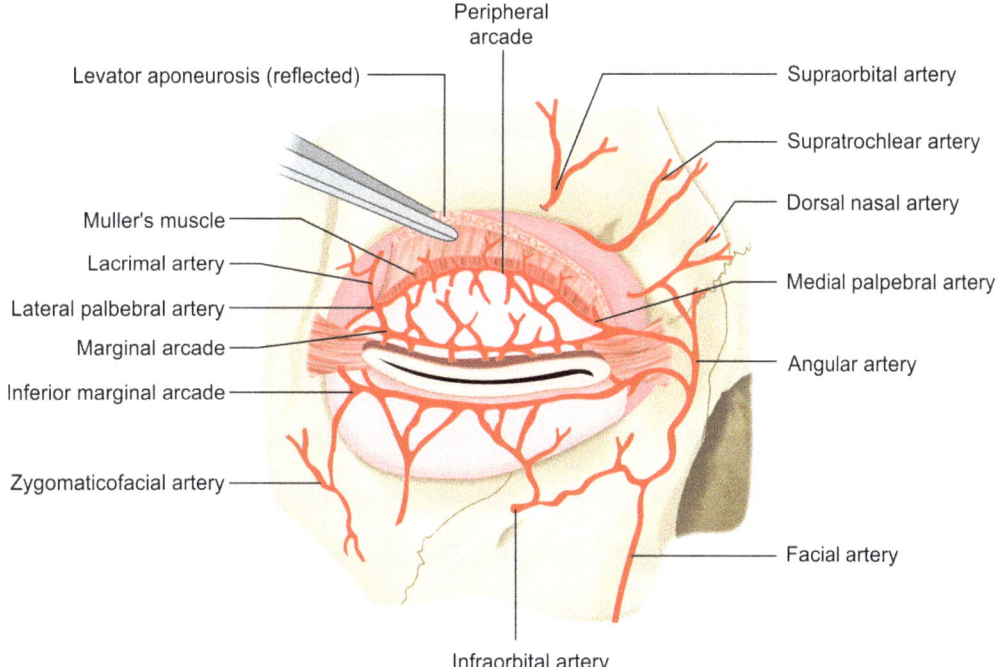

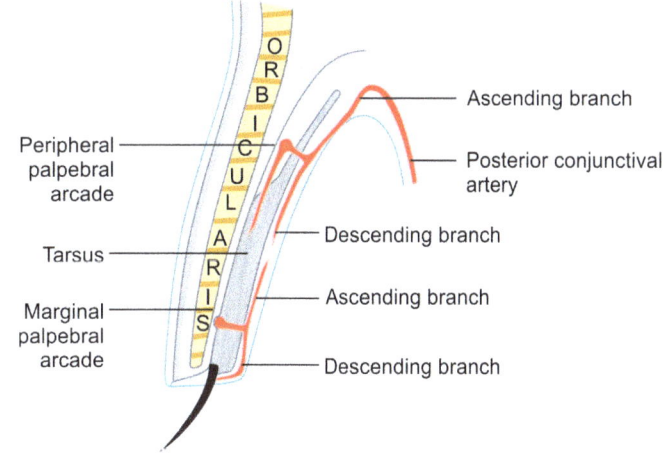

Each eyelid has a *marginal arcade*, which is found on the surface of the tarsus along the eyelid margin. The upper eyelid has an additional arterial supply known as the *peripheral arcade*, which lies between the levator aponeurosis and Muller's muscle.

Venous Drainage

- Preseptal tissues:
  - Superficial temporal vein laterally
  - Angular vein medially
- Postseptal tissues:
  - Orbital vein
  - Deeper branches of anterior facial vein
  - Pterygoid plexus.

Applied Anatomy

- Reconstructive flaps of eyelids rarely undergo failure due to ischemia due to rich vascular supply.
- The extensive blood supply of the periocular tissues allows incision and mobilization of the tissues of the glabellar flap (a random flap) without a specific arterial supply.
- Extensive anastomoses provide a rich blood supply to the tissues of the periocular area, which prevents infection and promotes healing after trauma.

Suggested Reading

1. Bron A, Tripathi RC, Tripathi B. Wolff's Anatomy of the Eye and Orbit. UK: Hodder Arnold; 1998.
2. Cantor LB, Rapuano C, Cioffi GA. Orbit, Eyelids, and Lacrimal System. Orbit, Eyelids and Lacrimal system. San Francisco: American Academy Ophthalmology; 2016-17.
3. Collin JR. A Manual of Systematic Eyelid Surgery. Philadelphia: Elsevier Health Sciences; 2006.
4. Leatherbarrow B. Oculoplastic Surgery. Boca Raton, FL: CRC Press; 2010.
5. Sevel D. Developmental and congenital abnormalities and diseases of the nasolacrimal apparatus and orbit in children. Curr Opinion Ophthalmol. 1990;1(6):602-6.
6. Tawfik H, Abdulhafez M, Fouad Y, Dutton J. Embryologic and fetal development of the human eyelid. Ophthalmic Plast Reconstr Surg. 2018;32:407-14.
7. Tyers AG, Collins JR. Colour Atlas of Ophthalmic Plastic Surgery. Hong Kong. 1995;159:128.

1.2 Eyelid Embryology and Congenital Eyelid Anomalies

Oshin Bansal, Jyoti Batra

Q 1. Describe the embryological development of eyelids in brief and enumerate four congenital anomalies of eyelids.

Origin of Eye Lid Tissue

The eyelids develop from both secondary mesenchyme (mesoderm invaded by cranial neural crest cells) and surface ectoderm **(Table 1)**.

TABLE 1: Development of eyelid structures.	
Surface ectoderm	• Conjunctiva • Skin epithelium • Hair follicles • Zeis glands • Glands of Moll • Meibomian glands
Mesenchyme	• Fibers of striated muscles • Endothelial lining of eyelid blood vessels
Neural crest cells	• Tarsal plate • Levator aponeurosis and Muller • Orbital septum • Eyelid melanocytes • Pericytes of eyelid blood vessels • Schwann cells and axons in eyelid nerves • Connective tissue components of the levator and orbicularis muscles

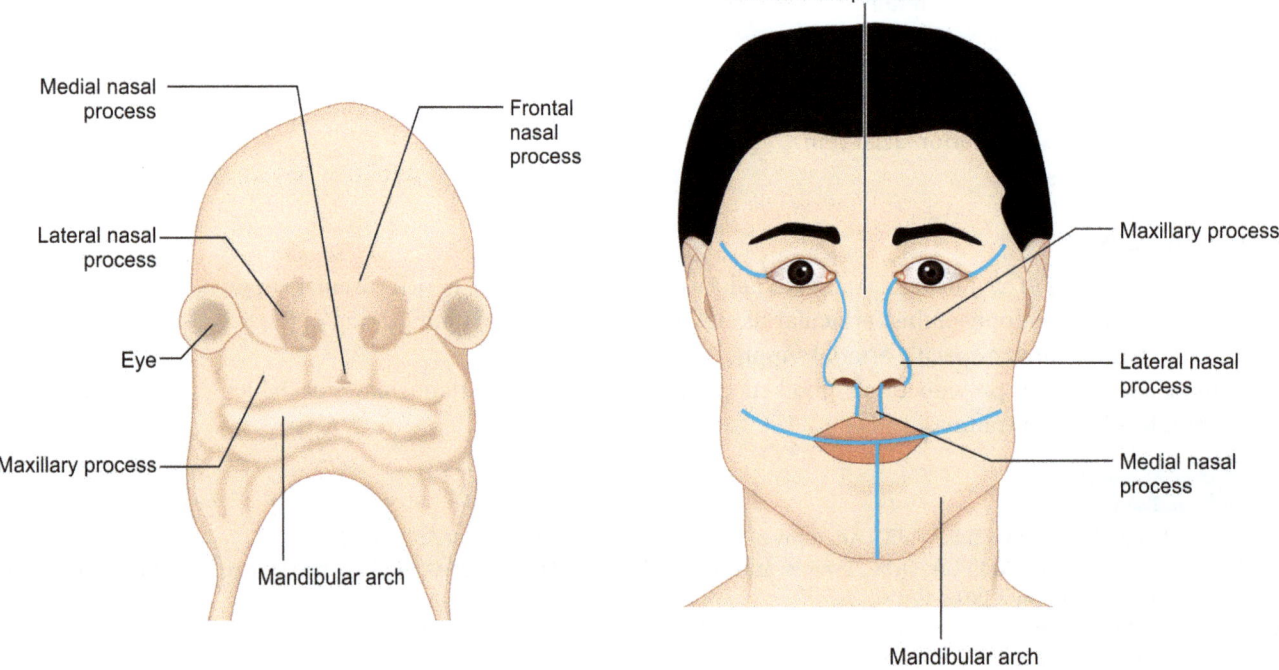

- Upper lid develops from fusion of medial and lateral nasal processes.
- Lower lid forms from extension of maxillary process.

There are five phases:
1. Eyelid formation
2. Fusion
3. Development
4. Separation
5. Maturation of eyelid structures.

At 6 weeks of gestational age:
    First indication of the embryonic eyelid development is seen.
    ↓
    Small grooves or depressions develop in the surface ectoderm immediately above and below the developing eye.
    ↓
    Rapidly deepen to form the eyelid folds (7 weeks)

Also during the seventh week, a solid cord of epithelial cells invaginates into the thickened mesenchyme in the medial one-sixth of the eyelid and bifurcates forming the precursors of puncta and canaliculi.

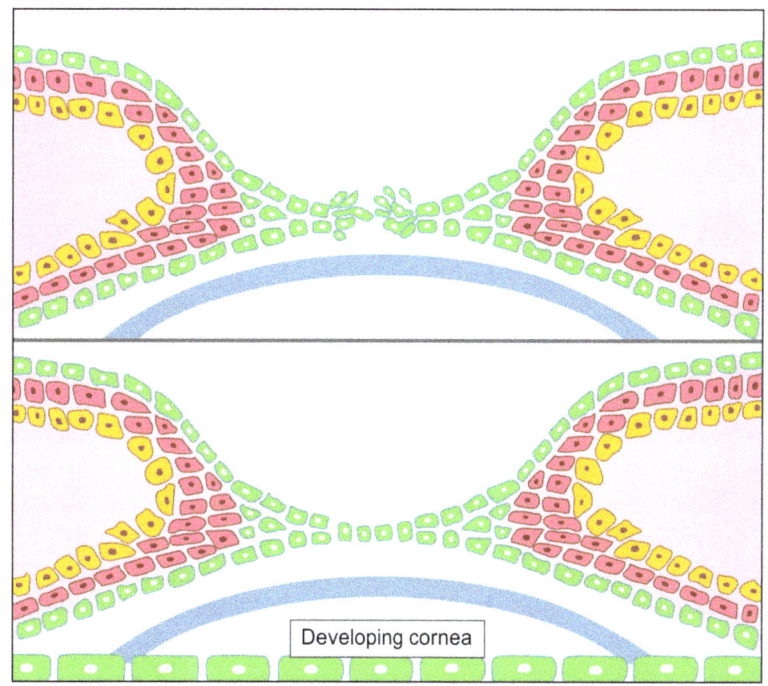

At the beginning of week 8:
    The gap between the upper and lower eyelid folds and the cornea is filled by epithelial migration and proliferation
    ↓
    Eyelid fusion

11 Weeks—Primordial tarsal plate, eyelash follicle anlages, primordial orbital septum, and meibomian gland

14th Week—The eyelid clearly divided into separate layers.

Rudimentary eyelashes, sebaceous, and sweat glands could be seen near the eyelid margin, and a primordial tarsal plate has formed.

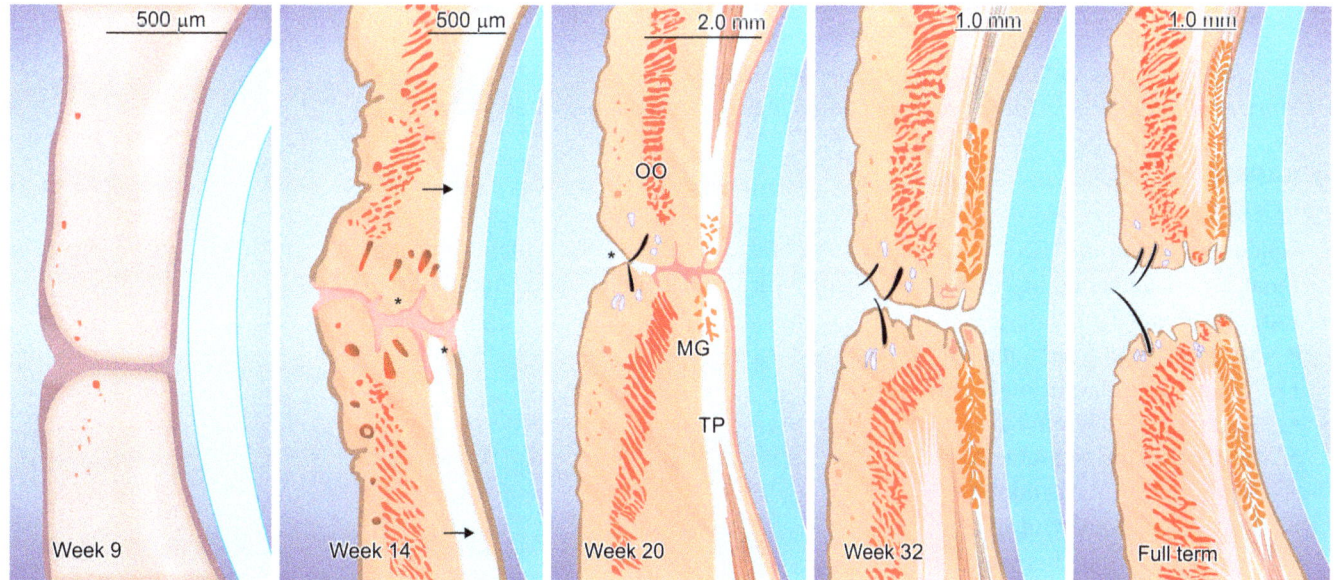

(MG: meibomian gland; OO: orbicularis oculi; TP: tarsal plate)

20th Week:
- Eyelid separation starts anteriorly.
- Meibomian gland branching is first observed.
- Tarsal plate lengthens significantly.
- Orbicularis oculi muscle looks more fully developed.
- Mature eyelash follicles about to pierce the eyelid margin.

32nd week:
- Nearly fully developed appearance
- Meibomian glands increase in length—present in two-thirds of the length of the tarsal plate
- The eyelids are fully separated.

Full term: Final appearance of the eyelids at birth, which is not dissimilar from the adult counterpart.

 2. Describe the common developmental anomalies of eyelids.

The common eyelid anomalies due to an anomaly in the process of development include the following:

Coloboma of the Lid

- An embryological cleft in the eyelid—usually isolated anomaly when it occurs in medial upper eyelid.
- If, in lower eyelid, it will be associated with other congenital conditions such as facial cleft and lacrimal deformities.
- Coloboma of the eyelid has a different embryologic origin from a coloboma of the globe. Although the sequence of eyelid development itself is induced by the developing globe, there is no clear evidence that eyelid coloboma results from globe abnormalities. Coloboma of the eyelid is along the spectrum of craniofacial clefts and can occur either as an isolated malformation or associated with ocular or systemic anomalies.
- Lid coloboma arises from defective eyelid development, either during fusion or during reseparation

Isolated Coloboma

- *Coloboma associated with corneopalpebral adhesion (CPA; cryptophthalmos):*
  - *Complete:* No discernible eyelid differentiation, and the eyes are completely covered with skin
  - *Incomplete:*
    - A skin-fold devoid of tarsus covers the medial aspect of the palpebral aperture
    - Significant CPA
    - Lower fornix and lateral upper eyelids usually spared
  - *Abortive type/congenital symblepharon variant (CSV):*
    - True coloboma of variable sizes with a diverse range of CPA
    - Lower fornix and lateral upper eyelids usually spared
- *Simple coloboma (SC):* Upper eyelid coloboma in isolation not associated with CPA.

Syndromic Variants

- Fraser syndrome
- Goldenhar syndrome (GS)/oculoauriculovertebral spectrum—GS is a pleiotropic condition with a spectrum of cardiac, renal, and skeletal manifestations besides the typical facial and vertebral anomalies.
- *Rare syndromes:*
  - Manitoba oculotrichoanal syndrome
  - Ablepharon-macrostomia syndrome
  - Nasopalpebral lipoma–coloboma syndrome
  - Amniotic band sequence
  - Oculoectodermal syndrome
  - Neurocutaneous syndromes
  - Encephalocraniocutaneous lipomatosis
  - Delleman syndrome or oculocerebrocutaneous syndrome
  - Linear nevus sebaceous syndrome
  - CHARGE syndrome.

Cryptophthalmos

- Characterized by partial or complete absence of eyebrow, palpebral fissure, eye lashes, and conjunctiva.
- The partially developed adnexa are fused to anterior segment of the globe and can be unilateral/bilateral.
- Histologically all eyelid structures are attenuated or absent. Underlying eye will be defective.
- *Types*:
  - *Complete (typical) cryptophthalmos:* The lids are replaced by a sheet of skin running from forehead to cheek with absence or poor development of the eyebrow. No lashes or gland structures can be identified. The covered globe gives rise to an elevation in the overlying skin which moves when eye movements occur. The skin is adherent to the underlying cornea, and there is no conjunctival sac. Microphthalmos is usual.
  - *Incomplete (atypical) cryptophthalmos:* Rudimentary lids are present, with a small conjunctival sac placed laterally. The palpebral aperture is about one third of normal length. The globe is usually small and almost completely covered by skin.
  - *Abortive form or congenital symblepharon:* The upper lid, without a defined margin, covers and adheres to up to 75% of the upper cornea. The lid has no punctum, and there is no upper conjunctival fornix. The free part of the cornea may be keratinized and opaque. The globe is usually of normal size but may be small.

The systemic associations of cryptophthalmos include abnormalities of head shape, nose and ears, meningoencephalocele, cleft lip and cleft palate, syndactyly, genital anomalies, and a miscellaneous group of defects including atresia of larynx, kidneys, bladder and anus, and umbilical hernia.

Epiblepharon

- Epiblepharon is characterized by redundant anterior lamella presenting as an abnormal horizontal skin fold overriding the eyelid margin, resulting in misdirected lashes toward the conjunctiva and cornea.
- Symptoms range from none to features of eye irritation. The severity of epiblepharon symptoms may be associated with the type and number of eyelashes irritating the eyes.
- Few and fine eyelashes are often less symptomatic than thick and plentiful lashes. Due to this variability, symptoms of epiblepharon may change with age.
- Child may develop decreased visual acuity due to the development of induced astigmatism.

Epicanthal Folds

Epicanthus is a medial canthal fold that may result from immature midfacial bones or a fold of skin and subcutaneous tissue. There are four types of epicanthi.

1. *Epicanthus tarsalis*—fold is more prominent in upper lid.
2. *Epicanthus inversus*—fold is more prominent in lower lid associated with blepharophimosis, ptosis, and epicanthus inversus syndrome (BPES).
3. *Epicanthus palpebralis*—fold involves upper and lower lid equally.
4. *Epicanthus superciliaris*—fold arises from eyebrow region and runs to lacrimal sac.

Suggested Reading

1. Bron AJ. Wolff's Anatomy of the Eye and Orbit. London; Weinheim; Tokyo: Chapman & Hall Medical; 1997.
2. Cantor LB, Rapuano C, Cioffi GA. Orbit, Eyelids, and Lacrimal System. San Francisco: American Academy Ophthalmology; 2016.
3. Collin JR. A Manual of Systematic Eyelid Surgery. Philadelphia, PA: Elsevier Health Sciences; 2006.
4. Leatherbarrow B. Oculoplastic Surgery. London: CRC Press; 2010.
5. Sevel D. Developmental and congenital abnormalities and diseases of the nasolacrimal apparatus and orbit in children. Curr Opinion Ophthalmol. 1990;1(6):602-6.
6. Tawfik H, Abdulhafez M, Fouad Y, Dutton J. Embryologic and fetal development of the human eyelid. Ophthal Plast Reconstr Surg. 2016;32(6):407-14.
7. Tyers AG, Collins JR. Colour Atlas of Ophthalmic Plastic Surgery. Hong Kong. 1995;159:128.

1.3 Blepharitis

Oshin Bansal, Jyoti Batra

Q 1. Discuss the classification, pathogenesis, risk factors, clinical features, and management of blepharitis.

Blepharitis is an inflammation of the eyelids. It can be classified in the following manner:

Anatomic Classification

Blepharitis can be divided into anterior and posterior according to the anatomic location, although there is considerable overlap between the two.

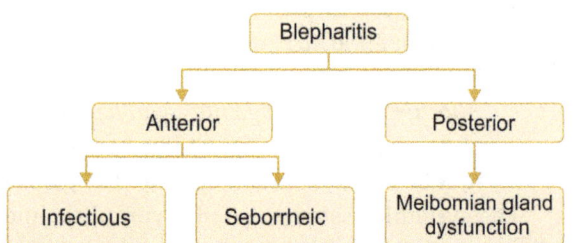

Anterior blepharitis affects the eyelid skin, base of the eyelashes, and the eyelash follicles. It occurs more commonly in young females.

It includes the following:
- Staphylococcal blepharitis
- Seborrheic blepharitis.

Posterior blepharitis affects mainly the meibomian glands and gland orifices, and the primary cause is meibomian gland dysfunction (MGD).

Based on the onset, it is divided into *Acute* and *Chronic*.

Acute Blepharitis

Acute blepharitis, also referred to as lid infection, may be bacterial, viral, or parasitic in etiology.

Acute blepharitis is subdivided into acute ulcerative (often secondary to staphylococcal or herpetic infection) and acute nonulcerative (typically allergic).

Chronic Blepharitis

The more common form is chronic blepharitis.

Earlier classification categorized chronic blepharitis into six entities: (1) Staphylococcal, (2) Seborrheic, (3) Staphylococcal/Seborrheic, (4) Meibomian seborrhea, (5) Secondary meibomian inflammation, and (6) Meibomian keratoconjunctivitis.

Recent classification [based on the American Academy of Ophthalmology (AAO) preferred practice pattern of blepharitis] of chronic blepharitis classifies it into three distinct categories:
↓
Staphylococcal, seborrheic, and MGD.

Other Types of Blepharitis

- *Angular blepharitis* tends to occur in the canthal region and may present independent of anterior and posterior etiologies.
- *Marginal blepharitis* has been referred to in recent literature as a collective term for involvement of both anterior and posterior blepharitis.

Risk Factors and Associated Conditions

- Dry eye is associated with staphylococcal blepharitis and posterior blepharitis. A decrease in local lysozyme and immunoglobulin levels associated with tear deficiency may alter resistance to bacteria, predisposing patients to the development of staphylococcal blepharitis.

In cases of posterior blepharitis, it results from increased tear film evaporation due to a deficiency in the lipid component of the tears as well as reduced ocular surface sensation.
- *Dermatological conditions:*
  - Acne rosacea is reported to be associated mainly with posterior blepharitis. Characteristic facial skin findings include erythema, telangiectasias, papules, pustules, and prominent sebaceous glands.
  - Seborrheic dermatitis, characterized by flaking and greasy skin on the scalp, retroauricular area, glabella, and nasolabial folds can predispose to the development of seborrheic blepharitis.
  - Atopic dermatitis

- *Demodicosis:* Demodex folliculorum is a parasite that resides in between the lashes and is reported to be associated with chronic blepharitis. Eyelashes with cylindrical dandruff or sleeves at the eyelash base are reported to be a sign of ocular Demodex infestation.
- Isotretinoin is an oral medication that is used to treat severe acne. This drug is associated with a significant increase in colonization of the conjunctiva with *Staphylococcus aureus*, blepharitis, and a disruption in tear function. Discontinuation of the medication itself leads to improvement in most cases.
- Giant papillary conjunctivitis (GPC)—Patients with contact lens–associated GPC have an increased frequency of MGD.

Pathophysiology

The exact pathogenesis of blepharitis is unknown but is considered to be multifactorial. Although a precise mechanism behind the development of anterior blepharitis is unclear, three convergent pathways likely underlie the pathophysiology.

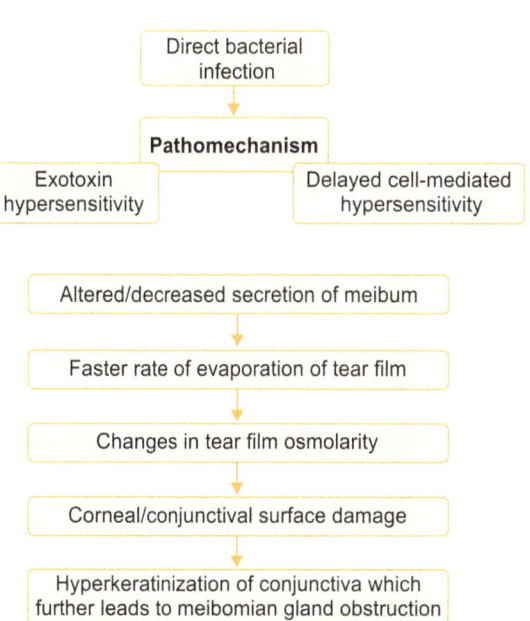

Staphylococcal Blepharitis

The mechanism by which the bacteria cause symptoms of blepharitis is not fully understood, and may include direct irritation from bacterial toxins or enhanced cell-mediated immunity to *S. aureus*. The most commonly identified species are *S. aureus* and *S. epidermidis*.

Others include *Propionibacterium*, *Corynebacteria*, and *Moraxella*.

Chronic forms of anterior blepharitis tend to be associated more with nonpathogenic flora. Chronic blepharitis is more associated with keratoconjunctivitis sicca, acne rosacea, and seborrheic dermatitis.

Meibomian gland dysfunction is characterized by functional abnormalities of the meibomian glands which tends to alter secretion of meibum.

Clinical Features

Symptoms
- Redness
- Burning sensation
- Irritation, itching
- Watering
- Eyelid sticking and crusting
- Visual problems—blurring of vision and photophobia.

Signs

Staphylococcal blepharitis:
- Erythema and edema of the eyelid margin
- Eyelash loss and/or misdirection
- Telangiectasia on the anterior eyelid
- Hard scales/collarettes encircling the lash base
- Corneal changes (infiltrates, phlyctenules)
- In severe and long-standing cases, eyelid ulceration, and corneal scarring may occur

Seborrheic blepharitis is differentiated by:
- Less erythema, edema, and telangiectasia of the lid margins
- An increased amount of oily scale and greasy crusting on the lashes

Posterior blepharitis/MGD:
- The meibomian glands may appear capped with oil, be dilated, or be visibly obstructed.
- The secretions of the glands are usually turbid and thicker than normal.
- The tear film will often have a foamy layer from the abnormal fatty acids, which can produce blurred vision.

- Severe cases will have posterior dragging of the meibomian gland orifices, and severe scarring can result. Telangiectasias and lid scarring may also be present in this area.
- Chalazia may be a cause or consequence of MGD.

Table 1 illustrates the differentiation of blepharitis among the three categories defined by the AAO.

TABLE 1: Categorization of blepharitis.			
	Infectious	*Seborrheic*	*Meibomian gland dysfunction*
Location	Anterior eyelid	Anterior eyelid	Posterior eyelid
Loss of lashes	Frequent	Rare	None
Lid margin	Hard, fibrinous scales with matted crusts	Oily or greasy	Unusual
Lid ulceration	Occasionally	None	None
Conjunctivitis discharge	Papillary with occasional purulent discharge	Follicular or papillary tarsal reaction with mild hyperemia	Papillary tarsal reaction with mild-to-moderate hyperemia
Keratitis	Inferior punctate erosions, marginal infiltrates, vascularization, phlyctenules	Inferior punctate erosions	Inferior punctate erosions, marginal infiltrates, vascular pannus
Tear film disruption	Occasional	Occasional	Occasional
Rosacea	Negative	15–25%	40–50%

Investigations

- There are no specific clinical diagnostic tests for blepharitis; however, cultures of the eyelid margins may be indicated for patients who have recurrent anterior blepharitis with severe inflammation as well as for patients who are not responding to the therapy.
- Since blepharitis is commonly associated with dry eye syndrome, the method most frequently used to assess tear film stability is to measure the tear break up time (TBUT; TBUT <10 seconds reflects tear film instability).
- Microscopic evaluation of epilated eyelashes may reveal Demodex mites, in few cases of chronic blepharitis. The specimen is prepared for microscopy by placing the explanted eyelashes on a glass slide, adding a drop of fluorescein, and securing the specimen beneath a cover slip.

  A biopsy of the eyelid may be indicated to exclude the possibility of carcinoma if the following features are present:

  - Unilateral blepharitis
  - Resistance to therapy
  - Unifocal recurrent chalazia
  - Loss of normal anatomy
  - Focal areas of madarosis

- If there are any signs of cicatrizing disease, always be suspicious about the possibility of ocular mucous membrane pemphigoid (OMMP) and the proper workup should be initiated, including immunofluorescence studies of the biopsy specimen.

Differential Diagnosis

Differential diagnosis of blepharitis presentation.	
Clinical condition	*Etiology*
Bacterial infection	• Impetigo • Erysipelas
Viral infection	• Herpes simplex virus • Molluscum contagiosum • Vaccinia
Parasitic infection	• *Pthirus pubis* • *Demodex*

Contd…

Contd...

Clinical condition	Etiology
Immune response related	• Atopic dermatitis • Contact dermatitis • Erythema multiforme • Ocular pemphigoid
Dermatoses	• Psoriasis • Ichthyosis
Benign lid tumors	• Pyogenic granuloma • Sebaceous cell hyperplasia • Actinic keratosis • Hemangioma
Malignant lid tumors	• Sebaceous carcinoma • Squamous cell carcinoma • Melanoma • Mycosis
Trauma	• Chemical • Thermal • Mechanical
Toxic	Medicamentosa

Management

Eyelid Hygiene

An initial step in treating patients who have blepharitis is to recommend eyelid hygiene, which includes warm compresses, eyelid massage, and eyelid scrubs. Eyelid cleansing is especially useful for anterior blepharitis, while warm compresses are especially helpful for posterior blepharitis and MGD.

Eyelid cleansing can be accomplished by brief, gentle massage of the eyelids. Cleaning the eyelid can be safely accomplished by having the patient gently rub the base of the eyelashes using either Blepharitis PPP 22 diluted baby shampoo or commercially available eyelid cleaner on a pad, cotton ball, cotton swab, or clean fingertip. Vertical eyelid massage can be performed to express meibomian secretions. Rubbing the eyelid margins from side to side removes crusting from the eyelashes.

Once- or twice-daily compresses and massage are generally adequate and have to be continued for 10–14 days.

Topical Antibiotics and Steroids

For anterior blepharitis, topical antibiotics have been found useful for symptomatic relief and effective in eradicating bacteria from the eyelid margins.

Oral antibiotics such as tetracyclines (tetracycline, doxycycline, minocycline) or macrolides (erythromycin, azithromycin) are recommended for patients with MGD not controlled with eyelid hygiene or patients with associated rosacea.

Short courses of topical steroids have been found beneficial for symptomatic relief in cases with clinically significant ocular inflammation. Corticosteroid drops or ointment can be applied several times daily to the eyelids or ocular surface until the inflammation is reduced. These agents can be tapered over time and gradually discontinued.

Topical Lubrication

Since most cases of blepharitis patients have associated dry eye problems, artificial tears may improve symptoms when used as an adjunct to eyelid cleansing and medications. If artificial tears are used more than four times per day, preservative-free tears should be preferred.

Seborrheic blepharitis is typically concomitant with seborrheic dermatitis, requiring simultaneous treatment of the underlying dermatological condition. Additional treatment options include *microblepharoexfoliation* and *antiseptic lid cleaning* for more moderate-to-severe cases.

Posterior Blepharitis

In the treatment of ocular surface disease secondary to posterior blepharitis, topical azithromycin has been demonstrated to improve patient signs and symptoms. Topical 1% azithromycin solution in combination with hyperthermic lid therapy was found to have increased effects when compared against hyperthermic lid therapy.

Newer Treatment Modalities

- Topical 0.05% cyclosporine is useful in MGD and posterior blepharitis, showing improved Schirmer scores, improved TBUT, and decreased patient symptoms when compared to tobramycin with dexamethasone.
- Increased intake of essential fatty acids, specifically omega-3 fatty acid, was recommended by the International Workshop on MGD for cases of mild-to-severe MGD. These essential fatty acids may be beneficial to anti-inflammatory processes and also reduce dry eye symptoms.
- For patients with Demodex infestation, 50% tea-tree oil eyelid scrubs and daily tea-tree-oil shampoo scrubs have been shown to be of some benefit when used for a minimum of 6 weeks. Oral ivermectin is useful in some cases of recalcitrant Demodex blepharitis.
- LipiFlow® (TearScience®, Morrisville, NC, USA) is a thermal pulsation system that applies heat and pressure to the eyelid tissue simultaneously to express the meibomian glands. LipiFlow system is proved to provide significant improvement in both signs and symptoms of MGD for up to 1 year.
- Intense pulse light (IPL) therapy for skin conditions such as rosacea is also noted to be beneficial in their MGD and dry eye symptoms. IPL is typically administered every 2–4 weeks for at least three sessions.

Prognosis

- Blepharitis is a chronic condition that has periods of exacerbation and remission.
- Patients should be informed that symptoms can frequently be improved but are rarely eliminated.

Complications

Rarely, severe blepharitis can result in permanent alterations in the eyelid margin or vision loss from superficial keratopathy, corneal neovascularization, and ulceration.

Suggested Reading

1. American Academy of Ophthalmology. Preferred Practice Pattern: Blepharitis. October 2012 revision. [online] Available from http://one.aao.org/preferred-practice-pattern/blepharitis-ppp--2013. [Last accessed May, 2022].
2. Bernardes TF, Bonfioli AA. Blepharitis. Semin Ophthalmol. 2010;25(3):79-83.
3. Bowman RW, Dougherty JM, McCulley JP. Chronic blepharitis and dry eyes. Int Ophthalmol Clin. 1987;27:27-35.
4. Geerling G, Tauber J, Baudouin C, Goto E, Matsumoto Y, O'Brien T, et al. The international workshop on meibomian gland dysfunction: report of the subcommittee on management and treatment of meibomian gland dysfunction. Invest Ophthalmol Vis Sci. 2011;52(4):2050-64.
5. Holzchuh FG, Hida RY, Moscovici BK, Villa Albers MB, Santo RM, Kara-José N, et al. Clinical treatment of ocular Demodex folliculorum by systemic ivermectin. Am J Ophthalmol. 2011;151(6):1030-4.e1.
6. Huber-Spitzy V, Baumgartner I, Bohler-Sommeregger K, Grabner G. Blepharitis: a diagnostic and therapeutic challenge. A report on 407 consecutive cases. Graefes Arch Clin Exp Ophthalmol. 1991;229(3):244-7.
7. Kanski JJ, Bowling B. Clinical Ophthalmology: a systemic approach, 7th edition. New York: Elsevier Saunders; 2011. pp. 34-9.
8. Kemal M, Sumer Z, Toker MI, Erdogan H, Topalkara A, Akbulut M. The prevalence of Demodex folliculorum in blepharitis patients and the normal population. Ophthalmic Epidemiol. 2005;12(4):287-90.
9. Lane SS, DuBiner HB, Epstein RJ, Ernest PH, Greiner JV, Hardten DR, et al. A new system, the LipiFlow, for the treatment of meibomian gland dysfunction. Cornea. 2012;31(4):396.
10. Luchs J. Efficacy of topical azithromycin ophthalmic solution 1% in the treatment of posterior blepharitis. Adv Ther. 2008;25(9):858-70.
11. McCulley JP, Dougherty JM, Deneau DG. Classification of chronic blepharitis. Ophthalmology. 1982;89:1173-80.
12. Putnam C. Diagnosis and management of blepharitis: an optometrist's perspective. Clin Optom (Auckl). 2016;8:71-8.
13. Rubin M, Rao SN. Efficacy of topical cyclosporine 0.05% in the treatment of posterior blepharitis. J Ocul Pharmacol Ther. 2006;22:47-53.
14. Seal D, Ficker L, Ramakrishnan M, Wright P. Role of staphylococcal toxin production in blepharitis. Ophthalmology. 1990;97(12):1684-8.
15. Shimazaki J, Sakata M, Tsubota K. Ocular surface changes and discomfort in patients with meibomian gland dysfunction. Arch Ophthalmol. 1995;113(10):1266-70.
16. Skuta GL, Cantor LB, Cioffi GA, et al. (Eds). American Academy of Ophthalmology Basic Clinical Science Course: External Disease and Cornea. Vol. 8. San Francisco, CA: American Academy of Ophthalmology; 2013. pp. 44-50, 58-66.
17. Toyos R, McGill W, Briscoe D. Intense pulsed light treatment for dry eye disease due to meibomian gland dysfunction; a 3-year retrospective study. Photomed Laser Surg. 2015;33(1):41-6.

Oculoplasty and Tumors

1.4 Blepharoptosis

Kavya B Madhuri, Devjyoti Tripathy

Q 1. Classify blepharoptosis and discuss its relevance to management and complication.

Blepharoptosis usually results from a congenital or acquired abnormality of the muscles that elevate the upper eyelid **(Figs. 1 and 2)**. Further classification of ptosis is helpful in recognizing the underlying cause, formulating an appropriate

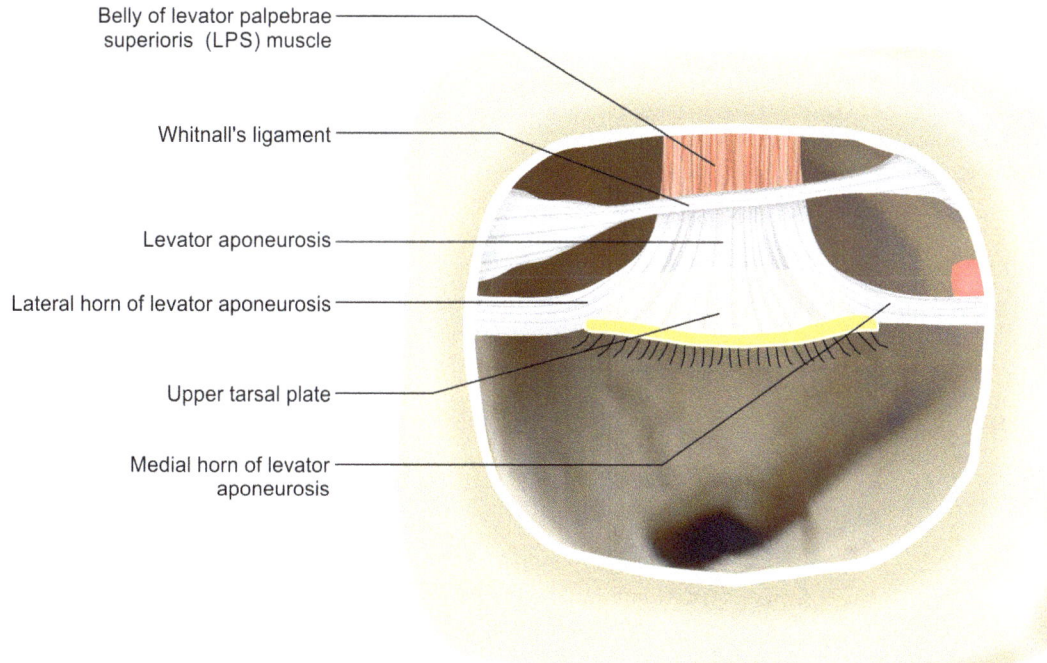

Fig. 1: The levator palpebrae superioris muscle arises from the lesser wing of the sphenoid bone, attaches to the fibrous levator aponeurosis in close proximity to Whitnall's ligament, and continues inferiorly to insert onto the anterior tarsal surface. The levator aponeurosis widens to form the medial and lateral levator horns as it passes inferiorly from Whitnall's ligament.

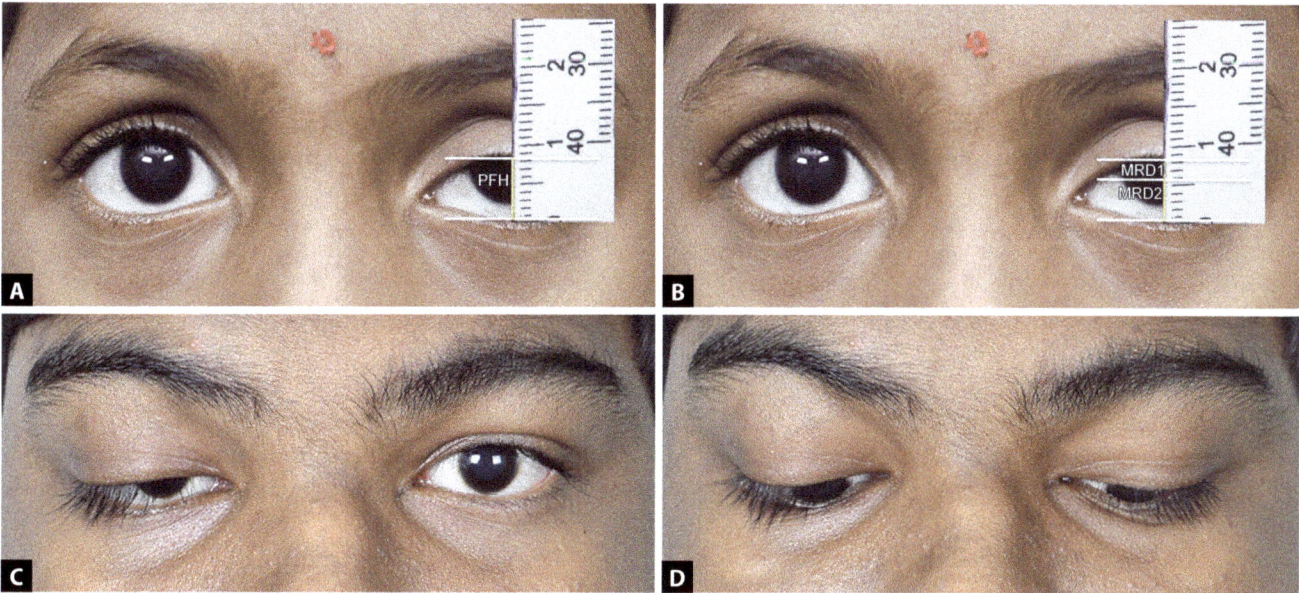

Figs. 2A to D: *Ptosis examination:* (A) PFH (palpebral fissure height) is the distance in millimeters measured between the upper and lower eyelid margins; (B) MRD_1 (margin reflex distance) is the distance from the corneal light reflex to the upper eyelid margin, MRD_2 is the distance of the lower eyelid from the corneal light reflex in primary gaze; (C) In simple congenital ptosis, eyelid crease is typically diminished; (D) the involved eyelid is higher than the uninvolved one in downgaze.

management plan, and minimizing the complications. Different classification systems exist for blepharoptosis. Here, the classification presented is based on the patient's clinical presentation and the need to select the appropriate surgical procedure for ptosis correction. Thus, blepharoptosis may be classified as follows.

Pseudoptosis

In a variety of conditions, the upper eyelid may appear to be ptotic even in the absence of true ptosis. These conditions mimic ptosis and should be differentiated from a true ptosis.

- *Contralateral widening of the lid fissure:* Contralateral proptosis, contralateral lid retraction
- *Lack of mechanical support:* Enophthalmos, phthisis bulbi, microphthalmos, anophthalmos, postenucleation socket syndrome, and superior sulcus defect
- *Globe displacement:* Ipsilateral hypotropia, double elevator palsy
- *Abnormal neurogenic innervations:* Duane's retraction syndrome, aberrant reinnervation of the facial nerve
- *Involuntary facial movements:* Hemifacial spasm, blepharospasm
- *Redundant skin:* Dermatochalasis, blepharochalasis, brow ptosis

True Ptosis

True ptosis, in turn, can be subdivided into congenital and acquired types.

Congenital Ptosis

Congenital ptosis can be further classified based on the etiopathogenesis:

- Simple congenital ptosis
- Monocular elevation deficit (MED)
- Marcus Gunn jaw-winking ptosis (MJWP)
- Blepharophimosis syndrome
- Congenital third cranial nerve palsy
- Congenital aponeurotic ptosis

Simple Congenital Ptosis

In simple congenital ptosis, the normal striated muscle fibers of levator palpebrae superioris (LPS) muscle are replaced by fibrous and adipose tissues in the muscle belly, thereby inhibiting the normal contraction and relaxation of the muscle. This condition is commonly called *congenital dysgenetic ptosis*. It is commonly noted during surgery in which the levator muscle is fibrotic and yellowish with fat deposition depending on the severity of the muscle dysgenesis.

Management
Congenital ptosis affects the patient physically (ptosis), functionally (amblyopia), and psychologically (psychosocial impact). It is relevant to understand when to intervene and how to repair the ptosis for an optimal outcome with minimal complications.

When to intervene?
- Generally, surgical intervention is planned before the child commences primary school in an attempt to minimize the psychosocial implications that can be associated with an asymmetric facial appearance while attending school. If not urgent, surgical correction of congenital ptosis is often delayed until the age of 3-4 years. Waiting until this age allows for a more accurate preoperative assessment.
- *Exception:* Surgery can be planned at an early stage in the following conditions:
  - *Abnormalities of visual development and function:* Amblyopia, strabismus, and refractive errors
  - *Ocular torticollis:* If not intervened early, the child develops compensatory chin-up head posture resulting in delayed milestones.

How to repair?
Selection of the appropriate surgical technique in simple congenital ptosis depends on the amount of levator function and the severity of ptosis. Depending on the clinical scenario, the following surgical techniques can be selected **Flowchart 1** in Management section.

Monocular Elevation Deficit

In this type of congenital ptosis, in addition to levator dysgenesis, there is an association of abnormal superior rectus muscle development which can be explained by their common embryological origin. The patient presents clinically with unilateral ptosis and limited eyeball elevation with poor Bell's phenomenon ("double elevator palsy").

Management

The elevation deficit needs to be corrected first to improve primary deviation and ocular motility followed by dysgenetic ptosis correction as mentioned above. Although the etiology is complicated, with the selection of a proper surgical approach, most cases with MED can achieve good therapeutic outcomes.
- If the forced duction test is positive, inferior rectus recession is the first choice of management.
- If the forced duction test is negative, the Knapp procedure could be considered, using either the standard or an augmented approach.
- For a vertical deviation of <30Δ, the standard Knapp procedure is preferred.
- For a larger deviation of 30Δ–40Δ, the foster procedure should be adopted.

Marcus Gunn Jaw-winking Ptosis

It is a peculiar type in which the congenital ptosis has association with a synkinetic jaw-winking phenomenon. There is an abnormal innervation of the levator muscle and the masticatory (external pterygoid) muscle. With mastication, the ptotic eyelid elevates abnormally with a jerky motion which is often seen in an infant while feeding.

Management

Depending on the amount of jaw-winking and degree of ptosis, several surgical techniques have been described for MJWP management:
- The milder forms of jaw winking (<2 mm) can be ignored, and the surgical correction is aimed to correct the ptosis.
- In moderate (2–4 mm) to severe (>4 mm) forms of jaw-winking associated with ptosis, frontal suspension with or without levator excision is preferred.

Blepharophimosis Syndrome

This is a genetically inherited disorder characterized by blepharophimosis (horizontal shortening of palpebral fissure), ptosis (drooping of upper eyelid), epicanthus inversus (upward fold of skin near medial canthus), telecanthus (increased inner intercanthal distance), hypoplasia of the nasal bridge, and superior orbital rim.

Management

Surgical management is aimed to correct the associated abnormalities first followed by ptosis correction.
- *First step:* The Mustarde's double "Z" plasty operation or a Y-V procedure can be performed for correction of epicanthal folds. Medial and lateral canthoplasties may help to increase the palpebral aperture width and telecanthus correction.
- Ptosis is usually left for the last as it may worsen following surgical intervention or other associated abnormalities. A bilateral frontalis sling is usually indicated for correction of ptosis.

Congenital Third Cranial Nerve Palsy

Congenital third cranial nerve palsy is discussed subsequently under the neurogenic ptosis section.

Congenital Aponeurotic Ptosis

It is a rarely described entity which may be attributed to perinatal events such as birth trauma resulting in partial or complete dehiscence or disinsertion of aponeurosis from its insertion. The patient presents clinically with mild-to-moderate ptosis, higher upper eyelid crease, and good levator action. It is essential to differentiate this from dysgenetic ptosis clinically as the management differs completely.

Management
- Surgical correction of the ptosis aims to address the aponeurotic defect and restore the aponeurosis to its normal anatomical position. Once the aponeurosis is repositioned, the levator function is restored and the ptosis is corrected.
  - In cases of levator disinsertion, a levator reinsertion procedure is recommended.
  - In patients with levator dehiscence, levator plication surgery is done.

Acquired Ptosis

It can be further divided under the following headings:

- Aponeurotic
- Myogenic
- Neurogenic
- Mechanical

Aponeurotic

Unlike the congenital aponeurotic ptosis, acquired aponeurotic ptosis is commonly encountered in clinical practice. The predisposing factors responsible for this acquired ptosis are ocular allergy, traumatic, surgical, or spontaneous. The degree of ptosis ranges from mild to severe depending on the levator disinsertion and dehiscence with relatively good levator function. The upper eyelid position is lower in downgaze, and multiple eyelid creases or higher eyelid crease are frequently associated.

Management

The dehisced or disinserted edge of levator aponeurosis is reattached to the anterior surface of the upper edge of the tarsus by a simple surgical procedure resulting in ptosis correction.

Myogenic

The myogenic ptosis types are usually recurrent and progressive despite multiple surgeries. Myasthenia gravis (MG) and chronic progressive external ophthalmoplegia (CPEO) are the most common myogenic ptosis types.

Acquired ptosis that is not associated with levator tendon dehiscence or trauma is a bigger challenge. MG, ocular-pharyngeal syndrome, idiopathic late-onset familial ptosis, and progressive external ophthalmoplegia fall into this category.

- MG:
  - The first line of treatment for ptosis in a patient of MG is with cholinesterase-inhibiting medications, immunosuppressive agents, and steroids. Dose titration and the drug combination need to be started along with the advice of an internist.
  - In refractory cases, a ptosis crutch spectacle may be tried, but some patients may not be very comfortable with these spectacles.
  - A silicone sling is usually reversible and could be a possibility for some patients in whom normal activities are being hampered. The basic aim is to lift the upper eyelid just clear of the optical axis.
- CPEO: Bell's phenomenon is absent in many patients with CPEO; therefore, ptosis surgery may be often contraindicated.
  - Initially, a ptosis crutch spectacle may be tried during his or her official activities, but some patients are not very comfortable with a crutch spectacle.
  - A silicone sling is usually reversible, so it could be a possibility for some patients, where normal activities are being hampered. The basic aim is to lift the lids just above the optical axis, so that the person can see. A higher correction can give rise to exposure keratopathy due to the absence of Bell's phenomenon. In some cases, this little correction may even have to be reversed back, if the patient starts to develop exposure keratopathy.

Neurogenic

Neurogenic ptosis is discussed subsequently under the neurogenic ptosis section.

Mechanical

Mechanical ptosis results secondary to excess eyelid skin (blepharochalasis) or eyelid lesions (stye, capillary hemangioma, neurofibroma, etc.) or orbital lesions causing the pressure over eyelid.

2. A 6-year-old child is brought to the Outpatient Department (OPD) by her parents with complaints of drooping of the left upper lid noticed 3 years ago. How would you evaluate this patient and decide on your course of management?

3. Describe the clinical features, evaluation, syndromic association, and management of congenital ptosis.

4. Discuss the management of a case of congenital ptosis.

 5. Evaluate in detail the surgical management and your criteria for decision-making in a case of congenital ptosis.

In congenital ptosis, abnormal drooping of upper eyelid is present since birth. The ptotic eye is recognized by the parents usually at birth or within infancy. There is preponderance of unilateral presentation without significant sex predilection.

Simple congenital ptosis is the most leading subtype of congenital ptosis with anomalous development of levator. The muscular and aponeurotic components of levator are supplanted by fibrous and adipose tissues. The magnitude of the ptosis depends on the extent of the myogenic dysgenesis resulting in variable clinical presentation: mild, moderate, and severe variants. (Refer to answer 1 for description of other subtypes of congenital ptosis.)

The disease onset is sporadic in majority of the patients. The autosomal dominant and recessive patterns of inheritance are seen less frequently. Some types of congenital ptosis are affected by variant syndromic associations **(Table 1)**.

TABLE 1: Syndromic associations of congenital ptosis.

Syndromic association	Etiology	Pathology	Clinical presentation
Isolated Duane syndrome	q arms of chromosome-2,8	Abnormal innervation of lateral rectus muscle by CN III	Drooping of upper eyelid on attempted adduction
Blepharophimosis-ptosis-epicanthus inversus syndrome (BPES)	*FOXL2* gene mutation	Abnormal proteins are expressed in the mesenchyme of eyelids in developmental stage	Bilateral ptosis associated with blepharophimosis
Lymphedema-distichiasis syndrome	*FOX2* gene mutation	Abnormal development of lymphatic vessels	Ptosis associated with distichiasis, lymphedema of extremities
Congenital fibrosis of the extraocular muscles (CFEOM)	• Autosomal dominant (types 1, 2) • Autosomal recessive (type 3)	Cranial dysinnervation	Ptosis associated with ophthalmoplegia
Congenital myasthenic syndrome	Autosomal recessive	Abnormal neuromuscular transmission	Ptosis associated with ocular signs and pulmonary dysfunction
Marcus Gunn syndrome	Sporadic	Abnormal connection between CN III and CN V	Variable ptosis with eye wink on jaw movement
Horner syndrome	Idiopathic	Abnormal sympathetic nerve pathway affecting Muller's function	Ipsilateral ptosis, miosis, anhidrosis

(CN: cranial nerve)

How to Distinguish Congenital Ptosis from Acquired Ptosis?

- Good history-taking
- Clinical examination.

History

- *Age of onset:* Birth; but it can be recognized by the parents at variable periods, ranging from birth to infancy.
- *Mode of onset:* Sudden/gradual/any precipitation factors
- *Duration:* Since birth in congenital type
- *Laterality:* Unilateral/bilateral
- Is the diagnosis simple congenital ptosis? The simple congenital ptosis is diagnosed by the absence of associated ocular or systemic associations.
- *Constant:* Extreme variation of the lid position by chewing, sucking, or other changes in jaw position suggests a synkinetic form of ptosis. Another variant of variable ptosis with ocular movements is seen in third nerve palsy with aberrant regeneration.
- *Intermittent/fatigue:* Any ptosis will be slightly worse when the patient is tired. Diurnal variation is typically absent in simple congenital ptosis.
- *Ocular history:* Prior usage of glasses, occlusion therapy, prisms, eye drops, ocular surgery
- *Medical history:* Birth weight, birth trauma, developmental delay, syndromic association, schooling, neurological, allergies, fatigability
- *Family history:* Congenital ptosis is predominantly sporadic. Familial inheritance is commonly seen in blepharophimosis syndrome. Often the parent bringing the child will have the syndrome.
- Review of old photographs

Clinical Examination

Refer to **Tables 2 and 3**.

TABLE 2: Clinical examination.

Clinical examination	Method	Interpretation

Vision	• Visual acuity:
	  – *Pre/nonverbal age:* Teller's acuity chart, preferential gaze testing
	  – *Verbal:* Pattern recognition cards, Allen cards, Snellen chart
	• Cycloplegic refraction
	• 10-Prism diopter test
		• Anisometropia
		• Amblyopia

Head posture	Inspection	• Abnormal head tilt • Chin elevation Developmental delay is noted in severe ocular torticollis with abnormal head tilt and extreme chin-up position
Facial symmetry	Inspection	*Eyebrow asymmetry:* Ipsilateral brow elevation due to frontal overaction is seen in ptosis patients
Extraocular muscle movements	Measure ductions and versions	Look for strabismus, superior rectus weakness, aberrant eyelid movements
Pupillary reaction	Direct, consensual, and accommodative reflex	Miosis is seen in Horner's syndrome
General ocular examination	Slit-lamp examination and fundus examination	• *Evert upper eyelid:* Look for tarsus height, papillary conjunctivitis, floppy eyelid syndrome • Eyelid laxity may need correction along with ptosis surgery • *Assess tear film, TBUT:* To look for dry eye syndrome • Corneal sensation • *Pigmentary retinopathy:* In CPEO
External photographs	Digital camera	Helpful in planning ptosis surgery

(CPEO: chronic progressive external ophthalmoplegia; TBUT: tear breakup time)

TABLE 3: Ptosis evaluation.

	Ptosis examination (**Fig. 2**)	
Clinical examination	Method	Interpretation
Palpebral fissure height (PFH)	Measure the distance (in millimeters) between upper and lower eyelid margin with physical ruler	• *Normal:* 9–10 mm • *Decreased PFH:* <9 mm • Reliable for ptosis diagnosis, only if lower eyelid is in normal position

Margin reflex distance (MRD)	• *Prerequisites:*
	  – *Position:* Patient seated at examiners eye level
	  – Relax patient's eyebrow by placing the hand on patient's forehead
	  – Patient's eye in primary gaze
	  – Ask patient to look at distant target
	  – At the level of patient's eye, shine penlight	

MRD_1	Measure the distance (in millimeters) between corneal light reflex to upper eyelid margin with physical ruler	• *Normal:* 4–5 mm • *Decreased:* <4 mm
MRD_2	Measure the distance (in millimeters) between corneal light reflex to lower eyelid margin with physical ruler	*Normal:* 4–5 mm
Levator palpebral superioris action (LPSA)	1. Measure the levator excursion (in millimeters) from extreme downgaze to extreme upgaze by placing the ruler over the lid in pupillary plane • *Prerequisite:* Immobilize the brow by holding with thumb 2. *Iliff's sign:* Evert the upper eyelid and ask the patient to look up	1a. *Poor:* ≤4 mm 1b. *Fair:* 5–7 mm 1c. *Good:* 8–11 mm 1d. *Excellent:* ≥12 mm • Child must be aged 3–4 years to obtain cooperation for this test 2. *Poor levator function:* If eyelid fails to flip back to its normal position

Contd...

Contd...

Clinical examination	Method	Interpretation

Margin crease distance (MCD)	Measure the distance (in millimeters) from upper lid margin to skin crease	• *Normal:* 8–10 mm (adult women), 6–8 mm (adult men)
		• *Absent/faint lid crease:* Indicates
		  – Poor LPS action (except patients of East Asian ancestry)
		  – Congenital ptosis with myogenic dysgenesis
		  – Elevated/multiple lid creases indicate aponeurotic dehiscence/disinsertion
		  – Choice of incision as it gives easy access to levator and leaves minimal scar at the wound site

Lid lag on downgaze	Compare the upper eyelid position in downgaze with the primary gaze	Lid lag with diminished amplitude of muscle action is typical of congenital ptosis
Lagophthalmos	Measure the distance (in millimeters) between upper and lower eyelid margin after eyelid closure	Impaired eye closure indicates poor orbicularis function, which may be exacerbated after ptosis correction
Hering's law	Lift the ptotic eye and look the contralateral upper eyelid position simultaneously	Hering's test is considered positive if contralateral eyelid drops down. Surgical correction of unilateral ptosis in these patients causes postoperative contralateral eyelid drooping
Bell's phenomenon	Hold the patient's upper eyelid, ask the patient to close the eyes, and look for eyeball movement	• *Normal:* If eyeball moves upward and outward • *Absent/poor:* Minimal or absent elevation of globe Consider absent Bell's phenomenon prior to ptosis surgery to estimate the risk of exposure keratopathy
Aberrant innervation	Ask the patient to perform oral or jaw movements	Eye wink is noted with jaw movements in Marcus Gunn jaw-winking ptosis

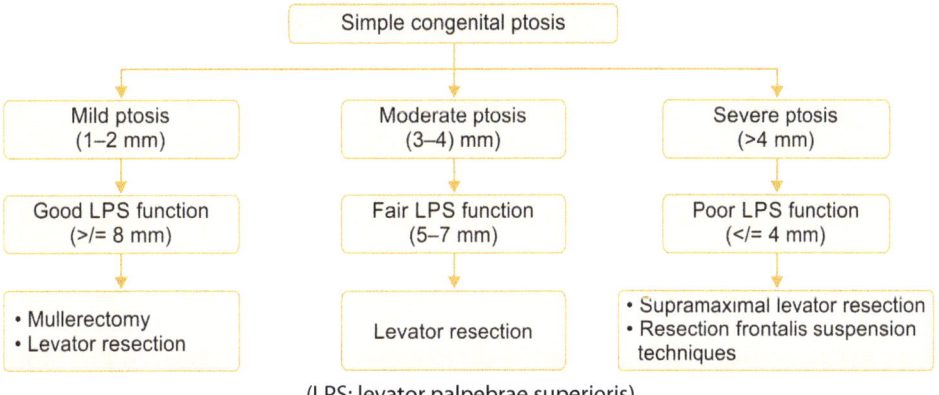

Flowchart 1: Management of congenital ptosis.

(LPS: levator palpebrae superioris)

Management

The procedure required for ptosis correction is planned based on the diagnosis of the subtype of congenital ptosis and the assessment of associated factors affecting the surgical outcome as discussed in the history taking and clinical examination.

In addition, the severity of ptosis and levator function plays a crucial role in selecting the surgery **(Flowchart 1)**. The levator function depends on the severity of ptosis which in turn depends on the proportion of levator dysgenesis.
- Mild myogenic dysgenesis is associated with mild ptosis (1-2 mm) and good to excellent levator function (>8 mm).
- Moderate myogenic dysgenesis has moderate ptosis (3-4 mm) with fair levator function (5-7 mm).
- Severe myogenic dysgenesis has severe ptosis (>4 mm) with poor levator function (<4 mm).

Mild Ptosis with Good Levator Action

Fasanella and Servat first described the surgical technique for correction of mild ptosis. In this technique, both the posterior lamella (conjunctiva, tarsus) and the middle lamella (Muller's levator) are excised in small bites. In view of associated complications with this technique, this procedure underwent many modifications. Out of these, Muller's muscle resection (MMR) is the most predictable technique and offers excellent results in mild ptosis with a positive phenylephrine test (refer to Section 1.6).

Moderate ptosis with fair to good levator action
In patients with moderate type of congenital ptosis with good levator function, levator resection is the procedure of choice (refer to Section 1.6).

How much Amount of Levator to Resect?

There are many techniques for estimating the amount of levator resection. All techniques are based on one of two well-known principles for estimating the amount of resection.

Levator Function Technique

In this technique, the amount of resection is determined intraoperatively. It assumes that the eyelid height, set during general anesthesia, will elevate or drop a predictable amount after the operation based on the patient's levator function. In this technique, the intraoperative height is adjusted based on the levator function **(Table 4)**.

TABLE 4: Levator function technique (based on Berke, 1959).

Levator function	Intraoperative lid height
2–3 mm (poor function)	At upper limbus
4–5 mm (poor function)	1–2 mm overlap
6–7 mm (fair function)	2 mm overlap
8–9 mm (good function)	3–4 mm overlap
10–11 mm (good function)	5 mm overlap

The easiest way to remember this is (Rule of Eight technique):
- If the levator function is 8 mm, set the intraoperative lid height at normal eyelid position.
- If the levator function is <8 mm, advance the aponeurosis more to set the lid height higher than the required postoperative level.
- For >8 mm of levator function, set the lid height lower, expecting that the levator will lift the lid more than the drop caused by the orbicularis muscle.

Margin Reflex Distance Technique

In this technique, amount of levator resection is determined based on the amount of ptosis preoperatively. With this technique, the levator is resected to a certain amount, depending on the preoperative margin reflex distance (MRD). There is no adjustment based on levator function. The amount of levator resection is increased in proportion to the severity of the ptosis **(Table 5)**.
- Although these two techniques seem quite different, they are similar in principle because the degree of ptosis is usually related to the amount of levator function. It is difficult to overcorrect congenital ptosis. A good rule to follow is to resect more if the eyelid position is not high enough intraoperatively.
- Posterior approach: In this type of ptosis correction, levator is approached through conjunctival route. Iliff's modified Blaskovics conjunctival approach is described for levator resection (refer to Section 1.6).

TABLE 5: Minimal residual disease technique.

Preoperative MRD$_1$	Amount of resection
3–4 mm (mild ptosis)	10–13 mm
2–3 mm (moderate ptosis)	14–17 mm
1–2 mm (marked ptosis)	18–22 mm
0–1 mm (severe ptosis)	>23 mm

Severe Ptosis with Poor Levator Action
Supramaximal levator resection and frontalis suspension techniques are described in patients with severe ptosis and poor levator function (refer to Section 1.6).

Q 6. Discuss the etiopathogenesis, clinical features, and management of unilateral ptosis with Marcus Gunn phenomenon or diagnosis and management of a case of unilateral ptosis with jaw-winking phenomenon.

It is a peculiar type in which the congenital ptosis has association with a synkinetic jaw-winking phenomenon.

Pathophysiology

There is an abnormal innervation of the levator muscle [cranial nerve III (CN III)] and the masticatory (external pterygoid) muscle (CN V). With mastication, the ptotic eyelid elevates abnormally with a jerky motion which is often seen in an infant while feeding.

Genetics

Unilateral ptosis is sporadic in nature.

Clinical Features

- *Laterality:* Usually unilateral.
- *Severity:* Mild-to-moderate ptosis.
- *Constant:* Variable ptosis in resting and primary position.
- *Time of onset:* It is usually diagnosed after birth, especially while feeding the infant by the mother.
- *Jaw wink:* Elevation of ptotic eyelid with oral or jaw movements **(Figs. 3A to D)**.

Gradation of Jaw-wink

- *Mild:* Elevation of ptotic eyelid ≤2 mm
- *Moderate:* Elevation of ptotic eyelid between 3 and 6 mm
- *Severe:* Elevation of ptotic eyelid ≥7 mm.

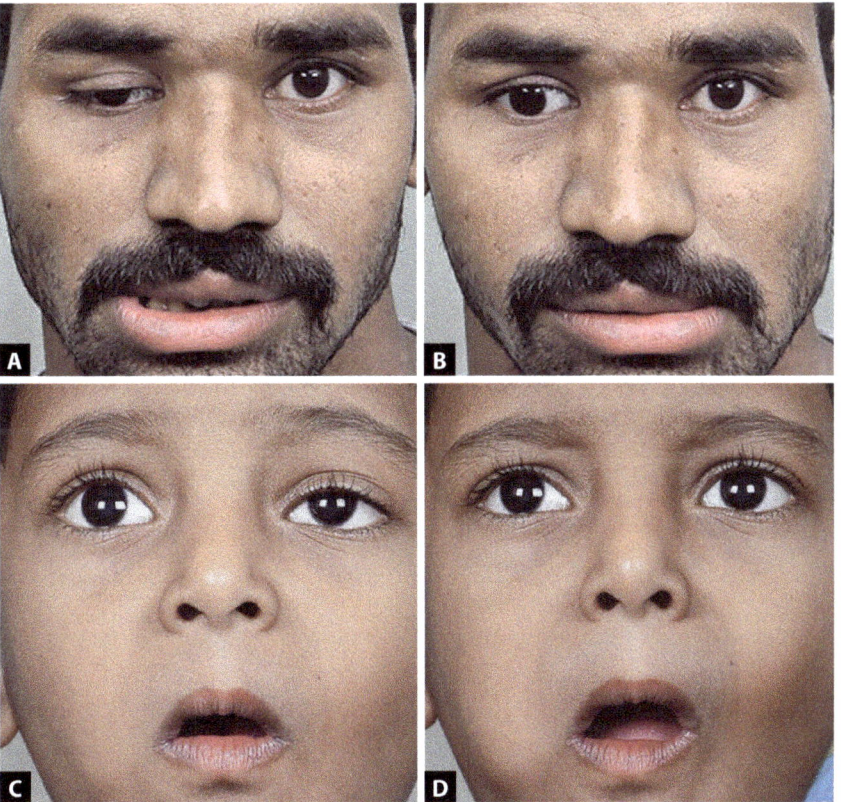

Figs. 3A to D: Patients with Marcus Gunn jaw-winking syndrome consist of a momentary upper eyelid retraction or elevation to an equal or higher level than the normal fellow eyelid upon stimulation of the ipsilateral pterygoid muscle. The wink phenomenon may be elicited by thrusting the jaw to the contralateral side (A and B) or by opening the mouth (C and D).

Other Associations

Strabismus is seen in more than half of the patients with MJWP followed by superior rectus palsy, anisometropia, and amblyopia.

Management

Refractive Errors

It is essential to correct the refractive errors and amblyopia management if required.

Strabismus

Squint correction must be addressed prior to any ptosis surgery.

Ptosis

Mild-to-moderate jaw wink
In Marcus Gunn jaw-winking phenomenon (MGJWP) patients with mild-to-moderate jaw wink, ptosis correction should be done in similar lines to simple congenital ptosis considering the severity of ptosis and levator function (refer to Section 1.6). The persistence of jaw wink even after ptosis correction should be explained to the patients prior to the surgery.

Severe Jaw Wink
Levator is disinserted followed by unilateral or bilateral frontalis suspension.

Other techniques:
- Levator muscle excision (Bullock)
- *Partial levator myectomy:* Anterior approach (Dillman and Anderson)
- *Partial levator myectomy:* Posterior approach (Bowyer and Sullivan)
- Fixation of transected levator to the superior orbital rim (Dryden)
- Bilateral levator excision and frontalis suspension (Beard)
- Ipsilateral levator excision and frontalis suspension (Kersten)
- Levator extirpation followed by frontalis flap suspension (Islam)
- Levator transection followed by brow suspension (Lemagne and Neuhaus).

 7. What are the components of blepharophimosis syndrome? Outline various principles in the complete management of this syndrome.

This is a genetically inherited disorder characterized by bilateral drooping of upper eyelid with horizontal shortening of palpebral fissure.

Genetics

Genetics involves mutation of *FOXL2* gene, on the long arm of chromosome 3 (3q23).

It is inherited as an autosomal dominant trait in both types of blepharophimosis, ptosis, and epicanthus inversus syndrome (BPES). Premature ovarian failure is typically seen in type I. It is more common in males compared to females.

Clinical Presentation (Fig. 4)

- *Blepharophimosis:* Abnormally narrow horizontal palpebral fissure
- *Ptosis:* Drooping of the upper eyelid
- *Epicanthus inversus:* A vertical fold of skin extending from the lower eyelid that stretches upward covering the inner canthus
- Absence of the eyelid fold.

Others

- *Telecanthus:* Widely spaced eyes with increased distance between the medial canthi
- *Microphthalmos:* Abnormally small eyes
- Displaced tear ducts

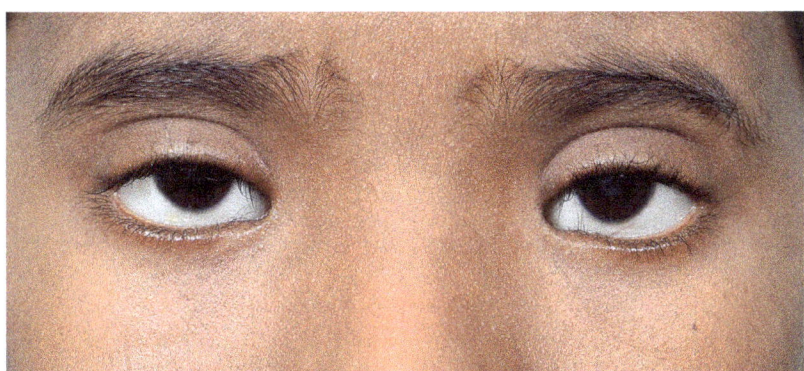

Fig. 4: Blepharophimosis syndrome is characterized by abnormally narrow horizontal palpebral fissure, drooping of the upper eyelid, and epicanthus inversus.

- Low bridge of the nose
- Developmental anomaly of the external ears
- Highly arched palate
- Infertility in females who are affected.

Management

Diagnosis

Blepharophimosis, ptosis, and epicanthus inversus syndrome is diagnosed based on the good history-taking and clinical evaluation.

Treatment

The surgical correction for BPES requires two stages:
- First stage involves correction of epicanthus, telecanthus, and blepharophimosis.
- Second stage is the correction of ptosis.
- Genetic counseling may be of benefit for patients and their families.

First Stage

Epicanthus
Epicanthus can be corrected by many procedures of which Mustarde's double Z-plasty/rectangular flap operation, or a Y-V plasty are the most popular procedures for correction of epicanthal folds and give good results.

Telecanthus
Medial canthal tendon shortening followed by transnasal fixation of the canthi reduces the intercanthal distance.

Blepharophimosis
Lateral canthotomy and cantholysis and new medial canthus with the correction of epicanthus inversus increase the palpebral aperture width horizontally.

Second Stage

Ptosis Correction
Ptosis should be carefully evaluated after the first stage of surgical correction. Ptosis correction should be done in similar lines to simple congenital ptosis considering the severity of ptosis and levator function (refer to Section 1.6).

 8. Explain the causes, pathophysiology, diagnosis, and management of acquired ptosis and senile ptosis.

 9. Explain the causes, pathophysiology, diagnosis, and management of senile ptosis.

Acquired ptosis is classified under the following headings depending on the etiopathogenesis:

- Aponeurotic
- Myogenic
- Neurogenic
- Mechanical

Aponeurotic

It is the most common type of acquired ptosis. It affects all the age groups.

Causes

- *Congenital:* Birth trauma
- *Acquired:*
  - Idiopathic
  - Involutional
  - Chronic inflammation or allergies with constant eye rubbing
  - *Chronic irritation:* Long-term use of contact lenses
  - Trauma
  - *Surgery:* Eyelid or intraocular surgery

Pathophysiology

Levator Dehiscence

In this type, LPS remains attached to the tarsal plate, but the aponeurotic fibers become stretched or elongated resulting in elevation of the lid crease.

Levator Disinsertion

In this type, there is thinning and stretching of the aponeurosis resulting in a complete or an incomplete disinsertion of the aponeurosis.

Clinical Features (Figs. 5A to D)

- *Laterality:* Unilateral or bilateral
- *Severity:* Ranges from mild to severe
- *Constant:* Ptosis is constant in all positions of gaze

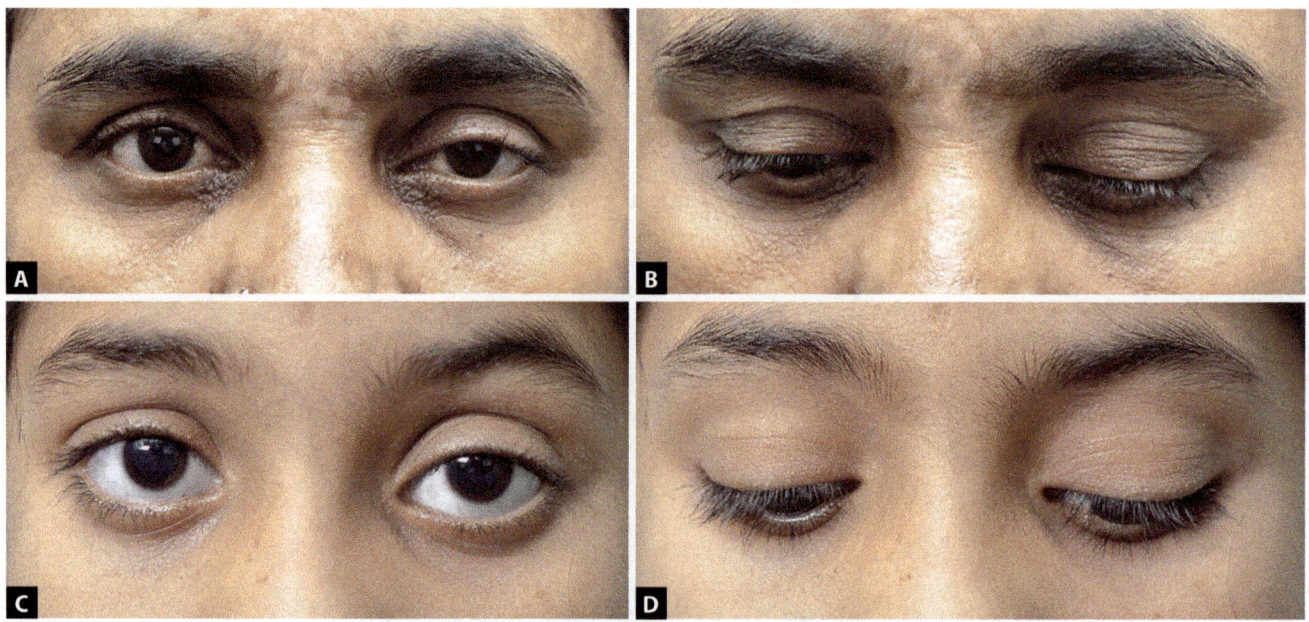

Figs. 5A to D: Aponeurotic ptosis is characterized by higher or multiple upper eyelid creases, lid drop on downgaze, and good levator function. It can be acquired (A and B) or congenital (C and D).

- *High skin crease:* In most of the patients with involutional ptosis, the upper eyelid crease will be higher than normal due to the upward drag of skin fibers by the levator aponeurosis. In some patients, multiple eyelid creases are noted.
- *Lid drop on downgaze:* In downgaze, the upper eyelid margin remains lower than the normal level. Contrast to this, lid lag on downgaze is noted in congenital ptosis due to the fibrotic levator muscle.
- *Good levator function:* The patients usually have normal or relatively normal levator function even though the eyelid droops. Though the aponeurosis has either slipped from its original insertion or has thinned and stretched, the muscle function remains normal.
- Visible iris sign is characteristically seen in aponeurotic ptosis with thinned-out eyelid skin and preaponeurotic fat atrophy.
- *Diurnal variation:* Patients complain of increase in intensity of the symptoms at the end of the day, mimicking ocular myasthenia.
- Normal extraocular motility.

Management

Levator advancement or reattachment is the treatment of choice in patients with aponeurotic ptosis. Levator muscle resection must never be attempted in these patients, as it leads to overcorrection of the ptosis (refer to Section 1.6).

Myogenic

Myasthenia gravis and CPEO are the most common causes of myogenic ptosis followed by myotonic dystrophy, facioscapulohumeral muscular dystrophy, oculopharyngeal muscular dystrophy, and congenital myopathies.

Myasthenia Gravis

Pathophysiology

It is an autoimmune disease in which abnormal antibodies are formed against the acetylcholine receptors resulting in blockage of neuromuscular transmission.

Clinical Presentation (Figs. 6A to E)

- *Onset:*
  - Neonates (transfer of maternal autoantibodies)
  - 20–30 years
  - Older than 50 years
- Unilateral or bilateral and usually asymmetrical.

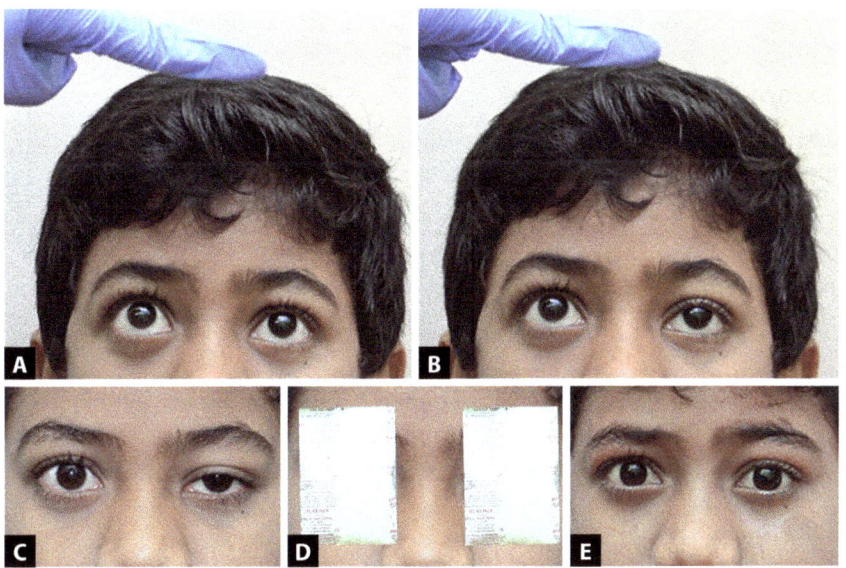

Figs. 6A to E: *Clinical tests for ocular myasthenia gravis:* (A) *Fatigue test:* Ask the patient to look in extreme upgaze for 1–2 minutes; (B) Worsening of ptosis by >2 mm is considered to be positive; (C to E) *Ice pack test:* It is considered positive if ptosis improves by 2 mm after 2 minutes.

- *Diurnal variation:* Worsening of the symptoms as the day progresses.
- Variable degree of ptosis
- Cogan's lid twitch sign can sometimes be demonstrated when the patient is asked to slowly look up from the downgaze.
- *Peek sign:* An attempt to open the eyes against forced eye closure cause the eyelid to drift apart making underlying sclera visible.
- Limited ocular motility and patient often complains of diplopia
- Difficulty in mastication and deglutition with involvement of pharyngeal muscles
- Generalized weakness
- Reduced exercise tolerance

Clinical Tests

- *Fatigue test:* Ask the patient to look in extreme upgaze for 1–2 minutes. Worsening of ptosis by >2 mm is considered to be positive.
- *Sleep test:* Look for resolution of ptosis and ophthalmoparesis after a period of rest of about 30 minutes.
- *Ice pack test:* It is based on the principle that cooling reduces the activity of acetylcholine-esterase, and it is considered positive if ptosis improves by 2 mm after 2 minutes and ophthalmoparesis after 5 minutes.

Other Tests

- *Pharmacological:* Edrophonium test (sensitivity 86%, specificity 97%) and neostigmine test (sensitivity 83%, specificity 97%) are performed to confirm the diagnosis of MG.
- *Immunological:* Acetylcholinesterase antibody (AChR-Ab) and antimuscarinic antibody (anti-MuSK Ab) tests are used to detect the abnormal acetylcholine receptor antibodies. AchR-Ab is present in 80–99% of patients with generalized myasthenia but only in about 50% of ocular myasthenia.
- *Electrophysiological:* Repetitive nerve stimulation (RNS) test (sensitivity 11–33%, specificity 89–98%) and single-fiber electromyography (sensitivity 85–100%, specificity 86–98%) may be helpful in detecting the ocular myasthenia.
- *Imaging:* Computed tomography (CT) or magnetic resonance imaging (MRI) of the chest must be done in patients with MG to screen for thymoma.

Management

- *Medical management:* Patients respond well to the medications with significant reduction or complete reversal of ptosis. Options are as follows:
  - Anticholinesterase agents
  - Systemic steroids
  - Immunosuppressants
  - Plasmapheresis
- *Surgical management:* Frontalis suspension with silicone sling is usually limited to the patients with poor response to medical management or with hampered normal daily activities. The basic aim is to lift the upper eyelids just above the visual axis so that the person can see. Thymectomy may be beneficial in patients with thymoma.

Chronic Progressive External Ophthalmoplegia

- It is a slowly progressive, symmetrical hereditary myopathy affecting the extraocular muscles.
- It is commonly manifested in younger population.

Pathophysiology

It is due to deletions of mitochondrial DNA (mtDNA) leading to impaired metabolic function.

Clinical Features

- Ptosis with abnormal head posture
- *External ophthalmoplegia:* It is usually symmetrical and progressive.
- *Others:* Facial and limb muscle weakness may be noted in up to 25% of the patients.

Management

Patients with CPEO are poor candidates for surgery because of the external ophthalmoplegia and progressive nature of the disease. These patients are more suitable for nonsurgical management, such as ptosis crutch glasses. A silicone sling is usually reversible, so it could be a possibility for some patients, where normal activities are being hampered. The basic aim is to lift the lids just above the optical axis, so that the person can see.

Neurogenic

Neurogenic ptosis is discussed in neurogenic section.

Mechanical

It occurs secondary to eyelid lesions that cause gravity-related ptosis.

Causes
- Eyelid lesions
- Orbital lesions
- Lesions causing adhesions between the eye and eyelid.

Management
The primary cause for ptosis must be treated in these patients.

 10. Discuss various modalities of management in a case of ptosis and their indications. Critically evaluate the operative procedures available and appropriate steps for prevention and treatment of postoperative problems.

Management Modalities

Ptosis repair is a challenging oculoplastic procedure, and the treatment options available can be divided into *nonsurgical* and *surgical* depending on the etiology and severity of ptosis.

Nonsurgical

When to prefer nonsurgical options in ptosis?
- Inappropriate candidates for ptosis correction
- Patients not keen for surgery.

Indications

When ptosis is accompanied with the following conditions:
- *Weakness of orbicularis muscle:* Ocular (myotonic dystrophy, CPEO) or generalized myopathies (myasthenia graves), combined CN III and CN VII palsies
- External or internal ophthalmoplegia to minimize exposure keratopathy, symptomatic diplopia, or photophobia.
- *Underlying pathology:* With uncertain disease process (myasthenia graves), transient disease (CN III palsy), and conditions (Tolosa–Hunt syndrome) suitable for medical management
- *Corneal hypoesthesia:* Isolated disease (viral keratitis) or combined cranial nerve palsies (CN III and CN V)
- Momentary phase secondary to botulinum toxin injections
- Ptosis with systemic morbidity.

Mechanical Measures
- *Lid crutches or ptosis crutch:* Spectacle frame with crutch to elevate the eyelid
- Eyelid taping is the simplest method of raising the eyelid by the use of adhesive tape to the upper eyelid.
- *Glues:* Redundant upper eyelid skin is glued to the subrow region
- Haptic contact lens is equipped with a shelf on which eyelid margin rests.

Medical Measures
- Topical medications (apraclonidine, oxymetazoline, phenylephrine, etc.) may be used in mild ptosis with sympathetic denervation of Muller's muscle, where the eyelid is elevated by nearly 2 mm.

- Botulinum toxin, though carries the risk of worsening the ptosis by weakening the levator palpebrae muscle, in fact serves to lessen the true ptosis temporarily by causing toxin-mediated paresis of orbicularis muscle.

Surgical

The following procedures are the most frequently used with which most of the ptosis patients can be corrected.
- MMR
- Levator muscle resection
- Levator aponeurosis repair (advancement)
- Frontalis suspension.

The key factors in choosing the appropriate operation are:
- Amount of ptosis
- Levator muscle function
- Ocular motility.

Muller's Muscle Resection

Muller's muscle resection is the most predictable technique and offers excellent results.

Indications
Mild ptosis of 2 mm with the levator function of at least 10 mm with positive phenylephrine test

Contraindications
- History of previous surgeries involving the tarsus
- Abnormalities of the posterior lamella
- Scarring of superior fornix or posterior lamella.

Phenylephrine test
Phenylephrine is an alpha-1 adrenergic agonist that stimulates Muller's muscle to contract.

How to perform the test?
Instill 10% phenylephrine into the superior fornix of both the eyes. Assess MRD_1 before and 5 minutes after phenylephrine instillation and note the response.

Interpretation
- *Good response:* Symmetry at a good height
- *Moderate or poor response:* Persistent or inadequate elevation.

Role in planning for surgery depending on the ptotic eyelid position
- *Rises to normal level:* 8 mm should be resected.
- *Rises higher than the expected:* Reduce the resection to 6.5–8 mm.
- *Remains lower than the expected rise:* Resect 8–9.5 mm.
- *Poor or absence of response:* Consider an alternative procedure (levator surgery).

Procedure
- *Type of anesthesia:* Local (+/− sedation) or general anesthesia
- Upper eyelid skin crease is marked.
- Subconjunctval infiltration of adrenaline mixed local anesthetic can be injected to improve hemostasis and for better plane of dissection.
- *Eyelid eversion:* Desmarres retractor or Cotton Tip Applicator is used for everting the eyelid.
- *Tissues to be resected:* Grasp the Muller's muscle-conjunctival complex, incorporate in Putterman clamp and resect the desired amount.
- The internal wound is closed with continuous nonabsorbable suture with exteriorization of suture knots.

Advantages
The procedure leaves minimal postoperative edema and no external scar and offers faster recovery period, with minimal effect on patient's blink rate.

Levator Muscle Resection

Levator muscle resection offers ptosis correction with shortening of levator–aponeurosis complex.

Indications
- Congenital ptosis with a moderate levator dysgenesis
- Acquired ptosis with a myopathic problem or scarring within the levator muscle
  In both of these situations, a reasonable amount of levator function must be present (at least >4 mm).

Contraindications
- Decreased corneal sensation, dry eye
- Absent Bell's phenomenon.

Procedure
- *Type of anesthesia:* Local (in adults) or general anesthesia (in children)
- *Incision:* Along the upper eyelid crease or presumed crease in symmetry to the contralateral eyelid
- *Exposure of levator:* Suborbicularis dissection is carried in preseptal plane till 10-15 mm superiorly. Extend transseptally and retract the preaponeurotic fact to expose the levator muscle till the Whitnall's ligament.
- *Tissues to be resected:* Grasp the levator–aponeurosis complex and resect the desired amount **(Tables 4 and 5)**.
- The wound is closed with continuous nonabsorbable suture.

Advantages
The procedure offers revision of surgery with ptosis suture adjustment.

Levator Aponeurosis Repair (Advancement)

Levator muscle resection offers ptosis correction with advancement of levator–aponeurosis complex.

Indications
- Senile involutional ptosis
- Ptosis secondary to trauma or chronic inflammatory changes resulting in levator dehiscence or disinsertion
- Congenital aponeurotic ptosis.

Contraindications
- Decreased corneal sensation, dry eye
- Absent Bell's phenomenon.

Procedure
- *Type of anesthesia:* Local (in adults) or general anesthesia (in children)
- *Incision:* Along the upper eyelid crease or presumed crease in symmetry to the contralateral eyelid
- *Exposure of levator:* Suborbicularis dissection is carried in preseptal plane till the preaponeurotic fat is visible through the orbital septum, extend transseptally and retract the preaponeurotic fact to expose the disinherited or dehisced edge of levator aponeurosis.
- *Tissues to be advanced:* Grasp the disinherited or dehisced edge of levator aponeurosis and fix to tarsal plate after achieving desirable upper eyelid height and contour.
- The wound is closed with continuous nonabsorbable suture.

Advantages
The procedure offers revision of surgery with ptosis suture adjustment.

Frontalis Suspension

This procedure offers ptosis correction by transferring the frontal action to the eyelid.

Indications
- Congenital and acquired ptosis with poor levator function of <4 mm.
- In a very young child with severe ptosis, when levator function cannot be measured, frontalis suspension can be used as a temporary measure.
- In patients with absent Bell's phenomenon, ptosis undercorrection can be attempted with frontalis suspension.

Relative Contraindications
- Decreased corneal sensation, dry eye
- Absent Bell's phenomenon

Variations of the frontalis suspension technique include the *type of suspensory material* employed, *configuration for implantation*, and the *surgical approach*.

Suspensory Materials
- *Autologous:* Fascia lata, palmaris longus tendon, deep temporal fascia
- *Allogenous:* Prolene, silicone, Supramid, Gore-Tex, Mersilene mesh.

Configuration of frontal suspension
Historically, a double rhomboid or double triangular (Crawford) configuration for frontalis suspension has been used. Now, the use of a single-strand configurations *(Trapezoid-Pentagon Fox technique)* are popular as the use of the two strands of suspensory material in the upper lid is unnecessarily cumbersome and introduces more bulk than is necessary.

Surgical approaches
- *Open approach:* In this type of approach, tarsus is exposed through skin crease incision and suspended to the frontalis muscle with suspensory material. This technique ensures greater stability of the suspension and reduces the risk of migration, but associated with the postoperative edema and lash ptosis.
- *Closed approach:*
  - Trapezoid-pentagon Fox technique
  - Double triangle (Crawford) technique.

Procedure
- *Type of anesthesia:* Local (+sedation in adults) or general anesthesia (in children).
- *Incisions:* Three sub-brow incisions (stab) and three eyelid incisions (nick)
- *Type of suspension:* Suspensory material is passed through brow-eyelid-skin incisions in pentagonal or double triangle fashion.
- Once the contour and desired height adjusted, the knot is placed in the suspensory material and the ends are tucked in a tunnel fashioned from the central brow incision superiorly.
- The forehead wound is then closed with interrupted 6/0 absorbable sutures. The eyelid wounds are left unsutured.
- A lower eyelid Frost suture is placed to prevent postoperative exposure keratopathy.

Advantages
The procedure can be reversible or readjustable.

 11. Complications of LPS resection in ptosis surgery.

 12. Outline your approach for the evaluation and management of a case of failed ptosis surgery.

 13. Outline your approach for the evaluation and management of failed ptosis.

The clinical examination and classification of ptosis plays a vital role in proper selection of surgical technique and thereby reducing the complication rate. In majority of the patients, complications of ptosis surgery results from inadequate assessment, improper diagnosis, or inadequate surgical correction. In this section, the different varieties of complications associated with ptosis surgery is discussed.

- Overcorrection
- Undercorrection
- Eyelid contour defects
- Skin crease defects
- Entropion
- Ectropion
- Infection and inflammatory reactions
- Late granulomatous inflammatory reactions
- Suture exposure

- Corneal abrasions
- Excess skin
- Exposure keratopathy
- Conjunctival prolapse
- Peaking of the lid
- Lash ptosis
- Lid lag and lagophthalmos
- Hemorrhage
- Double vision

Overcorrection

Etiology
- Inadvertent shortening of orbital septum
- Whitnall's ligament is fixed to tarsus instead of levator
- Excess levator advancement or levator resection in aponeurotic ptosis.

Management
In mild cases of overcorrection, lid pulling exercises can be advised to the patient during the second week of postoperative period. If there is significant overcorrection, ptosis suture adjustment is attempted in immediate postoperative period. Rarely, spacers or levator recession may be useful if there is persistent overcorrection even after applying all the necessary measures.

Undercorrection

It is most commonly noted following surgical repair of congenital ptosis.

Etiology
- Insufficient amount of levator resection
- Excess intraoperative hemorrhage
- Misplace or slippage of sutures.

Management
Significant undercorrection can be corrected only by revising the surgery with appropriate amount of levator resection or suture adjustment or proper hemostasis.

Eyelid Contour Defects

Etiology
- Inappropriate placement of cardinal sutures
- Improper tarsal bites.

Management
Eyelid pull can be attempted if there is mild peaking of eyelid contour. In severe cases or in flat contours, the sutures are readjusted selectively.

Skin Crease Defects

Skin crease defects are seen in patients with unaddressed blepharoplasty or improperly marked eyelid crease or failure to perform the lid crease forming sutures during ptosis surgery. It can be corrected by performing a blepharoplasty or formation of Pang sutures.

Entropion

Entropion is rarely seen in patients with redundant anterior lamella which can be reversed by resection of excess skin and formation of deep lid crease sutures.

Ectropion

Ectropion is seen in patients with excess resection of anterior lamella or highly placed lid crease, which can be corrected by wound undermining and inferior placement of lid crease.

Infection and Inflammatory Reactions

Infection and inflammatory reactions are seen in some patients with traumatic ptosis in which proper wound irrigation followed by wound exploration for foreign body needs to be done. It is also seen in frontalis suspension patients with allogenous suspensory materials.

Late Granulomatous Inflammatory Reactions

Late granulomatous inflammatory reactions are noted around the suture materials or suspensory materials, which should be treated with topical or intralesional steroids or removal of the suspensory material, respectively.

Suture Exposure

Suture exposure occurs with inadequate trimming of the suture ends at the surgical knot causing irritation.

Corneal Abrasions

Corneal abrasions are commonly seen in patients with lagophthalmos which can be avoided by applying frost sutures.

Excess Skin

Excess skin can be resected simultaneously during ptosis correction.

Exposure Keratopathy

Exposure keratopathy is commonly noted in congenital ptosis patients or acquired myopathies with lagophthalmos or poor Bell's phenomenon. Patient needs close monitoring with lubricants and frost suture application.

Conjunctival Prolapse

Conjunctival prolapse is associated with inadvertent intraoperative damage to check ligament or due to postoperative edema. The options available to correct the conjunctival prolapse is by repositioning of the conjunctival fornix or excision of the prolapsed tissue.

Peaking of the Lid

Peaking of the lid can occur with unevenly placed cardinal sutures, which can be corrected by revision of the surgery.

Lash Ptosis

Lash ptosis can be prevented by suturing the skin edges to the levator stump.

Lid Lag and Lagophthalmos

Lid lag and lagophthalmos is commonly seen in moderate-to-severe type of ptosis where frequent lubrication is advised in the immediate postoperative period.

Hemorrhage

Intraoperative and postoperative hemorrhage in ptosis surgery can be prevented by asking the patient to discontinue antiplatelet drugs 3–5 days before surgery, maintaining stable blood pressure levels, usage of subcutaneous injection of local anesthesia, and meticulous hemostasis during surgery.

Double Vision

Double vision is very rarely noted after ptosis repair, secondary to superior rectus, or superior oblique tendon injury, which may happen with surgeons having poor understanding of eyelid anatomy.

Suggested Reading

1. Albert DM, Lucarelli MJ. Ptosis. In: Clinical Atlas of Procedures in Ophthalmic Surgery. Chicago, IL: AMA Press; 2004.
2. Allen CE, Rubin PAD. Blepharophimosis-ptosis-epicanthus inversus syndrome (BPES): clinical manifestation and treatment. Int Ophthalmol Clin. 2008;48(2):15-23.
3. Anderson RL, Beard C. The levator aponeurosis: attachments and their clinical significance. Arch Ophthalmol. 1977;95(8):1437-41.
4. Anderson RL, Dixon RS. Aponeurotic ptosis surgery. Arch Ophthalmol. 1979;97(6):1123-8.
5. Anderson RL, Jordan DR, Dutton JJ. Whitnall's sling for poor function ptosis. Arch Ophthalmol. 1990;108(11):1628-32.
6. Anderson RL. Age of aponeurotic awareness. Ophthal Plast Reconstr Surg. 1985;1(1):77-9.
7. Baroody M, Holds JB, Vick VL. Advances in the diagnosis and treatment of ptosis. Curr Opin Ophthalmol. 2005;16(6):351-5.
8. Beard C. A new classification of blepharoptosis. Int Ophthalmol Clin. 1989;29(4):214-6.
9. Beard C. Ptosis. St Louis, MO: CV Mosby; 1981.
10. Ben Simon GJ, Lee S, Schwarcz RM, McCann JD, Goldberg RA. Muller's muscle-conjunctival resection for correction of upper eyelid ptosis: relationship between phenylephrine testing and the amount of tissue resected with final eyelid position. Arch Facial Plast Surg. 2007;9(6):413-7.
11. Berry-Brincat A, Willshaw H. Paediatric blepharoptosis: a 10-year review. Eye (Lond). 2009;23(7):1554-9.
12. Bowyer JD, Sullivan TJ. Management of Marcus Gunn jaw-winking synkinesis. Ophthal Plast Reconstr Surg. 2004;20(2):92-8.
13. Buckman G, Levine MR. Treatment of prolapsed conjunctiva. Ophthal Plast Reconstr Surg. 1986;2(1):33-9.
14. Carroll RP. Preventable problems following the Fasanella-Servat procedure. Ophthalmic Surg. 1980;11(1):44-51.
15. Cetinkaya A, Brannan PA. Ptosis repair options and algorithm. Curr Opin Ophthalmol. 2008;19(5):428-4.
16. Cetinkaya A, Brannan PA. What is new in the era of focal dystonia treatment? Botulinum injections and more. Curr Opin Ophthalmol. 2007;18(5):424-9.
17. Codère F, Tucker NA, Renaldi B. The anatomy of Whitnall ligament. Ophthalmology. 1995;102(12):2016-9.
18. Collin JR. Complications of ptosis surgery and their management: a review. JR Soc Med. 1979;72(1):25-6.
19. Dresner SC. Further modifications of the Müller's muscle-conjunctival resection procedure for blepharoptosis. Ophthal Plast Reconstr Surg. 1991;7(2):114-22.
20. Dutton JJ. Atlas of clinical and surgical orbital anatomy. Philadelphia, PA: WB Saunders; 1994.
21. Edmunds B, Manners RM, Weller RO, Steart P, Collin JR. Levator palpebrae superioris fibre size in normals and patients with congenital ptosis. Eye (Lond). 1998;12(Pt 1):47-50.
22. Fasanella RM, Servat J. Levator resection for minimal ptosis, with indications and reappraisal. Int Ophthalmol Clin. 1970;10(1):117-30.
23. Fasanella RM, Servat J. Levator resection for minimal ptosis: another simplified operation. Arch Ophthalmol. 1961;65:493-6.
24. Ficker LA, Collin JR, Lee JP. Management of ipsilateral ptosis with hypotropia. Br J Ophthalmol. 1986;70(10):732-6.
25. Frueh BR. The mechanistic classification of ptosis. Ophthalmology. 1980;87(10):1019-21.
26. George A, Haydar AA, Adams WM. Imaging of Horner's syndrome. Clin Radiol. 2008;63(5):499-505.
27. Georgescu D, Vagefi MR, McMullan TFW, McCann JD, Anderson RL. Upper eyelid myectomy in blepharospasm with associated apraxia of lid opening. Am J Ophthalmol. 2008;145(3):541-7.
28. Gundersen T. Conjunctival flaps in the treatment of corneal disease with reference to a new technique of application. AMA Arch Ophthalmol. 1958;60(5):880-8.
29. Jordan DR, Anderson RL. The aponeurotic approach to congenital ptosis. Ophthalmic Surg. 1990;21(4):237-44.
30. Juel VC, Massey JM. Myasthenia gravis. Orphanet J Rare Dis. 2007;2:44.
31. Khooshabeh R, Baldwin HC. Isolated Muller's muscle resection for the correction of blepharoptosis. Eye (Lond). 2008;22(2):267-72.
32. Koursh DM, Modjtahedi SP, Selva D, Leibovitch I. The blepharochalasis syndrome. Surv Ophthalmol. 2009;54(2):235-44.
33. Lane CM, Collin JR. Treatment of ptosis in chronic progressive external ophthalmoplegia. Br J Ophthalmol. 1987;71(4):290-4.
34. Lee MJ, Oh JY, Choung HK, Kim NJ, Sung MS, Khwarg SI. Frontalis sling operation using silicone rod compared with preserved fascia lata for congenital ptosis: a three-year follow-up study. Ophthalmology. 2009;116(1):123-9.
35. Leibovitch I, Selva D. Floppy eyelid syndrome: clinical features and the association with obstructive sleep apnea. Sleep Med. 2006;7(2):117-22.
36. Leone Jr CR, Shore JW. The management of the ptosis patient: part I. Ophthalmic Surg. 1985;16(10):666-70.
37. Lin LK, Uzcategui N, Chang EL. Effect of surgical correction of congenital ptosis on amblyopia. Ophthal Plast Reconstr Surg. 2008;24(6):434-6.
38. Malhotra R, Mahadevan V, Leatherbarrow B, Barrett AW. The post-levator aponeurosis fat pad. Ophthal Plast Reconstr Surg. 2015;31(4):313-7.
39. Malhotra R, Salam A, Then S-Y, Grieve AP. Visible iris sign as a predictor of problems during and following anterior approach ptosis surgery. Eye (Lond). 2011;25(2):185-91.
40. Manners RM, Rosser P, Collin JR. Levator transposition procedure: a review of 35 cases. Eye (Lond). 1996;10(Pt 5):539-44.
41. Manners RM, Tyers AG, Morris RJ. The use of Prolene as a temporary suspensory material for brow suspension in young children. Eye (Lond). 1994;8(Pt 3):346-8.
42. Martin Jr JJ, Tenzel RR. Acquired ptosis: dehiscences and disinsertions. Are they real or iatrogenic? Ophthal Plast Reconstr Surg. 1992;8(2):130-2, discussion 133.

43. McCord C (Ed). Complications of ptosis surgery and their management. In: Eyelid Surgery—Principles and Techniques. Philadelphia, PA: Lippincott-Raven; 1995. pp. 144-55.
44. McCord C (Ed). Decision making in ptosis surgery. In: Eyelid Surgery—Principles and Techniques. Philadelphia, PA: Lippincott-Raven; 1995. pp. 139-43.
45. McNab AA. The eye and sleep apnea. Sleep Med Rev. 2007;11(4):269-76.
46. McNab AA. The eye and sleep. Clin Experiment Ophthalmol. 2005;33(2):117-25.
47. Meyer DR, Linberg JV, Wobig JL, McCormick SA. Anatomy of the orbital septum and associated eyelid connective tissues. Implications for ptosis surgery. Ophthal Plast Reconstr Surg. 1991;7(2):104-13.
48. Michels KS, Vagefi MR, Steele E, Zwick OM, Torres JJ, Seiff SR, et al. Müller muscle-conjunctiva resection to correct ptosis in high-risk patients. Ophthal Plast Reconstr Surg. 2007;23(5):363-6.
49. Nerad J. Evaluation and treatment of the patient with ptosis. In: The Requisites—Oculoplastic Surgery. St Louis: Mosby; 2001. pp. 157-92.
50. Nerad JA, Carter KD, Alford MA. Disorders of the eyelid: blepharoptosis and eyelid retraction. In: Rapid Diagnosis in Ophthalmology—Oculoplastic and Reconstructive Surgery. Philadelphia: Mosby Elsevier; 2008. pp. 102-15.
51. Ortisi E, Henderson HWA, Bunce C, Xing W, Collin JR. Blepharospasm and hemifacial spasm: a protocol for titration of botulinum toxin dose to the individual patient and for the management of refractory cases. Eye (Lond). 2006;20(8):916-22.
52. Peter NM, Khooshabeh R. Open-sky isolated subtotal Muller's muscle resection for ptosis surgery: a review of over 300 cases and assessment of long-term outcome. Eye (Lond). 2013;27(4):519-24.
53. Putterman AM, Urist MJ. Müller muscle-conjunctiva resection. Technique for treatment of blepharoptosis. Arch Ophthalmol. 1975;93(8):619-23.
54. Putterman AM. Müller's muscle-conjunctival resection. In: Levine MR (Ed). Manual of Oculoplastic Surgery, 3rd edition. Boston, MA: Butterworth Heinemann; 2003. pp. 117-23.
55. Putterman AM. Müllers muscle-conjunctival resection ptosis procedure. Aust N Z J Ophthalmol. 1985;13(2):179-83.
56. Rose GE. The giant fornix syndrome: an unrecognized cause of chronic, relapsing, grossly purulent conjunctivitis. Ophthalmology. 2004;111(8):1539-45.
57. Shore JW, Bergin DJ, Garrett SN. Results of blepharoptosis surgery with early postoperative adjustment. Ophthalmology. 1990;97(11):1502-11.
58. Striph GG, Miller NR. Disorders of eyelid function caused by systemic disease. In: Bosniak S (Ed). Principles and Practice of Ophthalmic Plastic and Reconstructive Surgery. Philadelphia, PA: WB Saunders, 1996. pp. 72-93.
59. Wong VA, Beckingsale PS, Oley CA, Sullivan TJ. Management of myogenic ptosis. Ophthalmology. 2002;109(5):1023-31.
60. Woog JJ. Obstructive sleep apnea and the floppy eyelid syndrome. Am J Ophthalmol. 1990;110(3):314-5.
61. Yanovitch T, Buckley E. Diagnosis and management of third nerve palsy. Curr Opin Ophthalmol. 2007;18(5):373-8.

1.5 Entropion and Ectropion

Akruti Desai, Suryasnata Rath

1. Explain the etiopathogenesis, classification, preoperative assessment, and management modalities of different types of entropion.

The eyelid position is determined by various anatomic factors comprising anterior and posterior lamellae of eyelids, such as the orbicularis oculi muscle and eyelid retractors. Destabilization of eyelid margin may cause an inward rotation or outward rotation of the eyelid margin. Entropion is characterized by inward rotation of the eyelid margin. Patients with entropion tend to present early due to symptoms of foreign body sensation, irritation, watering, or redness.

Relevant Anatomy (Figs. 1A and B)

Classification

Entropion is classified as given in **Table 1**:

TABLE 1: Classification of entropion.	
Congenital	**Acquired**
	• Senile/involutional
	• Cicatricial
	• Spastic
	• Marginal

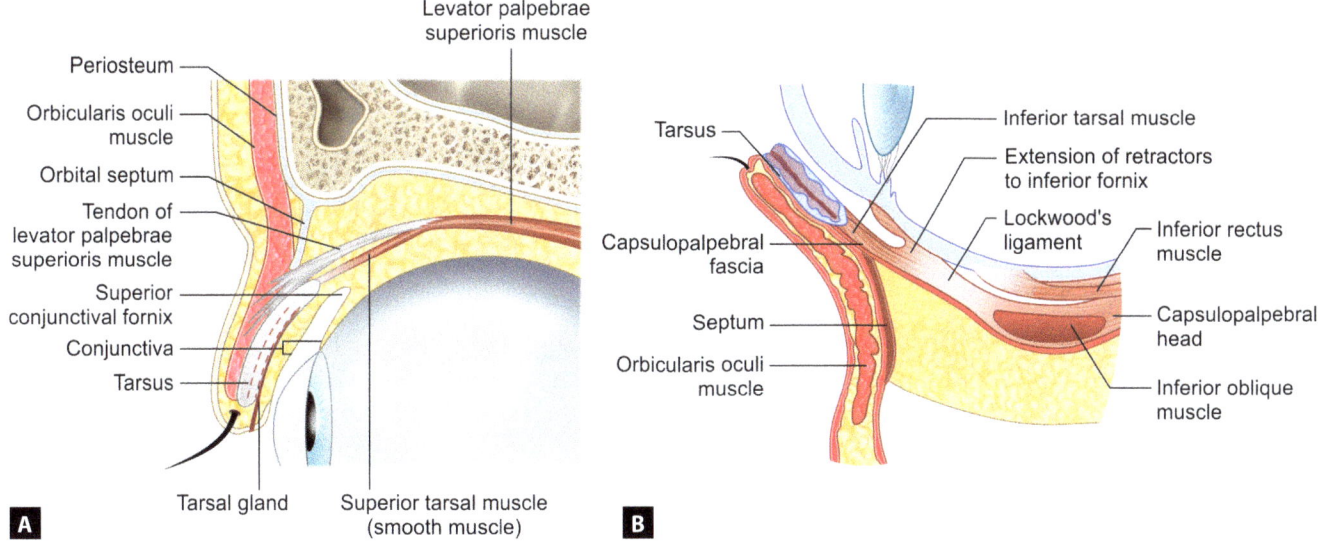

Figs. 1A and B: Cross-sectional diagrammatic representation of (A) upper and (B) lower eyelid.

Lower eyelid entropion is invariably involutional and upper eyelid entropion invariably cicatricial. Entropion is graded as per its severity.

Grading

TABLE 2: Grading of entropion.	
Grade 1	Only posterior lid margin is in-turned
Grade 2	In-turning of intermarginal strip
Grade 3	In-turning of anterior lid margin

Kemp and Collin's Grading

TABLE 3: Kemp's and Collin's grading of entropion.		
Mild	**Moderate**	**Severe**
Normal tarsal plate	Normal tarsal plate	Gross tarsal deformities
Conjunctivalization of eyelid margin	Conjunctivalization of eyelid margin	Marked conjunctival scarring
Lash-globe contact only on gaze toward involved eyelid	Lash-globe contact in primary position	

Clinical Features

Symptoms occur due to rubbing of eyelid margin and lashes on the cornea and conjunctiva (pseudotrichiasis).

TABLE 4: Signs and symptoms of entropion.	
Symptoms	**Associated signs**
Foreign body sensation	Punctate epithelial erosions
Lacrimation	Pannus formation
Irritation	
Photophobia	

One must always evert the eyelid to look for scarring before reaching a diagnosis **(Fig. 2)**. Now, let us study the characteristics of each type.

Involutional Entropion

It is the most common type of entropion. In lower eyelid, involutional changes lead to entropion or ectropion, whereas in upper eyelid involutional changes result in ptosis **(Fig. 3)**.

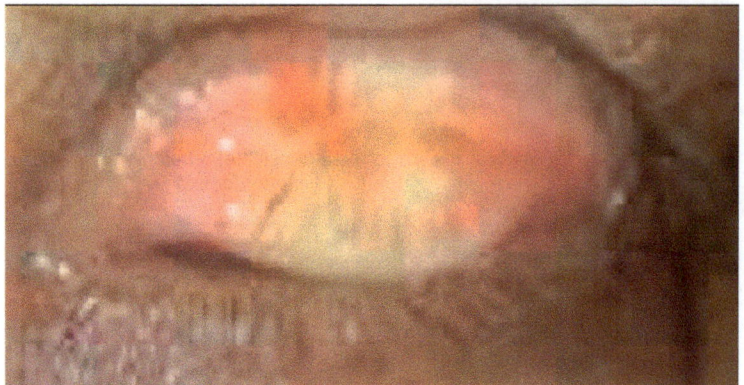

Fig. 2: Clinical photograph of everted upper eyelid showing scarring.

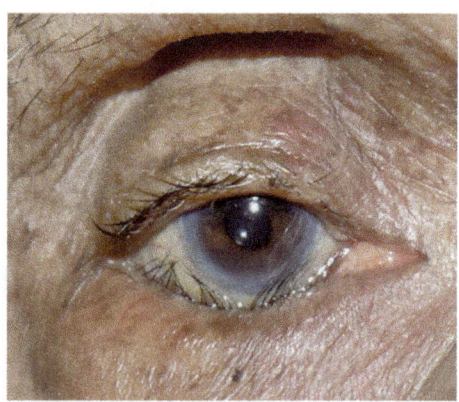

Fig. 3: Clinical photograph of severe right lower eyelid involutional entropion.

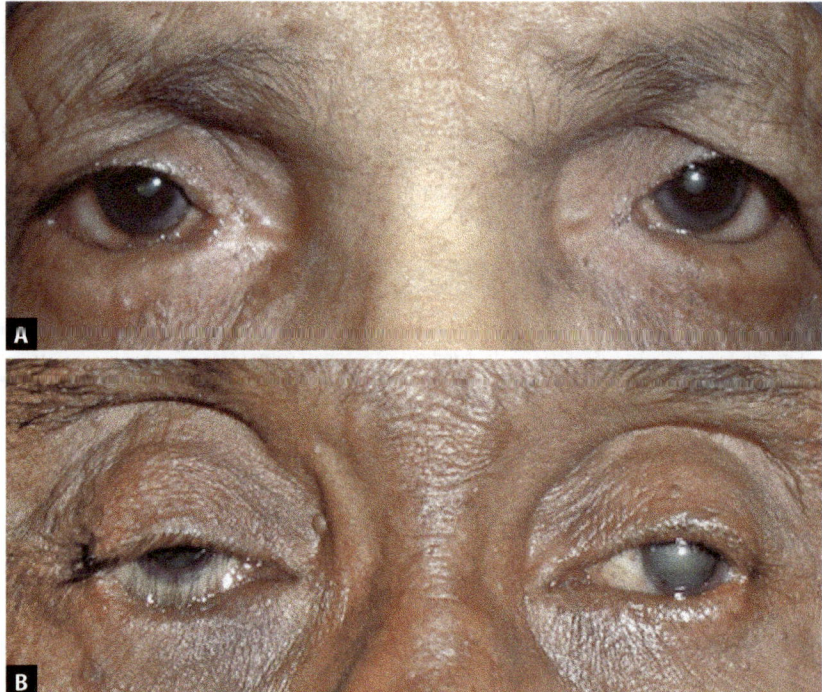

Figs. 4A and B: Clinical photograph of right lower eyelid entropion showing (A) medial canthal laxity and (B) lateral canthal laxity (rounding and medialization of lateral canthus).

Factors responsible for involutional entropion are:
- Vertical eyelid laxity (most important)
- Horizontal eyelid laxity **(Figs. 4A and B)**
- Overriding of preseptal orbicularis over pretarsal orbicularis muscle.
  Vertical eyelid laxity is caused by attenuation or dehiscence of lower eyelid retractors from their attachment to tarsus. On inspection, it can be noticed that excursion of lower eyelid when globe moves from up- to downgaze is reduced.

Clinical Tests **(Figs. 5A and B)**
- *Distraction test:* Anterior distraction of >6 mm is suggestive of excess horizontal laxity.
- *Lateral distraction test:* If lower puncta is pulled laterally and crosses mid-point between plica and corneal limbus, the test is positive. This indicates laxity of medial canthal tendon (MCT).
- *Medial distraction test:* If lower punctum is moved medially and crosses mid-point of lacrimal caruncle, test is positive. This indicates laxity of lateral canthal tendon.
- *Snap-back test:* When lower eyelid is pulled away from the globe, normally it snaps back and apposes to the globe. Incomplete or delayed return to normal position points toward reduced tone or orbicularis oculi.

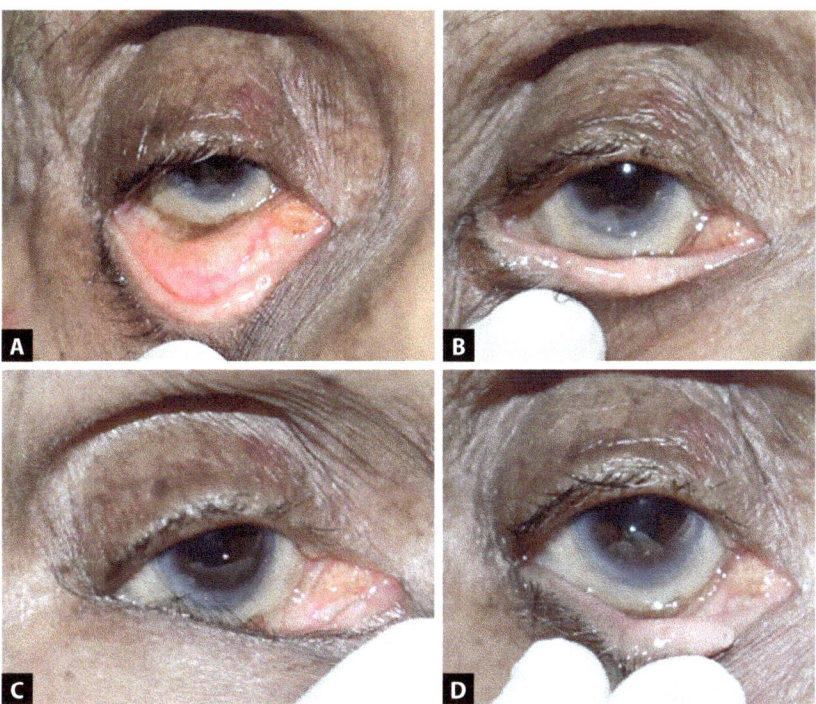

Figs. 5A to D: Clinical tests for entropion. (A) Distraction test; (B) Lateral traction test; (C) Medial traction test; (D) Snap-back test.

- Capsulopalpebral fascia disinsertion signs include:
  - Lower eyelid margin covering the inferior limbus in primary gaze resting position.
  - Inability of lower eyelid to retract downward in inferior gaze
  - White horizontal band seen in inferior fornix
  - Absent lower eyelid crease.

Management
- *Conservative measures:* These are directed toward protection of ocular surface and comprise lubricant eyedrops, soft bandage contact lens, and adhesive taping of lower eyelid.
- *Surgical procedures:*
  - *Lateral tarsal strip (LTS):* It is indicated in the presence of lateral canthal tendon laxity. A lateral canthotomy and inferior cantholysis are performed and lateral end of tarsus is fashioned to create a "tendon" of tarsal plate. This is attached to the inner lateral orbital rim at the desired height to maintain symmetry between two eyes. This is the most commonly performed procedure in which horizontal eyelid shortening is required to achieve optimal eyelid tightening.
    This procedure should be avoided in patients with a negative vector. A negative vector exists when the anterior projection of the globe (apex of cornea) lies anterior to malar eminence.
  - *Lateral canthal resuspension:* This procedure is less invasive and obviates the need of canthotomy-cantholysis. It is performed via a lateral upper eyelid crease incision by passing a prolene suture around the lateral canthal tendon, temporarily externalizing near the tendon's attachment to tarsus eventually anchoring it to lateral orbital rim **(Figs. 6A and B)**.
  - *Jones procedure:* It is also known as plication of lower eyelid retractors. An incision in made 4 mm below lash-line lateral to the punctum and inferior border of tarsus is reached. After retracting the skin, orbicularis, orbital septum, and fat, the lower eyelid retractors are identified as a visible white sheet of tissue **(Fig. 7)**. These are reattached/plicated to the anterior surface of the inferior tarsal border with sutures, thereby rectifying vertical eyelid laxity. A strip of preseptal orbicularis oculi can be excised before closing the incision to prevent overriding of preseptal orbicularis over pretarsal orbicularis muscle **(Figs. 8A and B)**.
  - *Weis procedure:* This involves creating a scar between lower eyelid retractors, inferior tarsal border, and anterior lamellae (skin and orbicularis) by combining a full-thickness blepharotomy (transverse lid split) at the inferior tarsal border with rotation sutures **(Figs. 9A and B)**. This prevents over-riding of preseptal over pretarsal orbicularis and in the modification described also tackles lower eyelid retractors. Recurrence rate is slightly higher with Weis procedure than Jones procedure.

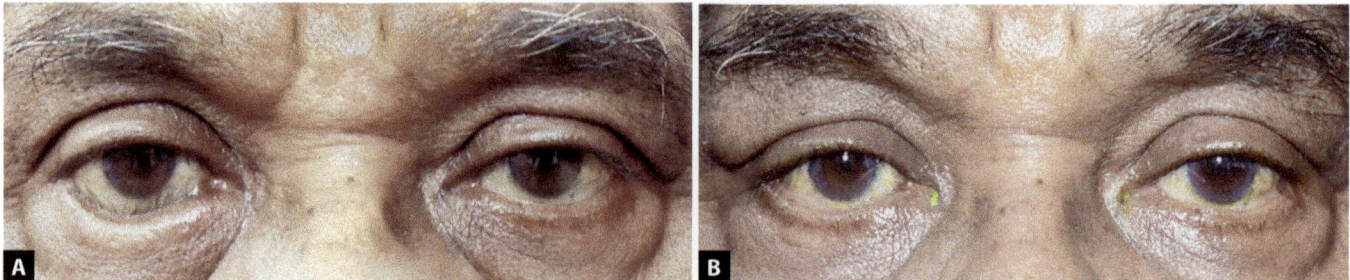

Figs. 6A and B: Clinical photograph showing (A) right lower eyelid entropion and (B) correction of right lower eyelid entropion post-lateral canthal resuspension.

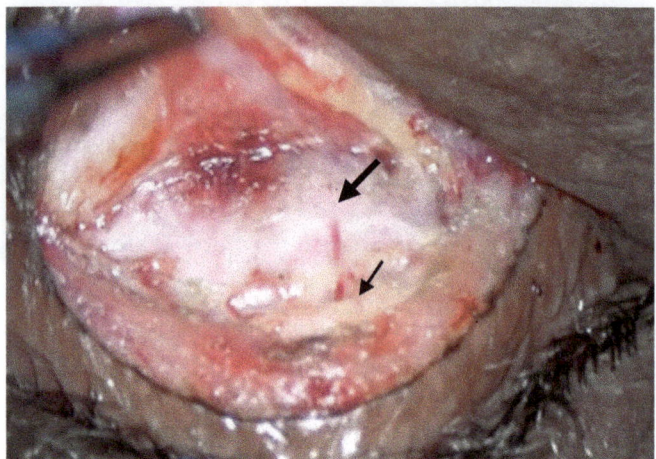

Fig. 7: Intraoperative photograph showing lower eyelid retractors as a whitish band (broad arrow) and inferior tarsal border (narrow arrow).

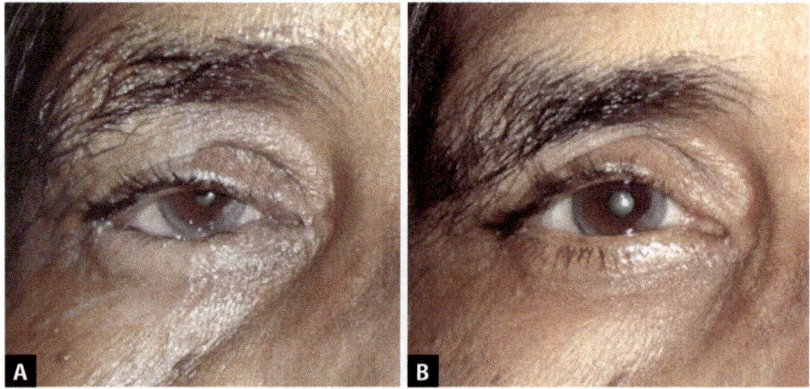

Figs. 8A and B: Clinical photograph showing (A) right lower eyelid involutional entropion (vertical laxity) and (B) post-Jones procedure for the correction of entropion.

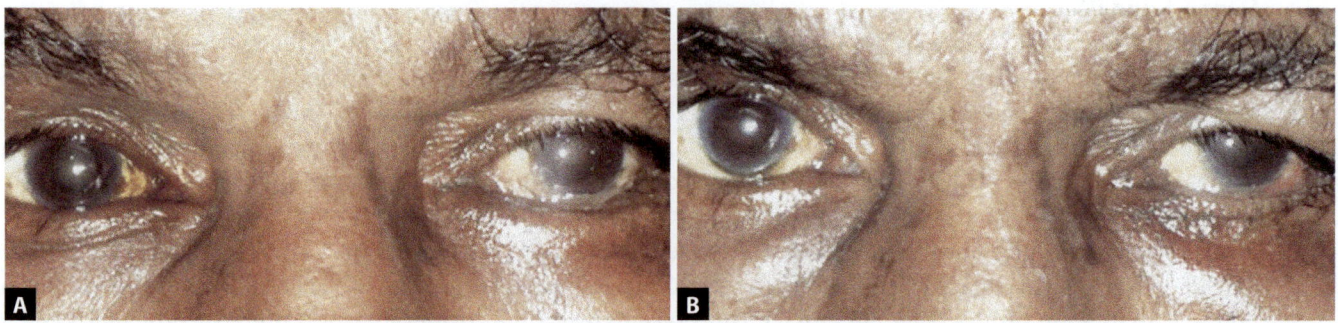

Figs. 9A and B: Clinical photograph showing (A) left lower eyelid entropion with over-riding of preseptal orbicularis over pretarsal orbicularis and (B) correction of entropion with Weis procedure combined with LTS.

A transconjunctival approach has also been used to advance lower eyelid retractors and address orbicularis.
- *Quickert procedure:* A procedure which combines Weis procedure along with a full-thickness wedge resection of the lateral segment of eyelid. This technique tackles horizontal as well as vertical eyelid laxity.
- *Everting sutures:* Quickert and Rathbun's suture technique comprised of creating a rotational vector similar to sutures passed in Weis procedure but without any incision on the eyelid. Three-double armed sutures passed from the conjunctiva closer to the inferior fornix and tied 1–2 mm below lash-line change the vector and helps evert eyelid. This can be a temporary measure used while awaiting definitive surgery or can be a useful measure to relieve symptoms in debilitated patients in whom incisional surgery is not possible.

A suitable technique or a combination of techniques needs to be chosen after assessing causative factors in a particular case as well as the surgeon's comfort and expertise.

Cicatricial Entropion

It is shortening of posterior lamella of eyelid due to a cicatrix causing in-turning of eyelid margin. Trachoma (caused by *Chlamydia trachomatis*) which has been endemic in some parts of the Indian subcontinent is a common cause of cicatricial entropion. Recurrent infection of conjunctiva leads to severe inflammatory process and subsequent scarring. Scarring of upper tarsal conjunctiva, known as *Arlt's* line, is a sequelae of trachomatous disease.

Cicatricial entropion is also often seen secondary to cicatrizing diseases such as Stevens–Johnson syndrome or ocular cicatricial pemphigoid. Medical management is optimized and surgical correction is deferred till the disease has stabilized.

Chemical burns of ocular surface, such as accidental fall of lime, can cause cicatricial entropion since they cause significant inflammation and loss of function of conjunctival epithelium and in chronic phase lead to scarring **(Box 1)**.

Clinical Assessment

An early sign could be anteriorization of mucocutaneous junction/apparent posterior migration of meibomian gland orifices. There could be associated eyelid retraction. Eyelid eversion will show conjunctival scarring. It is crucial to differentiate trichiatic lashes from entropion as both conditions need to be dealt with separate procedures.

Management

Management of cicatricial entropion is primarily surgical and the choice of the procedure depends on certain factors listed in **Box 2**.

Tarsal fracture: In mild degrees of lower eyelid entropion or in cases with the presence of posterior lid margin keratinization rubbing the ocular surface a technique—tarsal fracture and margin rotation (Trabut) can be used **(Fig. 10)**. On everting eyelid, a horizontal incision is given close to the inferior edge of tarsus/just posterior to keratinization and the fractured tarsus is rotated externally and fixed in place by three everting sutures.

BOX 1: Etiology of cicatricial entropion.
- Chemical burns
- Trachoma
- Cicatrizing conjunctivitis secondary to systemic conditions such as Stevens–Johnson syndrome and ocular cicatricial pemphigoid
- Iatrogenic, e.g., as a complication of conjunctival mullerectomy/Fasanella–Servat
- *Socket:* Chronic recurrent inflammation of anophthalmic socket

BOX 2: Factors guiding the choice of procedure for the management of cicatricial entropion.
- Underlying etiology
- Severity of entropion
- Presence/absence of keratin on posterior lamella
- Thickness of tarsal plate
- Presence of any associated eyelid retraction
- Presence of an anophthalmic socket + artificial eye

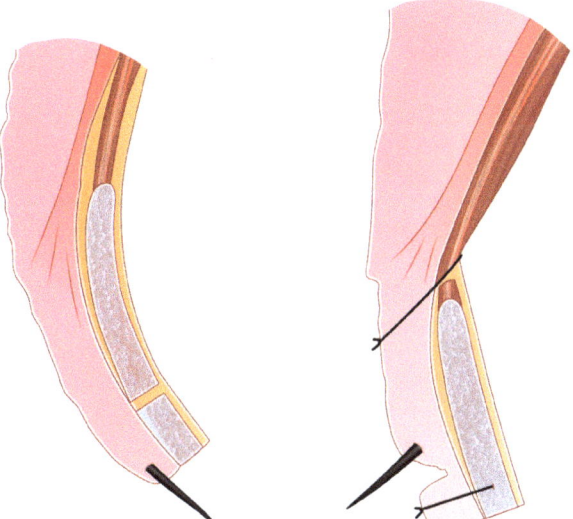

Fig. 10: Cross-sectional diagrammatic representation of marginal rotation procedure.

In cases with severe cicatricial entropion, there often is some eyelid retraction and need to be corrected by lengthening of posterior lamella. Oral mucous membrane graft, nasal mucoperichondrial graft, auricular cartilage, or lower eyelid hard palate mucoperichondrial graft could be used to supplement posterior lamellae.

- *Anterior lamellar reposition +/− lid split:* This procedure is an option for mild upper eyelid cicatricial entropion. A lid crease incision is made and suborbicularis dissection is done exposing the tarsus up to the level of hair follicles. The anterior lamella is then pulled up and eversion of margin assessed. A lid spilt at gray line may be added at the stage. Three mattress sutures are then passed through skin and orbicularis just above lashes and at a higher level through partial-thickness tarsus and back through skin and orbicularis just above eyelashes to draw the anterior lamella superior in relation to posterior lamella.
- *Wedge resection:* It is a variation of lamellar reposition indicated in mild-to-moderate cases of cicatricial entropion with a thick tarsus **(Fig. 11)**.
- *Lamellar division/anterior lamellar recession:* For severe upper eyelid entropion, division of anterior and posterior lamella with recession of anterior lamella is the preferred surgical technique. In this procedure, an incision is made along the length of the gray line and deepened in suborbicularis plane to expose the entire anterior surface of tarsal plate. Recession of retractors should be added to manage any associated eyelid retraction. The anterior lamellar margin is then sutured by means of three everting sutures to the superior margin of tarsus. The surface of tarsus may be allowed to heal by granulation or a thin mucous membrane graft may be placed over it **(Figs. 12A to C)**.

Spastic Entropion

Spams of orbicularis oculi are responsible for entropion in a few cases. Botulinum toxin works by breaking the vicious cycle of ocular surface irritation and increased spasm **(Figs. 13A to D)**. If the cause of ocular surface irritation like discomfort after an intraocular surgery can be corrected, a repeat injection of Botulinum toxin can be avoided. Some patients may need repeat injections. Quickert's everting sutures may also be used to mechanically tighten lower lid retractors, but they do not treat the spasms.

Congenital Entropion

Epiblepharon is most commonly mistaken for congenital entropion. In this condition, a fold of redundant lower eyelid pushes eyelashes toward the ocular surface. Usually, the child is asymptomatic but warrants intervention when ocular irritation is conspicuous **(Figs. 14A and B)**. Only when there is true inward rotation of eyelid margin since birth, it is termed

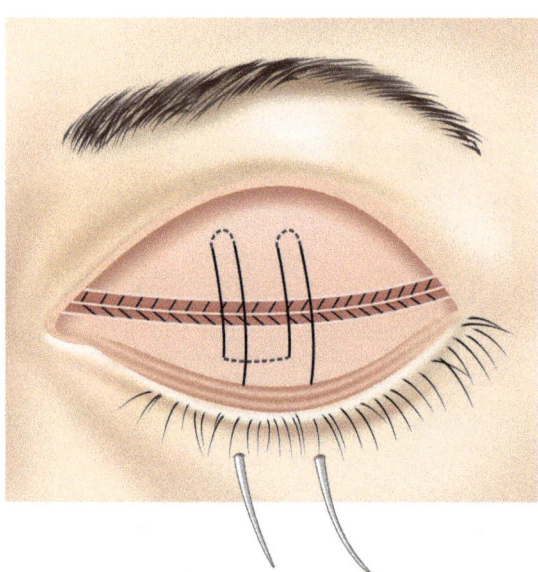

Fig. 11: Cross-sectional diagrammatic representation of wedge-resection procedure for upper eyelid cicatricial entropion.

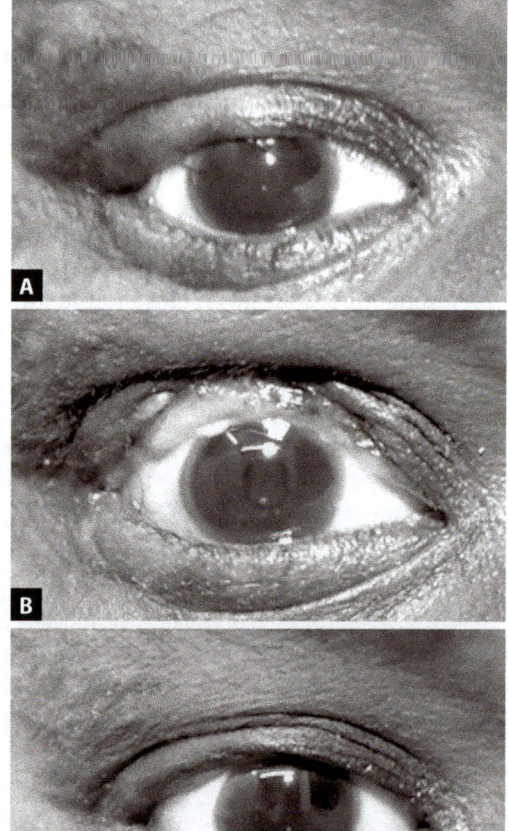

Figs. 12A to C: Clinical photograph showing (A) right upper eyelid entropion, (B) exposed tarsus after anterior lamellar recession, and (C) postoperative 6 weeks' photograph showing correction of entropion.

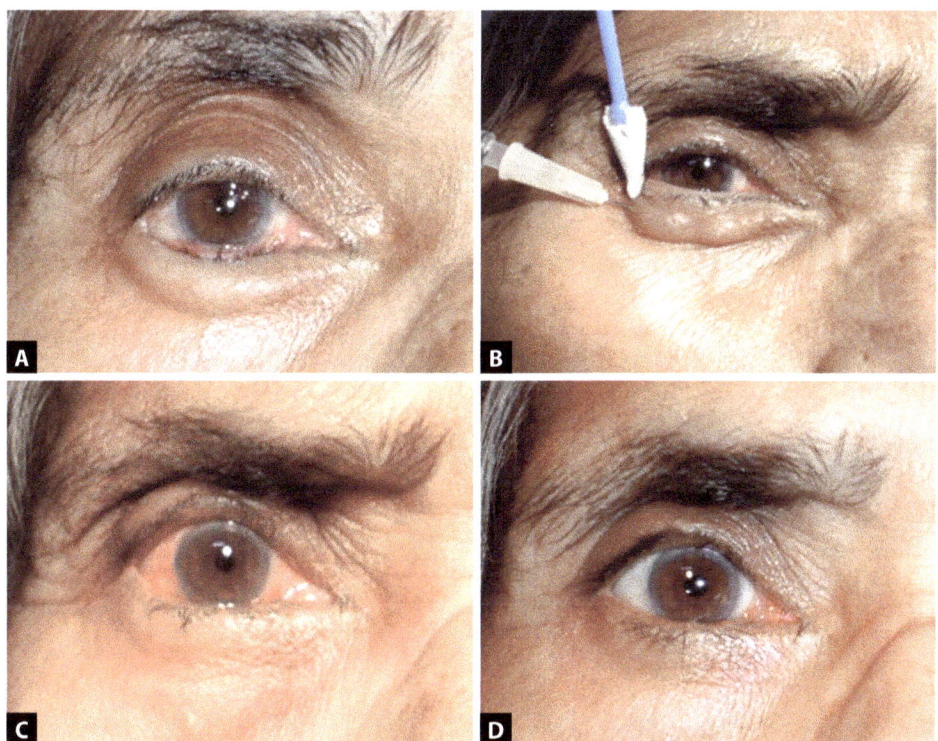

Figs. 13A to D: Clinical photograph showing (A) RE lower lid spastic entropion, (B) Inj botulinum toxin in preseptal orbicularis oculi and (C and D) Correction of entropion and no recurrence after resolution of ocular irritation.

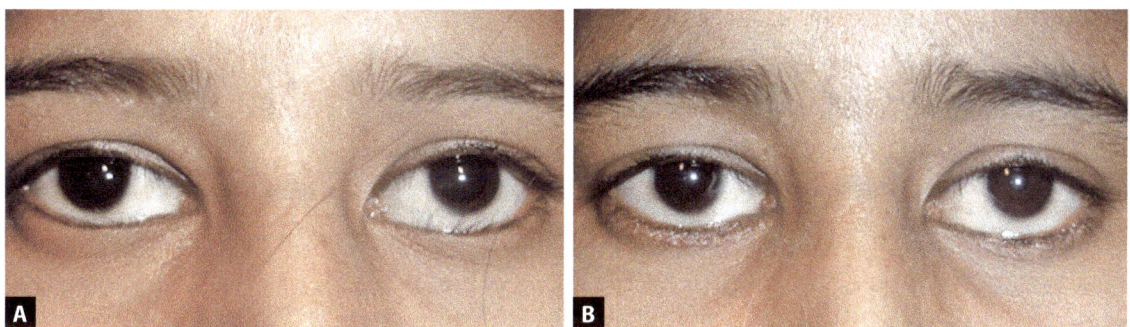

Figs. 14A and B: Clinical photograph showing (A) bilateral epiblepharon (L > R) causing ocular surface irritation and (B) post-Hotz procedure for epiblepharon correction.

congenital entropion. A rare congenital malformation known as tarsal kink syndrome is a severe form of entropion and needs to be surgically corrected.

Epiblepharon invariably self-corrects as the child grows. But when an epiblepharon warrants correction, a minimally invasive technique such as a hyaluronic acid filler is often useful. Rarely, a Hotz procedure in which the redundant eyelid fold is excised may be performed.

 2. Discuss the classification, preoperative assessment, and management modalities of different types of ectropion.

Out-turning of eyelid margin resulting in lack of apposition of eyelid margin to the globe is termed as ectropion. It is more often seen in the lower eyelid than the upper eyelid.

Classification (Table 5)

Congenital entropion is rare and results from deficiency of anterior lamellae. It is seen to be associated with Down syndrome or ichthyosis **(Fig. 15)**.

48 Oculoplasty and Tumors

TABLE 5: Classification of ectropion.	
Congenital	**Acquired**
	• Senile/involutional • Cicatricial • Paralytic • Mechanical

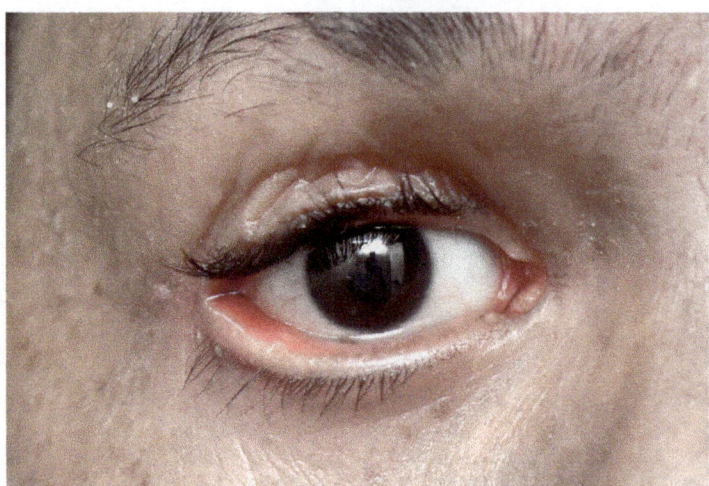

Fig. 15: Clinical photograph showing ichthyosis of skin resulting in right lower eyelid ectropion.

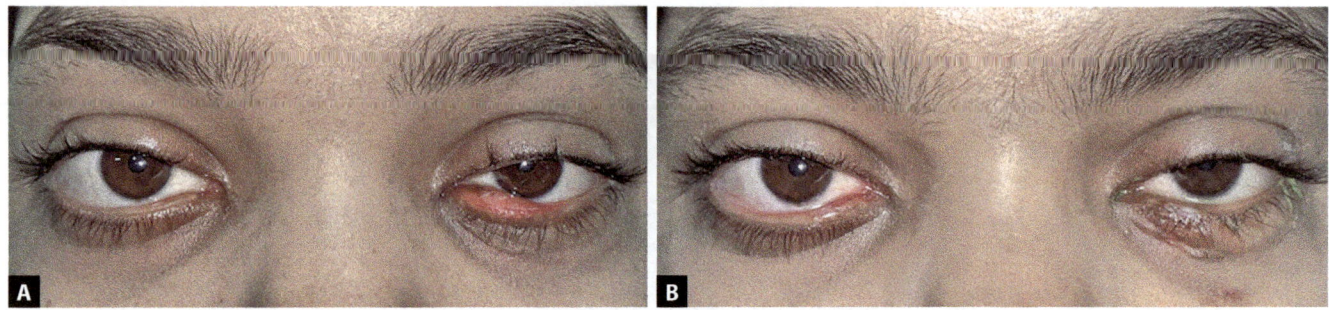

Figs. 16A and B: Clinical photograph showing (A) bilateral lower eyelid medial ectropion, left significantly more than right and (B) correction of left lower eyelid ectropion with medial canthal tendon (MCT) plication and diamond conjunctivoplasty.

Clinical Features

Symptoms of patients with ectropion are related to conjunctival exposure, lacrimal dysfunction, and cosmetic deformity. The exposed conjunctiva becomes inflamed, erythematous, and keratinized.

Watering in a case of ectropion is multifactorial.
- Secondary to exposure of conjunctival surface, poor blink, and superficial keratitis
- Mal-apposed punctum, which prevents lacrimal outflow. Punctal stenosis may be noted in cases with chronic ectropion.
- Lacrimal pump failure in cases with paralytic ectropion.

Preoperative Assessment

- *Eyelid puncta:* The normal position of punctum in primary gaze is in lacrimal lake and not visible unless medial eyelid is manually pulled down. If the punctum is visible in resting position, a medial ectropion could be present **(Figs. 16A and B)**.
- Distraction test (performed same as test for entropion)
- Medial and lateral distraction test to assess lateral and MCT laxity (as in tests for entropion). On inspection, a rounding of lateral canthal angle is a sign of lateral canthal tendon laxity.
- *Snap-back test:* Normally when eyelid is pulled away from the globe and released, it immediately snaps back and abuts the globe. The tone of orbicularis can be assessed based on how long does the eyelid take to return to normal position and whether or not it returns back after a blink.

- *Anterior lamella assessment:* It is an indispensable factor in the evaluation of cicatricial ectropion. Early signs of skin deficiency are poor superior excursion of lower lid in upgaze and eyelid lag of upper lid in downgaze. On mouth opening if there is eversion of lower eyelid, a cicatrix involving midface should be looked for. In severe cases, there can be tethering of the scar to orbital rim as well.

Management of Ectropion

- *Medial spindle:* This procedure can be performed as a standalone procedure in cases with only medial ectropion without any horizontal eyelid laxity or can be combined with LTS in those with associated horizontal laxity. A diamond-shaped excision of conjunctiva and subconjunctival tissue is done, lower eyelid retractors identified, and a double-armed mattress sutured passed with 6-0 vicryl to attach them to the inferior tarsal border.
- LTS corrects horizontal laxity and is performed in the same manner as for entropion.
- *Lazy-T procedure:* Few surgical techniques such as Kuhnt–Szymanowski procedure, which involves horizontal eyelid shortening + blepharoplasty (full-thickness pentagon excision is combined with excision of redundant skin), are less favored as better surgical techniques are now available. The Lazy-T procedure comprises medial spindle along with a medial wedge resection.
- *Bick's procedure:* In this, a full-thickness wedge excision of the eyelid is performed just medial to the lateral canthus. This may cause rounding and medial displacement of the lateral canthal angle.
- *Retractor reinsertion:* In involution or senile ectropion, there is likely a retractor dehiscence. Total tarsal ectropion may be noted in such cases. Reattachment of lower lid retractors to tarsus along the whole length of lower lid restores normal eyelid position. A horizontal eyelid shortening such as an LTS may be additionally needed **(Figs. 17A and B)**.
- Paralytic ectropion can be rectified with medial canthoplasty/MCT plication +/− lateral canthal resuspension +/− tarsorrhaphy depending on the preoperative clinical tests and the severity of ectropion.
- Mechanical ectropion can be correction by excision of tumor or eyelid mass causing eversion of eyelid due to gravitational pull on the mass. If there is associated horizontal laxity, the same can be tackled with a horizontal eyelid shortening procedure.
- *Cicatricial ectropion:* Causes of cicatricial ectropion could be:
  - *Trauma:* Mechanical, thermal (burns), or chemical
  - *Iatrogenic:* Postblepharoplasty
  - Dermatologic conditions.

Detailed evaluation of causative factor is essential as ectropion secondary to certain conditions such as allergic contact dermatitis in acute stage can be reversed by avoiding the offending agent **(Figs. 18A and B)**. Once a cicatrix has formed, the extent and location need to be evaluated.

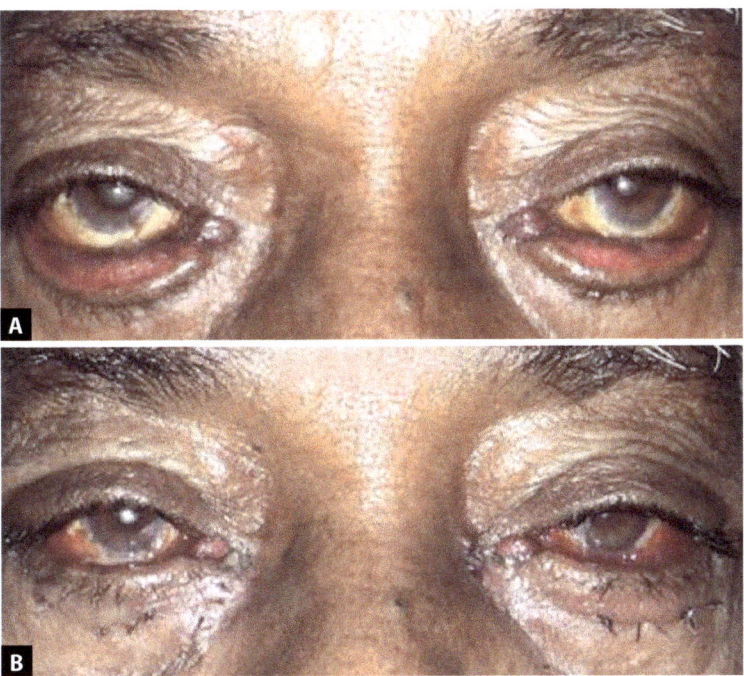

Figs. 17A and B: Clinical photograph showing (A) bilateral severe lower eyelid ectropion with total tarsal rotation and (B) correction of ectropion with reattachment of retractors and lateral tarsal strip (LTS).

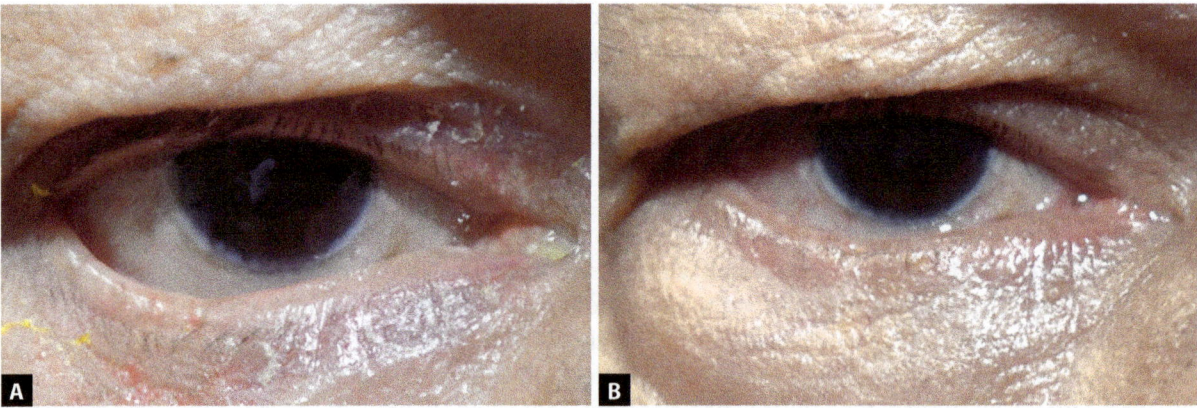

Figs. 18A and B: Clinical photograph showing (A) right lower lid dermatitis resulting in mal-apposed lower lid margin and (B) resolution of dermatitis and thereby ectropion by conservative management by stopping the offending agent.

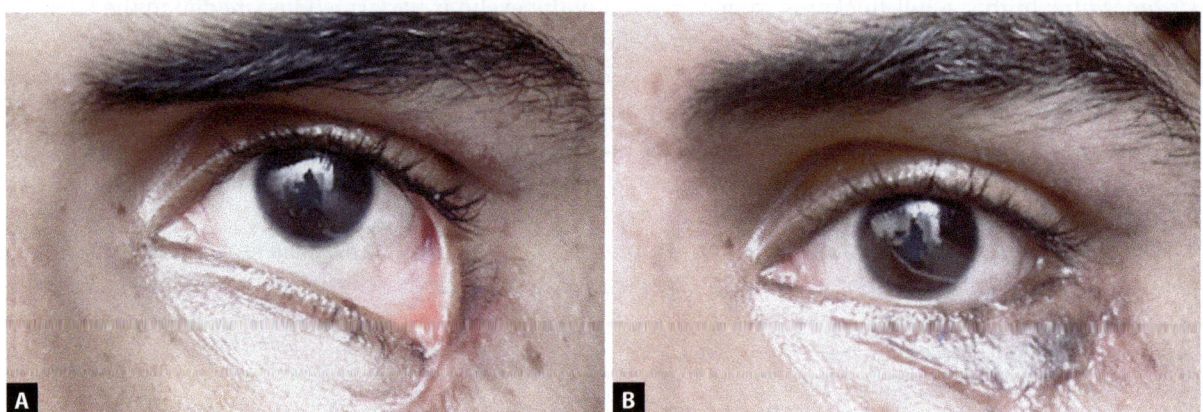

Figs. 19A and B: Clinical photograph showing (A) severe cicatricial ectropion of left lower eyelid and (B) correction of ectropion by means of a postauricular full-thickness skin graft.

Conservative Management

An early scar can be treated with (1) topical antiscar creams, (2) injections such as 5-fluorouracil or triamcinolone, and (3) occlusive dressings such as silicone gel sheet.

Surgical management is needed in advanced or nonresponsive cases.

- *Skin flaps:* Localized, limited, linear scars can be managed by redirecting periocular Langer's lines and lengthening anterior lamella. Z-plasty is one such technique. Multiple Z-plasties may be combined with the knowledge that length of the wound is improved by 30% with each Z-plasty. When midface ptosis is associated, a SOOF (suborbicularis oculi fat) or midface [superficial musculoaponeurotic system (SMAS)] lift made be added.
- *Full-thickness skin graft for anterior lamella:* Cicatrix released or excised and anterior lamella are replaced by means of a full-thickness skin graft **(Figs. 19A and B)**. Eyelid skin is the thinnest skin of the body and a suitable donor site must be chosen to ensure a good color and thickness match. Fellow upper eyelid is the most ideal site in patients with dermatochalasis. Other favored sites are retroauricular, preauricular, or supraclavicular skin.

In patients with diffuse shortage of lower eyelid skin, a subciliary incision is often used and in upper eyelid a lid crease incision is preferred whenever possible. Dissection is performed to release any deep cicatricial bands. After dissection is completed, one should be able to lift up the lower eyelid to the superior limbus and it should be possible to pull down the upper eyelid up to the inferior limbus. The defect site is then measured and a suitable donor site graft is marked with a skin marker. The donor graft should be slightly oversized to account for mild postsurgery contraction of the graft. The graft is then thinned and fashioned to suit the recipient bed and secured in placed with sutures. A tarsorrhaphy should be performed to keep the graft stretched and prevent wrinkling and fluid accumulation underneath the graft.

A combination of approaches would be needed in a mixed mechanism ectropion. A careful evaluation and diligent treatment would result in an acceptable outcome.

Suggested Reading

1. Anderson RL, Gordy DD. The tarsal strip procedure. Arch Ophthalmol. 1979;97:2192.
2. Boborridis K, Bunce C, Rose GE. A comparative study of two procedures for the repair of involutional lower lid entropion. Ophthalmology. 2000;107:959-61.
3. Dutton JJ, Fowler AM. Botulinum toxin in ophthalmology. Surv Ophthalmol. 2007;52:13-31.
4. Elder MJ, Collin R. Anterior lamellar repositioning and grey line split for upper lid entropion in ocular cicatricial pemphigoid. Eye (Lond). 1996;10(1):439-42.
5. Freuh BR, Schengarth LD. Evaluation and treatment of patient with ectropion. Ophthalmology. 1982;89:1049-54.
6. Jones LT, Reeh MJ, Wobig JL. Senile entropion: a new concept for correction. Am J Ophthalmol. 1972;74:327-9.
7. Kemp EG, Collin JR. Surgical management of upper lid entropion. Br J Ophthalmol. 1986;70:575-9.
8. Naik MN, Ali MJ, Das S, Honavar SG. Nonsurgical management of epiblepharon using hyaluronic acid gel. Ophthal Plast Reconstr Surg. 2010;26(3):215-7.
9. Nowinski TS, Anderson RL. The medial spindle procedure for involutional medial ectropion. Arch Ophthalmol. 1984;103:1750-53.
10. Quickert MH, Rathbun E. Suture repair of entropion. Arch Ophthalmol. 1971;85(3):304-5.
11. Schaefer AJ. Variation in the pathophysiology of involutional entropion and its treatment. Ophthalmic Surg. 1983;14(8):653-5.
12. Smith B. The "Lazy-T" correction of ectropion of the lower punctum. Arch Ophthalmol. 1976;94:1149.
13. Wies FA. Spastic entropion. Trans Am Acad Ophthalmol Otolaryngol. 1955;59:503-6.

1.6 Eyelid Reconstruction

Kavya B Madhuri, Anasua G Kapoor

 1. Describe and discuss the principles and techniques of eyelid reconstructions/principles and techniques of lid reconstruction.

 2. What are the principles of lid reconstruction? Discuss the indications, technique, and complications of Cutler–Beard operation.

Aim for eyelid reconstruction is to re-establish the normal eyelid function along with enhancement of the periocular cosmesis with least surgical damage.

Factors Affecting the Decision Making

- Type of the eyelid defect
- Age and systemic status
- Accessibility and durability of adjacent areas
- Visual performance of contralateral eye
- Skills and priorities of the surgeon.

Principles for Successful Eyelid and Periocular Reconstruction

Principles for successful eyelid and periocular reconstruction		
I. General		• No graft on graft • Measure the defect prior to direct closure • Balancing techniques
II. Periocular	Structural	• Match the tissue • Avoid eyelid tension • Adequate canthal fixation • Punctal apposition
	Functional	• Smooth mucosal lining of eyelid • Smooth eyelid margin • Adequate eyelid closure • Normal eyelid mobility
	Cosmesis	Good eyelid contour

General Principles

- *No graft on graft:* Never place graft over graft. At least one of the eyelid lamellae; either anterior or posterior must be replaced by a flap in full-thickness defects to promote vascular support for tissue viability.
- *Measuring the defect:* While assessing the wound size, it is always mandatory to approximate the wound edges and calculate the residual defect.
- *Balance the technique:* A wide range of surgical techniques are described for eyelid reconstruction. Techniques can be combined with good balance, especially in larger defects for better outcome.

Principles in Relation to Periocular Region

Structural

- *Match the tissue:* The donor tissue (flaps and grafts) should be identical to the recipient tissue (eyelid and periocular region) in terms of color, texture, thickness for ideal cosmesis, and good symmetry.
- *Avoid eyelid tension:* Avoid stretching of the wound margins by harvesting the adequate donor tissue while reconstructing the eyelid to reduce the tension over the tissues.
- *Adequate canthal fixation:* Appropriate fixation of canthi is essential to maintain the eyelid-globe apposition.
- *Punctal apposition:* If the normal position of puncta is not restored, it may result in epiphora.

Functional

- *Smooth mucosal lining of eyelid:* The reconstructed eyelid should have smooth lining to protect the ocular surface.
- *Smooth eyelid margin:* Look for smooth eyelid margin to avoid ocular surface damage from keratin and trichiasis.
- *Adequate eyelid closure:* Lagophthalmos may result in exposure sequelae.
- *Normal eyelid mobility:* It is important to avoid complications such as ptosis or lagophthalmos by maintaining normal upper eyelid movement.

Cosmesis

Eyelid contour: Maintain normal eyelid contour.

Techniques of Eyelid Reconstruction

A wide variety of modifications of eyelid reconstruction are described, but the basic techniques remain the same. The surgical technique depends upon the following:
- Size of the defect
- Extent of the defect.

Surgical technique		
Size of the defect	<25%	• Direct closure • Direct closure with undermining
	25–50%	• Direct closure with lateral canthotomy and cantholysis • Tenzel's semicircular flap • Sliding tarsal graft
	>50%	• Hughes tarsoconjunctival flap • Cutler–Beard procedure • Mustardé's "lid switch" procedure
Extent of the defect	Partial thickness	• Direct closure with or without undermining the tissue • Myocutaneous flaps • Tarsoconjunctival flaps • Skin grafts • Tarsal grafts
	Full thickness	• Lid-sharing procedures (Cutler–Beard procedure) • Tarsoconjunctival flap with skin graft • Myocutaneous flap with tarsal graft • Tarsoconjunctival flap with myocutaneous flap

Direct Closure

For outstanding results, the surgery should be simple with good cosmetic and functional results. This procedure is preferable in wound defects with adjacent excessive skin.

Indication: In eyelid defects of size <25%, either partial or full thickness, direct closure of the defect can be done.

Components affecting direct closure:
- Associated laxity of eyelid tissues including canthal tendons
- Inbuilt tissue resilience
- With direct closure of wound defect even under minimal tension, the eyelid tissue has the capability to expand in appropriate proportions postoperatively.

Reconstruction of eyelid margin (Figs 1A to D):
- *Align the eyelid margin:* The eyelid margin is aligned by passing the vertical mattress suture through the meibomian gland orifices. Leave the suture ends long to provide eyelid traction.
- *Suture the tarsal plate:* Once the eyelid margins are apposed together, partial-thickness bites are passed through the tarsal plate and placed together with interrupted sutures.
- *Suture the lid margin:* Then the eyelid margin anterior to gray line is sutured to align the lash line and to evert the eyelid margin.

Assessment of wound tension: Approximate the edges of wound defect gently with fixation forceps and determine the wound tension for direct closure of eyelid defect.

Techniques for minimizing high skin tension:
- In periocular region, the dissection should be carried out in the suborbicularis plane.
- To avoid wound tension in subcutaneous plane, subcutaneous tissues can be anchored to the periosteum with deep sutures.
- Undermining and mobilization of the adjacent tissues aids in reducing the wound tension in direct eyelid closure.
- "*Principle of mechanical creep*": The eyelid tissues have inherent capacity to expand over time resulting in tissue expansion and elongation when the defect is closed under minimal tension.

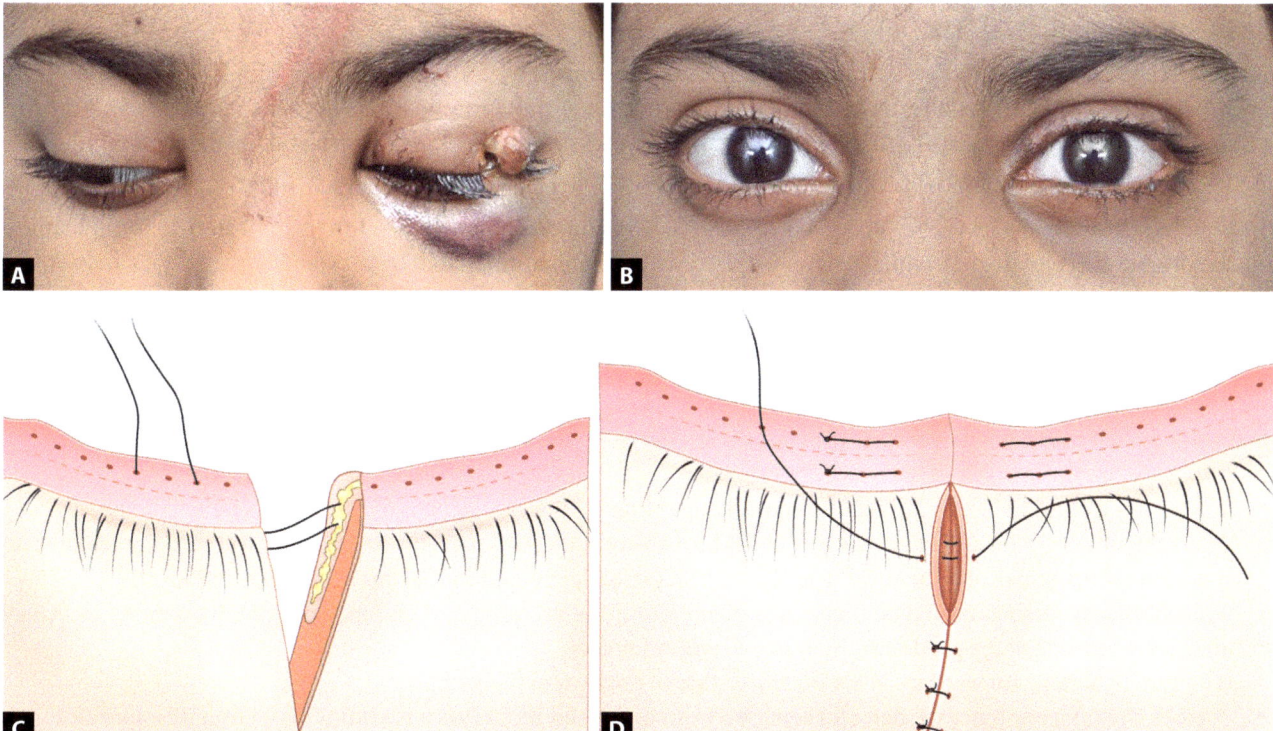

Figs. 1A to D: Before (A) and after (B) eyelid margin reconstruction. First suture is a vertical mattress (C) that is primarily based within the tarsus (and not the gray line). The remaining layers (tarsus, orbicularis, and skin) are then closed with partial-thickness 6-0 Vicryl sutures placed in such a way that no knots face the conjunctiva (D).

Lateral Canthotomy and Lateral Cantholysis (LC, LC)

This is an excellent option for moderate full-thickness eyelid defects and can be used as an adjunct to direct wound closure.

Indication: In eyelid defects of size 25–50%, either partial or full thickness, direct closure of the defect can be done.

Technique: Lateral canthotomy incision is given followed by disinsertion of inferior crus of lateral canthal tendon which "gives away" eyelid. Keep the superior crus of the canthal tendon intact to maintain the canthal configuration.

Tenzel Flap or Lateral Semicircular Skin Flap

If the wound tension still exists, convert the canthotomy incision into lateral semicircular skin rotation flap, i.e., Tenzel flap. This flap advances the periocular tissues lateral to the canthal region to the form the lateral eyelid and thereby allowing the residual eyelid tissue to mobilize centrally.

Indication: Though Tenzel flap is preferred in moderate eyelid defects of size <50%, it can be applied even in larger wound defects of up to 70% with additional severing of orbital septum and lower eyelid retractors from their attachments to lateral orbital rim.

The advantages are less noticeable scars, minimal horizontal wound tension, and avoids postoperative ectropion or flap necrosis.

Unlike lid-sharing procedures (Cutler-Beard, Hughes, etc.), it offers another advantage of avoiding the eye closure for several weeks and is preferable in single-eyed patients.

Technique:
- *Markings:* A semicircular marking is drawn with its proximal ascending limb extending from lateral canthus to the sub-brow region (halts just below the tail of the brow) and the distal descending limb extending 2 cm temporally.
- Incision is carried out along the semicircular marking.
- Dissect the myocutaneous flap till the superficial temporal fascia.
- Perform lateral canthotomy and lateral inferior cantholysis.
- Advance the flap medially, anchor the lateral canthus to the periosteum of the lateral orbital rim, and create the neo-lateral eyelid. The conjunctival lining is formed by mobilizing the inferior forniceal conjunctiva and by suturing to the flap.
- Excise if any dog-ear exists, and close the wound.

Hughes Tarsoconjunctival Flap

Dr Wendel Hughes first reported in 1937 and popularized this procedure for reconstruction of full-thickness lower eyelid defects. Later, this procedure underwent modifications to reduce the complications such as trichiasis and entropion, associated with the initial procedure. To maintain the upper eyelid stability, at least 4 mm tarsal height is required. With this principle, the following modified Hughes procedure is recommended.

Indication: In full-thickness lower eyelid defects of size >50%, modified Hughes procedure is preferred. It is applicable even in entire horizontal eyelid defects, which can be repaired with combination of local periosteal flaps.

Contraindication: As it occludes the eye temporarily for 3–10 weeks, it is better to avoid in one-eyed patients and in pediatric population which increases the risk of developing amblyopia. Single-stage procedures with local advancement flaps are preferable in them.

Technique **(Figs. 2A to D)**: It is a two-stage procedure:
- *First stage:*
  - Assess the wound defect by pulling the wound edges together.
  - Evert the upper eyelid and mark the incision 4 mm above the eyelid margin. To maintain the stability and to prevent vascular compromise of upper eyelid, at least 4 mm tarsal height and half of tarsal length is required.
  - Full-thickness tarsoconjunctival incision is given along the marking and extend horizontally parallel to the eyelid margin according to the predetermined size of wound defect.
  - Then vertical relieving cuts are given on either side of horizontal incision.
  - Elevate the tarsoconjunctival flap and separate from the eyelid retractors with blunt dissection till superior fornix.
  - Advance the flap inferiorly and suture to the residual lower eyelid to reconstruct the posterior lamella.
  - Anterior lamella is formed by local myocutaneous flaps or skin grafts.
  - Maximal Hughes procedure can be employed with the additional combination of periosteal flaps.

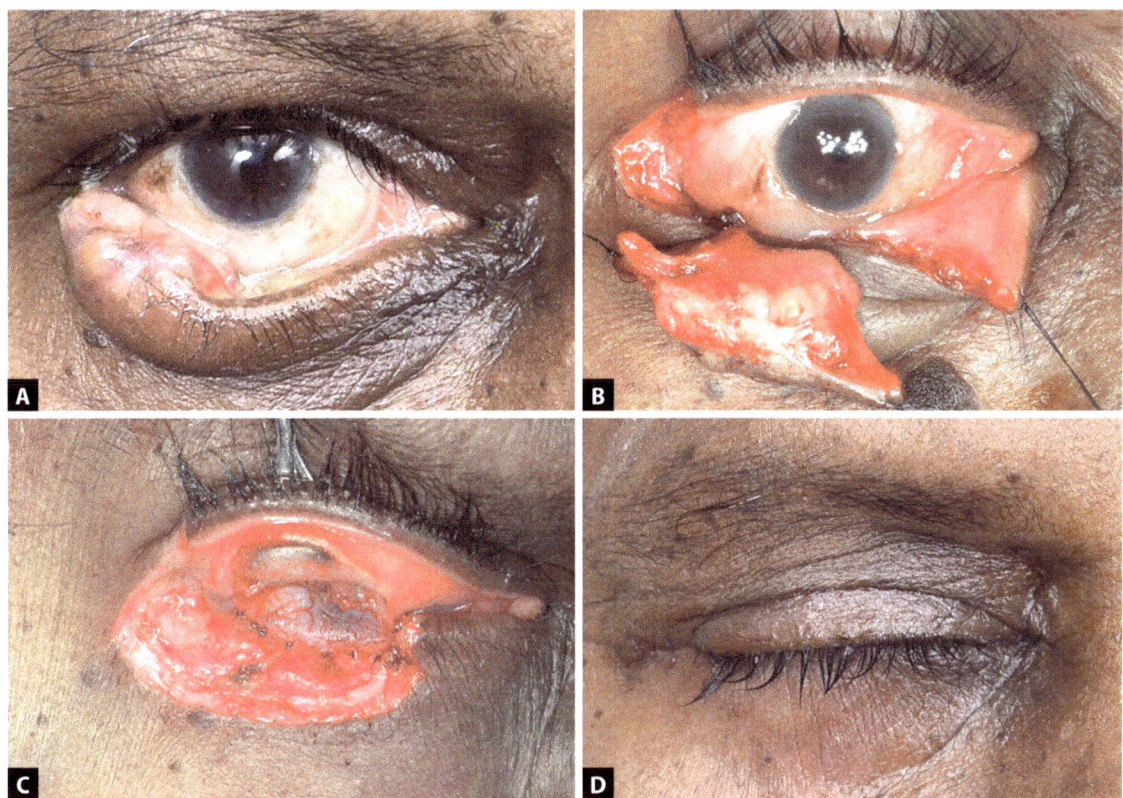

Figs. 2A to D: Right lower eyelid sebaceous gland cell carcinoma, involving the eyelid margin (A). Wide excision done around the lesion with 4-mm margin (B). Hughes tarsoconjunctival flap for posterior lamellar reconstruction (C) and anterior lamella reconstructed with advancement of adjacent skin (D).

- *Second stage:*
  - After 3–10 weeks, incise the flap along the intended new lower eyelid margin.
  - Mucocutaneous margin is reconstructed by draping the conjunctiva over the lower lid margin with the help of glue or suturing.
  - Evert the upper eyelid and trim the residual flap.

Complications:
- Lower eyelid retraction may result from insufficient anterior lamella or with early division of flap.
- Lower eyelid ectropion
- Erythematous eyelid margin
- Upper eyelid retraction is rarely seen when Muller's muscle is included in the tarsoconjunctival flap.
- Trichiasis and entropion may result from failure to maintain the sufficient tarsal height in upper eyelid.

These complications are minimized by adhering to the basic principles of eyelid reconstruction.

Cutler–Beard Technique

Cutler and Beard first reported in 1955 and popularized this procedure for the reconstruction of full-thickness upper eyelid defects. Modifications have been implemented for this procedure too for improving the eyelid stability. Marginal arcade lies 2 mm below the lower eyelid margin and absent or rudimentary peripheral arcade. With this anatomical landmark as background, the procedure is described as follows:

Indication: In full-thickness upper eyelid defects of size >50%, Cutler–Beard technique is preferred.

It is applicable even in entire horizontal eyelid defects, which can be repaired with combination of local myocutaneous flaps. Reverse Cutler–Beard technique been described for full-thickness defects of lower eyelid.

Technique **(Figs. 3A and B)***:* It is a two-stage procedure:
- *First stage:*
  - Assess the wound defect by pulling the wound edges together.

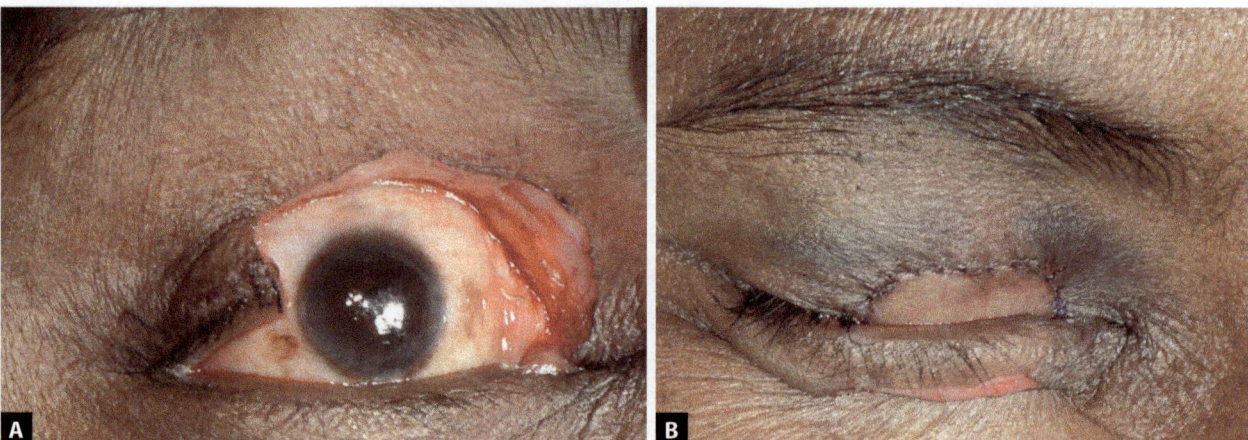

Figs. 3A and B: Final appearance upon closure of the full-thickness upper eyelid defect with Cutler–Beard technique.

- Mark the incision 3–4 mm below the lower eyelid margin to maintain the stability and to prevent vascular compromise of lower eyelid.
- Full-thickness cutaneotarsoconjunctival incision is given along the marking and extend horizontally parallel to the eyelid margin according to the predetermined size of wound defect.
- Then vertical relieving cuts are given on either side of horizontal incision and carried blunt dissection till inferior fornix.
- Advance the lower eyelid skin-muscle flap superiorly under the lower eyelid margin, which acts as bridge and suture with the residual upper eyelid edge to edge to reconstruct the neo upper eyelid.
- *Second stage:*
    - After 2–6 weeks, incise the flap along the intended new upper eyelid margin.
    - Mucocutaneous margin is reconstructed by draping the conjunctiva over the upper lid margin with the help of glue or suturing.
    - The residual flap is sutured back to the lower eyelid margin.

Complications:
- *Corneal abrasion:* As levator pulls the newer posterior lamella more than the newer anterior lamella, the fine hair over the neo upper eyelid margin rubs over the cornea resulting in corneal abrasions.
- Upper eyelid entropion
- Lid margin irregularity
- Loss of eyelash
- Eyelid retraction
- Bridge-flap necrosis if insufficient lower eyelid margin is left behind which compromises the vascular supply.

Skin Graft

It is a simpler technique when compared to the periocular flaps when good knowledge regarding the planes of dissection and anatomical landmarks are known. Though periocular flaps offer good cosmesis, skin graft remains the procedure of choice in particular case scenarios. Full-thickness skin graft (FTSG) is used in periocular region for eyelid reconstruction.

Indication: Anterior lamellar eyelid defects not amenable for direct closure.

Donor sites: Upper eyelid skin is the best donor site and used whenever available.

Other preferable donor sites are:
- Preauricular or postauricular areas
- Supraclavicular
- Inner brachial areas.

Upper eyelid skin is the best donor site for skin grafting in anterior lamellar reconstruction as it offers skin match and reduces the risk of graft-related complications such as contraction, scarring, and failure. To improve better graft survival and uptake, bolster can be used and small nicks can be made in larger skin grafts to prevent fluid accumulation. It is preferable to keep the pressure dressing for at least 24–48 hours.

Medial Canthal Plication

This would be suitable for severe medial laxity of medial canthal tendon (MCT).

Lower Eyelid Spacer Grafts

It comprises placement of spacer grafts between inferior border of tarsus and lower eyelid retractors. Autografts (hard palate mucosa, ear cartilage), allografts (preserved sclera, acellular human dermal matrix), and xenografts (acellular porcine dermis) have all been used for this purpose.

Indication
- Patients with negative vector
- Patients in whom horizontal lid tightening procedures fail to correct lower eyelid retraction adequately.

Long-term success of correcting lower eyelid position and function greatly depends upon correction of midface position.

Management of Epiphora

Medial Spindle Procedure

Indication
- Punctal eversion

Procedure
- A small diamond of tarsoconjunctiva is excised surgically or using laser or cautery conjunctivoplasty.

Periocular Adjunctive Procedures

Management of Brow Ptosis

Brow lift

Indication
Severe brow ptosis causing:
- Pseudoblepharoptosis
- Superior visual field defect
- Secondary misdirection of upper eyelid lashes with constant ocular irritation.

Approaches
- *Direct brow lift:*
  - Simple and effective
  - Often combined with upper eyelid blepharoplasty
- *Endoscopic brow lift:*
  - *Advantages:*
    - Incisional scars hidden behind hairline
    - Reduced risk of postoperative sensory loss in forehead
    - Faster postoperative recovery
  - *Disadvantages:*
    - Expensive
    - Chances of recurrence.

Management of Midface Ptosis

- Use of static sling using autogenous fascia lata to pull the lip and face upward toward the zygomatic arch
- Suborbicularis oculi fat (SOOF) or mid-face lift

  These procedures help to eliminate the inferior traction of the sagging face from the lower eyelid.

Management of Aberrant Regeneration

Jaw-winking Phenomenon/Narrowing of Palpebral Fissure with Lower Facial Movements
- Injection of very minimal doses of 1 and 3 units of onabotulinum A toxin (Botox) in the medial and lateral orbicularis oculi muscle, respectively.
- Risk of lagophthalmos with injection Botox into orbicularis oculi should be kept in mind.

Gustatory Lacrimation/Crocodile Tears
- Injection of 5 units of onabotulinum A toxin into the palpebral lobe of the lacrimal gland.
- Risk of ptosis to be explained to the patient before injection.

Summary of Management of Lagophthalmos

Summary of management of lagophthalmos is shown in **Table 4**.

TABLE 4: Summary of management of lagophthalmos.

Cicatricial lagophthalmos	Scar management			• Scar revision • Z-plasty • Full-thickness skin grafts
Nocturnal lagophthalmos	Conservative measures			• Lubricants • Eyelid taping • Moist chamber goggles
Paralytic lagophthalmos	Temporary measures			• Temporary suture tarsorrhaphy • Injection Botox to LPS • Injection fillers
	Brow ptosis			Brow lift
	Dermatochalasis			Upper eyelid blepharoplasty
	Upper eyelid retraction	Mild to moderate		• Mullerectomy • LPS recession
		Moderate to severe		LPS recession + upper eyelid gold weight
	Lower eyelid retraction + ectropion	Medial	• With MCT laxity	• MCT Plication
			• Without MCT laxity	• Lee's medial canthoplasty
		General	• With horizontal lengthening of lid	• Full-thickness wedge excision + lateral tarsal strip
			• Without horizontal lengthening of lid	• Lower eyelid spacer grafts + lateral tarsal strip
		Lateral	LCT laxity with horizontal lengthening of lid	Lateral tarsal strip
			LCT laxity without horizontal lengthening of lid	Lateral canthopexy
	Severe lagophthalmos with associated risk factors for exposure keratopathy			Medial or lateral tarsorrhaphy
	Epiphora		• Punctal ectropion	Medial spindle procedure
			• Recalcitrant epiphora due to lacrimal pump failure	CDCR/Jones tube
	Midface ptosis			Static sling using autologous fascia lata SOOF lift
	Aberrant regeneration		• Narrowing of palpebral fissure with lower facial movements	• Injection Botox to orbicularis oculi
			• Crocodile tears	• Injection Botox to palpebral lobe of lacrimal gland

(CDCR: conjunctivodacryocystorhinostomy; LCT: lateral canthal tendon; LPS: levator palpebrae superioris; MCT: medial canthal tendon; SOOF: suborbicularis oculi fat)

Suggested Reading

1. Allam G, Biousse V, Gwathmey K, Newman N. Section 1. Cranial nerve and neuroophthalmologic disorders. In: Jones HR, Burns TM, Aminoff MJ, Pomeroy SL (Eds). The Netter Collection of Medical Illustrations—Nervous System, Part II: Spinal Cord and Peripheral Motor and Sensory Systems, 2nd edition, volume 7. Philadelphia, PA: Elsevier; 2013. pp. 1-48.

2. Bosniak S (Ed). Principles and Practice of Ophthalmic Plastic and Reconstructive Surgery. New York, NY: W.B. Saunders; 1996. p. 473.
3. Gausas RE. Facial paralysis: a comprehensive approach to current management. In: Guthoff RF, Katowitz JA (Eds). Essentials in Ophthalmology: Oculoplastics and Orbit. Germany: Springer; 2006. pp. 191-204.
4. Holds JB. Facial palsy: periocular management. In: Black EH, Nesi FA, Calvano CJ, Gladstone GJ, Levine MR (Eds). Smith and Nesi's Ophthalmic Plastic and Reconstructive Surgery, 3rd edition. New York: Springer; 2012. pp. 332-43.
5. Homer N, Fay A. Management of long-standing flaccid facial palsy: periocular considerations. Otolaryngol Clin North Am. 2018; 51:1107-18.
6. House JW, Brackmann DE. Facial nerve grading system. Otolaryngol Head Neck Surg. 1985;93:146-7.
7. Latkany R, Lock B, Speaker M. Nocturnal lagophthalmos: an overview and classification. Ocul Surf. 2006;4:44-53.
8. Leatherbarrow B, Jones PF. Oculoplastic Surgery, 2nd edition. New York, NY: Informa Healthcare; 2011. pp. 192-204.
9. May M, Klein SR. Differential diagnosis of facial nerve palsy. Otolaryngol Clin North Am. 1991;24:613-45.
10. Monkhouse, S. Cranial Nerves: Functional Anatomy. New York, NY: Cambridge University Press; 2006. p. 133.
11. Pereira MVC, Glória ALF. Lagophthalmos. Semin Ophthalmol. 2010;25:72-8.
12. Rahman I, Sadiq SA. Ophthalmic management of facial nerve palsy: a review. Surv Ophthalmol. 2007;52:121-44.
13. Tyers AG. Seventh nerve palsy and corneal exposure. In: Collin R, Rose G (Eds). Fundamentals of Clinical Ophthalmology Plastic and Orbital Surgery. London: BMJ Books; 2001. pp. 67-77.
14. Yücel OE, Artürk N. Botulinum toxin-A-induced protective ptosis in the treatment of lagophthalmos associated with facial paralysis. Ophthal Plast Reconstr Surg. 2012;28:256-60.

1.10 Anatomy of Lacrimal System

Priyanka V Walvekar, Nandini Bothra

 1. Describe the anatomy of the lacrimal system.

The lacrimal apparatus is a system involved in the production and conduction of tears. It is broadly divided into the secretory system and excretory system.

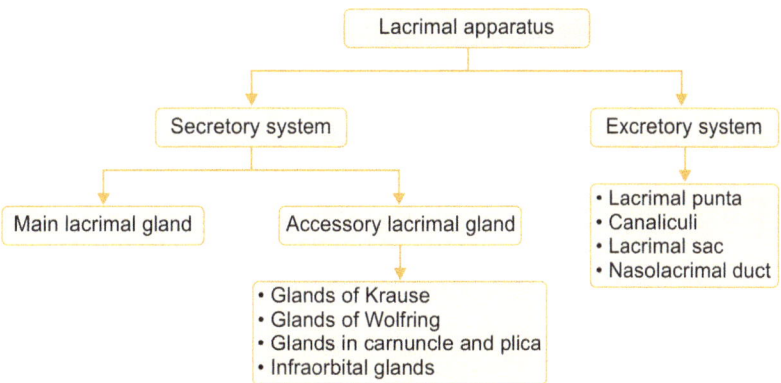

Lacrimal Secretory System

Lacrimal Gland

- The lacrimal gland is the main component of the secretory system. It develops from ectodermal buds in the anterior superolateral orbit. These buds branch and canalize, forming ducts and alveoli.
- The lacrimal glands are small and do not function fully until approximately 6 weeks after birth. Hence, newborn infants do not produce tears when crying.
- The main lacrimal gland is an exocrine gland located in the superior lateral quadrant of the orbit within the lacrimal gland fossa.
- The lateral horn of the levator aponeurosis indents the lacrimal gland and divides it anteriorly into orbital and palpebral lobes.

> Removal of (or) damage to the palpebral portion of the gland can seriously reduce secretion from the entire gland. This is the reason that biopsy of the lacrimal gland is generally performed on the orbital lobe.

- 8–12 major lacrimal ducts empty into the superior cul-de-sac approximately 5 mm above the lateral tarsal border after passing posterior to the aponeurosis.
- The ducts from the orbital portion run through and join the ducts of the palpebral lobe.

Glands of Krause and Wolfring

The accessory exocrine glands of Krause and Wolfring are located deep within the superior fornix and just above the superior border of the tarsus, respectively.

Aqueous Lacrimal Secretion

Tear secretion is a complex, multifactorial process and dysfunction of any component of the ocular surface system can result in tear film instability and hyperosmolarity with resultant dry eye disease. The tear film is primarily composed of lipids, aqueous, and mucins, with aqueous accounting for a majority of its thickness. The aqueous is produced by the main lacrimal gland, accessory lacrimal glands, corneal, and conjunctival epithelia. Although the main lacrimal gland has long been considered an indispensable source of the aqueous component of tears, there is evidence that adequate tear secretion can exist in the absence of the main lacrimal gland.

- Aqueous lacrimal secretion has traditionally been divided into basal low-level secretion and reflex secretion.
- Previously, it was argued that the accessory glands provided basal tear secretion and the lacrimal gland was responsible for reflex tearing.
- However, recent evidence suggests that all tearing may be reflex.

> Basal tear secretion in the absence of stimuli probably does not occur to a significant extent as evidenced by decreased tear secretion during sleep and under local and general anesthesia.

Understanding the Basics of Tear Secretion

- *The ocular surface system:* The lacrimal functional unit, an important subset of the ocular surface system, consists of the cornea, conjunctiva, meibomian glands, lacrimal glands, eyelid, and their interconnected nervous system. The lacrimal functional unit highlights the main structures responsible for tear secretion and the blink reflex. Dysfunction of any component of the ocular surface system can result in abnormalities of the tear film and loss of the smooth refractive tear film.
- *Tear secretion:* It is a multifactorial process that involves the nervous, muscular, endocrine, vascular, and immune systems. It is a reflex response initiated by stimulation of the ocular surface or nasal mucosa. The polymodal nociceptors of the cornea are the primary sensory fibers responsible for initiating tear secretion. These sensory fibers relay signals to the spinal trigeminal nucleus where information is processed and relayed to the superior salivary nucleus of the pontine tegmentum. Preganglionic parasympathetic neurons originating from the superior salivary nucleus project to the pterygopalatine ganglion. Postganglionic parasympathetic neurons then project to the lacrimal glands, and also presumably to the goblet cells and meibomian glands, where they release neurotransmitters such as acetylcholine and vasoactive intestinal peptide that stimulate tear secretion.

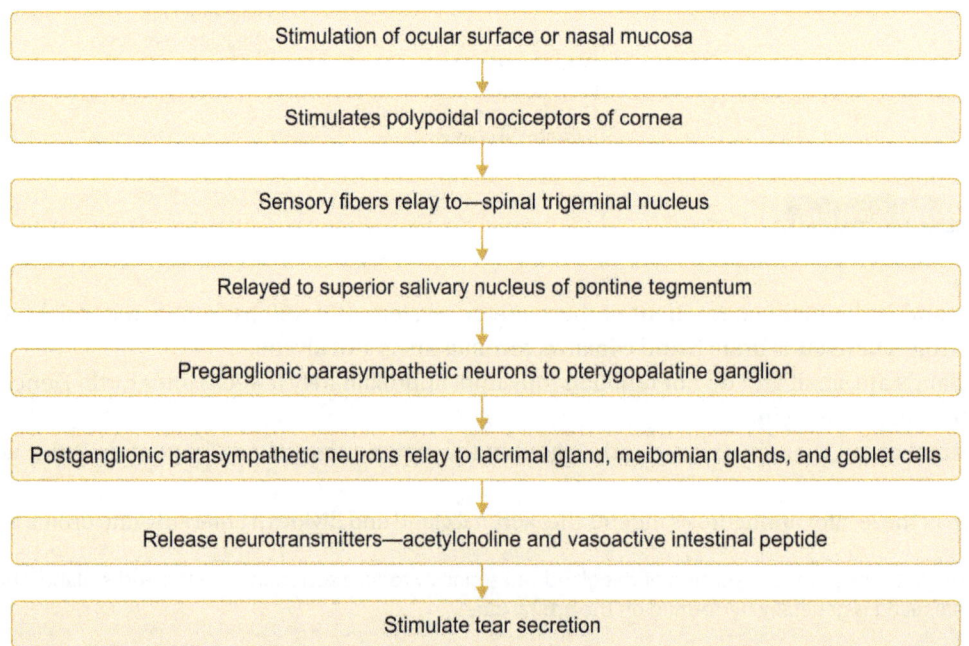

- The blink reflex, also known as the trigeminofacial reflex, is critical for tear secretion and function. Blinking stimulates the release of lipids from the meibomian glands and replenishes the tear film with tears from the inferior tear meniscus.

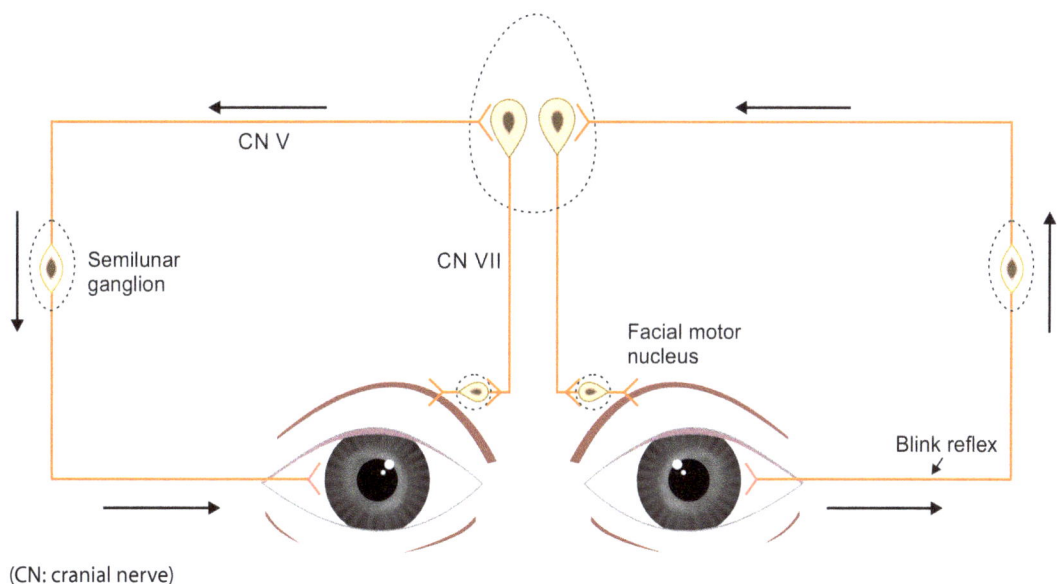

(CN: cranial nerve)

Lacrimal Excretory System

This system mainly comprises the puncta, the canaliculus, the lacrimal sac, and the nasolacrimal duct (NLD).

Puncta
- The lacrimal punctum lies on a small fibrous mound, called the "lacrimal papilla." Diameter of its opening is 0.2–0.3 mm and directs posteriorly toward the lacrimal lake.
- The inferior punctum lies 0.5–1.0 mm more temporally than the superior one because the maxillary process in embryonic life grows faster than the lateral nasal process.
- The inner epithelium is lined by nonkeratinized stratified squamous epithelium.

Upper and Lower Canaliculus

Each punctum leads to its respective canaliculus.
- Each canaliculus is divided into the vertical and horizontal portions.
- The length of the vertical portion is 2 mm and that of the horizontal part is 10 mm. The medial most 2 mm of the horizontal portion mostly forms the common canaliculus and more than half of this part runs in the wall of the sac.
- The punctum and vertical canaliculus are encircled by a similar hard fibrous tissue. This fibrous tissue in the vertical canaliculus contains skeletal muscle fibers, called the muscle of Riolan.
- Vertical canaliculus ends in a dilated segment called ampulla before transitioning to the horizontal canaliculus.
  - *Applied anatomy:* It is the ampulla which contains a lot of secretions in canaliculitis and is important to remove all the secretions from the ampulla for rapid recovery.
- The diameter of the canaliculus is usually 0.3–0.6 mm, but it can be expanded to over 1.0 mm owing to the elastic fibers in its wall. The temporal four-fifths part is directed posteronasally and surrounded by the Horner's muscle, occasionally called the lacrimal part of the orbicularis oculi muscle.
- The superior canaliculus courses almost straight to the internal common ostium, but the inferior canaliculus changes its course before joining the superior canaliculus.

Common Canaliculus
- More than 95% of the upper and lower canaliculi join to become the common canaliculus to reach the common internal ostium.
- The canaliculi empty into the sinus of Maier and those independently pouring into the sac are <2%. The common internal ostium is the part where the common canaliculus pours to the sac.
- The common canaliculus has a non-keratinized stratified squamous epithelium.

Sinus of Maier: Represents a laterally bulged portion of the sac which is formed around the common internal ostium and some canaliculi empty to this portion. An expanded common canaliculus can also be called the sinus of Maier.

Valve of Rosenmüller

- A protuberance (fold) is present, although in only half of the cases, at the junction between the common canaliculus and the sac called the valve of Rosenmüller (VOR).
- The part around the common internal ostium needs a structure dealing with nasal movement of the ostium during eye closing and this may be the real reason for a valvular presence in this region.

Valve of Rosenmüller (VOR): Study by Ali described two types of VOR. Type 1 is a freely mobile, elliptical fold arising from the superior portion of the medial edge of the internal common ostium. Type 2 is group of folds arising from the superior and inferior portions of the medial edge of the ostium. The same study proposed that the valve of Huschke was a misnomer and when present, is a part of VOR.

The Lacrimal Sac

- Lies in the lacrimal sac fossa which is bound by the anterior and posterior lacrimal crests.
- The length of the lacrimal sac is around 12-15 mm. The part of the sac superior to the medial canthal tendon (MCT) is called the fundus, with its vertical length of 3-5 mm. The body of the sac, inferior to the MCT, is about 10 mm in length.
- The anterior and posterior crus of the MCT encircle the fundus of the lacrimal sac and attach to the anterior and posterior lacrimal crests, respectively.
- The deep head of preseptal orbicularis oculi (Horner's muscle) helps in pumping the tears accumulated in the lacrimal sac. The lateral aspect of the sac wall is covered by a fascia, and its posterior portion is a common fascia with the Horner's muscle which is called the "lacrimal diaphragm."
- The sac is lined by stratified columnar epithelium and contains goblet cells, cilia, and serous glands.

Horner's or the Horner-Duverney's Muscle
Although William Edmonds Horner has been credited to the detailed description of the Horner's muscle in 1824, the first ever description of this muscle was given by French anatomist Jaques Francois Marie Duverney way back in 1730.

Nasolacrimal Duct

- The lacrimal sac and the NLD are a continuous tissue, and anatomically, the "nasolacrimal duct" (mucosal portion) is the part inferior to the superior opening of the nasolacrimal canal (bony portion).
- The nasolacrimal canal is formed by the lacrimal bone superonasally, the inferior turbinate bone inferonasally, and the maxillary bone temporally.
- The superior opening is about 6 mm in diameter and the superoinferior length of the canal is about 12 mm. Although the longitudinal axis of the canal directs about 20° posteriorly, it directs almost vertically in most cases.
- The nasolacrimal canal empties into the superior part of the inferior meatus. The NLD opens into the nose through an ostium under the inferior turbinate, which is usually partially covered by a mucosal fold called the valve of Hasner.
- Failure of this ostium to develop is, in most cases, the cause of congenital NLD obstruction.
- The lining epithelium of the NLD is a stratified columnar epithelium, similar to the lacrimal sac, and contains goblet cells and serous glands.

 2. Describe the structural and functional aspects of lacrimal pump mechanism.

Physiology of Tear Drainage

- Approximately 10-20% of tear drainage is carried out by evaporation. Most of the tear flow from the eye to nose through the nasolacrimal system is by an active pump mechanism of orbicularis oculi **(Fig. 1)**.
- With each blink the orbicularis contracts and thus squeezes the lacrimal sac, forcing out the tears collected before the blink, down the NLD. During the blink, both the puncta remain apposed to the lid margin thus preventing any backward regurgitation of tears.
- As the eye opens up after the blink, both the puncta open up and the tear gets sucked in the lacrimal sac by the negative pressure or capillary action. The same cycle continues on with each blink.

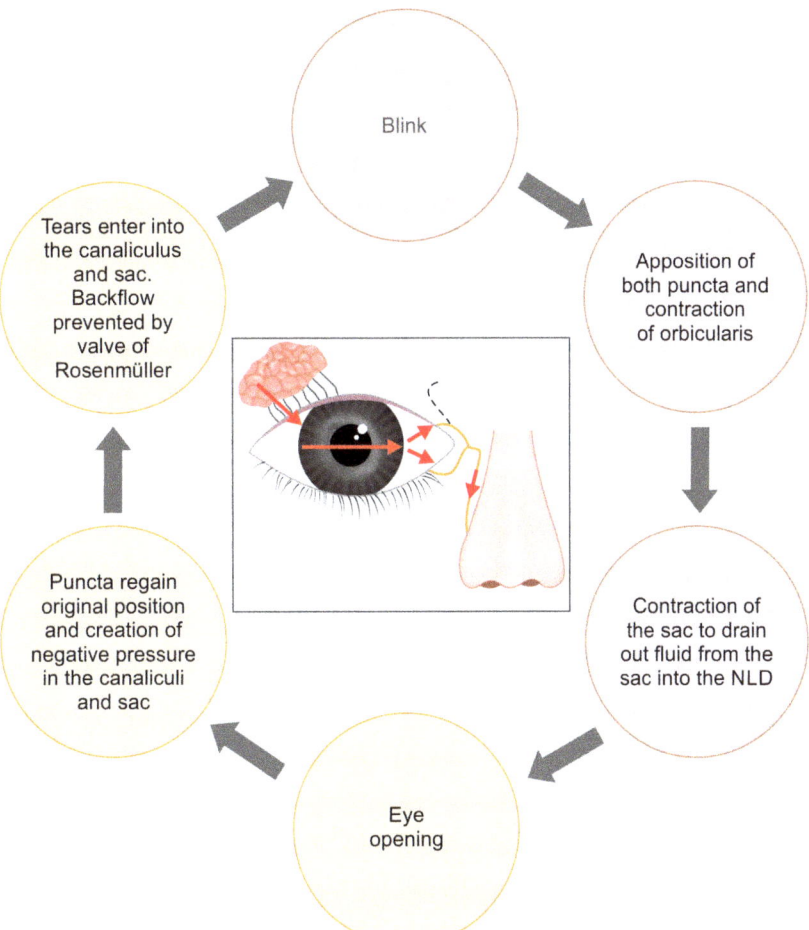

Fig. 1: Lacrimal pump mechanism.
(NLD: nasolacrimal duct)

The Krehbiel flow is a special type of lacrimal fluid drainage. This is a phenomenon in which a lacrimal fluid aspiration from the lacus lacrimalis into the punctum continues for a considerable period during eye opening (without blinking). Although all the cases do not show this phenomenon, 25% of the lacrimal passage with 45° posterior inclination demonstrate it. The Krehbiel flow is believed to occur by a lower intrasac pressure against a canalicular pressure, namely by a pressure gradient from the canaliculus to the sac.

- Present evidence supports the crucial role of the palpebral-canalicular pump mechanism in lacrimal elimination.
- All efforts should be made to preserve the lacrimal canaliculi. Repeated instrumentation of the lacrimal system or NLD probing is unlikely to help the underlying pathology and may injure the canaliculi thus permanently impairing lacrimal elimination.
- Very little can be done to restore scarred fibrosed canaliculi. Frieberg has used a manometer to measure a pressure gradient within the canaliculi and lacrimal sac. This pressure gradient cannot be produced if the canaliculus is slit open.
- Thus, overly aggressive procedures on the lacrimal outflow system, such as aggressive "three-snip" punctoplasties or aggressive surgical treatment of canaliculitis should be avoided.
- Experimental and clinical studies show that tear elimination is equivalent through the upper and lower canalicular systems.
- Therefore, equal consideration to be given to a patient with lacerations of either the upper or lower canaliculus. Traditional teachings that upper eyelid canalicular lacerations are unimportant are simply not true.

Applied Aspect

The lacrimal outflow system may be anatomically patent to irrigation yet be functionally inadequate in terms of normal lacrimal elimination.
- Facial nerve paresis is among the most common situations in which lacrimal pump failure is present despite patency of the membranous lacrimal conduit.
- Any condition that impairs the normal contractile and elastic properties of the palpebral-canalicular pump mechanism can cause epiphora.

- These conditions include scleroderma, radiation fibrosis of the eyelids, and cutaneous burns or trauma of the periocular region.
- Chronic or recurrent canaliculitis may leave the canaliculi anatomically patent yet functionally impaired.

Suggested Reading

1. Albert DM, Jakobiec FA (Eds). Principles and Practice of Ophthalmology, 3rd edition. Philadelphia, PA: Elsevier; 2008. pp. 3497-501.
2. Ali MJ (Ed). Textbook of Principles and Practice of Lacrimal Surgery. Singapore: Springer; 2019.
3. American Academy of Ophthalmology. Basic and Clinical Course. Section 7, Orbit, Eyelids and Lacrimal System. San Francisco, CA: American Academy of Ophthalmology; 2008–2009. pp. 259-64.
4. Spalton DJ, Hitchings RA, Hunter PA (Eds). Atlas of Clinical Ophthalmology, 2nd edition. Mosby Wolfe; 1993.
5. Stevenson W, Pugazhendhi S, Wang M. Is the main lacrimal gland indispensable? Contributions of the corneal and conjunctival epithelia. Survey Ophthalmol. 2016;61(5):616-27.

1.11 Congenital Disorders of the Lacrimal System

Priyanka V Walvekar, Nandini Bothra

Q 1. Describe the etiology, clinical features, differential diagnosis, and management of congenital nasolacrimal duct obstruction.

Q 2. Outline the differential diagnosis and management of watering of eye in children.

Q 3. Congenital abnormalities of the lacrimal drainage system and their management.

Congenital disorders of the lacrimal system can be broadly divided into developmental disorders of the secretory system and the excretory system.

Developmental Disorders of the Lacrimal Secretory System

Congenital abnormalities of the lacrimal glands are relatively rare and include hypoplasia or agenesis of the lacrimal gland. Occasionally, children are born with ectopic lacrimal glands and lacrimal gland fistula.

Lacrimal Gland Agenesis

- Congenital lacrimal gland agenesis is a rare cause of dry eye syndrome in childhood. Lacrimal gland agenesis may occur as an isolated condition or it may accompany salivary gland agenesis and atresia of lacrimal drainage system.
- Isolated form of congenital lacrimal gland agenesis is a rare condition but should be considered in the differential diagnosis of childhood dry eye syndrome. In children with dry eye syndrome without any systemic findings, it should be emphasized that noninvasive measures such as magnetic resonance imaging (MRI) can be primarily undertaken for the possible diagnosis of lacrimal gland agenesis before performing any invasive procedure.

Lacrimal Gland Aplasia/Hypoplasia

- Congenital alacrima is a form of primary lacrimal deficiency characterized by aplasia or hypoplasia of the lacrimal gland. The puncta and salivary glands may also be aplastic.
- Autosomal dominant aplasia of lacrimal and salivary glands is rare and characterized by irritable eyes, epiphora (constant tearing) and xerostomia (dryness of the mouth).
- Aplasia of the lacrimal and major salivary glands (ALSG) has variable expressivity and affected individuals may have aplasia or hypoplasia of the lacrimal, parotid, submandibular, and sublingual glands and absence of the lacrimal puncta.

Ectopic Lacrimal Glands

- Ectopic lacrimal gland tissue is rare but should be considered in the differential diagnosis of masses in the epibulbar conjunctiva, eyelid, orbit, and lacrimal sac, particularly in childhood.
- It can undergo neoplastic transformation in the same way as can the lacrimal gland and incomplete excision can result in recurrence.

- The most common location for ectopic lacrimal gland tissue is epibulbar conjunctiva, other locations include orbit, eyelid, intraocular, lacrimal sac, and nasal mucosa.
- Ectopic lacrimal glands on the bulbar conjunctiva within the uveal tract and on the surface of the cornea are a well-recognized source of choristomatous tumors, which are usually identified in early childhood.

Developmental Disorders of the Lacrimal Excretory System

Developmental abnormalities (major) of the lacrimal excretory system can be classified as follows:

Puncta and canaliculus	*Lacrimal sac*	*Nasolacrimal duct*
• Punctal agenesis • Incomplete punctal canalization (IPC) • Canalicular agenesis and dysgenesis • Canaliculops • Supernumery puncta and canaliculi	• Lacrimal anlage duct or lacrimal fistula • Lacrimal sac diverticula	• Congenital nasolacrimal duct obstruction • Congenital dacryocele • Congenital absence of valves

Developmental abnormalities include duplication of puncta, punctual aplasia and hypoplasia, congenital lacrimal cutaneous fistula, congenital nasolacrimal duct obstruction (CNLDO), and dacryocele among others. CNLDO is the most common developmental abnormality of the lacrimal excretory system.

Ectopic Caruncle and Canaliculus

An ectopic canaliculus opens on an ectopic caruncle due to common developmental origin of the lower eyelid and caruncle.

Punctal Agenesis

It can be defined as the absence of punctum occurring secondary to a failure of embryogenesis.
- The basic etiopathogenesis of punctal agenesis is failure of canaliculi outbudding from the upper end of the solid lacrimal cord in an embryo of 18–24 mm.
- Agenesis has important associated ocular and systemic associations such as lacrimal fistula, blepharitis, distichiasis, eyelid tags, absence of caruncle, and divergent strabismus.
- Punctal agenesis has well-known association with systemic syndromes such as ectodermal dysplasia, Hay–Wells syndrome, and Levy–Hollister syndrome.

Hay–Wells syndrome: It is also known as ankyloblepharon-ectodermal-dysplasia-clefting syndrome and is characterized by ectodermal dysplasia, alopecia, cleft lip, and punctal agenesis

Levy–Hollister syndrome: It is also known as lacrimo-auriculo-dento-digital syndrome and is characterized by anomalies of lacrimal and salivary glands as well as ducts, ears, dentition, and extremities.

- The term punctal atresia has been used interchangeably with punctal agenesis as well as for a spectrum of punctal disorders varying from a fine membrane in the punctum to its absence itself.
- The diagnosis of punctal agenesis should include a careful history and examination.
- Single missing puncta may not present with gross epiphora. But when associated with discharge and gross epiphora, suspect underlying nasolacrimal duct (NLD) obstruction also.
- *Symptomatology:* History of epiphora with no mucoid/mucopurulent discharge. Presence of epiphora since birth.
- *Signs:* Eyelashes on the pars lacrimalis portion of the eyelid (extension of the eyelashes medial to the site of the expected puncta), absence of the punctal papilla, a subtle depression in the canalicular portion of the eyelid when it is associated with canalicular agenesis (which is common).
- Management of punctal agenesis is challenging. Patients who have a single punctum missing and are asymptomatic may be observed without any intervention. However, probing is warranted in those who have associated NLD obstruction.
- *Patients with involvement of both punctum:* The management is difficult and we can opt for lacrimal gland botulinum toxin injection or lacrimal gland debulking if the epiphora is troublesome. Some have advocated conjunctivodacryocystorhinostomy (CDCR) with Lester-Jones tubes to treat this condition and establish an alternative pathway for tear drainage.

Incomplete Punctal Canalization

Incomplete punctal canalization (IPC) is a term that refers to a form of punctal dysgenesis with membrane. This term was described by Ali et al.

- *Pathogenesis:* It is believed to either represent failed dehiscence of epithelium overlying the normally formed canaliculi or failure of canalization of the most proximal part of lacrimal apparatus.
- May be associated with canalicular stenosis.
- No systemic association is known.
- *Clinical diagnosis:* High degree of suspicion, clear epiphora without discharge (usually when both puncta are involved), and slight avascular dimple at the site of the puncta
- *On slit-lamp examination:* A translucent membrane is seen, sometimes with a vessel seen traversing across the membrane.
- *Two types of membranes are seen:* IPC external membrane (IPC-EM) and internal membrane (IPC-IM).
- *IPC-EM type:* External type will cover the external surface of the puncta and the punctal opening is hidden beneath the membrane (appears like punctal agenesis). On closer observation, we can notice a vessel traversing over the translucent membrane.
- *IPC-IM type:* Here the punctal margins are made out although blurred, and the membrane can be seen dipping into the punctal opening. Also, the vessel traversing the membrane can be seen dipping into the punctal opening.
- Management of IPC is usually simple. A membranotomy using a slow taper punctum dilator is almost always helpful. If associated with canalicular stenosis, mini-monoka stent can be placed in the canaliculus and when associated with NLD obstruction, probing can be carried out.

Canalicular Agenesis

This results from failure of outpouching of epithelial buds from the upper end of lacrimal cord or abrupt halt in migration toward eyelids immediately following outpouching.
- Canalicular agenesis is associated with punctal agenesis.
- Signs and symptoms are similar to punctal agenesis.
- *Treatment:* If the symptoms are minimal or if only one canaliculus is involved, patient can be observed.
- If both canaliculi are involved then, lacrimal gland measures (botulinum toxin/debulking) can be attempted to reduce epiphora. CDCR is another option in these cases.

Canalicular Wall Dysgenesis

Ali et al. introduced the term canalicular wall dysgenesis and its eight subtypes of aplasia (nondevelopment of the wall/complete dehiscence) and hypoplasia (thinning of the wall).
- Its etiopathogenesis is unknown but is believed to occur during the embryonic stages (Carnegie stages 18 or 22) or during the early fetal life.
- The canaliculus is believed to have four walls: Roof, floor, anterior, and posterior walls. Roof is parallel to the lid margin and posterior wall is parallel to palpebral conjunctiva.
- It can involve single wall or can involve multiple walls of the canaliculus. Also, it can either involve a small part of the wall or the complete wall (focal/diffuse involvement). Accordingly it is classified as follows:
  - *Single canalicular wall dysgenesis (SCWD):*
    - *Single canalicular wall hypoplasia (SCWH):*
      - Focal
      - Diffuse
    - *Single canalicular wall aplasia (SCWA):*
      - Focal
      - Diffuse
  - *Multiple canalicular wall dysgenesis (MCWD):*
    - *Multiple canalicular wall hypoplasia (MCWH):*
      - Focal
      - Diffuse
    - *Multiple canalicular wall aplasia (MCWA):*
      - Focal
      - Diffuse
- *Diagnosis:* It is made on slit-lamp biomicroscopy. Place a probe in the canaliculus. If a wall is aplastic, complete dehiscence of the wall with direct visualization of the underlying probe within the canaliculus will be noted. However, if the wall is hypoplastic, then the probe will shine through a thin mucosal lining of the canaliculus.
- Most common involvement in a study by Ali et al., has been found to be SCWD involving the roof (around 71%). Hypoplasia (57%) is more common than aplasia (43%).
- *Lacrimal associations:* Punctal agenesis, IPC, CNLDO, punctal stenosis, and agenesis.

- *Symptoms:* Epiphora usually accompanies these anomalies. These patients generally do well once the underlying lacrimal association is taken care of. However, some weakness of the lacrimal pump is expected, more so when multiple canalicular walls are involved.
- *Caution:* While irrigation or probing, care should be taken to avoid aggressive movement within the lacrimal drainage system as these walls are weak and there is a tendency to rupture. During probing, the probe should be turned 90° slowly and with care so as to prevent rupture of the hypoplastic walls.

Supernumerary Puncta and Canaliculi

These may result from multiple epithelial buds developing from the upper end of lacrimal cord during the embryonic period of development.
- *Incidence:* 1 in 60,000
- *Lacrimal associations:* Lacrimal fistula and lacrimal sac diverticulum
- *Systemic associations:* Down syndrome and preauricular sinus.

Canaliculops

Canaliculops or canaliculocele is a term used for a noninfectious and noninflammatory distention of a localized segment of the canaliculus with accumulation of serous fluid within the lumen.
- *Predisposing factors:* Trauma, surgeries, or past infections. These can also be present with punctal agenesis.
- It is a painless, translucent, and slow-growing medial eyelid cystic lesion. Transillumination is generally positive since it is filled with serous fluid.
- *Investigations:* Usually, clinical examination is enough for diagnosis but can be supplemented with ultrasonography and anterior segment ocular coherence tomography.
- *Treatment:* Usually these cysts have a blind medial end, making it difficult to have a patent lacrimal drainage pathway. In these cases, marsupialization of the cyst for cosmetic reasons can be attempted.
- If the medial end is patent, careful removal of the cyst with Monoka stent through the canaliculus and suturing the ends of the canaliculus over the stent is needed. Stent extubation to be done at the end of 4–6 weeks.
- Histopathological analysis is needed for definite diagnosis. The cyst wall is lined by the canalicular epithelium—multilayered nonkeratinizing stratified squamous epithelium. Immunohistochemistry is confirmatory—superficial epithelial layer staining by cytokeratin 7 (CK-7).

Lacrimal Anlage Duct or Lacrimal Fistula

Lacrimal fistula is an accessory or an anlage duct communicating with the skin on one side and the canaliculus, lacrimal sac, or NLD on the other.
- Autosomal inheritance pattern has been reported for congenital lacrimal fistulas.
- Congenital lacrimal fistulae are usually asymptomatic.
- *Signs:* Small, lack pigmentation, or other skin changes around it and are usually located inferomedial to the medial canthal angle.
- *Treatment:* Symptomatic ones may have an underlying transient functional or anatomical NLD obstruction. Treatment is observation for asymptomatic cases and management of underlying pathology with fistulectomy for symptomatic ones or cosmetic concerns.

In contrast, the acquired fistulas may be irregular, large with surrounding scarring, and without any probable fixed location.

Lacrimal Sac Diverticula

Lacrimal diverticula are cystic outpouchings, most commonly seen arising from the lacrimal sac.
- *Most common site:* The inferolateral wall of the lacrimal sac since resistance to any expansion is least in this region as compared to other walls of the sac.
- It can cause stagnation of secretions in the diverticula causing diverticulitis/acute dacryocystitis/abscess formation.
- *Diagnosis:* It usually needs dacryocystography for diagnosis.
- *Treatment:* Symptomatic cases will need dacryocystorhinostomy (DCR).

Congenital Nasolacrimal Duct Obstruction

- It is a common cause of epiphora in children with incidence of symptoms ranging from 1.2% to 30%.
- It is usually caused by a membranous block at the level of the valve of Hasner covering the nasal end of the NLD.

- During the development of the lacrimal system, the canalization begins in the lacrimal sac at the 10th month of the fetal stage. This canalization then proceeds proximally and distally. At seventh month of intrauterine life, the eyelids separate and the puncta open in the surface. However, at the caudal end at the junction of the lacrimal cord and inferior meatal lamina, apoptosis of the cells begins to form the lacrimal passage but is completed few weeks or months after birth. Therefore, the caudal end of the NLD is the last to canalize. Sometimes, this membrane persists at the caudal end causing CNLDO.
- *The obstruction can be of two types:* Simple CNLDO or complex CNLDO.
  1. *Simple CNLDO:* Membranous obstruction at the lower end of the NLD/at the valve of Hasner. Also presence of canalicular valves where resistance is felt while bypassing them (not a true obstruction) is also classified as simple CNLDO.
  2. *Complex CNLDO:* All the other variations such as buried probe, misdirected opening of the NLD anywhere other than in the inferior meatus or nondevelopment of the NLD. Also variations such as impacted anterior end of the inferior turbinate, lacrimal drainage pathways stenosis are included in complex CNLDO.
- *Symptoms: Classical triad:* Watering, discharge, matting of eyelashes.
- Epiphora with mucoid/mucopurulent discharge, sac swelling. Sometimes can present with acute infections with pain, redness, and swelling in the lacrimal sac region.
- *Signs:* Raised tear meniscus height, matted lashes, delayed fluorescein dye disappearance test, ROPLAS (regurgitation on pressure on the lacrimal sac) is generally positive.

Nasolacrimal Duct Variations in Congenital Nasolacrimal Duct Obstruction
1. Nasolacrimal duct does not open into inferior meatus and may end abruptly onto the vault of the meatus or get buried in the lateral wall.
2. Nasolacrimal duct ending blindly into the inferior turbinate.
3. Nasolacrimal duct ending blindly into the medial maxillary sinus wall.
4. Nasolacrimal duct ending in a bony, noncanalized nasolacrimal canal.
5. Absence of nasolacrimal duct

Treatment

- *Spontaneous resolution:* It is believed that respiratory efforts, crying, and sucking create negative pressure within the nose which helps to break the membrane present at the NLD opening. This spontaneous perforation usually occurs by 3–4 weeks of age, but if it fails, manifestations of CNLDO are seen. Natural history of the disease favors spontaneous remission rate by 1 year of age (in almost 96% cases).
- *Lacrimal sac compressions (Crigler massage):* These compressions create hydrostatic intraluminal pressure in the NLD by obstructing the common canaliculus and increasing the pressure downward causing the rupture of the membranous obstruction. Earlier the compressions are advocated, more are the chances of resolution as per studies. Recent evidence suggests resolution of CNLDO until 18 months of age with lacrimal sac compressions when correct technique is practiced (Bansal et al.).

Method

Parents should wash hands and make sure the nails are trimmed. Using the index finger, pressure is directly applied inside the anterior lacrimal crest, below the medial canthal tendon, directly onto the lacrimal sac without compressing the bone or the eye. Pressure is applied in the inward and medial direction and slightly downward. Ten such compressions every sitting and four such sittings/day to be done until resolution of the obstruction.

Irrigation and probing: If the CNLDO fails to resolve with lacrimal sac massage, therapeutic probing of the NLD is carried out. If lacrimal sac compressions fail to relieve the obstruction till 1 year of age, then irrigation and probing under endoscopic guidance is advocated.

Early probing (less than a year old child): Indications:
1. Acute dacryocystitis/lacrimal abscess
2. Congenital dacryocele
3. Need for an early intraocular surgery
4. *Relative:* Extremely dilated lacrimal sac, mucocele

Technique

Instil topical anesthetic eyedrops (2% proparacaine eyedrops). Child is in reclining position and is under general anesthesia. Upper punctum is generally preferred for the procedure as it is believed to be in direct communication with lacrimal sac and prevents injury to the lower lacrimal drainage pathways which is believed to drain more fluid as compared to the upper lacrimal drainage pathway. Pull the upper eyelid up and lateral such that the lacrimal canaliculus is at a stretch and is partly straightened. Punctal dilatation with slow-taper Nettleship's punctal dilator is done directing the dilator perpendicular to the punctal opening till the ampulla (approximately 2 mm) and then directing it horizontal and parallel to the lid margin so as to follow the canalicular anatomy slowly rotating the dilator. Now gently insert the 1 cc syringe mounted lacrimal cannula in the opposite fashion as the dilator and irrigate the lacrimal passages. Once the obstruction is confirmed by noting the mucoid/mucopurulent regurgitation from the opposite punctum, Bowman's lacrimal probe "0" (for neonates) and "1" (for other children) is inserted in a similar fashion as the cannula. Once hard stop is felt, it is gently rotated by 90° and then directed laterally, backward and downward along the NLD. Endoscope is introduced in the nose, inferior turbinate is medialized, and inferior meatus is viewed. The probe is then gradually advanced under direct visualization to open into the inferior meatus. Irrigation is then repeated and free flow of the fluorescein-stained saline into the nose seen endoscopically confirms that the obstruction has been overcome.

Guidelines for choosing the size of Bowman's lacrimal probe:
- Neonate   #00
- Infants   #0
- 1–4 years #1
- >4 years   #1 or #2

- *Balloon dacryoplasty or balloon catheter dilatation:* Although a few practice, this modality as the primary procedure, it is mostly indicated in the following cases:
  Indications: Previous failed probing:
  - Failed intubation
  - Complex CNLDO
  - Complex CNLDO with syndromic associations
  - Older age groups.

Technique: Usually a 2-mm size balloon for children <30 months and 3-mm size balloon for children >30 months of age is used. Initial technique is similar to irrigation and probing, the passage of probe is confirmed in the inferior meatus. The balloon catheter is then lubricated and passed in the similar fashion as the probe. There are two markings on the catheter—15 mm and 10 mm. The catheter is passed till 15 mm mark reaches the punctum. The balloon is then inflated and deflated for two cycles: first cycle at 8 atm of pressure for 90 seconds and then again for 60 seconds. Now, the catheter is withdrawn till the 10 mm mark reaches the puncta and the process of inflation and deflation is repeated. Irrigation is confirmed by the passage of fluorescein-stained saline in the nose.

Recently introduced percutaneous transluminal coronary angioplasty balloons for balloon dacryoplasty has helped reduce the cost of the balloons from around 350$ to 90$ with similar safety profile and success rates.

- *Silicone intubation:* Usual indications include cases of failed probing and complex CNLDO, but some use it as primary treatment modality. Monocanalicular and bicanalicular intubation have the same success rates. Common stents used for monocanalicular intubation are Monoka-Crawford and mini-monoka stents. Advantages of these stents over bicanalicular stents are easy removal in the OPD under topical anesthesia. Commonly used bicanalicular stents are Crawford silicone stent. They need sedation or general anesthesia for removal.

  Stent extubation is generally done at 4–6 weeks. Various studies debate the timing of stent removal and the timing can be as late as 6 months according to various studies.

  Complications are rare, but can include spontaneous stent extubation, nasal bleed, injury to the floor of the nose and the inferior meatus, punctal cheese-wiring, corneal abrasion, pyogenic granuloma, etc.
- *Dacryocystorhinostomy:* DCR is a procedure in which the normal lacrimal pathway is bypassed and an alternative drainage pathway is surgically created which opens into the middle meatus. The procedure is generally performed after 5 years of age. It is indicated in cases in which probing, intubation, and balloon dacryoplasty have failed or where probing cannot be done because of a bony block or extensive developmental abnormalities of the drainage pathway.

Congenital Dacryocele
- The pathogenesis in dacryocele is believed to be persistent noncanalization of the lower end of NLD along with a functional obstruction at the valve of Rosenmüller. This is thought to cause sufficient pressure to dilate the entire sac and in many cases the membranous part of the NLD, leading to formation of an intranasal cyst.
- Earlier was also known as amniontocele as it was believed that this cyst was filled with amniotic fluid.

- Seen in neonates usually in the first 1–2 months of life.
- *Symptoms:* Epiphora, mucoid/mucopurulent discharge
- *Signs:* Bluish swelling in the lacrimal sac area, raised tear meniscus height, matted lashes, and delayed fluorescein dye disappearance test. Sometimes can present with difficulty in breathing especially during breast-feeding.
- *Treatment:* Early irrigation and probing under endoscopic guidance. Presence of intranasal cyst in the inferior meatus will need cruciate marsupialization of the cyst along with probing.

> *Difficulty in breathing:* Occurs due to the presence of intranasal cyst; generally during feeding as neonates are nasal breathers. Cyst can be small or large (occupying >50% of the nasal cavity).
> - Bilateral large cyst can be potentially life-threatening.

Congenital Absence of Lacrimal Valves

Absence or defective development of the lacrimal valves may result in few uncommon conditions.
- Absence of the valves in the NLD will cause retrograde passage of air from the nose especially during sneezing or blowing of the nose causing pneumatocele of the lacrimal sac.
- *Absence of valve of Rosenmüller and Hasner:* Retrograde passage of air from nose to the ocular surface resulting in dry eyes and abnormalities of the ocular surface.

Suggested Reading

1. Ali MJ. Disorders of upper lacrimal system. In: Ali MJ (Ed). Principles and Practice of Lacrimal Surgery. Singapore: Springer; 2018. pp. 133-46.
2. Bansal O, Bothra N, Sharma A, Ali MJ. Congenital nasolacrimal duct obstruction update study (CUP study): paper II—profile and outcomes of complex CNLDO and masquerades. Int J Pediatr Otorhinolaryngol. 2020;139:110407.
3. Bansal O, Bothra N, Sharma A, Walvekar P, Ali MJ. Congenital nasolacrimal duct obstruction update study (CUP study): paper I-role and outcomes of Crigler's lacrimal sac compression. Eye (Lond). 2021;35:1600-4.
4. Kamal S, Ali MJ, Gauba V. Congenital nasolacrimal duct obstruction. In: Ali MJ (Ed). Principles and Practice of Lacrimal Surgery. Singapore: Springer; 2018. pp. 147-61.
5. Wladis EJ, Aakalu VK, Yen MT, Bilyk JR, Sobel RK, Mawn LA. Balloon dacryoplasty for congenital nasolacrimal duct obstruction: a report by the American Academy of Ophthalmology. Ophthalmology. 2018;125:1654-7.

1.12 Acquired Lacrimal Disorders

Richa Dharap Wagh, Swati Singh, Nandini Bothra

 1. Management of chronic dacryocystitis OR What are the different types of dacryocystorhinostomy (DCR) surgeries and their advantages and disadvantages? OR Endoscopic lacrimal surgeries or Common causes of severe bleeding during external DCR OR Failed DCR—causes and management.

Long-standing inflammation of the lacrimal sac (LS) in the presence of nasolacrimal duct obstruction (NLDO) causes stasis of tears and accumulation of secretions in the sac that predisposes to bacterial colonization, and leads to chronic dacryocystitis. There is a female preponderance, mostly in the fifth to sixth decades of life. The NLDO can further be divided into primary or secondary depending upon the underlying cause.

Primary acquired nasolacrimal duct obstruction (PANDO)	Idiopathic
Secondary acquired lacrimal drainage obstruction (SALDO)	- Infectious - Traumatic - Mechanical - Neoplastic

Pathophysiology

Numerous factors are believed to contribute to the etiopathogenesis of PANDO. The basic pathogenesis is the long-standing inflammation causing vascular congestion, mucosal edema, which overtime will lead to fibrosis, obstruction, and stasis. Initial theories contemplating the role of anatomical factors such as longer, thinner, irregular, and tortuous nasolacrimal

lacrimal duct in females is more prone for to develop NLDO does not appear to play a significant role. There is no convincing data to substantiate nose as the site of disease origin and nasal factors appear to be comorbidities. Hormonal mechanisms are more evidence-based but can only partly explain the pathogenesis. Studies have shown that in the postmenopausal age group the expressions of estrogen alpha and beta, CYP19, oxytocin, and prolactin in the LS and NLD was more in normal males compared to normal females and it was grossly reduced in patients with PANDO. Thus, lower levels of hormones deprives the local microenvironment from the protective and anti-inflammatory effects of these hormones, lower levels of oxytocin expression in the vessels of the LS and NLD predispose to cavernous body malformation leading to vascular stasis and mucosal edema and lastly, the loss of prolactin causes glandular dysfunctions and loss of immunomodulatory benefits. Vascular theories are based on the behavior of perilacrimal cavernous bodies, their autonomic control, and additional structural changes in the helical patterns of connective tissue fiber arrangements. Repeated vascular malfunction leads to structural epithelial and subepithelial changes leading to the development of NLDOs. Tear proteomics holds a promise in decoding the etiopathogenesis of PANDO, at least in part.

Diagnosis

Diagnosis is usually based on clinical findings. This includes eliciting history of trauma, surgery, sinus disease, and systemic granulomatous diseases. Any history of previous sac swelling associated with inflammatory signs suggestive of acute dacryocystitis should be asked for.

Symptoms usually include epiphora, watery or mucoid or mucopurulent discharge, and swelling over the LS area (mucocoele). Rarely patients may themselves elicit a positive regurgitation test with expression of discharge. Typically, the watering is present for 6 months to 1 year prior to presentation. Presence of a raised tear meniscus height, matted lashes, and sac swelling must raise the suspicion of an underlying NLDO. Eliciting regurgitation on pressure over the lacrimal sac (ROPLAS) is the easiest maneuver to confirm the diagnosis. Regurgitation from opposite punctum with a hard stop on lacrimal drainage system (LDS) irrigation is another common method to diagnose NLDO. Rarely, a patent system on irrigation, with subsequent sac swelling, is suggestive of atonicity of the sac wall to conduct tears down the NLD, and can mimic a mucocele. ROPLAS would be positive in a mucocele, whereas the discharge will drain down the NLD easily on manual pressure in an atonic sac. A thorough examination of the puncta is a must in all cases of epiphora.

Complications of chronic dacryocystitis
- Acute dacryocystitis
- Lacrimal abscess
- Acquired lacrimal fistulas
- *Orbital cellulitis (rare)*
- Cavernous sinus thrombosis

Acute dacryocystitis is defined as "A medical urgency which is clinically characterized by rapid onset of pain, erythema, and swelling, classically below the medial canthal tendon with or without preexisting epiphora mainly resulting from the acute infection of the LS and perisac tissues." This is clinically characterized by tender sac swelling with overlying erythema, with variable amount of lid swelling. The skin may have a pus point suggestive of a lacrimal abscess and an evolving lacrimal fistula.

Imaging in the form of computed tomography (CT) scans—dacryocystogram is usually required in cases where SALDO is suspected. Sudden onset of unilateral epiphora in a younger individual having a history of facial trauma or surgery warrants imaging to rule out any secondary cause.

It is ideal to include nasal endoscopy as a part of preoperative examination, for examining the nasal anatomy, to rule out any granulomas/polyps/gross septal deviations or hypertrophic turbinates that may cause a hindrance to surgery. It is a must in every case of failed DCR to evaluate the ostium in detail to find the cause of failure.

Indications of Treatment

Patient related	• *Severity of symptoms:* Constant epiphora, frequent dabbing • Motivation
Severity of disease	• Partial PANDO/mild cases may not opt for surgical management • *Acute dacryocystitis:* Urgent medical management and definitive surgery in the early course of disease • *Chronic dacryocystitis:* Elective surgery
Other ocular comorbidities	Need for intraocular procedures, e.g., cataract surgery, as a part of microbial keratitis management.

Preoperative Workup

Detailed ocular workup is required, to rule out any coexisting ocular pathologies. A thorough systemic workup including complete blood picture, bleeding time, clotting time, viral screening, and echocardiography in consultation with the physician.

Treatment

Medical Management

It is indicated in case of acute dacryocystitis, to decrease the infective load and to reduce the inflammation prior to surgery. Usually, the acute episode is resolved using broad-spectrum antibiotic course along with anti-inflammatory agents and application of hot fomentation in over 94% of cases. Early endoscopic DCR is curative in such situations to provide alternative channel for pus drainage and is helpful to prevent recurrences.

Surgery

Surgery is the definitive treatment for any case of chronic dacryocystitis. It includes:

- Dacryocystectomy (DCT) is complete surgical extirpation of the LS. Preferred route for the surgery is external. An external incision is used to approach the anterior lacrimal crest, identify and dissect the sac from all sides, avulse it from the LS fossa, separate it from NLD, and excise it.
    Life-long persistent epiphora is the most troublesome side effect of this surgery.
    - *Absolute indications:*
        - LS neoplasm
    - *Relative indications:*
        - Patients awaiting urgent intraocular surgery, e.g., one-eyed, total cataract, therapeutic keratoplasty
        - Older individuals with multiple systemic comorbidities, bleeding diathesis
        - Severe dry eyes like in patients with Stevens–Johnson syndrome
        - Patients with predisposing conditions causing nasal scarring such as cicatricial pemphigoid, systemic lupus erythematosus (SLE), and Crohn's disease
        - Multiple times failed DCR
        - Severe atrophic rhinitis
- *Dacryocystorhinostomy:* It can be done by the external or endonasal endoscopic approach. As the name suggests, it involves creating an anastomosis between the LS and the nasal mucosa via a bony ostium.
    - *External DCR:* This involves using an external skin incision to create an anastomosis between the LS and nasal mucosa. The preferred incision site is along the anterior LS. When the incision is taken along the subciliary plane, the surgery is believed to be more cosmetically appealing but requires a longer learning curve.
    Surgical steps:
        - Incision along the anterior lacrimal crest
        - Orbicularis fibers are separated using tenotomy scissors.
        - The underlying periosteum is exposed and incision taken on the periosteum along the anterior lacrimal crest.
        - Periosteum is reflected till the crest and sac are reflected from the LS fossa.
        - Bony osteotomy is initiated by perforating the thin lacrimal bone.
        - Osteotomy is expanded to allow complete exposure of the LS. The boundaries of the osteotomy—anteriorly till the punch cannot be inserted between the bone and the nasal mucosa, posteriorly till removal of aerated ethmoid, superiorly till 5 mm above the common canaliculus, and inferiorly till the NLD is deroofed.
        - H-shaped nasal mucosal and LS flaps are created.
        - Adjuvants such as 0.02% mitomycin-C (MMC) and bicanalicular intubation can be used at this stage.
        - Mucosal flap anastomosis is performed
        - Orbicularis and skin are closed using sutures.
    - *Endoscopic DCR:* Endoscopic DCR gained popularity in the last 2 to 3 decades with the advent of rigid fiber-optic endoscopes. The endonasal endoscopic DCR avoids an external incision, preserves the medial canthal tendon, prevents injury to terminal branch of facial nerve, and prevents a full-thickness ring contracture over the osteotomy site, which may lead to lacrimal pump failure despite anatomical patency.
    Success rates comparable to that of external DCR (>95%) has been shown in recent studies indicating better understanding of nasal anatomy and endoscope and mucosal handling.

Various types of endoscopic endonasal surgeries are:
- *Primary endonasal endoscopic surgery:*
  - Can be done under local or general anesthesia
  - Nasal cavity is decongested with nasal packs soaked in 2% xylocaine with 1:200,000 adrenaline.
  - Posterior based nasal flap 10 mm superior and 10 mm anterior to the axilla of the middle turbinate is made and reflected.
  - Bony osteotomy is initiated using bone rongeur at the inferior most point on the maxillary line—at the junction of the sac and NLD.
  - Osteotomy is then enlarged to expose the sac completely. Powered instruments such as drills may be used in this step to complete the osteotomy and obtain adequate exposure. Boundaries of the osteotomy endoscopically are superoanteriorly, the orbicularis oculi muscle is exposed, superoposteriorly the Agger nasi cell is entered to ensure complete exposure of the fundus and posteriorly a limited anterior ethmoidectomy may be needed depending on the exposure of the sac.
  - LS flaps are then fashioned and reflected posteriorly and anteriorly.
  - Adjuvants such as 0.02% MMC and bicanalicular intubation are performed.
  - Nasal and lacrimal flap anastomosis is established and can be secured with glue or sutures.
- *Ultrasonic endoscopic DCR:*
  - Ultrasonic DCR was introduced by Krasnov in 1971.
  - This technique uses piezoelectric or ultrasonic waves in the range of 20–30 kHz to cut mineralized tissues, sparing the soft tissues.
  - The principle is that alternate current is used to cause vibrations, contractions, and expansion of piezoelectric element or quartz particles, which cause microvibrations which causes inserts to vibrate linearly between 60 and 210 µm. The piezo element thus generates ultrasonic vibrations transmitted to the tips causing bone fragmentation by acoustic and jackhammer effects.
  - The technique is essentially similar to primary endonasal endoscopic DCR except that the osteotomy is performed using the piezoelectric probe (Synthes piezoelectric system).
  - A diamond cutting tip at a flow rate of 30 mL/min with D2 program and power of 5 is used initially to begin osteotomy at the inferior end of maxillary line. A trench is created by placing the tip perpendicular to the bone and moving in brush-stroke fashion. The entire bone is emulsified till NLD is visible. Osteotomy is then enlarged to expose the entire sac.
  - The procedure is then completed as described above.
- *Primary endocanalicular laser DCR:*
  - In 1992, the technique of DCR using laser was described by Levin and Silkiss in cadavers and was performed for the first time using argon laser by Christenbury.
  - Success rates with this technique have been consistently low and are reported between 47% and 97% in various studies.
  - A laser fiber-optic is inserted in the punctum and passed through canaliculus into the LS. A nasal endoscope is used to visualize the glow from the nasal side. Then, laser fiber-optic is utilized to puncture onto the nasal cavity, creating an osteotomy. The bone, LS, and nasal mucosa in front of the common canaliculus and around it are ablated and an opening is created. There are no flaps created in this technique.
  - The surgical success will depend on proper patient selection, through preoperative nasal endoscopy, appropriate laser machine, and good technique.

Advantages and disadvantages:

	External DCR	**Endoscopic DCR**
Advantages	• Ideal for any patient having contraindication to general anesthesia • Lacrimal sac anatomy better delineated, allows easier biopsy of mass lesions • Preferred in cases of traumatic SALDO with abnormal bony anatomy • Short learning curve • Cheaper instrumentation	• No cutaneous scar • Better visualization of nasal anatomy • Simultaneous correction of nasal abnormalities, e.g., large septal deviations or hypertrophied middle turbinate obstructing the lacrimal sac opening, etc. • Lesser postoperative recovery time • Can be performed in acute setting • Lesser time for surgery • Good approach for addressing ostium in case of failed DCRs

Contd...

Contd...

	External DCR	*Endoscopic DCR*
Disadvantages	• Cutaneous scar • Damage to facial nerve branch and orbicularis weakness • More chances of bleeding • No visualization of nasal details	• Steep learning curve • Damage to nasal mucosa and synechiae formation • Orbital fat prolapse (rare) • Damage to medial rectus (rare) • Expensive instrumentation

Other variations include nonendoscopic endonasal (NEN) DCR and balloon-assisted DCR.

Complications of DCR surgery: Intraoperative complications include bleeding, inappropriate incision placement, inadvertent trauma to the LS or the nasal mucosa, cerebrospinal fluid (CSF) leak, opening the ethmoid or maxillary sinus, fat prolapse, breach of the periorbita, inadvertent anastomosis between the ethmoid and sac mucosa, incomplete opening up of the sac, damage to the common canalicular opening, inadvertent trauma to the septum, middle turbinate, and punctal cheese wiring during fixing of the stent.

Bleeding: It is the most common complication and one must be aware of its causes and further management. Causes (in order of encounter in external DCR) include the following:

- *Angular vein:* It passes 6–8 mm from the medial canthal tendon. Any variation in anatomy, or incorrect incision placement can lead to injury to the angular vein and torrential bleeding. Accurately identifying the vessel and cauterizing or ligating it is required in order to proceed.
- *Muscular branches:* Vessels within the orbicularis can sometimes cause a continuous ooze and may need to be cauterized. This usually happens due to decreased orbicularis tone or increased pulse pressure.
- *Bone bleeding:* Sutura notha or the false suture actually houses a branch of the infraorbital artery, the nutrient artery, which can bleed. It is more common in osteoporotic bones. Fulguration of the site is ideal. If that fails to prevent it, proceeding further using a suction cannula to perform osteotomy and crush the bone (and the artery in it) is another measure that can be taken.
- *Nasal mucosa:* It is another common cause of bleeding, and best prevented. The bleeding can occur while performing the osteotomy where there is inadvertent damage to the nasal mucosa, or due to uncontrolled intraoperative blood pressure, where the mucosa bleeds on touch with the most minimal handling.

A good preoperative nasal packing consisting of anesthetic and vasoconstrictors, and a slight head-up position during surgery are useful to prevent and counter the nasal bleeding.

- *Ethmoid mucosa:* The anatomic position of the ethmoid sinus in relation to the sac varies greatly, and can sometimes be encountered during DCR surgery. This mucosa is thinner and more friable, and bleeds very easily. Using a cottonoid pledget over the mucosa, while proceeding with the surgery is helpful.
- *Miscellaneous factors:* Systemic diseases such as uncontrolled or labile hypertension, use of antiplatelet drugs or anticoagulants, preexisting coagulopathy. A thorough workup of the systemic comorbidities and medications used for the same, blood pressure evaluation, and a basic screening for coagulopathies is mandatory prior to DCR surgery.

The general principles to achieve hemostasis during DCR surgery include appropriate preoperative assessment of systemic conditions, using vasoconstrictors such as adrenaline or oxymetazoline cottonoids along with local anesthetics when not contraindicated, adequate nasal decongestion, keeping a head-up table position, avoiding known blood vessels, well-powered suction, use of cautery when appropriate, keeping materials such as gelfoam or bone wax handy. Intravenous agents such as tranexamic acid should be kept handy in case of uncontrolled bleeding. Another useful tip is to sit 45° toward the site of surgery to get maximum visualization.

Postoperative complications:

Early (1–4 weeks)	*Intermediate (1–3 months)*	*Late (>3 months)*
Epistaxis	Stent displacement	Webbed facial scar
Wound infection	Intranasal synechiae	Ostial fibrosis
Wound dehiscence	Ostium granulomas	Medial canthal distortion
Ostium crusting	Prominent facial scar	Failed DCR
Stent prolapse	Nonfunctional DCR	Sump syndrome
Lagophthalmos		

Failed DCR: Evidence of persistent/recurrent epiphora with or without discharge, with nonpatency of the ostium after DCR surgery is defined as failed DCR. Failure is more likely to occur in cases of congenital NLDO or traumatic SALDO.

Causes: The most common causes of failure include inadequate osteotomy, incomplete sac marsupialization, and cicatricial closure of the ostium. Other uncommon causes scarred common canaliculus, obstructed distal canaliculi, organizing granulomas, intervening ethmoids, sump syndrome, turbinoseptal synechiae, and internal ostium stenosis. Rare causes include occult carcinoma, bony obstruction related to Paget's disease, or granulomatous inflammations. Intraoperative factors leading to failures can be related to incorrect localization of the sac, inappropriate osteotomy, inadequate sac opening leading to sump syndrome, prolapse of orbital fat, prolonged operative time, active inflammation, significant septal deviations, and concha bullosa.

Time to failure is usually during the early-intermediate postoperative period, with a mean of 4.9 months, usually related to obstruction proximal to the internal common opening (ICO). Rarely, an asymptomatic individual can have recurrence of symptoms after more than 12 months after surgery, and these are usually associated with a common canalicular obstruction.

Diagnosis: Presence of raised tear meniscus, positive ROPLAS test, and regurgitation on irrigation of lacrimal passage are indicative of an unfavorable outcome. Nasal endoscopy is done to examine the area and dimensions of the ostium, the ICO and its dynamicity, eliciting the fluorescein endoscopic dye test (FEDT) to check for the time taken for dye to egress internally, to look for presence of any granulomas, synechiae, ostial stenosis, or ostium cicatrization.

Revision surgery is based on the following principles:
- A thorough understanding of intranasal endoscopic anatomy including the location and extent of the LS
- An efficient bone removal to expose LS completely
- A complete incision and marsupialization of the LS mucosa
- Complete excision of the cicatrix
- Use of circumostial MMC, stents, and balloon as and when indicated

Surgery can be done using an external or an endoscopic approach. The success rates are usually lower as compared to primary surgeries, especially in cases of cicatrization.

Summary

Chronic dacryocystitis is one of the most common lacrimal disorders that is seen in clinical practice. Having adequate knowledge about the entity, diagnosis, and its treatment is imperative for a satisfactory outcome. It is important to address the primary complaint of the patient. Certain patients who are mainly concerned about their vision owing to a dense cataract, are referred to the oculoplasty service for the incidentally detected PANDO. In such situations, performing a DCT reduces their recovery time and their time to cataract surgery, with a minor concern of postoperative epiphora; whereas a patient who may or may not have cataract, but has visited the clinic with the primary complaint of watering is unlikely to be benefit with DCT, and DCR is an appropriate intervention to address his chief complaint.

2. What are the etiological factors for canaliculitis? Describe the clinical features and management.

Canaliculitis is the inflammation of the lacrimal canaliculus. It can be primary or secondary to an identifiable precedent cause. Canaliculitis is often misdiagnosed as chronic conjunctivitis and treated improperly.

Etiologies

- Infection (bacterial, viral, and fungal)
- As a complication of punctal plug insertion or migration
- Secondary to intubation.

Although commonly the involved pathogen is bacteria, there are few reports of herpes simplex virus DNA detection in concretions on electron microscopy studies.

Epidemiology

Lacrimal canaliculitis usually affects middle-aged adults and has female preponderance (5:1, female:male ratio). There are no significant racial or ethnic variations.

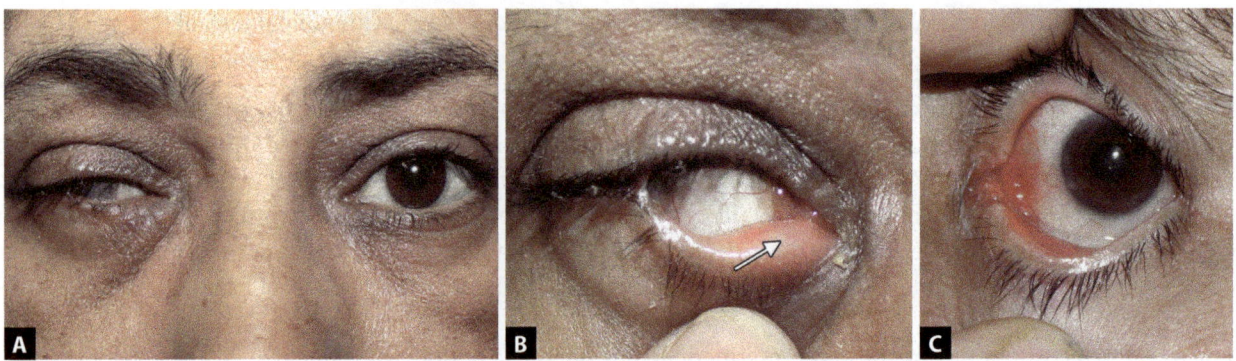

Figs. 1A to C: Shows the classic presenting signs of canaliculitis-Medial lower lid swelling, discharge, pouting puncta and non-resolving conjunctivitis.

Clinical Features

The classic presenting symptoms are epiphora, medial canthal swelling, swollen, pouting punctum, with or without mucopurulent discharge, and nonresolving or recurrent conjunctivitis **(Figs. 1A to C)**. The conjunctival inflammation is more prominent in medial bulbar and palpebral conjunctiva. The concretions can be expressed by applying pressure over the medial canthal/canalicular swelling, which are diagnostic of canaliculitis. These concretions are made of bacterial aggregates along with debris.

A careful routine slit-lamp examination of the upper and lower eyelids and medial canthus clinches the diagnosis. The misdiagnosis often results in inappropriate treatment with broad-spectrum topical antibiotics as for a conjunctivitis case, which may transiently improve the symptoms, but without providing a lasting cure. Hence, clinical examination is crucial for making the diagnosis. The lacrimal system is usually patent to irrigation, which helps in differentiating it from dacryocystitis.

Investigations

Samples taken from the punctal discharge, concretions recovered via massage or curettage are sent for microbiological evaluation. *Actinomyces israelii* is the most common pathogen seen in concretions. It characteristically appears as branching gram-positive filaments. Recent publications report greater rates of infection with streptococcal, and staphylococcal species than *Actinomyces*. Almost 21% of reported cases fail to show any microorganism.

The concretions are mostly yellow, cheese-like granules with a gritty consistency, considered the pathologic hallmark of *A. canaliculitis*. Histopathology reveals the sulfur granules to be basophilic masses originating from aggregated gram-positive filamentous bacteria with peripheral club-like eosinophilic structures. Other commonly reported organism is streptococci species.

Employed imaging techniques in canaliculitis are macrodacryocystography, high-resolution ultrasound, and dacryoendoscopy. These are usually not necessary to make diagnosis but have been reported in literature. An X-ray due to their amorphous nature does not pick concretions. Ultrasound might show reflective structures such as sulfur granules measuring 12 mm in diameter, which are pathognomonic for canaliculitis. The negative cultures, refractory to antibiotics, and resolution following stent removal suggest secondary canaliculitis due to an immune reaction to the stent.

Management

Conservative management with warm compresses, digital massage, and topical and systemic antibiotics fails to achieve complete cure. The thick granular debris formed within the canaliculus may prevent the antibiotics to penetrate and act. Simple curettage alone or incision and curettage achieves clinical cure in 80–90% patients. Dilation of the punctum allows enough space to insert curette and express all the concretions.

Canaliculotomy offers greater access and easier curettage of canalicular contents. There is debate whether canaliculotomy should be performed or not due to the fear of loss of lacrimal pump, canalicular scarring, and fistula formation. However, long-term follow-up revealed no persistent epiphora in eyes postcanaliculotomy (Anand et al.). One should not do forceful irrigation since mucosa is inflamed so chances of bleeding and injury are increased. Also, it can push the concretions more distally. Irrigation should be performed after curettage with antibiotic solution.

Recurrence

The recurrent canaliculitis, due to trapped residual concretions, are seen in up to 21–26% cases. Canaliculostomy can effectively manage the recurrences. Recently, intracanalicular antibiotic injections or irrigation with fortified antibiotics such as cefazolin has been tried as a treatment modality. Usually a mean number of four injections are required for achieving complete cure and surgical intervention can be avoided. The choice of antibiotic depends on the antibiotic sensitivity results.

3. Discuss the management of canalicular obstruction.

Canalicular obstructions can be anatomically divided into proximal, mid, and distal obstructions. This classification not only helps in the diagnosis but also with the management. The etiology and management of each subtype is as follows:

- Proximal canalicular obstructions typically occur within the first 4 mm of the canaliculi. The different causes are punctal stenosis, drug induced, cicatrizing surface disorders, idiopathic, infectious, canalicular inflammatory disorders, post-trauma, and postpunctal cauterization. These obstructions are difficult to manage. The existing treatment options are:
    - *Conjunctivo-DCR with a Lester Jones tube:* This is the classical way of managing proximal bicanalicular obstruction, provided the medial canthal anatomy is not grossly distorted. The basic principle of this surgical procedure is to bypass the canalicular obstruction in a way to allow a direct communication of the inferomedial conjunctival fornix with that of the nasal cavity. This is achieved using either the Pyrex Lester Jones tubes or the modified Gladstone-Putterman tubes **(Fig. 2A)**. The outcomes are satisfactory. Most complications are related to either tube migration or tube loss.
    - *Lacrimal gland-based therapies:*
        - Botulinum toxin injection into the lacrimal gland
        - Needling of lacrimal gland
        - Debulking of the orbital lobe of the lacrimal gland

    Lacrimal gland-based modalities are used as a primary option in refractory proximal bicanalicular obstructions or in cases where conjunctivo-DCR failed, or if the patient prefers a minimally invasive option **(Fig. 2B)**. Only symptomatic epiphora affecting one's daily activities is advised for surgical options. The most common amongst these therapies is the use of intraglandular botulinum toxin-A (BTX-A), which is usually injected transconjunctivally, directly into the lacrimal gland. The usual dose is 2.5 U/0.1 mL. It is important to monitor the patient for complication of BTX-A–like ptosis or strabismus.

- Mid-canalicular obstructions are those which are encountered between 4 and 8 mm from the punctal opening. These are often are secondary to viral infections, mismanaged or unmanaged canalicular trauma, infective or noninfective canaliculitis, or medications. These fair slightly better than proximal obstructions in surgical outcomes. Management options are:
    - *Canalicular trephination and intubation:* This is the most common approach in mid canalicular obstructions. The trephines commonly used are the Sisler trephines. These trephines are accompanied by stylets, and are specifically designed for the human lacrimal canaliculus. Following a successful recanalization, it is mandatory to place a silicone stent. The choice of stent depends on whether the trephination was performed for a single canaliculus or

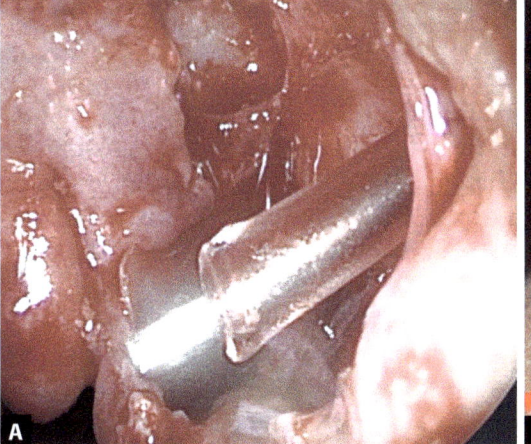 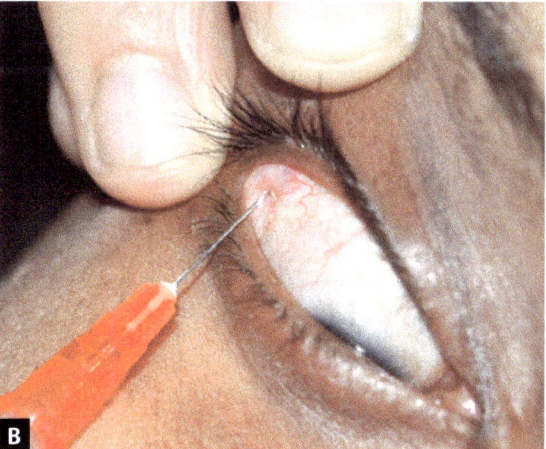

Figs. 2A and B: (A) Shows in conjunctivo-DCR direct communication of the infero-medial conjunctival fornix is established with the nasal cavity using the Pyrex Lester-Jones tubes; (B) shows Botulinum toxin being injected into the lacrimal gland with 29G needle in refractory proximal bicanalicular obstruction.

both canaliculi. Single canalicular trephination can be followed by a mini-monoka stent, monoka-Crawford stent, or a Masterka stent. The duration of stent retention is anywhere between 4 and 6 weeks.
- *Canaliculoplasty using dacryoendoscopy-guided microdrill:* The advent of dacryoendoscopy allows the surgeon to visualize the obstruction directly and under direct guidance either a trephine or a microdrill can be used to overcome the obstruction followed by intubation as discussed earlier.
- Refractory mid canalicular obstructions can be managed as for bicanalicular proximal canalicular obstructions.

Distal obstructions, more so the ones near the common canaliculus, are often mucosal folds (valve of Rosenmüller or canalicular-LS mucosal folds) where the common canaliculus opens into the LS. Besides, LS infections, trauma or iatrogenic injury may result in distal canalicular obstruction. Distal obstructions occur beyond 8 mm from the punctum. These have the best prognosis of all canalicular obstructions. The existing surgical options are:
- *Canalicular trephination and intubation:* The principles of canalicular trephination and intubation remain the same as for mid-canalicular obstructions, but care has to be taken to avoid additional damage to the ICO of the canaliculus into the LS.
- Canalicular trephination and DCR

In some of the cases, following a canalicular trephination, the surgeon can identify the status of the NLD. In the event of a coexisting NLD obstruction, the canalicular trephination is combined with an external or an endoscopic DCR. The principles of intubation remain the same as for those trephinations without a DCR surgery.

 4. Write a short note on dacryocystography.

Dacryocystography (DCG) refers to the radiological technique of imaging LDS. First DCG was performed in 1909 using bismuth subnitrate, and since then it has undergone progressive refinements in terms of contrast media, acquisition time, resolution, and radiation exposure. The conventional plain DCG (CDCG) or digitally subtracted DCG (DS-DCG) uses X-rays for capturing the lacrimal system after filling it with contrast media. CT-DCG is the term used when DCG is performed using CT scanning. It provides information about the surrounding bony structures. The information on the dynamic tear flow can be obtained by CT-DCG or magnetic resonance-DCG (MR-DCG).

The primary purpose of DCG is to localize the LDS and study the pathologies and their locations. It has also been utilized for evaluating the dynamic changes in canaliculus and LS in various physiological states, and for the demonstration of valves in the lacrimal system.

Indications

- Complex lacrimal disorders such as secondary acquired NLDO and syndromic CNLDO
- Suspected lacrimal diverticula
- Tumors of LDS
- Partial NLDO
- Unexplained epiphora
- Navigation-assisted lacrimal surgeries.

Types of Dacryocystography and Contrast Media

Conventional and Digitally Subtracted Dacryocystography

Currently DS-DCG remains the standard examination technique for the assessment of obstructions of the LDS. DS-DCG produces bone-free images of LDS, mainly performed to locate the site of common canaliculus obstruction. It has been utilized for localizing the site of obstruction in patients with epiphora, differentiating canalicular from proximal sac obstructions, and to visualize the stenotic segments. However, proximal LDS is better visualized with dacryoendoscopy.

The radiation dose exposure received during DS-DCG (mean 0.68 mSv) was found to be much less as compared to the CDCG (mean 1.53 mSv).

The available contrast media for CDCG, DS-DCG, and CT-DCG include oil-soluble (like lipiodol) and water-soluble media (such as iohexol, iopamidol, sinografin). The image quality is better with oil-soluble media like lipoidal; however, media with high iodine content like iohexol, iopamidol 300 fair closely to oil-soluble media. Disadvantages of oil-soluble media are its viscous nature, immiscible with tears, and the rare chances of a granuloma formation following accidental extravasation. The contrast can be used as a drop or cannulation method. The iodine-containing media are currently used more commonly. The average dimensions of normal LS are 2.4 mm in lateral diameter and 4.0 mm in anteroposterior diameter.

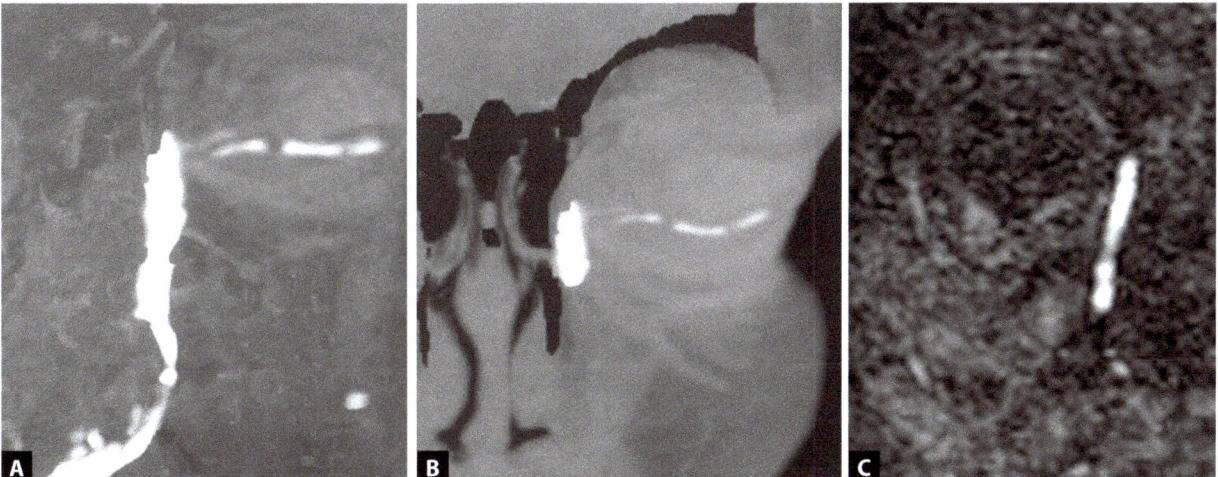

Figs. 3A to C: (A and B) Shows CT-DCG documentation of adjacent bony and soft tissues structures; (C) shows Tear flow assessment using real time MR-DCG in normal individuals.

The lacrimal system can be normal in 54% (85/158) of symptomatic patients and among the abnormal DCGs (73/158), NLD stenosis or obstruction is the most common (56%, 41/73) finding, followed by common canalicular obstruction (CCO) (37%, 27/73) and LS stenosis (7%, 5/73). Interestingly, there are discrepancies between lacrimal irrigation and DCG findings in 36% patients (obstructed LDS on irrigation but patent on DCG). A direct comparison between fluorescein dye disappearance test (FDDT), Jones test, dacryoscintigraphy (DSG), and DS-DCG revealed imaging to have no decisive role in the diagnosis of partial NLDO or functional epiphora.

Computed tomographic-dacryocystography: CT-DCG allows for documentation of adjacent bony and soft tissues structures apart from the LDS **(Figs. 3A and B)**. The role of CT-DCG lies in complex orbitofacial trauma and lacrimal drainage tumors. First CT-DCG was performed in 1990 almost 81 years after the first DCG. CT-DCG involves use of contrast media (lipiodol, iohexol, omnipaque) either in drop form or injection via inferior (or superior) canaliculus followed by imaging. The topical method involves instillation of iodinated contrast medium every minute for 5 minutes or 3 times at 0, 5, and 10 minutes. The 3D helical CT-DCG introduced in 2002, revealed a better agreement between CT-DCG and irrigation findings in the partial and complete lacrimal obstructions. However, the agreement was poor in freely patent systems. While operating with navigation assistance in complex facial trauma, 3D CT-DCG guidance helps in dacryolocalization in secondary acquired lacrimal duct obstructions. Another modification, cone beam CT-DCG (CBCT-DCG) can be performed in sitting position and uses limited field of view with 0.5 mm slices at 0.5-mm intervals providing clearer images.

Magnetic resonance DCG: The first MR-DCG was performed in 1993 using 0.5% gadolinium (1:100 dilution) contrast media. The main advantages of MR-DCG are ability to provide functional and morphological aspects of lacrimal pathways without any radiation exposure, and capturing the series of images in real time. However, the high cost, longer acquisition time, and motion artifacts are the limitations of this technique. MR-DCG is performed using 1, 1.5, or 3-T MR scanners. Images are enhanced by fat suppression and dedicated surface coils. Both cannulation and topical method can be used. MR-DCG has the advantage of determining the timing of contrast clearance across lacrimal system. Gadolinium, a paramagnetic substance, is used as contrast media and no adverse effects have been reported so far. Normal saline alone or in combination with 0.5% lidocaine can also be used.

Topical drops are instilled every minute for 5 minutes or one drop every 3 minutes for 15–20 minutes. Dynamic MR-DCG allows for the capture of passage of contrast media across the LDS; oblique coronal and sagittal plane represent the whole LDS in one image. Tear flow was assessed using real-time MR-DCG in normal individuals **(Fig. 3C)**. The mean transit time for contrast to appear in LS was 15.2 seconds (9.4–66 seconds), 50.4 seconds for NLD (18.9–151), and 150.5 seconds for inferior meatus (37.8–490). Its exploration in diseased system would help in differentiating lacrimal pump failure from stenosis and true obstruction.

 5. Describe the techniques for repair of a canalicular injury.

Any laceration medial to the punctum should be assumed to involve the canaliculus until proven otherwise **(Fig. 4A)**. The most commonly injured structure in lacrimal trauma is lacrimal canaliculi (lower, upper, and bicanalicular) followed by

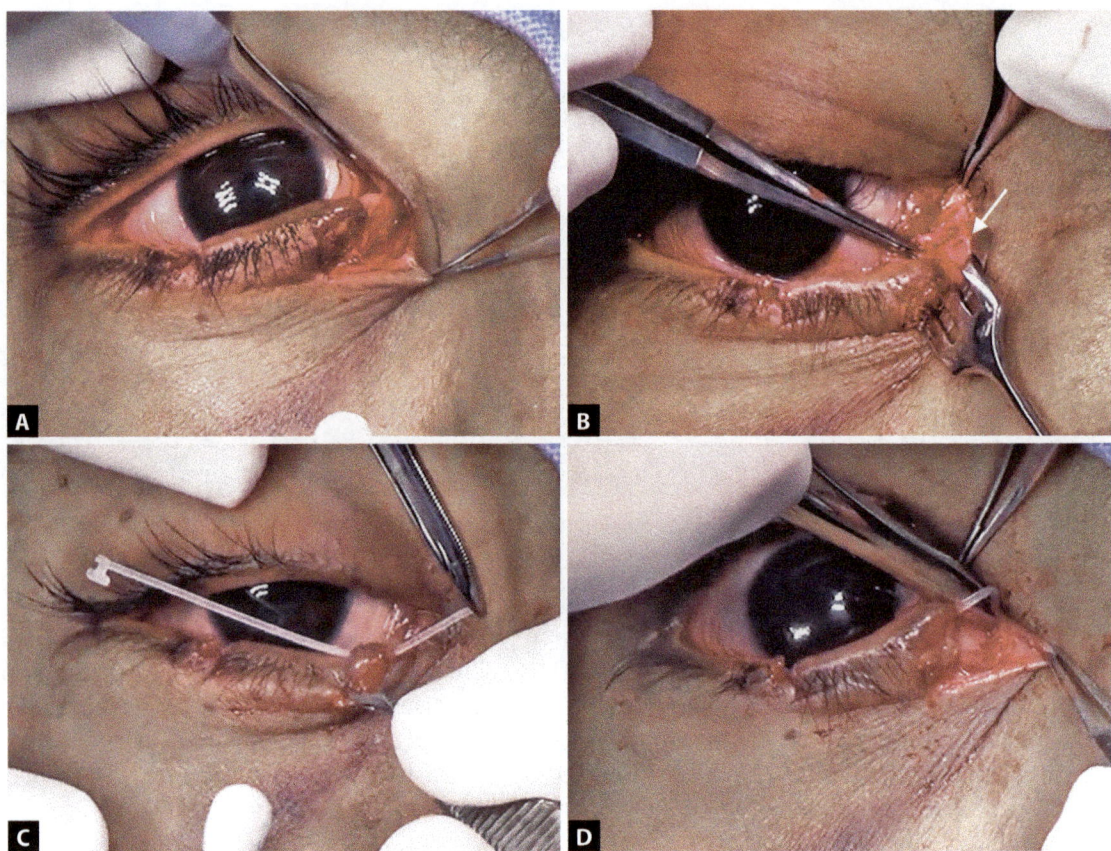

Figs. 4A to D: (A) Any laceration medial to the punctum should be assumed to involve the canaliculus until proven otherwise; (B) Canalicular mucosa appears smooth, whitish elevated structure at the cut- calamari ring sign; (C and D) Once confirmed, monocanalicular stent (Mini-Monoka) is being introduced with nontraumatic forceps.

NLD, LS/naso-orbit-ethmoid (NOE) fractures. One should attempt to repair canaliculus irrespective of whether lower or upper is involved.

The surgical steps are listed here.
- Surgery can be performed under general or local anesthesia depending upon the age, extent of injury, and associated orbital trauma. Repair should be performed using an operating microscope for easy identification of lacerated end.
- Thorough wound toileting is performed with 5% betadine followed by syringing via opposite uninvolved canaliculi to check for patency of the lacrimal system. The medial end of the canaliculus retracts posteriorly and inward (toward the posterior lacrimal crest).
- The cut end of the canaliculus can be identified via many ways: (1) Canalicular mucosa appears smooth, whitish elevated structure at the cut end typically resembling the ring of a "calamari" and hence known as calamari sign **(Fig. 4B)**; (2) Using pigtail probe passed through the uninvolved canaliculus; (3) Use of air or fluorescein stained viscoelastic or methylene blue as an irrigation solution; and (4) Use of endoilluminator light pipe for examining the deeper tissues at higher magnification.
- After identifying cut ends, punctum is dilated and probe is passed through identified medial cut end of canaliculus to confirm hard stop. Syringing can be done through the medial cut end of canaliculus to confirm the lacrimal patency. Once confirmed, monocanalicular stent (Mini-Monoka/Aurostent/20G silicone rod) **(Figs. 4C and D)** is introduced with nontraumatic forceps. Bicanalicular stent can be used if both canaliculi are involved. The intubation is inspected for proper fitting of the stent. The cut ends of the canaliculus are then sutured together over the stent.
- Pericanalicular tissue is approximated with 6-0 Vicryl in horizontal mattress manner. There have been reports of successful repair with direct suturing of the canalicular mucosa. Medial canthal tendon is repaired thereafter with 5-0 prolene followed by orbicularis and skin closure using 6-0 Vicryl or 5-0 silk.

Postoperative Care

Postoperatively, topical antibiotics and lubricants are administered for 1–2 weeks. Stent is removed at 6 weeks or 3 months. Lacrimal irrigation is performed thereafter, which indicates anatomical success. Functional success is documented with negative FDDT and epiphora resolution.

Variations in Repair Technique

Traditionally, pigtail probe is used for identifying the canaliculus and bicanalicular intubation is performed. The risk of injury to the uninvolved canaliculus is high with intubating or manipulating the uninvolved canaliculus especially in inexperienced hands. The timing of stent removal varies in different series, and is influenced by the material and the type of fixation used, and surgeon's preference. There are successful reports with an early removal at 6 weeks as well as late removal at 15 weeks.

Complications

The stent-related complications are:
- Premature stent loss
- Stent migration
- Granuloma formation.

The reported rates vary from 0% to 29% premature stent loss and 14% cases of stent migration. The chances are more with pediatric patients.

Suggested Reading

1. Alam MS, Poonam NS, Mukherjee B. Outcomes of canaliculotomy in recalcitrant canaliculitis. Saudi J Ophthalmol. 2019;33(1):46-51.
2. Ali MJ, Naik MN, Honavar SG. External dacryocystorhinostomy: tips and tricks. Oman J Ophthalmol. 2012;5(3):191.
3. Ali MJ. Primary external dacryocystorhinostomy. In: Principles and Practice of Lacrimal Surgery. Singapore: Springer; 2018. pp. 189-95.
4. Anand S, Hollingworth K, Kumar V, Sandramouli S. Canaliculitis: the incidence of long-term epiphora following canaliculotomy. Orbit. 2004;23:19-26.
5. Dave TV, Mohammed FA, Ali MJ, Naik MN. Etiologic analysis of 100 anatomically failed dacryocystorhinostomies. Clin Ophthalmol (Auckland, NZ). 2016;10:1419.
6. Freedman JR, Markert MS, Cohen AJ. Primary and secondary lacrimal canaliculitis: a review of literature. Surv Ophthalmol. 2011;56(4):336-47.
7. Guzek JP, Ching AS, Hoang TA, Dure-Smith P, Llaurado JG, Yau DC, et al. Clinical and radiologic lacrimal testing in patients with epiphora. Ophthalmology. 1997;104(11):1875-81.
8. Kamal S, Ali MJ. Primary acquired nasolacrimal duct obstruction (PANDO) and secondary acquired lacrimal duct obstructions (SALDO). In: Principles and Practice of Lacrimal Surgery. Singapore: Springer; 2018. pp. 163-71.
9. Li E, Yuen H, Ali MJ. Revising a failed dacryocystorhinostomy. In: Principles and Practice of Lacrimal Surgery. Singapore: Springer; 2018. pp. 271-83.
10. Liarakos VS, Boboridis KG, Mavrikakis E, Mavrikakis I. Management of canalicular obstructions. Curr Opin Ophthalmol. 2009;20(5):395-400.
11. Litwin A, Malhotra R. The great debate: external versus endonasal dacryocystorhinostomy. In: Principles and Practice of Lacrimal Surgery. Singapore: Springer; 2018. pp. 477-85.
12. Naik MN, Kelapure A, Rath S, Honavar SG. Management of canalicular lacerations: epidemiological aspects and experience with Mini-Monoka monocanalicular stent. Am J Ophthalmol. 2008;145(2):375-80.
13. Reifler DM. Management of canalicular laceration. Surv Ophthalmol. 1991;36(2):113-32.
14. Singh S, Ali MJ, Paulsen F. A review on use of botulinum toxin for intractable lacrimal drainage disorders. Int Ophthalmol. 2018;38(5):2233-8.
15. Singh S, Ali MJ, Paulsen F. Dacryocystography: from theory to current practice. Ann Anat. 2019;224:33-40.
16. Singh S, Dhull A, Selva D, Ali MJ. Tear transit time evaluation using real-time technique for dynamic MR dacryocystography. Orbit. 2021;40:34-8.
17. Singh S, Ganguly A, Hardas A, Tripathy D, Rath S. Canalicular lacerations: factors predicting outcome at a tertiary eye care centre. Orbit. 2017;36(1):13-8.
18. Singh S, Nair AG, Alam MS, Mukherjee B. Outcomes of lacrimal gland injection of botulinum toxin in functional versus nonfunctional epiphora. Oman J Ophthalmol. 2019;12(2):104-7.
19. Wladis EJ, Aakalu VK, Tao JP, Sobel RK, Freitag SK, Foster JA, et al. Monocanalicular stents in eyelid lacerations: a report by the American Academy of Ophthalmology. Ophthalmology. 2019;126(9):1324-9.
20. Yip CC. Management of distal common canalicular obstruction: internal or external approach? Asia Pac J Ophthalmol (Phila). 2013;2(2):73-5.

1.13 Evaluation of Epiphora

Nandini Bothra

1. Explain clinical evaluation in a case of epiphora.

Watering from eye can be due to multiple reasons. But it is important to distinguish between epiphora and pseudoepiphora/hyperlacrimation.

True Epiphora

True epiphora is secondary to lacrimal drainage system obstruction. Obstruction can be anatomical or functional. Anatomical obstruction refers to physical block in the lacrimal drainage system pathway, e.g., punctal effacement, canalicular obstructions, and nasolacrimal duct obstructions. Functional obstruction, by definition, is epiphora without a detectable lacrimal drainage system obstruction. It implies an anatomically patent lacrimal passage with a physiological dysfunction. Different reasons have been cited in the literature, including partial obstruction of nasolacrimal duct, which is patent upon positive-pressure irrigation through the canaliculus, lacrimal pump failure due to eyelid laxity, conjunctivochalasis, megalocaruncle, or caruncular edema occluding the puncta, punctal as well as medial eyelid ectropion preventing punctal apposition to the lacrimal lake and causes like facial palsy.

Hyperlacrimation

Hyperlacrimation is excessive watering to the reflex irritation of the corneal and conjunctival surfaces. Causes of hyperlacrimation include:
- *Supranuclear etiologies:* Emotional distress, central nervous system disorders
- *Infranuclear etiologies:* Aberrant regeneration, cerebellopontine angle tumors
- *Reflex lacrimation:* Keratoconjunctivitis, tear film abnormality, corneal foreign body
- *Direct lacrimal gland stimulation:* Inflammation, tumor

Evaluation of epiphora has to done under following headings:
- *History:*
  - It is important to elicit the history with regards to onset, frequency, discharge, pain, swelling, intermittency, laterality of the symptoms, trauma, previous interventions, etc. These can give a clue to the underlying condition.
  - Onset of watering from a birth or a few days after birth may point toward a congenital nasolacrimal duct obstruction.
  - Continuous epiphora from the eye associated with discharge may point toward obstruction in the lacrimal drainage system. Only epiphora may point to proximal lacrimal drainage system obstruction whereas that associated with discharge may point to distal lacrimal drainage system obstruction.
  - Pain and swelling in the lacrimal sac area associated with history of epiphora may point to acute dacryocystitis or a lacrimal abscess.
  - An infant with a bluish swelling in the lacrimal sac area points to a dacryocele, which needs immediate intervention. Associated history of difficulty in feeding, difficult respiration with stertor points to an intranasal cyst with dacryocele. This warrants immediate treatment.
  - Intermittent epiphora associated with upper respiratory tract infection may be secondary to nasal mucosal edema and may be observed.
  - History of trauma to the eye and adnexa followed by epiphora may indicate to an underlying naso-orbito-ethmoid fracture or direct damage to lacrimal drainage apparatus.
  - History of previous interventions to the nose or sinuses associated with epiphora can indicate a traumatic nasolacrimal duct obstruction.
  - History of previous lacrimal intervention will help planning further interventions.

  Thus, eliciting correct history helps in narrowing the possible diagnosis.
- *Local examination:*
  - Inspection of the eye and adnexa will give important clues to the underlying condition. Look at the face and ocular adnexa—symmetry of the face, gross malformations on the face and eyelid, orbital or nasal malformations, eyelid position (entropion, ectropion, lagophthalmos, and retraction), misdirected eyelashes, punctal position (punctal ectropion, puncta away from the ocular surface), swelling and redness in the lacrimal sac area, associated facial palsy, and proptosis of the globe.

- Palpation of the eye and adnexa—eyelid laxity and lacrimal pump function (eyelid lateral distraction test and eyelid snap test), palpation of the swelling in the lacrimal sac area (mucocele, lacrimal sac mass), and ROPLAS (regurgitation on pressure over the lacrimal sac).
- ROPLAS is an important sign which will give a clue to the underlying obstruction. It is important to elicit ROPLAS in the lacrimal sac area, i.e., just beyond the anterior lacrimal crest toward the nose and directed inferomedially. The interpretation can be as follows:

ROPLAS	Possible interpretation
Mucoid, mucopurulent, purulent, or watery discharge regurgitation on pressure	Distal lacrimal drainage system obstruction
Bloody discharge	Dacryolith or lacrimal sac malignancy or rhinosporidiosis
No discharge from punctum but contents emptying into the nose and mouth	Atonic sac
No regurgitation and no reduction in size of the lacrimal sac swelling	Encysted mucocele or lacrimal sac mass

- Slit-lamp evaluation of the eyelids (presence of blepharitis or meibomitis, position of eyelids with respect to the ocular surface), eyelashes (misdirected or not), punctum (punctal position and opening—normal, stenosed, edematous or effaced, presence and absence of membranes, punctal pouting, and discharge), peripunctal area (edema, telangiectatic vessels), caruncular edema and position with respect to the puncta, and ocular surface (corneal or conjunctival foreign bodies, lack of luster of the surface, conjunctival papillae, corneal defects, and erosions).

- *Clinical evaluation:* The tests for clinical evaluation can be secretary or excretory tests which aid in determining the anatomical site of obstruction that can influence the mode of management. The excretory tests check for the anatomical patency and functioning of the lacrimal outflow pathway, while the secretory tests check for causes that can be incite reflex hypersecretion.
  - *Lacrimal irrigation:* This is by far the most important test for lacrimal drainage system assessment which when performed correctly can give us the important interpretations.
    - *Instrumentation:* 1 cc syringe, 26G straight lacrimal cannula, distilled water.
    - *Technique:* Instill topical anesthetic eyedrops (2% proparacaine eyedrops). Patient is in reclining position and should be comfortable. Upper punctum is generally preferred for the procedure as it is believed to be in direct communication with lacrimal sac and prevents injury to the lower lacrimal drainage pathways which is believed to drain more fluid as compared to the upper lacrimal drainage pathway. Pull the upper eyelid up and lateral such that the lacrimal canaliculus is at a stretch and is partly straightened. Punctal dilatation with Nettleship's punctal dilator can be done directing the dilator perpendicular to the punctal opening till the ampulla (approximately 2 mm) and then directing it horizontal and parallel to the lid margin so as to follow the canalicular anatomy slowly rotating the dilator. Now gently insert the 1 cc syringe mounted lacrimal cannula in the same fashion as the dilator.
    - If canalicular stenosis is encountered, small amount of fluid is injected to dilate the canaliculus as we advance the cannula through the canaliculus. Once the insertion is complete, small amount of fluid is gently injected and the interpretation is as follows:
    - *Interpretation:*

Finding	Interpretation
Soft stop (also note the movement of the eyelid with the attempted advancement of the cannula), clear regurgitation from the same puncta	Individual canalicular obstruction
Soft stop (also note the movement of the eyelid with the attempted advancement of the cannula), clear regurgitation from the same puncta	Common canalicular obstruction
Hard stop (hits the bone in the lacrimal sac fossa) with clear, mucoid, or mucopurulent regurgitation from opposite puncta	Nasolacrimal duct obstruction
Hard stop with clear, mucoid, or mucopurulent regurgitation from same puncta	Nasolacrimal duct obstruction with canalicular obstruction of the opposite pathway
Hard stop with no regurgitation but sac swelling (Note: on pressing the dilated lacrimal sac, the contents empty into the nasal cavity with minimal spillage into the cul-de-sac)	Atonic lacrimal sac
Hard stop with partial regurgitation of clear or mucoid fluid from opposite punctum	Partial nasolacrimal duct obstruction

- *Diagnostic probing:* This is generally done to confirm the site of upper lacrimal drainage pathway obstruction. The technique is similar to lacrimal irrigation. After dilatation of the puncta with Nettleship's punctal dilator, a Bowman's lacrimal probe is advanced into the lacrimal canaliculus in a similar fashion as the irrigation lacrimal cannula.
  - *Interpretation:* Soft stop or hard stop
  - *Soft stop:* Spongy feel against the probe anywhere along the canaliculus. Note the movement of the medial canthus and the eyelid when advancement of the probe is attempted beyond the site of obstruction. The site of obstruction can be measured by measuring the length of probe within the canaliculus and the obstruction classified as proximal (2–4 mm), mid (4–6 mm), and distal (>6 mm). The management of canalicular obstruction will depend on above classification.
  - *False soft stop:* The eyelid traction laterally during probing will stretch the canalicular pathway making it straight and removing kinks. Sometimes a kink at the junction of the sac and common canaliculus will give rise to a false soft stop by pushing the roof of the common canaliculus against the lateral wall of the sac.
  - *Hard stop:* Indicates the probe has crossed the common canaliculus and is now in the lacrimal sac. This implies that the upper lacrimal drainage pathway does not have any obstruction.
- *Fluorescein dye disappearance test (FDDT):* This is a physiological noninvasive test with high specificity (94.8%) and high positive predictive value (93.5%). This test is particularly useful in children where other invasive procedures are not possible. This test is a good screening tool for epiphora but does not distinguish between anatomical and functional obstructions. Further, it does not give information on the site of obstruction. Positive test (dye retention) then needs further procedures such as irrigation and diagnostic probing to confirm the obstruction.
  - *Technique:* A drop of 2% fluorescein is placed in the conjunctival cul-de-sac without instilling topical anesthetic drops. Patient is asked to blink normally without rubbing or dabbing the eye. Residual fluorescein should be looked for using cobalt blue filter at the end of 5 minutes. Normally, all the fluorescein should drain into the nose at the end of 5 minutes, any retention points to a possible obstruction of the lacrimal drainage system.
  - *Grades:* Using the slit lamp and cobalt blue filter, the height of the stained tear film can be measured. Grading is done from grade 0 to grade 4. Grade 0–1 is when there is no or a very thin stained tear film strip. This indicates a negative test. Grade 2–3 indicates a positive test with retention of fluorescein-stained tear film strip.
  - *False negative test:* In cases of large mucocele or lacrimal sac diverticula, the dye may pool within the sac giving a false negative result.
  - *Variation: Fluorescein endoscopic dye test (FEDT):* This test is used to assess the anatomical and functional outcomes post-dacryocystorhinostomy (DCR) surgery using the endoscopes. 2% fluorescein is placed in conjunctival cul-de-sac and the patient is asked to blink normally. The passage of dye into the DCR ostium is noted. Visualization of dye in the nose indicates anatomical and functional success of the procedure.
- *Jones dye test:* This test is almost obsolete as the above-mentioned three tests are usually enough to diagnose the cause of epiphora. Also, high number of false positive and false negative results limit the utility of this test.
  - *Technique:* Instill 2% fluorescein dye in the conjunctival cul-de-sac. Patient is asked to blink normally and not rub the eyes. A cotton-tipped applicator coated with local anesthetic is placed in the nasal cavity.
  - *Interpretation:*
    - *Jones 1 test:* At the end of 5 minutes, the dye is expected to reach the nasal cavity and hence stain the cotton-tipped applicator. If case of no staining (negative test) indicates nonspecific drainage abnormality and Jones 2 test is performed.
    - *Jones 2 test:* The cul-de-sac is cleared of any residual fluorescein dye. Then using 1 mL syringe mounted with lacrimal cannula, irrigation is done through the canalicular system at increased physiologic pressures. The cotton-tipped applicator is placed in the nasal cavity.

Finding	Interpretation
No irrigant is retrieved	Anatomical obstruction of the lacrimal drainage pathway
Irrigant without fluorescein staining of the cotton-tipped applicator	Functional obstruction of the proximal lacrimal drainage system
Irrigant with fluorescein staining of the cotton-tipped applicator	Functional obstruction of distal lacrimal drainage system allowing pooling of the dye in the lacrimal sac (e.g., atonic sac)

- *Dacryocystography (DCG):* This is a radiological test to assess the lacrimal drainage system.
  - *Technique—Drop method and cannulation technique:* Drop method is physiological, and mostly done in patients uncooperative for irrigation and in children. In the cannulation technique, the contrast dye is injected within

the lacrimal drainage system. Contrast dye (lipiodol, omnipaque, or gadobutrol) 1 mL is injected in the lacrimal drainage system. As the dye is being injected, serial scans [X-ray/computed tomography (CT) scan/magnetic resonance imaging (MRI) scans] are taken.
- When X-rays are used, it is called DS-DCG (digital subtraction dacryocystography). This was first described by Galloway et al. in 1984. Images are captured every second till about 10 seconds. Images are acquired in anteroposterior, oblique and frontal projections, and off-lateral views for better delineation. This helps to distinguish between presacchal and postsacchal stenosis, diagnose lacrimal sac diverticula, dacryoliths, lacrimal drainage system obstructions and can also be used for postoperative analysis of DCR ostium.
- *CT-DCG:* It gives better delineation of the bony structures around the lacrimal system along with some soft tissue study. It was first described in 2002. Serial axial and coronal images (2 mm cuts) of the lacrimal area are acquired. *Absolute contraindications:* Pregnancy and iodine allergy. *Relative contraindication:* Children and uncooperative patients. This is mainly helpful is delineating bony abnormalities causing epiphora and planning the management in such cases along with the sac abnormalities as mentioned above.
- *MR-DCG:* It was first described by Goldberg et al. in 1993. It offers superior soft tissue delineation and can differentiate lacrimal system fluid signals from surrounding tissues. Dye used is 0.5% gadolinium meglumine. Higher image acquisition time, no bony details, and it being an expensive procedure limit its use in routine practice. However, it offers advantages such as high tissue contrast, imaging in any obliquity as desired, and nonionizing radiation.
- *Dacryoscintigraphy (DSG):* This technique of radionucleotide evaluation of lacrimal system was first described by Rossomondo et al. in 1972. This is a physiological test and is useful for assessing flow dynamics.
  - *Technique:* 10 μL of technetium 99m pertechnetate is instilled in the conjunctival cul-de-sac. Patients are instructed to blink normally and not to rub the eyes. The passage of dye is traced through the lacrimal system using a pinhole-collimated gamma camera. Images are acquired in real time for up to 30 minutes. End point of image acquisition is detection of the dye in the nasal cavity (usually about 10–20 minutes).
  - *Interpretation:* The time taken and quantity of dye in the areas of interest can be plotted on the time-activity scale. In case of obstruction, the slope would be flat on the time-activity scale.
  - *Disadvantages:* Poor anatomical details, poor resolution, and variable transit times throughout the lacrimal system.
- *Nasal endoscopy:* It is important to assess nasal pathologies (deviated nasal septum, turbinate hypertrophy) which can be a reason for epiphora and have a bearing on the surgical management. Certain granulomatous infections and tumors of the nasal cavity can cause obstruction of the nasolacrimal duct and can be diagnosed only with nasal endoscopy. It is very important for evaluation of cases with failed DCR.
- *Secretory tests:* These are done to rule out any reflex cause of watering and to look for any evidence of dry eyes. It includes tests such as Schirmer's test, tear film break-up time, and rose Bengal staining of the ocular surface.

Suggested Reading

1. Das S. Evaluation of epiphora. In: Ali MJ (Ed). Principles and Practice of Lacrimal Surgery. Singapore: Springer; 2018. pp. 69-82.
2. Gokhale SM. Dacryoscintigraphy: a pictorial essay. Indian J Nucl Med. 2018;33:214-7.
3. Karlin JN, Mustak H, Gupta A, Ramos R, Rootman DB. Cone beam computerized tomography dacryocystography (CBCT DCG) for the evaluation of lacrimal drainage system dysfunction. Ophthalmic Plast Reconstr Surg. 2020;36:549-52.
4. Mandeville JT, Woog JJ. Obstruction of the lacrimal drainage system. Curr Opin Ophthalmol. 2002;13:303-9.
5. Paramanathan N, Nemet A, Lee SE, Benger RS. A modified Jones test: lacrimal scintigram correlation. Ophthalmic Plast Reconstr Surg. 2011;27:81-6.
6. Singh S, Ali MJ, Paulsen F. Dacryocystography: from theory to current practice. Ann Anat. 2019;224:33-40.

1.14 Tumors of the Eyelids

Vijitha S Vempuluru, Shruthi Gunda, Anasua G Kapoor

1. Benign eyelid tumors—classification. Write a note on the clinical features, differential diagnosis, management, and histopathology of common benign eyelid tumors.

Tumors of the eyelid can be classified based on the origin or by nature, i.e., benign or malignant **(Figs. 1 and 2) (Tables 1 and 2)**.

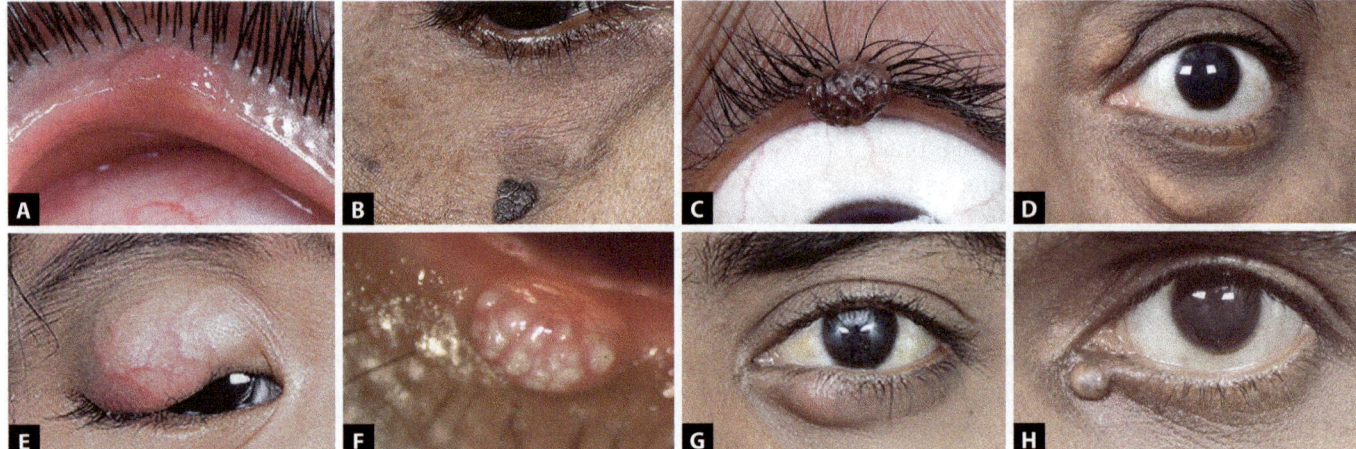

Figs. 1A to H: Common benign eyelid lesions: (A) Squamous papilloma of the upper lid, (B) seborrheic keratosis over lower lid, (C) upper eyelid nevus, (D) xanthelasma over upper lid and lower lid, (E) capillary hemangioma of upper lid in a child, (F) molluscum contagiosum of lower lid magnified view, (G) lower lid chalazion, and (H) epidermoid cyst of lower lid near medial canthus.

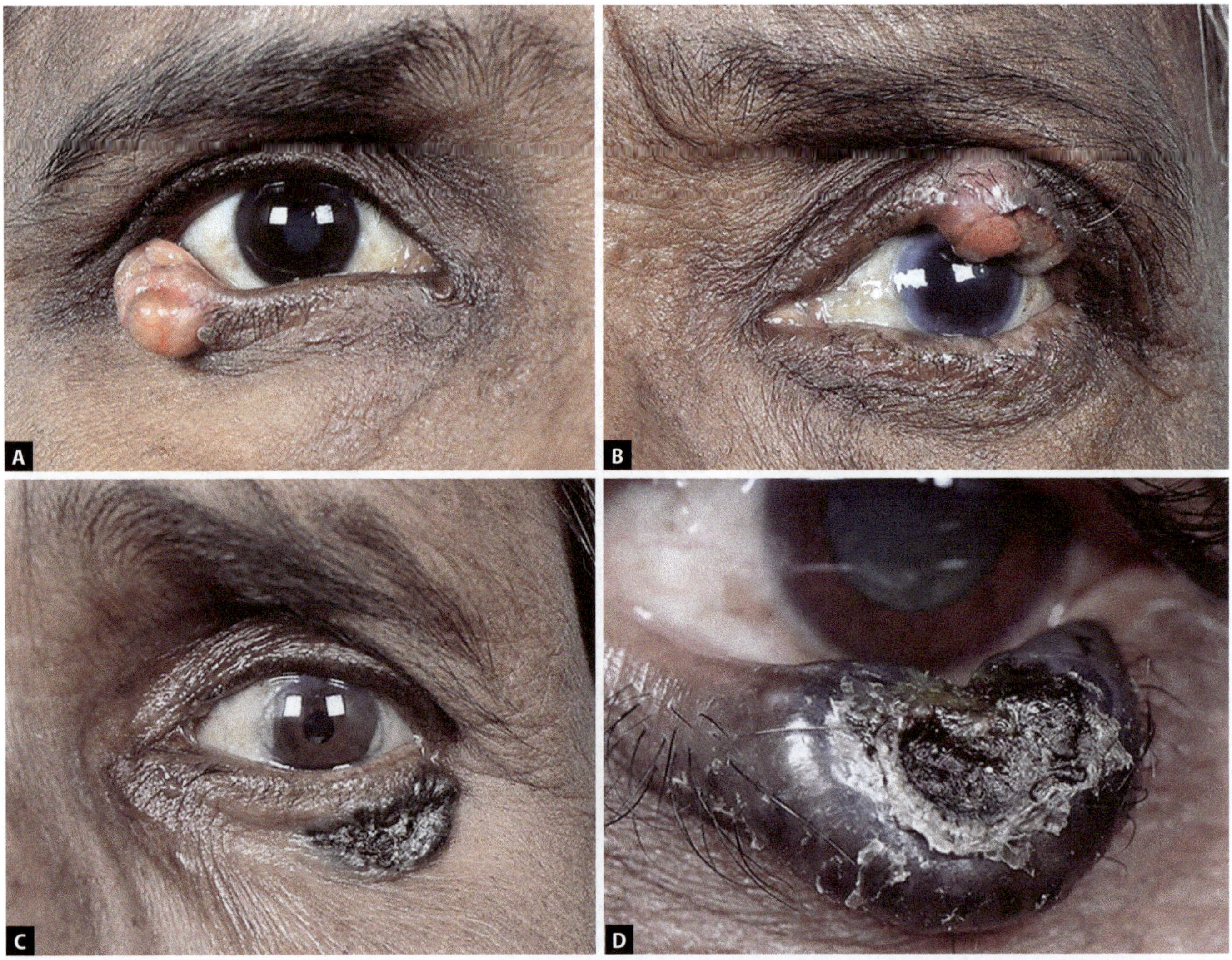

Figs. 2A to D: Common malignant eyelid tumors: (A) Sebaceous gland carcinoma of lower lid lateral canthus, (B) squamous cell carcinoma of upper lid, (C) basal cell carcinoma noduloulcerative form, pigmented variant of lower lid near lateral canthus, and (D) malignant melanoma of lower lid.

TABLE 1: List of benign and malignant eyelid tumors with tissue of origin.

Origin	Benign	Premalignant	Malignant
Epidermal	• Squamous papilloma* • Seborrheic keratosis* • Pseudoepitheliomatous hyperplasia • Keratoacanthoma	• Actinic keratosis • Sebaceous nevus (of Jadassohn)	• Basal cell carcinoma* • Squamous cell carcinoma*
Sebaceous glands	• Sebaceous hyperplasia • Sebaceous adenoma	–	Sebaceous carcinoma*
Sweat glands	• Syringoma* • Eccrine acrospiroma* • Syringocystadenoma papilliferum • Pleomorphic adenoma	–	Sweat gland adenocarcinoma
Hair follicle	• Trichoepithelioma • Trichofolliculoma • Trichilemmoma • Pilomatrixoma*	–	–
Melanocytic	• Nevus* • Nevus of Ota* • Blue nevus	• Congenital dysplastic nevus • Lentigo maligna	Melanoma
Neural	• Neurofibroma • Neurilemmoma (Schwannoma) • Neurothekeoma	–	Merkel cell carcinoma
Vascular	• Congenital capillary hemangioma* • Acquired hemangioma • Nevus flammeus* • Varix • Lymphangioma* • Glomus tumor	–	• Kaposi's sarcoma • Angiosarcoma
Fibrous/fibrous histiocytic	• Xanthelasma* • Xanthoma • Xanthogranuloma • Necrobiotic xanthogranuloma • Angiofibroma • Nodular fasciitis • Juvenile fibromatosis • Fibrous histiocytoma	–	Fibrosarcoma
Smooth and skeletal muscles	• Leiomyoma • Rhabdomyoma	–	• Leiomyosarcoma • Rhabdomyosarcoma
Fat	Lipoma	–	Liposarcoma
Hamartomas, choristoma, and others	Myxoma	–	
Lymphoid, plasmacytic	–	–	• Lymphoma • Plasmacytoma
Metastatic	–	–	Primary from breast*, lung, cutaneous melanoma, and stomach

Tumor-like conditions

Cysts • Eccrine hidrocystoma • Apocrine hidrocystoma • Sebaceous (pilar) cyst • Epidermoid cyst • Dermoid cyst	*Infections* • Molluscum contagiosum* • Fungal infections • Chronic bacterial infection	*Granulomatous diseases* • Sarcoidosis • Granulomatosis polyangiitis • Pseudorheumatoid nodule	*Inflammations/miscellaneous conditions* • Chalazion* • Amyloidosis* • Lipoid proteinosis

*Common.

TABLE 2: Common benign eyelid tumors: Clinical features, differential diagnosis, management, and histopathology.

Diagnosis	Clinical features	Differential diagnosis	Management	HPE
Squamous papilloma	Wart-like fleshy lesion arising from the epidermis	Basal cell carcinoma, seborrheic keratosis, and sessile lesions can simulate melanocytic nevus	Observation or excisional biopsy for cosmetic concerns. Other options: CO_2 laser, argon laser, photodynamic therapy, topical imiquimod	Connective tissue comprising fibrovascular cores covered by acanthotic epithelium
Melanocytic nevus	• *Congenital:* Present at birth *Acquired:* Apparent in childhood and evolves through stages of junctional nevus, compound nevus, and dermal nevus • Well-defined cutaneous lesions with variable pigmentation. Periocular cutaneous nevi can also involve mucocutaneous junction and conjunctiva. "Kissing nevus" involves both the eyelids	Pigmented basal cell carcinoma	• Observation or excisional biopsy for cosmetic concerns • Depending on the lamellar involvement of the eyelid, surgical options include shave excision or lamellar to full-thickness resection with reconstruction	• *Stages of nevus: Junctional:* Nests of nevus cells in the basal layers • *Compound:* Comprises junctional and intradermal components • *Intradermal:* Within the dermis
Seborrheic keratosis (basal cell papilloma, seborrheic wart)	• Usually solitary, can be multiple. The sudden appearance of multiple lesions: Sign of Leser-Trelat seen in visceral malignancies • Elevated hyperpigmented plaques to dome-shaped lesions with rough surfaces and fissures	Pigmented basal cell carcinoma, melanocytic nevus, melanoma	Observation or excisional biopsy (shave biopsy/excision with primary closure) for cosmetic concerns. Smaller lesions can be treated with liquid nitrogen or curettage	Benign proliferation of basal cells with hyperkeratosis, acanthosis, papillomatosis, and intraepithelial keratin deposits (horn cysts/pseudohorn cysts)
Sebaceous/pilar cyst	Focal nodular lesion, underneath the skin. Often possess a central comedo plug	Epidermal inclusion cyst	Observation or complete excisional biopsy for cosmetic concerns of when large enough to cause mass effect	Cystic lesion with epithelium lacking intercellular bridges
Epidermal inclusion/epidermoid cyst	Freely mobile, soft subcutaneous lesion. Ruptured cysts can have associated inflammation	Other cystic lesions such as sebaceous cyst, rarely dermoid cyst	Excisional biopsy	Lined by keratinizing epithelium and contain keratin
Dermoid cyst	A smooth subcutaneous cystic lesion, usually around suture lines and may be tethered to the underlying bone	Subcutaneous cystic lesions	Excisional biopsy	Lined by stratified squamous epithelium. Wall also contained adnexal structures such as glandular elements
Pilomatrixoma (pilomatricoma, calcifying epithelioma of Malherbe)	Subcutaneous nodule with a bluish hue, usually located below the eyebrow	Subcutaneous cystic lesions	Excisional biopsy	Proliferating basaloid cells, shadow cells, and the presence of calcification

(HPE: histopathologic examination)

 2. Discuss capillary hemangioma of the eyelid.

Nomenclature

Capillary hemangiomas of the eyelid can be congenital or acquired.

Congenital capillary hemangioma = strawberry hemangioma, infantile hemangioma, benign hemangioendothelioma, strawberry nevus

Acquired hemangioma = cherry hemangioma, senile hemangioma

Congenital Capillary Hemangioma

Etiopathogenesis

- Benign vascular tumor present at birth or develops in the first few weeks of life
- Can be superficial, deep, or combined.
- *Associations with hemangiomatosis can exist:* Kasabach–Merritt syndrome, posterior fossa anomalies, hemangioma, arterial anomalies, cardiac anomalies, and eye anomalies (PHACE) syndrome.

Clinical Features

- *Superficial:* Well-defined reddish skin lesion involving the eyelid or periocular area.
- *Deep:* Located within the subcutaneous tissue, appears bluish, and can cause proptosis if orbital extension is present.
- Both superficial and deep can coexist and have a similar course: progressive increase in size (up to 3-6 months), stabilizes (12–18 months), and involutes (90% by 7 years of age) spontaneously.
- Eyelid lesions can cause mechanical ptosis and induce astigmatism or obscure visual axis, both of which can cause amblyopia.

Differential diagnosis: Diagnosis of superficial lesions is straightforward. Differentials of deep lesions include other pediatric orbital tumors.

Histopathology: Capillary lobules are seen separated by fibrous septa. The endothelial cells lining the capillaries are abundant in proliferating phase and reduce in number as the lesions involutes.

Management: Visual acuity and refraction should be assessed and closely monitored during follow-up visits.
Obscuration of the visual axis and induced astigmatism threatening vision are indications for treatment.

- *Medical management:*
  - Oral/topical propranolol
  - Intralesional corticosteroids
- *Minimally invasive:*
  - Intralesional steroids, propranolol
- *Surgical management:* Rarely indicated for eyelid lesions. Considered in well-defined deeper eyelid lesions with rapid progression.

Acquired Capillary Hemangioma

- Common in middle-aged adults
- Can be single or multiple
- Seen as a dome-shaped red mass, usually small in size, and often unnoticed.
- Increase in size may be noted in pregnancy.
- Usually observed; treatment is rarely indicated in large lesions with cosmetic concern or suspicion of malignancy.
- Excision biopsy is preferred.

 3. List the various malignant eyelid tumors. Elaborate on clinical features and management of squamous cell carcinoma (SCC), sebaceous gland carcinoma (SGC), and basal cell carcinoma (BCC).

- Primary eyelid malignancies can arise epidermis, glands within the eyelid, connective tissues, or lymphocytes.
- Common eyelid malignancies include SGC, BCC, and SCC.
- Less common tumors are malignant melanoma, Merkel cell carcinoma, and malignant sweat gland tumors.
- Sebaceous carcinoma is the most common eyelid malignancy in the Asian and Asian-Indian populations, whereas in Caucasians, BCC is the most common eyelid tumor **(Table 3)**.

Management of eyelid malignancies depends on the type, size, and extent in terms of anterior or posterior lamellar involvement, orbital extension, and presence of locoregional or systemic metastasis.

TABLE 3: Clinical features of common eyelid malignancies.

Clinical features	SGC	BCC	SCC
Age	60–70 years	50–80 years	Elderly
Gender	Female > male	No predilection	Males > females
Risk factors	• Irradiation • Acne	Sun exposure, increased age, immunosuppression, light skin, arsenic exposure, irradiation, immune suppression	Fair skin, sun exposure, immune suppression, albinism
Syndromic associations/systemic disease	–	• Xeroderma pigmentosum Gorlin–Goltz syndrome (Nevoid basal cell carcinoma syndrome) • Sebaceous nevus of Jadassohn	Xeroderma pigmentosum
Clinical features	Can be a discrete lesion of diffuse thickening of the tarsus *Associated features:* • Loss of lashes • Thickening of lid margin with loss of normal contour • Ulceration • Adjacent conjunctival involvement	• Usually a pearly waxy nodule • *Associated features:* Ulceration, telangiectasia, pigmentation, loss of lashes • *Most common location:* Medial canthus > lower eyelid > upper eyelid > lateral canthus • *Types:* Nodular, noduloulcerative, cystic, morpheaform, superficial	• *Keratotic lesion:* Plaque or nodule • *Associated features:* Ulceration, telangiectasia, loss of lashes, pigmentation
Differential diagnosis	• Chalazion • Blepharoconjunctivitis • Squamous cell carcinoma • Merkel cell carcinoma	Keratoacanthoma, melanoma, seborrheic keratosis	• *Malignant:* BCC, SGC, Merkel cell carcinoma • *Benign:* Actinic keratosis, seborrheic keratosis, inverted follicular keratosis, pseudoepitheliomatous hyperplasia, keratoacanthoma
Propensity to spread	Pagetoid spread, when present, can involve the entire ocular surface and orbit, rarely the cranium	*Locally invasive:* Can involve the orbit, nasolacrimal system, and brain	Aggressive lesions can invade orbit. Also, show neurotropism
Lymph node involvement	More common than SCC and BCC (16%)	Uncommon	Can be present (2–24%): Preauricular, submandibular, and anterior cervical nodes may be involved
Systemic metastasis and sites	More common than SCC and BCC (13%)	Uncommon	Uncommon

(BCC: basal cell carcinoma; SCC: squamous cell carcinoma; SGC: sebaceous gland carcinoma)

Assessment of Local Invasion

- Thorough clinical examination including the extent of lamellar involvement in the eyelids, entire ocular surface, limits of the lesion, and possible extension to orbit.
- Computed tomography scan of the orbits with or without brain is indicated in lesions where posterior extension is not made out.

Assessment of Locoregional Metastasis

- Clinical examination/ultrasound examination to look for regional lymphadenopathy
- Fine needle aspiration cytology or biopsy of suspicious lymph nodes.

Assessment of Systemic Spread

Complete systemic assessment by whole-body positron emission tomography is indicated for all SGC and SCC with orbital/lymph node involvement.

Surgical Aspects of Management

Excisional Biopsy Principles

- All malignant lesions of the eyelid are excised with a 4 mm margin of normal tissue.
- Complete resection can be confirmed by evaluation of the margins, which can be done by standard histopathology, frozen sections, or Mohs micrographic surgery.
- Obtaining negative margins is crucial to prevent recurrences.
- The residual eyelid defect can be reconstructed adhering to principles of eyelid reconstruction.
- In cases of advanced tumors with orbital invasion, exenteration may be needed.

Other Considerations

- Involvement of regional lymph nodes warrants surgical excision with irradiation.
- Neoadjuvant chemotherapy has a role in extensive SGC/SCC not amenable to surgical resection.
- Small/multiple BCC can be treated with topical imiquimod/vismodegib.
- Follow-up after treatment is essential to detect early recurrences/metastatic disease.

4. Give a differential diagnosis for a painless nodular progressively increasing swelling of the lower lid in a 60-year-old male. Describe in detail the management of a BCC 5 mm in diameter, located in the center of the lower lid margin.

Or

A 60-year-old patient presents with noduloulcerative lesion involving central lower lid. Discuss differential diagnosis, evaluation, and management of such a case.

Differentials of a progressive nodular lesion in an elderly patient **(Table 4)**:
- *BCC:* Pearly nodule with rolled out edges, may be pigmented
- *SCC:* Ulceroproliferative nodular lesion with keratin

TABLE 4: Differential diagnosis of painless lower eyelid nodules with their characteristic clinical features.

Diagnosis	Clinical features
Chalazion	• Well-circumscribed round to ovoid lesion within the tarsus or overlying the same and fixed to it • Usually painless and nontender unless inflamed or accompanied by secondary infection • Associated meibomitis may be present • Does not show a progressive increase in size
Eyelid cyst	• Well-defined lesion • Epitarsal cysts may be adherent to tarsus • Do not show rapid growth
Benign eyelid tumors (refer **Table 1**)	• Well-circumscribed lesions • Signs of eyelid malignancy are usually absent
Malignant eyelid tumors	One or more signs of eyelid malignancy are usually seen: • Ulceration • Bleeding • Telangiectasia • Loss of lashes • Distorted eyelid margin architecture • Obliteration of meibomian orifices • Orbital extension • Regional lymphadenopathy

- *Malignant melanoma:* Usually pigmented nodule with variegated pigmentation and irregular borders
- *SGC:* Noduloulcerative lesion arising from the tarsus.

Management of Basal Cell Carcinoma (5 mm, Lower Eyelid)

Clinical Assessment

- Lamellar involvement in breadth and height is to be assessed.
  - If only anterior lamella is involved, differential excision sparing the tarsus may be feasible ensuring that the base is free after excision.
  - In case of bilamellar involvement, full-thickness excision with 4 mm margins should be performed.
- Surgical resection is to be combined with frozen section of margins or Moh's micrographic surgery.
- If either Moh's or frozen section cannot be performed, the eyelid defect can be temporarily closed to avoid corneal exposure and reconstruction can be taken up once histopathology of margins is found to be clear.
- In cases where the posterior extent of the lesions is not palpable, a computed tomography scan is mandatory.

Factors Involved in the Planning of Reconstruction of the Defect

- Width of the defect with respect to the width of the eyelid, i.e., half or one third to full length
- Uni- or bilamellar tissue loss
- Laxity of eyelids
- With a 5 mm tumor in the lower eyelid, the residual defect after margin clearance is likely to be one third to half.
- Reconstruction options include the following:
  - Anterior lamella: Undermining of adjacent skin, Tenzel semicircular flap, or skin graft
  - Posterior lamella: Hughes tarsoconjunctival flap or free tarsal graft
  - Combination of flap + flap or flap + graft can be used for either lamella but graft over graft should be avoided.

 5. Discuss the differential diagnosis and management of a growth on the lateral aspect of eyelids.

- Differential diagnosis includes benign lesions such as a dermoid cyst, epithelial inclusion cyst, or sebaceous cyst and malignant lesions such as BCC, SCC, SGC, and melanoma.
- A benign lesion can be excised in toto while a malignant lesion would require additional margin clearance.
- Systemic workup is essential in all malignant tumors.

Reconstruction principles remain the same for either (refer Question 4).
- *Defect in the lateral aspect of the upper or lower eyelids:*
  - Combination of Tenzel semicircular flaps and lateral periosteal flap or free tarsal graft
- *Defect lateral to lateral canthus:*
  - Direct closure with mobilization or skin graft
- *Defect involving lateral canthus:*
  - Attempt should be made to form a lateral canthal angle.
  - Combination of the lateral periosteal flap, McGregor's flap, or Mustarde's flap for very large defects may be chosen.

 6. A 65-year-old Asian-Indian lady presents with progressively increasing upper lid mass (15 × 10 × 10 mm). Discuss differential diagnosis and management.

Common differential diagnoses of a noduloulcerative lesion in the upper eyelid include malignancies such as:
- Sebaceous carcinoma
- SCC
- BCC.
  Clinical features that aid in distinguishing these tumors are described in **Table 3**.

Other uncommon eyelid lesions that can present as noduloulcerative lesions include tumors such as malignant melanoma, Merkel cell carcinoma, Kaposi's sarcoma, angiosarcoma, inflammatory lesions such as sarcoidosis, chronic bacterial infection, fungal infection (blastomycosis, mucormycosis, coccidiomycosis), and eyelid amyloidosis.

Management for a Malignant Tumor of the Upper Eyelid

Excisional Biopsy Principles

- All malignant lesions of the eyelid are excised with a 4 mm margin of normal tissue.
- Complete resection can be confirmed by evaluation of the margins which can be done by standard histopathology, frozen sections.
- Obtaining negative margins is crucial to prevent recurrences.
- The residual eyelid defect can be reconstructed adhering to principles of eyelid reconstruction.
- In cases of advanced tumors with orbital invasion, exenteration may be needed.
- Map biopsy is mandatory in all SGCs to rule out pagetoid spread.

Other Considerations

- Involvement of regional lymph nodes warrants surgical excision with irradiation.
- Neoadjuvant chemotherapy has a role in extensive SGC/SCC not amenable to surgical resection.
- Small/multiple BCC can be treated with topical imiquimod/vismodegib.
- Follow-up after treatment is essential to detect early recurrences/metastatic disease.

Factors Involved in the Planning of Reconstruction of the Defect

- Width of the defect with respect to the width of the eyelid, i.e., half or one third to full length
- Uni- or bilamellar tissue loss
- Laxity of eyelids
- A 15 mm tumor in the upper eyelid is likely to cause a near full-length defect and bilamellar loss considering an SGC.
- Reconstruction options include the following:
  - Cutler-Beard procedure:
    - Full-thickness flap from lower eyelid which usually serves as a substitute for both anterior and posterior lamella although it lacks tarsus
    - Patient has to be counseled that lashes lost in the upper eyelid cannot be replaced.
  - Free tarsal graft from contralateral upper eyelid + Fricke's flap/Hemi-Tripier flap
  - Other substitutes for posterior lamella include mucoperiosteum and sclera.

 7. (a) Enumerate malignant tumors of the eyelid (refer **Table 1**). (b) Describe the clinical features and histopathology of sebaceous cell carcinoma (refer **Table 3**). (c) Histopathology of sebaceous gland carcinoma. (d) Outline the management strategy for 20 mm-sized (horizontal) sebaceous cell carcinoma of upper eyelid (refer Question 6).

Histopathology of Sebaceous Gland Carcinoma

- SGC can arise from meibomian glands, glands of Zeis, and caruncular sebaceous glands (rare).
- Tumor cells form lobules and sheets similar to normal sebaceous glands.
- They lack peripheral palisading, with large pleomorphic and hyperchromatic nuclei and abnormal mitoses.
- Cytoplasm is foamy due to the presence of lipid.
- Necrotic areas may be present within the lobules.
- *Pagetoid spread:* A characteristic feature of SGC is to involve even the entire ocular surface epithelium, which can be seen even with small tumors, hence, the importance of a map biopsy.
- Fat stains such as oil red O can demonstrate intracytoplasmic lipid, which must be performed on frozen sections.

- Histopathological factors, which herald poor prognosis include upper eyelid origin, diameter >10 mm, meibomian gland origin, duration >6 months, infiltrative pattern, poor differentiation, extensive pagetoid invasion, and invasion of vessels, lymphatics, and orbital invasion.

Suggested Reading

1. Chaugule SS, Honavar SG, Finger PT. Surgical Ophthalmic Oncology. New York: Springer Open; 2019.
2. Eagle Jr RC. Eye Pathology: An Atlas and Text, 2nd edition. Philadelphia: Wolters Kluwer; 2011.
3. Kaliki S, Bothra N, Bejjanki KM, Nayak A, Ramappa G, Mohamed A, et al. Malignant eyelid tumors in India. A study of 536 Asian Indian patients. Ocul Oncol Pathol. 2019;5(3):210-9.
4. Pe'er J, Singh AD, Damato B. Clinical Ophthalmic Oncology: Eyelid and Conjunctival Tumors, 3rd edition. New York: Springer Nature; 2019.
5. Savar A, Esmaeli B. Management of primary eyelid cancers. In: Esmaeli B (Ed.). Ophthalmic Oncology, MD Anderson Solid Tumor Oncology Series. New York: Springer; 2011.
6. Shields JA, Shields CL. Eyelid, Conjunctival, and Orbital Tumors. An Atlas and Textbook, 3rd edition. Philadelphia: Wolters Kluwer; 2015.

1.15 Orbital Anatomy

Akruti Desai, Anasua G Kapoor

 1. Discuss the functional and surgical anatomy of the orbit along with their development, their various important disorders, and anomalies.

Orbit is a pyramidal-shaped confined space consisting of the eyeball, the extraocular muscles, fat, and a complex of secretory, vascular, and neurological structures anteriorly bound by the eyelids, superiorly by bone and intracranial contents, medially and nasally by bone and sinuses, and laterally largely by bone and temporalis muscle. The superior orbital fissure (SOF) and the optic canal form the apex of this pyramid. The volume of the eyeball is 7 cm^3, while that of the orbit is 30 cm^3.

The medial walls of both orbits are about 2.5 cm apart and measure 4.5–5 cm. It is the thinnest wall of the orbit. Anterior ethmoidal foramen is 24 mm behind the anterior lacrimal crest (ALC) at the level of frontoethmoidal suture. The posterior ethmoidal foramen lies 12 mm behind this, and the optic canal lies 6 mm behind the posterior ethmoidal foramen (24-12-6 rule). The anterior and posterior ethmoidal foramina transmit the anterior and posterior ethmoidal vessels which need to be diligently cauterized during exenteration and even medial wall orbital decompression surgeries. The lateral wall is the strongest wall of the orbit and is at 45° angle to medial wall **(Fig. 1)**. The lateral wall is separated from floor by inferior orbital fissure (IOF) and from the roof by SOF. The IOF lies about 2.5–3 cm posterior to inferior orbital rim. The infraorbital canal is part of the floor and at 2.5 cm from orbital rim forms infraorbital sulcus. The infraorbital foramen lies 5–7 mm below inferior orbital rim. Trauma to infraorbital nerve during exploration of the orbit can cause hypoesthesia of lower eyelid, cheek, lateral side of nose, and also anterior teeth.[1] The thinnest part of the floor is posteromedial portion medial to the infraorbital sulcus. Orbital blowout fractures are commonly located in this area.

Surface Anatomy

Inferior orbital rim proceeds medially to become ALC. The superior orbital rim proceeds to become posterior lacrimal crest (PLC) medially **(Table 1)**.

TABLE 1: Bones forming walls of the orbital pyramid.	
Medial wall	Maxillary, lacrimal, ethmoid, sphenoid
Lateral wall	Zygomatic bone, greater wing of sphenoid
Roof	Frontal bone, lesser wing of sphenoid
Floor	Maxillary, zygomatic, palatine bones

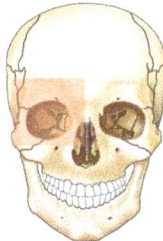
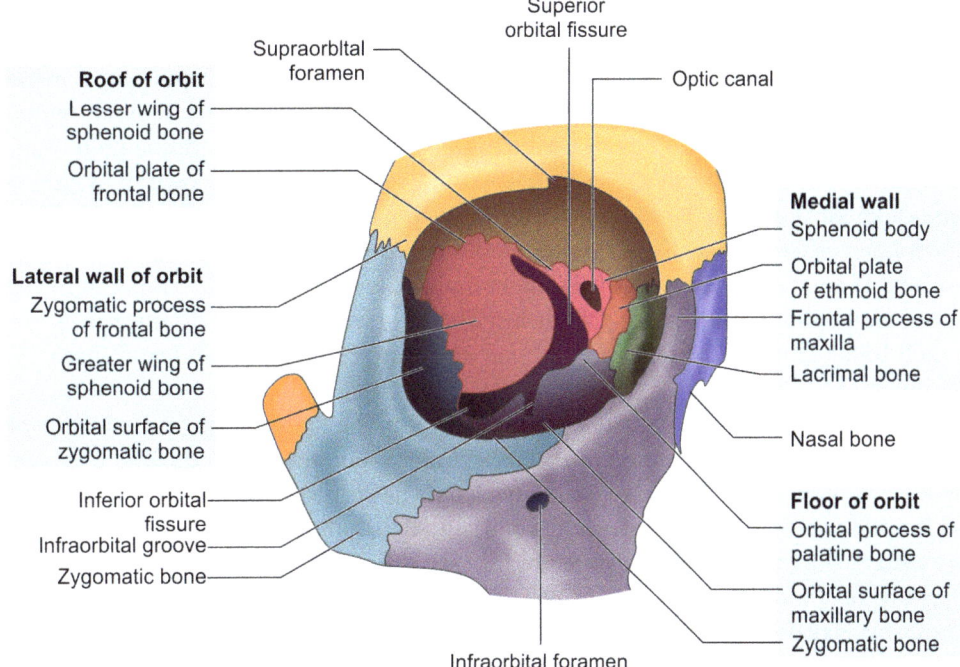

Fig. 1: Bony walls of the orbit.

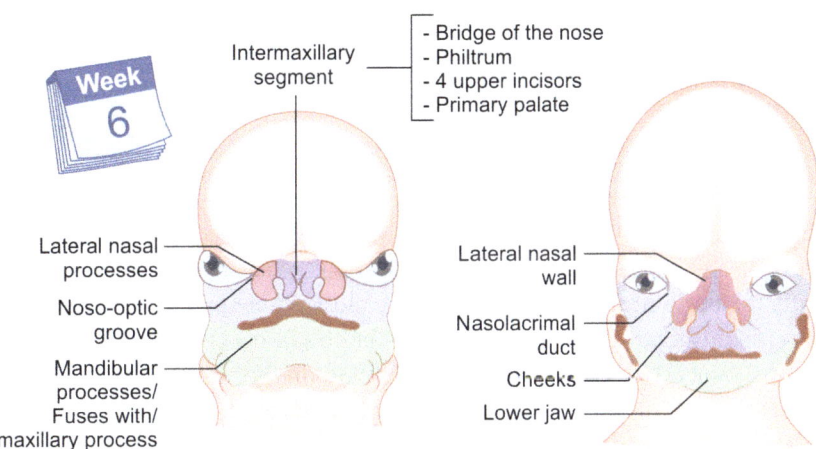

Fig. 2: Development of face.

Development of Orbit

Most of the embryonic face is formed by 8 weeks of gestation. The lateral margins of embryonic neural folds consist of neural crest cells. The neural crest cells lie between the surface ectoderm and underlying neural tube. By fourth week of gestation, pharyngeal arches begin to form. Majority of the face develops from the first pharyngeal arch. Five prominences of the pharyngeal arch are—two paired: maxillary and mandibular and one unpaired: frontonasal prominence. The nasal placodes are formed in the fifth week of gestation by thickening of surface ectoderm of frontonasal process on its ventrolateral aspect. Then medial and lateral nasal prominences develop from the nasal placode **(Fig. 2)**. The nasolacrimal drainage system is formed by fusion of the lateral nasal prominence and the maxillary prominence. During fusion two layers of epithelium get trapped. Initially, this epithelial cell cord is directed horizontal, but gets oriented vertically with further development of maxillary process. Canalization of the cord occurs near birth and failure to canalize completely leads to congenital nasolacrimal duct obstruction. Treacher Collins syndrome (mandibulofacial dysgenesis) and Tessier clefts are related to this stage of development of midface.

The development of bony skull is from the mesenchyme of neural crest. Its two parts are membranous and cartilaginous neurocranium. Foci of ossification develop in mesenchyme of membranous neurocranium. These develop into calvarial bones, which are attached to each other by intervening dense connective tissue membranes that comprise the sutures. Multiple forces are responsible or the growth of skull. Craniosynostosis is caused by premature fusion of sutures of the calvarium. Out pouches of ectoderm trapped into bony sutures (commonly at frontozygomatic suture) develop into dermoid cysts. Encephaloceles seen usually at frontoethmoid junction are due to entrapment of neuroectoderm in orbital space. Fronto-orbital fibrous dysplasia is a developmental disorder of bone due to mutation in G protein leading to inability to develop into mature bone. The resulting tissue has islands of woven bone in fibrous tissue.

The skull base (sphenoid bone, ethmoid bone, sella turcica, nasal concha, and septum) is formed from cartilaginous neurocranium.

Optic vesicles evolve from diverticula of the forebrain. The optic cup is formed by invagination of optic vesicle. The lens placode is formed by invagination of surface ectoderm into the optic cup. The edges of optic cup move forward and lens placode is nipped into the vesicle forming the lens. The cornea is formed by the surface ectoderm which subsequently overlies the optic cup. In the sixth week, cranial and caudal to the evolving cornea twofolds of ectoderm with mesenchyme at their core begin to be formed. They migrate toward each other and fuse. Till fifth to seventh month, they remain fused after which they divide to form upper and lower eyelids. Cryptophthalmos is a condition in which the eyelids fail to form.

A normal eye development is vital to the development of the orbit. Neural crest cells which surround the optic cup lead to shaping of orbital walls. Orbital angle starts decreasing as rest of the face develops and is 68° in an adult.

Periorbita

Periorbita is the fibrous tissue that covers the orbital bones. Periorbita is loosely attached to the bones except at (1) suture lines, (2) orbital rim, (3) orbital fissures, and (4) lacrimal crest. The periorbital tissue thickens along orbital rim at arcus marginalis. The orbital septum has its origin at arcus marginalis and attaches to anterior surface of tarsus (eyelid). At SOF and optic canal, the periorbita is continuous with dura mater.

Orbital Fascia

Connective tissue network in the orbit helps to support orbital contents. Koornneef has extensively described the complex arrangement of orbital connective tissue. To simplify the network, it can be divided into three sections: (1) Tenon's fascia/fascia bulbi, (2) extraocular muscle fascia, (3) check ligaments. Tenon's fascia extends posteriorly from just behind corneal limbus to the dura covering the optic nerve where it enters the globe. It separates the eyeball from intraconal fat of the orbit. The septa segregating orbital fat are attached to posterior Tenon's fascia **(Fig. 3)**. Fascia covering extraocular muscles extends to fibrous septa segregating orbital fat on inner aspect and to orbital walls on its external aspect. These extensions from muscle fascia to orbital walls are thickened anteriorly and are identified as check ligaments.

Clinical importance: Postenucleation orbital implants are placed invariably deep to the posterior layer of tenons—inside the muscle cone.

Contents of Orbit

- Extraocular muscles (covered in strabismus section)
- Lacrimal system
- Vascular anatomy
- Optic nerve and peripheral nerves
- Contents of orbital fissures and canal.

Lacrimal System

Lacrimal fossa is a shallow depression in superolateral orbit (frontal bone) **(Fig. 4)**. In this lies the lacrimal gland which measures 20 × 12 × 5 mm and is divided by the lateral horn of levator muscle into a larger orbital and a smaller palpebral lobe. The lacrimal gland is a serous gland. The 10–12 lacrimal ducts traverse through the palpebral lobe and open into lateral conjunctival fornix about 5 mm from the upper edge of superior tarsus.

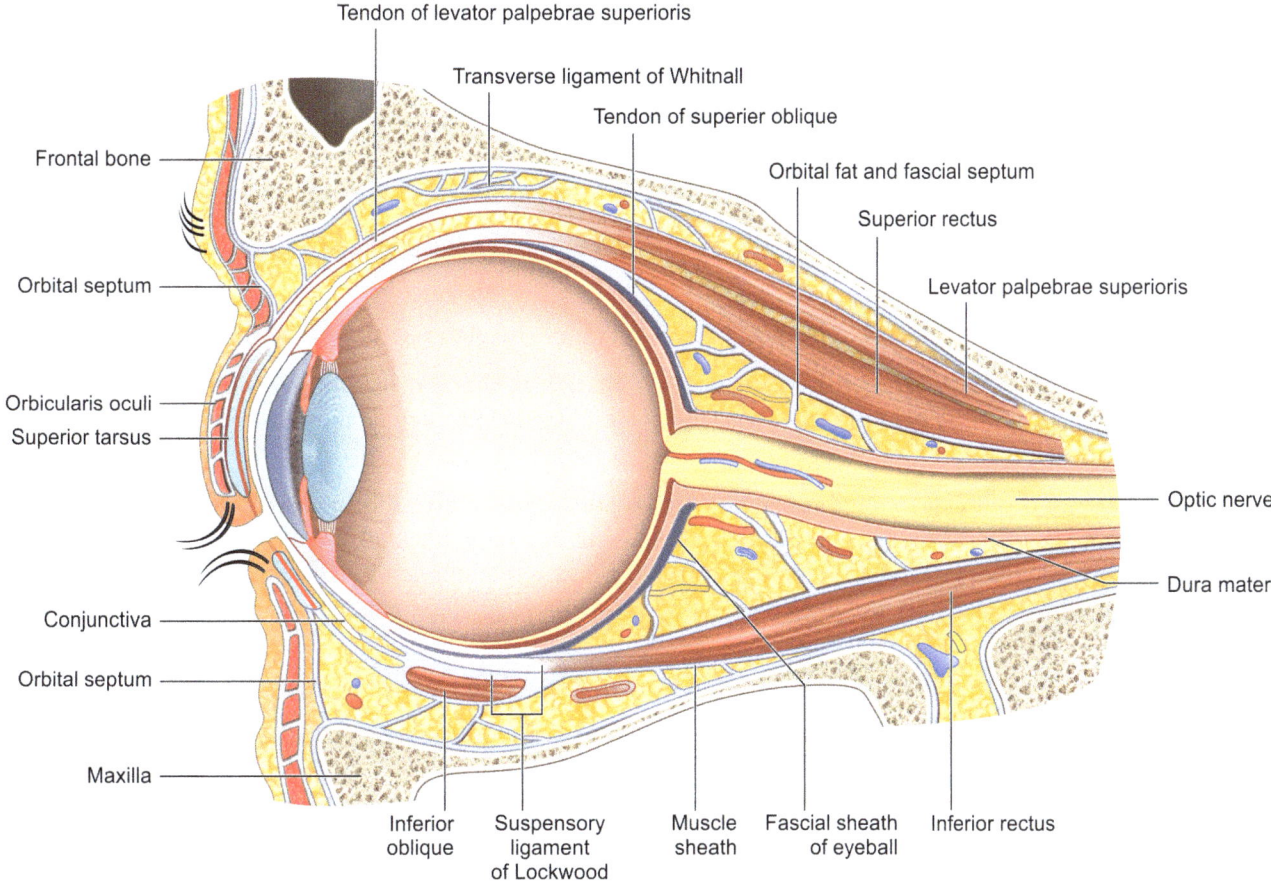

Fig. 3: Orbital fascia.

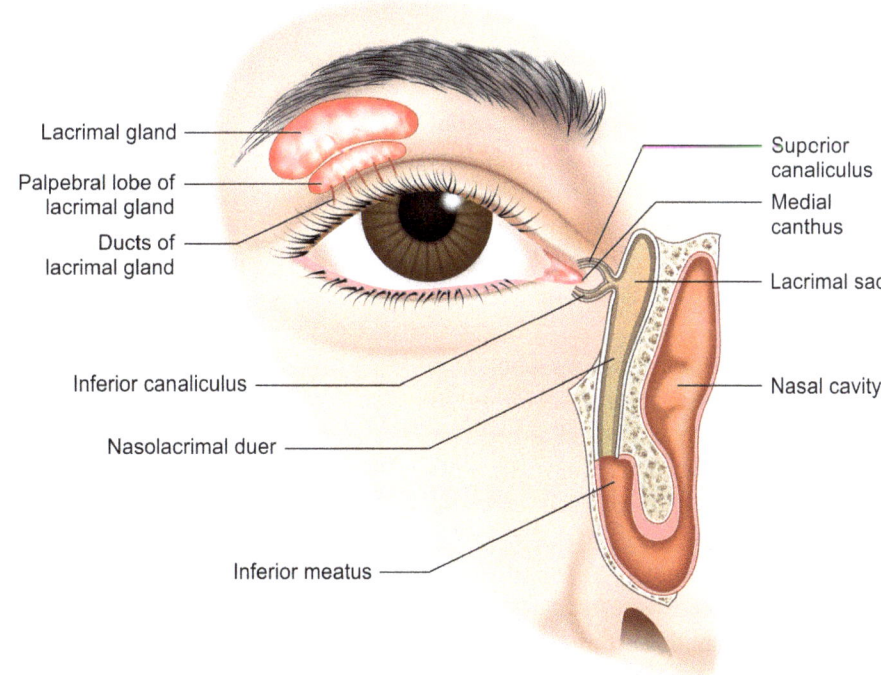

Fig. 4: Lacrimal gland anatomy.

The lacrimal gland in bound on all sides as below (**Table 2**):

TABLE 2: Boundaries of the lacrimal gland.	
Medial	Superior rectus, eyeball
Inferior	Lateral rectus
Anterior	Orbital septum
Posterior	Orbital fat
Superolateral	Lacrimal fossa

Clinical importance: Excision of palpebral lobe destroys secretory function of the gland.

The glandular branch of lacrimal artery runs along superior margin of lateral rectus muscle along with lacrimal nerve. It further branches variably either before or after entry into lacrimal gland through its posterior surface. The lacrimal vein drains into the ophthalmic vein.

Innervation: Sensory innervation in the lacrimal nerve which is a branch of ophthalmic nerve which is a branch of trigeminal nerve. *Parasympathetic innervation:* Greater petrosal, then nerve of pterygoid canal which synapses in pterygopalatine ganglion. Postganglionic fibers stimulate secretion from the gland. Sympathetic fibers from superior cervical ganglion are carried by internal carotid plexus and deep petrosal nerve to join parasympathetic fibers in pterygoid canal and then innervate lacrimal gland to inhibit its secretion.

Vascular Anatomy

The vascular supply of the orbit is intricate with multiple individual variations. The ophthalmic artery is the chief arterial supply of the orbit. It invariably arises from the internal carotid artery inferomedial to optic nerve and rarely from the middle meningeal artery. It normally lies within the dural sheath of optic nerve and courses anterolaterally in optic canal. In the orbital portion, after piercing the dura, it usually crosses over the optic nerve to medial orbit. In the superomedial orbit, it lies underneath superior oblique and over medial rectus muscles and eventually passes under the trochlea before dividing into its terminal branches. The branches of ophthalmic artery are as follows (**Fig. 5**):

- *Central retinal artery:* Supplies not only the optic nerve but also inner six to seven retinal layers. It is most commonly the first branch of ophthalmic artery crossing over the optic nerve. It runs inferolateral to optic nerve and pierces the dura of optic nerve 5–15 mm behind the globe. *Clinical importance:* In enucleation for retinoblastoma, >15 mm optic nerve stump is necessary.
- *Posterior ciliary:* These divide further into long and short posterior ciliary vessels. They pierce the eyeball lateral to the optic nerve and supply sclera, choroid as well as anterior aspect of the globe. The long posterior ciliary arteries traverse the muscle suprachoroidal space to end at the sclerocorneal junction by contributing to major anterior circle of iris.
- Lacrimal artery is one of the largest branches of ophthalmic artery and commonly arises from the segment crossing over the optic nerve. The branches of lacrimal artery are meningeal, zygomatic, glandular, and lateral palpebral. Zygomatic branch further divides into zygomaticotemporal and zygomaticofacial which exit the orbit through its inferolateral wall. Lacrimal artery primarily supplies the lacrimal gland but also supplies eyelids and conjunctiva.
- *Muscular:* Branches often accompany oculomotor nerve to provide blood supply to extraocular muscles. Of the two major muscular branches, the lateral branch supplies the levator, superior rectus, and superior oblique while the medial supplies inferior rectus and oblique and medial rectus. Arteries of recti anterior divide into two anterior ciliary arteries.

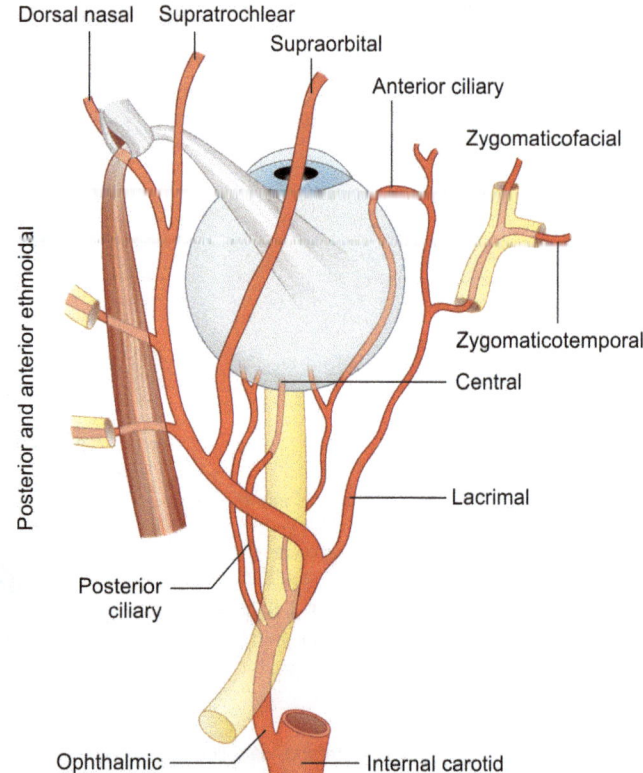

Fig. 5: Ophthalmic artery branches.
Source: Anderson JE (Ed). Grant's Atlas of Anatomy, 8th edition. Lippincott: Williams and Wilkins; 1983. pp. 7-56.

- Supraorbital artery is formed after the ophthalmic artery crosses over optic nerve to medial orbit. It has an orbital portion with gives branches to superior rectus and levator palpebrae superioris after which it exits the orbit through supraorbital foramen along with supraorbital vein and nerve after which it supplies the periosteum, skin, and muscles of forehead.
- *Posterior ethmoidal:* It passes through posterior ethmoidal canal into anterior cranial fossa. It supplies posterior ethmoidal air cells and then give off meningeal branches in anterior cranial fossa.
- *Anterior ethmoidal:* It enters anterior ethmoidal foramen along with nasociliary nerve and supplies falx cerebri, dura, and gives branches that passes through cribriform to supply anterior and middle ethmoidal cell mucosa, part of septum and lateral nasal wall.
- *Palpebral:* Medial palpebral artery arises just superior to trochlea and further divides into superior and inferior branches to supply the upper and lower eyelid, respectively.
  - The medial (branch of ophthalmic A) and lateral (branch of lacrimal A) palpebral arteries form eyelid marginal arcades which are situated 4 mm from upper and 2 mm from lower eyelid margin.
- Supratrochlear
- Dorsal nasal } Terminal branches

The terminal branches emerge at the superomedial edge of the orbit. Supratrochlear artery exits the orbit medial to supraorbital notch, ascends superiorly, and provides blood supply to forehead. Doral nasal artery has branches that supply lacrimal sac and dorsum of nose. Through some of its branches the ophthalmic artery anastomose with external carotid artery. In the orbit, ophthalmic artery also gives areolar branches to orbital fat.

External carotid artery: Its contribution to blood supply of the orbit is small. The infraorbital artery and orbital branch of middle meningeal artery are branches of external carotid artery.

Venous Drainage of the Orbit

The superior ophthalmic vein formed by supraorbital and angular veins begins at the trochlea and courses posteriorly along medial border of levator muscle. It then enters the muscle cone and runs below the superior rectus muscle in middle third of the orbit. In posterior third of the orbit, the vein lies between superior rectus and lateral rectus origin and enters anteroinferior portion of cavernous sinus through SOF. Its tributaries are:
- Medial palpebral
- Superior vortex
- Anterior ethmoidal
- Lacrimal
- Central retinal
- Muscular
- Inferior ophthalmic vein.

Inferior ophthalmic vein originates in anteromedial portion of orbital floor. Lower eyelid, lacrimal sac, inferior vortex veins, and inferior rectus and oblique muscles drain into a plexus which then drains into inferior ophthalmic vein. The inferior ophthalmic vein traverses the inferior orbit on surface of inferior rectus close to the orbital floor and drains into the superior ophthalmic vein or pterygoid venous plexus or cavernous sinus directly **(Fig. 6)**.

There are also a few inconstant veins in the orbit, namely: middle ophthalmic vein which lies over the inferior rectus, medial ophthalmic vein seen in about 40% cases coursing along orbital roof and medial wall and collateral veins which connect the superior venous system to inferior venous system. In addition, there are orbital venous plexuses (anteroinferior, posteroinferior, and superior have been described).

Clinical importance:
- *Radiological sign:* Dilatation of superior ophthalmic vein in carotid-cavernous fistulas
- Optic nerve sheath meningioma close to the exit of central retinal vein causes gradual central retinal vein occlusion (CRVO) and subsequently retinociliary collaterals develop over the optic disc (clinical sign of optic nerve sheath meningioma).

Orbital lymphatic drainage: A network of vessels lined by endothelium which transport the extravasated protein and fluid venous drainage are termed lymphatic vessels. It was stated by Duke-Elder that "in the orbit there are no lymphatic nodes, and no lymphatic vessels have been demonstrated." He had come to the conclusion that main lymphatic drainage of the orbit accompanies venules in perivascular channels through "the IOF to internal maxillary lymph nodes, thence to the superior cervical lymph nodes." In spite of their debatable existence, it is likely they do exist since pathologies such as orbital venolymphatic malformations (lymphangiomas) do occur.

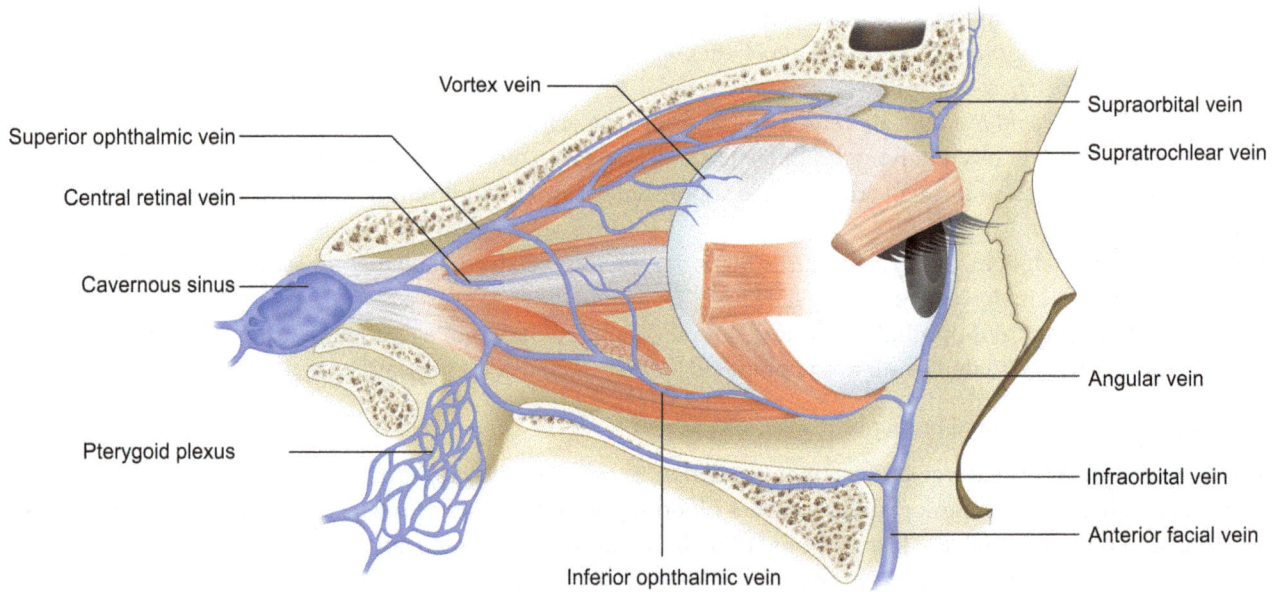

Fig. 6: Orbital venous drainage.

Optic and Peripheral Nerves

Out of the 12 cranial nerves (CNs), 5 innervate the orbit (optic, oculomotor, trochlear, first and second division of trigeminal and abducens). In addition to this, parasympathetic and sympathetic nerves also supply the orbit.

- *Optic nerve* extends from the eyeball to the optic chiasm. The two optic nerves diverge into the orbit at the optic chiasm where the angle between the two is about 68°. Optic nerve is about 5 cm long and 4 mm in diameter and is divided into intracranial (10 mm), intracanalicular (9 mm), intraorbital (24–30 mm), and intraocular (1 mm) segments. In its intracanalicular segment, the ophthalmic artery is encased in the dura but artery pierces the dura soon as the optic nerve enters the orbit. The distance between the optic foramen and back of the globe is about 18 mm, while the length of intraorbital portion of optic nerve is longer and thereby making the course of nerve sinuous. *Clinical importance:* Severe proptosis or recurrent globe luxation causes excessive stretch on the optic nerve and may result in visual loss. The central retinal artery pierces the optic nerve inferomedially about 10–15 mm behind the globe.
- *Oculomotor nerve:* It enters the orbit through the SOF (within annulus of Zinn) as superior and inferior division of oculomotor nerve. The nasociliary and abducens nerve lie between the two divisions of 3rd CN. The superior division is small and lies underneath the superior rectus muscle. It supplies the superior rectus and levator palpebra superioris. The larger inferior division further divides into three branches. Its first branch travels below the optic nerve to pierce the medial rectus muscle (posterior one-third) through its lateral surface. Second branch traverses anteriorly overlying the inferior rectus to enter the inferior rectus muscle approximately in its middle third. The third branch travels anteriorly and penetrates the middle segment of inferior oblique on its upper surface. Its motor root then joins the ciliary ganglion (lateral to optic nerve). *Clinical importance:* Clinical signs of oculomotor nerve injury within the orbit depend on the level of injury to the nerve. For example, inferior division disruption affects the pupil since pupillary branches are received from branch to inferior oblique. Also, oculomotor palsy can be a sign of diabetes mellitus and is usually pupil sparing. Whereas compressive lesions such as those due to an aneurysm involve the pupil as pupillary fibers lie superficial in the nerve trunk. Total loss of function of 3rd CN results in a complete ptosis with downward and outward deviation of the eye.
- *Trochlear nerve* (4th CN) provides motor supply to superior oblique muscle. It arises from the dorsal aspect of the brainstem, even though it is the smallest CN, it has the longest intracranial course (40 mm). It traverses the superolateral portion of SOF to enter the orbit and courses anteromedially over the levator and superior rectus muscle before entering posterior one-third of superior oblique along its upper border. It is the only motor nerve in the orbit that does not pierce the extraocular muscle through its intraconal surface.
- *Trigeminal nerve* **(Fig. 7)** has a small motor root and a larger sensory root. In the cavernous sinus, the ophthalmic division of trigeminal nerve divides into: (1) lacrimal, (2) frontal, and (3) nasociliary branches. The lacrimal and frontal branches enter the orbit superolateral to the annulus of Zinn, while the nasociliary branch enters via the annulus.

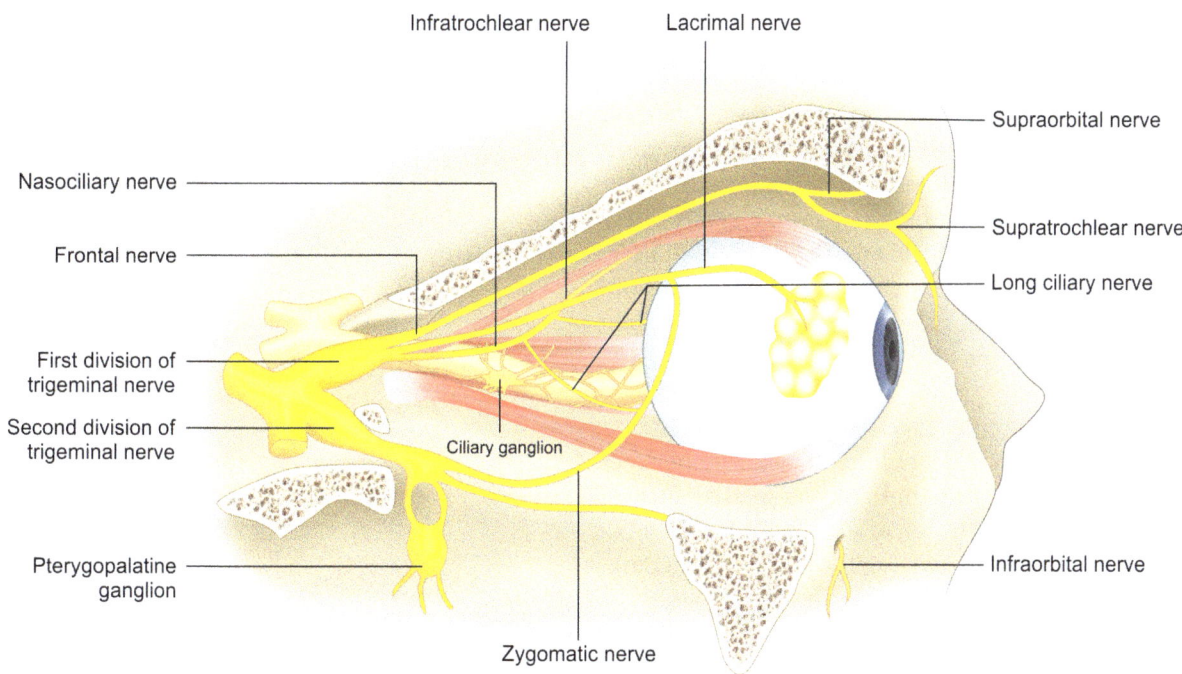

Fig. 7: Intraorbital trigeminal nerve and branches.

The lacrimal division traverses anteriorly over the lateral rectus muscle and is joined by the zygomaticotemporal nerve (parasympathetic supply) before it innervates the lacrimal gland. The lacrimal nerve not only supplies the gland but also the conjunctival and skin of lateral one-third of upper eyelid. The frontal division traverses anteriorly along the roof of the orbit above the levator muscle. It further divides into supraorbital and supratrochlear nerve prior to its exit from the orbit. The supraorbital branch transmits sensory signals from the forehead, scalp, middle two-thirds of the upper eyelid, and conjunctiva as well as frontal sinus. The supratrochlear nerve innervates the skin of forehead and medial one-third of the upper eyelid.

The nasociliary nerve upon entering the orbit gives off a sensory root to the ciliary ganglion. The long ciliary branches of nasociliary nerve travel along the medial and lateral surface of the globe to enter the sclera. These branches in addition to sensory input carry sympathetic efferent fibers to dilator pupillae. The anterior and posterior ethmoidal nerves (which pass through ethmoidal foramina) are branches of the nasociliary nerve. The nasociliary nerve then ends as infratrochlear nerve which courses along superior border of the medial rectus to supply medial conjunctiva, caruncle, nasolacrimal sac, and lateral aspect of nose (The anterior ethmoidal nerve enters the cranium, over the cribriform plate and enters the nasal cavity to form internal nasal nerve, which gives off medial and lateral internal nasal branches and a third branch, which continues as external nasal nerve supplying the nasal tip). *Clinical importance:* Hutchinson's sign of Herpes Zoster Ophthalmicus. The involvement of tip of the nose and the ocular signs reflect the distribution of nasociliary nerve.

Note on Ciliary Ganglion

The ciliary ganglion is situated in the loose retrobulbar fat in posterior orbit lateral to the optic nerve. Ciliary ganglion receives: (1) motor root carrying parasympathetic fibers from inferior division of 3rd CN; (2) sensory root from nasociliary; and (3) sympathetic root from sympathetic plexus of carotid and cavernous sinus. In the ciliary ganglion the preganglionic fibers of the motor root synapse with postganglionic fibers, which supply the sphincter pupillae and ciliary muscle through short ciliary nerves. Sensory root carries sensations from cornea, iris, and ciliary body, and these fibers do not synapse in the ciliary ganglion. The sympathetic root carrying postganglionic fibers from superior cervical ganglion too do not synapse in ciliary ganglion and get distributed through short ciliary nerves supplying vessels of the eyeball.

The maxillary division of 5th CN provides sensation to lower eyelid, side of the nose, mid-face, upper lip, teeth, mucous membrane of maxillary sinus, nasopharynx, tonsils, soft palate, and upper gingiva. It exits the cranial cavity via foramen rotundum and reaches the pterygopalatine fossa. Few sensory roots extend to the sphenopalatine ganglion, while parasympathetic fibers are received from the ganglion which are later responsible for the secretomotor function of lacrimal gland (via zygomaticotemporal branch fibers to lacrimal nerve). The zygomatic nerve enters the orbit through IOF overlying the lateral wall and eventually forming zygomaticotemporal and zygomaticofacial nerves innervating temporal fossa and skin of the cheek. The main maxillary nerve comes into the orbit through the IOF and is termed as the infraorbital nerve on entering the infraorbital groove which anteriorly forms the infraorbital canal and the nerve exits from the orbit about 10 mm below the inferior orbital rim. *Clinical importance:* (1) Infraorbital local anesthesia infiltration for dacryocystorhinostomy and (2) In blowout fractures of orbital floor involving infraorbital groove/canal, numbness of the cheek, teeth, etc. along the distribution of infraorbital nerve can be a symptom.

- *Abducens nerve:* It enters the orbit via the annulus in the SOF and pierces the lateral rectus muscle between its middle and posterior thirds on its medial surface. It is responsible for abduction of the eye. Abducens nerve palsy can be one of the early signs of raised intracranial tension.

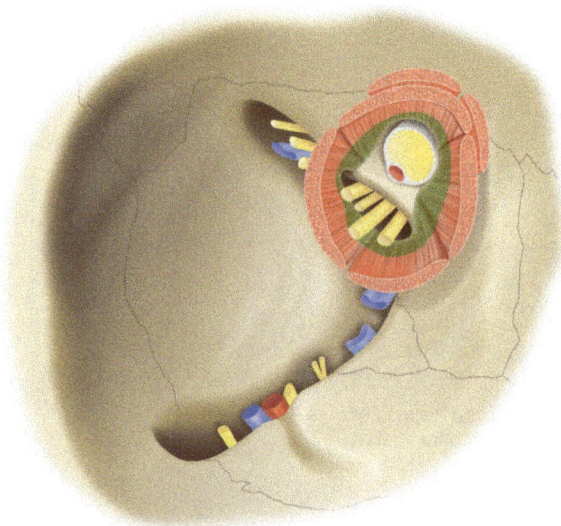

Fig. 8: *Orbital apex:* Superior orbital fissure, annulus of Zinn (common tendinous ring), optic canal, and inferior orbital fissure with contents.

Orbital Canal and Fissures

Orbital apex is a busy zone of the orbit since it is the origin of most extraocular muscles and a conduit for neurovascular structures **(Fig. 8)**.

The sphenoid bone is the keystone to the bony orbit. The canals and fissures at the orbital apex include the following:

- *SOF:* It lies between greater and lesser wings of sphenoid and is about 22 mm in length. The annulus of Zinn divides the SOF into three segments: (1) *Superolateral segment* (outside the annulus of Zinn) transmits the lacrimal, frontal, and trochlear nerves and superior ophthalmic vein. *Note:* At the anterior end of cavernous sinus, the ophthalmic division of the trigeminal nerve divides into lacrimal, frontal, and trochlear branches; (2) Central segment enclosed by annulus of Zinn. (3) *Inferomedial segment:* Superior division of inferior ophthalmic vein passes inferior to annulus of Zinn in the SOF. Annulus of Zinn (common tendinous ring) is a fibrous ring enclosing an area called oculomotor foramen which opens into middle cranial fossa. It transmits the following:
  - Superior and inferior division of CN III
  - Nasociliary division of CN V
  - Cranial nerve VI
  - Sometimes orbital branch of middle meningeal artery
  - Sympathetic nerve fibers
- IOF is the space between floor and lateral wall of the orbit. It lies between orbital plate of maxillary bone and palatine bone (part of the floor), greater wing of sphenoid, and zygomatic bone laterally. It communicates with the pterygopalatine, SOF, and infratemporal fossa. IOF transmits the following:
  - Maxillary division of trigeminal V2 (branch: infraorbital nerve)
  - Infraorbital artery
  - Branches of inferior ophthalmic vein to pterygoid plexus
  - Branches of sphenopalatine ganglion
  - Zygomatic nerve
- Optic canal lies in the lesser wing of sphenoid bone. It is bound by the lesser wing of sphenoid superiorly, sphenoid body medially, and by optic strut inferolaterally. It is about 12 mm in length and contains the optic nerve and ophthalmic artery.

Clinical importance: (1) SOF syndrome (Rochon-Duvigneaud syndrome) comprises followings features: upper eyelid ptosis, proptosis, ophthalmoplegia, fixed dilatation of the pupil, and hypoesthesia or anesthesia of the upper lid and forehead. (2) Orbital apex syndrome implies a constellation of symptoms and signs such as visual deficit along with features of SOF syndrome (due to involvement of II, III, IV, first two division of V and VI CN).

Suggested Reading

1. Acartürk S, Seküçoğlu T, Kesiktäs E. Mega dose corticosteroid treatment for traumatic superior orbital fissure and orbital apex syndromes. Ann Plast Surg. 2004;53:60-4.
2. Bergen MP. A literature review of the vascular system in the human orbit. Acta Morphol Neerl Scand. 1981;19:273.
3. Conlon MR, Sutula FC. Congenital eyelid anomalies. In: Albert DM, Jakobiec FA (Eds). Principles and Practice of Ophthalmology. Philadelphia, PA: WB Saunders; 1994. pp. 1693-4.
4. Dickinson AJ, Gausas RE. Orbital lymphatics: do they exist? Eye (Lond). 2006;20:1145-8.
5. Dolman PJ, Glazer LC, Harris GJ, Beatty RL, Massaro BM. Mechanisms of visual loss in severe proptosis. Ophthal Plast Reconstr Surg. 1991;7:256.
6. Duke-Elder S, Wybar KC. The Anatomy of the Visual System. St. Louis: CV Mosby; 1961. p. 479.
7. Dutton JJ. Atlas of Clinical and Surgical Orbital Anatomy. Philadelphia: WB Saunders; 1994. p. 116.
8. Hayreh SS. The ophthalmic artery. III. Branches. Br J Ophthalmol. 1962;46:212.
9. Hornblass A. Pupillary dilation in fractures of the floor of the orbit. Ophthalmic Surg. 1979;10:44.
10. Koornneef L. Orbital septa: anatomy and function. Ophthalmology. 1979;86:876.
11. Lang J, Kageyama I. The ophthalmic artery and its branches, measurements and clinical importance. Surg Radiol Anat. 1990;12:83-90.
12. Leatherbarrow B. Applied Anatomy. Oculoplastic Surgery, 3rd edition. London: Thieme; 2019. pp. 33-83.
13. Mann I. The Development of the Human Eye. New York: Grune & Stratton; 1950.
14. Natori Y, Rhoton AL. Microsurgical anatomy of the superior orbital fissure. Neurosurgery. 1995;36:762.
15. Piest KL. Embryology and anatomy of the developing face. In: Katowitz JA (Ed). Pediatric Oculoplastic Surgery, 1st edition. New York: Springer; 2001. pp. 11-28.
16. Schendel SA, Tessier P, Tulasne JF. Facial clefting disorders and craniofacial synostoses: skeletal considerations. In: Turvey TA, Vig KWL, Fonseca R (Eds). Facial Clefts and Craniosynostosis. Philadelphia: WB Saunders; 1996. pp. 3-27.
17. Sulik KH, Johnson MC, Smiley S, Speight HS, Jarvis BE. Mandibulofacial dysostosis (Treacher Collins syndrome): a new proposal for its pathogenesis. Am J Med Genet. 1987;27:359-72.
18. Sutton JE. The fascia of the human orbit. Anat Rec. 1920;18:141.
19. Whitaker LA, Katowitz JA, Randall P. The nasolacrimal apparatus in congenital facial anomalies. J Maxillo Facial Surg. 1974;2:59-63.
20. Whitnall SE. The Anatomy of the Human Orbit and Accessory Organs of Vision, 2nd edition. New York: Oxford University Press; 1932.
21. Yeh S, Foroozan R. Orbital apex syndrome. Curr Opin Ophthalmol. 2004;15:490-8.

1.16 Orbital Fracture

Adit Gupta, Prerana Tahiliani, Manpreet Singh

1. How will you approach and manage a case of orbital fracture presenting to the emergency department?

Orbital fractures are commonly referred to ophthalmologists in a polytrauma setting. They are frequently associated with other panfacial fractures, and collaborations with a maxillofacial surgeon might be needed. From an ophthalmologist's point of view, it is very important to triage these patients in the emergency room and decide further course of action based on specific clinico-radiological findings.

Blowout Fracture of the Orbit

This is the most common orbital fracture seen by an ophthalmologist. In a typical blowout fracture, a fragment of the orbital wall is displaced outward and away from the orbital cavity. The most common involved walls are the medial and inferior orbital walls. It is further classified as:

- *Pure blowout fracture:* Involves only the orbital wall and spares the orbital rim
- *Impure blowout fracture:* Involves the orbital rim along with other fractures
- *Trapdoor fracture:* Involves entrapment of orbital contents (muscle/fat) between bone fragments
- *Open door fractures:* Orbital fractures with prolapse of tissues without entrapment.

There are two main theories explaining the pathophysiology of a blowout fracture:
1. *Hydraulic theory (Pfeiffer):* Increased intraorbital pressure due to object larger than orbital dimensions causing displacement of globe backward and give way at the weakest point **(Fig. 1)**
2. *Buckling theory:* Direct trauma to the orbital wall causing transmission of force along the orbital rim to the walls (This supported Le Fort's theory as well) **(Fig. 2)**.
   However, multifactorial pathogenesis of orbital fractures can explain it better.

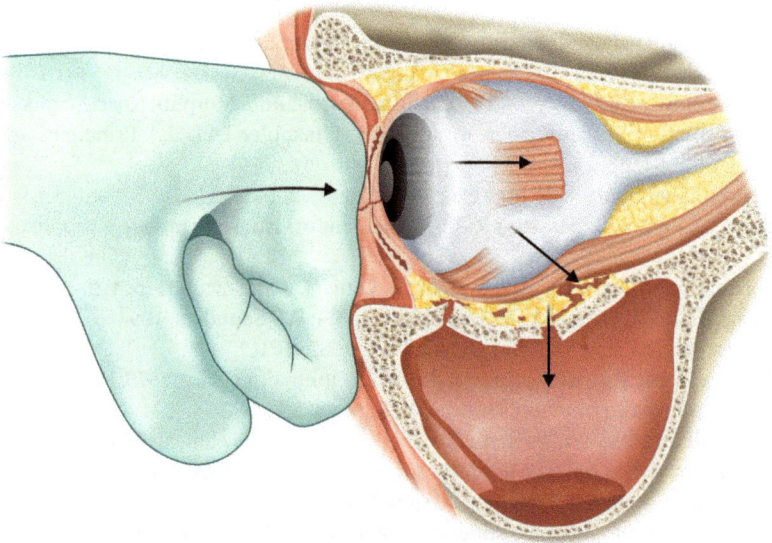

Fig. 1: Hydraulic theory demonstrating how an object larger than orbital dimensions causes increase intraorbital pressure and force transmission to the orbital wall causing a fracture.

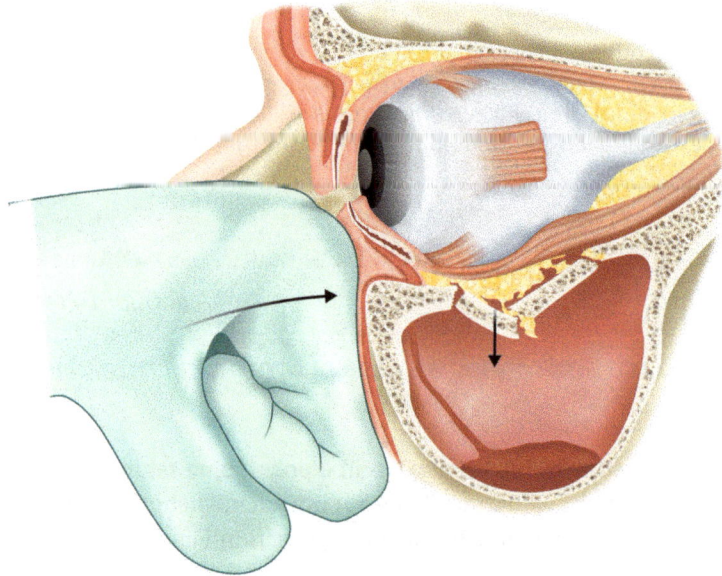

Fig. 2: Direct trauma causing transmission of force from the rim to the orbital wall and fracture.

Relevant Orbital Anatomy

Orbital Floor

Bones: Three, i.e., zygomatic, palatine, and maxillary
The shortest orbital wall (approximately 35 mm anteroposteriorly).

Vital structures: Infraorbital nerve and vascular bundle (in infraorbital groove and canal), and inferior rectus muscle (commonly involved in orbital floor fractures).

Medial Wall

Bones: Four, i.e., lacrimal, frontal process of maxilla, orbital plate of ethmoid, and sphenoid.

Lamina papyracea: A thin bone separating the orbit from the ethmoid sinuses, the thinnest part of the medial wall (0.2–0.4 mm), most common site for medial wall fractures.

Vital structures: Anterior and posterior ethmoidal foramen (at the junction of the medial wall and orbital roof), anatomical landmarks during medial orbitotomy. The medial rectus muscle is commonly entrapped in medial wall fractures causing abduction limitation.

Lateral Wall

Bones: Two, i.e., zygomatic and maxillary

The lateral orbital wall fractures usually cause flattening of the malar eminence and trismus as masseter and temporalis muscles are attached to the zygoma. Tripod fractures are most commonly associated with lateral orbital fractures.

Vital structures: The terminal branch of the facial nerve is in close relation with the zygoma.

Orbital Roof

Bones: Two, i.e., orbital plate of frontal and lesser wing of sphenoid

It separates the cranial cavity from the orbital cavity. Orbital roof requires significant amount of force to fracture. These fractures are more commonly seen in children as pneumatization of the frontal sinus is incomplete.

Vital structures: The frontal sinus lies within the roof of the orbit and offers an additional layer of protection.

Clinical Evaluation of Orbital Trauma

Signs and Symptoms

- Ecchymoses and swelling of the eyelid (s)
- Emphysema of eyelid and crepitus due to air trapped in subcutaneous tissues
- Pain
- Restriction of ocular movement due to entrapment of muscle/orbital tissues
- Diplopia due to entrapment of extraocular muscle or paralysis of muscles
- Nose bleed/cerebrospinal fluid (CSF) leaking medial wall fractures
- Enophthalmos due to increased bony orbital volume and prolapse of orbital contents
- Exophthalmos (rare) due to orbital hemorrhage and edema can be the initial presenting feature.
- Decreased sensation in the infraorbital (V2) dermatome due to injury to infraorbital neurovascular bundle.
- Trismus or inability to open mouth with associated zygomatic/mandible fractures
- Palpable "step-deformity" or tenderness of the orbital rim
- Decreased vision due to concomitant intraocular/optic nerve injury
- Bradycardia and vomiting due to the oculocardiac reflex
- Facial symmetry and displacement of lateral canthus as a fracture of the zygomatic complex can cause flattening of malar eminence.

Pediatric Orbital Fractures/White Eye Blowout Fracture

In children, orbital floor fractures can occur with minimal signs of trauma and thus called as white-eyed fractures. The bones are malleable and flexible in children so entrapment of extraocular muscles occurs most commonly due to trapdoor mechanism.

A high index of suspicion has to be maintained in a child with a history of trauma regarding this condition.

(**Figure 3** is an example of a young girl who had an orbital floor fracture with entrapment of inferior rectus. There are minimal signs of trauma or inflammation. She has restriction of elevation. Postsurgery photo shows improved elevation after release of inferior rectus muscle.)

Indications for Orbital Fracture Repair

The timing and need for intervention is based on certain clinical and radiological signs in cases of orbital fractures.
- Diplopia that persists beyond 7–10 days
- Obvious signs of entrapment
- Relative enophthalmos >2 mm
- A fracture that involves >50% of the orbital floor area
- Entrapment that causes an oculocardiac reflex with resultant bradycardia and cardiovascular instability
- Progressive numbness in the infraorbital area.

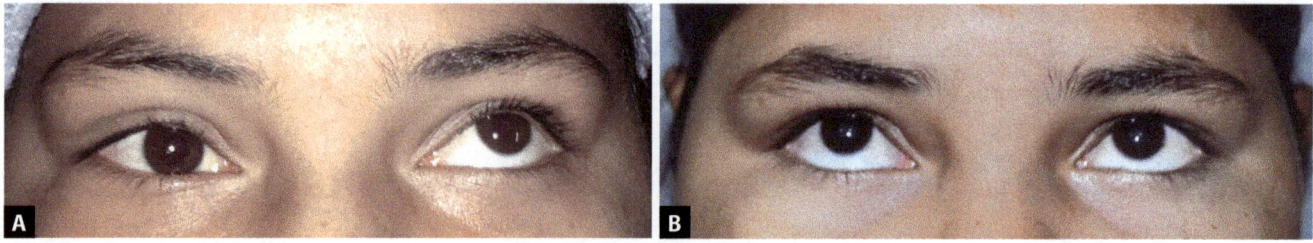

Figs. 3A and B: White eye blowout fracture of the right orbit in a 5-year-old girl showing restriction in elevation. Note the lack of inflammation or signs of trauma. She presented with vomiting and dizziness as the main complaints.

TABLE 1: Summarizing the planning in a case of orbital fracture.	
Immediate	• Diplopia present with CT evidence of an entrapped muscle or periorbital tissue associated with a nonresolving oculocardiac reflex: bradycardia, heart block, nausea, vomiting, or syncope • "White-eyed blowout fracture." Young patients (<18 years), history of periocular trauma, little ecchymosis or edema (white eye), marked extraocular motility vertical restriction, and CT examination revealing an orbital floor fracture with entrapped muscle or perimuscular soft tissue • Early enophthalmos/hypoglobus causing facial asymmetry
Within 2 weeks	• Symptomatic diplopia with positive forced ductions, evidence of an entrapped muscle or perimuscular soft tissue on CT examination, and minimal clinical improvement over time • Large floor fracture causing latent enophthalmos • Significant hypo-ophthalmos • Progressive infraorbital hypesthesia
Observation	Minimal diplopia (not in primary or downgaze), good ocular motility, and no significant enophthalmos or hypo-ophthalmos

Source: Burnstine MA. Clinical recommendations for repair of isolated orbital floor fractures: an evidence-based analysis. Ophthalmology. 2002;109:1207-12.

These indications can be further classified into those needing immediate versus delayed intervention (<2 weeks; **Table 1**).

Observation is warranted in the following situations:
- Minimal diplopia (not in primary or downgaze)
- Good ocular motility
- No significant enophthalmos or hypoglobus
- Vitals stable.

Investigations and Workup

Computed Tomography Scan

A computed tomography (CT) scan with bone window is the investigation of choice in cases of orbital trauma. A CT scan of orbits with 1–2 mm cuts should be requested along with paranasal sinus scans to delineate the site and size of the fracture.

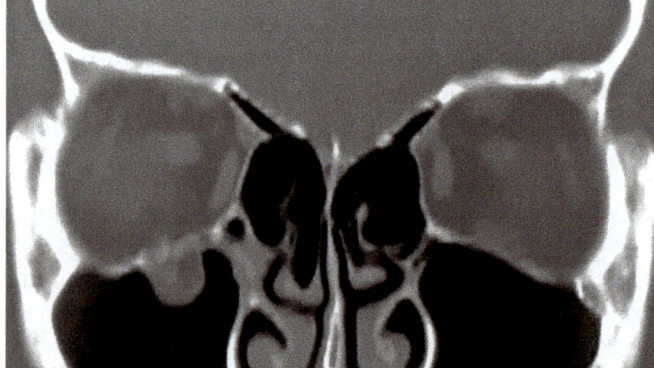

Fig. 4: Corresponding CT scan showing inferior orbital fracture with the classical "teardrop sign" seen in entrapment of inferior rectus muscle and orbital contents prolapsing in the maxillary sinus.

Axial, coronal, and sagittal cuts with 3D rendering help in formulating a plan for the management. A typical orbital fracture of the floor of the orbit will reveal the "tear-drop sign" which signifies prolapse of inferior rectus muscle with or without orbital contents via a defect in the orbital floor into the maxillary sinus (**Fig. 4**).

Screening cuts of the brain should also be included if clinical signs of neural involvement are suspected.

X-ray Orbits and Paranasal Sinus

An X-ray gives a rough idea about orbital and sinus anatomy and was used in earlier days before CT scan became readily available. However, it is a sensitive investigation to rule out a radiopaque foreign body associated with orbital trauma.

Diplopia Charting

This is done usually to determine and document the amount of diplopia preoperatively.

Forced Duction Test

This is performed to differentiate between restrictive versus paralytic etiology in the case of orbital fractures. If the forced duction test (FDT) is positive, it points toward muscle entrapment and is an indication for early surgery.

Exophthalmometry

This test is done to quantify the amount of enophthalmos due to trauma with respect to the normal eye.

Management

The assessment and treatment of systemic, facial, and neural injuries take precedence in case of orbital trauma. Once the patient is stabilized, orbital fractures can be managed.

Initially, a course of oral anti-inflammatory medicines, steroids, and local medications is prescribed to accelerate the reduction of swelling and ecchymoses. Globe injuries following orbital trauma is very common and range from 7% to 30%. Injuries to the eye should be managed before any intervention for orbital fractures.

Surgical Management

If surgical repair is indicated, the orbital floor can be approached via either a transconjunctival incision or a subciliary incision. A transconjunctival incision is preferred as it does not leave a visible scar and the chances of eyelid retraction with ectropion are minimal. A wider exposure can be achieved by adding a lateral canthotomy and inferior cantholysis.

The routine steps of surgery are as follows:
1. Incision of the conjunctiva in the fornix beneath the tarsus (transconjunctival) or incision of the skin 4 mm from the eyelash line (subciliary) **(Fig. 5)**
2. Blunt dissection to reach the orbital rim with a scissors
3. Incision on the periorbita 4–5 mm outside the rim to facilitate closure at the end
4. Reflection of the periorbita from the floor till the fracture site is visualized.
5. Periorbita around the fracture site reflected all around to delineate the incarcerated tissues
6. Release of incarcerated tissues and repositioning back into the orbit
7. Minimal damage to surrounding sinus mucosa
8. FDT to ascertain release of tissues
9. Measure the size of orbital floor defect with a template to choose appropriate size and material of implant
10. Placement of implant and securing it with either screw or glue
11. Closure of periorbita to over anterior part of implant with absorbable polygalactin sutures
12. Closure of incision.

Placement of a drain is usually not needed if proper hemostasis is maintained. Care has to be taken to avoid damage to the infraorbital neurovascular bundle during dissection.

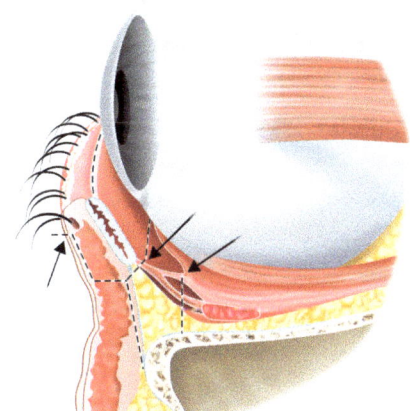

Fig. 5: Incisions used to approach a case of orbital fracture, the external subciliary incision, and the internal transconjunctival incision (preseptal and postseptal).

The patient should avoid blowing the nose for couple of weeks after surgery and should be on antibiotic cover to avoid infections.

Complications

- *Hemorrhage:* This is a serious complication and should be recognized immediately and treated. It usually happens within the first 48 hours after surgery. Urgent orbital decompression by performing a canthotomy and expressing the blood clot is needed.
- *Infraorbital hypoesthesia:* It is due to trauma to the infraorbital nerve as it traverses through the floor of the orbit. It usually recovers over a period of 3–6 months.

- *Diplopia:* This is commonly seen postoperative due to edema or damage to the extraocular muscle. It usually recovers with anti-inflammatory medicines. If it persists beyond 6 weeks, rehabilitation in the form of prism glasses or strabismus surgery is advised.
- *Infection:* It is common due to communication with the sinus cavity and so antibiotic cover is necessary postoperative.
- *Implant related migration/extrusion/cyst formation:* These are late postoperative complications and are less common with biointegrated orbital implants. Seen more commonly with silicone implants. Removal with replacement of implant is warranted in these cases **(Fig. 6)**.
- *Cerebrospinal fluid leak:* CSF leaks occur more commonly in medial orbital fractures where roof of the ethmoid bone, cribriform plate is also fractured at the time of trauma.
- *Eyelid malposition:* It is due to improper incision or cicatrix formation at the incision site. Aggressive cautery to the eyelid tissue also can cause eyelid malposition.

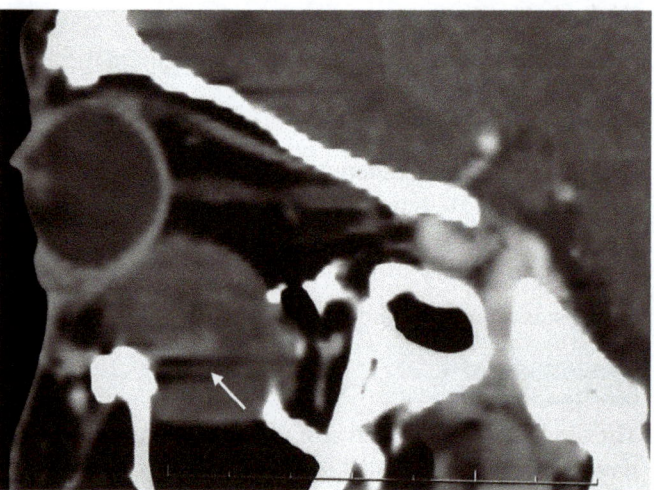

Fig. 6: CT scan showing formation of a cyst surrounding the implant 8 years after the surgery. Arrow shows the radiolucent implant within the cyst.

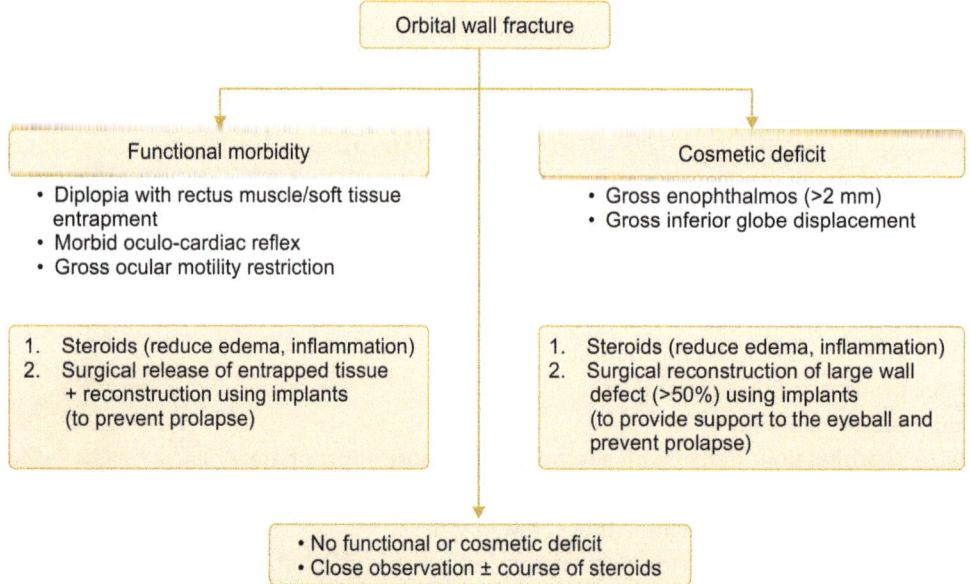

Q2. What are the various orbital implants available for the reconstruction of orbital fractures?

The choice of orbital implant used while reconstructing a defect in the orbital wall determines the long-term success of rehabilitation of the patient. An ideal implant should have the following characteristics:
- Inert and biocompatible
- Durable, pliable, easy to insert, good memory
- Cost-effective and easily available
- Strong to provide support
- Minimal extrusion rate
- Minimal infection rate
- Should have a smooth surface
- Radiopaque for postoperative imaging
- Provide volume to correct enophthalmos.

It is very difficult to simulate all these characteristics in an orbital implant, but with modern technologies and 3D printing, the search for an ideal orbital implant will soon end.

Implants can be classified into the following, depending on the source.

Autogenous	Allogenic	Alloplastic
• Calvarial graft • Iliac crest • Conchal/septal cartilage • Fibula graft	• Banked bone • Lyophilized dura • Lyophilized cartilage	Nonresorbable: • Titanium • Silicone sheet • Porous polyethylene • Hydroxyapatite Resorbable: • Polycaprolactone • (Osteomesh©) • Polygalactin

Advantages and Disadvantages

Autogenous	Alloplastic
Advantages: • Biocompatibility • Low infection rate • Easy integration Disadvantages: • Prolonged surgical time • Donor site morbidity	Advantages: • Surgical time shortened • Moldable • No donor site problems Disadvantages: • Higher infection rates • Expensive

Silicone

Silicone implants have been used for orbital reconstruction for a long time. They are cheap and easily available. They are available as sheets or slabs. The sheets can be cut depending on the size of the defect. The slabs available can be carved with a knife. The downside is the number of complications associated with the use of this implant material. Implant extrusion and migration is very common. Implant-related inclusion cysts are also commonly associated.

Titanium

It is the most biocompatible of all the alloplastic implants. It can be easily contoured, and due to fibrovascular ingrowth, there are fewer chances of extrusion. It also adheres to the bone firmly. The disadvantages are strong fibrotic reaction causing adhesions between the implant and the orbital tissue leading to ocular motility restriction and diplopia.

Recently, titanium implants are being fashioned in a way that fibrovascular adhesion is minimal. Also, 3D printing and rapid prototyping technology is used to design customized implant which conforms closely to the individual orbital cavity. The cost-effectiveness of this technology is still a concern **(Fig. 7)**.

Porous Polyethylene (Medpor)

Porous polyethylene is a high density, nonresorbable, and flexible implant that allows contouring to the orbital bones. It is very biocompatible with an adequate pore size (250 μ) to allow fibrovascular ingrowth and mineralization. This helps in long-term assimilation of the implant within the defect. This implant has shown lesser complication rates as compared to silicone implants. It is radiolucent, so postoperative imaging is not possible.

Composite Implants

A hybrid implant (Medpor Titan©) comprising porous polyethylene embedded in a titanium mesh is being used frequently in orbital reconstructions. It combines the qualities of both implants and offers more strength in reconstructions **(Fig. 8)**.

Polyglycolic Acid/Polycaprolactone

These are bioresorbable materials with osteoinductive properties. Copolymers have been used now, which include poly-L-lactic/polyglycolic acid sheet (LactoSorb) and polycaprolactone (Osteomesh). These can be molded when inserted in a hot

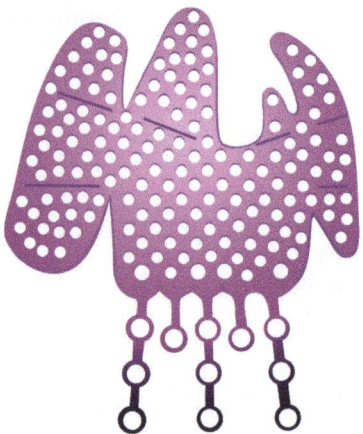

Fig. 7: Orbital floor titanium implant.

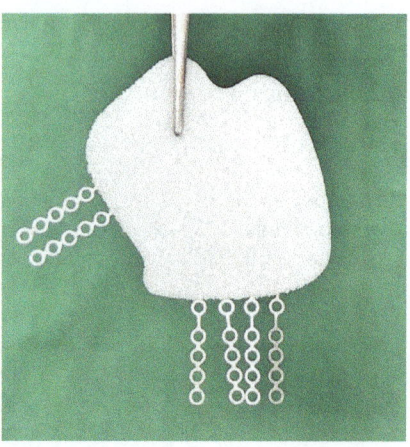

Fig. 8: Composite orbital floor implant made of porous polyethylene embedded in titanium mesh.

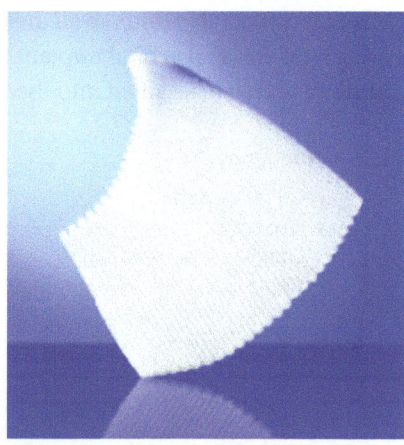

Fig. 9: Osteomesh® orbital implant made of polycaprolactone. This implant can be molded after heating it in a water bath to conform to the orbital floor defect.

water bath intraoperatively. Also the resorption time is between 12 and 18 months and is fairly predictable. They are in the true sense, integrated implants and provide the least rates of extrusion and infection **(Fig. 9)**.

Autogenous Bone

Bone harvested from the iliac crest, calvarium, and nose has been used in the past for reconstruction of orbital defects. Bone has good acceptance, low infection rates, and almost no extrusion, but it is less pliable and resorption rates are variable.

Bone grafts are better suited for secondary reconstructions and fixing fractures that need volume restoration as well. Increased surgical time and donor site morbidity has to be kept in mind while using this modality.

Suggested Reading

1. Boyette JR, Pemberton JD, Bonilla-Velez J. Management of orbital fractures: challenges and solutions. Clin Ophthalmol. 2015;9:2127-37.
2. Bratton EM, Durairaj VD. Orbital implants for fracture repair. Curr Opin Ophthalmol. 2011;22(5):400-6.
3. Grob S, Yonkers M, Tao J. Orbital fracture repair. Semin Plast Surg. 2017;31(1):31-9.
4. Joseph JM, Glavas IP. Orbital fractures: a review. Clin Ophthalmol. 2011;5:95-100.
5. Oppenheimer AJ, Monson LA, Buchman SR. Pediatric orbital fractures. Craniomaxillofac Trauma Reconstr. 2013;6(1):9-20.
6. Wei LA, Durairaj VD. Pediatric orbital floor fractures. J AAPOS. 2011;15(2):173-80.

1.17 Proptosis

Nirav Raichura, Savari T Desai

Q 1. Differential diagnosis of a patient with proptosis/unilateral proptosis/bilateral proptosis.

The first most important clinical decision is to differentiate between a true proptosis and pseudoproptosis **(Flowchart 1)**.

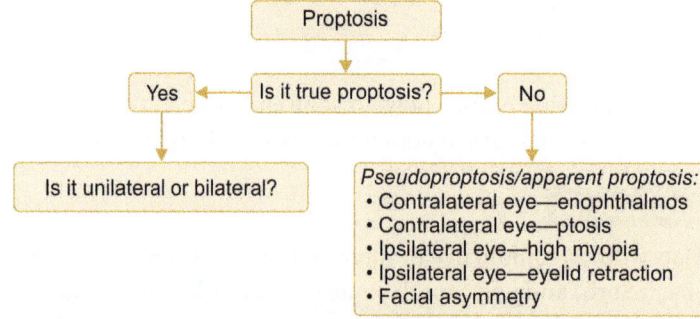

Flowchart 1: Proptosis vs. pseudoproptosis.

The differential diagnosis of true proptosis is based on: Laterality (unilateral or bilateral) and etiology **(Table 1)**.

TABLE 1: Differential diagnosis in a patient with proptosis.

Unilateral proptosis	Bilateral proptosis

• *Inflammatory:*
  – TED
  – IOID
  – Specific causes of inflammation:
    - Sarcoidosis
    - Wegener's granulomatosis
• *Cystic:*
  – Sinus mucocele extending into orbit
  – Dermoid cyst
  – Parasitic cysts
• *Infection:*
  – Orbital cellulitis:
    - Bacterial
    - Mycobacterial/TB
    - Fungal
    - Parasitic
• *Vascular:*
  – Lymphangioma (venolymphatic malformation)
  – Capillary hemangioma
  – Cavernous hemangioma
  – Varices
  – AVM
• *Neoplastic:*
  – *Neural:*
    - ON glioma
    - ON meningioma
    - Schwannoma
  – *Mesenchymal:*
    - Rhabdomyosarcoma
    - Fibro-osseous lesions
    - Hemangiopericytoma/SFT
  – *Secondary—spread from adjacent structures/metastasis:*
    - Orbital retinoblastoma
    - Leukemia
    - Metastatic neuroblastoma
    - Nasopharyngeal carcinoma
    - Visceral malignancies
  – *Other neoplasia:*
    - Lymphoma and lymphoproliferative lesions
    - *Lacrimal gland tumors:*
      - Pleomorphic adenoma
      - Adenoid cystic carcinoma
    - *Histiocytic lesions:*
      - Langerhans cell histiocytosis
      - Non-Langerhans histiocytosis
	• *Inflammatory:*
	  – TED
	  – Sarcoidosis
	  – Wegener's granulomatosis (rare)
	  – IOID (infrequently causes bilateral involvement)
	• *Neoplastic:*
	  – Lymphoma
	  – Chloroma/granulocytic sarcoma
	  – Secondaries/metastasis
	  – Xanthogranuloma
	  – Fibrous dysplasia
	• *Vascular:*
	  – Carotid cavernous fistula
	  – Cavernous sinus thrombosis
	• *Structural/skeletal:*
	  – Craniosynostosis

(AVM: arteriovenous malformation; IOID: idiopathic orbital inflammatory disease; ON: optic nerve; SFT: solitary fibrous tumors; TB: tuberculosis; TED: thyroid eye disease)

2. Describe the causes, type, investigation, and management of a case of unilateral axial proptosis in adult.

Etiology/causes of unilateral axial proptosis in an adult are given in **Box 1**.

Proptosis is abnormal protrusion of globe from the bony socket. When protrusion is purely in the posteroanterior direction, without any vertical or horizontal displacement of the globe, it is termed as axial proptosis.

Axial proptosis is seen in intraconal space-occupying lesions and diseases such as thyroid orbitopathy and inflammatory conditions that affect the extraocular muscles. Thyroid eye disease (TED) should be considered as a differential diagnosis

> **BOX 1:** Etiology/causes of unilateral axial proptosis in an adult.
>
> - *Neural:*
>   - ON glioma
>   - ON meningioma
>   - Schwannoma (intraconal)
> - *Vascular:*
>   - Cavernous hemangioma
>   - Varices
>   - Lymphangioma (solitary intraconal)
>   - Carotid cavernous fistula (commonly bilateral)
> - *Mesenchymal:*
>   - Hemangiopericytoma/solitary fibrous tumor
>   - Fibro-osseous lesions
> - *Inflammatory:*
>   - TED
>   - IOID
>   - *Autoimmune disease:*
>   - Sarcoidosis
>   - Wegener's granulomatosis
> - *Infection:*
>   - Orbital cellulitis:
>   - Bacterial
>   - Mycobacterial/TB
>   - Fungal
>   - Parasitic
> - Secondary/orbital metastasis
> - *Cystic:*
>   - Parasitic cysts—intraconal/apical
> - *Other neoplasia:*
>   - *Histiocytic lesions:*
>   - Langerhans cell histiocytosis
>   - Non-Langerhans histiocytosis
>
> (IOID: idiopathic orbital inflammatory disease; ON: optic nerve; TB: tuberculosis; TED: thyroid eye disease)

even in patients with unilateral proptosis as involvement may be asymmetric and more pronounced unilaterally. TED is the most common cause of unilateral or bilateral proptosis.

Types of unilateral axial proptosis are:
- *Pulsatile proptosis:*
  - Carotid cavernous fistula
  - Neurofibromatosis with absent sphenoid wing
  - Meningocele/encephalocele
  - Traumatic/postsurgical deficiency of orbital roof
  - Arteriovenous fistula
- *Intermittent proptosis:*
  - Orbital varices—with bending forwards or on Valsalva maneuver
  - Solitary lymphangioma—with episodes of upper respiratory tract infection
  - Capillary hemangioma—on crying
- *Painful proptosis:*
  - Infections
  - Inflammatory lesions
  - Traumatic conditions
  - Certain neoplastic conditions with neural infiltration.

Investigations

- *Imaging:* It is a crucial part of assessment in a case of proptosis. Generally, imaging is required unless the cause of proptosis is very obviously TED. **Table 2** gives an overview of imaging features of common causes of unilateral proptosis in adults.

TABLE 2: Imaging features of adult orbital lesions.

	CT scan	MRI T1W image	MRI T2W image	Contrast enhancement	Special features
Cavernous hemangioma	Homogeneous, well-defined, isodense	Isointense	Hyperintense	Late, but marked enhancement, may be patchy	Phleboliths may be present
Thyroid eye disease	Enlarged EOM	Isointense	Hyperintense (in active stage)	Present	EOM bellies enlarged with sparing of tendons
IOID	Enlarged EOM/ posterior scleritis/ mass	Isointense, becomes hypointense with chronicity	Hyperintense in acute phase, hypointense with increasing chronicity due to fibrosis	Moderate to marked	EOM enlargement involving tendons
Optic nerve sheath meningioma	Smooth, tubular enlargement of optic nerve, calcification may be present	Isointense	Heterogeneous; CSF— hyperintense, calcification— hypointense	Marked	Tram-track appearance on CT due to calcification

(CSF: cerebrospinal fluid; EOM: extraocular muscles; IOID: idiopathic orbital inflammatory disease)

- Computed tomography (CT) scan provides excellent view of orbital bones and bony lesions. Soft-tissue orbital masses also are seen well on CT scan as they stand out against the radiolucent (black) orbital fat.
- Magnetic resonance imaging (MRI) provides greater detail of soft tissue masses, especially, those located at the apex and those with intracranial extension.
- CT/MR angiography are used to visualize the blood supply of vascular tumors and to diagnose arteriovenous malformations.
- Ultrasonography (USG)—Useful in selective cases such as diagnosis and follow-up in a case of orbital cysticercosis, carotid cavernous fistula (dilated superior ophthalmic vein)
- *Laboratory investigations:*
  - Complete blood count (CBC)—leukocytosis in orbital cellulitis/infectious etiology
  - Erythrocyte sedimentation rate (ESR)—raised in infections and inflammatory conditions
  - Blood sugar—especially in diabetic patients with suspected orbital infections. Uncontrolled diabetics are prone to orbital fungal infections.
  - Thyroid function tests—in suspected thyroid orbitopathy with or without past history of thyroid disease
  - Autoimmune profile—antinuclear antibody (ANA), antineutrophil cytoplasmic antibody (ANCA), serum angiotensin-converting enzyme (ACE)—for autoimmune causes of orbital inflammation like Wegener's granulomatosis, sarcoidosis.

Management of Unilateral Axial Proptosis

Management begins with history-taking and clinical evaluation. **Flowcharts 2 to 4** represent the pertinent points to be kept in mind while assessing the clinical history examination and management of an adult patient with unilateral proptosis.

Treatment

Treatment depends on the cause of proptosis. It may be possible to diagnose the etiology based on clinical features and investigations alone. An incisional biopsy of an orbital mass may be indicated when diagnosis is uncertain. An algorithm is presented in **Flowchart 2**.

Treatment of common causes of unilateral axial proptosis in an adult is discussed below.

Cavernous Hemangioma

It is the most common benign orbital tumor in adults. It is usually intraconal. Observation is an option if the hemangioma is small and not causing compression of optic nerve. Excision should be performed if it is causing visual disturbance or proptosis that is severe or not acceptable to the patient. Stereotactic radiotherapy is an option for tumors located at the orbital apex to reduce the risk of surgical damage to vital structures.

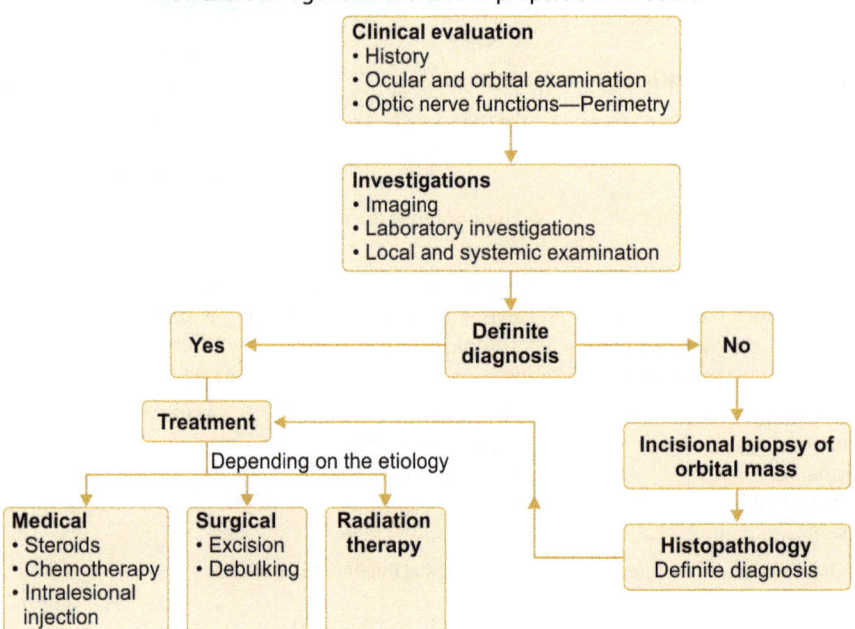

Flowchart 2: Algorithm in a case of proptosis in an adult.

Thyroid Eye Disease

- Medical management
- Radiation
- Surgery.

Treatment depends on "activity" and "severity" of the disease. "Activity" is an indicator of active ongoing inflammation. Active TED needs intervention mostly in the form of systemic steroids. Intravenous pulsed therapy with once weekly injection of methylprednisolone for 12 weeks is the preferred therapy as per the European Group on Graves' Orbitopathy (EUGOGO) guidelines. Inactive disease is managed with topical lubricants and regular monitoring of visual functions. In "severe" disease threatening the vision due to compressive optic neuropathy, aggressive medical therapy with intravenous steroids (1 g methylprednisolone) for 3 days is initiated. If response to therapy is adequate, systemic (oral) steroids may be continued. If there is progressive optic neuropathy despite aggressive medical therapy, urgent surgical decompression of the orbital apex is indicated. Decompression is also indicated in patients with severe proptosis and exposure keratopathy threatening vision. Patients with inactive disease but cosmetically unacceptable proptosis are also offered orbital decompression to reduce proptosis. Patients may also need correction of associated squint and eyelid retraction which have to be planned as secondary procedures. The order of corrective surgery in TED should be—decompression → squint correction → eyelid surgery.

Optic Nerve Sheath Meningioma

- *Observation:* If there is no visual loss and a very close follow-up can be maintained. Most will progress, though slowly, and eventually affect vision (either visual acuity or fields) indicating need for intervention.
- *Surgery:* It was the treatment of choice in the past. Invariably surgery is associated with a decrease in vision that is severe to the extent of no perception of light in a large number of patients. Surgery is performed in patients with complete loss of vision or when tissue diagnosis is required.
- *Radiotherapy:* It is now the treatment of choice. Several modalities of radiotherapy are available. Fractionated external beam radiotherapy is widely used but has higher complication rate. 3D conformal radiotherapy or stereotactic radiotherapy delivers intended radiation dosage to the lesion with minimal damage to the surrounding structures decreasing the chances of radiation-related side effects.

Idiopathic Orbital Inflammatory Disease

- *Steroids:*
  - First-line therapy
  - *Starting dose:* 1 mg/kg body weight/day methylprednisolone
  - *Taper:* Gradually over 6–8 weeks

- Recurrences can occur after stopping or during tapering phase
- May not be tolerated by few patients
■ *Steroid-sparing agents:*
  - In patients who cannot tolerate steroids or when steroids are contraindicated.
  - In patients who are nonresponsive to steroids.
  - As steroid sparing treatment when long-term treatment is required.
  - *Antimetabolites:* Methotrexate, azathioprine, mycophenolate mofetil
  - *Alkylating agents:* Cyclophosphamide, chlorambucil
  - *Calcineurin inhibitors:* Cyclosporine A
  - *B-lymphocyte inhibitor:* Rituximab
  - *Tumor necrosis factor-α inhibitors:* Infliximab, adalimumab
■ *Radiotherapy:*
  - As an adjunct to steroids/medical therapy
  - 1,000–3,000 cGy in fractions.

Solitary Fibrous Tumor
- It is a tumor of mesenchymal origin and has a spectrum from benign to malignant.
- Complete excision is the treatment of choice.
- Residual tumor if left behind leads to recurrence and possible malignant transformation.
- Radiation is used in case of incomplete excision and recurrences.

 3. Discuss the etiology and management of pediatric proptosis.

The causes of pediatric proptosis are diverse and range from very benign to highly malignant, from not-so-harmful to life-threatening pathologies. Common causes of pediatric proptosis depending on age and laterality are enlisted in **Tables 3 and 4**, respectively.

TABLE 3: Causes of pediatric proptosis based on age.

Birth to 1 year	1–5 years	>5 years of age
- Capillary hemangioma - Lymphangioma - Dermoid cyst - Teratoma - Chloroma/granulocytic sarcoma - Craniosynostosis - Optic nerve glioma - Orbital cellulitis - Meningocele/encephalocele - Neurofibromatosis	- Orbital cellulitis - Capillary hemangioma - Lymphangioma - Rhabdomyosarcoma - Granulocytic sarcoma - Optic nerve glioma - Orbital retinoblastoma - Neurofibromatosis - Secondaries/metastasis - Metastatic neuroblastoma	- Orbital cellulitis - Lymphangioma - Rhabdomyosarcoma - Granulocytic sarcoma - Thyroid eye disease - Idiopathic orbital inflammatory disease - Fibrous dysplasia - Secondaries/orbital metastasis - Meningioma (rare in pediatric age group)

TABLE 4: Causes of pediatric proptosis based on laterality.

Unilateral	Bilateral

- Capillary hemangioma
- Lymphangioma
- Dermoid cyst
- Rhabdomyosarcoma
- Teratoma
- Optic nerve glioma
- Orbital cellulitis
- Neurofibromatosis
- Orbital retinoblastoma
- Idiopathic orbital inflammatory disease
- Encephalocele
	- Granulocytic sarcoma
	- Craniosynostosis
	- Thyroid eye disease
	- Fibrous dysplasia (can be unilateral or bilateral)
	- *Secondaries:*
	  – Neuroblastoma
	  – Orbital retinoblastoma (rarely bilateral)

Management of Pediatric Proptosis

Management begins with history taking and clinical evaluation. Apart from the routine, relevant and significant information that needs to be obtained from the patient's parent/guardian includes the following:

- *Time since proptosis:* Was there proptosis at birth?
  If yes, differential diagnosis is limited in this clinical setting and includes:
  - Congenital capillary hemangioma
  - Lymphangioma
  - Craniosynostosis
  - Orbital dermoid cyst
  - Teratoma
- *Onset and progress of proptosis:* Development of proptosis may range from rapid development within minutes to slow prolonged progression over years. **Table 5** gives a brief overview of likely diagnosis depending on the onset and progress of proptosis.
- *Is there a change on crying?*
  Venous malformations are known to fill and expand on Valsalva maneuver causing increase in proptosis. Similar effect is obtained when patient cries/strains. A capillary hemangioma may also increase in size when the patient cries thus expanding the orbital lesion or associated superficial eyelid lesion.
- *Is there an increase in proptosis with episodes of upper respiratory tract infection?*
  If yes, it indicates a diagnosis of lymphangioma.
- *What are the associated ocular symptoms?*
  Presence of squint and ptosis may indicate visual impairment and risk of amblyopia. Such patients require early intervention. Older children may complaint of decrease in vision or diplopia. Complaint of leukocoria points to a diagnosis of retinoblastoma.
- *Are there any associated systemic symptoms?*
  History of fever favors a diagnosis of infection/orbital cellulitis. History of swellings elsewhere in the body may point to diagnosis of neurofibromatosis or metastasis or secondaries.

Examination

Refer to **Flowcharts 3 and 4**.

Orbital examination should include inspection of the face, eyelids and adnexa, and globe position. Proptosis evaluation should also include inspection to look for visible pulsations. In children, neurofibromatosis with absence of sphenoid wing is the most common cause of pulsatile proptosis. Insinuation along the orbital rims and between the globe and rims can be performed to palpate lesions located in the deep anterior orbit.

One must also palpate for the presence of regional lymph nodes. Exophthalmometry should be performed to document the degree/severity of proptosis whenever possible in older children. Auscultation with bell of stethoscope will elicit a bruit in cases of carotid cavernous fistula or arteriovenous malformation.

Local examination should be followed by systemic evaluation to look for associated systemic features that may point to a diagnosis or draw attention to associated systemic complication.

TABLE 5: Differential diagnosis of proptosis.

Time	Hyperacute/catastrophic (within minutes to hours)	Acute (within days)	Subacute (weeks to months)	Chronic (months to years)
Cause/mechanism of proptosis	Bleeding/hematoma	Infection/inflammation	Chronic inflammation/fast-growing tumors	Tumors
Examples	• Bleeding in a pre-existing lymphangioma • Traumatic or spontaneous orbital hematoma	• Orbital cellulitis • Thyroid eye disease • Idiopathic orbital inflammatory disease • Ruptured dermoid	• Rhabdomyosarcoma • Granulocytic sarcoma • Secondary neuroblastoma • Capillary hemangioma (rapid growth phase) • Idiopathic orbital inflammatory disease	• Neurogenic tumors • Lymphangioma • Optic nerve glioma • Fibrous dysplasia

Oculoplasty and Tumors

Flowchart 3: Salient aspects of clinical history in a patient with proptosis.

- **Proptosis clinical history**
  - **How fast is it progressing**
    - Rapidly progressing → Inflammation/infection
    - Gradually progressing → Neoplasia
  - **Is it acute/subacute/chronic**
    - Hyperacute → Bleed within a pre-existing lesion
    - Acute → Infection / Inflammation
    - Subacute → Inflammation / Fast growing tumors
    - Chronic → Slow growing tumors
  - **Is it painful?**
    - Painless → Neoplasia
    - Painful → Inflammation / Infection / Neural infiltration in certain → Adenoid cystic carcinoma
  - **Is there change with postition/change with valsalva?**
    - Yes → Varices
    - No
  - **Is there an increase with URTI episodes?**
    - Yes → Lymphangioma/VLM
    - No
  - **Is there a history of systemic disease?**
    - Uncontrolled diabetes mellitus → Fungal orbital cellulitis
    - Thyroid disease → Thyroid eye disease
    - Malignancy elsewhere → Secondaries in orbit
    - Tuberculosis → Orbital TB
    - Auto-immune disorders → Orbital inflammatory disease
    - Neurofibromatosis → Meningioma
  - **What are associated systemic symptoms?**
    - Fever → Orbital cellulitis
    - Swelling in the neck or elsewhere → Malignancy
  - **Is there loss of weight/appetitie?**
    - Yes → Malignancy / Orbital TB
    - No
  - **History of head injury in the past?**
    - Yes → Carotid-cavernous fistula
    - No
  - **Is it pulsatile?**
    - True pulsations → Carotid-cavernous fistula
    - Transmitted pulsations → Traumatic/post-surgical deficiency of orbital roof
  - **What are the associated ophthalmic symptoms?**
    - Diplopia
      - Restriction of ocular movements → Thyroid orbitopathy / Orbital SOL
      - Paralysis of ocular movements → Cavernous sinus lesion / Orbital apex lesion
    - Diminution/loss of visiosn → Comprehensive optic neuropathy / Primary optic nerve tumor
    - Dryness → Thyroid eye disease
  - **Did diminution of vision precede or follow proptosis?**
    - Proceed → Primary optic nerve tumor-like meningioma / Lesion originating at orbital apex
    - Followed

(SOL: space occupying lesion; TB: tuberculosis; URTI: upper respiratory tract infection; VLM: venous lymphatic malformation)

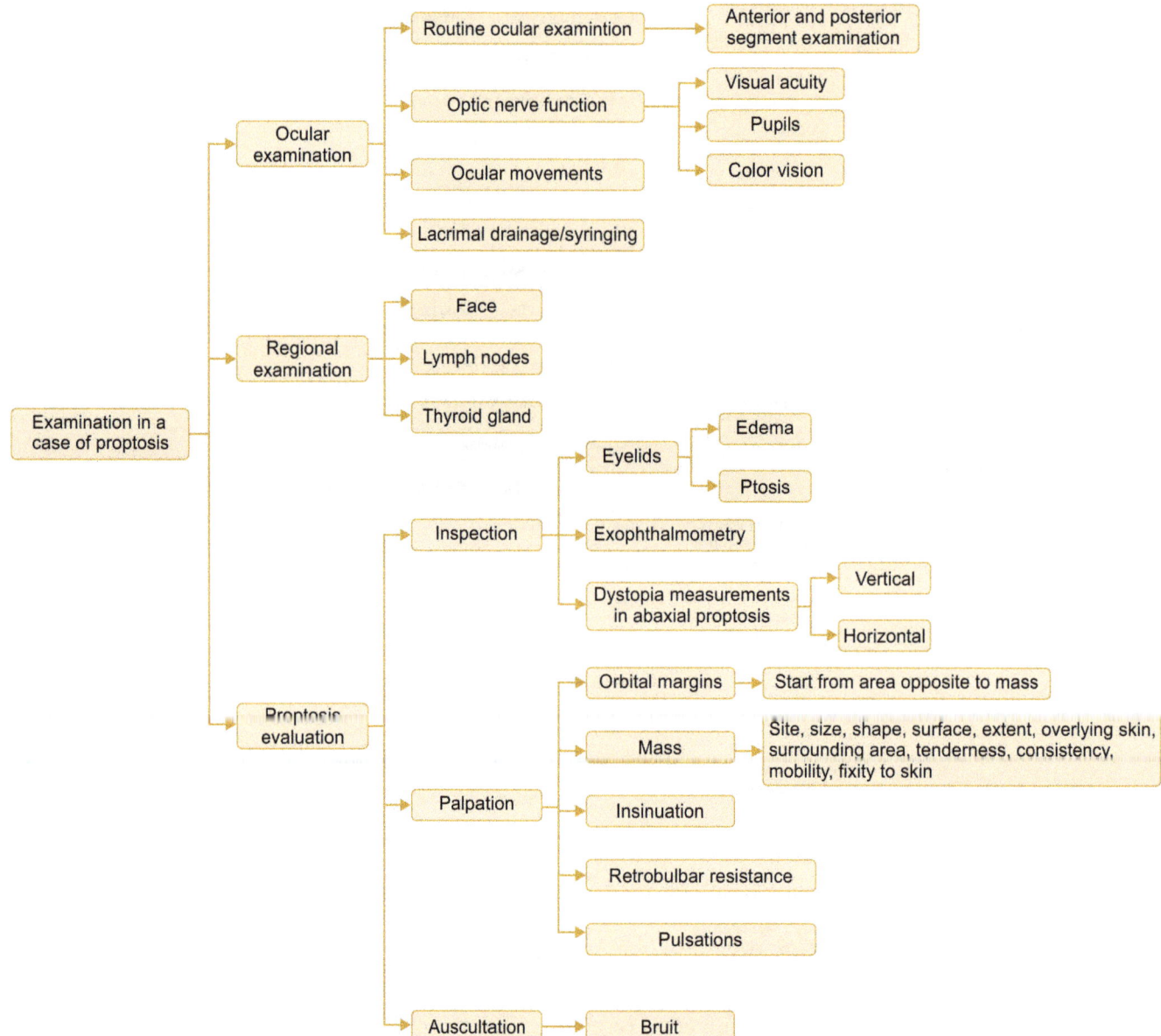

Flowchart 4: Salient aspects of clinical examination in a case of proptosis.

- *Neurofibromatosis:* Café-au-lait spots
- *Capillary hemangioma:* Rule out PHACE syndrome and Kasabach–Merritt syndrome.

Investigations

- *Imaging:* Orbital imaging modalities include CT scan, MRI, and USG. **Table 6** gives a comparative overview of these modalities. The imaging features of common pediatric orbital lesions are represented in **Table 7**.
- *Laboratory investigations and other investigations:*
  - CBC—leukocytosis in orbital cellulitis/infectious etiology
  - ESR—raised in infections and inflammatory conditions
  - Peripheral blood smear—should be performed in all cases of sudden onset proptosis or orbital mass in children. It is a useful tool in diagnosing leukemia and associated orbital granulocytic sarcoma.
  - Chest X-ray/CT scan and abdominal USG/CT scan—to look for metastasis in case of malignant neoplasms.

Treatment

The treatment of pediatric proptosis depends on and varies with etiology of proptosis. It may be possible to identify an etiology based on clinical features and investigations alone. But, if that is not possible and whenever in doubt, a biopsy

TABLE 6: Orbital imaging modalities—pediatric considerations.

	CT scan	MRI	USG
Advantages	• Short acquisition time • Bony lesions and calcification are visualized better	• No risk of exposure to harmful radiation • Characteristics of soft tissue lesions are better defined • Best for visualizing apical lesions and intracranial extensions	• No need for sedation/general anesthesia • Good to visualize cystic lesions • Can be used intraoperatively to guide during intralesional injection therapy
Disadvantages	• Risk of inducing cancer due to radiation exposure—best to avoid until 5 years of age	• Acquisition time is longer than CT • Requires intravenous sedation/general anesthesia in infants and toddlers • Higher cost	• Cannot be used for very deep orbital lesions • Limited information regarding lesion characteristics

TABLE 7: Imaging features of common pediatric orbital lesions.

	CT scan	MRI T1W image	MRI T2W image	Contrast enhancement	Special features
Capillary hemangioma	Homogeneous, generally well defined	Hypointense to intermediate intensity	Hyperintense	Marked enhancement	Flow voids, internal septae
Lymphangioma	• Heterogeneous, irregular, ill-defined, infiltrating transcompartmental lesion • Hypodense cystic areas • May extend to sinuses, subcutaneous area of face • May show enlargement of bony orbit	Isointense	Hyperintense	No enhancement	• Micro-/macrocystic • Fluid level within cysts • Internal septations • No flow voids
Orbital cellulitis	• Opacification of sinuses • Lid edema, fat stranding	• *Subperiosteal abscess:* Intermediate signal • *Orbital cellulitis:* Diffuse isointense signal	• *Subperiosteal abscess:* Hyperintense • *Orbital cellulitis:* Diffuse hyperintense signal	Rim enhancement in subperiosteal and orbital abscess	• *Orbital abscess:* Well-defined lesion, necrotic center, and enhancing rim • *Subperiosteal abscess:* Dome-shaped homogeneous lesion along orbital wall adjacent to opacified sinus
Rhabdomyosarcoma	Moderately well defined, heterogeneous (due to areas of focal necrosis), isodense to muscle	Isointense	Hyperintense	Moderate to marked	

of an orbital mass must be performed to ascertain the diagnosis on histopathology. Treatment will then depend on final histopathological diagnosis and may include one or more of—observation, conservative medical management, intralesional injections, and surgery (excision or debulking).

Treatment of common causes of pediatric proptosis is discussed below.

Capillary Hemangioma

Infantile capillary hemangioma are the most common benign orbital tumors of pediatric age group. Infantile hemangiomas have a tendency for spontaneous regression making conservative management possible in many cases. Indications for intervention include very large hemangiomas and risk of amblyopia due to severe ptosis, induced anisometropia, and strabismus. Currently, the preferred first-line management is systemic propranolol (starting with 0.5 mg/kg/day and increased to 2 mg/kg/day) which should be given under care of a pediatrician. Other options include intralesional steroids and systemic steroids.

Lymphangioma

Treatment options include:
- *Surgical debulking/removal:* Generally, not possible to completely remove due to infiltrative nature of disease and risk of damage to vital structures. Recurrences are common.
- *Sclerosant therapy:* Safer and preferred treatment option. Various sclerosants have been used—bleomycin, OK-432, sodium morrhuate, sodium tetradecyl sulfate.
- Systemic steroids.

Orbital Cellulitis

Chandler's classification divides orbital cellulitis into:
- *Group 1:* Preseptal cellulitis
- *Group 2:* Orbital cellulitis
- *Group 3:* Subperiosteal abscess
- *Group 4:* Intraorbital abscess
- *Group 5:* Cavernous sinus thrombosis.

Treatment of orbital cellulitis is summarized in **Flowchart 5**.

Rhabdomyosarcoma

Rhabdomyosarcoma is the most common primary malignant orbital tumor in children.
- *Surgical excision:* When rhabdomyosarcoma is suspected clinically and radiologically, a complete excision biopsy should be attempted.
- *Further treatment:* Depends on whether tumor-free margins are obtained on biopsy and includes chemotherapy or a combination of chemotherapy and radiotherapy.

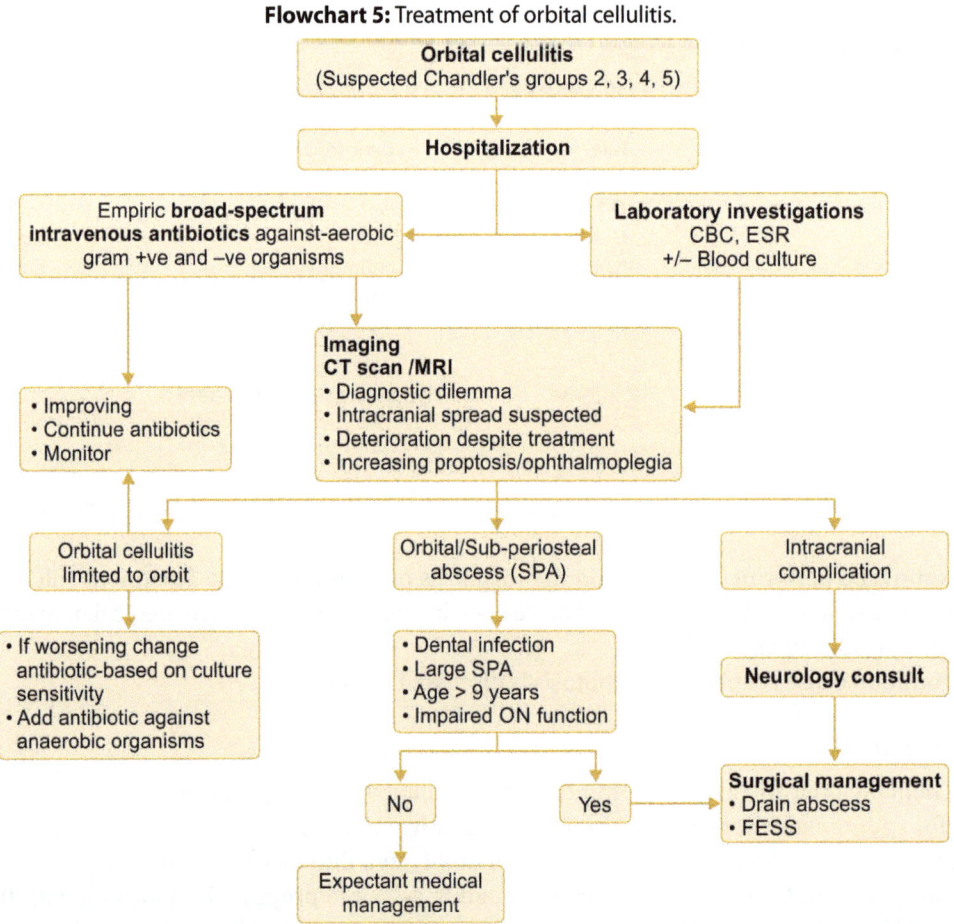

Flowchart 5: Treatment of orbital cellulitis.

(CBC: complete blood count; ESR: erythrocyte sedimentation rate; FESS: functional endoscopic sinus surgery; ON: optic nerve)

- *Chemotherapy:* Vincristine, actinomycin D, cyclophosphamide, ifosfamide, etoposide
- *Radiotherapy:* 4,000–5,000 cGy over 6 weeks.

 4. A middle-aged female presents with unilateral proptosis of 1 year duration. Discuss differential diagnosis, evaluation, and management.

For differential diagnosis, **Box 2**.

BOX 1: Differential diagnosis of unilateral proptosis.

- *Inflammatory:*
  - TED
  - IOID
  - *Specific causes of inflammation:*
    - Sarcoidosis
    - Wegener's granulomatosis
- *Vascular:*
  - Cavernous hemangioma
  - Varices
  - AVM
- *Neoplastic:*
  - Lymphoma and lymphoproliferative lesions
  - *Lacrimal gland tumors:*
    - Pleomorphic adenoma
    - Adenoid cystic carcinoma
  - *Neural:*
    - ON meningioma
    - Schwannoma
  - *Mesenchymal:*
    - Fibro-osseous lesions
    - Hemangiopericytoma/SFT
  - *Secondary/metastasis:*
    - Breast carcinoma
    - Thyroid carcinoma
    - Pulmonary carcinoma
    - Nasopharyngeal carcinoma
    - Visceral malignancies
  - *Histiocytic lesions:*
    - Langerhans cell histiocytosis
    - Non-Langerhans histiocytosis

(AVM: arteriovenous malformation; IOID: idiopathic orbital inflammatory disease; ON: optic nerve; SFT: solitary fibrous tumors; TED: thyroid eye disease)

For management and evaluation, refer to **Flowcharts 2 to 4**.

 5. A 50-year-old female presents with abaxial proptosis. Discuss differential diagnosis, evaluation, and management.

Refer to **Flowchart 6** for details on differential diagnosis, and **Flowcharts 2 to 4** for details on evaluation and management.

 6. Discuss the differential diagnosis of pulsatile proptosis. Outline your approach to their investigation and management.

The differential diagnosis of pulsatile proptosis is:
- Carotid cavernous fistula
- Neurofibromatosis
- Meningocele

Flowchart 6: Differential diagnosis of abaxial proptosis.

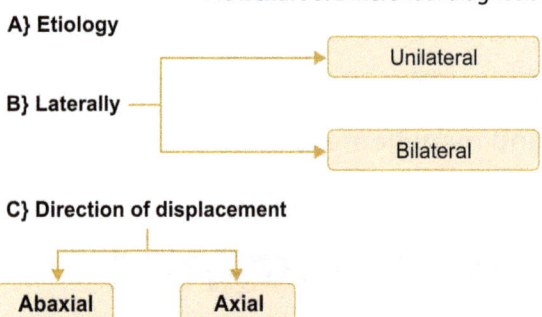

A} Etiology
B} Laterally
- Unilateral
- Bilateral

C} Direction of displacement
- Abaxial
- Axial

Abaxial (Non Axial) proptosis is the displacement of the eyeball in the direction opposite from the lesion.

Inferior displacement
- Lacrimal gland lesions/tumors—benign/mixed tumor or lymphoid tumor
- Frontal sinus lesions/mucocoele
- Sphenoid wing meningioma
- Orbital roof fracture (Blow in fracture)
- Enchephalocele

Lateral displacement
- Lacrimal sac lesions
- Ethmoid sinus mucocele/abscess
- Ethmoid sinus carcinoma

Superior displacement
Maxillary sinus carcinoma/lymphoid tumor

Medial displacement
Lacrimal gland lesions/tumors

Flowchart 7: Approach to pulsatile proptosis.

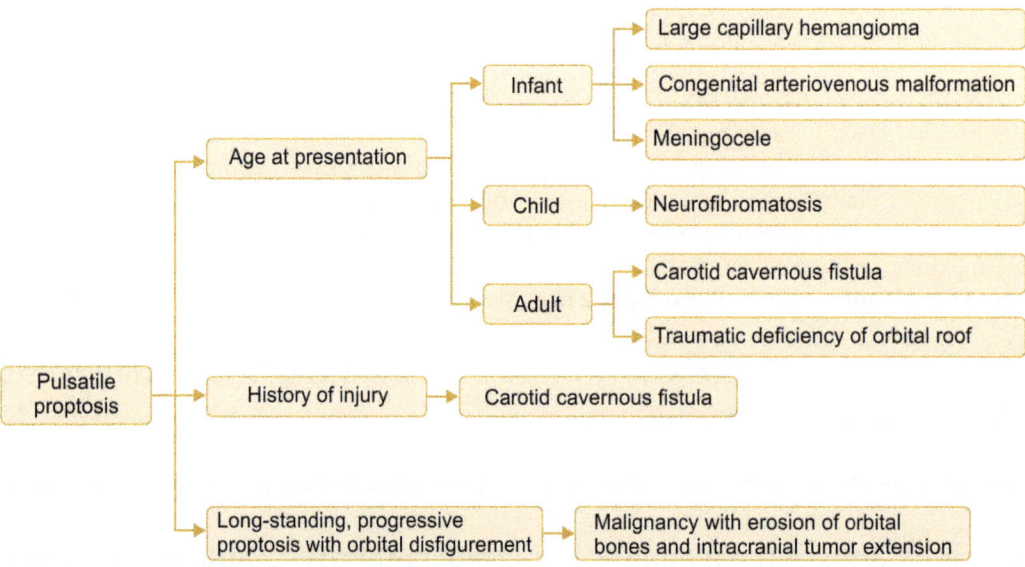

- Erosions in chronic infections/malignancies
- Large capillary hemangioma
- Traumatic/operative deficiency of orbital roof

The approach and investigations for pulsatile proptosis are shown in **Flowcharts 7 and 8.**

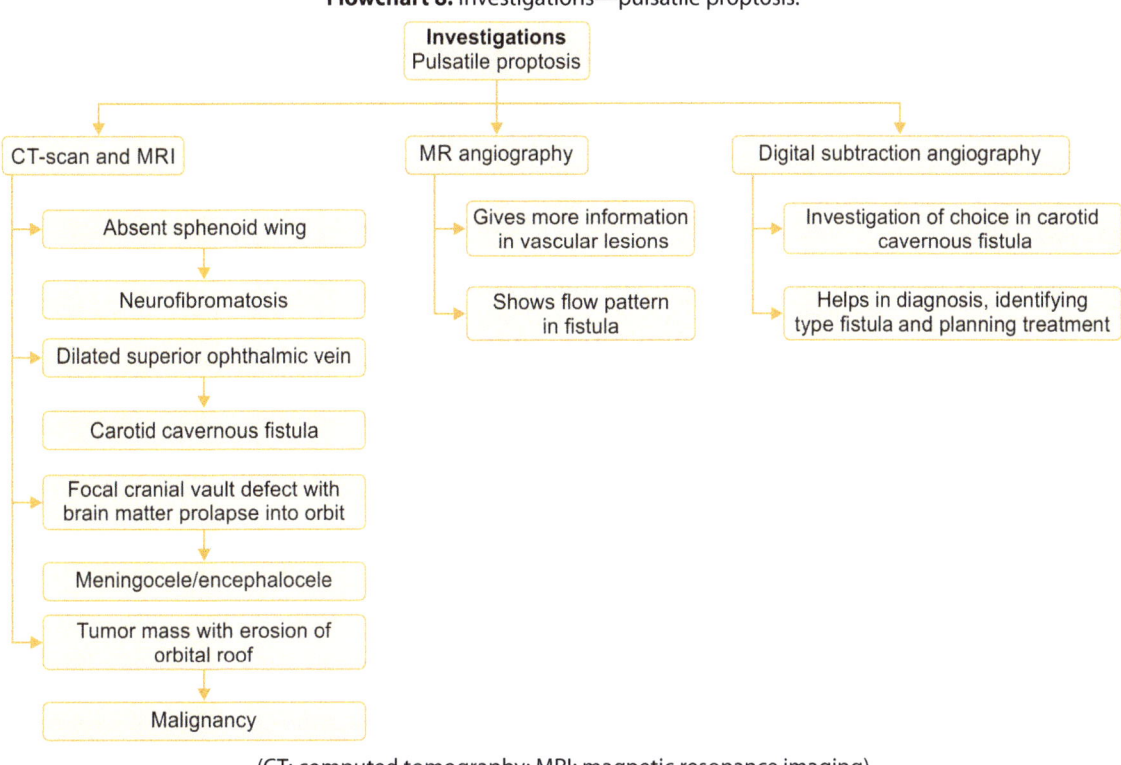

Flowchart 8: Investigations—pulsatile proptosis.

(CT: computed tomography; MRI: magnetic resonance imaging)

Q 7. Explain exophthalmometry.

Proptosis is defined as the prominence of the eye or eyes, secondary to an orbital space-occupying lesion other than dysthyroid orbitopathy.

Exophthalmos has been used interchangeably with proptosis, though Henderson et al. used it to describe prominent eyes secondary to dysthyroid orbitopathy.

Exophthalmometry is the measurement of the amount of proptosis.

Importance of Exophthalmometry

- Presence of proptosis/enophthalmos
- Differentiate between true and pseudoproptosis
- Progression of proptosis
- Response of proptosis to treatment
  All instruments are used to measure the distance between the lateral orbital rim and the lateral orbital wall.

Classification of Exophthalmometry

- *Clinical—Nafziger's sign:* The patient sits on a chair and tilts his head backward and looks upward. The clinician stands behind the patient. He adjusts the head of the patient to a position, where the upper and lower orbital rim align. The protrusion of the corneal apex in relation to the orbital rim is reviewed for proptosis.
- *Proptometry:* A transparent scale/ruler is used to measure the amount of proptosis. The edge of the ruler is placed at a point on the deep lateral orbit wall and the distance between this point and the apex of the cornea is measured.
- *Instrument exophthalmometry:* Various instruments are used to measure the amount of proptosis.

Types of Exophthalmometers

- *Lueddes:* This consists of a transparent arrow-shaped ruler with markings on it. It eliminates parallax and allows the clinician to directly measure the amount of protrusion.

- *Naugles:* This exophthalmometer rests its footplate on the superior and inferior orbital rim. Due to this, it can measure proptosis even in a patient who has undergone lateral orbitotomy.
- Zehenders, Gormaz
- Hertel exophthalmometer—most commonly used
- *Radiological—CT scan orbits:* A special contact lens with a central radiopaque dot is placed on the cornea. The measurement from the apex of the cornea to the anterior clinoid process of the sella is done.

Types of Measurement

- *Absolute exophthalmometry:* The reading is compared with a known normal value.
- *Comparative exophthalmometry:* The reading is compared from time to time.
- *Relative exophthalmometry:* The reading is compared between the two eyes.

Inference of Measurement

- Value of >21 mm in an eye indicates proptosis
- Value <10–12 mm indicates enophthalmos
- A difference between the two eyes of 2 mm is also indicative of proptosis.
  Interobserver variability is seen when measuring proptosis with a Hertel exophthalmometry, though it is a reliable tool.

Procedure

- The two edges or footplates are placed on the orbital rim. There are internal mirrors with millimeters scales on the right and left sides. The red lines are made to coincide into one, and its distance from the corneal apex is noted for each eye.
- The examiner sits opposite to the patient at eye level.
- To have comparative readings in the future, the baseline measurement is kept constant. The parallax and the resting of the footplate on the lateral orbital rim are some of the disadvantages of the Hertel exophthalmometer.
- Hertel is the most commonly used exophthalmometer.

Suggested Reading

1. Bartalena L, Baldeschi L, Boboridis K, Eckstein A, Kahaly GJ, Marcocci C, et al. The 2016 European Thyroid Association/European Group on Graves' Orbitopathy Guidelines for the management of Graves' orbitopathy. Eur Thyroid J. 2016;5(1):9-26.
2. David L. Disorders of orbit. In: Harley's Pediatric Ophthalmology, 6th edition. Philadelphia, PA: Lippincott Williams & Wilkins; 2013.
3. Kashkouli MB, Beigi B, Noorani MM, Nojoomi M. Hertel exophthalmometry: reliability and interobserver variation. Orbit. 2003; 22(4):239-5.
4. Murthy R, Vemuganti GK, Honavar SG, Naik M, Reddy V. Extramedullary leukemia in children presenting with proptosis. J Hematol Oncol J Hematol Oncol. 2009;2:4.
5. Nerad JA (Ed). Techniques in Ophthalmic Plastic Surgery: A Personal Tutorial. Philadelphia, PA: Saunders, Elsevier; 2010.
6. Rootman DB, Rootman J, Gregory S, Feldman KA, Ma R. Stereotactic fractionated radiotherapy for cavernous venous malformations (hemangioma) of the orbit. Ophthal Plast Reconstr Surg. 2012;28(2):96-102.
7. Tasman W, Jaeger EA, Duane TD. Introduction to orbital disease. In: Duane's Clinical Ophthalmology on CD-ROM. Philadelphia, PA: Lippincott Williams & Wilkins; 2006.

1.18 Thyroid Eye Disease

Varshita H Vasanthapuram, Kavya B Madhuri

 1. Discuss the etiopathogenesis, clinical features, diagnosis, indication for intervention, and management of thyroid-related ophthalmopathy.

Thyroid-related ophthalmopathy or thyroid eye disease (TED) or thyroid-associated ophthalmopathy (TAO) or Graves' ophthalmopathy (GO) is characterized by the pathological changes that occur in periocular and orbital tissue as an effect of dysthyroidism. It is an immunomediated inflammatory disorder that produces expansion of the extraocular muscles (EOMs) and fat in the orbit. It may occur in patients with hyperthyroid, euthyroid, or hypothyroid autoimmune disorders. The clinical spectrum of presentation is wide and varied ranging from mild symptoms to sight-threatening condition.

Etiopathogenesis

Thyroid eye disease is a chronic autoimmune inflammatory disorder affecting a variety of tissues that include the periorbital skin, EOMs, orbital fat, and lacrimal gland. It promotes tissue expansion from glycosaminoglycan (GAG) deposition and edema, as well as fibrosis from collagen production and myofibroblastic proliferation.

The pathogenesis can be described under three main phenomena:
1. *Inflammation* of the periorbital soft tissues
2. Overproduction of *GAGs* by orbital fibroblasts
3. *Hyperplasia* of adipose tissue.

Cellular and Molecular Mechanisms

The following changes at the histological level lead to the above-mentioned phenomena:

Principal target is the *orbital fibroblast*. It is the thyroid-stimulating hormone receptor (TSHR)-expressing cell against which the autoimmune process is targeted in TED. They also express high levels of insulin-like growth factor-1 receptor (IGF-1R).

Autoantibodies against TSHR (present on thyroid follicular cells) bind to the TSHR expressed on orbital fibroblasts. There is *activation of helper T-cells* recognizing TSHR peptides presented by orbital fibroblasts or resident antigen-presenting cells leading to the local secretion of inflammatory cytokines and chemokines.

Further, ligation of TSHR on orbital fibroblasts by circulating autoantibodies results in *increased hyaluronan production and enhanced adipogenesis* within the orbital fibroblast population **(Fig. 1)**.

There is mononuclear cell infiltration in the EOM, levator muscle, lacrimal gland, and adipose tissue in active disease, i.e., CD4+ T-cells primarily with minor population of CD8+ cells, B-cells, plasma cells, and macrophages.

In early disease, type 1 helper T-cells predominate which secrete interleukin-2 (IL-2), interferon (IFN) gamma, and tumor necrosis factor (TNF), indicating ongoing cell-mediated immunity within the orbit.

In longer duration disease, type 2 helper T-cells dominate which produce IL-4, -5, -10, transforming growth factor (TGF-β), and propagate autoantibody production **(Fig. 2)**.

Mechanism Underlying Fat or Muscle Predominant Disease

Based on the presence or absence of cell surface glycoprotein CD90 (thymocyte antigen-1 or Thy-1), the orbital fibroblasts can be classified as Thy-1+ and Thy-1–. The relative proportions of these two types of fibroblasts and their degree of exposure to TGF-β determines whether muscle or fat expansion predominates and the extent of fibrosis. The adipogenic potential of orbital fibroblasts decreases with age. There is relative predominance of Thy-1+ fibroblasts in older patients **(Fig. 3)**.

The role of mi-RNA 21 expression has also been implicated in the promotion of fibrosis in orbital fibroblasts in TED.

Clinical Features

The clinical manifestations of TED are a direct consequence of the soft tissue changes which take place at the histological level, i.e., GAG deposition, edema during the active phase and fibrosis in the inactive phase.

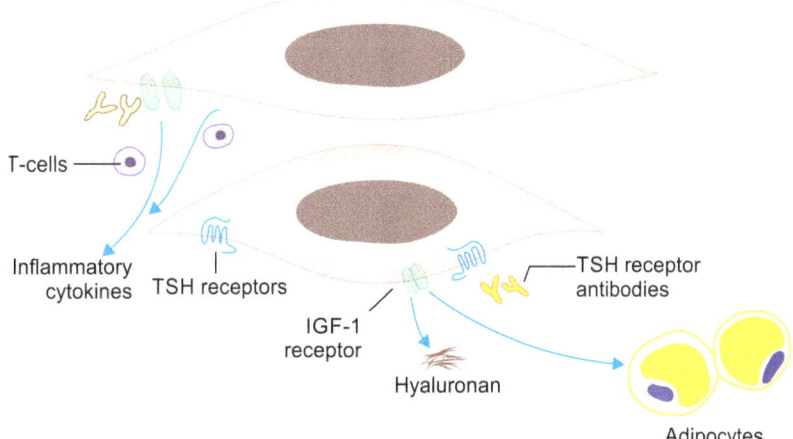

Fig. 1: Pathophysiology of thyroid eye disease: Interplay of cellular and molecular mechanisms.
(IGF-1: insulin-like growth factor 1; TSH: thyroid-stimulating hormone)

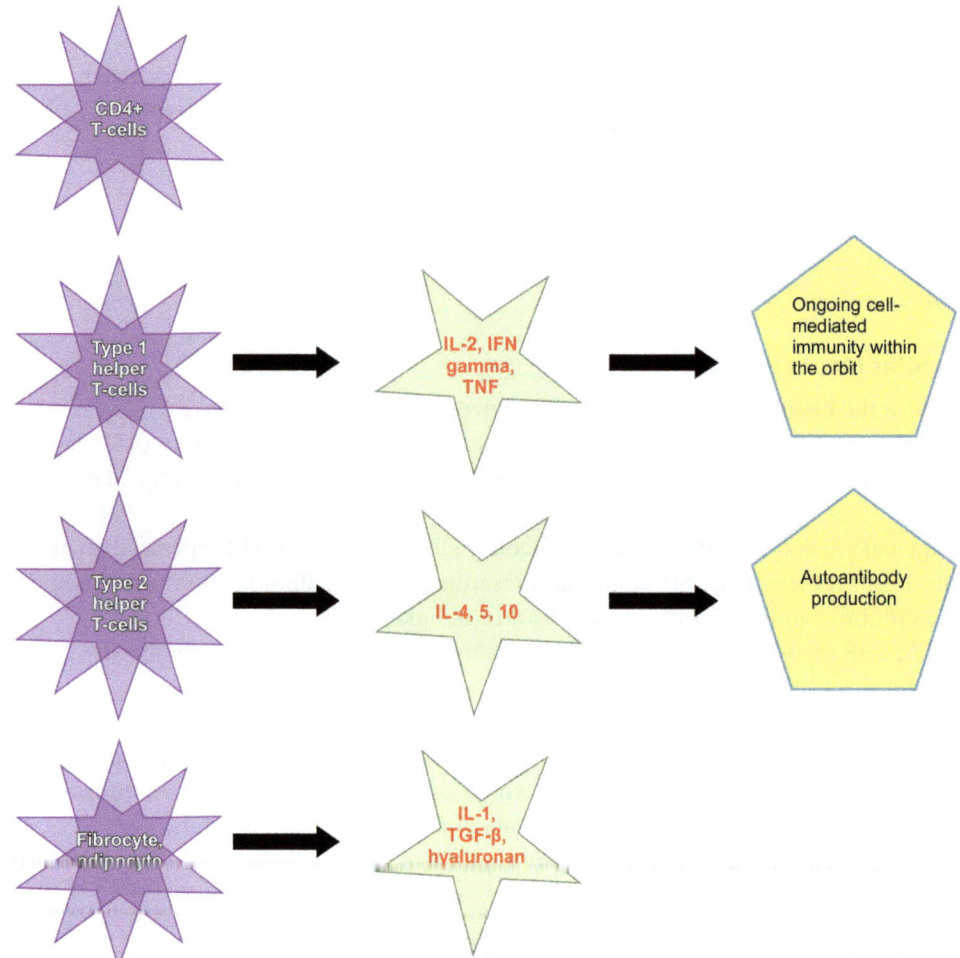

Fig. 2: Role of T helper cells in pathogenesis of thyroid eye disease.
(IFN: interferon; IL-2: interleukin-2; TGF: transforming growth factor; TNF: tumor necrosis factor)

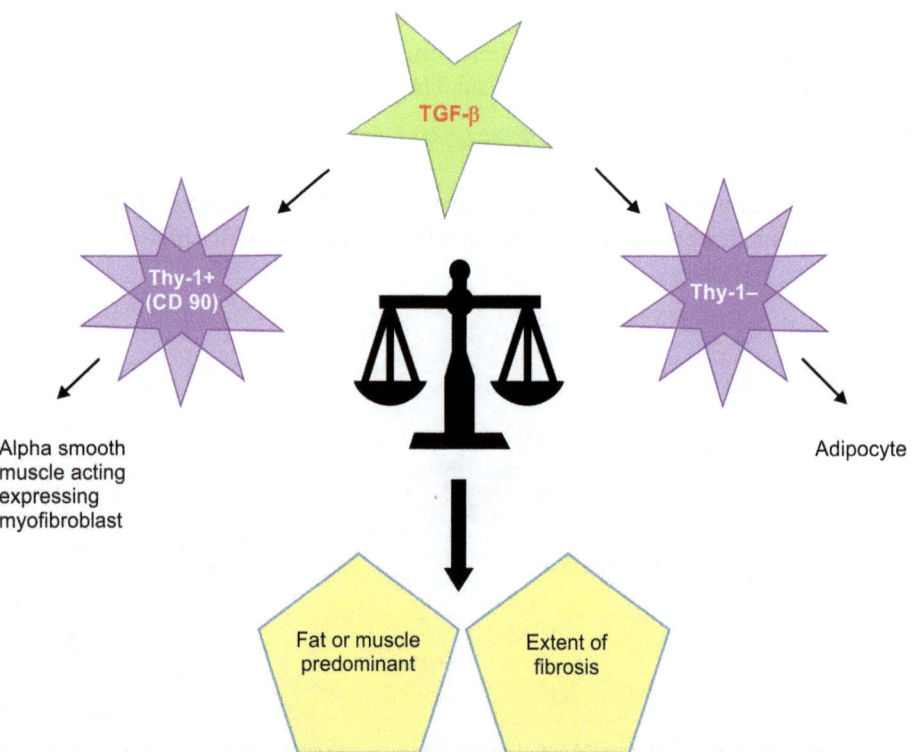

Fig. 3: The two subgroups of orbital fibroblasts and their role in development of a fat predominant or a muscle predominant disease.
(TGF: transforming growth factor)

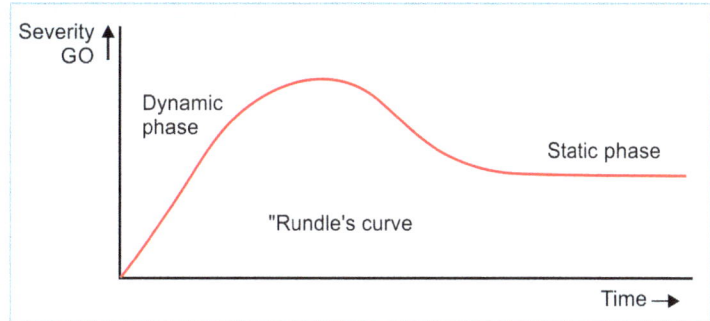

Fig. 4: The Rundle's curve. (GO: Graves' ophthalmopathy)

Timeline of the Changes

The Rundles curve: Francis Felix Rundle was the first to describe "the behavior of the principal ocular changes during the dynamic phase of protrusion and recession" of GO through "ideal and theoretical curves" through his astute observations which he published in several papers the 1940s. This is what we know today as the Rundle's curve. The curve represents the timeline of TED. Severity of GO plotted on the y axis against time on x axis. The curve has a peak which is the dynamic phase or the active phase followed by a plateau which is the static phase or the inactive phase **(Fig. 4)**. Active phase typically lasts 12–18 months but may extend up to 36 months in smokers.

Clinical Features

- Proptosis and eyelid retraction are the most common presenting signs.
- Upper eyelid retraction is more common in the Caucasians, whereas lower eyelid retraction is more common in Asians and Indians.
- Axial proptosis together with eyelid retraction gives rise to dry eyes and cause troublesome exposure-related symptoms.
- Approximately up to 5% patients can have optic neuropathy.
- Others include diplopia and motility limitation. A small proportion of patients present with blepharoptosis and microbial keratitis.

In the active phase, the signs and symptoms are secondary to inflammation and tissue expansion in the orbit leading to increased intraorbital pressure.

The cardinal signs of inflammation (rubor, calor, tumor, dolor, function laesa) are manifested as lid swelling and erythema, conjunctival congestion and chemosis, proptosis, motility limitation, and orbital pain. The secondary effects include exposure keratopathy, microbial keratitis, corneal breakdown, ocular hypertension (HTN), and secondary glaucoma. The latter can partly be attributed to increased venous pressure.

Periocular features such as glabellar lines, prominent brows, prominent eyelid fat pads, and malar festoons, are also seen.

Atrophy, fibrosis, and sclerosis in various tissues in the aftermath of inflammation give rise to the signs in the static or inactive phase.

There is either a fat disease or a muscle predominant disease or mixed disease. Patients under the age of 40 years tend to have fat expansion, whereas those >60 years of age have more EOM expansion.

Diagnosis

Gorman and Bartley proposed the criteria for diagnosing TED in 1995.

Graves' ophthalmopathy is considered to be present if eyelid retraction occurs in association with objective evidence of thyroid dysfunction or abnormal regulation, exophthalmos (>20 mm Hertel exophthalmometry measurement), optic nerve dysfunction, or EOM involvement [either restrictive myopathy or evidence of enlarged muscle on imaging computed tomography (CT)/ magnetic resonance imaging (MRI)/ultrasonography (USG)].

The ophthalmic signs may be unilateral or bilateral, and confounding causes must be excluded. If eyelid retraction is absent, then GO may be diagnosed only if exophthalmos, optic nerve involvement, or restrictive extraocular myopathy is associated with thyroid dysfunction or abnormal regulation and if no other cause for the ophthalmic feature is apparent.

Indications for Intervention

A patient of TED should be assessed for activity (refers to the inflammatory process) and severity (refers to the quality of life or the risk of vision loss). Intervention is based on degree of severity and activity.

TABLE 1: Clinical Activity Score (CAS) (amended by EUGOGO after Mourits et al.).	
For initial CAS, only score items 1–7	
1	Spontaneous orbital pain
2	Gaze-evoked orbital pain
3	Eyelid swelling that is considered to be due to active GO
4	Eyelid erythema
5	Conjunctival redness that is considered to be due to active GO
6	Chemosis
7	Inflammation of caruncle OR plica
Patients assessed after follow-up (1–3 months) can be scored out of 10 by including items 8–10	
8	Increase of >2 mm in proptosis
9	Decrease in uniocular ocular excursion in any one direction of >8°
10	Decrease of acuity equivalent to 1 Snellen line
(GO: Graves' ophthalmopathy)	

There are several assessment protocols for the same namely the NO SPECS Classification by Werner, Clinical Activity Score (CAS) by Mourits, VISA (Vision, Inflammation, Strabismus, Appearance) classification, and European Group on Graves' Orbitopathy (EUGOGO) classification.

The NO SPECS classification grades clinical severity and the CAS grades the activity, whereas the VISA and EUGOGO classifications assess the signs of activity and the degree of severity. They help in guiding the treatment of TED.

European Group on Graves' Orbitopathy Classification

First established in 1999, it uses the modified CAS for assessing the clinical activity (amended by EUGOGO after Mourits et al.). One point is given for the presence of each of the parameters assessed **(Table 1)**. The sum of all points defines clinical activity: active ophthalmopathy if the score is above 3/7 at the first examination or above 4/10 in successive examinations.

As per EUGOGO, the severity of disease is divided as mild, moderate-to-severe, and sight-threatening:

- *Mild:* Characteristics of GO have a minimum impact on the patient's life. They usually present one or more of the following signs:
  - Minor lid retraction (<2 mm).
  - Mild soft tissue involvement.
  - Exophthalmos <3 mm (above the normal range for the race and gender).
  - Transient or no diplopia.
  - Corneal exposure responsive to lubricants.
- *Moderate to severe:* Patients without sight-threatening GO whose eye disease has sufficient impact on daily life to justify the risks of immunosuppression (if active) or surgical intervention (if inactive). Patients usually present one or more of the following signs:
  - Lid retraction (>2 mm).
  - Moderate or severe soft tissue involvement.
  - Exophthalmos ≥3 mm (above the normal range for the race and gender).
  - Inconstant or constant diplopia.
- *Sight-threatening GO:* Patients with dysthyroid optic neuropathy or corneal breakdown due to severe exposure. Other infrequent cases are ocular globe subluxation, severe forms of frozen eye, choroidal folds, and postural visual darkenings. This category warrants immediate intervention.

As a rule of thumb, all patients who do not have a mild or a sight-threatening ophthalmopathy are categorized as moderate-to-severe disease.

VISA Classification

It was developed by Dolman and Rootman in 2006.

The VISA system is based on symptoms and signs inputs. It assesses four severity parameters **(Table 2)**: V (vision); I (inflammation/congestion); S (strabismus/motility restriction); and A (appearance/exposure).

TABLE 2: The VISA system (developed by Dolman and Rootman in 2006).

Sign or symptom	Score
Caruncular edema	• 0: Absent • 1: Present
Chemosis	• 0: Absent • 1: Conjunctiva lies behind the gray line of the lid • 2: Conjunctiva extends anterior to the gray line of the lid
Conjunctival redness	• 0: Absent • 1: Present
Lid redness	• 0: Absent • 1: Present
Lid edema	• 0: Absent • 1: Present but without redundant tissues • 2: Present and causing bulging in the palpebral skin, including lower lid festoon
Retrobulbar ache • At rest • With gaze	 • 0: Absent; 1: present • 0: Absent; 1: present
Diurnal variation	• 0: Absent • 1: Present

(VISA: Vision, Inflammation, Strabismus, Appearance)

Each feature is considered and graded independently.

A global severity grade (maximum score is 20 points) is the sum of each of the involved systems graded independently: vision: 1 point; inflammation/congestion: 10 points; strabismus: 6 points (diplopia: 3 points plus restriction: 3 points); appearance/exposure: 3 points.

Vision (V): Assessed through visual acuity, pupillary reflexes, color vision, visual fields, optic nerve examination, and visual evoked potentials.

Inflammation (I): Soft tissue inflammation is graded according to the worst score for the eye or the eyelid as per the inflammatory index.

Patients with moderate inflammatory index (<4 of 10) are managed conservatively. Patients with high scores (>4 of 10) or with evidence of progression in the inflammation are offered a more aggressive therapy.

Strabismus/motility restriction (S) is documented by three aspects:
1. Diplopia that is graded from 0 to 3 (0 = no diplopia, 1 = diplopia with horizontal or vertical gaze, 2 = intermittent diplopia in straight gaze, and 3 = constant diplopia in straight gaze).
2. Ocular ductions are measured to the nearest 5° in four directions using the corneal light reflex technique. Any change of ≥12° in any direction can be considered progression.
3. Ocular restriction can be graded from 0 to 3 based on the range of ductions (0 = duction >45°, 1 = 30–45°, 2 = 15–30°, and 3 = <15°).

Appearance/exposure (A) symptoms include appearance concerns, i.e., bulging eyes, eyelid retraction, and fat pockets and those due to ocular exposure, i.e., gritting sensation, photophobia, dryness, and secondary tearing. Signs include measurements of eyelid retraction (millimeters from the pupillary light reflex to the lid margin); scleral show (millimeters from the limbus to the lid margin); levator palpebrae superioris function; lagophthalmos (incomplete eyelid closure); and proptosis with Hertel exophthalmometer.

Management

- *Investigations:*
  - *Blood investigations specific to TED:*
    - Thyroid function test (TFT)—free T3, free T4, TSH
    - Antibody assays—TRAb (thyroid receptor antibody)

    (Refer Answer 2 for more description)

- *Imaging:* Various imaging modalities are used in the assessment of TED: Orbital ultrasonography, CT and MRI. CT is widely used in the clinics. MRI with diffusion-weighted imaging (DWI) has recently been proven to be useful in the objective assessment of activity.

  Imaging helps in:
  - Determining the type of orbitopathy—type 1 orbitopathy (lipogenic variant) or type 2 orbitopathy (myogenic variant) is differentiated depending on which component is predominant.
  - Assessing the optic nerve, stretch due to proptosis, and compression in apical crowding due to enlarged EOM in optic neuropathy
  - Assessing the bony orbit, sinuses, and surgical planning for orbital decompression

- *Treatment:* TED is treated based on the severity of disease. There are various medical and surgical modalities of management. Medical therapy is the first line in the treatment of active disease. Surgical intervention is usually performed in inactive or stable phase unless indicated.

  However, the following measures apply to all cases of TED:
  - Restoration of systemic euthyroid levels and stabilizing the same. Monitoring should be performed every 4-6 weeks during the initial period. Uncontrolled thyroid dysfunctions are prone to develop severe TED.
  - Cessation of active or passive smoking.
  - General measures—sleeping with head end elevated, use of artificial tears, sunglasses, and nocturnal ointment in cases of incomplete eyelid closure helps.
  - Treatment of comorbidities like diabetes mellitus (DM).

Medical Treatment

- Medical treatment includes use of topical lubricating drops to address dry eye and exposure keratopathy symptoms; parenteral or oral steroids to address inflammation; certain immunosuppressive drugs; and orbital radiotherapy.
- Newer biological agents which include teprotumumab and tocilizumab.

The treatment strategies for different severity of disease are described here (as per EUGOGO protocol):

- *Mild disease:*
  - Artificial tears
  - Sunglasses
  - Head of the bed slightly elevated
  - Selenium (200 µg daily ~6 months)
  - Fresnel-type prisms
  - Botulinum toxin in Müller muscle
- *Moderate-to-severe disease:*
  - *Intravenous (IV) methylprednisolone:*
    - 1st, 500 mg/week ~6 weeks
    - 2nd, 250 mg/week ~6 weeks
    - 3rd, if activity persists: Consider prolongation of treatment up to 8 g of maximum cumulative dosage
    - 4th, if nonresponsive after 6 weeks, change the treatment.
  - *Patients resistant to glucocorticoids:*
    - Association of cyclosporin A (5 mg/kg/day in two doses) plus oral glucocorticoids, methotrexate (7.5-10 mg/week), tocilizumab (8 mg/kg/every 4 weeks), and rituximab (500-1,000 mg)
    - *If muscular involvement predominates:* Orbital radiotherapy (20 Gy) (not in <35 years or diabetic patients)
  - Consider botulinum toxin in EOMs if with diplopia (medial rectus or inferior rectus)
- *Sight-threatening disease:*
  - *Dysthyroid optic neuropathy:*
    - Methylprednisolone 1 g intravenously for 3 days, repeat after a week.
    - *If nonresponsive:* Urgent orbital decompression (deep orbital medial wall +/− glucocorticoids intravenously if still active +/− radiotherapy).
  - *Severe exposure keratopathy:* Intravenous methylprednisolone when relevant orbital inflammation; palpebral closure, lubrication, tarsorrhaphy, botulinum toxin in Müller muscle; and orbital decompression if other measures are inefficient.

Orbital Radiotherapy

- Orbital radiotherapy is a second-line therapy. It does not show benefits during the early phase of treatment but have long-lasting effects.
- The lymphocytes which infiltrate the orbital soft tissue are radiosensitive, radiotherapy acts by nonspecific anti-inflammatory effects and reduce the secretion of proinflammatory cytokines from activated lymphocytes.
- It also targets orbital fibroblasts inducing terminal differentiation in progenitor fibroblasts, suppressing the downstream consequences of fibroblast activation by reducing their capability to synthesize and secrete GAGs.
- The treatment regimen is 20 Gy in 10 divided doses over 2 weeks. Systemic steroids should be given during radiotherapy.
- Indications include active TED, muscle predominant disease. Diabetes is a relative contraindication. Patients with uncontrolled HTN and DM are poor candidates.
- Side effects include radiation retinopathy (1%), cataract, and dry eye.

Immunotherapies in Thyroid Eye Disease

(Refer to answer 6 for description).

Surgery

Surgical rehabilitation is aimed at addressing proptosis, strabismus, eyelid abnormalities, and cosmetic concerns and usually performed in the inactive phase. However, there are a few procedures which should be performed in the *active phase* as follows:

- *Tarsorrhaphy:* Exposure keratopathy, microbial keratitis, corneal breakdown. In cases of severe eyelid retraction or proptosis, tarsorrhaphy can be combined with levator palpebrae superioris (LPS) recession or botulinum toxin injection.
- *Orbital decompression:* In cases of sight-threatening TED, i.e., dysthyroid optic neuropathy or severe exposure keratopathy, two-wall or three-wall orbital decompression can be performed. Medial wall decompression can be performed via transcaruncular approach or endoscopic approach.
- *As temporary measures: Local steroid/botulinum toxin injection/fillers:* Intraorbital injection of steroid, steroid injection in the upper eyelid. Botulinum injection into the LPS can induce ptosis and improve exposure keratitis.

Surgical rehabilitation during *inactive phase* is aimed to address the four aspects, i.e., proptosis, restrictive strabismus, eyelid abnormality (retraction), and cosmetic concerns (fat bags, rhytids).

They are addressed in a staged manner. Traditionally, the orbital surgery is performed first followed by strabismus correction and eyelid correction.

In select cases, a customized orbital decompression is performed addressing the proptosis and eyelid/strabismus in a single session.

- *Orbital decompression:*
  - Depending on the degree of proptosis, graded one-wall/two-wall/three-wall or a four-wall decompression can be planned as follows:
    - *First wall:* Fat 2–3 mm
    - *Second wall:* Lateral wall 3–6 mm
    - *Third wall:* Medial wall 4–7 mm
    - *Fourth wall:* Orbital floor 5–9 mm

  Decompression of the roof is also described but reserved in extreme cases owing to the risk and complications involved.
  - *Approaches:* Various approaches to orbital decompression include:
    - *Transorbital:* Eyelid crease incision, inferior transconjunctival incision, lateral canthotomy, swinging eyelid incision.
    - *Coronal:* Simultaneous bilateral orbital decompression can be performed.
    - *Endoscopic:* Preferred for emergency orbital decompression in cases of optic neuropathy. Medial wall and floor decompression can be performed via this approach.
    - *Transantral approach:* Via the maxillary sinus through an intraoral incision
- *Strabismus surgery:*
  - Diplopia is the most disabling effect of TED and the most challenging to manage. Asymmetric fibrosis of the recti results in strabismus.
  - Most favorable results are obtained if operated in the inactive stable phase of the disease after ensuring stable measurements over a 6-month period.

- Surgical goal is to provide binocular single vision for maximum range as possible, particularly in the primary gaze and downgaze.
- Preoperative orthoptic measurements should be noted in all gazes, any secondary muscle involvement should be noted.
- Intraoperative forced duction test should be performed.
- In case of more than single muscle involvement in each eye, surgery should be performed in two stages, the first addressing the largest deviation—horizontal or vertical.
- Adjustable surgery improves outcomes.
- Most commonly, recession of EOMs is performed, though rarely muscles may be resected.
- Recession of the Tenon capsule along with recession of the muscle is effective in prevention of limited globe rotation.

- *Eyelid surgery:* Eyelid surgery is mainly directed at correcting eyelid retraction.
Various procedures are described which may be performed either via the anterior transcutaneous approach or posterior transconjunctival approach, namely—
  - Müllerectomy
  - Levator recession
  - Combination of the above with or without partial or complete lateral horn division (of the levator)
  - Levator recession with spacer grafts and adjustable sutures has also been described.

  Upper eyelid retraction: Graded surgery can be performed depending on the degree of eyelid retraction:
  - *Mild:* Müllerectomy (1–2 mm)
  - *Moderate:* Levator recession +/– müllerectomy
  - *Severe:* Levator recession + müllerectomy with lateral horn division or Koorneef blepharotomy

  Lower eyelid retraction:
  - Lower eyelid retractor release
  - Recession with spacer graft—sclera or dermal fat graft or mucus membrane or upper eyelid tarsus in severe cases

- *Cosmetic concerns:* Cosmetic concerns include eyelid fat bags, periorbital hollows, and rhytids such as glabellar folds. These issues are addressed at the fourth stage of surgical rehabilitation toward the end with an individualistic approach to restore the normal appearance.

Several options are available in the armamentarium, which include blepharoplasty, botulinum toxin, and fillers. Lacrimal gland can be addressed during decompression by performing lateral wall decompression or can also be fixed to the periosteum by lacrimal gland fixation procedure.

 2. Describe various thyroid function tests; give clinical picture and management of hyperthyroidism with special regard to ocular involvement/thyroid ophthalmopathy.

Autoimmune thyroid disease (AITD) is a spectrum of thyroid-related autoimmune disorders ranging from Hashimoto's hypothyroidism to Graves' thyrotoxicosis including euthyroid or subclinical variants of Hashimoto's and Graves', lymphocytic thyroiditis, postpartum thyroiditis, and fibrous variants. The pathogenesis and outcome of AITD are multifactorial with genetic and environmental influences.

Hyperthyroidism

- Hyperthyroidism is a pathological condition characterized by increased thyroid hormone synthesis and secretion by thyroid gland leading to excess circulating thyroid hormones resulting in a clinical syndrome called thyrotoxicosis.
- The important causes are Graves' disease, toxic nodular goiter, thyroiditis, iodine-induced and drug-induced thyroid dysfunction, and factitious ingestion of excess thyroid hormone.
- A normal or high thyroid radioactive iodine update differentiates true hyperthyroidism from thyrotoxicosis without hyperthyroidism wherein there is an extra-thyroid source of thyroid hormone.
- *Hyperthyroidism may be overt or subclinical:*
  - *Overt:* Low-serum TSH; raised T3 and/or T4
  - *Subclinical:* Low-serum TSH; normal T3 and T4
- *Epidemiology:* Female preponderance, increased incidence in whites, iodine-deficient areas.
- *Etiology:* Graves' disease, toxic multinodular goiter, solitary toxic adenoma

Graves' Disease

- The etiology of Graves' disease is multifactorial with genetic and environmental influences.
- There is loss of immunotolerance and development of autoantibodies that stimulate thyroid follicular cells by binding to the TSH receptor.
- Genes involved are immune-regulatory genes (HLA region, CD40, CTLA4, PTPN22, and FCRL3) and thyroid autoantigens such as thyroglobulin and TSH receptor genes.
- Nongenetic influences include psychological stress, smoking, and female gender.
- Infection has also been implicated especially *Yersinia enterocolitica* due to molecular mimicry with TSH receptor.
- Other causes include vitamin D deficiency, selenium deficiency, thyroid damage, and immunomodulating drugs.
- The onset of TED and hyperthyroidism may be simultaneous in about a third of cases, precedes hyperthyroidism in about 7–8% cases, and follows it in 60% cases.
- *Clinical presentation:*
  - Symptoms include palpitations, fatigue, tremor, anxiety, disturbed sleep, weight loss, heat intolerance, sweating, and polydipsia.
  - Some of the signs include tachycardia, tremor of the extremities, and weight loss. The excessive circulating thyroid hormones affect every system in the body **(Table 3)**.
  - Extrathyroid manifestations of Graves' disease after from TED include thyroid dermopathy which occurs in 1–4% of patients with TED. Lesions are characterized by slightly pigmented thickened skin, primarily involving the pretibial area. Acropachy is the rarest manifestation wherein there is clubbing of fingers and toes.

Diagnosis

Thyroid Function Tests

Physiology:
- The hypothalamus releases thyrotropin-releasing hormone (TRH) which stimulates the pituitary to release thyroid-stimulating hormone (TSH). TSH regulates the steps involved in the production of thyroid hormones, T3 and T4.
- T4 (thyroxine) is 85% of the released hormone and T3 (triiodothyronine) constitutes 15%.
- The hormones are protein bound (99.8%) and only the free components (free T3 and T4) bind to the receptors in the tissues.
- The active hormone is the free T3. In the periphery, T4 gets converted to the active T3.

Serum Thyroid-stimulating Hormone

- Has the highest sensitivity and specificity, hence should be measured first.
- The relationship between TSH and free thyroid hormones is log-linear, i.e., any small changes in free T3 or T4 will result in large changes in TSH. But any small changes in TSH will cause only minute changes in T3 and T4. So, any changes

TABLE 3: Systemic manifestations of Graves' disease.

	Symptoms	Signs
Constitutional	Weight loss despite increased appetite; heat-related symptoms (heat intolerance, sweating, and polydipsia)	Weight loss
Neuromuscular and skeletal	Tremor; nervousness; anxiety; fatigue; weakness; disturbed sleep; poor concentration	Tremor of the extremities; hyperactivity; hyperreflexia; pelvic and girdle muscle weakness (osteoporosis)
Cardiovascular	Palpitations	Tachycardia; systolic hypertension; irregular heartbeat (atrial fibrillation)
Pulmonary	Dyspnea, shortness of breath	Tachypnea
Gastrointestinal	Hyperdefecation; nausea, vomiting	Abdominal tenderness
Skin	Increased perspiration	Warm and moist skin
Reproductive		Menstrual disturbances and decreased fertility in women, gynecomastia in males (long-standing)
Ocular (Graves')	Diplopia; sense of irritation in the eyes; eyelid swelling; retro-orbital pain; or discomfort	Proptosis; eyelid retraction and lag; periorbital edema; conjunctival injection and chemosis; ophthalmoplegia

in the T3 or T4 within the normal range, reflects in an abnormal change in the TSH level. This makes TSH as a highly sensitive marker of thyroid function in the absence of hypothalamic or pituitary disease.
- As per an analysis of the National Health and Nutrition Examination Survey (NHANES) III database, the upper limit of normal for TSH at the 97.5th percentile is 3.5 mIU/mL for 20–29 year olds increasing to 4.5 mIU/mL for 50–70 year olds and 7.5 mIU/mL for those over the age of 80 years.

Free Thyroxine

- Measurement of free T4 by equilibrium dialysis is considered the gold standard but, it is of limited availability. Most laboratories utilize the direct analog immunoassay (IA) for the measurement of free T4.
- The accuracy of the free T4 level is highly dependent on the method of assay employed which unfortunately has questionable reliability owing to poor accuracy and high false-positive results.
- Hence, there are limited indications for ordering free T4:
  - Assess the degree of hyperthyroidism when TSH is suppressed.
  - To confirm the diagnosis of subclinical hypothyroidism in the setting of a mildly elevated TSH.
  - Monitor response to antithyroid drug therapy and radioiodine (TSH may not be reliable in the initial months after therapy).
  - Monitor L-thyroxine therapy in patients with known pituitary disease (TSH is not reliable).
  - Single assessment to assure TSH is a reliable indicator of thyroid function.

Antithyroid Peroxidase Antibodies (Anti-TPO Ab)

- Thyroid peroxidase is one of the key enzymes involved in catalyzing many steps in the synthesis of T3 and T4.
- Anti-TPO antibodies indicates AITD, especially Hashimoto's thyroiditis, postpartum thyroiditis, and Graves' disease.
- It predicts the risk of developing overt hypothyroidism in euthyroid and subclinical hypothyroid patients.
- Lymphocytic infiltration of thyroid gland gives rise to anti-TPO Ab.
- Indications for ordering its levels include:
  - *Pregnancy:* Performed only for women at risk for hypothyroidism, i.e., with positive family history or personal history or any other associated autoimmune disease
  - Infertility and frequent miscarriages.

Other Thyroid Tests

- *Free T3:* To determine the degree of hyperthyroidism when TSH is suppressed (sometimes used in conjunction with free T4).
- *Reverse T3:* No clinical utility (elevated in nonthyroidal illness).
- *Free thyroxine index:* Evaluation and management of hyperthyroidism during pregnancy.
- *Thyroid-stimulating immunoglobulin and TSH receptor antibodies:* Evaluation of the cause of hyperthyroidism (used in conjunction with thyroid uptake and scan and/or at times when radioiodine scanning cannot be performed, i.e., pregnancy).
- *Thyroglobulin:* Follow-up of differentiated thyroid cancer.
- *Antithyroglobulin antibodies:* Only useful in conjunction with thyroglobulin (to assure reliability of thyroglobulin result).
- *Total T3 and T4:* No clinical utility with the availability of assays for free hormone levels.
- *Free T4 by equilibrium dialysis:* Considered the gold standard for free T4 measurement.

Interpretation of TFT (Table 4)

Flowchart 1 shows the investigation and diagnosis in a case of hyperthyroidism.

TABLE 4: Interpretation of thyroid function tests.

TSH	Free T3 and/or free T4	Diagnosis
Within normal range	Within normal range	Euthyroidism
Increased	Within normal range	Subclinical hypothyroidism
Increased	Decreased	Overt hypothyroidism
Decreased	Within normal range	Subclinical hyperthyroidism
Decreased	Increased	Overt hyperthyroidism

(TSH: thyroid-stimulating hormone)

Flowchart 1: Flowchart to proceed in diagnosing a case of hyperthyroidism.

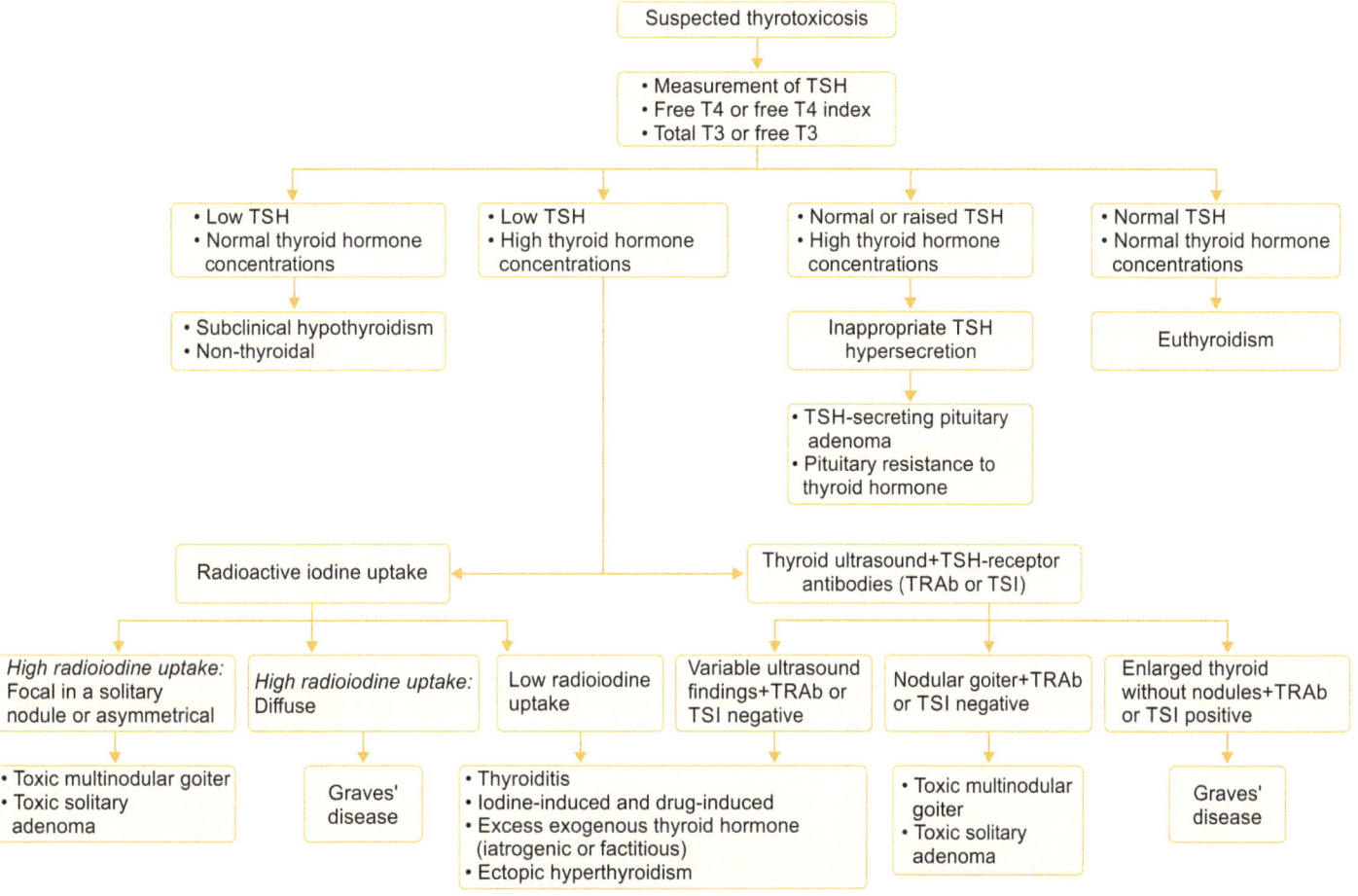

(TRAb: TSH receptor antibody; TSH: thyroid-stimulating hormone; TSI: thyroid stimulating immunoglobulins)

Treatment

The modalities for treatment of hyperthyroidism include antithyroid drugs (ATDs), radioactive iodine ablation, and surgery. Beta blockers help in relieving symptoms of thyrotoxicosis.

Antithyroid Drugs

- The drugs are propylthiouracil, thiamazole, and carbimazole.
- All are actively transported into the thyroid where they inhibit iodide oxidation and organification by inhibiting thyroid peroxidase and the coupling of the iodotyrosines to synthesize T4 and T3.
- Propylthiouracil also decreases the conversion of T4 to T3 in peripheral tissues by inhibiting the outer ring deiodinase of T4.
- Thiamazole is recommended drug in Graves' disease with exceptions during first trimester of pregnancy. Thiamazole has better efficacy, longer half-life, and duration of action compared to propylthiouracil, also less severe side effects.
- *Thiamazole dosage:* Mild hyperthyroidism and small gland 10–15 mg daily
- Severe hyperthyroidism and large gland 20–40 mg daily.
- *Propylthiouracil:* Starting dose 50–150 mg three times daily (starting dose).
- The two approaches to the treatment of Graves' disease are titration, block, and replace. With titration, the dose of antithyroid drugs (ATD) is titrated over time to the lowest dose needed for maintaining a euthyroid state.
- *Block and replace regimen:* A higher dose of ATD is used with concurrent replacement with levothyroxine. Both regimens are equally effective but the titration method has lesser side effects.
- TFT should be performed every 4–6 weeks after initiation of therapy and every 2–3 months after achieving euthyroid state. TSH might remain suppressed for several months, which is why serum T4 and T3 should be monitored to assess efficacy of therapy.

- *Drawback:* High rate of relapse after discontinuation. Relapse is more frequent in the first year after therapy. Assessment of TRAb concentrations at the end of treatment might be useful to identify patients in whom hyperthyroidism will recur after discontinuation of therapy
- Side effects include pruritus, arthralgia, gastrointestinal distress, agranulocytosis, hepatotoxicity, and rarely vasculitis.

Radioactive Iodine Therapy (RAI)

- 10-15 mCi is the dose for treating Graves' disease and 10-20 mCi for toxic nodular goiter when using fixed doses.
- *Contraindications:* Pregnancy, breastfeeding, planning pregnancy, and inability to comply with radiation safety recommendations, thyroid nodule biopsy samples suspicious, or diagnostic of thyroid cancer
- There is increased risk of worsening of TED in those who receive radioactive iodine as compared to ATD or surgery; hence, it is contraindicated in patients with active moderate-severe TED. RAI-induced cell death releases antibodies which worsens the TED.
- Prophylactic steroids should be given in patients with mild active TED starting 1-3 days after initiating radioactive iodine tapered over 3 months.
- RAI can be given in inactive TED without corticosteroid coverage.
- Risk factors for the development and worsening of TED on RAI include smoking, high pretreatment T3 concentration, high TRAb titers, and untreated hypothyroidism post-RAI.
- After RAI, thyroid function should be monitored every 1-2 months. Thyroid replacement should be started as soon as hypothyroidism sets in.

Thyroidectomy

- It is the most successful treatment for Graves' hyperthyroidism. It is recommended in patients with large goiters or low uptake of radioactive iodine (or both); suspected or documented thyroid cancer; moderate-to-severe ophthalmopathy, for which RAI is contraindicated.
- Pregnancy is a relative contraindication.
- Pretreatment with ADT is necessary to achieve euthyroidism before surgery.
- Postsurgery thyroid replacement therapy should be initiated and TSH monitored 6-8 weeks after surgery.
- Side effects include hypocalcemia due to hypoparathyroidism and recurrent laryngeal nerve injury.

 3. Enumerate the ocular changes in thyroid dysfunction and its management.

Thyroid eye disease has various ocular manifestations. The underlying anatomical changes that give rise to the ocular features are enumerated.
- *Eyelid:*
  - *Retraction:* Etiology of upper eyelid retraction is multifactorial:
    - Mechanical factor related to globe proptosis with the upper eyelid draping over the protruding corneal surface.
    - Müller muscle and the inferior tarsal muscle have sympathetic innervation. Sympathetic overaction is a contributing factor to eyelid retraction.
    - Inflammation, fibrosis, and fat infiltration in the Müller muscles have been attributed to be a contributory factor.
    - Lateral flare in the upper eyelid retraction is due to the lateral extension of the Müller's smooth muscle fibers accompanying the lateral horn of the LPS aponeurosis between lobes of lacrimal gland.
    - Levator muscle enlargement or hypertrophy has been proposed to be a likely cause of retraction.
    - Inferior rectus muscle restriction causes overaction of superior rectus and levator muscles from Hering's law.
    - Levator connective tissue system fibrosis and of the suspensory ligaments of the superior conjunctival fornix is contributory.
    - Weakened tone of the orbicularis has also been demonstrated in animal studies. The weakened tone allows overaction of the less opposed levator muscle.
    - *Management:* (Refer to Answer 1 for description)
  - *Eyelid edema:* Histology of edematous eyelid skin shows dilated lymphatic vessels, perivascular cellular infiltrates predominantly lymphocytic, in the dermis, but no deposition of mucopolysaccharide. The mechanism has been attributed to reduced lymphatic flow secondary to reduced ocular motility; and periorbital venous stasis.

- Ocular surface changes lead to unstable tear film and severe dry eye symptoms. Ocular surface inflammation has been implicated in causing increased conjunctival squamous metaplasia associated with a decreased Schirmer tear test and increased tear film break up time.

   Incomplete blink and lagophthalmos also contribute to dry eye symptoms. Topical lubricating drops are the mainstay in management, tarsorrhaphy helps in reducing the lagophthalmos. Eyelid procedures described above can also help in decreasing the palpebral fissure height.
- *EOM:*
  - The EOM are functionally and anatomically distinct from the other striated muscles. Enlargement results in restrictive strabismus. The medial rectus, the inferior rectus muscles, and the superior rectus-levator complex are commonly involved muscles, but all muscles can be enlarged.
  - Histologically, EOMs show focal or diffuse infiltration of CD4+ T-cells, with some B-cells, plasma cells, and macrophages. GAG infiltration, mostly hyaluronan, is a major component, with significant edema resulting from its hydrophilic nature and consequent osmotic pressure.
  - Accumulation of collagen fibrils and GAGs, predominantly hyaluronan. The polyanionic charge and high osmotic pressure renders it hydrophilic resulting in accumulation of fluid. Muscle bodies enlarge to many times their size.
  - Enlarged EOMs typically involve the muscle bellies, a minority of cases show tendon enlargement as well.
  - In the inactive phase, there is atrophy and fibrosis of muscle bundles.
- *Orbital bones:*
  - Orbital soft tissue remodeling is a major feature of TED and includes enlargement of EOMs, adipogenesis, cellular infiltration, and GAG deposition and edema, all of which expand the orbital soft tissue compartment.
  - The enlarged soft tissue prolapse through the anterior deficient portion of the bony orbit manifesting as proptosis.
  - The orbital volume varies from 18.9 to 33.4 mL, and the globe volume from 6.0 to 10.1 mL across individuals. The orbital apex cone angle varies from 39.7 to 65.7°. A narrower cone angle means a narrower area between the expanded EOM and the optic nerve translating to increased risk of optic nerve compression.
  - Increased orbital volume, congestion increases the soft tissue hydrostatic pressure. Soft tissue enlargement can have remodeling effect on the bone. Spontaneous decompression from orbital fractures can occur rarely.
  - The angle between the medial wall and the floor is increased in TED. The medial wall angle from the sagittal plane is decreased. Bony remodeling renders a protective mechanism against dysthyroid optic neuropathy.
  - Orbital decompression expands the bony confines of the orbit opening into the adjacent sinuses—ethmoid and maxillary.
- *Orbital fat:*
  - One of the aspects of TED pathophysiology is adipogenesis.
  - The circulating autoantibodies to TSHR bind to the TSHR present on orbital fibroblasts which stimulate adipogenesis, T-cell infiltration, cytokine release, and hyaluronan deposition.
  - IGF-1 also influences the pathway and enhances the adipogenesis. Hypoxia too enhances adipogenesis through activating hypoxia-inducible factor-1-dependent pathways in orbital fibroblasts. Cigarette smoke extract elevates hypoxia-inducible factor-1 in orbital fibroblasts.
  - In about a fourth of patients, small tongues of fat prolapse through the superior orbital fissure. In a small proportion of patients, extraconal fat can prolapse anteriorly through the Tenon capsule presenting as a superotemporal yellow subconjunctival mass.
  - Fat decompression is performed alone in mild proptosis or in conjunction with bony orbital wall decompression (medial, lateral wall, or floor).
- *Dysthyroid optic neuropathy:*

  The pathophysiology is complex and multifactorial:
  - *Compression:*
    - Enlarged EOM bellies result in crowding at the orbital apex and direct compression of the optic nerve.
    - In early stages of compression, decreased vision is attributed to disruption of axonal transport which can be reversed with corticosteroids or orbital decompression.
    - In late chronic phase, there is permanent visual loss from atrophy of the ganglion cells.
  - *Vascular compromise:*
    - During the active phase of TED, there is vascular compression and reduced flow in the orbital vessels, especially the superior ophthalmic vein owning to its anatomy. As it passes from medial to lateral between the optic nerve and superior rectus muscle, it gets compressed from the enlarged muscle.

- *Stretching of the nerve:*
  - In longer orbit, shorter nerve and significant proptosis, stretching of the nerve can result in ischemic visual loss.
  - Stretching may also result in nerve compression by the myelin sheath on nerve fibers and pial vessels.

Management

Management depends on the degree of compression and vision loss. Early stages can be treated with IV glucocorticoids (as per EUGOGO protocol) which helps reduce edema and congestion. In case of unfavorable response to steroids, orbital decompression is performed. Radiotherapy and immunosuppressive therapy are employed in severe cases. Orbital decompression either bone or fat or both helps reduce the orbital soft tissue volume, prolapse into the sinuses, and expand the bony compartment.

(Refer to Answers 1 and 4 for description)

 4. Orbital decompression techniques in thyroid ophthalmopathy.

- Orbital decompression involves decreasing the orbital pressure and soft tissue volume by planned removal of either fat or bone or both and expanding the confines of bony orbit into the adjacent paranasal sinus, i.e., ethmoid and maxillary sinus.
- There is a decrease in the venous congestion and mechanical pressure on the optic nerve and proptosis reduction.
- Orbital decompression is performed in the inactive phase for disfiguring proptosis; in the active phase it is performed for dysthyroid optic neuropathy and severe exposure keratopathy.
- Four walls of the bony orbit can be decompressed: medial, lateral, floor, and roof.

Preoperative Planning

- *History:* A detailed history of the onset of TED symptoms, systemic thyroid status, any comorbid conditions such as DM or myasthenia gravis are noted.
- Comprehensive ocular examination documenting the vision, pupillary reaction, relative afferent pupillary defect (RAPD), visual fields, ocular alignment and extraocular motility, degree of exophthalmos, the fundus, and optic nerve status. Measurement of eyelid-related parameters: margin to reflex distance (MRD), the palpebral fissure height, tarsal plate show, degree of upper and lower eyelid retraction, superior and inferior scleral show, and lagophthalmos. Interpupillary distance (IPD) can also be noted. Lastly, periocular features such as eyelid fat bags, glabellar lines, and periocular hollows should be documented.
- Premorbid full face photographs can help in customized staged surgical rehabilitation aimed at addressing the cosmetic concerns.
- Preoperative photographs—standard, nine gaze photos, worms view, and side facial profiles.
  - *Imaging:* CT orbit with 2 mm intervals, axial and coronal sections, soft tissue, and bone window is requested. In cases wherein navigation technology–assisted surgery is planned, 1 mm section is requested.
  - *Points to note before surgical planning:*
    - *Type of disease:* Fat or muscle predominant disease
    - Degree of proptosis.
    - *Apex:* EOM thickening, degree of crowding
    - *Optic nerve:* Stretch, compression
    - *Cribriform plate:* Position and relation with the medial wall
    - Ethmoid sinus/maxillary sinus
    - Infraorbital canal location
    - *Lateral wall:* Thickness
    - *Orbital floor:* Thickness
- Preanesthetic work-up and fitness for surgery under for general anesthesia.

Surgical Approaches

As a thumb rule, however, each orbital wall provides approximately 2 mm reduction in proptosis, and fat alone provides approximately 2 mm reduction.
- *Transorbital:* Eyelid crease incision, inferior transconjunctival incision, lateral canthotomy, swinging eyelid incision **(Fig. 5)**.

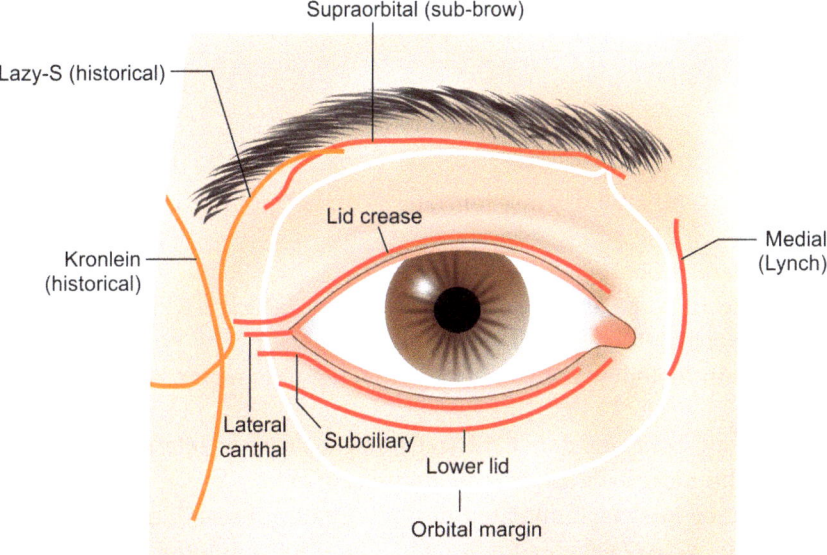

Fig. 5: Various approaches to orbital decompression.

- *Coronal:* Simultaneous bilateral orbital decompression can be performed.
- *Endoscopic:* Preferred for emergency orbital decompression in cases of optic neuropathy. Medial wall and floor decompression can be performed via this approach.
- *Transantral approach:* Via the maxillary sinus through an intraoral incision (Caldwell-Luc).

Fat Decompression

- Fat is considered as the "first wall." It can improve double vision, reduce congestive orbitopathy, proptosis, and compressive optic neuropathy. It is suitable for mild proptosis.
- Fat can be approached transconjunctivally or transcutaneously.
- The fat in TED is vascular, hemostasis achievement is essential during surgery. Fat removal should be performed under direct visualization to minimize the risk of damage to vital structures.
- Fat from the intraconal and/or extraconal compartments can be removed. Fat is usually removed from the inferotemporal quadrant where it is abundant with minimal risk to damage to vital structures. The superomedial quadrant has smaller volume of fat and carries risk to the ethmoidal and supratrochlear neurovascular bundles.
- For every milliliter of fat removal, there is reduction of approximately 0.93 mm of proptosis.
- Decompression can be performed in isolation or can be combined with bony decompression.
- In a muscle predominant disease, fat decompression can be challenging as the fat expansion is minimal and fat is fibrotic. There is increased risk of damage to the enlarged muscle.

Medial Wall

- *Approach:*
  - *Transorbital:* Medial transcaruncular incision, Lynch incision
  - Transantral (Caldwell-Luc), transnasal endoscopic, coronal
- *Bones removed:* Ethmoid
- Medial orbital wall decompression is graded and includes removal of the ethmoid bone, the palatine and posterior infraorbital strut are also removed in cases of apical crowding causing optic neuropathy or orbital congestion and in cases requiring maximal proptosis reduction.
- The anterior limit is the posterior lacrimal crest, posterior limit can extend up to the anterior wall of the sphenoid sinus.
- Anterior strut sparing reduces risk of postoperative diplopia.
- *Superior extent:* Frontoethmoidal suture. The surgeon should be mindful of the skull base anatomy and position of the cribriform plate to avoid inadvertent entry into the cranial cavity through the fovea ethmoidalis.
- *Inferior limit:* The inferomedial strut posteriorly should be removed. The orbital process of the palatine forms the posterior inferomedial strut. Removal of this strut allows for the maximal decompression reduction.
- Navigation technology also aids in safely performing bony decompression in critical areas such as orbital apex and medial wall.

- Periosteal incision is particularly important for preventing postoperative diplopia. In endoscopic surgeries, a strip of periosteum is left intact over the medial rectus.

Lateral Wall

Approaches: Coronal Incision

- *Transorbital:* Eyelid crease incision, sub-brow incision, lateral canthal incision. En-bloc removal of lateral orbital rim was described by Dollinger.
Rose described creating a lateral orbital window.
The transorbital ab-interno technique was popularized by Goldberg, which is widely followed now.
- *Bones removed:* The greater wing of the sphenoid, frontal, and zygomatic.
- "Deep" lateral decompression includes removal of the diploe of the greater wing of the sphenoid with substantial reduction in axial proptosis.
- *Areas:* lacrimal keyhole (yellow), sphenoid door jamb (red), and basin of the inferior orbital fissure (green) **(Fig. 6)**.
- Mechanical or piezoelectric burr is usually used for the thinning of bone.

Orbital rim around the lacrimal fossa is thinned to improve visualization and instrumentation access to deep orbital drilling. Diploe within the greater wing of sphenoid is entered after drilling anterior and superior to the tip of the inferior orbital fissure. The diploic space is then followed superiorly to the region of the superior orbital fissure. Finally, the pocket of thick bone extending anterior from the tip of the superior orbital fissure to the frontozygomatic suture is removed. Part of this area involves sections of the zygomatic and/or frontal bone.
- In the technique described by Rose, the orbital rim is exposed and the periorbita and temporalis muscle are reflected medially and laterally. A window is then created, and the thin anterior portion of the lateral orbital wall is exposed. This bone is then removed with a rongeur.
- There is an average decompression of 4.5 mm with deep lateral wall decompression.
- *Advantages:* Reduced risk of new onset strabismus and sinusitis. Faster resolution of postoperative strabismus and is especially useful for woody/fibrotic orbits.

Floor

- Floor decompression is usually performed along with medial wall.
- *Approaches:* Transorbital: transcutaneous-subciliary, inferior transconjunctival, transcaruncular, swinging eyelid and lateral orbital; coronal approach; transnasal endoscopic; transantral (Caldwell-Luc).

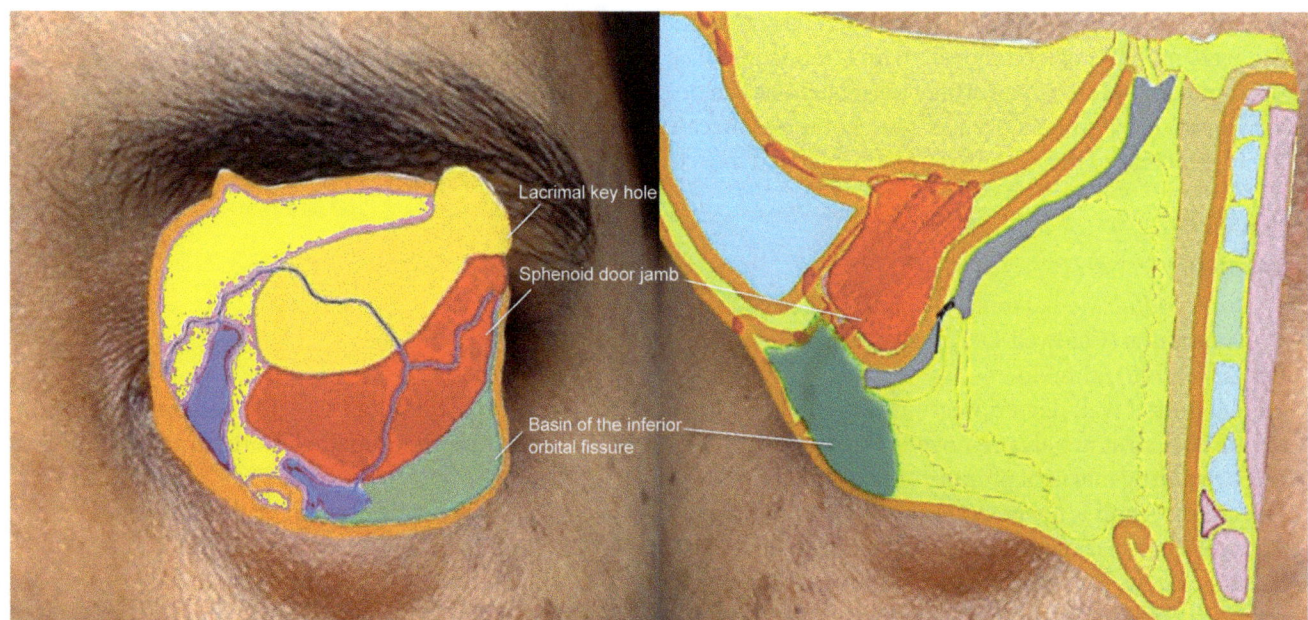

Fig. 6: The deep lateral wall decompression: lacrimal keyhole (yellow), sphenoid door jamb (red), and basin of the inferior orbital fissure (green).

- *Bones removed:* Maxillary, palatine
- Bone is removed medial to the infraorbital canal with care to avoid damage to the neurovascular bundle. Bone lateral to the canal can also be removed to obtain greater reduction.
- Anteromedial strut of bone left intact to avoid hypoglobus and strabismus.
- Posterior part of the floor is formed by the orbital process of the palatine bone. This is removed in cases of dysthyroid optic neuropathy.
- Bone removal can be performed with rongeurs or with mechanical/piezoelectric burr.
- The inferior scleral show reduces in floor decompression postoperatively. This is employed customized decompression of eyes with proptosis and lower eyelid retraction/scleral show. Mild retraction can be rectified.
- Infraorbital anesthesia can be avoided by using piezoelectric technology for bone removal which avoids soft tissue damage.

Balanced, Unbalanced, and Three-Wall Orbital Decompression

- *Balanced decompression:*
  - Performed in moderate-to-severe proptosis
  - Lateral wall and medial wall addressed
  - Believed to prevent inferomedial displacement of globe produce an equal prolapse of the medial and lateral rectus muscles into the surrounding space
  - Proposed to reduce postoperative strabismus
- *Unbalanced decompression: medial wall and floor:*
  - Performed in moderate-to-severe proptosis
  - Floor and medial wall addressed
  - Advantage of this technique is the use of routine instruments for bone removal. Use of specialized instruments such as mechanical drill can be avoided
  - Significant chances of new-onset diplopia and globe dystopia noted with the transantral approach. However, this can be prevented by preserving the anteromedial strut.
- *Three-wall decompression:*
  - Performed in severe proptosis (exophthalmometry >26 mm)
  - Medial wall, floor, and lateral wall are addressed along with intraconal fat removal.

Customized Orbital Decompression

- With the advent of minimally invasive techniques, surgical rehabilitation is now individualized on a case-by-case basis.
- Orbital decompression can be combined with eyelid surgery in the same sitting to improve the prominence and eyelid contour or can be combined with strabismus surgery.
- Floor decompression can be performed in cases with inferior scleral show in unilateral cases.
- In cases with excessive upper eyelid retraction and proptosis, deep lateral wall decompression via an eyelid crease incision can be performed and levator can be simultaneously recessed.
- In patients prone to scarring, transcutaneous incisions can be avoided and transconjunctival approaches can be employed.

Complications

- *Intraoperative:* Hemorrhage, cerebrospinal fluid (CSF) leak: medial wall and lateral wall decompression
- *Early:* Infection (<1%), hemorrhage (<1%)
- *Late complications:* Supraorbital anesthesia at 1.5–6% (in fat decompression), new onset diplopia, ectropion, lower eyelid retraction in lower eyelid subciliary approach, entropion.
  - *Coronal incision:* Skin necrosis, alopecia, and anesthesia.
  - *Medial wall decompression:* Cerebrospinal fluid leak, epistaxis, eyelid and conjunctival swelling, sensory anesthesia, orbital hemorrhage, infection, and sinusitis.
  - *Lateral wall decompression:* CSF leak (intraoperative), temporalis muscle wasting, and oscillopsia (ab-externo technique).
  - *Floor decompression:* Sensory anesthesia and paresthesia over the cheek.

5. Indications of orbital decompression. Importance of medial wall in orbital decompression.

Orbital decompression has TED and non-TED indications:
- *TED:* Orbital decompression in TED is performed in the inactive fibrotic stage or active stage:
  - Disfiguring proptosis
  - Dysthyroid optic neuropathy
  - Severe exposure keratitis or corneal breakdown
  - Customized decompression—mild-to-moderate retraction with scleral show
- *Non-TED:* The functional and cosmetic aspects in certain conditions with pseudoproptosis and non-TED causes of proptosis can be addressed with orbital decompression:
  - *Negative vector:*
    - To address pseudoproptosis due to high axial myopia
    - Malar hypoplasia with scleral show
    - *Shallow orbits like in Crouzon syndrome:* Can protect from keratopathy and globe luxation
  - *Inflammatory orbitopathy:* Cosmetic correction of disfiguring proptosis in inflammatory orbital diseases such as orbital vasculitis, granulomatosis with polyangiitis, xanthogranulomatosis, and idiopathic orbital inflammation has been described.
  - *Orbital tumors:* Proptosis correction in cases of sphenoid wing meningioma, lymphangioma, and lymphoma has been described.

Importance of Medial Wall Decompression

Enlarged recti muscles cause crowding at the orbital apex and cause compressive optic neuropathy. The medial wall removal releases pressure over the optic nerve by prolapsing the enlarged medial rectus in the ethmoid sinus. When combined with floor decompression, further release of the compressive effect is obtained.

In active TED with optic neuropathy, emergency decompression of the medial wall is performed owing to easy access and immediate release of compression due to enlarged medial wall.

The various approaches include transorbital, coronal, transantral, and transnasal endoscopic.

Transnasal endoscopic approach has various advantages:
- Absent external scar
- Good and direct visualization during bone removal close to vital anatomical locations such as anterior wall of the sphenoid sinus, close to optic canal
- Better apical decompression
- Faster postoperative recovery and comfort.

The limitations include need for equipment for endoscopic surgery, longer learning curve, and limited control over intraorbital bleeders.

(Refer to Answer 4 for preoperative planning, description of medial wall decompression)

 6. Write a note on the various immunotherapies in the treatment of TED. What are the newer drugs available?

- TED is an autoimmune disease with a complex pathophysiology. The mainstay of management in active TED is corticosteroids for immunosuppression. About a fourth of severe TED patients have an unfavorable response to steroids, some relapse on withdrawal. Systemic adverse effects also limit the use of steroids, necessitating steroid-sparing alternate immunosuppressive drugs.
- Steroids suppression is generalized on the adaptive immunity and nonspecific increasing the risk of unwanted side effects.
- Various drugs are now available which are employed targeting the specific cell populations, molecules, or checkpoints in the immune pathomechanism, sparing the components of adaptive immune system uninvolved **(Table 5)**.

TABLE 5: Immunosuppressive drugs.	
Nonspecific immunosuppressants	**Specific immunosuppressants**
Glucocorticoids	Rituximab
MMF	Teprotumumab
Cyclosporine	Tocilizumab
Azathioprine	Anti-TNF alpha drugs
Methotrexate	
(MMF: mycophenolate mofetil; TNF: tumor necrosis factor)	

Nonspecific Immunosuppressants

Glucocorticoids

- Steroids are the mainstay of therapy. They inhibit lymphocyte recirculation, interfere with inflammation, and autoantigen release. They act by three mechanisms:
    1. *Direct genomic effects:* The binding of glucocorticoid receptors to glucocorticoid-responsive elements.
    2. *Indirect genomic effects:* These are on gene expression through the interactions of glucocorticoid receptors with other transcription factors.
    3. *Nongenomic mechanisms:* Glucocorticoid receptor–mediated effects are on a second-messenger cascades.
- They can be administered via oral, IV, retrobulbar, or subconjunctival routes.
- The cumulative dose of IV methylprednisolone is 6–8 g, liver function should be monitored apart from being mindful of other complications such as bone resorption, psychosis, and flare of infection.
- The risk factors for adverse effects from IV methylprednisolone are dose, age older than 53 years, daily pulses, and preexisting hepatitis.
- As per EUGOGO recommendations, for moderate-to-severe TED is weekly doses of 500 mg for 6 weeks followed by 250 mg weekly doses for a further 6 weeks.

Cyclosporine

- It is a lipophilic cyclic polypeptide which inhibits calcineurin and prevents secretion of IL-2 by CD4+ T-cells. It interferes in the amplification of immune response and prevents the reactivation of the cycle of autoimmunity making it an ideal drug to maintain remission of the disease. It also inhibits release of TNF-alpha from CD4+ cells and macrophages.
- It is effective when administered along with steroids at a starting dose of 2 mg/kg twice daily, then tapered over 2 years.
- Side effects include HTN, irreversible rise in plasma creatinine.

Mycophenolate

- The active metabolite of mycophenolate mofetil (MMF) is mycophenolic acid, which is the product of hydrolysis of MMF by esterase. It inhibits the de novo pathway for guanosine monophosphate synthesis, thereby inhibiting lymphocytic proliferation. It has cytostatic effect on lymphocytes, suppresses antibody formation, and inhibits leukocyte recruitment.
- Randomized trials comparing MMF with steroid in the treatment of active moderate-to-severe TED showed better CAS, improvement in diplopia, and proptosis in the MMF group at 24 weeks.
- *MINGO trial:* Mycophenolate plus methylprednisolone versus methylprednisolone alone in active, moderate-to-severe Graves' orbitopathy. It was a randomized, observer-masked, multicentric trial, which suggested that addition of mycophenolate to treatment with methylprednisolone improved rate of response to therapy by 24 weeks in patients with active and moderate-to-severe Graves' orbitopathy, i.e., there was improvement in quality of life, ophthalmic signs, and symptoms.

Azathioprine

- It is a cytostatic drug and acts by inhibiting purine synthesis. It is effective when combined with radiotherapy or steroid therapy. Studies have shown improved long-term clinical outcome in combination therapy and a potential role in preventing TED relapse.
- Side effects include nausea, vomiting, and bone marrow suppression.

Methotrexate

It inhibits dihydrofolate reductase enzyme, leading to the inhibition of the DNA, RNA, and protein synthesis. It is an effective steroid-sparing agent in patients of active TED intolerant to steroids. Studies have shown improved CAS and ocular motility at 12 months. It is administered at a weekly dose of 7.5 or 10 mg depending on the weight.

Specific Immunosuppressants

Rituximab

- A biological agent, it is a chimeric mouse-human monoclonal antibody that targets CD20 on B-cells. It reduces the antigen-presenting capacity of B-cells by B-cell depletion thereby causing decreased T-cell activation and halting the inflammatory process.
- There have been conflicting studies regarding the efficacy of rituximab. Better outcome has been noted if it was administered during the early active phase of the disease. At present, rituximab is suggested as a second-line option in patients with active disease who do not tolerate or fail to respond to IV steroids.

Teprotumumab

- It is a recombinant, fully human monoclonal antibody of the immunoglobulin G1 subclass and binds to IGF-1R, blocking its activation. IGF-1R is overexpressed by orbital fibroblasts, T-cells and B-cells in GD.
- IGF-1R acts as a bridge between immune cells and orbital fibroblasts and the molecular pathways leading to proliferation and differentiation of orbital fibroblast, the secretion of HA and adipogenesis.
- The Food and Drug Administration (FDA) approved the drug for the treatment of TED in adults on January 21, 2020 under the brand name Tepezza and received a "breakthrough therapy" designation.
- The approval was based on the results of two studies (study 1 and 2) consisting of a total of 170 patients with active TED who were randomized to either receive Tepezza or a placebo. Of the patients who were administered Tepezza, 71% in study 1 and 83% in study 2 demonstrated a >2 mm reduction in proptosis as compared to 20% and 10% of subjects who received placebo, respectively.
- Side effects include muscle spasm, nausea, alopecia (hair loss), diarrhea, fatigue, hyperglycemia (high blood sugar), hearing loss, dry skin, dysgeusia (altered sense of taste) and headache. Pregnancy is a contraindication.

Tocilizumab

- It is an anti-IL-6 receptor monoclonal antibody and binds to both soluble and membrane bound IL-6 receptors.
- IL-6 is a cytokine secreted by T-cells, macrophages, fibroblasts, and endothelial cells. Its role includes activation of B-cells and plasma cells.
- In a prospective, randomized study with active steroid resistant TED patients, tocilizumab was administered at a dose of 8 mg/kg (minimum 480 mg) every 4 weeks for at least four cycles. Treatment was stopped when CAS was 1 or less or thyroid-stimulating immunoglobulin was negative. Improved CAS, reduced proptosis, improved motility, and resolved diplopia were noted. Mild and transient adverse effects were noted.

Antitumor Necrosis Factor-Alpha

- *Etanercept:* TNF-alpha receptor blocker. It has been shown to be useful in mild–moderate TED in improving CAS. *Dosage:* 25 mg etanercept twice weekly for 12 weeks.
- *Adalimumab:* It is fully human monoclonal antibody against TNF. It is a longer acting drug which is effective in improving inflammatory scores in TED. Infliximab has also been reported in treatment of TED.

Other Potential Targets in Thyroid Eye Disease

- *Anakinra:* IL-1 receptor antagonist
- *Lerdelimumab, GC1008:* TGF-β–specific monoclonal antibodies
- *ChAglyCD3:* Fc-mutated CD3-specific monoclonal antibody
- *Abatacept:* CTLA-4–immunoglobulin recombinant protein
  IDEC-131: Humanized CD154-specific monoclonal antibody
- *Selective peroxisome proliferator-activated receptor (PPAR) modulators:* Novel selective PPAR-γ antagonists
- *NIDDK/CEB-52:* Low-molecular-weight thyrotropin-receptor antagonist

Suggested Reading

1. Bahn RS. Graves' ophthalmopathy. N Engl J Med. 2010;362(8):726-38.
2. Bahn RS, Kazim M. Thyroid eye disease. In: Fay A, Dolman PJ (Eds). Diseases and Disorders of the Orbit and Ocular Adnexa. Edinburgh: Elsevier; 2017. pp. 478-516.
3. Barrio-Barrio J, Sabater AL, Bonet-Farriol E, Velázquez-Villoria Á, Galofré JC. Graves' ophthalmopathy: VISA versus EUGOGO classification, assessment, and management. J Ophthalmol. 2015;2015:249125.
4. De Leo S, Lee SY, Braverman LE. Hyperthyroidism. Lancet. 2016;388(10047):906-18.
5. Dutton JJ. Anatomic considerations in thyroid eye disease. Ophthalmic Plast Reconstr Surg. 2018;34(4S suppl 1):S7-12.
6. Kahaly GJ. Immunotherapies for thyroid eye disease. Curr Opin Endocrinol Diabetes Obes. 2019;26(5):250-5.
7. Limongi RM, Feijó ED, Rodrigues Lopes E Silva M, Akaishi P, Cruz AAVE, Pieroni-Gonçalves AC, et al. Orbital bone decompression for non-thyroid eye disease proptosis. Ophthalmic Plast Reconstr Surg. 2020;36(1):13-6.
8. Naik MN, Nair AG, Gupta A, Kamal S. Minimally invasive surgery for thyroid eye disease. Indian J Ophthalmol. 2015;63(11):847-53.
9. Naik MN, Vasanthapuram VH, Joseph J, Murthy SI. Microbial keratitis in thyroid eye disease: clinical features, microbiological profile, and treatment outcome. Ophthalmic Plast Reconstr Surg. 2019;35(6):543-8.
10. Rootman DB. Orbital decompression for thyroid eye disease. Surv Ophthalmol. 2018;63(1):86-104.
11. Sheehan MT. Biochemical testing of the thyroid: TSH is the best and, oftentimes, only test needed: a review for primary care. Clin Med Res. 2016;14(2):83-92.

1.19 Orbital Cellulitis

Ashi Morawala, Anasua G Kapoor

 1. What is orbital cellulitis? Explore its etiologies. What are the classification systems to grade this entity?

The orbital septum is a condensation of connective tissue that theoretically holds back the orbital fat.[1] Orbital cellulitis is the inflammation of the postseptal region of the orbit which includes all the orbital contents behind the eyelids. This is in contrast to preseptal cellulitis, which is the inflammation of the contents in front of the orbital septum, essentially the eyelid tissues. It is a multilaminated structure that attaches circumferential to the periosteum of the orbital margin to form the arcus marginalis.

The cause of orbital cellulitis differs in the pediatric age group as compared to adults. In the pediatric group, 91% of cases of orbital cellulitis may have radiologically confirmed sinus disease, most commonly ethmoidal and maxillary sinusitis. This implies that sinusitis is the most common etiology for orbital cellulitis in children. In adults as well, the most common etiology is adjacent sinus infection. However, other causes such as trauma associated with retained foreign bodies or orbital fractures, are to be kept in mind.

Causes of orbital cellulitis are:
- Spread of infection from the paranasal sinuses
- Trauma
- Spread of infective focus from teeth, particularly after dental surgeries
- Spread from the lacrimal drainage system—acute dacryocystitis
- Spread from intraocular source—endophthalmitis leading to panophthalmitis
- Secondary infection within a tumor
- Retained foreign body
- Distant hematogenous spread from an infective focus elsewhere in the body, particularly in diabetics, patients on dialysis, and immunocompromised patients.

An important point to note is that with regard to sinusitis-induced orbital cellulitis, the focus of infection in children is more commonly the maxillary and ethmoid sinuses, because they complete pneumatization early, while in adults it is the frontoethmoidal complex. Children in the first decade of life are likelier to have sinusitis induced by a single species of aerobic pathogens with good response to medical therapy. Older children and adults most often show polymicrobial infection with poorer response to antibiotics and are therefore likelier to require surgical drainage of the orbital abscess, if any.

The Chandler classification grades orbital inflammation in terms of severity of the complications to help determine the appropriate treatment. It is important to note that the Chandler classification is not a temporal one, meaning that the grades mentioned do not necessarily progress in the same order.

The Chandler classification is as below:

Grade I	Preseptal cellulitis
Grade II	Orbital cellulitis
Grade III	Subperiosteal abscess
Grade IV	Orbital abscess
Grade V	Cavernous sinus thrombosis

Another classification to note is the Jain–Rubin classification which was proposed to overcome the *absence of temporal progression* noted in Chandler's classification.

The Jain–Rubin classification brought out the progression of a cellulitis stage to a frank abscess stage.

The Jain–Rubin classification is as below:

The important pearl to keep in mind is that preseptal cellulitis, which has traditionally been understood as a benign entity can evolve into orbital cellulitis if not treated effectively.

 2. Give a brief overview of the applied anatomy of the orbit in the context of orbital cellulitis.

As previously mentioned, orbital cellulitis is the presence of inflammation within the structures that lie posterior to the orbital septum. There are four main surgical spaces within the orbit—the extraconal, intraconal, subperiosteal, and sub-Tenon's spaces. Infection of any space may lead to spread into adjoining spaces and involvement of the entire orbit at a later stage.

The Extraconal and Intraconal Spaces

The four recti muscles arise from the annulus of Zinn at the orbital apex and course anteriorly to insert onto the sclera. The intermuscular septum between the recti form a cone that divides the orbit into intraconal and extraconal compartments. In the posterior orbit, these intermuscular fascial connections are thin, and sometimes incomplete, hence infective or inflammatory foci may spread between the intraconal and extraconal spaces.

The extraconal space lies between the bony orbital walls and the annulus of Zinn.

It contains:
- Lacrimal gland
- Superior and inferior oblique muscles
- Trochlea
- Extraconal orbital fat
- Superior and inferior ophthalmic veins
- Blood vessels and nerves

The intraconal space lies within the annulus, extending form the retrobulbar surface to the orbital apex. It contains:
- Optic nerve
- Intraconal orbital fat
- Blood vessels and nerves.

The Subperiosteal Space

This is a potential space between the periorbita and the bony orbital walls. The periorbita is loosely attached to the orbital bones except at the suture lines and the orbital margin. This space may be enlarged with blood in the form of a subperiosteal hematoma following trauma or with pus in a subperiosteal abscess following orbital cellulitis. A characteristic *dome-shaped* configuration is noted when the periorbita is lifted off the bones, which is bound by the bony suture lines.

The Sub-Tenon's Space

This is a potential space between the globe and the Tenon's capsule. The Tenon's capsule of fascia bulbi is a fibroelastic membrane that extends from the dura of the optic nerve to the globe, over the conjunctiva, to fuse with it just behind the corner-scleral limbus. It separates the globe from the intraconal orbital fat. The rectus muscles penetrate the Tenon's capsule posterior to the equator of the globe, as do nerves and vessels en route to the globe. This space may be enlarged with fluid as

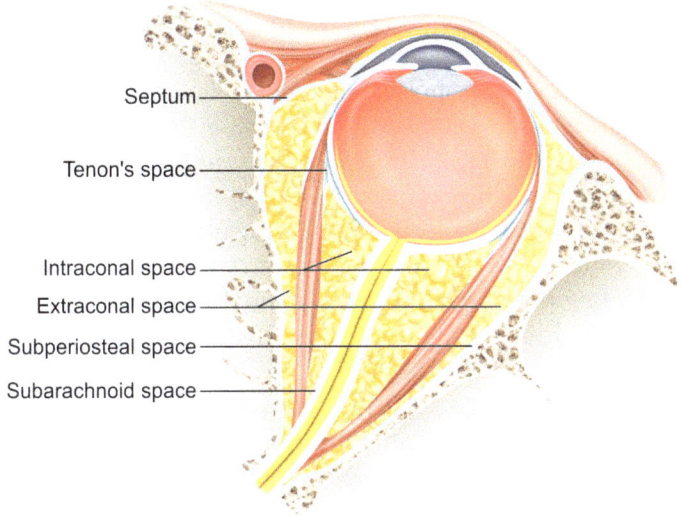

Fig. 1: The surgical spaces of the orbit.
Source: Adapted from Leatherbarrow (2010).

in posterior scleritis or air after trauma or by tumor infiltration such as in choroidal melanoma. These contents are detectable by B-scan ultrasonography (USG).

The Paranasal Sinuses

Orbital cellulitis secondary to sinusitis is the most common etiology. The paranasal sinuses include frontal, ethmoidal, maxillary, and sphenoid sinuses. They are air-filled cavities within the skull bones that decrease the relative weight of the skull and provide a buffer against facial trauma. They humidify and heat the inspired air and form a line of immunological defenses.

- *Frontal sinuses:* Located superior to the eyes, within the frontal bone. Begin pneumatization at 5–6 years of age.
- *Maxillary sinuses:* Located within the maxillary bones, under the eyes—the largest of all the sinuses. Begin pneumatization in utero; the first sinuses to fully pneumatize.
- *Ethmoid sinuses:* Formed by many separate air cells, within the ethmoid bone, between the eyes. Composed of three to four air cells by birth, continue to expand, and pneumatize till adulthood.
- *Sphenoid sinuses:* Located within the sphenoid bone. Start pneumatization at 3 months of age, and reach full size by 12 years.

The reasons why spread of infection occurs easily from the ethmoid sinuses to the medial orbit are:
- Thin lamina papyracea
- Multiple foramina for passage of blood vessels and nerves
- Valveless veins between the orbit and adjacent structures allowing for bidirectional passage of pathogens
- Congenital and acquired bony defects; the congenital defects are known as Zuckerkandl dehiscences.

Ethmoid sinusitis results in medial orbital cellulitis or a medial subperiosteal abscess collection. This can then spread further to the rest of the orbital tissues and spaces. Maxillary sinusitis may result in a subperiosteal abscess involving the orbital floor, which is also composed of relatively thin bone. Abscesses that involve the roof of the orbit, such as in case of frontal sinusitis, have a higher tendency of intracranial extension and life-threatening sequelae.

Venous drainage from the paranasal sinuses and the mid-face is from the orbital veins. These veins are valveless and communicate with the cavernous sinus and the pterygoid plexus. The lack of valves may allow the spread of infectious processes both in an antegrade or retrograde manner. Thus complications such as cavernous sinus thrombosis (CST), meningitis, and intracerebral abscess are seen in severe orbital cellulitis. Infectious processes within the cavernous sinus can involve the structures contained within it including the oculomotor nerve, the trochlea nerve, the abducens, the internal carotid artery, and the sympathetic nerve plexus. The infection can also spread to the contralateral cavernous sinus, the pituitary gland, and the meninges leading to life-threatening sequelae.

3. What are the pathogens commonly implicated in bacterial orbital cellulitis?

Haemophilus influenzae was the most commonly implicated pathogen in orbital cellulitis before the introduction of the *H. influenzae* type B (HiB) vaccine in 1985. Most commonly now, *Staphylococcus aureus* including methicillin-resistant *S. aureus* (MRSA) are implicated as the causative organisms. *Staphylococcus epidermidis* is the next most common pathogen. *Streptococcus pneumoniae* is rare, again due to increased vaccination against pneumococci in infants. The microbiological profile is thus variable and depends on the community pattern and expansion of childhood vaccination. Diphtheroids and anaerobic bacteria have also been implicated in orbital cellulitis. Anaerobic infections are less common in the pediatric age group. *Pseudomonas* and fungal infections primarily occur in immunocompromised hosts. Gram-positive organisms are most common etiological agents in orbital cellulitis, as compared to gram-negative organisms, which however are associated with more sequelae.

In most cases of orbital cellulitis, blood cultures are negative (yield <2%), implying a low rate of bacteremia. However, more invasive surgical procedures such as drainage of an orbital or epidural abscess and even sinus cultures yield higher positive cultures. Still, studies have shown no growth in up to 25% of orbital abscesses, indicating that these may be a spillover of orbital inflammation and not representative of true orbital infection.

The complexity of pathogens and the response to antibiotic therapy appears to be age related. Children in the first decade of life are likelier to have sinusitis induced by a single species of aerobic pathogens with good response to medical therapy. Older children and adults most often show polymicrobial infection with poorer response to antibiotics and are therefore likelier to require surgical drainage of abscesses. As the sinuses expand in size, the ostium becomes comparatively narrower. Utilization of oxygen by aerobic microbes, created oxygen deficiency, which in turn provides a suitable environment for the growth of anaerobes. Anaerobes produce β-lactamase, which renders antibiotics less effective leading to infection which is unresponsive to medical therapy. Infectious orbital cellulitis in young children is thus more amenable to conservative management, while older children and adults may require surgical intervention.

 4. What are the clinical features of orbital cellulitis? How does preseptal cellulitis differ from orbital cellulitis clinically?

Like an inflammatory pathology in the body, orbital cellulitis is primarily diagnosed by the presence of the five cardinal signs of inflammation:
1. Calor: warmth
2. Dolor: pain
3. Rubor: redness
4. Tumor: swelling
5. Functio laesa: loss of function.

Symptoms typically include pain, swelling, and redness of periorbital tissues. In advanced cases, an outward bulging of the eye with diminution of vision may be the presenting complaints. The patient may also complain of pain on eye movements and diplopia. A past history of common cold and trauma should be elicited to determine causality. It is important to check vital signs and note the presence of constitutional symptoms such as malaise and loss of appetite.

For each clinical feature, it is important to document the location, type, severity, and exacerbating/relieving factors. Fever and tachycardia indicate the presence of the infectious focus in the body. Signs of inflammation include lid edema, conjunctival congestion, and chemosis. Proptosis is also noted which indicates orbital pathology. The kind of proptosis present will give a clue as to the location of an orbital abscess. Intraconal abscesses typically present with axial proptosis while extraconal abscesses present with abaxial proptosis. The globe is dystopia, in a direction opposite to the abscess site. Extraocular motility restriction may be present. This may be mechanical due to volume expansion, but may also be due to the associated inflammation of the extraocular muscles. Advanced cases of orbital cellulitis can have cranial nerve palsies, which may also contribute to motility restriction. Both the amount of proptosis and degree of extraocular motility restriction must be measured and documented. Hypoesthesia of the trigeminal nerve may be noted.

Diminution of vision indicates that the inflammation is severe with compression of the globe or the optic nerve, or spread of inflammation to the optic nerve. Loss of vision in orbital cellulitis may be reversible if it is due to spread of inflammation or infection to the neural tissue. However, in case of vascular thrombosis or compression, as seen in some etiologies such as mucormycosis, the visual compromise may be irreversible. It is important to note that orbital inflammation leading to cellulitis may occur as an extension of intraocular pathology. Clinical examination must include testing for relative afferent pupillary defect, color vision, and fundus examination to rule out the presence of disc edema. A detailed examination of the globe and the ocular adnexal is essential, especially if there is a positive history of trauma.

Periocular vascular congestion may indicate superior ophthalmic vein thrombosis. CST can present with high fever, headache, severe vision loss, and total ophthalmoplegia, with features progressing to the contralateral side. Intracranial involvement is heralded by the appearance of neurological signs such as altered mental status, meningismus, neurological deficits, and seizures.

A history of immunosuppression such as diabetes mellitus or long-term use of corticosteroids is useful to point to a possible etiology of mucormycosis and other fungal infections leading to orbital cellulitis. Evaluation of necrotic tissue and histopathological examination of such specimens can yield the causative organism.

Distinguishing preseptal cellulitis from orbital cellulitis requires noting three important clinical features that are present in orbital pathologies and absent in a condition like preseptal cellulitis that involves only anterior tissues. These are proptosis, extraocular motility restriction, and diminution of vision. Eyelid edema and even conjunctival congestion may be present in both conditions. Preseptal cellulitis typically occurs from an infected stye, trauma to the eyelids, infection of adjacent skin, and even via spread from paranasal sinuses.

Clinical features	*Preseptal cellulitis*	*Orbital cellulitis*
Eyelid edema	+	+
Conjunctival congestion	+	++
Proptosis	–	+
Vision diminution	–	+
Ophthalmoplegia	–	+

5. What are the investigative modalities that may be used to diagnose orbital cellulitis? Give a brief overview of the findings seen.

A computed tomography (CT) scan is the essential investigation in all cases of suspected orbital cellulitis, particularly in cases where examination may be limited as in children or with severe periorbital edema. All patients of suspected orbital cellulitis must undergo a CT scan to detect the presence of an abscess. Diminution of vision, proptosis, and extraocular motility restriction in particular are indicators to requisition a CT scan.

A noncontrast CT scan is excellent to detect the spread of infection, the condition of paranasal sinuses, and to detect the presence of subperiosteal or orbital abscesses. It helps distinguish between preseptal and orbital cellulitis. Retained foreign bodies, location, and extent of abscesses can be determined. A CT scan can help determine the etiology of the inflammation such as a tumor or a vascular malformation. Worsening of clinical picture while on treatment for a confirmed infection, also warrants imaging. It helps plan timing and approach of surgical intervention.

A magnetic resonance imaging (MRI) is more expensive, and does not outline the bony orbit well. MRI with fat saturation and gadolinium contrast is reserved for patients with intracranial abscesses or suspected cavernous sinus or venous thrombosis or aggressive fungal infection. It is also useful in the identification of nonmetallic foreign bodies. For suspected CST, an MR venography is the investigation of choice. The inflamed sinus shows a loss of convexity and an absence of filling on the affected side.

An orbital abscess appears as an ill-defined, homogeneous or heterogeneous mass within the orbit. It may show gas-fluid levels in the orbit, and has a contrast-enhancing margin. It is commonly seen in pediatric patients. Subperiosteal abscess have a dome-shaped configuration with the collection located between the bone and the periosteum. Adjacent sinuses may show pacification. An abscess may initially appear to increase in size while the patient is actually improving clinically. Therefore, the size of the abscess in isolation is not a reliable factor to determine the efficacy of the administered treatment.

Ultrasonography is another investigative modality, which while not widely used in diagnosing cases of orbital cellulitis, can still be used as a bedside modality for preliminary investigation. USG can be used for risk stratification, to distinguish between preseptal and orbital cellulitis, and to detect the presence of an abscess. It can detect muscle inflammation and orbital foreign bodies. The resolution of the posterior orbit is poor; however, there is no visualization of the intracranial contents. Orbital abscesses are seen as medium–low echogenic lesions on USG. They may be noted against the adjacent orbital wall which can be visualized.

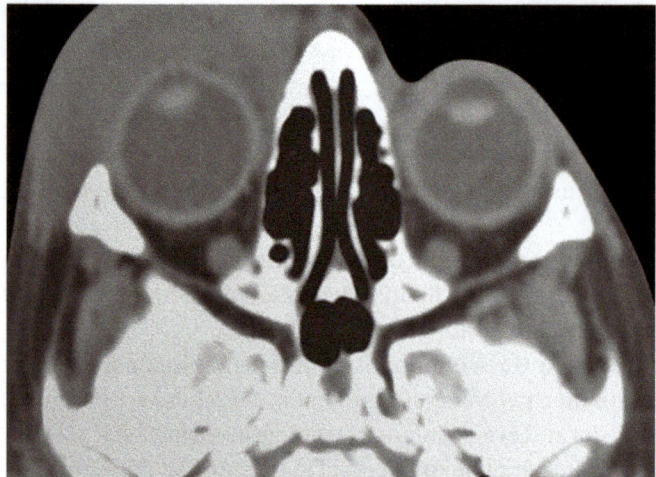

Fig. 2: A mid-axial cut of a computed tomography (CT) scan in a patient with preseptal cellulitis.

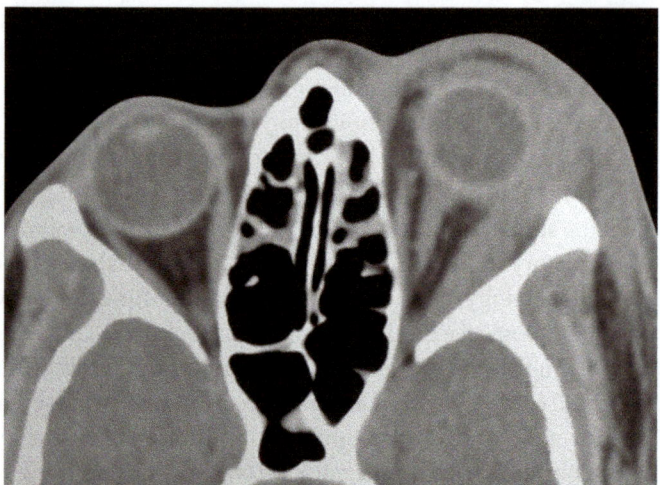

Fig. 3: An orbital abscess in the temporal extraconal space of the orbit. Infection began in the upper eyelid. Incision and drainage of the infective focus was done.

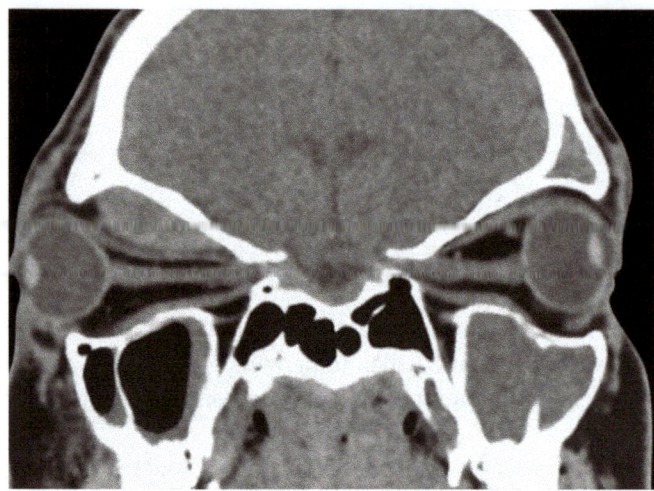

Fig. 4: A dome-shaped collection in the superior subperiosteal space in a patient with orbital cellulitis which indicates a subperiosteal abscess.

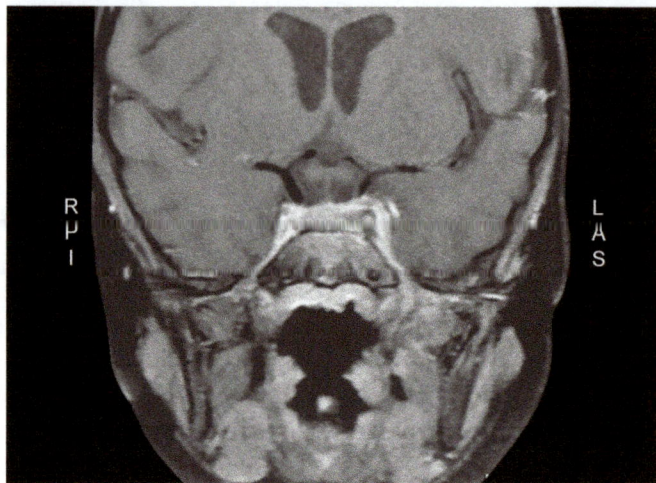

Fig. 5: Left-sided cavernous sinus thrombosis. Note the loss of convexity of the normal sinus, which is evident on the normal contralateral side.

6. How is bacterial orbital cellulitis managed in a pediatric patient?

All cases of suspected orbital cellulitis must be hospitalized and started on intravenous antibiotics without delay. A multispeciality approach requiring an ophthalmologist, an otorhinolaryngologist, and an infectious disease specialist is ideal.

Fever and tachycardia should prompt testing of the complete blood picture including total and differential leukocyte count. The white blood count is significantly higher in orbital cellulitis than in preseptal cellulitis.

Indications of medical therapy	Indications of surgical therapy
Preseptal cellulitis	Subperiosteal/orbital abscess in older children and adults
Empirical therapy in orbital cellulitis	Orbital abscess associated with frontal sinusitis
Subperiosteal abscess in young children	• Worsening of vision/proptosis/ophthalmoplegia • Intracranial complications • No response to medical therapy

Blood cultures should be obtained before starting antibiotics therapy. However, since they are positive, in less than one-third of cases, starting empirical therapy while awaiting results is advised to prevent worsening of the clinical picture. The overall yield is <2% for cases with orbital cellulitis. However, for children younger than 4 years of age, the yield can be up to 33%. This indicates that young children with orbital cellulitis have a much higher prevalence of bacteremia than older children and adults. Intranasal swabs to collect pus from infected sinuses yields higher positive cultures and directs medical therapy. This is because there is a strong correlation between the organisms that cause sinusitis and those that cause orbital cellulitis in the same patient. Cultures from the source of infection: sinuses in sinusitis, dental abscess in anaerobic infections, etc. allow more accurate antibiotic selection. Administering the correct antibiotic early, prevents progression from the cellulitis stage to a frank abscess. Lumbar punctures to obtain cerebrospinal fluid (CSF) for analysis is not routinely indicated and is reserved only for patients who show signs of neurological involvement.

Empirical antibiotic therapy is directed against common sinus pathogens and organisms that commonly cause abscesses. A trial of medical therapy may be initiated for 48 hours. If no response is noted, or if there is worsening of visual function, surgical intervention must be considered.

Broad-spectrum antibiotics commonly used:
- *Gram-positive coverage:* Amoxicillin clavulanate
- *Gram-positive + gram-negative coverage:* Cephalosporins (second and third generation)
- *MRSA:* Vancomycin is reserved for patients with MRSA, necrotizing infections or if warranted by culture and sensitivity results or for patients with penicillin allergy.
- *Vancomycin-resistant S. aureus (VRSA):* Linezolid
- *Gram-negative coverage:* Aminoglycosides
- *Broad-spectrum combinations:* Piperacillin–Tazobactam; Ticarcillin–Clavulanate
- *Anaerobic coverage:* Metronidazole.

Resistance is being increasingly noted with the use of amoxicillin clavulanate, fluoroquinolones, and crystalline penicillin. Recent studies suggest that broad-spectrum antibiotics such as ciprofloxacin, which have similar bioavailability in their oral as well as intravenous forms, can be used as oral medications in select patients. Antibiotics are commenced on an empirical basis and can then be altered based on bacteriology results. Usually a 48-hour window period is used to assess improvement before considering a change in regimen. Oral antibiotics, such as amoxicillin–clavulanate combination, are continued for another 1–3 weeks after discharge from the hospital. The goal is to continue until all signs of infection have completely subsided.

Systemic corticosteroids whether oral or intravenous can be used to curb inflammation which can otherwise persist for weeks or even months. Curbing inflammation should prevent a rise in pressure within the closed space of the orbital compartment and prevent undue compression on the optic nerve. In addition, the fibroblast inhibitory characteristics of corticosteroids may prevent scarring and long-term sequelae.

The benefit of oral corticosteroids may be evident in pediatric cases with subperiosteal abscesses. Reported benefits include earlier resolution of eyelid edema, ocular motility, proptosis, and a faster return to baseline vision. The length of hospital stay is also reduced.

Some studies have used oral steroids after the initial improvement noted with antibiotic administration, but some others have begun intravenous dexamethasone concurrently with intravenous antibiotics. Both types have seen improvement in clinical picture with few or no side effects. It is important to note that corticosteroid use is associated with impaired immune function against infective organisms. It may cause rapid progression in fungal or atypical infection.

Additionally, adjunctive treatment of sinusitis can promote the drainage of sinuses and may have a favorable impact on subperiosteal abscesses. Nasal decongestion and saline irrigation as well as intranasal corticosteroids help to reduce mucosal edema and facilitate drainage of the sinuses. Functional endoscopic sinus surgery (FESS) is an important adjunct treatment in cases of chronic sinusitis. It is a safe and effective means of acute drainage of infected ethmoidal and maxillary sinuses. The main objective here is drainage and obtaining material for culture.

Surgical management includes the drainage of orbital abscesses. The argument remains between early drainage of orbital abscesses to prevent complications versus the possibility of seeding of the infection with early surgery. The presence and location of an orbital abscess do not necessarily correlate with disease severity or prognosis.

It is important to know when urgent drainage (within 24 hours) is indicated:
- Large orbital abscess, particularly superior or inferior orbital abscess
- Presence of frontal sinusitis—due to increased risk of intracranial spread
- Intracranial complications at the time of presentation

- Anaerobic infection
- Any abscess compressing on the optic nerve cause visual dysfunction
- Inadequate/absence of response on medical therapy—deterioration despite 48 hours of medical therapy or no response 72 hours after initiating therapy
- To obtain a sample for culture and sensitivity
- Orbital abscess—orbital apex or intracranial extension.

In certain situations, a subperiosteal abscess may be observed and managed with conservative treatment. Subperiosteal abscesses can be treated medically in younger patients (<9 years of age), particularly with medial or inferior abscesses, in whom simple (single-organism, aerobic) infections are suspected without any vision loss of intracranial spread. In older individuals, the likelihood of polymicrobial disease and presence of anaerobic infection is greater. Such cases have an increased chance of antibiotic resistance as well and early evacuation of a subperiosteal abscess and drainage of sinuses aids quicker recovery. Abscesses not secondary to sinus infection may require more aggressive therapy, including early surgical intervention or foreign body removal.

Any abscess adjacent to the frontal sinus, whatever the age group may be, must be drained to prevent intracranial spread. Large volume abscesses (>3.8 mL) must be promptly drained. Those with associated intracranial complications must also be surgically managed. It is important to note that change/reduction in the size of the abscess or extent of inflammation as seen on imaging may lag behind clinical improvement—so even if the patient appears to be improving clinically, imaging findings may take longer to show objective improvement.

7. What are the complications of orbital cellulitis? Outline their management.

The venous drainage of the orbit is via two major veins, the superior and inferior ophthalmic veins, of which the superior is the larger. It has connections to the cavernous sinuses through the superior orbital fissure. The inferior ophthalmic vein has anastomoses with the superior ophthalmic vein and also connects to the pterygoid plexus. A branch of, or the entire inferior ophthalmic vein may also drain into the cavernous sinus in some cases. The cavernous sinus itself drains into the superior and inferior petrosal veins. Connections between the cavernous sinuses on both sides exist via the valveless anterior and posterior intercavernous sinus and the basilar plexus. These connections explain the routes of spread of infection in a case of orbital cellulitis from the orbit, to the cavernous sinuses, and further into the meninges and intracranial spaces.

Complications of orbital cellulitis	
Corneal involvement	Exposure keratopathy, neurotrophic keratitis
Intraocular involvement	Endophthalmitis, septic uveitis, elevated intraocular pressure
Posterior orbital changes	Optic neuritis, compressive optic neuropathy, vessel thrombosis, globe tenting, extraocular motility deficits
Intracranial complications	Cavernous sinus thrombosis, meningitis, intracranial abscess formation

Cavernous Sinus Thrombosis

Posterior extension of infection may lead to CST which can be life-threatening. Such patients can present with fever, nausea, headache, and ophthalmoplegia which is out of proportion to the severity of orbital cellulitis. Cranial nerve palsies, conjunctival congestion, and severe vision loss accompany these symptoms. The contralateral side may get involved as the infection progresses.

Investigation of choice in suspected CST is magnetic resonance (MR) venography. It shows absence of filling of the sinus on the affected side. Treatment includes intravenous antibiotics with good central nervous system (CNS) penetration such as high-dose third-generation cephalosporins in combination with vancomycin, and metronidazole for suspected anaerobic organisms, along with immediate drainage of the orbital abscess. With regards to anticoagulant use in the treatment of septic CST, the anticoagulant benefits of arresting further clot formation and facilitating lysis must be balanced by the risk of intracranial bleed, which depends on the severity of the disease.

Intracranial Abscess

An intracranial abscess is a rare complication of orbital cellulitis. More commonly it is caused by sinus infection—particularly frontal sinusitis or a superior subperiosteal abscess. The patient may present with epidural empyema or an abscess, meningitis, venous sinus thrombosis, or a brain abscess. Neurological symptoms may not be present initially, particularly

Oculoplasty and Tumors

Flowchart 1: Approach to a case of pediatric orbital cellulitis.

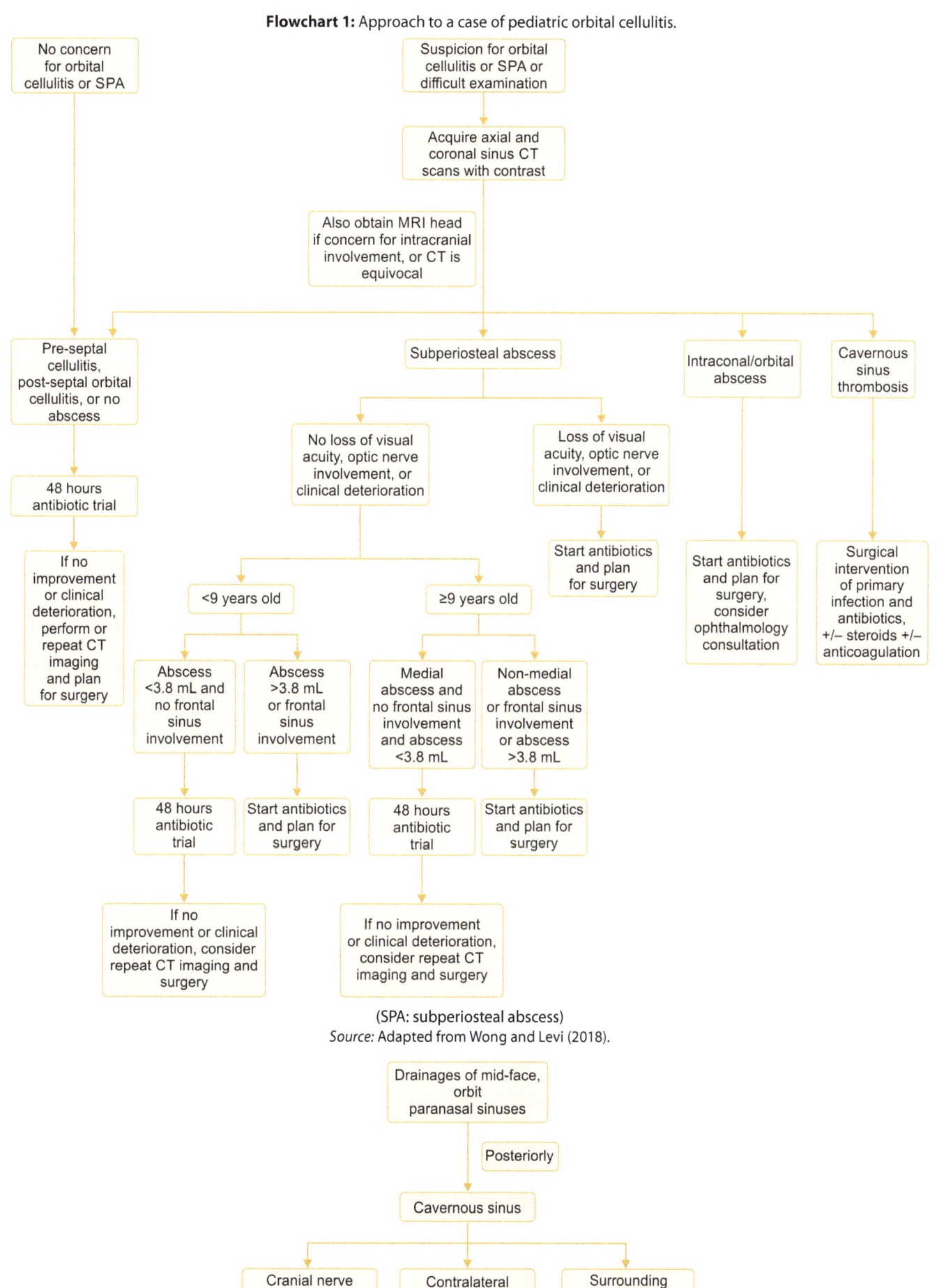

(SPA: subperiosteal abscess)
Source: Adapted from Wong and Levi (2018).

in the pediatric age group. These include fever, an altered sensorium, and seizures. Spread occurs either through direct extension or retrograde venous spread.

Treatment is immediate drainage of abscess and intravenous antibiotics—good anaerobic coverage and adequate CNS penetration. Concordance has been noted between the sinus flora and that within the intracranial abscess; therefore, sinus cultures can be useful in choosing the right antibiotic. Corticosteroid use can help reduce cerebral edema and encapsulation of the abscess; however, stopping them may lead to rebound edema.

Other complications include spread to adjacent adnexal structures leading to facial cellulitis, acute dacryocystitis, thrombosis of superior ophthalmic vein, retinal vessels, and meningitis. Proptosis may cause corneal exposure and lead to keratopathy and ulceration.

 8. What are the distinguishing features of fungal orbital cellulitis? What is the management?

Fungal infections are often associated with immunocompromised states. This is because while healthy individuals can clear the fungal spores easily by phagocytosis, immunocompromised hosts cannot prevent germination and hyphae formation by the fungal pathogen.

Immunocompromised states predisposing to invasive fungal infection	
Aspergillosis	*Mucormycosis*
Prolonged neutropenia	Diabetes mellitus with ketoacidosis
AIDS	Hematological malignancies
Organ transplantation/hematopoietic stem cell transplantation	Renal disease
Advancing age	
Diabetes mellitus	

Fungal infection leads to vascular invasion. This causes occlusion of blood vessels, particularly arterioles, resulting in soft tissue ischemia and necrosis. The acidic environment thus created, potentiates the growth of the organism and the cycle continues. Spread of the infection can occur via the lungs to the upper airway and then to the sinuses—especially the posterior ethmoid and sphenoid sinuses. Other routes include hematogenous spread and spread from adjacent sinuses. Involvement of the orbit can occur via all these routes. The two common causative species include *Aspergillus* and *Mucor*.

Features of Aspergillus:
- Commonly found in soil—saprophytic by nature
- Colonize sinuses
- **Septate hyphae, which branch at 45°**
- Aspergillosis is the *most common* mycosis caused by filamentous fungi.
- *Noninvasive colonization:* Sinonasal fungal ball, allergic sinusitis
- *Invasive colonization:* Involving soft tissue and bone, commonly in immunocompromised individuals

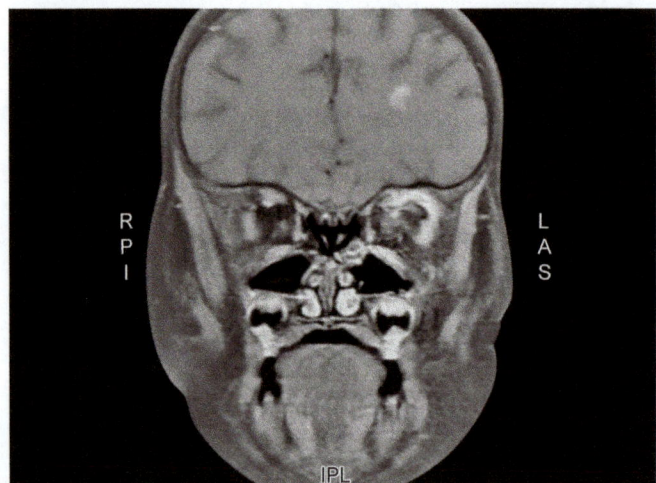

Fig. 6: An intracranial frontal lobe abscess in a patient with orbital cellulitis.

Clinical Features

Fungal orbital cellulitis may demonstrate an indolent course with minimal signs of inflammation, while bacterial disease typically has an acute presentation with prominent signs of inflammation. Mild fever, cough, and dyspnea may occur in cases with concomitant pulmonary aspergillosis as systemic features. Fungal sino-orbital disease mimics bacterial orbital cellulitis and nonspecific orbital inflammation or neoplastic disease as well. The posterior ethmoids and sphenoid sinuses are commonly involved in fungal sinusitis, while ethmoid and maxillary sinuses are most commonly involved in bacterial infections. Ophthalmoplegia and orbital apex syndrome, sometimes without features of orbital cellulitis may be the presenting manifestations. Mucormycosis may initially present with nasal mucosal ulceration, periorbital and facial swelling, proptosis, ophthalmoplegia, and vision loss. In mucormycosis, sinus infection can spread to the orbit and the cranium, via the orbital vessels, the cribriform plate, and the superior orbital fissure. Cavernous sinus involvement can progress to carotid artery occlusion and stroke. Necrosis and the classical black eschar formation (necrotizing fasciitis) occurs in advanced mucormycosis, over the skin, hard palate, and nasal mucosa. This is pathognomonic but a late finding. The causes of sudden visual loss in mucormycosis may stem from central retinal artery or vein occlusion, posterior ciliary artery occlusion, infarction of the intraorbital part of the optic nerve, and from direct invasion of the intracranial optic nerve or the optic chiasm.

Features of Mucor:
- *Class:* Zygomycetes; *Order:* Mucorales; *Species:* Rhizopus
- Colonize nose, mouth, throat, and stool of healthy individuals
- Mucormycosis is the second most common mycosis caused by filamentous fungi.
- **Broad, nonseptate hyphae, which branch at 90°**
- *Rhino-orbital mucormycosis:* Most common disease manifestation

Imaging

Imaging findings in fungal orbital cellulitis are often subtle and nonspecific. Imaging allows determining the sinuses involved, extent of orbital and adjacent structure involvement, and intracranial invasion (if any). It also allows for surgical planning. In case of mucormycosis, imaging may reveal mucosal thickening within the sinuses, bony necrosis involving the infratemporal and pterygoid fossa and thrombosis of superior ophthalmic vein. Intracerebral fungi appear as hypodense masses with peripheral enhancement—a ring abscess. The scans may reveal findings ranging from hyperintensity in T2-weighted images, to marked hyperintensity in all sequences. In case of aspergillosis, heterogeneous masses, with calcification and bony erosion may be noted. In aspergillosis, MRI shows contrast-enhancing lesions which are hypointense both on T1 and T2, unlike bacterial infections which usually show hyperintensity on T2-weighted scans.

Treatment

Treatment of fungal sino-orbital disease is based on the following principles:
- Early diagnosis
- Reversal of predisposing factors

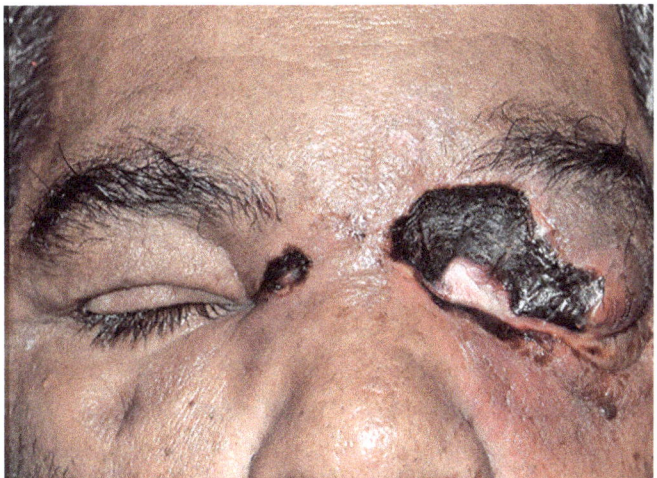

Fig. 7: Sino-orbital mucormycosis with black periorbital eschar seen due to occlusive vasculitis.

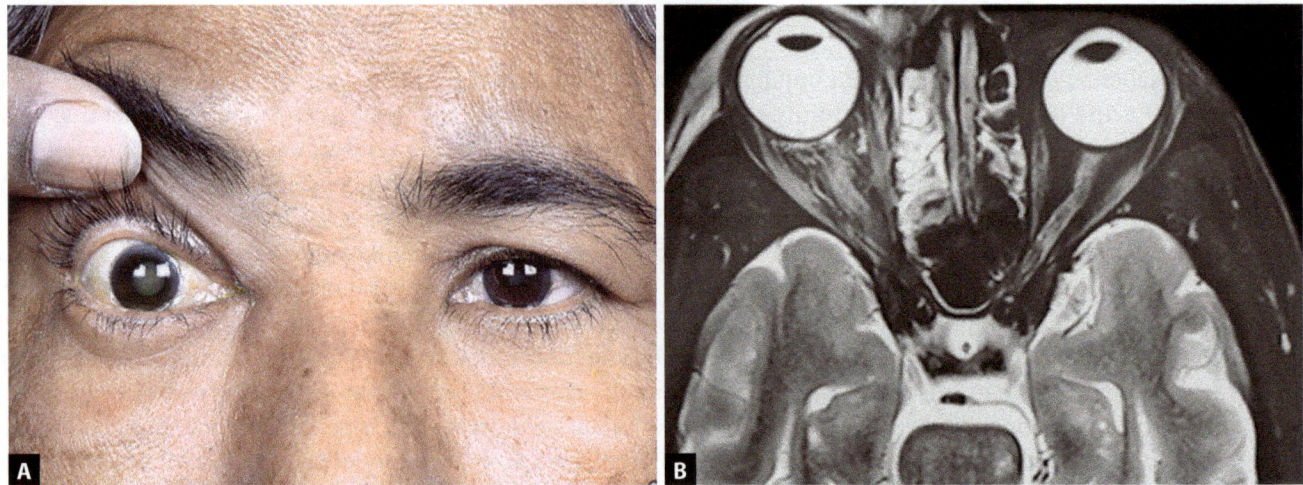

Figs. 8A and B: (A) Case of fungal orbital cellulitis in a patient with uncontrolled diabetes, presenting with complete external ophthalmoplegia. (B) MRI scans revealed orbital cellulitis secondary to ethmoid sinusitis.

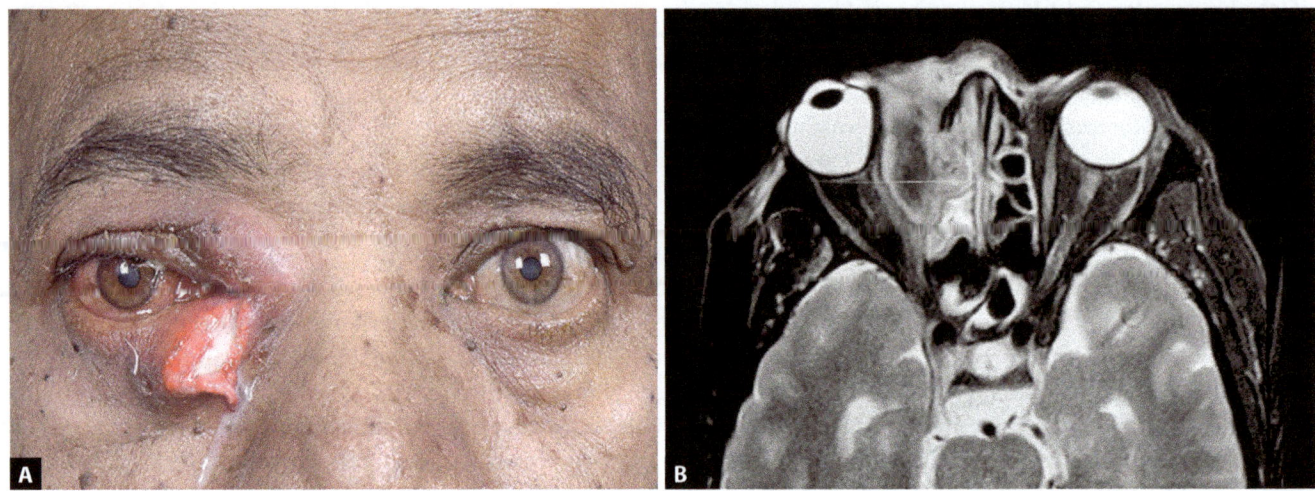

Figs. 9A and B: (A) Case of rhizopus-induced orbital cellulitis with a burst abscess. (B) MRI scans revealed a large medial subperiosteal abscess secondary to ethmoid sinusitis.

- Wide local debridement of necrotic tissue
- Establishing adequate sinus drainage
- Systemic antifungals.

Systemic antifungals include intravenous amphotericin B in a dose of 0.7–1 mg/kg with a cumulative dose of 2–4 mg (<5 mg, in some studies). Liposomal amphotericin B (AMB) has the advantage of reduced renal toxicity. It is more efficacious in rhino-orbital mucormycosis and is the drug of choice. It is given in a dose of 5 mg/kg/day, up to a maximum dose of 10 mg/kg/day. Topical AMB can be used for local treatment of the involved sites. The dose is 1 mg/mL. Nephrotoxicity is an important dose-limiting adverse effect of amphotericin B. It manifests as azotemia, hypokalemia, and hypomagnesemia. Its administration requires regularly monitoring of serum creatinine and blood urea nitrogen throughout the length of treatment. Other alternative/adjunctive drugs include posaconazole, caspofungin, and voriconazole, which is useful in the treatment of invasive aspergillosis. Timely treatment of fungal infections requires a high degree of suspicion due to the often nonspecific and subtle clinical features. Although rare, they cause significant morbidity and mortality. The diagnosis must be considered in all patients of orbital cellulitis, not responding to standard therapy.

Q 9. What are the differential diagnoses of orbital cellulitis?

In a child, the differential diagnosis of orbital cellulitis includes those conditions that can present with proptosis and signs of inflammation. The following table enumerates a list of causes but is not exhaustive.

Oculoplasty and Tumors

Causes of proptosis in a child	
Infection	Orbital cellulitis, orbital cysticercosis
Neoplasm	Rhabdomyosarcoma, neuroblastoma, intraocular tumors
Trauma	Subperiosteal hematoma, pneumo-orbit
Congenital vascular malformation	Lymphangioma
Inflammation	• Ruptured dermoid cyst • Eosinophilic granuloma

Preseptal Cellulitis

Preseptal cellulitis is an infection of the eyelid and periorbital soft tissues without involvement of the orbit and globe. It is important to distinguish preseptal cellulitis, where inflammation is confined to the eyelids, from postseptal (orbital) cellulitis. A lack of clinical signs of proptosis, ophthalmoplegia, or diminution of vision point to preseptal cellulitis. Appearance of these symptoms indicates progression from preseptal to postseptal cellulitis.

Preseptal cellulitis usually occurs from an infected stye or a traumatic wound to the eyelids. Mild cases are treated with oral antibiotics. In severe cases and in children less than a year old, treatment is with intravenous antibiotics.

Rhabdomyosarcoma

Rhabdomyosarcoma is a primitive round cell tumor of mesenchymal origin. It is the most common primary orbital malignancy in children. It presents with unilateral, acute, and rapidly progressive proptosis and globe dystopia, lid edema,

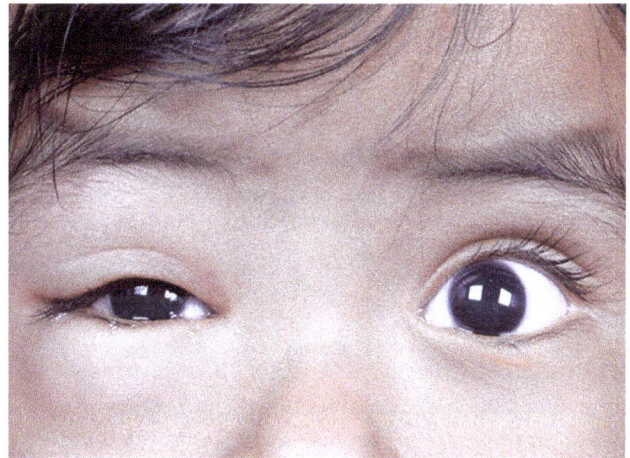

Fig. 10: Preseptal cellulitis in a 2-year-old child secondary to an upper eyelid stye.

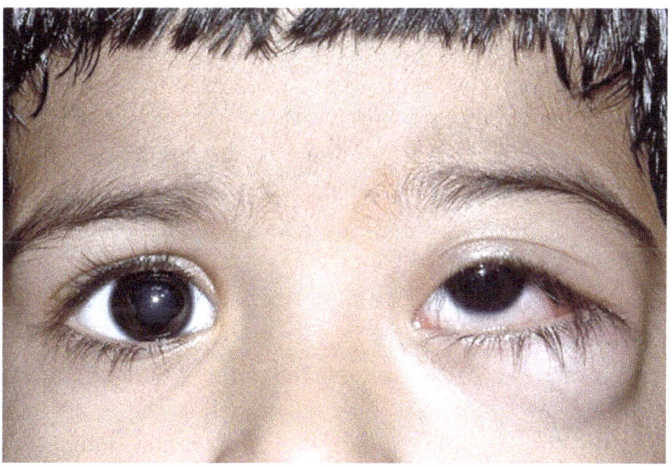

Fig. 11: Clinical picture of an RMS tumor in the left eye of a 3-year-old boy, causing globe dystopia.

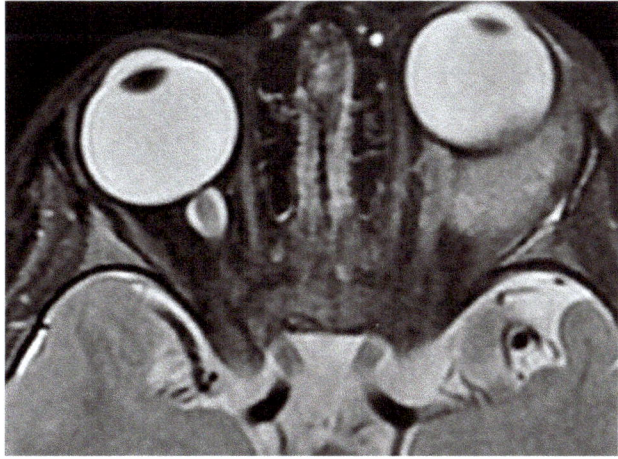

Fig. 12: Noncontrast MRI scan of the patient above, in the mid-axial cut showing an ill-defined mass in the temporal orbit, extending into the intraconal and extraconal space.

and conjunctival chemosis in children—males in the first decade of life are typically affected. Thus, it is a tumor that is often accompanied by signs of inflammation, which confound the clinician as to whether the etiology of the inflammation is infection or something more sinister, such as a life-threatening tumor, in case of rhabdomyosarcoma (RMS). Treatment is debulking and radiotherapy with systemic chemotherapy depending upon the stage of the tumor.

Orbital Lymphangioma

They are congenital lymphatic malformations that often have a variable-sized venous component. They may be superficial, deep, combined, and complex (involving other head and neck structures) depending on their location in the orbit and periocular tissues. Children present with acute, often severe proptosis with conjunctival chemosis and even diminished vision if there is optic nerve compression. They often give a history of antecedent upper respiratory tract infection (URTI) or trauma. Mechanism of proptosis is sudden rupture of a chocolate cyst with exsanguination of contents into the orbital tissues. It is important to treat this acute stage to prevent damage to the optic nerve. Treatment is multipronged with debulking and use sclerotherapy such as bleomycin or sodium tetradecyl sulfate.

On contrast scans, lymphangiomas present as mildly enhancing cystic lesions. If there is a venous component associated, enhancement may be variable. They are often poorly defined and extend between the various surgical spaces, reflecting the lack of a histological capsule. Without contrast, they appear as heterogeneous lesions of soft-tissue attenuation. Areas of hemorrhage may show rim enhancement of the cysts. The cysts themselves may be hypointense on MRI/hypodense on CT unless there is a recent bleed. Areas of dystrophic calcification may be noted.

Orbital Retinoblastoma

Occasionally, a large retinoblastoma can become necrotic and present with signs of inflammation mimicking bacterial preseptal and orbital cellulitis. There may or may not be extraocular extension of the tumor in such cases. Imaging will reveal an intraocular mass with or without extraocular extension. An antecedent history of leukocoria is a clue in such cases. Treatment includes combinations of enucleation, systemic chemotherapy, and external beam radiotherapy.

Clinical photograph of a 1-year-old girl presenting with a history of leukocoria and sudden onset redness and outward bulge of the eye. Axial MRI scans reveal a large intraocular tumor filling the affected globe. Enucleation and histopathological analysis of the sample revealed a retinoblastoma.

In adults, some common differential diagnoses of orbital cellulitis can include preseptal cellulitis, cellulitis following trauma, and orbital cysticercosis.

Orbital Cysticercosis

Orbital cysticercosis is an infection of the orbital tissues by the larval form of the cestode *Taenia solium*. Patients usually present with acute periorbital inflammation and proptosis which may be axial or abaxial depending upon location of the lesion within the orbit. Diminution of vision may indicate compression on the optic nerve. Extraocular motility restriction may indicate extraocular muscle involvement by the cyst. The superior rectus is most commonly involved. Inflammation of the lacrimal gland or dacryoadenitis may present as a mass in the superotemporal orbital region.

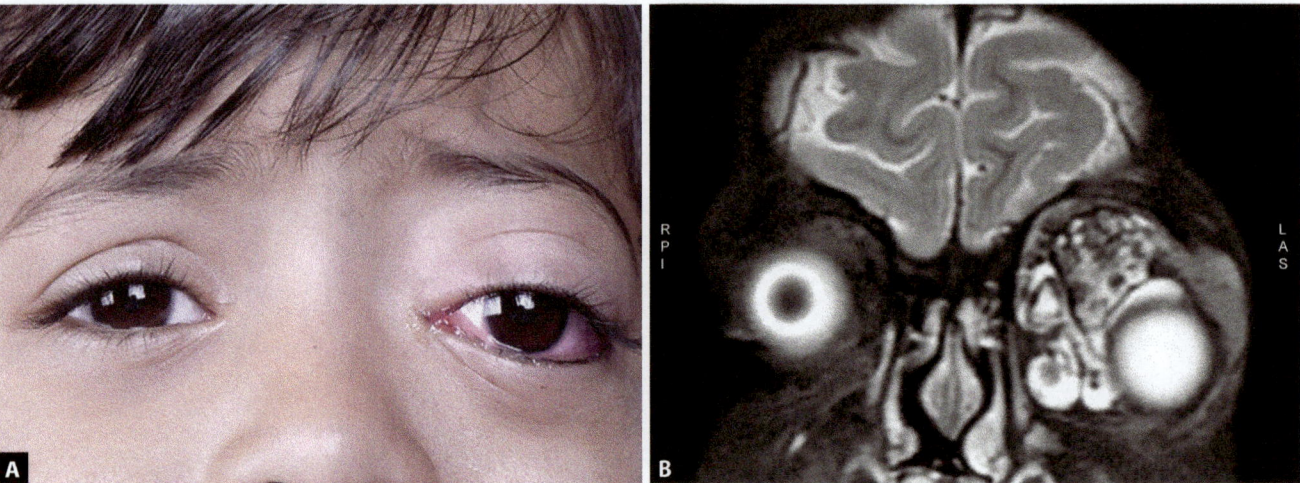

Fig. 13: Clinical picture of a young child with acute proptosis and inferotemporal globe dystopia. MRI scans reveal a multilobulated ill-defined lesion with heterogenous contrast enhancement suggestive of a lymphangioma.

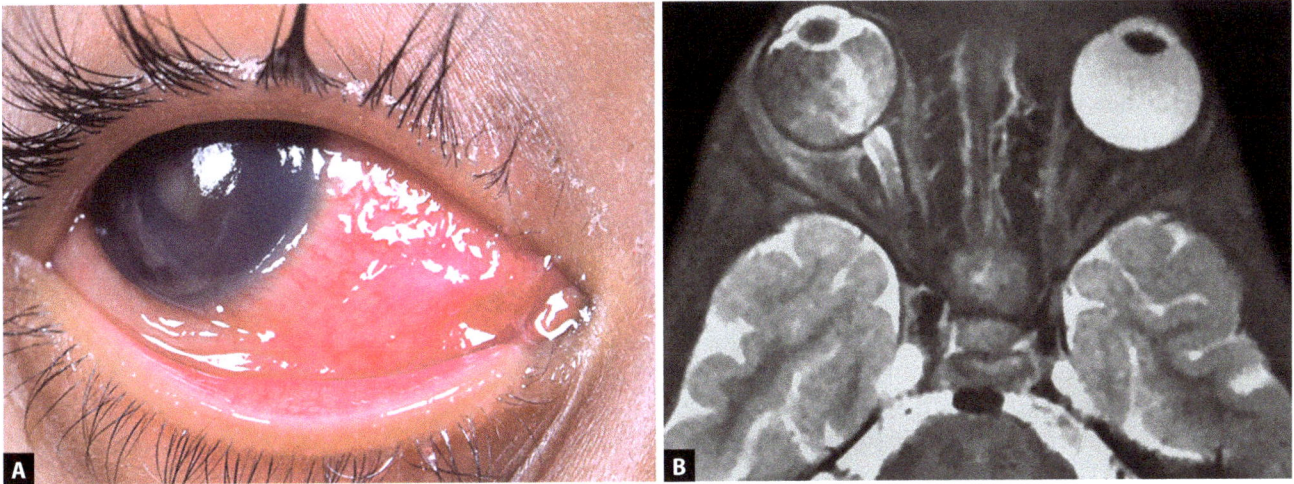

Figs. 14A and B: (A) Clinical photograph of a 1-year-old girl presenting with a history of leukocoria and sudden onset redness and outward bulge of the eye. (B) Axial MRI scans reveal a large intraocular tumor filling the affected globe. Enucleation and histopathological analysis of the sample revealed a retinoblastoma.

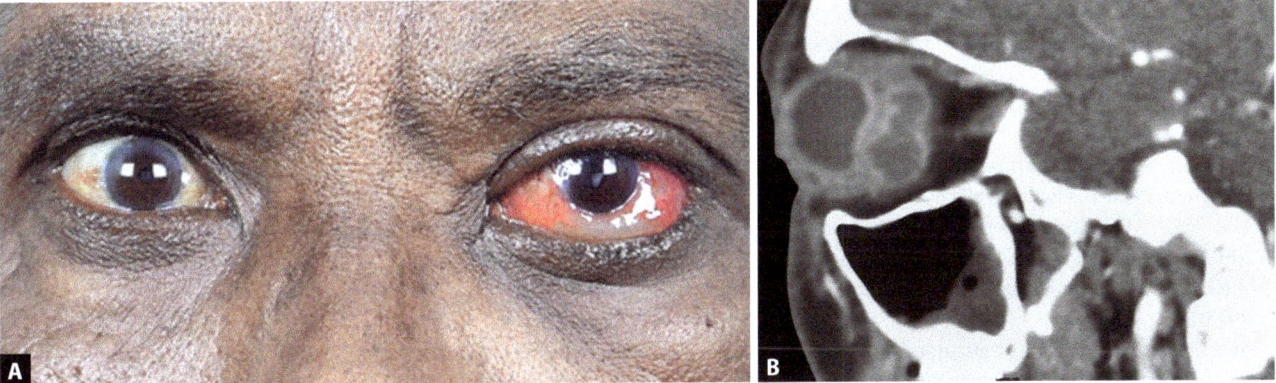

Figs. 15A and B: (A) Clinical photograph of a 45-year-old male presenting with proptosis accompanied by conjunctival congestion and chemosis. (B) Sagittal CT scan reveals a retrobulbar bilobed cystic lesion with intralesional hyperdense foci suggestive of a scolex within a cyst.

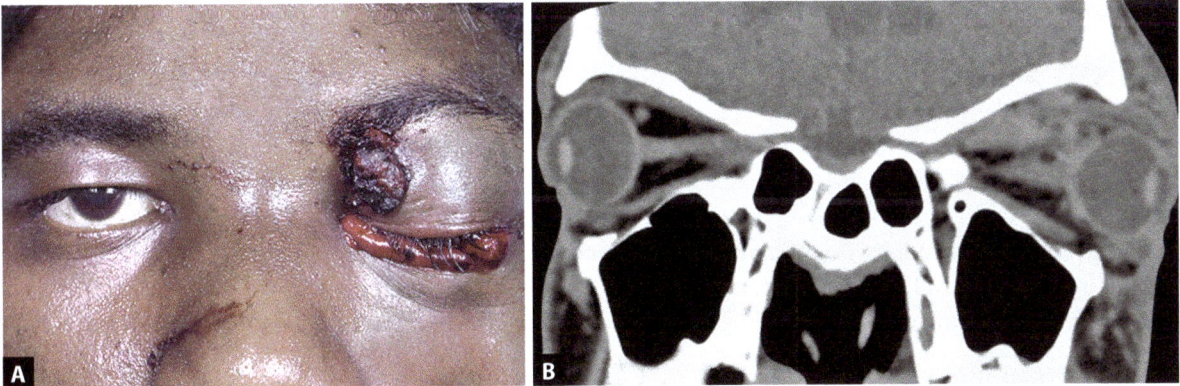

Figs. 16A and B: (A) 20-year-old male with clinical features of orbital cellulitis secondary to trauma. (B) Reconstructed sagittal CT scan reveals an apical foreign body, likely responsible for the orbital inflammation.

Ultrasonography typically shows an area of hypoechogenicity indicating the cyst, within which is a hyperechogenic focus—the scolex. An MRI better delineates the cystic lesion as compared to a CT scan due to superior soft tissue detailing. Treatment is via larvicidal drugs including albendazole or praziquantel with adjunct corticosteroids to reduce the accompanying inflammation. Surgical excision of the lesion particularly if occurring in the subconjunctival space is a viable option.

Trauma

Orbital inflammation following trauma can often mimic orbital cellulitis. Retained intraorbital foreign bodies can cause sterile inflammation which mimics bacterial cellulitis. A post-traumatic subperiosteal hematoma can cause lid edema and proptosis. Pneumo-orbit caused by fracture of medial orbital wall with entry of air from sinuses into the orbit can lead to progressive proptosis.

Suggested Reading

1. Basily A, Mansukhani S, Anzeljc A, Gutierrez P. Orbital cellulitis—when computed tomography imaging is falsely reassuring. Pediatr Emerg Care. 2021;37(1):e48-50.
2. Black EH, Nesi FA, Calvano CJ, Gladstone GJ, Levine MR. Smith and Nesi's Ophthalmic Plastic and Reconstructive Surgery, 3rd edition. New York: Springer; 2012.
3. Bodh SA, Kamal S, Kumar S, Goel R, Nagpal S, Aditya K. Orbital Cysticercosis. DJO. 2012;23:99-103.
4. Cappello ZJ, Dublin AB. Anatomy, Head and Neck, Nose Paranasal Sinuses [Updated October 27, 2018]. In: StatPearls [Internet]. Treasure Island, FL: StatPearls Publishing; 2019.
5. Chandler JR, Langenbrunner DJ, Stevens ER. The pathogenesis of orbital complications in acute sinusitis. Laryngoscopes. 1970;80:1414.
6. Chaudhry IA, Al-Rashed W, Arat YO. The hot orbit: orbital cellulitis. Middle East Afr J Ophthalmol. 2012;19(1):34-42.
7. Chen L, Silverman N, Wu A, Shinder R. Intravenous steroids with antibiotics on admission for children with orbital cellulitis. Ophthalmic Plast Reconstr Surg. 2018;34(3):205-8.
8. Dhiman R, Devi S, Duraipandi K, Chandra P, Vanathi M, Tandon R, et al. Cysticercosis of the eye. Int J Ophthalmol. 2017;10(8):1319-24.
9. Graeb A, Rootman J. Orbital lymphangiomas: clinical, radiologic and pathologic characteristics. Radiology. 1990;175:417-21.
10. Jain A, Rubin PA. Orbital cellulitis in children. Int Ophthalmol Clin. 2001;41(4):71-86.
11. Jurdy L, Merks JH, Pieters BR, Mourits MP, Kloos RJHM, Strackee SD, et al. Orbital rhabdomyosarcomas: a review. Saudi J Ophthalmol. 2013;27(3):167-75.
12. Kang TL, Seif D, Chilstrom M, Mailhot T. Ocular ultrasound identifies early orbital cellulitis. West J Emerg Med. 2014;15(4):394.
13. Leatherbarrow B. Oculoplastic Surgery, 2nd edition, Informa Healthcare; 2010.
14. Lee S, Yen MT. Management of preseptal and orbital cellulitis. Saudi J Ophthalmol. 2011;25(1):21-9.
15. Mukherjee B, Raichura ND, Alam MS. Fungal infections of the orbit. Indian J Ophthalmol. 2016;64(5):337-345.
16. Pushker N, Tejwani LK, Bajaj MS, Khurana S, Velpandian T, Chandra M. Role of oral corticosteroids in orbital cellulitis. Am J Ophthal. 2013;156:178-83.
17. Shields JA, Shields CL. Intraocular Tumors: An Atlas and Textbook, 3rd edition. Philadelphia, PA: Wolters Kluwer; 2008.
18. Suneetha N, Battu RR, Thomas RK, Bosco A. Orbital abscess: management and outcome. Indian J Ophthalmol. 2000;48:129.
19. Wong SJ, Levi J. Management of pediatric orbital cellulitis: a systematic review. Int J Pediatr Otorhinolaryngol. 2018;110:123-9.
20. Woo YJ, Kim CY, Sgrignoli B, Yoon JS. Orbital lymphangioma: characteristics and treatment outcomes of 12 cases. Korean J Ophthalmol. 2017;31(3):194-201.

1.20 Intraocular Tumor

Vijitha S Vempuluru, Vishal Raval, Anasua G Kapoor

 1. Classify extraocular and intraocular tumors with a note on their prognosis.

Classification of intraocular tumors is summarized in **Flowchart 1**. Extraocular tumors of the eye can be classified into: orbital, eyelid, and conjunctival tumors. Refer to respective Chapters for the same.

Prognosis of common intraocular tumors: Prognosis of common intraocular tumors has been summarized in **Flowchart 2**.

 2. Describe investigations for intraocular malignancies in an adult and options for their management.

Differential diagnosis of intraocular tumors in an adult: Refer **Flowchart 2**. Salient features of individual tumors have been summarized in **Table 1**.

Investigations for Intraocular Tumors

- Investigations for any intraocular tumor are tailored according to the location and tissue of origin after a detailed clinical examination.

Flowchart 1: Classification of intraocular tumors.

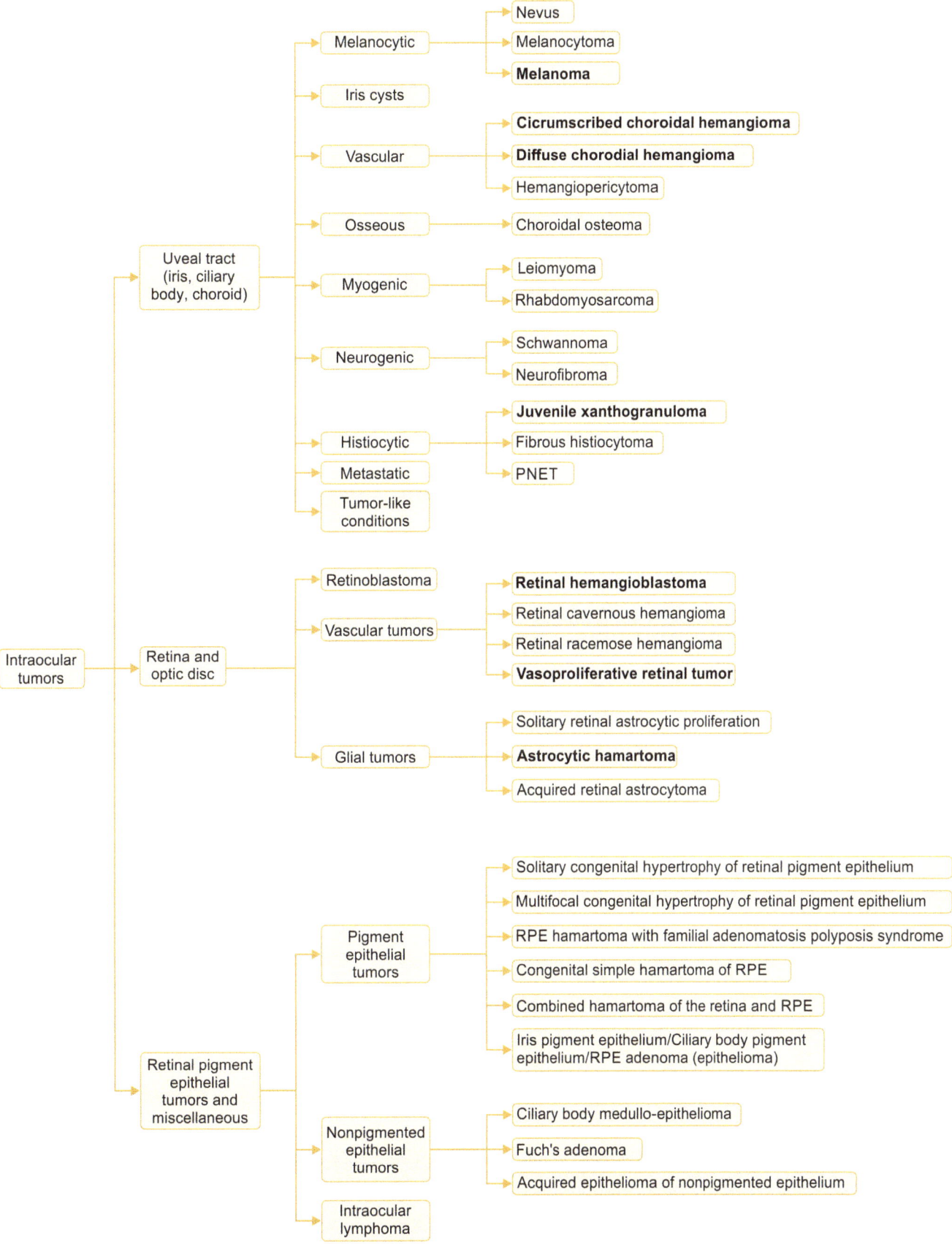

(PNET: primitive neuroectodermal tumor; RPE: retinal pigment epithelium)

Flowchart 2: Summary of prognosis of common intraocular tumors.

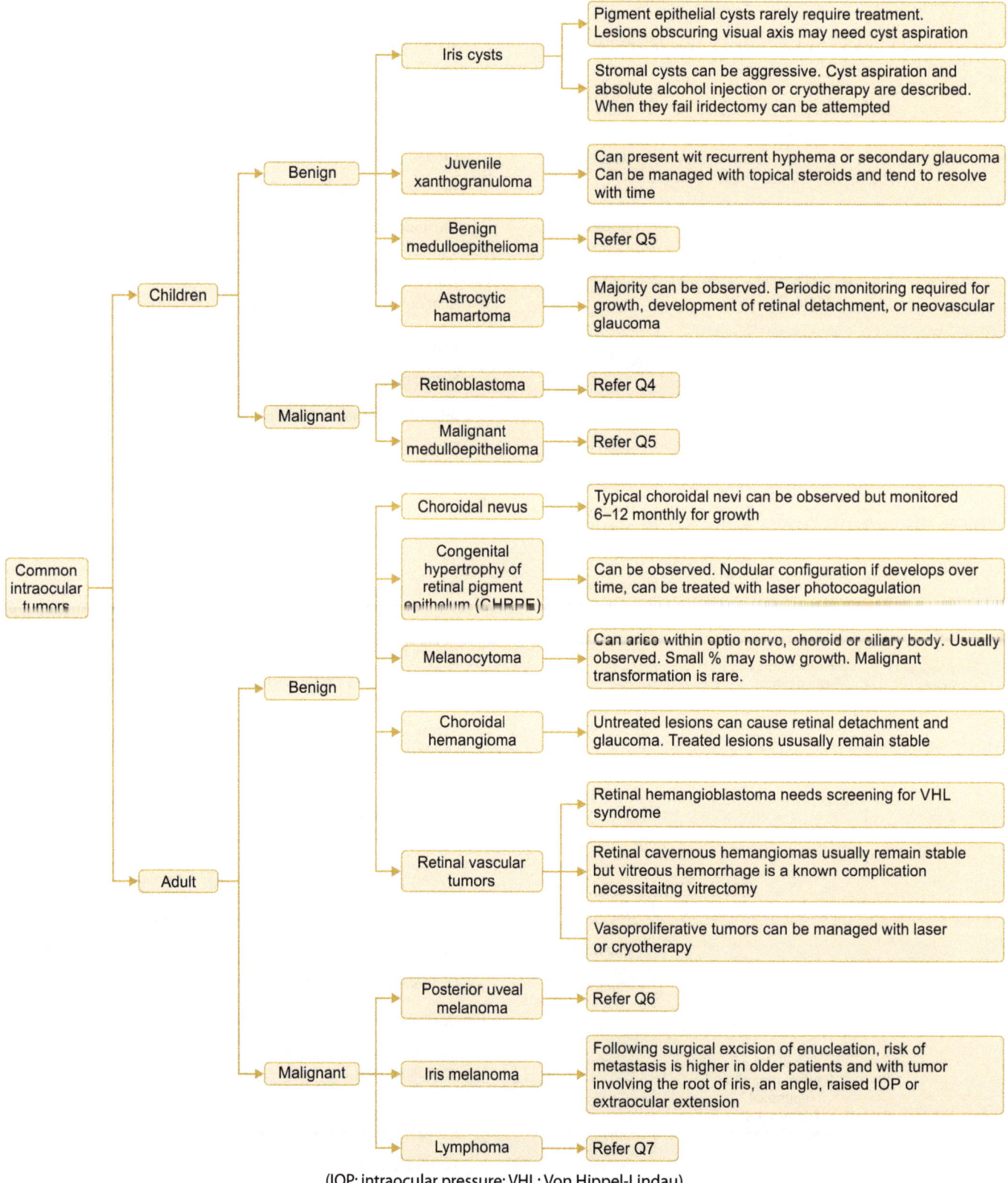

(IOP: intraocular pressure; VHL: Von Hippel-Lindau)

- They help in differentiating between tumors or from simulating tumor-like conditions, i.e., establishing the diagnosis.
- Aid in monitoring response to medical/laser/systemic therapy.

TABLE 1: Salient features of common intraocular tumors on clinical examination and common investigative modalities.

Tumor	Clinical feature	A scan	B scan	Optical coherence tomography	Fluorescein angiography
Choroidal melanoma	Usually pigmented, brown elevated choroidal lesion	Low-to-moderate spike	Mushroom/collar stud appearance, choroidal excavation, acoustic hollowing	Serous detachment, shaggy photoreceptors	Early hypofluorescence with late pin-point leakage; double circulation may be evident
Choroidal hemangioma	Red-orange, smooth choroidal lesion—diffuse or circumscribed	High-amplitude broad-based spike	Fusiform/biconvex	Subretinal fluid, intraretinal edema, photoreceptor loss	Early filling with late diffuse staining
Choroidal metastasis	Yellowish orange flat lesion with subretinal fluid that may be out of proportion to the size of lesion	Moderate-to-high spike	Dome-shaped/polygonal with retinal detachment or choroidal detachment	Thickened RPE, highly reflective subretinal deposits	Early hypofluorescence; later persistence hyperfluorescence with pin-point leakage
Choroidal osteoma	Orange-yellow with indistinct borders	High spike	Plaque-like with shadowing	Latticework reflective pattern	Early patchy hyper-fluorescence, late staining

(RPE: retinal pigment epithelium)

Common investigations employed for the diagnosis and/or follow-up of intraocular tumors include the following:
- *Anterior segment:*
  - Ultrasound biomicroscopy (UBM)
  - Anterior segment optical coherence tomography (OCT)
  - Anterior segment fluorescein angiography
- *Posterior segment:*
  - Ultrasound A and B scan
  - Optical coherence tomography (with enhanced depth imaging for choroidal tumors)
  - Autofluorescence
  - Fluorescein angiography and indocyanine green angiography
  - Computed tomography and magnetic resonance imaging (MRI) are performed in select cases with suspected extraocular extension.

General Principles of Management

- Benign tumors can be observed unless vision is threatened or secondary glaucoma ensues or a malignant transformation is seen.
- Malignant tumors warrant systemic work-up for metastasis in addition to ocular investigations.
- Treatment options vary between tumors and include the following:
  - Laser therapy (laser photocoagulation, transpupillary thermotherapy, photodynamic therapy)—small choroidal melanomas, circumscribed choroidal hemangioma, choroidal metastasis, retinal hemangioblastoma
  - Cryotherapy—vasoproliferative tumor of retina
  - *Radiotherapy:*
    - Plaque brachytherapy—choroidal melanoma, choroidal metastasis, circumscribed choroidal hemangioma, vasoproliferative tumor of retina
    - External beam radiotherapy—diffuse choroidal hemangioma, primary vitreoretinal lymphoma (PVRL)
  - *Chemotherapy:*
    - *Intraocular injections:* Intravitreal methotrexate, rituximab for PVRL
    - *Systemic chemotherapy:* Metastatic tumors, uveal lymphoma
  - *Enucleation:*
    - Indicated for advanced malignant tumors such as large uveal melanomas that cannot be successfully managed by other methods or painful blind eye with intractable glaucoma in eyes with benign tumors
    - Gentle handling of the globe is warranted throughout the surgery to avoid inadvertent globe rupture and extraocular seeding of tumor cells.
  - *Exenteration:* Reserved for cases with massive extraocular extension such as uveal melanomas
- Lifelong surveillance is warranted in malignant tumors to detect recurrence or metastasis.

3. Describe the methods, benefits, and risks of tumor biopsy of extraocular and intraocular tumors.

(Refer to Chapters on Eyelid, Conjunctival, and Orbital Tumors for biopsy techniques of extraocular tumors)

Biopsy for Intraocular Tumors

- Biopsy of intraocular tumors is attempted only when all ancillary investigations fail to establish a definitive diagnosis, most often to rule out melanoma or in case when the primary tumor remains undetected.
- Technique used is vitreous biopsy or fine needle aspiration biopsy (FNAB) for solid tumors. The approach used is either through transscleral or transvitreal route using indirect ophthalmoscopy or vitrectomy system.
- A fine needle is passed into the lesion of interest to obtain cells from the same.
- For iris tumors, the needle is passed through the corneoscleral limbus under microscopic visualization directly into the tumor.
- Retinochoroidal biopsy when mandated is performed after pars plana vitrectomy with necessary steps taken to prevent retinal detachment (laser, oil/gas tamponade).

Risks

- Most dreaded complication includes extraocular extension of tumor/tumor seeding through the biopsy route, which can be avoided by use of a fine needle and applying cryotherapy at the biopsy site.
- Risks of intraocular complications such as vitreous hemorrhage, retinal detachment, and endophthalmitis.

Benefits

Aids in the establishment of diagnosis and decision making regarding eye salvage in select cases.

 4. Discuss the clinical features and differential diagnosis of retinoblastoma (RB). What is International Classification of Retinoblastoma (ICRB) and outline the treatment of RB?

Retinoblastoma is the most common intraocular malignancy of childhood usually presents within 3 years of age.

Clinical features: The clinical features are summarized in **Table 2**.

Differential diagnosis: Differential diagnosis of RB is summarized in **Table 3**.

TABLE 2: Clinical features of retinoblastoma (RB).

Symptoms	Signs: examination under anesthesia
• Leukocoria • Strabismus • Red eye • Lid edema, proptosis • Poor vision • Sometimes asymptomatic or unnoticed by parents and incidentally detected by screening of retinoblastoma affected family members or routine screening	• Exophytic or endophytic white tumor • Can be unifocal or multifocal, unilateral, or bilateral • Can be associated with vitreous, subretinal seeding, retinal detachment • Advanced cases may have cataract, neovascular glaucoma, megalocornea, corneal scarring

TABLE 3: Differential diagnosis of retinoblastoma (RB).

Leukocoria	Vitreous disease	Retinal tumor
• Coats' retinopathy • Persistent hyperplastic primary vitreous • Retinopathy of prematurity • Familial exudative vitreoretinopathy • Ocular toxocariasis • Incontinentia pigmenti • Norrie's disease	• Endophthalmitis • Uveitis	• Astrocytoma • Medulloepithelioma (anterior tumors) • Toxocara granuloma

Diagnosis of Retinoblastoma

- Diagnosis is based on classical clinical features.
- Ultrasonography B scan shows well-defined intraocular mass with intratumoral hyperechogenic foci corresponding to calcifications.
- MRI is warranted for all cases with clinically evident optic nerve involvement and advanced tumors.
- Computed tomography is best avoid in view of risk of secondary cancers in children with RB1 mutations.
- Bone marrow aspiration and cerebrospinal fluid (CSF) cytology are performed in advanced tumors to look for systemic spread of disease.

Classification of Retinoblastoma

The ICRB (Shields) is summarized in **Table 4**.

Treatment Modalities for Retinoblastoma

- *Focal:*
    - *Transpupillary thermotherapy:*
        - Allows destruction of tumor cells by raising temperature within the tumor
        - Performed under indirect ophthalmoscopic guidance using 810 nm diode laser
        - Utilized for small posterior tumors (primary, recurrent, subretinal seeds) and also as an adjuvant to chemotherapy
    - *Cryotherapy:*
        - Useful in treating anteriorly located tumors
        - Performed under indirect ophthalmoscopic visualization
        - Triple free-thaw technique is employed
    - *Laser photocoagulation:* Acts by coagulating the blood supply to the tumor
- *Chemotherapy:*
    - *Intravenous chemotherapy:*
        - Drugs vincristine, etoposide, and carboplatin are used
        - Given as standard-dose or high-dose regimes
    - *Intra-arterial chemotherapy:* Superselective form of chemotherapy where in the drug is delivered to the eye through ophthalmic artery.

TABLE 4: International Classification of Retinoblastoma (Shields).

Group	Features
A	*Small tumor:* RB ≤ 3 mm in basal diameter/thickness
B	*Larger tumor:* • RB >3 mm in basal diameter/thickness • Macular location (≤3 mm to *foveola*) • Juxtapapillary location (≤1.5 mm to disc) • Clear subretinal fluid ≤3 mm from margin
C	*Focal seeds:* • *C1:* Subretinal seeds ≤3 mm from RB • *C2:* Vitreous seeds ≤3 mm from RB • *C3:* Both subretinal and vitreous seeds ≤3 mm from RB
D	*Diffuse seeds:* • *D1:* Subretinal seeds >3 mm from RB • *D2:* Vitreous seeds >3 mm from RB • *D3:* Both subretinal and vitreous seeds ≤3 mm from RB
E	*Extensive RB:* • Occupies >50% globe • Neovascular glaucoma • Opaque media from hemorrhage in vitreous, anterior chamber, or subretinal space • Invasion of postlaminar optic nerve, choroid, sclera, anterior chamber

(RB: retinoblastoma)

- *Intravitreal:*
  - Predominantly employed for vitreous seeds
  - Drugs utilized include melphalan and topotecan
- *Periocular:* Sub-Tenon carboplatin for primary or recurrent tumors, usually as an adjunct therapy
- Radiotherapy:
  - *Plaque brachytherapy:* Usually reserved for solitary group B/C tumors or recurrent tumors
  - *External beam radiotherapy:* Crucial for the management for orbital RB
- *Surgery:* Enucleation for advanced intraocular tumors

Treatment Choice, Follow-up, and Prognosis

- Choice of treatment modalities depends on a variety of factors such as tumor location, laterality, grouping socioeconomic status, primary or recurrent tumor, compliance for treatment, and follow-up of the caregivers.
- When treated in early stages, prognosis for survival is excellent for RB.
- Globe salvage for groups A, B, and C is excellent (>95%) and is improving over the past decades for groups D and E as well with advances in therapeutics.
- Lifelong surveillance is warranted for detection of second cancers and metastatic disease.
- Screening of family members must be emphasized in cases where genetic testing is not done.

5. Discuss the clinical features, differential diagnosis, and management of medulloepithelioma.

Medulloepithelioma is a primary intraocular neoplasm which arises from primitive medullary epithelial cells of embryonic cup.

Clinical features. The various clinical manifestations are summarized in **Table 5**.

Diagnosis

- As visualization may not be possible in cases due to anterior location, UBM plays an important role in the diagnosis of medulloepithelioma.
- Tumor being frequently cystic, hypoechogenic areas within a tumor arising from ciliary body is suggestive of medulloepithelioma.
- Differential diagnosis include anterior RB, amelanotic melanoma, leiomyoma, and juvenile xanthogranuloma.

Management

- *Systemic work-up:*
  - Medulloepitheliomas can be locally invasive and extraocular ocular extension if present warrants systemic screening for metastasis.
  - Systemic associations include pleuropulmonary blastoma family tumor and dysplasia syndrome with propensity to develop pleuropulmonary blastoma of lung, ovarian tumors, cystic nephroma, and other cystic lesions in various parts of the body. *DICER1* gene has been implicated and screening for the same is beneficial.

TABLE 5: Clinical manifestations of medulloepithelioma.

Symptoms	Signs
• Red eye • Altered iris color • Rarely visible tumor through pupil or iris	• Sectoral cataract • Raised intraocular pressure • Neovascularization of iris/angle • When large, a tan white tumor arising from ciliary body may be visualized on indirect ophthalmoscopy by visualization • Sectoral loss of zonules • Lens subluxation • Lens coloboma

- *Diagnostic intervention:* When other differential diagnoses cannot be ruled, fine needle aspiration cytology can be employed to establish the diagnosis.
- *Treatment:*
  - Plaque brachytherapy or localized iridocyclectomy for small tumors offer globe and vision salvage.
  - For advanced tumors, uncertain diagnosis and painful blind eye enucleation is the treatment of choice.
- *Prognosis and outcome:*
  - Intraocular tumors treated at an early stage have good prognosis for life.
  - Extraocular extension is a risk factor for metastasis.
  - Syndromic patients need follow-up for systemic tumors.

6. Discuss the clinical features, differential diagnosis, and management of posterior uveal melanoma.

Posterior uveal melanoma refers to melanoma arising from the ciliary body and choroid.

Clinical features: The various clinical manifestations are summarized in **Table 6**.

Investigations

- *Ultrasonography B scan:*
  - Solid, acoustically hypoechoic mass with a biconvex/collar stud/mushroom-shaped tumor with choroidal excavation
  - Trans-scleral or extrascleral invasion may be seen.
- *Fluorescein angiography:*
  - *When the Bruch's membrane is not breached:* Early hypofluorescence with evident large caliber vessels within the tumor. Late phases show leakage of dye into subretinal space. Pinpoint foci of accumulation of the dye at the level of retinal pigment epithelium (RPE) may be seen.
  - In tumor with breach of Bruch's membrane, intralesional vessels are prominent during the early phases which leak profusely in late phase and result in staining of tumor.
- *Indocyanine angiography:* Tumors show hypocyanescence with well-defined intralesions large caliber vessels.
- *Computed tomography or magnetic resonance imaging:* Indicated for tumors with suspected or clinically evident extraocular extension
- *Systemic evaluation:* Whole-body positron emission tomography (PET) computed tomography (CT) is mandated for the detection of metastasis.

Treatment

- *Small-size tumors:* Laser therapy (transpupillary thermotherapy, photodynamic therapy)
- *Medium-size tumors:* Plaque brachytherapy
- *Larger size tumors:* Plaque brachytherapy or enucleation
- *Tumors with extraocular extension or orbital disease:* Extended enucleation or exenteration
- Lifelong surveillance is warranted to detect metastasis disease (liver most common followed by lung, risk greater with thicker or larger size tumors and the presence of extraocular extension) which determines the prognosis for life.

TABLE 6: Clinical manifestations of posterior uveal melanoma.

Symptoms	Signs
• Can be asymptomatic (small lesions) • Vision loss • Field defect • Flashes • Floaters	• Solid, dark brown elevated tumor arising from choroid or ciliary body • Retinal invasion when present manifests as a dark brown component with no overlying retinal vessels • Lipofuscin when present appears as orange pigment clumps • Subretinal fluid is often present especially with larger tumors • Vitreous hemorrhage is a variable feature • Signs of neovascular or angle-closure glaucoma may be seen with advanced tumors

7. Discuss the clinical features, differential diagnosis, and management of primary intraocular lymphoma.

- Primary intraocular lymphoma refers to PVRL and uveal lymphoma.
- While uveal lymphoma is considered a manifestation of systemic non-Hodgkin's lymphoma, PVRL is considered a subtype of primary central nervous system (CNS) lymphoma (PCNSL) also referred to as PCNSL with ocular involvement (PCNSL-O).

Clinical features: The various clinical manifestations are summarized in **Table 7**.

TABLE 7: Clinical manifestations of primary intraocular lymphoma.

Symptoms	Signs
• Usually nonspecific • Common in older age groups and immunosuppressed (HIV+) • Floaters may be present • Known to masquerade as uveitis with nonresponse or frequent relapses on steroid therapy	• *Uveal lymphoma:* Creamy thickening of choroid usually diffuse or multifocal • *PCNSL-O:* Subretinal yellowish white infiltrates which represent clusters of lymphomatous cells

(HIV: human immunodeficiency virus; PCNSL-O: primary central nervous system lymphoma with ocular involvement)

Differential diagnosis:

PCNSL-O	Uveal lymphoma
• Chronic idiopathic vitritis • Amyloidosis • Pars planitis • Choroiditis	• Metastasis • Choroiditis • Benign reactive lymphoid hyperplasia • Bilateral diffuse uveal melanocytic proliferation

(PCNSL-O: primary central nervous system lymphoma with ocular involvement)

Management

- Systemic assessment is crucial for uveal lymphoma as well as PCNSL-O.
- Options for management of isolated PCNSL-O include the following:
  - Intravitreal methotrexate
  - Intravitreal rituximab
  - External beam radiotherapy
- Even with PCNSL-O (absence of CNS involvement at presentation) surveillance for CNS disease through periodic CSF tap and MRI brain and spine is mandated (every 6 months).
- CNS involvement has overall worse prognosis for survival.

Suggested Reading

1. Berry JL, Kim JW, Damato BE, Singh AD. Clinical Ophthalmic Oncology: Retinoblastoma. Switzerland: Springer Nature Switzerland; 2019.
2. Kapoor AG, Kaliki S, Vempuluru VS, Jajapuram SD, Ali MH, Mohamed A. Posterior uveal melanoma in 321 Asian Indian patients: analysis based on the 8th edition of American Joint Committee Cancer Classification. Int Ophthalmol. 2020;40(11):3087-96.
3. Perry JD, Singh AD. Clinical Ophthalmic Oncology: Orbital Tumors, 2nd edition. Berlin Heidelberg: Springer-Verlag; 2014.
4. Shields JA, Shields CL (Eds). Intraocular Tumors: An Atlas and Textbook, 3rd edition. China: Wolters Kluwer; 2016.
5. Singh AD, Damato BE. Clinical Ophthalmic Oncology, 3rd edition. Switzerland: Springer Nature Switzerland AG; 2019.
6. Vempuluru VS, Jakati S, Krishnamurthy R, Senthil S, Kaliki S. Glaucoma as the presenting sign of intraocular tumors: beware of the masquerading sign. Int Ophthalmol. 2020;40(7):1789-95.
7. Yanoff M, Duker JS. Ophthalmology, 4th edition. Chicago: Elsevier; 2014.

1.21 Conjunctival Pigmented Tumors

Shweta Gupta, Anasua G Kapoor

1. What are the pigmented conjunctival lesions and discuss in details about the classification of the conjunctival melanocytic proliferations?

Pigmented lesions that arise from conjunctiva are the most common tumors of the conjunctiva, accounting for up to 53% of all conjunctival neoplasms.

These lesions arise from the melanocytes of the conjunctiva and episclera. Conjunctival melanocytic proliferations are classified into two categories: benign and malignant lesions. The most important benign lesions include nevus, complexion-associated melanosis (CAM), and primary acquired melanosis (PAM), and the malignant one is conjunctival melanoma.

It is very important to differentiate among various pigmented conjunctival lesions as management varies depending on the diagnosis along with different ocular and systemic prognoses. The diagnosis of these lesions is usually made based on the clinical features and frequently confirmed with unique histopathologic findings. These conjunctival lesions can be diagnostic challenge, but better understanding of these lesions helps in the identification of the previously undiagnosed cases as well as to avoid aggressive management in benign lesions.

The various pigmented conjunctival lesions are as follows:
- *Conjunctival nevus:* It presents as well circumscribed, variably pigmented, flat to slightly elevated lesion which usually appears in young white individuals during the first or second decade of life.
- *CAM/racial melanosis:* It is flat conjunctival pigmentation at the limbus in both the eyes found most frequently in dark-skinned individuals.
- *PAM:* It is flat pigmented lesion of the conjunctiva near the limbus with poorly defined margins, appearing unilaterally, typically occurring in white patients.
- *Ocular melanocytosis:* It is a congenital pigmentary condition involving the sclera, which appears as a gray, flat lesion, and often associated with periocular skin pigmentation.
- *Conjunctival melanoma:* It is a condition that commonly presents as a well-defined, elevated, pigmented lesion and usually affects elderly white individuals **(Table 1)**.

TABLE 1: Differential diagnosis of pigmented epibulbar lesions.

Condition	Anatomical location	Color	Depth	Margins	Laterality	Other features	Progression
Nevus **(Fig. 1A)**	Interpalpebral limbus usually	Brown or yellow	Stroma	Well defined	Unilateral	Cysts	<1% Progress to conjunctival melanoma
Racial melanosis **(Fig. 1B)**	Limbus bulbar palpebral conjunctiva		Epithelium	Ill defined	Bilateral	Flat, no cysts	Very rare progression to conjunctival melanoma <1% progress to uveal melanoma
Ocular melanocytosis	Bulbar conjunctiva	Brown Gray	Episclera	Ill defined	Unilateral more so than bilateral	Congenital, usually 2 mm from limbus, often with periocular skin pigmentation	Progresses to conjunctival melanoma in nearly 50% cases that show cellular atypia
Primary acquired melanosis (PAM) **(Fig. 1C)**	Anywhere, but usually bulbar conjunctiva	Brown	Epithelium	Ill defined	Unilateral	Flat, no cysts Waxing and waning	32% develop metastasis by 15 years
Malignant melanoma **(Fig. 1D)**	Anywhere	Brown or pink	Stroma	Well defined	Unilateral	Vascular nodule, dilated feeder vessels, may be nonpigmented. Involvement of tarsal conjunctiva, fornix, and caruncle by pigmented lesion always rule out melanoma	

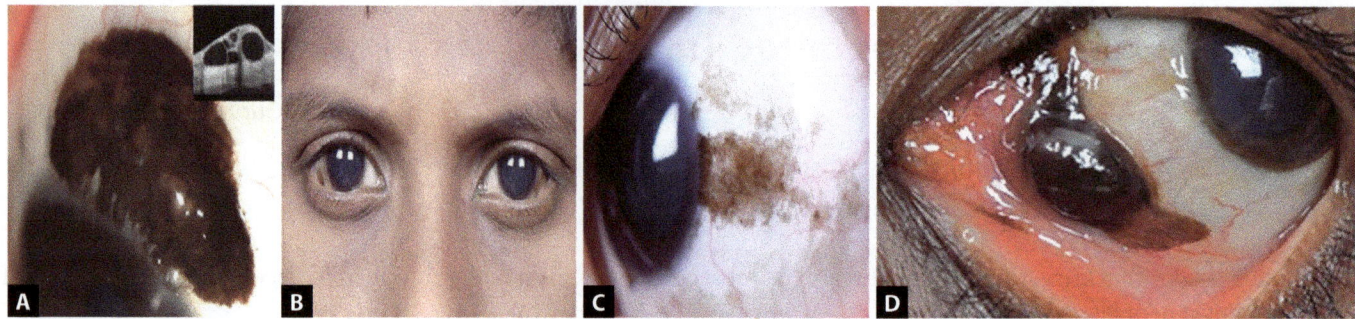

Figs. 1A to D: (A) Clinical photograph showing well-defined unilateral pigmented lesion with prominent cysts in a child suggestive of conjunctival nevus (Inset highlights the cysts on anterior segment OCT); (B) Clinical photograph showing bilateral cobblestone-like perilimbal pigmentation with microfolds suggestive of complexion-associated melanosis; (C) Clinical photograph in a middle-aged individual with unilateral flat peppery pigmentation with no cyst suggestive of primary acquired melanosis; (D) Clinical photograph showing unilateral elevated pigmented lesion involving plica semilunaris and extending to inferior forniceal conjunctiva. (OCT: optical coherence tomography)

2. What are the differential diagnosis for the conjunctival/epibulbar pigmented lesions or enumerate the conditions that can simulate conjunctival melanocytic tumors?

The differential diagnosis of various pigmented conjunctival lesions is an important step to plan further management.

Epibulbar melanocytic lesions include conditions of the conjunctival epithelium, stroma, and sclera. Melanosis can be primary or secondary (such as in Addison's disease), and congenital (such as CAM) or acquired. The most common form of melanosis is primary and acquired.

The neoplastic causes for the conjunctival pigmentation include benign lesions such as nevus, CAM, PAM, and the malignant lesions such as conjunctival melanoma. Other pigmented epibulbar mass, include pigmented squamous cell carcinoma of the conjunctiva and extraocular extension of a uveal melanoma.

There are several benign, non-neoplastic conditions that can resemble conjunctival melanocytic tumors. These include the following:
- Pingueculum
- Pterygium
- Axenfeld nerve loops at the site of a scleral emissarial canal
- Mascara deposition in the inferior fornix
- Silver deposition on the entire conjunctival surface after argyrol eyedrops
- Gunpowder deposition in patients exposed to gunpowder explosions
- Adrenochrome pigment in the inferior fornix in patients using epinephrine eyedrops
- Hemorrhagic conjunctival cyst following previous surgery
- Prolapsed uveal tissue through partial wound dehiscence of a cataract incision can simulate
- Pigmented cells trapped within a nonmelanocytic tumor (fellow travelers)
- Ochronosis pigmentation at the site of muscle insertion
- Pingueculum in patients with alkaptonuria
- Calcified Cogan's scleral plaque at the horizontal rectus muscle insertions in older adults.

The clinical features of these pigmented conditions occasionally overlap and cause diagnostic confusion. Therefore, clinicians managing patients with conjunctival malignancies should have exhaustive understanding and recognition of these pseudomelanomas.

3. Discuss in details about the clinical features and management of conjunctival nevus.

Nevus is a common benign melanocytic proliferation of the conjunctiva, accounting for 28% of all conjunctival tumors and 52% of the melanocytic tumors.

Clinical Features

It can manifest with a spectrum of signs and symptoms. The diagnosis is typically made based on the classic clinical features using slit-lamp biomicroscopy. These lesions most commonly arise in the bulbar conjunctiva, caruncle, or plica semilunaris.

It is typically located in the interpalpebral bulbar conjunctiva close to the limbus and remains relatively stationary throughout life with <1% risk for transformation into malignant melanoma. The interpalpebral location is very classic to nevus such that in any pigmented lesion in fornix, tarsus, or cornea, it is suggested to suspect PAM, racial melanosis, or malignant melanoma.

Nevi on the bulbar conjunctiva move freely over the sclera and appear well circumscribed without extension into the cornea. Conjunctival nevi generally stop abruptly at the limbus and typically do not involve the corneal epithelium or stroma. Overhang of the cornea from a large conjunctival nevus is possible, but invasion of the cornea by a nevus would be distinctly unusual. On the other hand, conjunctival melanoma often grows beyond the limbus into the cornea. Corneal involvement from a pigmented conjunctival lesion suggests PAM or racial melanosis if the conjunctival pigmentation is within the epithelium, but conjunctival melanoma should be suspected if the conjunctival pigmentation has thickness and extends into the stroma.

It usually appears in the first or second decade of life, most common in young white individuals, with a mean age at presentation of about 32 years. Majority of the patients report a spot on the eye, few notice inflammation or pain while others can be asymptomatic. It presents clinically as well circumscribed, variably pigmented, sessile, flat to slightly elevated lesion. Nevi in children are often inapparent and nonpigmented and usually increase in size and acquire pigmentation during puberty or pregnancy. However, up to 30% of nevi remain amelanotic. A common and characteristic feature of conjunctival nevi is the presence of fine clear intralesional cysts on slit-lamp biomicroscopy.

It remains relatively stationary throughout life with the risk of malignant transformation from a conjunctival nevus to a conjunctival melanoma <1%. However, 25% of conjunctival melanomas follow a conjunctival nevus.

Histopathologic Features

Histologically, conjunctival melanocytic nevi are classified as junctional, compound, and subepithelial nevi similar to cutaneous nevi. These benign melanocytes can be organized into intraepithelial nests, sheets, and spindle-like cells in the stroma near the basal layers of epithelium. Compound nevi are the most common type of conjunctival nevus, comprising about 70–78% of all nevi.

A very characteristic and diagnostically useful feature of conjunctival nevi is induction of epithelial protrusions into the lamina propria and formation of intralesional epithelial cysts lined by conjunctival epithelium and goblet cells. These stromal cysts are present in 50% of cases. It seems that cyst formation is a function of time, as they are less frequent in early lesions. In rare, longstanding nevi, cysts may occupy most of the volume of the lesion prominent and the melanocytic component may not be apparent. In contrast, conjunctival cysts are extremely rare in PAM and melanoma.

Treatment

Management of choice is periodic observation with slit-lamp measurements and serial photographic comparison every 6–12 months in order to detect any changes in size or color. Conjunctival nevi do not require treatment if clinically stable. On follow up, excision is recommended in lesions which show clinical characteristics of possible malignancy such as change in size, shape, or color, rapid growth, and recurrence after prior excision. At the time of excision, the entire mass is removed without leaving any residue using the no touch technique and if it is adherent to the globe, then a thin lamella of underlying sclera is removed intact with the tumor. Standard double freeze–thaw cryotherapy is applied to the remaining conjunctival margins. These precautions are taken to prevent recurrence of the nevus and also to prevent recurrence if the histopathology suggests a melanoma **(Box 1)**.

BOX 1: Indications for excision of a conjunctival nevus.

- Distinct onset in middle age or later in life
- Unusual location in the fornix or palpebral conjunctiva
- Lesion >10 mm in diameter
- Exuberant feeder blood vessels
- Exuberant intrinsic vascularity and hemorrhage
- Lesions with no cysts
- Lesions with dark uniform pigmentation
- Corneal epithelial invasion >3 clock hours and 3 mm from the limbus
- Episcleral fixity
- Cosmetic concern

 4. Write a short note on complexion-associated melanosis (CAM)/racial melanosis and ocular melanocytosis.

Complexion-associated Melanosis (CAM)/racial Melanosis

It is a relatively common condition of bilateral flat conjunctival pigmentation found in darkly pigmented individuals.

Clinical Features

This pigment is more concentrated at the limbus, often for 360° and a variable pigmentation can be noted on the perilimbal bulbar conjunctiva and cornea. Uncommonly, this pigment involves the fornix and rarely the palpebral conjunctiva. This pigmentation is generally flat uniform but can occasionally be mottled with a patchy appearance. It is extremely rare for conjunctival melanoma to arise from racial melanosis.

Histopathologically, the pigmented cells are benign melanocytes located in the basal layer of the epithelium.

Management

The recommended management is periodic observation.

Ocular Melanocytosis

Ocular melanocytosis is a congenital pigmentary condition of the periocular skin, sclera, orbit, meninges, and soft palate.

Clinical Features

It appears as flat, gray–brown irregularly scattered scleral and episcleral pigmentation posterior to the limbus visualized through the thin overlying conjunctival tissue. Typically, there is no conjunctival pigment but it can masquerade as conjunctival pigmentation. Since it is episcleral involvement, it does not move with manipulation of the conjunctiva. However, this condition is commonly confused with PAM because of their similar appearance. If associated with the dermal component, it is known as oculodermal melanocytosis or nevus of Ota.

It can involve the underlying uveal tract which can present with similar increased pigment. There is 1 in 400 risk for the development of uveal melanoma and not conjunctival melanoma. It is mandatory that all patients with oculodermal melanocytosis undergo fundus examination to exclude uveal melanocytosis or melanoma. Associated hairline pigmentation predisposes them for meningeal melanoma and palate pigmentation to esophageal melanoma; therefore, these signs should be elicited with appropriate referrals when needed.

Management

Affected patients should be followed once or twice yearly for the development of uveal, orbital, or meningeal melanoma.

 5. Discuss in details about the clinical features, histopathology, and management of primary acquired melanosis.

Primary acquired melanosis is an important benign conjunctival pigmented condition that can give rise to conjunctival melanoma. It comprises 21% of conjunctival melanocytic tumors. By definition, PAM is an acquired lesion that does not have an inciting event, is not congenital, and is not a secondary melanosis due to inflammation or a systemic disease.

Clinical Features

It is usually unilateral, flat, diffuse or multifocal, patchy pigmented, noncystic lesion most commonly occurring on the bulbar conjunctiva. It is most common in middle-aged or elderly white individuals. The melanosis can extend to the skin if the lesion involves the palpebral conjunctiva. The pigmentation in PAM may wax and wane over time and even disappear. Sunlight exposure may play a role in the development of PAM. It has also been seen in patients with neurofibromatosis. A slit-lamp examination may reveal subclinical melanosis around the clinically visible lesion. Occasionally, PAM may also be amelanotic, and thus clinically indistinct.

Differential Diagnosis

- PAM can be distinguished from CAM/racial melanosis because the latter is found commonly in dark-skinned individuals and shows bilateral involvement. In addition, pigmentation in CAM usually does not change over time.
- In contrast to conjunctival nevus, it is acquired in middle age and appears diffuse, patchy, flat, and noncystic.
- In contrast to ocular melanocytosis, the pigment is acquired, located within the conjunctiva, and appears brown, not gray, in color. The pigmentation can wax and wane over time.

> **BOX 2:** Indications for biopsy of PAM.
> - Lesion diameter >5 mm
> - Documented progression
> - Thickening of the involved conjunctiva
> - Distal nodule arising within the lesion
> - Nutrient vessels
> - Involvement of the cornea
> - Involvement of the tarsus, caruncle, or forniceal conjunctiva
> - Dysplastic nevus syndrome in the patient/close relative
> - Personal history of cutaneous/uveal melanoma

Histopathologic Features

Histopathologically, PAM is characterized by the presence of abnormal melanocytes near the basal layer of the epithelium. Based on the atypical melanocytic morphology and pattern of growth, melanocytes are further classified into PAM with atypia and PAM without atypia which are clinically indistinct. Histopathological examination is essential to determine the type of PAM and the risk of progression to melanoma. PAM with atypia has been associated with a 36–75% risk of progression to melanoma, whereas PAM without atypia is not believed to be a precursor lesion. However, it is important to realize that a diagnosis of PAM without atypia does not entirely rule out progression to PAM with atypia, as patients with a history of melanoma often have features of PAM without atypia on biopsies of recurring pigmented lesions. Clinically, larger the extent of PAM, greater is the risk of malignant transformation.

Management

The management of PAM depends on the extent of involvement and the association with melanoma.
- If there is only a small region of PAM, occupying <2 clock hours of the conjunctiva, then periodic observation is recommended.
- If the PAM occupies >2 clock hours, complete excision with wide margins and excision edge double freeze–thaw cryotherapy is recommended. For a larger lesion incision biopsy establishing diagnosing followed by complete excision can also be planned.
- If the patient has a history of previous or current conjunctival or cutaneous melanoma or if there are areas of nodularity or vascularity within the presumed PAM that are suspicious for melanoma, then a more aggressive approach is warranted with complete excisional biopsy with wide margins of the suspicious areas using the no touch technique. Additional small incisional map biopsies should be performed in the regions of flat PAM and even in the apparently uninvolved quadrants of the bulbar conjunctiva to determine if there are melanocytes with atypia. Cryotherapy should be applied to all remaining pigmented areas. Oral mucosal or amniotic membrane grafting may be required to fill defects after larger excisions.
- *Diffuse/unresectable PAM with atypia, recurrent corneal PAM:* Topical mitomycin C (MMC) can be considered. However, MMC is not as effective for PAM as it is for squamous epithelial neoplasia.
- If there is recurrent PAM on follow-up, prompt excisional biopsy and cryotherapy10,13 and close clinical follow-up is advised. At least 35% of PAM lesions will progress clinically and at least 11% will develop into a melanoma within 10 years. The extent of PAM, measured in clock-hours, best correlates with the risk of transformation into melanoma **(Box 2)**.

6. Discuss in details about the clinical features, classification, and management of conjunctival melanoma.

Conjunctival melanoma is rare and accounts for only 2–3% of ocular cancer, 12% of conjunctival melanocytic tumors, and about 1% of noncutaneous malignant melanoma. It is more common in light-skinned individuals and is epidemiologically associated with ultraviolet light exposure. Other risk factors are dysplastic nevus syndrome, neurofibromatosis, and xeroderma pigmentosum. About 75% of conjunctival malignant melanomas arise from PAM with atypia, 20% of cases are associated with a nevus, and the remaining 5% of conjunctival malignant melanomas arise de novo.

Clinical Features

Conjunctival melanomas are more common in middle age or elderly, with the mean age at presentation of 50–60 years, but rare cases of conjunctival melanoma in children have been recognized. Conjunctival melanoma shows considerable clinical variability. Conjunctival melanoma presents as an asymptomatic elevated pigmented lesion or tumor ranging in size from millimeters to large tumor masses often surrounded by flat PAM lesions. As a variant, it may appear as diffuse or multifocal with ill-defined margins particularly if arising from PAM. The color ranges from light to dark brown pigmented, sparsely pigmented, and rare amelanotic lesions. It is typically amelanotic, fleshy, and vascular when it recurs after prior excision. The clinical features suggestive of melanoma include large size, variegated appearance, lack of mobility in relation to the sclera, extension onto cornea, presence of large feeder vessels, and evidence of canalicular obstruction.

The most common location of the lesion is the bulbar conjunctiva close to the limbus. Melanoma involving the caruncle or the forniceal or palpebral conjunctiva is less common.

However, any pigmented lesion in these locations must be biopsied, as malignant melanoma is the most likely diagnosis. It may extend to cover the cornea or even arise as a primary corneal tumor. Conjunctival melanoma may rarely develop secondary to continuous touch from an eyelid margin melanoma (implantation melanoma). Upon diagnosis, conjunctival melanomas should be differentiated from other types of melanomas, such as uveal melanomas and metastatic melanomas.

Conjunctival melanoma is classified according to the American Joint Committee on Cancer (AJCC) classification **(Table 2)**.

Histologic Features

Histopathologically, conjunctival melanoma is composed of variably pigmented malignant melanocytes within the conjunctival stroma. There may be microscopic evidence of PAM or a nevus. Immunohistochemical studies for melanocytic markers such as S100, HMB-45, HMB-50, tyrosinase, melan-A, and MART-1 may help in the differential diagnosis of small round blue cell tumors in the conjunctiva. Worse prognosis has been described to be associated with tumor thickness of >2 mm, pagetoid growth pattern, high mitotic activity, mixed cell type (other than spindle cell) morphology, and the absence of an inflammatory response.

Management

The management of conjunctival melanoma varies with the extent of the lesion. Adjuvant cryotherapy, irradiation, or topical chemotherapy help in reducing the risk of recurrence.

TABLE 2: American Joint Committee on Cancer (AJCC) classification of conjunctival melanoma.

Primary tumor (T)	
Tx	• Primary tumor cannot be assessed
T0	• No evidence of primary tumor
T(is)	• Malignant melanoma confined to conjunctival epithelium
T1	• Malignant melanoma of the bulbar conjunctiva
T1a	• <1 Quadrant
T1b	• >1 But <2 quadrants
T1c	• >2 But <3 quadrants
T1d	• >3 Quadrants
T2	• Malignant melanoma of palpebral conjunctiva, forniceal conjunctiva, and/ or caruncle
T2a	• <1 Quadrant but not involving caruncle
T2b	• >1 Quadrant but not involving caruncle
T2c	• <1 Quadrant and involving caruncle
T2d	• >1 Quadrant and involving caruncle
T3	
T3a	• Malignant melanoma with local invasion
T3b	• Globe
T3c	• Eyelid
T3d	• Orbit
	• Paranasal sinus
T4	• Malignant melanoma with intracranial invasion
Regional lymph node (N)	
Nx	• Regional lymph nodes cannot be assessed
N0a	• No regional lymph node metastasis, biopsy done
N0b	• No regional lymph node metastasis, no biopsy done
N1	• Regional lymph node metastasis
Distant metastasis (M)	
M0	• No distant metastasis
M1	• Distant metastasis

- Complete excision in the episcleral plane with 4 mm clinically clear margins and no touch technique
- Absolute alcohol keratoepitheliectomy of the corneal epithelial component
- Partial lamellar sclerokeratectomy if sclera or corneal stroma are involved
- Double freeze-thaw cryotherapy to the excision edge, excision base cryotherapy if sclera is involved and the extent of involvement is <3 clock hours
- Postoperative adjuvant plaque brachytherapy if excision base is clinically detected to have been involved >3 clock hours and if the excision base is positive for tumor cells on histopathology. Since conjunctival melanoma is not radiosensitive, brachytherapy is not used as a sole treatment
- Extended enucleation with en-bloc excision if the tumor has deep corneal or sclera invasion or intraocular extension
- Extensive excision with tumor free margins encapsulating the tumor—larger lesions that extend into the forniceal region. Closure is achieved by primary apposition of conjunctiva or with conjunctival rotational flaps, mucous membrane graft from the opposite eye or buccal mucosa, or amniotic membrane transplantation
- Eyelid-sparing exenteration if the tumor extends into the orbit. Palliative therapy with proton beam radiotherapy may be used as an alternative and/or adjunct to exenteration
- Systemic chemotherapy is administered with combination of interferon (IFN) and interleukin-2 in disseminated melanoma.

Sentinel lymph node biopsy has been suggested in melanomas with a high risk for local metastases, such as those >10 mm in diameter and 2 mm in thickness and in nonlimbus locations to accurately remove lymph nodes. However, conjunctival melanoma of any thickness can metastasize because of the close proximity of lymphatic channels to the superficial substantia propria.

Prognosis

Despite excellent microscopic excision of the mass, further disease can develop from associated PAM in 26% of patients by 5 years, local recurrence after therapy is as high as 50–70% at 10 years. Metastasis was noted in 16% of patients, exenteration was required in 8% of patients, and death 7%. Overall mortality rate is 25% in 10 years and >30% in 15 years.

Conjunctival melanoma AJCC-tumor, node, metastasis (AJCC-TNM) staging predicts the prognosis and outcome. Clinical features predictive of local tumor recurrence and distant metastasis following resection include extralimbal (fornix, palpebral, caruncle) location, thickness (0.8–4 mm) tumor extending to surgical margin histopathologically pathology findings (de novo melanoma without PAM). Corneal invasion does not affect prognosis. Regional metastases usually involve ipsilateral preauricular, intraparotid, and submandibular lymph nodes. Fatal conjunctival melanoma is associated with distant metastasis to the liver, lung, brain, skin, bone, and peritoneum, most common sites.

Suggested Reading

1. Buckman G, Jakobiec FA, Folberg R, McNally LM. Melanocytic nevi of the palpebral conjunctiva: an extremely rare location usually signifying melanoma. Ophthalmology. 1988;95(8):1053-7.
2. Conjunctival Melanocytic Proliferations. In: The Melanocytic Proliferations. 2014.
3. Folberg R, Jakobiec FA, Bernardino VB, Iwamoto T. Benign conjunctival melanocytic lesions: clinicopathologic features. Ophthalmology. 1989;96(4):436-61.
4. Gerner N, Nørregaard JC, Jensen OA, Prause JU. Conjunctival naevi in Denmark 1960-1980. A 21-year follow-up study. Acta Ophthalmol Scand. 1996;74(4):334-7.
5. Gloor P, Alexandrakis G. Clinical characterization of primary acquired melanosis. Investig Ophthalmol Vis Sci. 1995;36(8):1721-9.
6. Honavar SG, Manjandavida FP. Tumors of the ocular surface: a review. Indian J Ophthalmol. 2015;63(3):187-203.
7. Kurli M, Finger PT. Melanocytic conjunctival tumors. Ophthalmol Clin North Am. 2005;18(1):15-24.
8. Marr BP, Shields JA, Shields CL, Materin MA, Tuncer S. Uveal prolapse following cataract extraction simulating melanoma. Ophthalmic Surg Lasers Imaging. 2008;39(3):250-1.
9. Roth M. Eyelid, Conjunctival, and Orbital Tumors. In: Shields JA, Shields CL (Eds). Intraocular Tumors: An Atlas and Textbook, 3rd edition. Wolters Kluwer; 2015. p. 824.
10. Sharara NA, Alexander RA, Luthert PJ, Hungerford JL, Cree IA. Differential immunoreactivity of melanocytic lesions of the conjunctiva. Histopathology. 2001;39(4):426-31.
11. Shields CL, Demirci H, Karatza E, Shields JA. Clinical survey of 1643 melanocytic and nonmelanocytic conjunctival tumors. Ophthalmology. 2004;111(9):1747-54.
12. Shields CL, Fasiudden A, Mashayekhi A, Shields JA. Conjunctival nevi: clinical features and natural course in 410 consecutive patients. Arch Ophthalmol. 2004;122(2):167-75.
13. Shields CL, Kaliki S, Al-Dahmash SA, Lally SE, Shields JA. American Joint Committee on Cancer (AJCC) clinical classification predicts conjunctival melanoma outcomes. Ophthal Plast Reconstr Surg. 2012;28(5):313-23.

14. Shields CL, Kaliki S, Livesey M, Walker B, Garoon R, Bucci M, et al. Association of ocular and oculodermal melanocytosis with the rate of uveal melanoma metastasis analysis of 7872 consecutive eyes. JAMA Ophthalmol. 2013;131(8):993-1003.
15. Shields CL, Shields JA, Gündüz K, Cater J, Mercado GV, Gross N, et al. Conjunctival melanoma: risk factors for recurrence, exenteration, metastasis, and death in 150 consecutive patients. Arch Ophthalmol. 2000;118(11):1497-507.
16. Shields CL, Shields JA. Tumors of the conjunctiva and cornea. Indian J Ophthalmol. 2019;67(12):1930-48.
17. Shields CL, Shields JA. Tumors of the conjunctiva and cornea. Surv Ophthalmol. 2004;49(1):3-24.
18. Shields JA, Shields CL, De Potter P. Surgical management of circumscribed conjunctival melanomas. Ophthal Plast Reconstr Surg. 1998;14(3):208-15.
19. Shields JA, Shields CL, Eagle RC, Singh AD, Demirci H, Wolf MA. Pigmented conjunctival squamous cell carcinoma simulating a conjunctival melanoma. Am J Ophthalmol. 2001;132:104-6.
20. Shields JA, Shields CL, Mashayekhi A, Marr BP, Benavides R, Thangappan A, et al. Primary acquired melanosis of the conjunctiva: risks for progression to melanoma in 311 eyes. The 2006 Lorenz E. Zimmerman lecture. Ophthalmology. 2008;115(3):511-9.e2.
21. Singh AD, De Potter P, Fijal BA, Shields CL, Shields JA, Elston RC. Lifetime prevalence of uveal melanoma in white patients with oculo (dermal) melanocytosis. Ophthalmology. 1998;105(1):195-8.

1.22 Orbital Imaging

Samir Mahapatra, Sanjana M

 1. What are the different imaging modalities for orbital diseases? What are the principles of X-ray and clinical applications in orbital pathology?

Patients with orbital diseases pose a challenge to the clinicians, as the interior of the orbit cannot be seen directly. This limitation in the clinical evaluation often necessitates orbital imaging to diagnose orbital disease, delineate orbital lesions, and decide upon various treatment modalities.

The various modalities for imaging the orbit are **(Table 1)**:
- Computed tomography (CT)
- Magnetic resonance imaging (MRI)
- Ultrasonography (USG)
- X-ray
- Positron emission tomography (PET) scan.

TABLE 1: Different orbital imaging modalities.

	X-ray	CT scan	MRI scan
Principle in medical imaging	Attenuation of X-rays as they pass through human tissues	Attenuation of X-rays as they pass through human tissues	Magnetization and decay of energy of protons in human tissues on exposure to strong magnetic field
Nature of scan	Two-dimensional scan	• Cross-sectional • Three-dimensional scan	• Cross-sectional • Three-dimensional scan
Image acquisition	Photographic emulsion is ionized on a sheet of photographic film to create an image	Computer screen	Computer screen
Image quality	• Flat image • Superimposition of all structures in a three-dimensional space • Depth information is lost	• Image acquired as multiple thin slices • No superimposition • Image acquired as thin slices • Depth information available	• Image acquired as multiple thin slices • No superimposition • Image acquired as thin slices • Depth information available
Image distortions	Objects farther away from the X-ray source are enlarged more than those closer to the source	• Both the X-ray source and detectors rotate 360° in the gantry around the patient • No image distortion	• The tissue of interest is exposed to a gradient of magnetic field strength • No image distortion
Resolution and contrast imaging	Poor resolution and contrast ability	Better contrast and high resolution	Best contrast and higher resolution

Contd...

Contd...

	X-ray	CT scan	MRI scan
Soft tissue detail	Poor detail	Better than X-ray	Best detail
Bone detail	Excellent detail	• Excellent detail • Better than X-ray	Poor detail
Cost	Cheaper	Cheaper than MRI	Expensive
Utility	Screening and localization of metallic FB	Orbital fractures and other pathologies	Contraindicated in metallic FB, more useful for soft tissue tumors and vascular imaging
Time	2–3 minutes	3–7 minutes	30–45 minutes
Radiation exposure	0.15 mSv; low	10 mSv; higher	No radiation exposure

(CT: computed tomography; FB: foreign body; MRI: magnetic resonance imaging)

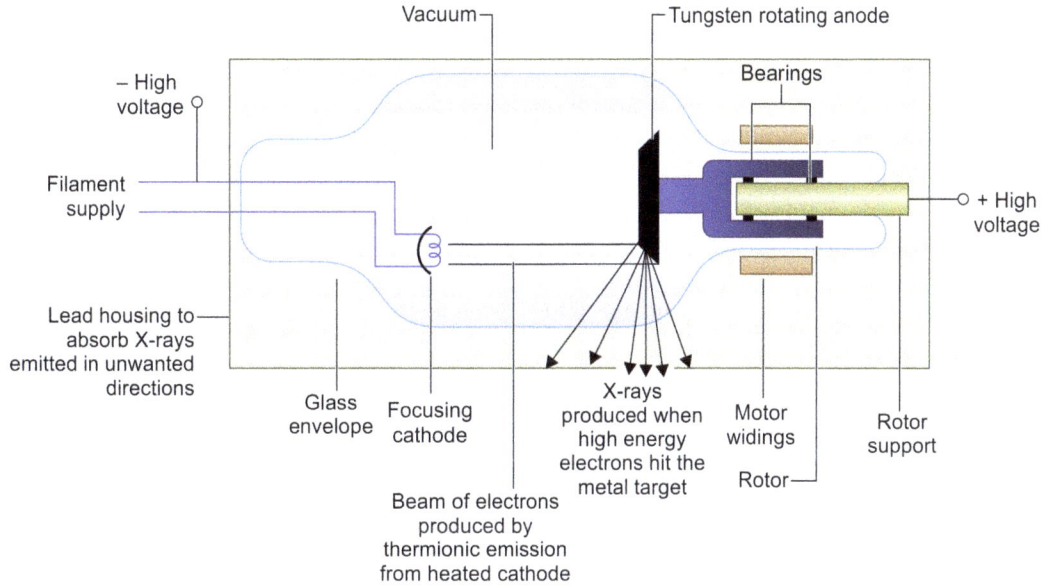

Fig. 1: Principle of X-ray.

Principles of X-ray (Fig. 1)

- The German physicist Wilhelm Conrad Röntgen, who discovered X-rays in 1895, described the basic principles of medical imaging.
- An object when irradiated with photons generated in an X-ray tube, they traverse the material and depending on the intensity of the photon beam and the nature of the material imaged, some of the energy is lost or attenuated. The amount of energy that emerges from the other side of the object can ionize a photographic plate and create an image.
- Mechanism of X-ray generation involves a cathode tube, tungsten filament, and an electric source **(Fig. 1)**. When high voltage electric current pass through cathode (negative charge) end of an X-ray tube, electrons are emitted and move toward a target material known as anode (positive end). This is called thermionic emission. When the electrons collide with the target material (tungsten metal disc), it causes electrons to expel from the outer orbits of atoms releasing an X-ray photon. These X-rays then travel through a focusing cup, which focuses and accelerates the photons toward the area of the body to be imaged. The photographic plate, a double emulsion film containing silver nitrate, is placed behind the part to be imaged.
- *The image of the part created depends on the tissue density:*
  - *High-density tissues (bone):* Absorbs X-ray to a greater degree and appear white on the film
  - *Low-density tissues (lungs):* Absorbs X-rays to a lesser degree and appear black on the film
  - *Intermediate-density tissues (muscle and fat):* Appear as shades of gray on the film

Clinical Applications of X-ray in Orbit Pathology

- Plain X-ray of orbits can delineate bony details of the orbit and face along with moderate soft tissue changes. Used as screening tool particularly in localizing orbital foreign bodies and fractures and complement the use of newer imaging technique.
- Orbit is in close proximity to larger bones of the skull; multiple shadows overlap and obscure some radiographic details. This is due to superimposition of all the structures in a three-dimensional (3D) space. So, the depth of information is lost.
- X-rays have a very narrow contrast capability (up to 2%). So, soft tissues are barely seen. Numerous radiologic projections are attempted to eliminate the obvious overlapping shadows.
- Since there is a single X-ray source, objects farther from the source are enlarged proportionately more than those closer to the source, resulting in image distortion. Thus, the distance of the object to the X-ray cassette should be minimized, and the distance between the subject and the X-ray beam should be maximized to have the maximal image clarity. Posteroanterior (PA) view is thus recommended; an X-ray comes from the posterior side, and the image plate is on the anterior side.

Projections or Standard Orbital Views (Table 2)

To increase the clarity of image and depth perception, X-ray images are taken in several projections:

- *Waters view:*
  - Improve the visualization of maxillary and ethmoid sinuses, orbital rim, floor, zygomatic bones, lesser wing of sphenoid, and infraorbital foramen.
  - Clinically helpful for orbital floor fracture assessment (anterior and middle portion of the floor): Floor of the orbit forms a continuous radiographic line with the lateral wall of the orbit. A soft tissue density at the roof of the maxillary sinus or opacification of the floor of the sinus suggests an orbital floor disruption.
- *Caldwell projection:*
  - Provides an excellent view of the frontal and ethmoid sinus. It also provides a good view of the orbital rim, greater and lesser wing of the sphenoid bone, lacrimal gland fossa, medial orbital wall, and both superior and inferior orbital fissures.
  - The innominate line is prominent in this view: Lack in continuity of the innominate line suggests a fracture of the lateral orbital wall.
  - Provides detailed imaging of the posterior medial orbital wall
- *Lateral projection:*
  - View of the sagittal plane of the skull
  - The structures that are best visualized are sphenoid, frontal, ethmoid and maxillary sinuses, sella turcica, the anterior and posterior clinoid process, the cribriform plate, and the nasopharynx and the orbital roof.

TABLE 2: Summary of radiographic projections and structures.

Projection	Structures	Pathology
Waters	Orbital floor (anterior two thirds)	Blow-out fracture
	Maxillary sinus	Maxillary sinus disease
Caldwell	Frontal and ethmoid sinus	Sinus disease (mucocele)
	Innominate line	Medial and lateral wall fracture
	Sphenoid bone	
	Orbital floor (posterior one third)	Meningioma of sphenoid wing
Lateral	Orbital roof	Orbital roof fracture
	Sella turcica	Frontal sinus disease
	Sinus air-fluid levels	Pituitary disease
Basal	Sphenoid and ethmoid sinus	Sinus disease
		Lateral wall fractures
	Lateral wall of orbit	Zygomatic arch fractures
	Zygomatic arch	
Optic foramen (Rhese)	Optic canal	Apex tumors
		Optic nerve tumors

- *Basal projection:*
  - Evaluation of sphenoid sinus and skull base
  - It shows the lateral orbital walls and the maxillary sinuses.
- *Rhese position:*
  - For evaluation of the ethmoid sinus and the optic foramen
  - Allows assessment of the orbital apex, optic foramen, and the upper ethmoid sinus.

2. Describe the physics and principles of CT imaging. What are the clinical applications in orbital pathology? Describe its advantages and disadvantages in comparison to other imaging modalities.

Computed tomography scan is an indispensable imaging modality used in the evaluation of orbital lesions. This allows to precisely localize the lesion, its extent, configuration, mass composition, and its effect on adjacent structures. It utilizes X-rays to generate cross-sectional, two-dimensional (2D) images of the body.

Physics and Basic principles of Computed Tomography Scan

- Electromagnetic radiations include gamma rays, X-rays, ultraviolet light, visible light, infrared light, microwaves, and radio waves. These consist of elementary particles called photons. An X-ray is a form of electromagnetic radiation with a wavelength in the range of 0.01–10 nm; for clinical radiology, X-rays with a wavelength of 0.01–0.1 nm are used.
- Photons have no net mass; they travel at the speed of light in vacuum, can be refracted by a lens, and transfer energy to other particles.
- X-rays are ionizing radiations as they have high energy and can ionize (detach) an electron from an atom when they interact with the matter.
- In CT scan, the X-ray tube is rotated around the patient for 360°. A series of thin collimated X-ray beams (1–10 mm) are passed through the body along one plane, and on interaction with body tissues of different densities, these X-ray beams are attenuated and are detected by an array of special detectors as they exit from the tissues **(Fig. 2)**.
- X-ray photons generate electrical signals in these detectors that are reconstructed into 2D images on a computer.
- Both the X-ray tube and the detectors rotate simultaneously to complete one rotation around a predetermined slice of tissue and then move the body in small increments to acquire the next slice images; images of one slice at a time are acquired.
- Tissues of lower density, such as muscle, cause less attenuation and allow more X-rays to pass through them and produce a darker image. Tissues of greater density, such as bone, cause attenuation of more X-rays and produce a brighter image **(Fig. 3)**.
- The attenuation value is expressed on a scale named Hounsfield units (HU), which ranges from +1,000 HU for bone (white on final image) to –1,000 HU for air (black on final image). The entire span of numbers that are selected to display the given image is the window width and the midpoint of the window width is the window level. So, window width can be 2,000. Water appears gray with an attenuation value of 0 HU.

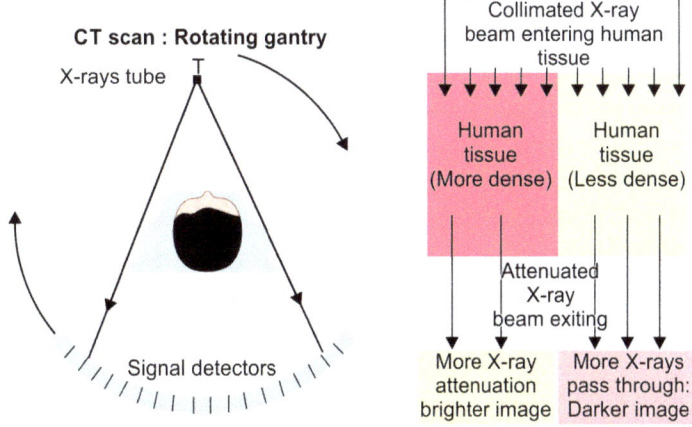

Fig. 2: Principle of computed tomography (CT) scan.

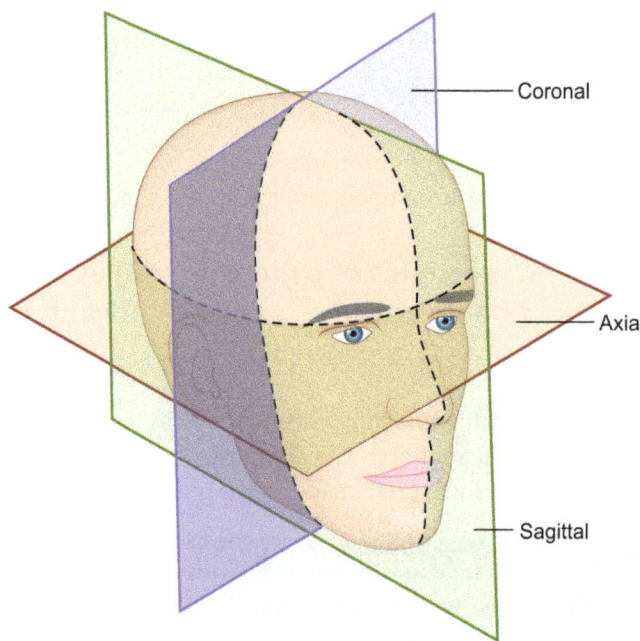

Fig. 3: Imaging planes.

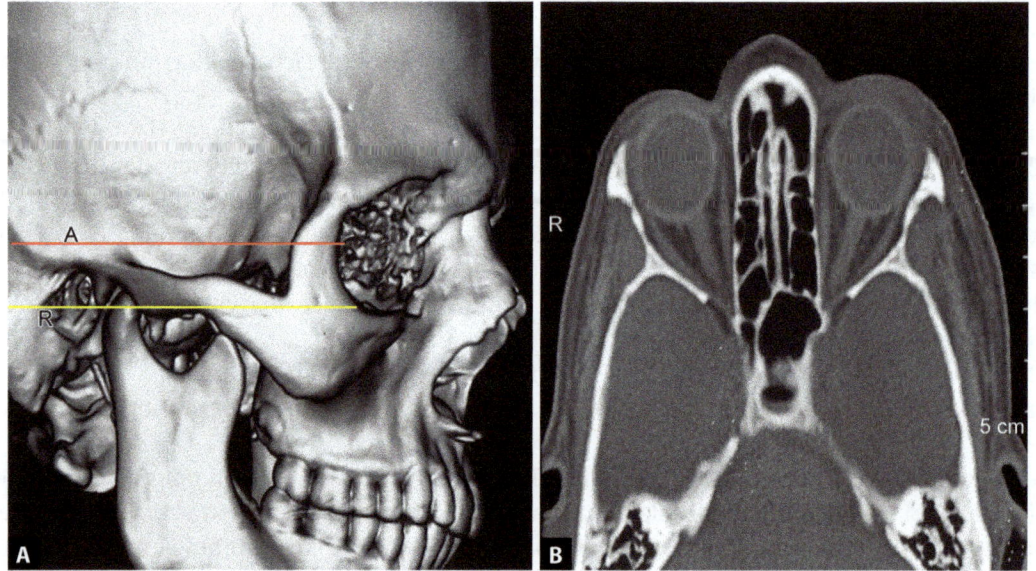

Figs. 4A and B: (A) Computed tomography (CT) orbit three-dimensional (3D) reconstructed model showing R (Reid's baseline) and A (axial plane). (B) Midaxial plain CT.

Imaging Planes

Standard CT scan of the orbit have the following planes:
- *Reid's baseline:* The line that extends from the inferior orbital rim to the external auditory meatus. This is considered as zero plane in CT imaging.
- *Axial plane:* Plane parallel to the Reid's baseline **(Figs. 4 and 5)**
- *Coronal plane:* Plane placed perpendicular to the axial scan but angled slightly obliquely **(Figs. 6 and 7)**
- Sagittal reformatted views **(Fig. 8)**
- 3D reconstructed views **(Figs. 9A and B)**.

Slice Thickness

- The slice thickness varies from 1 to 10 mm.
- Spatial resolution of CT depends on the slice thickness: Thinner the slice, better is the resolution.
- Thinner slices need higher radiation doses and greater scan time.

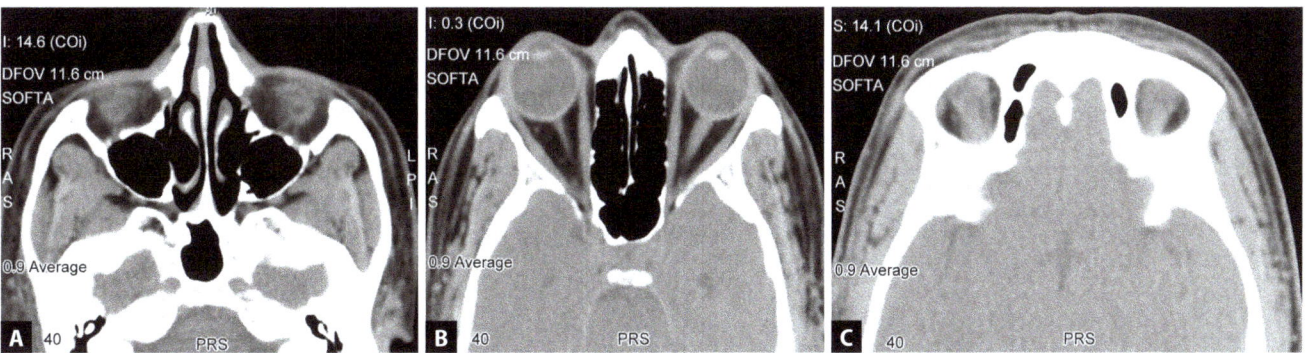

Figs. 5A to C: Computed tomography (CT) orbit posterior to anterior cuts of axial scan where on. (A) Posterior cut, we see nose is prominent. (B) Midaxial cut showing nucleus. (C) Anterior cuts showing more of brain parenchyma.

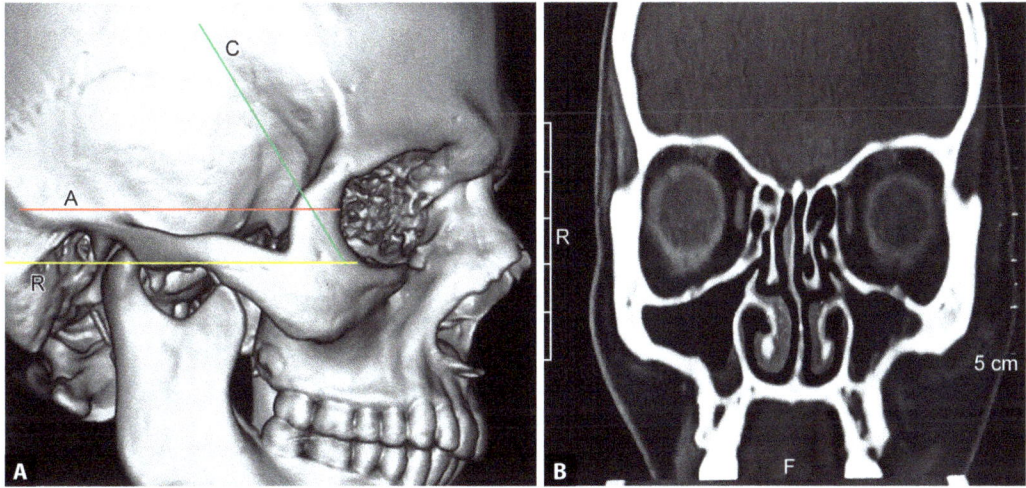

Figs. 6A and B: (A) Computed tomography (CT) orbit three-dimensional (3D) reconstructed model showing R (Reid's baseline), A (axial plane), and C (coronal plane). (B) CT orbit mid coronal plain CT.

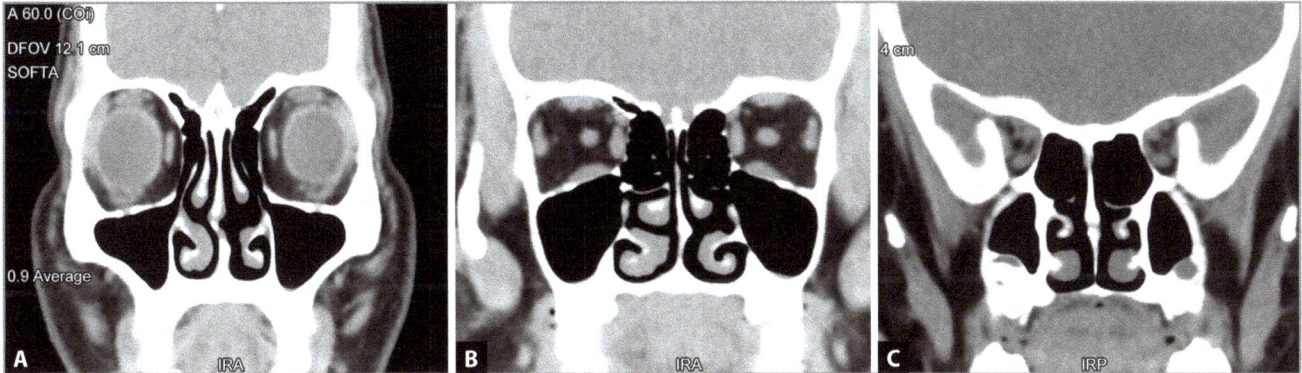

Figs. 7A to C: Computed tomography (CT) orbit anterior to posterior coronal cuts. (A) Anterior coronal cut showing maximum globe diameter. (B) Posterior coronal cut showing extraocular muscles and optic nerve. (C) Most posterior cut where the orbital cavity reduces.

- 2 mm cuts are optimal for ocular and orbital imaging; 1 mm slices are more informative for evaluation of optic nerve and orbital apex.

Clinical Applications

Indications

- Unexplained proptosis, ophthalmoplegia, or ptosis
- Palpable orbital mass

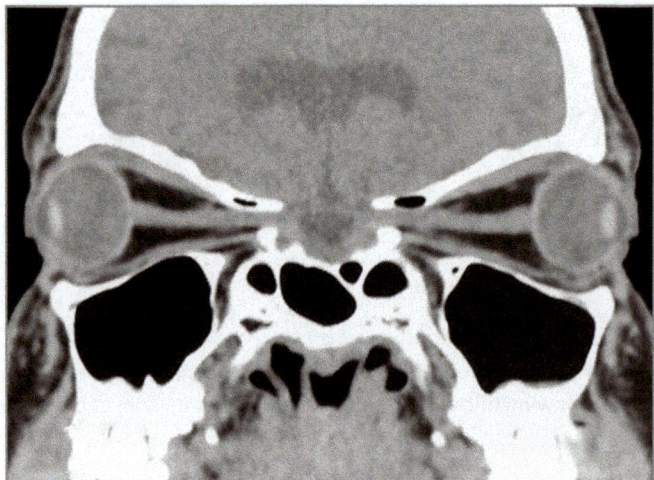

Fig. 8: Computed tomography (CT) orbit sagittal reformed view.

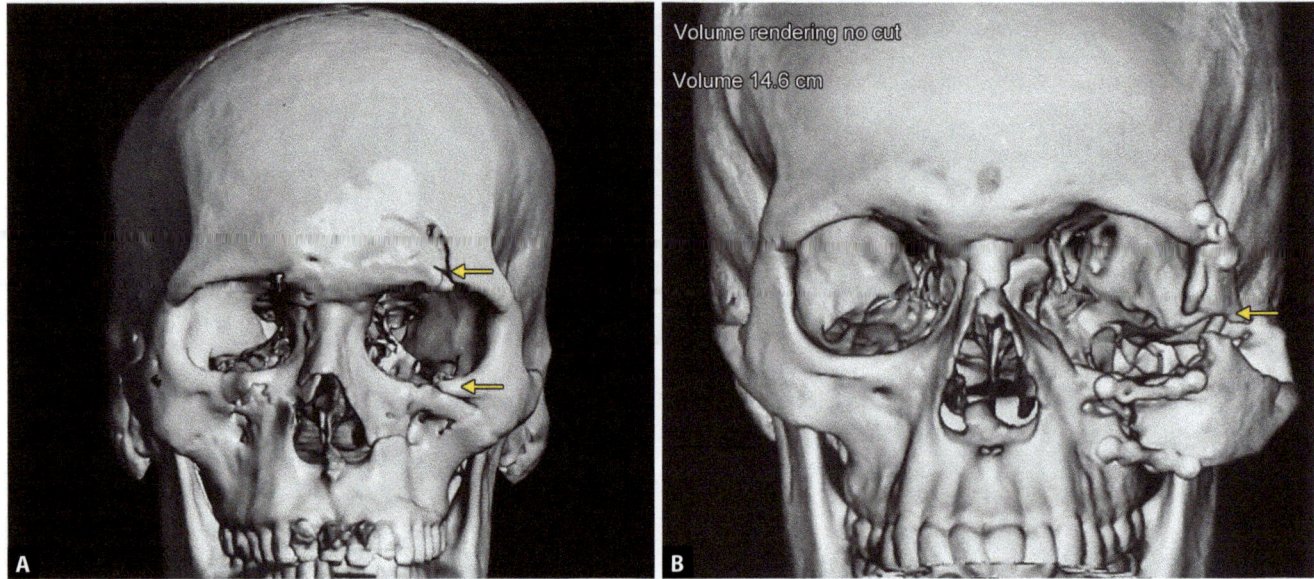

Figs. 9A and B: (A) Computed tomography (CT) orbit three-dimensional (3D) reconstructed view showing left orbital floor and roof fracture. (B) 3D reconstructed view showing left medial and lateral wall fracture with displacement of zygoma inferiorly and laterally repaired elsewhere with plates.

- Orbital signs of paranasal sinus disease
- Unexplained efferent pupillary dysfunction
- Ocular surface or eyelid tumor with suspected orbital spread
- Intraocular tumor with proptosis
- Orbital trauma **(Figs. 10A and B)**
- Preseptal cellulitis and orbital abscess.

Clinical Applications
- To delineate the location and extent of the tumor in a specified surgical space, which helps in determining the appropriate orbitotomy approach to ensure easy and safe access and complete removal. **(Figs. 11A and B)**
- To identify the tissue of origin of the tumor, look at the size, shape, and location of the tumor. Enlarged orbital structure may also give a clue to the origin and suspected pathology of the tumor **(Figs. 12A to C)**
- To assess the biologic behavior of the tumor as infiltrative or malignant and well circumscribed or smooth as in benign lesions **(Figs. 13A and B)**

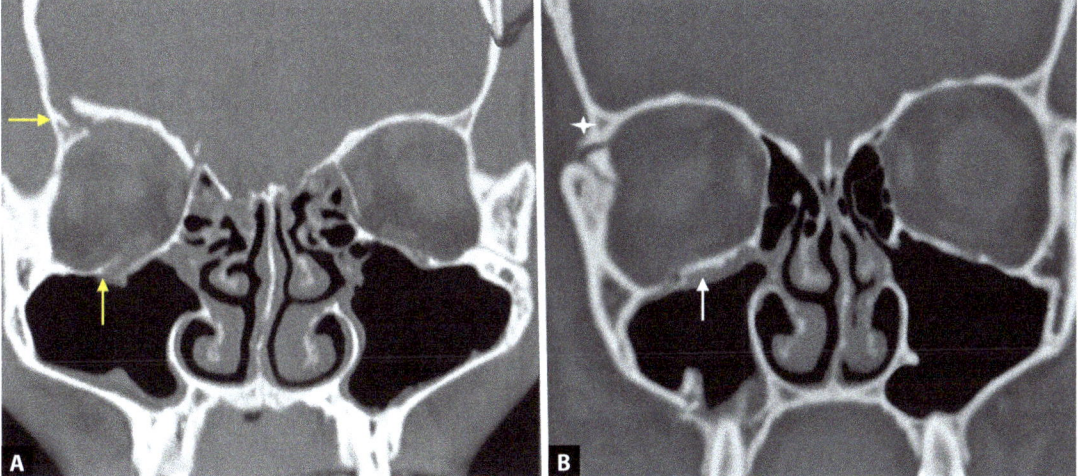

Figs. 10A and B: (A) Computed tomography (CT) orbit coronal view, bone window showing right eye superior, medial and inferior orbital wall fracture. (B) CT orbit coronal view, bone window showing right eye inferior and lateral wall fracture.

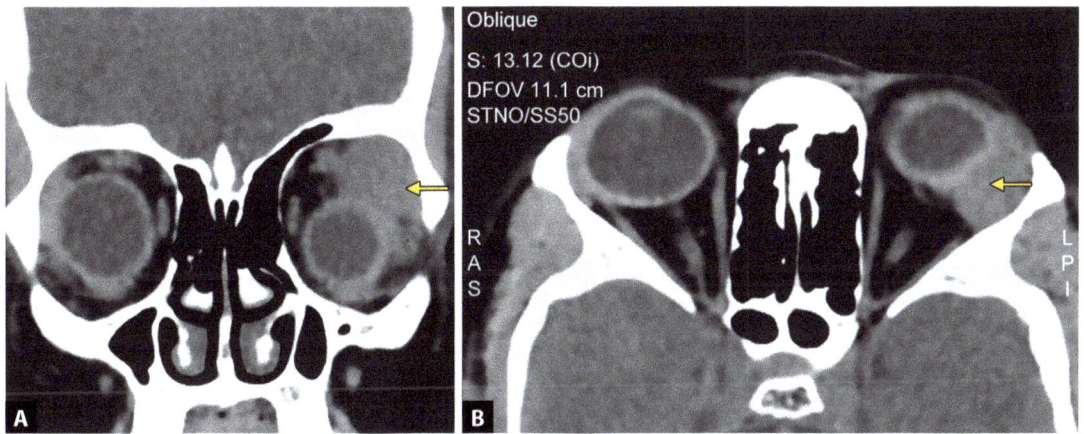

Figs. 11A and B: (A) Computed tomography (CT) orbit coronal cut showing superotemporal homogenous mass pushing the globe down and in. (B) CT orbit axial cut showing left eye homogenous extraconal mass in the lacrimal gland area.

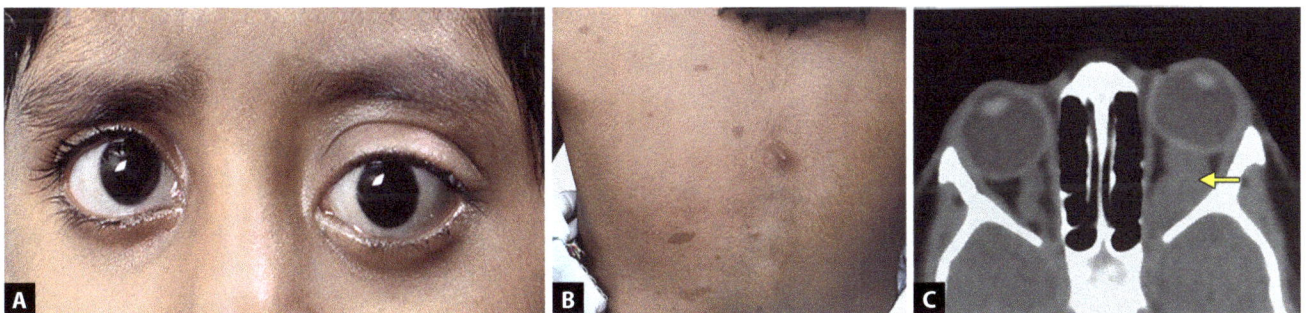

Figs. 12A to C: (A) Child presenting with left eye axial proptosis. (B) Multiple café au lait spots on the back. (C) Computed tomography (CT) orbit axial view, soft tissue window showing homogenous mass arising from optic nerve—suspicion of optic nerve glioma in a child with neurofibromatosis.

- To find out the relationship of the tumor to the adjacent bone (fossa formation vs. bone lytic lesions) and to differentiate between malignant and benign lesions **(Figs. 14A to D)**
- To look for specific diagnostic patterns in relation to its homogenous or heterogeneous internal consistency which may help arriving at a provisional diagnosis and suspected pathology **(Figs. 15A and B)**
- To look for presence of intratumoral calcification or localized hyperostosis which may point to the aggressive behavior of the tumor and its spread to adjacent structures **(Figs. 16A and B)**

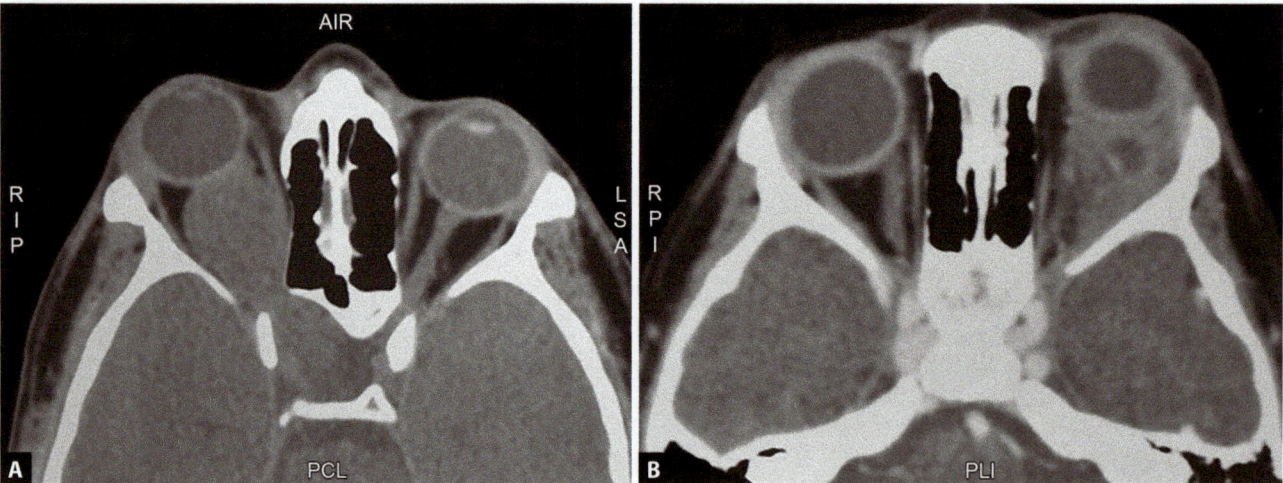

Figs. 13A and B: (A) Computed tomography (CT) orbit axial plane, soft tissue window showing right eye well-defined intraconal mass, with regular margins—suspicion of benign cavernous haemangioma. (B) CT orbit axial plane, soft tissue window showing left eye heterogenous lesion with irregular margins extending intracranially—disorder of malignant lymphoma.

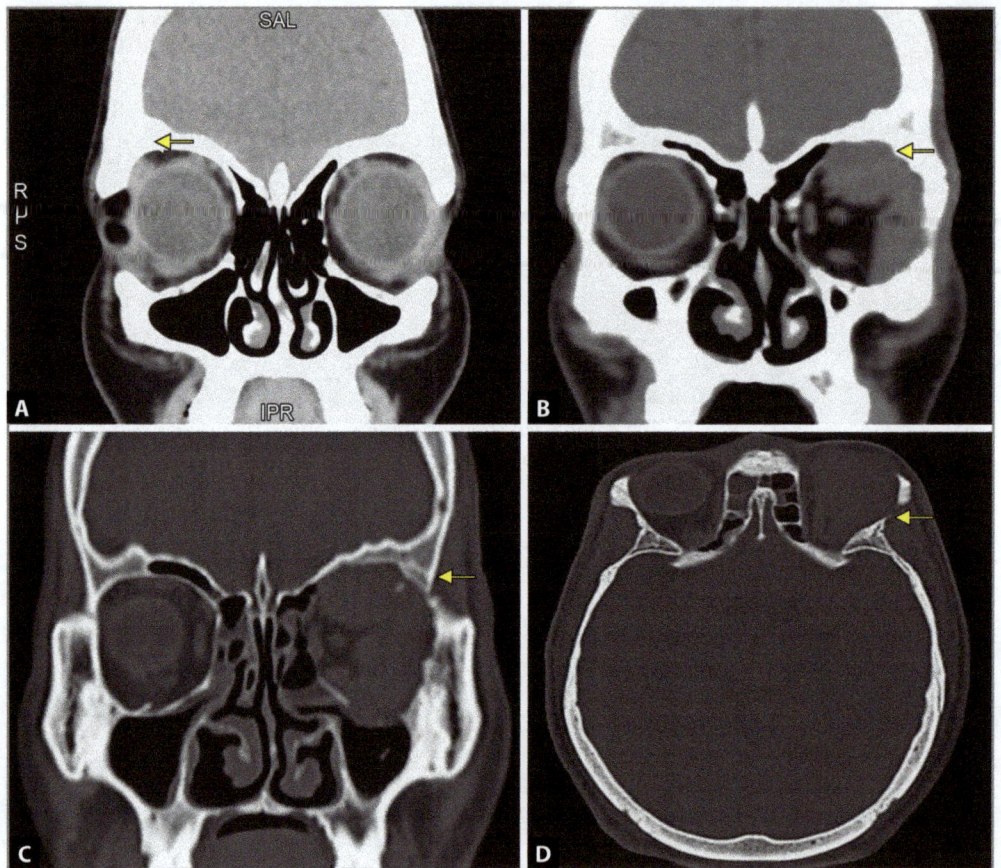

Figs. 14A to D: (A) Computed tomography (CT) orbit coronal view showing superotemporal hypodense lesion causing bone fossa formation—suspicion of dermoid. (B to D) CT coronal view, soft tissue window showing left eye temporal homogenous lesion with irregular margins; on bone window, we see the same lesion causing frontal bone and zygomatic bone lysis.

- Contrast enhancement may be helpful in differentiating vascular lesions, inflammatory lesions which may otherwise have an indolent course.
- To look at muscle enlargement and arrive at a diagnosis of inflammatory versus neoplastic versus infective etiology **(Figs. 17A and B)**
- Measurement of proptosis **(Fig. 18)**.

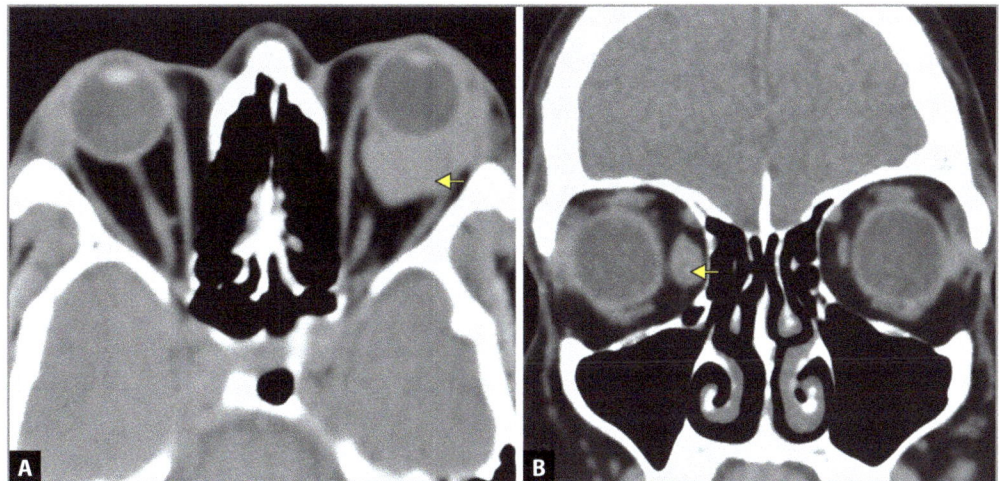

Figs. 15A and B: (A) Computed tomography (CT) orbit axial plane, soft tissue window showing a left homogenous mass molding around the globe—suspicion of lymphoma. (B) CT orbit coronal view, soft tissue window showing homogenous enlargement of right eye medial rectus with central hyperdensity suggestive of scolex in case of myocysticercosis.

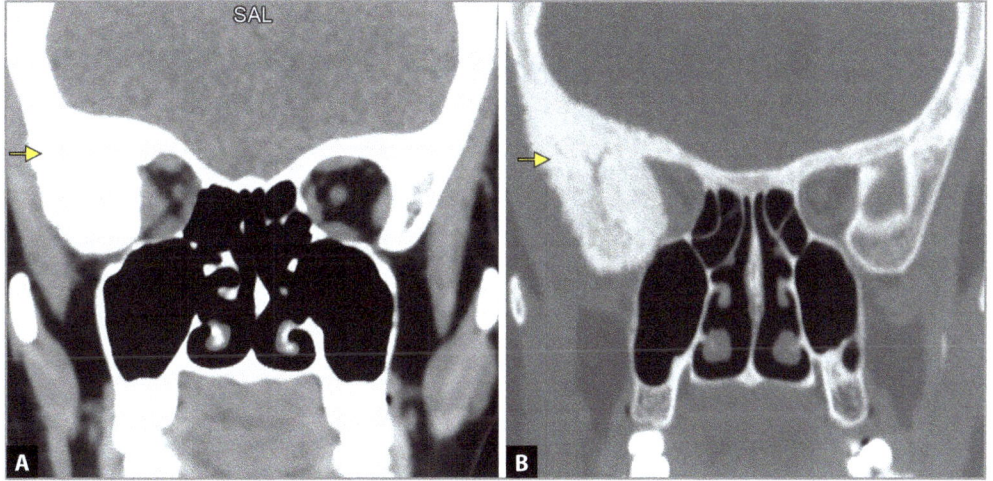

Figs. 16A and B: Computed tomography (CT) orbit showing hyperostosis of right eye zygomatic and orbital surface of frontal bone suggestive of osteoma as seen on soft tissue and bone window, respectively.

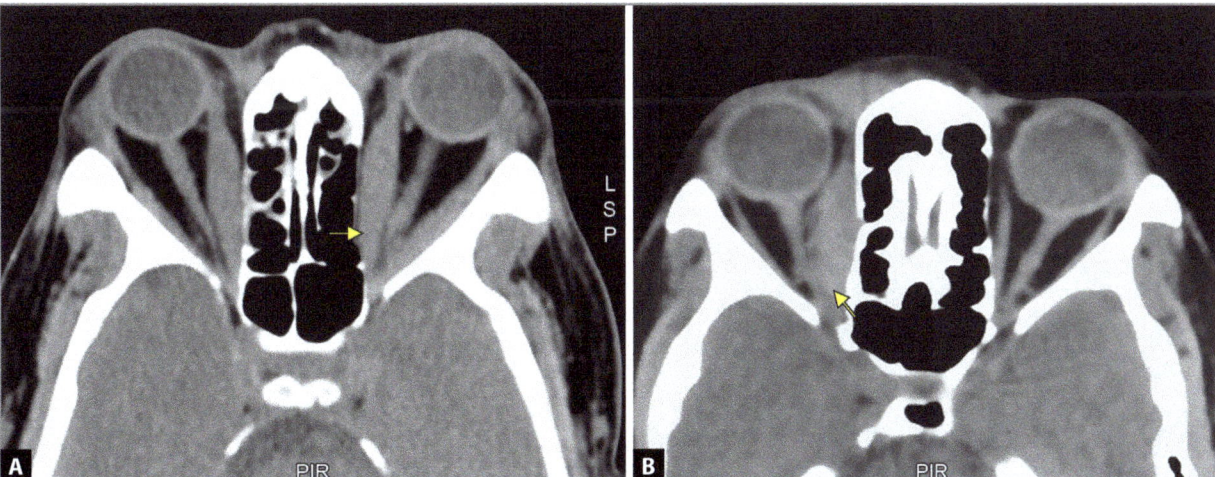

Figs. 17A and B: (A) Computed tomography (CT) orbit axial plane, soft tissue window showing both eyes enlargement of medial rectus with tendon sparing—suspicion of thyroid eye disease. (B) CT orbit axial plane, soft tissue window showing right eye enlargement of medial rectus involving the entire muscle with irregular margins—suspicion of infiltration in case of lymphoma.

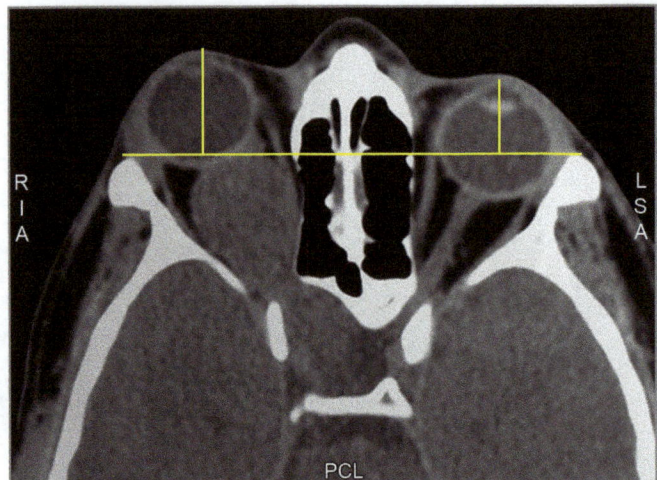

Fig. 18: Measurement of proptosis using Hilal and Trokel method: Midaxial computed tomography (CT) scan image, baseline between the tips of the lateral orbital rims, draw a perpendicular from each corneal apex to this line. An asymmetry of >2 mm between the two is considered significant proptosis.

 3. Discuss the common artifacts in CT imaging of the orbits. What are the modifications or technological advancements for better resolution of CT images?

Artifacts

Artifacts represent features that appear on the final image but which were not actually present in the tissue sample. The common artifacts in CT scans of orbits are:

- *Motion artifact:* Result from patient movement during scan acquisition. It appears as blurring or streaking of the image **(Fig. 19)**.
- *Streak or metallic artifacts:* Caused by dense objects that do not transmit X-rays, in case of metallic foreign bodies. Streaks or lines radiate away from the sharp corners and are seen behind the dense objects **(Fig. 20)**.
- *Partial density averaging:* Results when the scanner cannot distinguish a small amount of high-density material, such as bone, against a large amount of low-density material. The image appears as blurring at the edges while the denser tissue appears prominent.
- *Noise artifact:* Appears as graining on the image that is created by a low signal-to-noise ratio or when insufficient energy is used for penetration of the tissues **(Fig. 21)**.

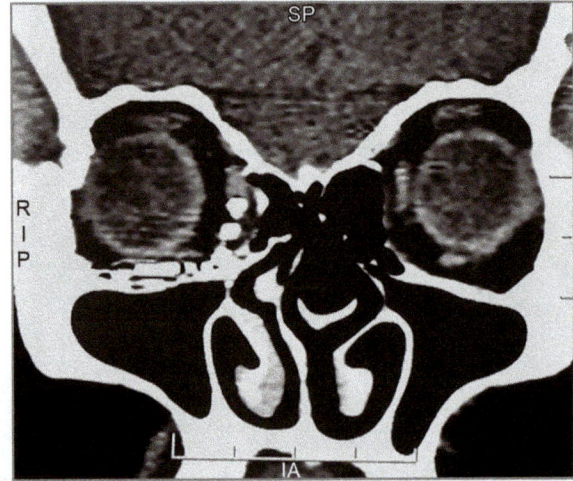

Fig. 19: Computed tomography (CT) orbit showing right eye inferior and medial motion artifact.

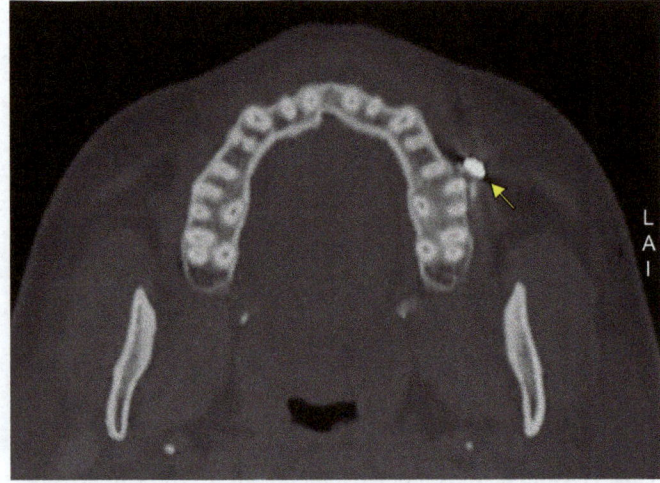

Fig. 20: Computed tomography (CT) orbit showing left-sided metallic artifact.

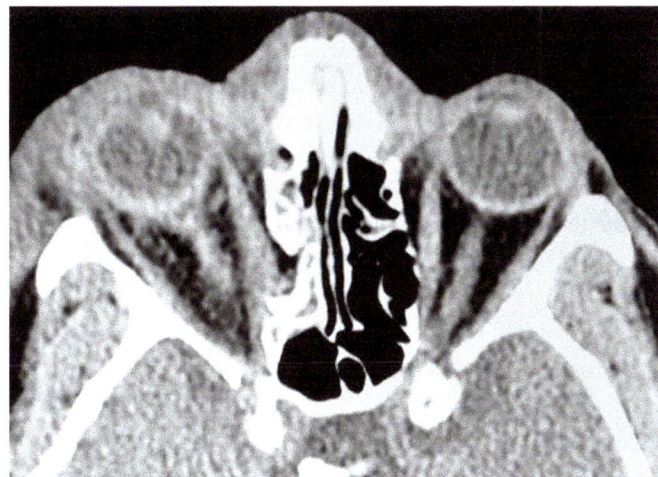

Fig. 21: Computed tomography (CT) orbit showing noise artifact.

- *Beam hardening:* It occurs when heterogonous X-ray beam passes through dense tissue such as a thick bone. Low-energy photons are absorbed, and high-energy photons pass through.

Modifications in Standard Computed Tomography

The various modifications in the standard CT imaging protocol, which are needed for better resolution of images, are:
- *Contrast-enhanced CT scan (CECT):* Tissues that do not differ significantly in their relative densities may not be different in contrast, and some important details may be lost. To overcome this limitation, various contrast agents with high molecular weights are injected intravenously, which increase the attenuation value of certain organs and tissues. These agents are called contrasts and are usually iodine based. These are used to increase the density of the vascular system and evaluate vascular tumors, inflammatory lesions.
- *Spiral or helical CT:* X-ray source rotates continuously in one direction along with the detectors as the patient moves forward along the head-to-toe axis. Continuous data are acquired in a very short period of time, thus reducing movement artifacts.

4. What is emission CT or PET scan? What are its clinical applications?

- Emission CT scan is a form of scintigraphy that uses radioactive tracer substances as the radiation source for imaging. It follows the principle of positron annihilation.
- It evaluates the rates of metabolism in body tissues. The radioactive tracer, when injected into the body, accumulates in metabolically active tissues such as tumors or areas of inflammation.
- These radioactive tracers, on decay, release small amount of energy in the form of gamma rays. These gamma rays are detected by a rotating gamma camera, which contains an array of detectors. These detectors contain a series of scintillation crystals. Each detector is connected to a photomultiplier tube that converts and amplifies the energy to electrical signals, which are processed, to clinical images by a computer.
- Depending on the rate of metabolic activity, areas within the body appear as hot spots (higher metabolism, more radioactive tracer accumulation) or cold spots (lower metabolism, smaller concentration of radiotracer)
- [^{18}F]Fluoro-2-deoxy-D-glucose (FDG) is the most commonly used radioactive tracer. The crystals present in the gamma-ray detectors are composed of lutetium–yttrium oxyorthosilicate (LYSO). These tracers measure the glycolytic activity of tumor cells. The most commonly used positron-emitting nuclides are carbon and fluorine.

Clinical Applications

- It has high sensitivity and high specificity in detecting neoplastic diseases.
- It is helpful in diagnosis, staging of cancers as well as evaluating the response to treatment and the prognosis.
- PET scan can be combined with CT (PET/CT) or MRI (PET/MRI) to provide both anatomical and functional imaging of tissues. This is called fusion imaging.

- It also provides the images of blood flow.
- The fluorine isotope can pass through the blood–brain barrier. So, it is particularly useful in imaging the brain tumors.
- Ocular malignancies such as uveal melanoma and squamous-cell carcinoma demonstrate intense FDG uptake on PET scan.
- It has more limited role for orbital lesions because of high signal from the adjacent brain. Primary orbital tumors such as lymphoma and adenoid cystic carcinoma of the lacrimal gland show intense FDG uptake on PET scan. It can also detect metastatic tumors in the orbit due to primary lung cancer in males or breast cancer in females.
- Optic nerve sheath meningioma and optic nerve glioma, ocular and ocular prosthesis show no uptake of FDG on PET scan.
- PET scan has low resolution in contrast to CT/MRI.

5. What are the principles of MRI and its clinical application? What are the modifications in MRI for orbital imaging?

Magnetic resonance imaging is the technique of generating a cross-sectional image of the body based on the magnetic resonance of atomic nuclei.

Basic Physics and Principles (Flowchart 1)

- Most of the human body is made up of water molecules in normal tissues; the nucleus of hydrogen atom contains a single proton with a positive charge and with a single electron with negative charge orbiting around the proton. The proton has spin or angular movement along an axis and is randomly oriented in space. The proton behaves like tiny magnets and is very sensitive to magnetic fields. Medical MRI utilizes hydrogen as the resonating nucleus of interest.

Flowchart 1: Principle of magnetic resonance imaging (MRI).

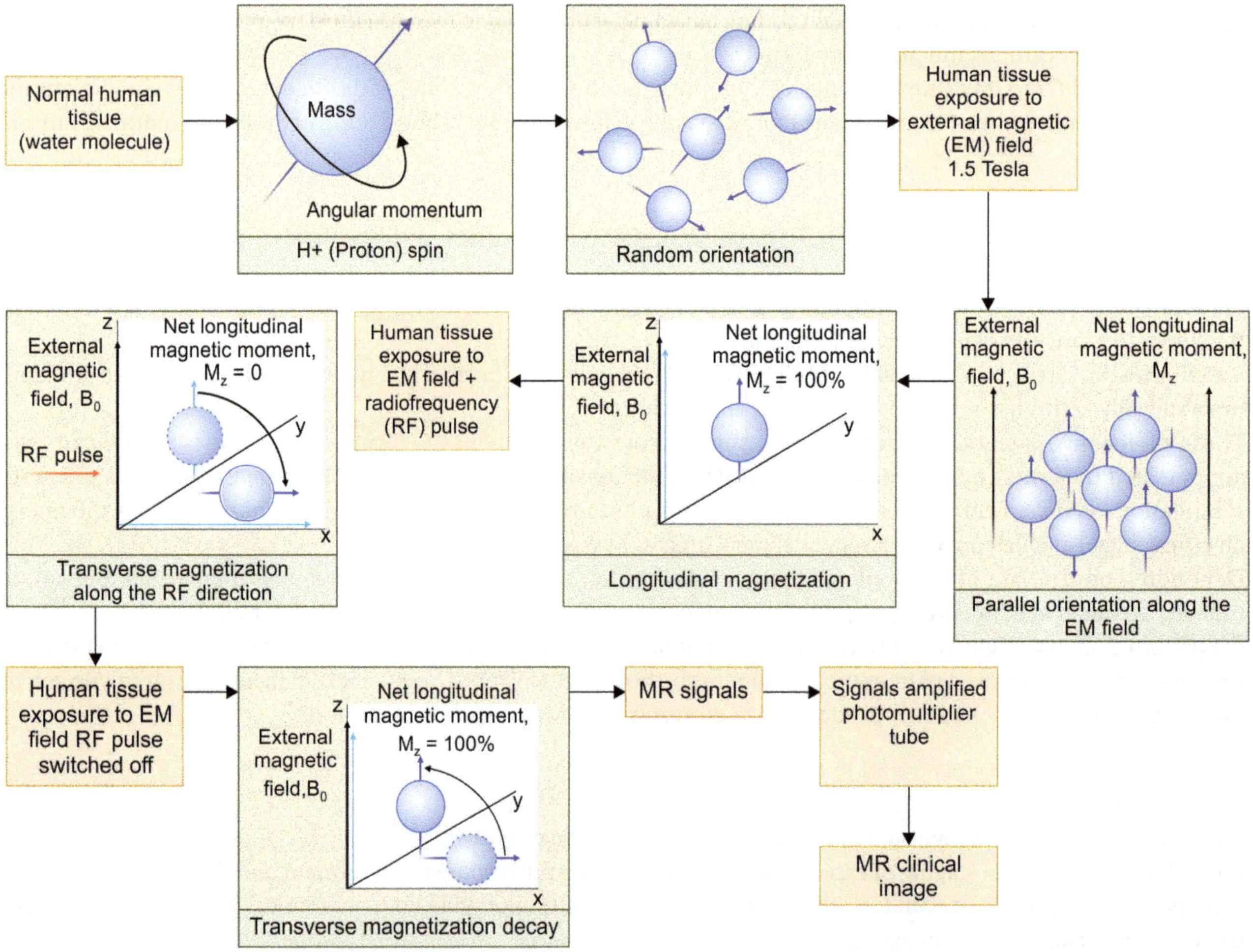

- *Longitudinal magnetization:* The proton when placed in a strong external magnetic field, the randomly oriented spinning protons align in the direction of the external magnetic field. This creates a stable system and a net magnetic field called longitudinal magnetization.
- *Transverse magnetization:* The stable system when subjected to activation by electromagnetic radio waves at 90° to the external magnetic field, the longitudinal magnetization decreases and the proton tilts to the direction of the radiofrequency (RF) wave. This net magnetization is called transverse magnetization.
- *T1 relaxation or recovery:* When the RF excitation is turned off, the transverse magnetization decays to zero and the longitudinal magnetization recovers to 100%. The protons gradually realign with the external magnetic field. The time taken for this transition from transverse to longitudinal magnetization is the T1 relaxation time or spin–lattice relaxation. In this process, the protons lose energy to the surrounding molecules and relax. The energy released during this time is measured as resonance signal.
- *T2 relaxation or recovery:* When the RF excitation is turned off, the protons lose their coherence and relax. The net transverse magnetization reduces to zero. There is no recovery of longitudinal magnetization. The time taken for this relaxation is called the T2 relaxation time or spin–spin relaxation. In this process, the protons exchange energy among themselves and do not lose energy to the surrounding molecules. T1 relaxation is always longer than T2 except in pure water, in which T1 = T2.
- This sequence of events is repeated several times, and the sum total of decay of transverse magnetization of all the protons in the magnetic fields gives rise to the magnetic resonance signals in the form of a voltage which is received by the receiver coil and an image of the tissue is reconstructed by the computer.

Major Components of Magnetic Resonance Imaging System

- A large magnet that provides the primary external magnetic field (1.5 T for medical imaging)
- Shim coils to correct any inhomogeneities in the field.
- RF coil to transmit RF waves to the imaged tissue.
- A receiver coil to detect the returning radio magnetic resonance (MR) signals.
- Gradient coils to provide spatial localization.
- Computer to reconstruct the signals into a final MR image.

Clinical Applications

- The contrast of the image can be distinguished by differences in T2 relaxation time, T1 relaxation time, the density of protons within the tissues, and the time interval between successive excitations.
- *T1-weighted image:*
  - Image acquired with short repetition time
  - Tissues with short T1 relaxation (fat, white matter, bone marrow, proteinaceous fluids): Generate a strong MR signal and a bright image with low contrast.
  - Tissues with long T1 relaxation [air, water, cerebrospinal fluid (CSF), vitreous, bone, calcium, metal, muscle, cortical gray matter]: Generate a weak signal and a darker image with high contrast.
- *T2-weighted image:*
  - Image acquired with long echo time
  - Tissues with short T2 relaxation time (muscle, fat, optic nerve, cortical white matter): Generate weak MR signals and a dark image.
  - Tissues with long T2 relaxation time (CSF, proteinaceous fluid, water and vitreous, cortical gray matter): Generate a strong MR signal and a bright image.

Modifications for Orbital Imaging

Magnetic resonance imaging is useful in the evaluation of all lesions of the orbit except in cases of suspected metallic foreign body, patients with metallic implants, pacemakers, and pregnant females. As orbit is predominantly composed of fat in different compartments, various techniques are used to suppress the bright signals from fat and increase the contrast of lesions in the intraconal and extraconal compartments, particularly in T1-weighted images. The modifications are:

- *Contrast MRI:*
  - Contrast agents are metal ion compounds with unpaired electrons in the outer shell (cobalt, iron, gadolinium, manganese)

- After intravenous administration, it becomes distributed in the vascular and extracellular compartments.
- Results in faster T1 relaxation and more rapid dephasing. Blood will show high signal intensity and brighter image in T1-weighted images and reduced signal intensity and darker image in T2-weighted images.
- It does not enhance the flow of blood; thus, it has limited usefulness in visualizing vascular lesions.
- Useful in fat suppression sequences
- It does not cross blood–brain barrier. In pathological conditions, there is a break in the blood–brain barrier, and the contrast agent diffuses into the interstitial space giving increased signal intensity.

- Short T1 inversion recovery (STIR) sequences
- Chemical shift imaging

Q6. What are the surgical spaces of the orbit? What is the role of CT/MRI in the diagnosis of orbital and ocular lesions? What are the surgical approaches to the orbit?

The orbit is conceptually and anatomically divided into surgical spaces. The surgical spaces of the orbit are shown in **Figure 22**.

The Intraconal Space (Central Surgical Space)

- Contains the optic nerve and orbital fat
- Common lesions include the optic nerve glioma and optic nerve meningioma.

The Extraconal Space (Peripheral Surgical Space)

- Contains the lacrimal gland, the superior oblique muscle, trochlea, nerves, and vessels
- Tumors of the lacrimal gland are common in this space; pleomorphic adenoma, adenocystic carcinoma.

The Extraocular Muscles

A fibrous membrane, the intermuscular septum, extends between the anterior portion of the extraocular muscles separating the intraconal and extraconal spaces. Muscles can be involved in inflammatory or neoplastic conditions such as thyroid orbitopathy, myositis, and metastatic lesions.

The Subperiosteal Space

- Potential space between the orbital bones and the periorbita
- Hematoma can collect in this space due to fracture of orbital bone or an abscess may form due to accumulation of pus adjacent to an infected paranasal sinus.

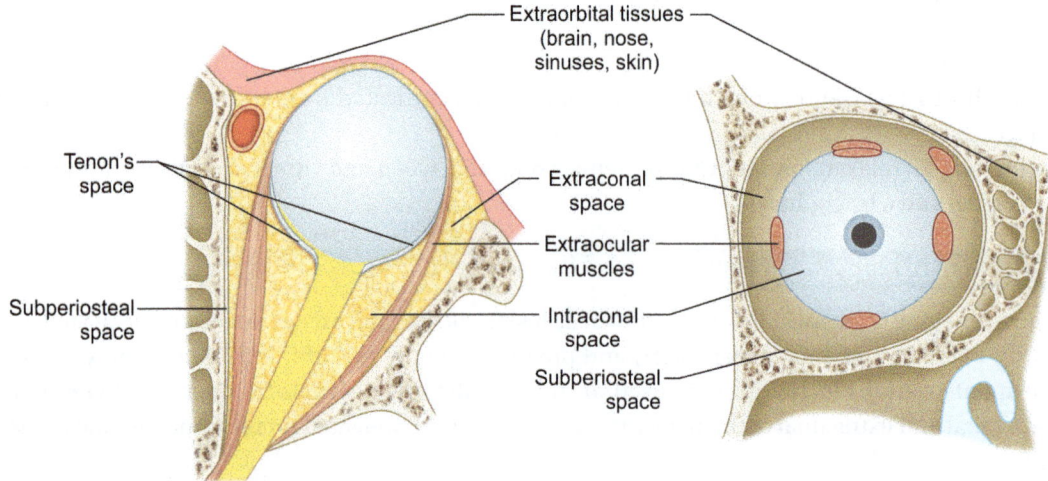

Fig. 22: Surgical spaces of orbit.

The Tenon's Space

- The Tenon's space lies between the eye and the fibrous Tenon's capsule.
- This space is rarely involved in orbital pathologies; the most common lesion being extraocular extension of choroidal melanoma.

The Extraorbital Space

The extraorbital space constitutes the bones and other adnexal structures.

Surgical Approaches to Orbit (Fig. 23)

Access to the orbital contents depends on the following factors:
- *Anterior or deep location:*
  - Tumors/lesions anterior to the equator of the eye: Anterior orbitotomy approach
  - Tumors/lesions posterior to the equator of the eye: Deep orbitotomy approaches
- *Position related to the optic nerve:*
  - Orbitotomy approach should avoid crossing the optic nerve
  - Tumors lateral to the optic nerve: Lateral orbitotomy
  - Tumors medial to the optic nerve: Transcutaneous or transconjunctival medial orbitotomy
  - Posterior one third of the orbit, optic canal chiasm: Transcranial orbitotomy
- The surgical space occupied
- *Goal of surgery:* Excision biopsy/incision biopsy

The various orbitotomy approaches are:
- *Anterior orbitotomy:*
  - Approach is from the front of the orbit.
  - *No bone resection:*
    - Upper eyelid skin crease or blepharoplasty incision:
      - Cosmetically appealing
      - Plane of dissection between the skin, orbicularis and the orbital septum and finally between the septum and the bone depending on the surgical indication
    - Lateral brow incision:
      - Incision is hidden in the hair-bearing skin of the lateral brow.
      - Less cosmetic result
- *Lateral orbitotomy:*
  - Approach is from the lateral side of the orbit.
  - Lateral orbital bony rim is removed.
    - Lateral brow incision extending up to the lateral canthus (Stallard–Wright) incision

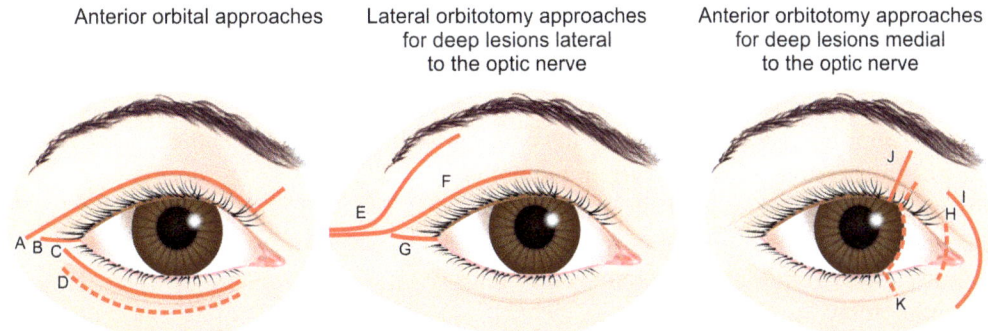

Fig. 23: Surgical approaches to orbit. Surgical incisions for orbitotomy. Anterior orbital approaches: (A) Upper lid skin crease incision. (B) Lateral canthotomy incision. (C) Lower lid transcutaneous incision. (D) Lower lid transconjunctival incision. *Lateral orbitotomy approaches for deep lesions lateral to the optic nerve.* (E) Stallard–Wright lateral orbitotomy incisions. (F) Upper lid skin crease incision with lateral canthal extension. (G) Modified lateral canthotomy incision. *Anterior orbitotomy approaches for deep lesions medial to the optic nerve.* (H) Transcaruncular incision. (I) Frontoethmoidal Lynch incision. (J) Vertical lid split incision. (K) Transconjunctival medial orbitotomy incision.

- Upper eyelid crease incision extending up to the lateral canthus
- Modified lateral canthotomy incision
- *Coronal/hemicoronal incision:*
  - To approach the superior orbit with robust exposure of the medial and lateral orbital walls up to the root of the zygoma
  - Gives wide exposure
  - Gives good cosmetic results
  - Provides access to multiple osteotomies
  - Plane of dissection is in the subpericranial plane below the scalp.
  - Injury to damage the facial and the supraorbital nerves
- *Inferior and anterior orbitotomy approach:*
  - To approach the inferior and lateral orbit:
    - *Transcutaneous approach:*
      - *Subciliary incision:* 2 mm inferior and parallel to the free margin of the lower lid
      - *Subtarsal incision:* 6-7 mm inferior to the free lid margin
  - Plan is between the skin–orbicularis and the septum and finally incising the periosteum over the inferior orbital rim.
  - Disadvantages of developing ectropion and having a prominent scar
    - *Transconjunctval approach:*
      - Approach to inferior, lateral, and medial orbital wall
      - Often combined with lateral canthotomy to improve the surgical exposure.
      - Inferior forniceal transconjunctival incision plane is 2-3 mm below the tarsus; dissection up to the inferior orbital rim can be done preseptally or postseptally.
      - Inferior oblique muscle should be protected by locating the incision along the anterior inferior rim.
- *Medial orbitotomy approaches:*
  - *Transconjunctival medial orbital approach or transcaruncular incision:*
    - Approach to the medial orbit
    - Plane of dissection is between the plica semilunaris and caruncle, extended into the superior and inferior fornices and directly posteriorly toward the posterior lacrimal crest.
    - Cosmetically acceptable
  - *Transcutaneous medial orbital approach (Lynch incision):*
    - Approach to medial orbit
    - Curvilinear skin incision placed anterior to the medial canthus on the frontal process of the maxilla, extending superiorly to the nasofrontal suture and inferiorly to the orbital rim.
    - It may require disinsertion and reattachment of the medial canthal tendon
  - *Vertical lid split incision:*
    - Anterior orbitotomy approach to the anterior intraconal tumors and medial orbital lesions that are medial to the optic nerve.
  - *Transnasal endoscopic approach:*
    - For approaches to deep medial orbit in orbital decompressions, ethmoidectomies, optic nerve sheath fenestrations and incision biopsy of lesions medial to the optic nerve
- *Transcranial orbitotomy:*
  - Provides improved access to the orbital apex and optic canal for:
    - Deep orbital tumors medial to the optic nerve
    - Tumors of the optic nerve with deroofing of the optic canal and exploration of the chiasm
    - Debulking of an extensive sphenoid wing meningioma
    - Extensive orbitocranial extension of any tumor
  - Three transcranial approaches are used to approach the orbit:
    - Frontal transcranial orbitotomy (panoramic orbitotomy)
    - Pterional craniotomy
    - Eyebrow craniotomy
- *Combined orbitotomies:* A combination of orbitotomies in addition to lateral canthotomy are used:
  - *Orbital fracture repair:* Medial and inferior orbitotomies
  - *Orbital decompression for thyroid eye disease:* Transcaruncular medial orbitotomy + lateral orbitotomy + burring away of the body of sphenoid.

7. What are the principles of USG of orbital and ocular lesions? Describe the indications, advantages, and clinical applications of USG.

Ultrasonography is an ancillary test for clinical evaluation of opaque ocular media and abnormal orbit.

Principles

Ultrasound is an acoustic wave with a frequency >20 kHz. For imaging the posterior segment of the eye and orbit, the frequencies used in ultrasound are 8–25 MHz. For imaging the anterior segment of the eye, the frequency required is 50 MHz.

The basic principles involved in clinical diagnostic ultrasound are:
- Pulse echo technology
- Tissue acoustic impedance.

Piezoelectric crystals in the transducers produce ultrasound waves. These waves, as they pass through the ocular structures, are absorbed, reflected, refracted, or scattered. Some of these sound waves return to the transducer and are called echoes.

Echoes are generated at the adjoining tissue interfaces that display differences in the acoustic impedances or densities; greater the difference stronger the echo.

These reflecting echoes are retrieved at the transducer, amplified and electronically processed and displayed in visual format as A scan or B scan images. The imaging zones can be hyperechoic, hypoechoic, or anechoic.

Higher frequency waves penetrate less into the tissue and have better resolution. Lower frequency waves penetrate more deeply but have worse resolution.

A scan (time amplitude) is used for tissue characterization and interpretation. These are generated at 8 MHz and converted to spikes that correspond to tissue interfaces.

B scan (intensity or brightness amplitude modulated) provides a cross-sectional image of the globe and the orbit and topographic information. These are generated at 10 MHz.

The display images are presented horizontally in contact scanning and vertically with water bath (immersion scanning).

Clinical Applications

Ossoinigs standardized echography stages:
- Screening for lesion detection (A + B scans)
- *Topographic echography:* Characterization of lesion in terms of location, shape, margins, and extension (A + B scans)
- *Quantitative echography:* Assessment of the internal structure of the lesion, its reflectivity and absorbance/attenuation of ultrasound waves (A scan). Wave attenuation is evaluated on the basis of angle kappa; angle kappa >45 denotes high echo attenuation, angle kappa = 45 denotes moderate echo attenuation, and angle kappa <45 denotes low echo attenuation. Angle kappa in a normal healthy orbit is >45.
- *Kinetic echography:* Information on lesion mobility, elasticity, and vascularity (A + B scans, color Doppler scan)

Measurement of globe length for lens power calculation and implant size determination:
- Diagnosis and measurement of tumors such as choroidal melanoma
- Detection of retinal detachment
- Visualization of the fundus and ocular structures in case of opaque media
- Localization of orbital and intraocular foreign bodies
- Localization of vascular lesions such as lymphangioma and hemangioma and USG-guided injection of sclerosants into these lesions
- USG-guided use of injectable fillers
- Color Doppler ultrasound is an adjunct to ultrasound to evaluate blood and better characterization of orbital vessels and vascular lesions.
- Measurement of thicknesses of extraocular muscles. In normal orbits, the differences in the thickness values between individual muscles are not >0.5 mm and the differences in the sum of the muscle thicknesses between two orbits do not exceed 1.2 mm.
- Evaluation of cystic lesions of the orbit

Advantages

- No exposure to ionic radiations, safer, cheaper, and repeatable
- Noninvasive and widely accessible
- Provides dynamic real-time information on orbital and ocular lesions (kinetic scan).

Disadvantages

- High level of interoperator variability
- Imaging through ultrasound is limited to a depth of 2 cm. Therefore, it does not allow for visualization of the orbital apex.
- It has poor resolution compared to CT/MRI.
- It has limited ability to image bony walls of the orbit.

Suggested Reading

1. Aviv RI, Casselman J. Orbital imaging: part 1. Normal anatomy. Clin Radiol. 2005;60(3):279-87.
2. Cohen LM, Yoon MK. Update on current aspects of orbital imaging: CT, MRI, and ultrasonography. Int Ophthalmol Clin. 2019;59(4): 69-79.
3. Dutton JJ. Computed tomography. Radiology of the Orbit and Visual Pathways. Philadelphia: Saunders Elsevier; 2010. pp. 1-8. Chapter 1.
4. Dutton JJ. Magnetic resonance imaging. Radiology of the Orbit and Visual Pathways. Philadelphia: Saunders Elsevier; 2010. pp. 9-29. Chapter 2.
5. Goh PS, Gi MT, Charlton A, Tan C, Gangadhara Sundar JK, Amrith S. Review of orbital imaging. Eur J Radiol. 2008;66(3):387-95.
6. Naik MN, Tourani KL, Sekhar GC, Honavar SG. Interpretation of computed tomography imaging of the eye and orbit. A systematic approach. Indian J Ophthalmol. 2002;50(4):339-53.
7. Nelson CC, Cartwright MJ. Orbital diagnosis and imaging. Curr Opin Ophthalmol. 1992;3(5):623-31.
8. Nerad JA. Surgical approaches to the orbit. Techniques in Ophthalmic Plastic Surgery: A personal Tutorial, 2nd edition. Philadelphia: Saunders Elsevier; 2010. pp. 429-61. Chapter 15.
9. Turvey TA, Golden BA. Orbital anatomy for the surgeon. Oral Maxillofac Surg Clin North Am. 2012;24(4):525-36.

1.23 Congenital Lesions of Orbit

Vijitha S Vempuluru, Anasua G Kapoor

 1. Discuss hypertelorism. How does it differ from telecanthus?

Definition: Orbital hypertelorism, also called teleorbitism, is a craniofacial malformation characterized by an increase in the interorbital distance, that is, the distance between the inner canthi (intercanthal distance) and the eyeballs (interpupillary distance) is increased.

Evaluation:
- Increased intercanthal (medial and lateral) distance
- Increased interpupillary distance
- *Increased intercrestal distance:* Distance between the posterior lacrimal crests on radiography **(Table 1)**.

Management

Principle of surgery: To achieve medialization of the orbits by osteotomy and bone removal, avoiding damage to the soft tissue and vital structures. Coronal flap is usually utilized for both subcranial and intracranial approaches **(Flowchart 1)**.

TABLE 1: Grading of hypertelorism (Gunther et al.).

Grade	Intercrestal distance (adults) (mm)
Normal	*Females:* 20–26 (mean, 25) *Males:* 21–28 (mean, 26)
Grade I	28–34
Grade II	34–40
Grade III	>40

Note: Expansive midline lesions (e.g., frontonasal meningoencephalocele) can falsely increase the intercrestal distance without the presence of true hypertelorism.

Flowchart 1: Management of hypertelorism.

```
                    ┌─→ Extracranial ──→ Grade 1 ──→ Cribriform plate
                    │   (subcranial)     hypertelorism   not descended
                    │                                    >10 mm from the
                    │                                    upper orbital rim
         Approach ──┤
                    │                ┌─→ Grade II
                    │                │   hypertelorism
                    └─→ Intracranial ┤
                                     │
                                     └─→ Grade III
                                         hypertelorism
```

Telecanthus

- *Telecanthus* is the presence of abnormally widely placed medial canthi.
- The intercanthal distance is increased in telecanthus when compared to normal population due to the presence of excess soft tissue at the medial canthus.
- *In contrast to hypertelorism, the interpupillary distance is normal.*
- Correction is rarely indicated and can be achieved by shortening of the medial canthal tendons and repositioning of medial soft tissue which can be achieved by transnasal wiring or fixation with screws.

 2. Discuss craniosynostosis and the eye.

Definition: Heterogenous group of disorders characterized by premature closure of suture lines, thus preventing growth perpendicular to the suture line and allowing the same in a direction parallel to the suture line. Craniosynostosis can be syndromic or nonsyndromic **(Tables 2 and 3)**. Both forms have been associated with mutations in the *FGFR* gene.

Depending on the site of premature closure, various forms of anomalous skull shapes can result **(Figs. 1 and 2A to F)**.

Management is complex and should be led by a multispecialty team consisting of craniofacial surgeon, neurosurgeon, oculoplastic surgeon, pediatric ophthalmologist, otolaryngologist, geneticist, pediatrician, physical anthropologist, orthodontist and pedodontist, psychologist, radiologist, speech therapist, anesthesiologist, and patient care coordinators.

 3. Explain cryptophthalmos, anophthalmos, microphthalmos, and congenital cystic eye with a note on the normal development of the eye. Elaborate on management.

Development of the Eye

Development of the eye begins in the day-22 embryo on either side of the forebrain, starting as shallow grooves which turn into outpouchings known as the optic vesicles. Contact of these optic vesicles with the surface ectoderm induces further changes which lead to the development of optic cup, invagination of lens placode, formation of a lens vesicle, and further differentiation of the embryonic eye. The surface ectoderm migrates over the lens vesicle which heralds the development of

TABLE 2: Manifestations of craniosynostosis.

Deformity	Sutures affected
Oxycephaly	Multiple (coronal and sagittal)
Brachycephaly	Bilateral coronal
Acrobrachycephaly	Bilateral coronal; patent anterior fontanelle
Plagiocephaly	Unilateral coronal
Scaphocephaly	Interparietal sagittal
Trigonocephaly	Metopic
Triphyllocephaly	Lambdoidal and coronal

TABLE 3: Syndromic craniosynostosis and clinical features.

Syndrome	Pathology	Systemic features	Craniofacial features	Ophthalmic features
Crouzon syndrome	Autosomal dominant; *FGFR2* gene mutation	Seizures CNS anomalies, musculoskeletal and vision anomalies	Acrobrachycephaly, oxycephaly, midface retrusion, widespread orbits	Hypertelorism, proptosis, megalocornea, microcornea, keratoconus, aniridia anisocoria, blue sclera, cataract, corectopia, ectopia lentis, glaucoma, iris, coloboma, nystagmus, optic nerve hypoplasia, strabismus
Apert syndrome	Autosomal dominant, *FGFR* gene family mutations	Medial deviation of great toe, syndactyly of hands and feet, Byzantine arch-shape palate, cleft soft palate, bifid uvula, dental anomalies, cardiovascular and genital anomalies	Oxycephaly, parrot beak nose, low set ears	Proptosis, hypertelorism, strabismus, refractive error, amblyopia, keratoconus, ectopia lentis, congenital glaucoma, oculocutaneous albinism
Pfeiffer syndrome	Autosomal dominant, *FGFR* gene family mutations	• Flat occiput, high forehead, small nose, low nasal bridge, midface hypoplasia, high arched palate, malocclusion of teeth, enlarged thumb • Type 1 or classic: Brachycephaly, midface hypoplasia, finger and toe anomalies • Type 2: Cloverleaf skull skeletal abnormality, developmental delay • Type 3: Type 2 without cloverleaf skull		Moderate to severe proptosis, hypertelorism, lateral canthal dystopia, papilledema optic atrophy, microcornea, corectopia, glaucoma
Saethre–Chotzen syndrome	Autosomal dominant; *TWIST1* gene mutation	Cognitive limitation, schizophrenia, seizure disorder, brachydactyly, clinodactyly	Bilateral coronal craniosynostosis, peace sign synostosis	Ptosis, down-slanting palpebral fissures, lacrimal duct obstruction, strabismus, refractive error, optic atrophy
Muenke syndrome	Autosomal dominant; *FGFR3* gene mutation	Broad toes, mental retardation, developmental delay, epilepsy, sensorineural hearing loss	Cloverleaf skull or tower-shape skull, flat forehead, deviated nasal root, anteriorly displaced ears	Hypertelorism, telecanthus, natural cancel dystopia, ptosis, optic atrophy
Carpenter syndrome	Autosomal recessive; *RAB23* gene mutation	CNS abnormalities, hydrocephalus, congenital heart disease, hypogonadism, obesity, umbilical hernia	Shallow supraorbital ridges, mid facial hyperplasia depressed nasal bridge, upturned nose, micrognathia	Hypertelorism, epicanthal folds

(*CNS*: central nervous system)

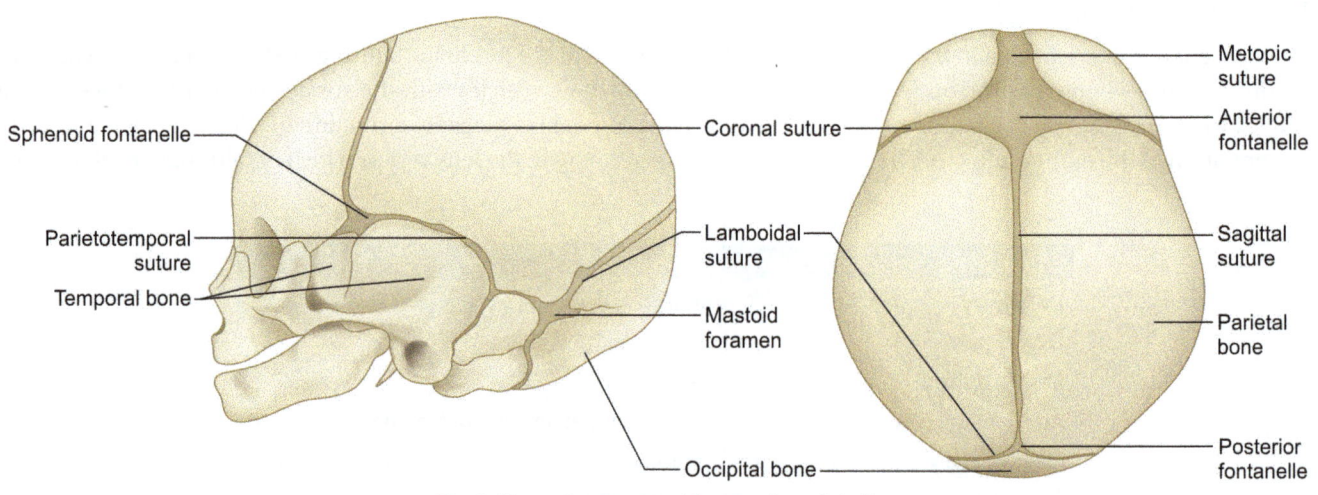

Fig. 1: Normal sutures and fontanelles of skull.

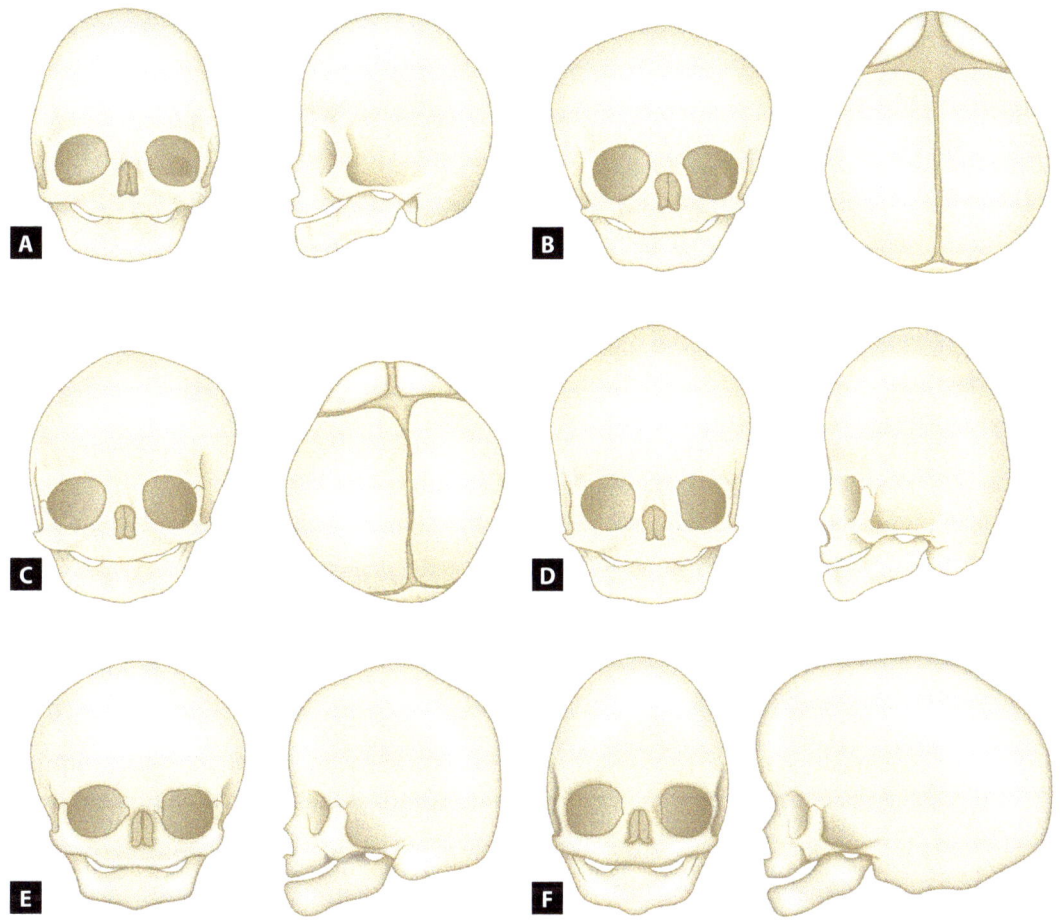

Figs. 2A to F: (A) Oxycephaly; (B) trigonocephaly; (C) plagiocephaly; (D) acrocephaly; (E) brachycephaly; (F) scaphocephaly.

eyelids in a 6-week fetus. Primitive eyelids are merely circumferential folds overlying the optic vesicle. Further development of the eyelids occurs by proliferation of the mesenchyme.

- *Cryptophthalmos (hidden eye):* Congenital eyelid abnormality characterized by failure of the eyelid folds to fuse.
  - *Types:* Complete, partial, and abortive (congenital symblepharon)
  - In complete cryptophthalmos, a uniform fold of skin can be seen extending from forehead to cheek. When only the medial aspect of the globe is covered by the skin and rest of the palpebral fissure can be made out, it is termed incomplete cryptophthalmos.
  - Abortive or congenital symblepharon form is characterized by formed eyelids which are adherent to ocular surface with no fornices and poor closure.
  - Depending on the type of symblepharon, ocular surface when exposed is of primary concern which is to be addressed with copious lubricants.
  - Visual evoked potentials are useful in determining the presence of visual potential. When there is possibility of useful vision, eyelid reconstruction may be attempted.
  - Syndromic associations with Fraser and Manitoba syndrome are known; hence, genetic screening is warranted.
- *Anophthalmos (absence of eye) and microphthalmos (small eye)*
  - Anophthalmia and microphthalmia lie within the same spectrum of disorders of development of the eye.
  - They may be isolated or associated with other systemic anomalies, especially the head and neck; hence, systemic evaluation is a mandate.
  - Congenital anophthalmia
    - Rare anomaly where there is no ocular tissue due to arrested development in embryogenesis as early as the formation of optic vesicle
    - Clinical anophthalmia is a more relevant term where no discernable ocular structures are present.

TABLE 4: Differentiating features.

Microphthalmos with cyst	Congenital cystic eye	Teratoma
• Bilateral or unilateral • Typically inferior in location • Bulges through lower eyelid • Small deformed globe is present • Enlarged orbit may be seen	• Usually unilateral • Central or bulges through upper eyelid • No discernible globe • Normal sized orbit	• Unilateral • Can extend into maxillary sinus • Normal globe • Normal to enlarged orbit

- Microphthalmia
    - Presence of small disorganized globe resulting from defective development of optic cup or obliteration of the embryonic fissure
    - It may be isolated, associated with a coloboma, colobomatous cyst, or orbitopalpebral cyst.
- Assessment of visual potential can be challenging in young children but is an important factor in planning further management; visual evoked potentials are a useful modality for the same.
- Since the eyeball plays an important role in the development of orbitofacial skeleton, assessment of the socket is crucial in cases of microphthalmos with no useful vision.
- Timely expansion procedures, wherever necessary, can avoid hemifacial microsomia. In the presence of orbitopalpebral or orbital cysts, orbital imaging can help assess for any communication with the globe.
- Treatment options include cyst aspiration, injection of sclerosants, and excision or removal of the rudimentary eye followed by socket reconstruction.
- *Congenital cystic eye*
    - Rare developmental anomaly characterized by partial or complete failure of invagination of the primary optic vesicle
    - On examination, the eyeball is replaced by a cystic swelling which is usually central and bulges through the upper eyelid.
    - Size of the cystic eye depends on the patency of the optic stalk. Patent optic stalk allows flow of cerebrospinal fluid; hence, the cyst is small.
    - Large cysts can cause expansion of bony orbit.
    - *Differential diagnosis:* Microphthalmos with cyst, orbital tumors such as teratoma, neuroblastoma, capillary hemangioma, lymphangioma, rhabdomyosarcoma, or encephalocele. Close differentials in a newborn are listed in **Table 4**.

Management

- Thorough assessment for other ocular, facial, and systemic anomalies
- Aims toward rehabilitation of the socket and maintains symmetrical development of the face.

Suggested Reading

1. Chung SA, Yun IS, Moon JW, Lee JB. Ophthalmic findings in children with nonsyndromic craniosynostosis treated by expansion cranioplasty. J Craniofac Surg. 2015;26(1):79-83.
2. del Campo AF. Orbital hypertelorism: surgical management. In: Greenberg AM, Prein J (Eds). Craniomaxillofacial Reconstructive and Corrective Bone Surgery. New York: Springer; 2002.
3. Gunther H. Konstitutionelle Anomalien der Augenabstandes und der Interorbitalbreite. Virchows Arch Pathol Anat. 1933;290:373.
4. Hayashi N, Repka MX, Ueno H, Iliff NT, Green WR. Congenital cystic eye: report of two cases and review of the literature. Surv Ophthalmol. 1999;44(2):173-9.
5. Helveston EM, Malone Jr E, Lashmet MH. Congenital cystic eye. Arch Ophthalmol. 1970;84(5):622-4.
6. Katowitz JA, Katowitz WR. Pediatric Oculoplastic Surgery, 2nd edition. New York: Springer; 2017.
7. Katowitz JA. Developmental eyelid abnormalities. In: Foster JA, Katowitz JA (Eds). Pediatric Oculoplastic Surgery. New York: Springer-Verlag; 2002. pp. 213-15.
8. Mauriello Jr JA, Caputo AR. Treatment of congenital forms of telecanthus with custom-designed titanium medial canthal tendon screws. Ophthalmic Plast Reconstr Surg. 1994;10(3):195-9.
9. Newman SA. Ophthalmic features of craniosynostosis. Neurosurg Clin N Am. 1991;2(3):587-610.
10. Ragge NK, Subak-Sharpe ID, Collin JR. A practical guide to the management of anophthalmia and microphthalmia. Eye (Lond). 2007;21(10):1290-300.
11. Sadler TW. Langman's Medical Embryology. Philadelphia: Lippincott Williams & Wilkins; 2012. pp. 329-34.

1.24 Orbital Cysts and Tumors

Vijitha S Vempuluru, Anasua G Kapoor, Shruthi Gunda

 1. Lacrimal gland lesions: Describe in detail the clinical features, differential diagnosis, and management of lacrimal gland swellings.

Lacrimal Gland Lesions: Approach, Clinical features, Differential Diagnosis, and Management

Differential Diagnosis

Clinical examination is aimed at distinguishing *inflammatory or neoplastic* etiology **(Table 1)**. Differential diagnosis of lacrimal gland tumors includes lesions of epithelial and nonepithelial origin **(Flowchart 1)**.

Management

Investigations

- Computed tomography (CT) of the orbit is the first line of investigation as it allows identification of lesion location, extent as well as associated features such as *bony abnormalities*.
- Magnetic resonance imaging (MRI) of the orbit can be requested in cases where soft tissue detail is inadequate **(Table 2)**.
- Chest X-ray, Mantoux, QuantiFERON gold, serum calcium, serum angiotensin-converting enzyme (ACE), immunological profile [antinuclear antibody (ANA), antineutrophil cytoplasmic antibody (ANCA), antiphospholipid antibody (APLA) as applicable]

Diagnostic Workup of Lymphoproliferative Lesions and Suspected Malignant Tumors (Table 3)

Complete physical examination with assessment of lymph nodes, complete blood picture, serum protein electrophoresis (where applicable—suspected paraproteinemia/multiple myeloma), and CT of chest, abdomen, and pelvis.

Treatment

Primary aim of clinicoradiological examination is to identify benign or malignant etiology to decide on medical or surgical management **(Flowchart 2)**.

TABLE 1: Clinical features of lacrimal gland lesions.

	Inflammatory (dacryoadenitis)	**Neoplastic (tumors)**
Age	• 3rd–4th decades: Viral/bacterial adenitis • 5th–6th decades: Autoimmune, idiopathic (NSOID)	4th–5th decades and beyond
Symptoms	• Pain • Swelling • Usually not associated with vision loss • Fever • Bilateral involvement	*Benign (pleomorphic adenoma) or lymphomatous lesions:* • Gradually progressive course • Prominent eye • Drooping of eyelid • Palpable mass *Malignant:* • Rapidly progressive proptosis • Vision loss • *Pain after the onset of proptosis*
Signs	• Eyelid edema • Erythema • Chemosis • Tenderness • Local warmth • Pain with extraocular movements	• S-shaped ptosis • Globe dystopia (inferior or inferonasal) • Proptosis • Palpable mass • Resistance to retropulsion • Limitation of ocular motility • *Signs of globe/optic nerve compression:* RAPD, disc edema, exudative detachment

(NSOID: nonspecific orbital inflammatory disease; RAPD: relative afferent pupillary defect)

Flowchart 1: Approach to common lacrimal gland lesions, based on origin.

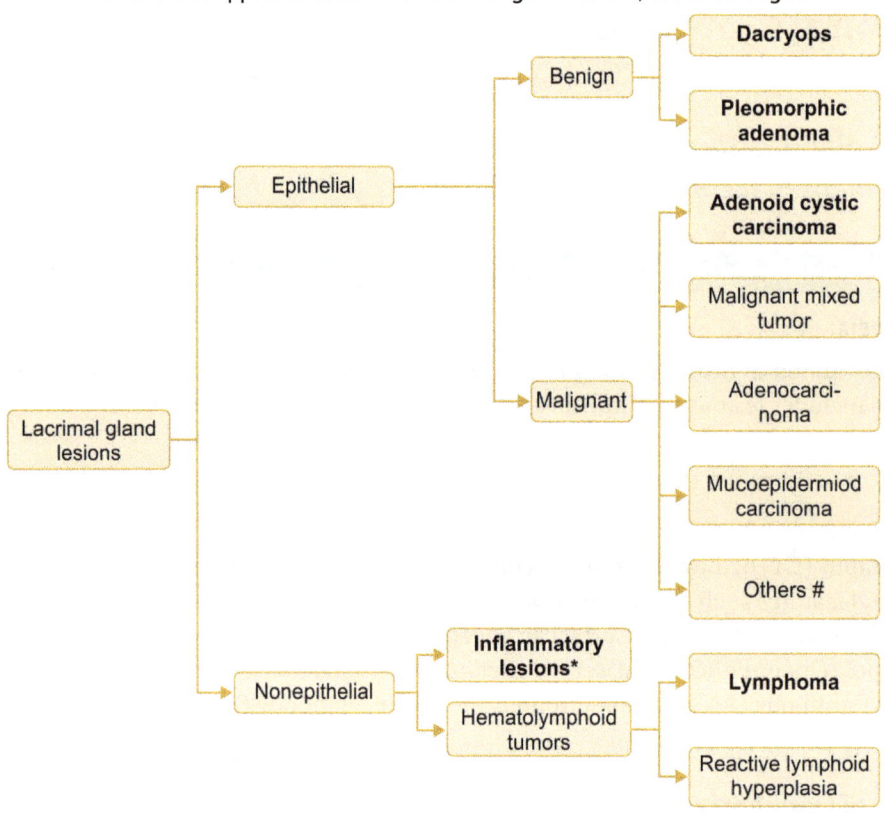

*Infectious (viral, bacterial), autoimmune (Sjögren's syndrome, sarcoidosis, granulomatosis with polyangiitis), and idiopathic [nonspecific orbital inflammatory disease (NSOID)].
†Squamous cell carcinoma, malignant oncocytoma, acinic cell carcinoma, and myoepithelial carcinoma.
Note: Based on etiology, about 50% of lacrimal gland lesions are inflammatory and 50% are neoplastic, with the most common primary neoplasms being pleomorphic adenoma and adenoid cystic carcinoma (Figs. 1A and B).

Lesion	Computed tomography (CT)	Magnetic resonance imaging (MRI)
Pleomorphic adenoma	• Variable attenuation: Highly cellular lesions, more homogenous • Nonhomogeneous areas due to mesenchymal stroma, cystic degeneration, necrosis, mucinous or serous collection	• Small tumors: T1—low signal intensity and T2—high signal intensity • Large tumor (containing hemorrhage and necrotic areas): Heterogenous signal intensities
Adenoid cystic carcinoma	Contrast enhancing soft tissue mass; bone erosion	Gadolinium-enhancing hyperintense (T1) lesion, perineural and intracranial extension can be seen
Lymphoid tumors	Can be bilateral; diffuse involvement of orbital and palpebral lobes; mold around the globe with a concave configuration	Homogenous lesion with contrast enhancement
Dacryoadenitis	Unilateral or bilateral; enlarged lacrimal glands with contrast enhancement	As in CT
Nonspecific orbital inflammatory disease	Enlarged lacrimal gland or soft tissue density lesion	Iso to hypointense on T1 and relatively hypointense on T2. Variable contrast enhancement

TABLE 2: Radiological features of common lacrimal gland lesions.

Indications for medical management:
- *First episode of dacryoadenitis:* Nonsteroidal anti-inflammatory drugs (NSAIDs), steroids, immunosuppression/immunomodulation
- Systemic inflammatory disorders/vasculitides
- Tuberculosis

TABLE 3: Diagnostic workup for inflammatory lesion of the lacrimal gland (or orbit).

Infections	Specific inflammations	Nonspecific inflammations	Collagen vascular disorders
• Tuberculosis • Lyme disease • Dacryoadenitis	• Sarcoidosis • Crohn's disease • Sjögren's syndrome	• Orbital pseudotumor • Foreign body granuloma	• Wegener's granulomatosis • Polyarteritis nodosa • Churg–Strauss syndrome • Kimura's disease Behçet's disease • Lupus erythematosus • Dermatomyositis • Scleroderma • Rheumatoid arthritis • Amyloidosis

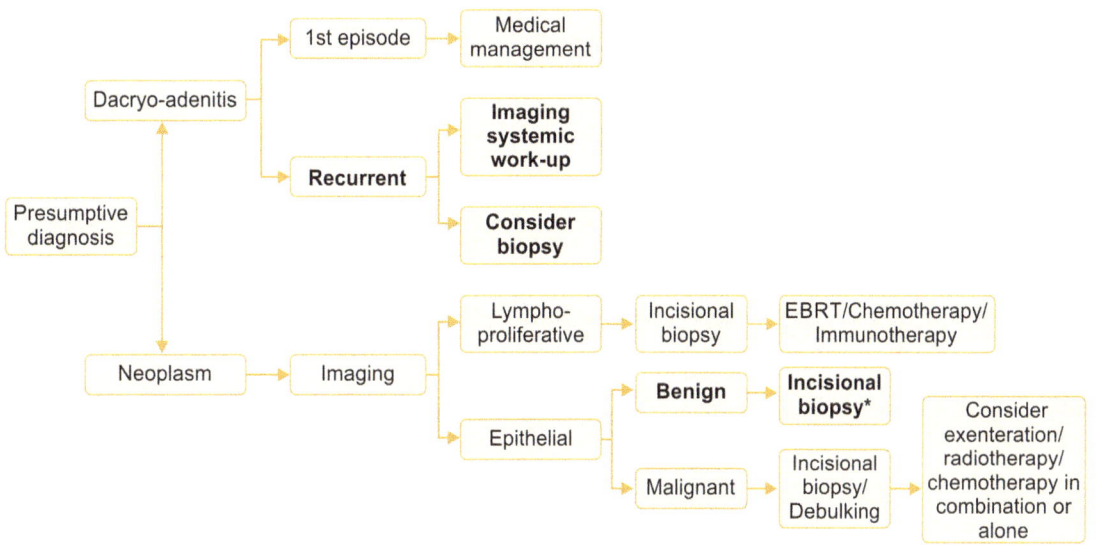

Flowchart 2: Summary of diagnostic and therapeutic lines of management.

*Incisional biopsy is strongly contraindicated in pleomorphic adenoma.
(EBRT: external beam radiation therapy)

Role of chemotherapy:
- Lymphoma with systemic disease (CHOP/R-CHOP regime)
- Neoadjuvant chemotherapy for lacrimal gland adenoid cystic carcinoma
- Adjuvant chemotherapy for gross residual disease in malignant tumors of lacrimal gland

Role of radiotherapy:
- Lymphoma localized to orbit
- Adjuvant radiation in residual tumor or most cases of adenoid cystic carcinoma with perineural invasion

Indications for surgical management:
- Excision of benign tumors
- Incisional biopsy or debulking of suspected malignant tumors

Principles of surgical management: Lacrimal gland lesions can be approached by a lateral orbitotomy (refer to Question 8).

2. Rhabdomyosarcoma (RMS): Discuss the clinical features and management.

Epidemiology

- Most common primary orbital malignancy in childhood
- Accounts for about 4% of pediatric orbital mass lesions and 1% of all orbital tumors
- Affects child in first and second decades, rarely adults.

Etiopathogenesis and Types

- Most cases are sporadic.
- *Known risk factors:* Exposure to radiation, genetic predisposition in familial cancer syndromes
- *Two major subtypes:* Alveolar RMS (ARMS) and embryonal RMS (ERMS). ERMS is more common, less aggressive, and has better prognosis than ARMS.

Clinical features of Rhabdomyosarcoma

Symptoms:
- Swelling
- Pain
- Vision loss
- Palpable mass

Signs:
- Anterior orbital or eyelid mass
- Proptosis and globe dystopia (tumors are usually extraconal and located in anterior to mid orbit)
- Chemosis
- Relative afferent pupillary defect
- Disc edema, choroidal folds

Note: It can have acute to subacute presentation with predominant inflammatory signs mimicking orbital cellulitis.

Management

The summary of diagnostic and therapeutic lines of management is shown in **Flowchart 3**.

Investigations

- *Orbital imaging:*
  - CT:
    - Well-circumscribed, isodense homogeneous lesion
    - Calcification in presence of bony destruction
    - Heterogeneous areas suggest tumor necrosis or hemorrhage.
    - Moderate to marked generalized enhancement with contrast
    - Preseptal soft-tissue changes may be seen with spillover inflammation.
  - MRI:
    - T1: Isointense; T2: Hyperintense

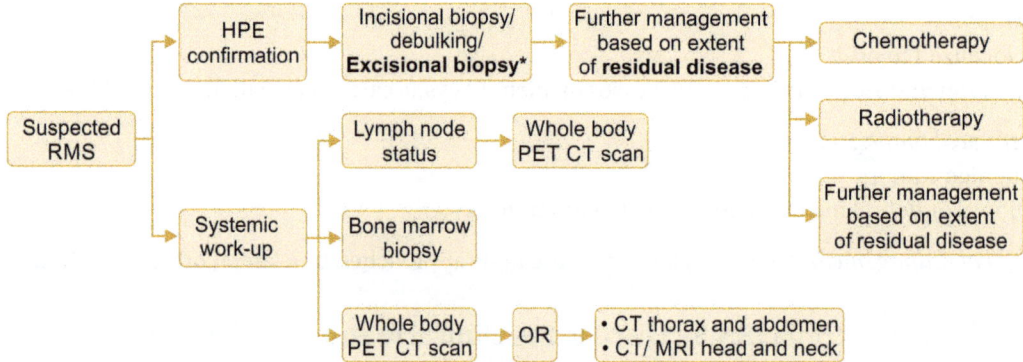

Flowchart 3: Summary of diagnostic and therapeutic lines of management rhabdomyosarcoma.

*Complete tumor removal has a favorable prognosis; however, it may not be possible in all cases due to potential damage to ocular and periocular vital structures.
(FNAC: fine needle aspiration cytology; HPE: histopathological examination; PET-CT: positron emission tomography-computed tomography; RMS: rhabdomyosarcoma)

- Moderate to marked uniform gadolinium enhancement
- Paranasal sinus involvement can be better delineated.
- *Systemic evaluation:*
  - Regional lymph node examination
  - Bone marrow biopsy
  - Whole body positron emission tomography-computed tomography (PET-CT) scan or CT chest, abdomen, and pelvis.

Grouping of Disease

The Intergroup Rhabdomyosarcoma Study Group (IRSG) grouping system is shown in **Table 4**.

Treatment

Surgery: Well-circumscribed lesions can be excised in toto by orbitotomy, but it is not always feasible. In cases with diffuse or ill-defined lesions, debulking can be performed.

Exenteration is reserved for recurrent tumors.

Chemotherapy: Adjuvant chemotherapy and radiotherapy are usually the norm following surgery to address residual disease. Follow-up of patients is crucial as recurrences can occur after completion of treatment.

3. What is a dermoid cyst? List systemic associations of dermoids. Discuss the differential diagnosis of epibulbar swellings.

- *Dermoid cyst* is a choristomatous lesion arising from ectodermal elements separated off at suture lines. Histopathologically, dermoid cyst shows hair follicles, keratin, sebaceous glands, macrophages, lipid, and calcium.
- Choristoma refers to presence of normal tissue in an abnormal location.
- Simple choristomas contain one type of tissue and complex choristomas contain more than one type of tissue.
- Dermoids can be located on the ocular surface (epibulbar dermoid), orbit (dermoid cyst), or rarely in the eyelids **(Tables 5 and 6)**.

Systemic Associations of Dermoids

- *Goldenhar syndrome:* Limbal dermoids, preauricular skin appendages, vertebral anomalies, eyelid coloboma, hearing loss, and mandibular hypoplasia
- *Gorlin syndrome or nevoid basal cell carcinoma syndrome:* Multiple basal-cell carcinomas of the skin; odontogenic keratocyst; intracranial calcification; skeletal abnormalities of face, mandible, spine, and ribs; and ovarian and cardiac fibromas
- *Klippel–Feil syndrome:* Scoliosis, spina bifida, cleft palate, anomalous dentition, cardiorespiratory anomalies, skeletal anomalies, Duane's syndrome
- *Organoid nevus syndrome:* Cutaneous sebaceous nevus, seizures, and epibulbar choristomas.

TABLE 4: Intergroup Rhabdomyosarcoma Study Group (IRSG) grouping system.

Group	Definition
I	*Localized tumor:* • Completely removed with *pathologically clear margins* • No regional LN involvement
II	*Localized tumor:* Grossly removed with • Microscopically involved margins • Involved, grossly resected regional LN, or • Both
III	*Localized tumor: Gross residual disease* after grossly incomplete removal, or biopsy only
IV	Distant metastases present at diagnosis

(LN: lymph node)

TABLE 5: Clinical features and treatment of ocular surface, adnexal and orbital dermoids.

	Clinical features	Treatment
Epibulbar dermoid	• Solid whitish-yellow or pigmented lesion with hair follicles • Can involve limbus or bulbar conjunctiva • Vision can be affected due to induced astigmatism *Grading of limbal dermoids*: • *Grade I*: <5 mm; localized to limbus • *Grade II*: Covers most of the cornea; extends down to stroma but Descemet's membrane is not involved • *Grade III*: Covers whole cornea and extends into the anterior chamber	• Small lesions can be observed • Excision biopsy for lesions causing astigmatism or cosmetic concerns • Need for lamellar or penetrating keratoplasty can be assessed by the depth of stromal involvement on anterior segment optical coherence tomography (ASOCT)
Orbit	• Can be superficial, deep, or a combination of both; present in childhood or in teens with painless swelling usually superotemporal in location • Nontender, slightly fluctuant cystic lesion, may be tethered to bone or suture lines • Deep lesions cause proptosis, diplopia, and motility limitation	• Conservative treatment: Foam sclerotherapy • Excision biopsy of orbital lesion • Deep lesions require removal by orbitotomy
Eyelids and adnexa	Rarely dermoids can be present in atypical locations such as within the eyelid or tarsus	Excision biopsy confirms the diagnosis and also addresses mechanical ptosis and cosmetic concerns

TABLE 6: Differential diagnosis of epibulbar swellings **(Figs. 2A to D)**.

Entity	Clinical features	Imaging	Histopathology
Epithelial inclusion cyst	Subepithelial, usually clear, smooth thin-walled lesion; can be pigmented from secondary melanosis	*ASOCT*: Subepithelial, usually homogenous hyporeflective lesion with a normal to thin epithelium	*Lining*: Conjunctival epithelium *Cavity*: Clear/mucin/epithelial debris or rarely keratin
Prolapsed orbital fat	Subconjunctival superotemporal or temporal yellowish lesion, may be lobulated, with a convex anterior border; enlarges with digital pressure over the globe and can be reposited with a Q tip	*ASOCT*: Subconjunctival homogenous hyporeflective lesion; back shadowing may be present *CT*: Well-defined lesion isodense to orbital fat and continuous with it	Adipose tissue
Dermoid	Yellowish-white solid lesion, usually at limbus; fine hairs may be present; can be pigmented; corneal involvement can be variable; *Ring dermoid syndrome*: Bilateral limbal dermoid with involvement of entire limbus	*ASOCT*: Hyper-reflective lesion with back shadowing	Lined by stratified squamous epithelium; substance can contain pilosebaceous glands, hair follicles or sweat glands, and fat
Dermolipoma	• Usually temporal in location • Concave anterior border • Cannot be reposited with a Q tip	*ASOCT*: Hyper-reflective lesion with back shadowing. Can appear heterogenous	Epidermal elements with fat
Osseous choristoma	Usually solitary superotemporal epibulbar lesion, hard in consistency; can involve extraocular muscle sheath	Calcification can be detected on ultrasound or CT	Composed of mature compact bone and connective tissue
Complex choristoma	Pedunculated mass which protrudes through palpebral fissure; color varies with tissue composition	Varies with tissue composition as described above	Presence of tissue elements of more than one germ layer, usually ectoderm and mesoderm

(ASOCT: anterior segment optical coherence tomography; CT: computed tomography)

 4. Phakomatoses: Discuss the definition, types, and ocular manifestations.

Definition

"A group of independent clinical syndromes characterized by multiple tumors or tumor-like lesions, some of which are or can become malignant and arise in disparate organs of the body, including the eye in a substantial proportion of patients."

Types (Table 7)

- Neurofibromatosis 1 (von Recklinghausen disease) and 2
- Von Hippel–Lindau disease
- Tuberous sclerosis (Bourneville disease)
- Sturge–Weber syndrome
- Wyburn–Mason syndrome
- *Others:* Louis–Bar syndrome (ataxia telangiectasia), Weskamp–Cotlier syndrome (retinal-neuro-cutaneous cavernous hemangioma syndrome), phakomatosis pigmentovascularis.

 5. What are the diagnostic criteria for neurofibromatosis (NF)? Describe the ocular features of neurofibromatosis types 1 and 2.

The diagnostic criteria of neurofibromatosis types 1 and 2 are shown in **Flowcharts 4 and 5**.

Ocular features of neurofibromatosis types 1 and 2 (refer to Question 6, Table 7).

 6. Discuss the management of ocular manifestations of neurofibromatosis.

The management of ocular manifestations of neurofibromatosis is shown in **Flowchart 6**.

TABLE 7: Features of common phakomatoses and their management.

Type	Inheritance	Ocular manifestations	Systemic manifestation	Management
Neurofibromatosis 1 (von Recklinghausen disease)	Autosomal dominant	Lisch nodules of the iris, subcutaneous pedunculated and plexiform neurofibromas of the eyelids, optic nerve gliomas, multifocal choroidal nevi	Café-au-lait spots, axillary and inguinal freckling, cutaneous neurofibromas, neurofibromas or other solid neoplasms of the central nervous system (CNS)	Systemic assessment; debulking of eyelid neurofibromas (refer to Question 9); optic nerve gliomas can be observed or may need surgery/chemotherapy/radiotherapy (refer to Question 8)
Neurofibromatosis 2	Autosomal dominant	Posterior subcapsular cataracts, cortical lens opacities, combined hamartomas of retina; less common: Lisch nodules of the iris, eyelid neurofibromas, and optic nerve gliomas	Bilateral vestibular schwannomas (acoustic neuromas), neurofibromas, meningiomas, gliomas, and schwannomas	
Von Hippel–Lindau disease	Autosomal dominant	Characteristic lesion, retinal hemangioblastoma is a well-reddish spherical lesion with feeding arteriole and draining venule, which may be dilated and tortuous. Intraretinal and subretinal exudation, exudative retinal detachment can be seen	Hemangioblastomas of brain and spinal cord; cysts of pancreas, kidney, and ovaries; other tumors: Renal cell carcinoma, pheochromocytoma, islet cell carcinoma, or cystadenoma of the pancreas	Ocular lesions can be treated with laser photocoagulation. Systemic assessment for tumors and cysts—treatment as indicated
Tuberous sclerosis	Autosomal dominant	Typical lesion is retinal astrocytoma or astrocytic hamartoma: Opaque white superficial retinal lesions which may be partially calcified and mulberry-like	Adenoma sebaceum, ash leaf spots, shagreen patches, subungual angiofibromas; tumors of heart, kidney, lungs, thyroid, and viscera	Periodic systemic monitoring. Observation for retinal lesions
Sturge–Weber syndrome	Sporadic	Navus flammeus—mostly unilateral legend; a long distribution of V1 and V2 branches of trigeminal nerve; diffuse choroidal hemangioma; glaucoma due to raised episcleral venous pressure	Leptomeningeal hemangiomatosis, seizures, and mental retardation	Treatment indicated for threatened vision: Photodynamic therapy (PDT) or radiation
Wyburn–Mason syndrome	Sporadic	Complex retinal arteriovenous malformations (AVMs)	Orbital, periorbital complex, ipsilateral midbrain AVM	Observe for retinal lesions. Cranial AVMs treated by resection embolization or irradiation

Flowchart 4: Diagnostic criteria: Neurofibromatosis (NF) type 1.

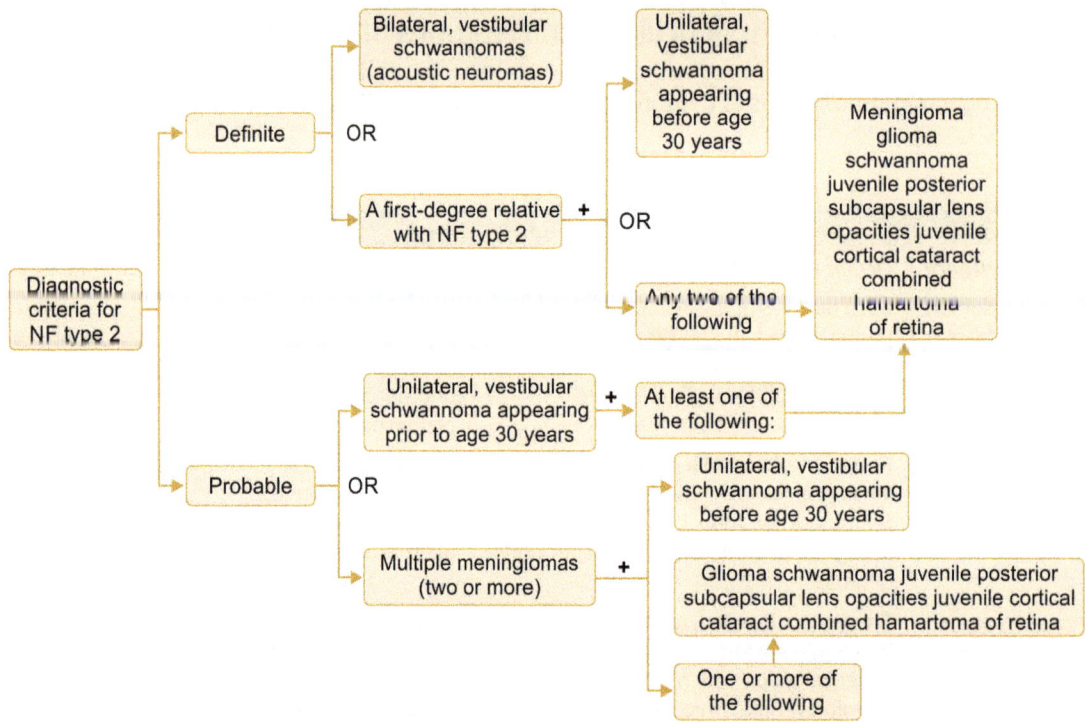

Flowchart 5: Diagnostic criteria for neurofibromatosis (NF) type 2.

Management of Eyelid Neurofibroma

Eyelid neurofibroma is also known as molluscum fibrosum or Quasimodo's tumor.

Eyelid neurofibromas can be:
- Plexiform [orbito-palpebral plexiform neurofibroma (OPPN)] or localized (can be treated by simple excision biopsy as they are well defined)
- Multifocal or solitary

Important surgical considerations for OPPN:
Dr J Conley states*:* "All results (of surgery in neurofibromatosis) are compromised by the very nature of the tumor, its *diffuse position*, its *widespread* involvement of *all the constituents of the region* or organ, and its *tendency to recur*."

Indication for surgery, timing, and possible need for multiple procedures should be carefully considered. Head, neck, and facial tumors have *twice the chance of recurrence* as compared to tumors in extremities.

Flowchart 6: Management of ocular manifestations of neurofibromatosis.

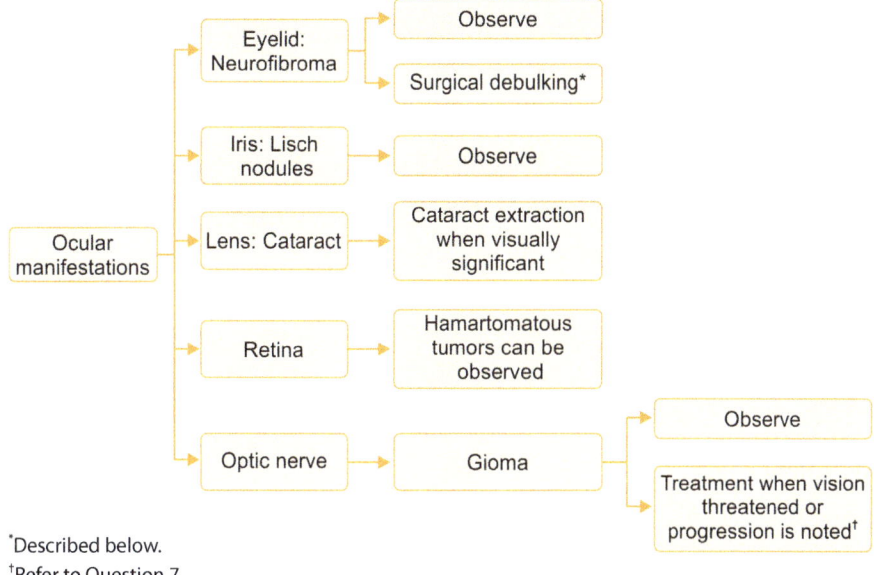

*Described below.
†Refer to Question 7.

Assessment of tissues involved:

Lee et al.	Jackson et al.
Brow ptosis	Soft tissue with a seeing eye
Upper lid infiltration with ptosis	Bone involvement with a seeing eye
Lower lid infiltration	Bone involvement with a nonseeing eye
Lateral canthal disinsertion	
Conjunctival infiltration	
Lacrimal gland infiltration	

Goals of surgery:
- Achieve clear visual axis
- Acceptable cosmesis (secondary)

Indications and timing:
Early surgery (<10 years) if there is:
- Risk of amblyopia
- Growth of tumor, likely to affect the orbitofacial development
- Psychosocial concerns

Surgical technique and principles:
- No definite plane of differentiation between the tumor and healthy tissue
- Amount of resection can be planned based on *template technique* based on the normal contralateral eyelid, usually excess skin, orbicularis is removed along with the tumor.
- Pinch technique is an alternate method for removal of excess involved tissue.
- Hemostasis can be difficult, which can be achieved with:
- Judicious use of cautery
- Use of CO_2 laser
- Hemostatic multiple figure-of-eight sutures in deeper planes
- Sequential multilayered hemostatic sutures cause collapse of the vessels by mechanical ligation and allow debulking in layers for larger tumors.
- Interrupted closure

- Additional procedures may be needed as appropriate:
- Full-thickness reduction by wedge resection
- Lateral canthopexy/canthoplasty
- Medial transnasal canthopexy in some cases
- Concerns of relapse or recurrence should always be emphasized.

 7. Discuss optic nerve glioma.

Optic pathways gliomas can involve the optic nerve, chiasm, or midbrain.

They arise from supporting astrocytes of the optic nerve. Histologically, most are benign pilocytic astrocytomas.

Clinical Features

- Can be asymptomatic
- Vision loss
- Optic disc edema and atrophy
- Proptosis
- Nystagmus
- Signs of raised intracranial tension.

Investigations

- *CT:* Well-defined intraconal mass which cannot be made or separated from the optic nerve or appears as a fusiform enlargement of the optic nerve. Posterior extension to chiasm and midbrain to be looked for.
- *MRI:* Hypo- to isointense on T1 and variable intensity on T2 with variable gadolinium enhancement.

Management

- Ocular and systemic evaluation to look for signs of neurofibromatosis
- Serial monitoring including clinical examination and imaging to note for progression
- If vision is stable, tumors can be observed.
- When vision loss, progression, or posterior extension is noted, chemotherapy or radiotherapy should be instituted to arrest disease progression.
- Chemotherapy is preferred in younger patients than radiation to avoid radiation-induced side effects (secondary tumors, radiation necrosis, Moyamoya disease).
- Prognosis depends on the location and optic nerve glioma has better prognosis.
- Resection is reserved for tumors confined to the optic nerve in eyes with no visual potential and disfiguring proptosis.

 8. Transfrontal orbitotomy: Discuss the procedure and indications.

Described by Naffziger

Indications

- Bilateral orbital decompression
- Orbital neurofibroma or meningioma with intracranial extension
- Intraconal or lateral posterior orbital tumors near optic foramen (since the structure beyond the superior orbital fissure cannot be approached by a lateral orbitotomy)
- Large schwannomas and optic nerve tumors.

Technique

Surgical steps are outlined below:

- Eyelids apposed after placing lubricating ointment
- Skin incision over the scalp down to the pericranium **(Fig. 3)** [extending from one ear to other in bilateral cases (Soutter scalp incision) and only till midline in unilateral cases]

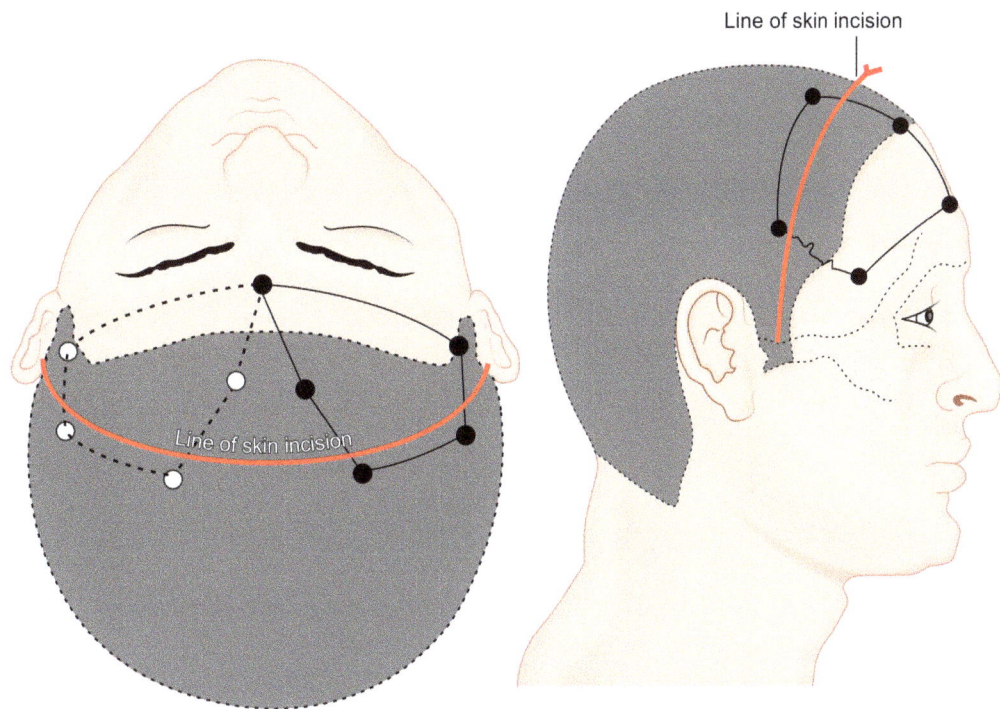

Fig. 3: Line of skin incision and bone flap used.

- Layers of scalp reflected
- Hemostatic sutures can be placed in multiple sites on either side.
- Quadrilateral bone flap created hinged at the temporal fossa **(Fig. 3)**. Alternatively, triangular flaps of bone may be raised. Flap is reflected away from the orbit.
- Dura is "peeled back" from the orbital roof.
- Bone removal performed as appropriate (limited for tumor removal, greater for decompression)
- Deep lateral wall removed
- Periorbital should not be damaged unless opening is mandated
- Biopsy taken when indicated
- Hemostasis should be meticulous.
- On closure, orbital content remains in contact with dura.
- Bone flaps replaced and positioned in place
- Scalp closure in layers
- Placement of a drain hinders formation of hematoma and is usually removed on second or third postoperative day.

Postoperative care:
- Hemorrhage is a dreaded complication and should be watched out for.
- In case of active bleeding, exploration and bipolar cauterization of vessels may be needed under careful visualization.
- Diplopia and ptosis (from levator injury) may be transient.
- Vision loss is a rare complication but can be irreversible.

Transfrontal orbitotomy has several disadvantages:
- Reported higher mortality
- Poorer localization of tumors
- Inadvertent trauma to frontal lobe
- Eventful postoperative course
- Ptosis and superior rectus weakness
- Cerebrospinal fluid (CSF) rhinorrhea and meningitis.

9. Discuss the different approaches of orbitotomy.

Each approach has its own set of advantages and disadvantages **(Tables 8 and 9)**. Primary considerations for choice of approach include the location, size, type of lesion, and diagnostic or therapeutic nature of intervention **(Figs. 4A to C)**.

TABLE 8: Comprehensive list of approaches to orbit.

Incision/approach	Described by/named after
Superior	
Sub-brow*	Benedict
Upper lid crease*	Harris
Vertical lid split*	Byron Smith
Transfrontal	Naffziger
Supraorbital	Maus and Goldman
Coronal	Stewart
Inferior	
Subciliary	Converse
Transconjunctival*	Bougert, later popularized by Tessier
Transconjunctival + lateral canthotomy (swinging eyelid)*	Tessier and Converse
Infraorbital	–
Transantral	Caldwell Luc
Lateral	
Lateral orbital (parallel to lateral orbital rim)	Classical Krönlein
Lateral canthal	Berke–Reese/Berke–Krönlein/modified by Krönlein
Superolateral hybrid orbital	Karagjozov
Medial	
Medial cutaneous (linear)	Lynch
Medial cutaneous (curved)	Gullwing
Transcaruncular*	Goldberg
Medial transconjunctival [limbal (anteromedial micro-orbitotomy)]	von Noorden
Transethmoidal	Patterson

*Commonly used approaches.

TABLE 9: Commonly used approaches and their indications, advantages, and disadvantages.

Approach	Visualization	Indications	Advantages	Disadvantages
Lateral	• Lateral, superior, and inferior intraconal compartments • Part of orbital apex	• Lacrimal gland lesions and lesions lateral to optic nerve • Decompression of deep lateral wall	Wide exposure to lateral orbit. Can be increased with removal of bony wall	Apical lesions and those with intracranial extension may be difficult
Superior	Superior and superonasal orbit	Superior orbital lesions: Schwannoma, tumors involving levator, superior rectus	Variable exposure based on approach; eyelid split offers excellent exposure	Paresthesia of forehead
Medial	• Medial orbital compartment • Medial aspect of orbital apex	• Medial extraconal or intraconal lesions • Optic nerve sheath fenestration • Medial decompression • Fracture repair of medial wall	No visible scar	• Limited exposure • Risk of cerebrospinal fluid (CSF) leak
Inferior	Inferomedial and lateral intraconal compartments	• Floor fracture • Floor decompression • Inferior orbital tumors, inferolateral extraconal tumors	• No visible scar in transconjunctival incisions • Allow access to maxillary sinus	• Lower eyelid retraction and scarring in subciliary approach • Infraorbital anesthesia

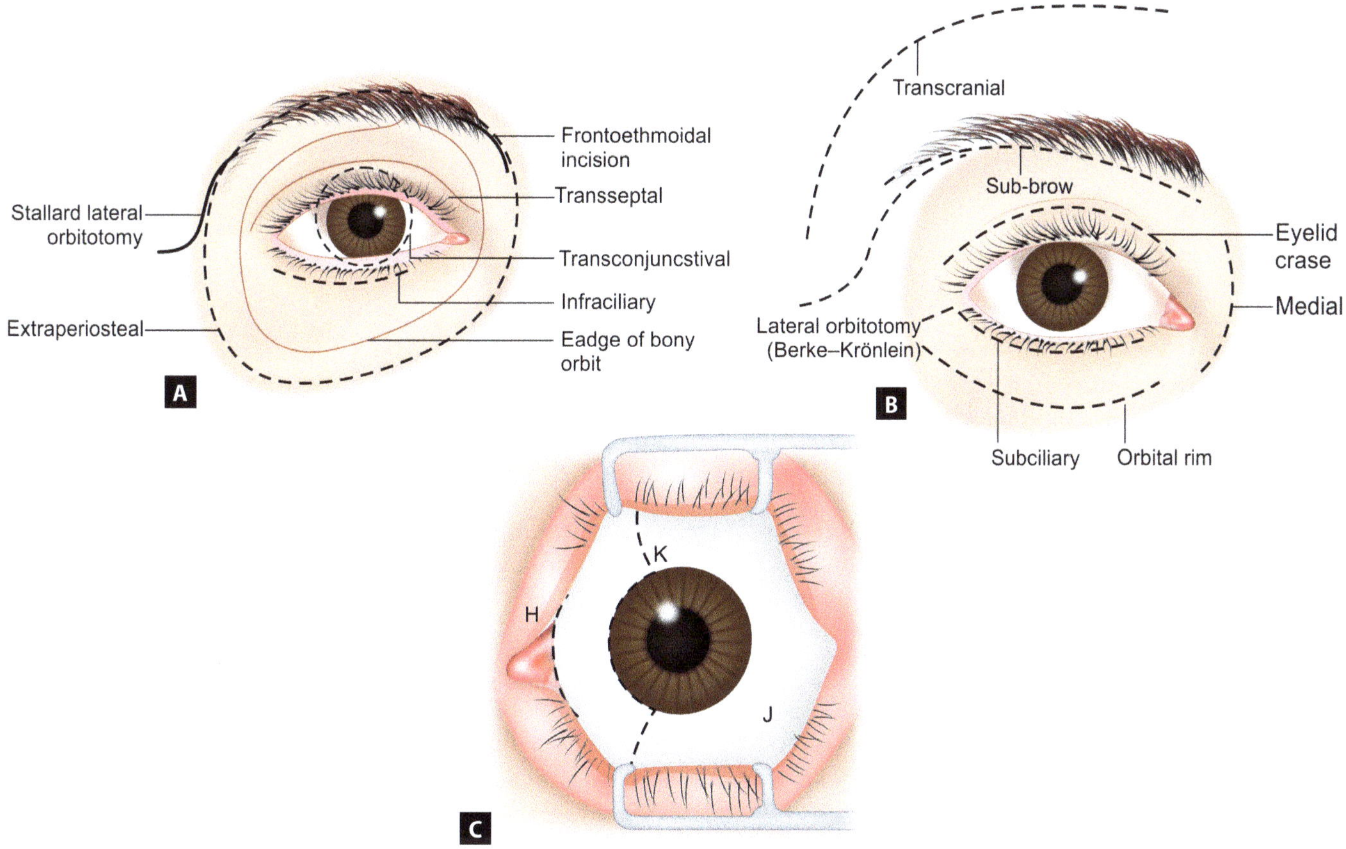

Figs. 4A to C: Incisions for orbitotomy. (J: swinging eyelid; K: medial transconjunctival; H: transcaruncular)

Based on location, space-occupying lesions of the orbit can be broadly divided into:
- *Intraconal lesions:* Cavernous hemangioma
- *Extraconal lesions:* Capillary hemangioma, dermoid cyst, neurofibroma, schwannoma, rhabdomyosarcoma, mucocele
- *Transcompartmental:* Lymphangioma
- *Optic nerve lesions:* Optic nerve glioma, meningioma, NSOID, orbital retinoblastoma
- *Lacrimal gland lesions:* Pleomorphic adenoma, adenoid cystic carcinoma
- *Extraorbital lesions extending into the orbit:* Sino-orbital mycosis, carcinoma of paranasal sinus with orbital invasion, primitive neuroectodermal tumors.

 10. Discuss the differential diagnosis of unilateral axial proptosis. Also, discuss the clinical features, histopathology, and management of cavernous hemangioma.

Axial proptosis results from diffuse orbital involvement or from space-occupying lesions within the intraconal space **(Tables 10 and 11)**.

TABLE 10: Causes of unilateral axial proptosis (Figs. 5A to H).

Vascular	Endocrine	Inflammatory/infectious	Neoplastic
• Carotico-cavernous fistula • Retrobulbar hemorrhage • Arteriovenous malformations • Varix	• Thyroid eye disease	• Myositis • Nonspecific orbital inflammatory disease (NSOID) • Orbital cellulitis • Intraconal abscess	• Cavernous hemangioma • Orbital retinoblastoma

TABLE 11: Causes of abaxial proptosis.			
Downward displacement	**Upward displacement**	**Medial displacement**	**Lateral displacement**
• Fibrous dysplasia • Frontal mucocele • Lymphoma • Neuroblastoma • Neurofibroma • Schwannoma • Subperiosteal hematoma	• Lacrimal sac tumors • Lymphoma • Maxillary sinus tumor	• Lacrimal fossa tumors • Sphenoid wing meningioma	• Ethmoid mucocele • Lacrimal sac tumors • Nasopharyngeal tumors • Rhabdomyosarcoma

CAVERNOUS HEMANGIOMA

- Most common benign orbital tumor in adults.
- Usually intraconal in location but can be extraconal, or rarely within lacrimal gland or intraosseous.

Clinical Features

- Manifests usually in adult between 40 and 60 years of age.
- Can be seen with Maffucci syndrome or blue rubber bleb nevus syndrome.
- Symptoms and signs depend on location of lesion.
- Most common symptom is painless progressive proptosis.
- Inflammation is typically absent.
- Proptosis or globe dystopia
- Visual acuity is usually normal but induced hyperopia, choroidal folds, or rarely optic nerve compression can compromise vision.
- Tumors are mostly unilateral but bilateral and multiple tumors can be seen in syndromic cases.

Management

Investigations

Ultrasonography: Sharply well-defined lesion with moderate acoustic echoes

Computed tomography: Well-circumscribed round to ovoid mass

Magnetic resonance imaging: Isointense on T1 and hyperintense on T2 with progressive enhancement with contrast due to pooling of contrast within the cavernous spaces within the lesion

Differential diagnoses include schwannoma and solitary fibrous tumor

Treatment

Posteriorly located asymptomatic lesions can be observed.

Excision biopsy is preferred for larger lesions by a cutaneous or transconjunctival approach depending on the location of tumor.

Assistance with a cryoprobe enables complete excision of tumor in to.

Intralesional sclerotherapy and propranolol administration have also been described.

Pathology of Cavernous Hemangioma

Gross Examination

- Purplish round to ovoid tumor with spongy feel
- Cut surface shows large vascular channels.

Microscopic Examination (Histopathology)

- Congested vascular channels
- Thin fibrous septae
- Flattened endothelium
- Occasional smooth muscle in the vessel walls

11. Discuss nonneoplastic vascular abnormalities (vascular lesions of the orbit).

Vascular anomalies of the orbit can occur in isolation as a part of congenital syndromes such as Sturge–Weber syndrome, Osler-Weber-Rendu disease, Klippel-Trénaunay syndrome, Wyburn-Mason syndrome, and blue rubber bleb nevus syndrome **(Table 12)**.

Though an anomaly of vascular development, they usually manifest later in life.

The International Society for the Study of Vascular Anomalies (ISSVA) proposed a more comprehensive classification of vascular anomalies **(Flowchart 7)**.

Principles of management of vascular anomalies:
- Lymphatic malformations can be microcystic (amenable to doxycycline, surgery) and macrocystic (more amenable to sclerotherapy: Bleomycin, sodium tetradecyl sulfate, picibanil)
- *Venous malformations:* Amenable to sclerosant therapy and surgical excision with intraluminal glue application
- Arteriovenous malformations embolization by balloons or platinum coils.

TABLE 12: The Orbital Society's hemodynamic classification and features.

	No flow (type 1)	Low flow (type 2)	High flow (type 3)
Pathology	• Lymphatic or combined lymphatic and venous malformations • Isolated from systemic circulation	Nondistensible venous, distensible venous, and distensible combined venous and lymphatic malformations	• Arteriovenous malformations • Detectable arterial flow
Clinical presentation	• Progressive proptosis • Can increase with respiratory infections • Spontaneous orbital hemorrhage, infection, ptosis, or strabismus can occur	Proptosis Can have spontaneous hemorrhage and thrombosis	Progressive swelling, proptosis, redness, pain, bruit Spontaneous hemorrhage can occur
Imaging	No venous or arterial flow	• Diffuse contrast enhancement Detectable venous flow • Can show distensibility, bone hypertrophy, or intraosseous extension	Arterial flow through dilated venous channels
Treatment	• Well-circumscribed lesions: Excision • Ill-defined diffuse lesions: Sclerotherapy (bleomycin) • Debulking	• Surgical excision can be difficult, can be attempted after ligation • Irradiation and electrocoagulation are other options • Sclerosant injection can cause intense inflammation	Endovascular embolization is the preferred technique as primary surgical excision can cause torrential bleeding and exsanguination

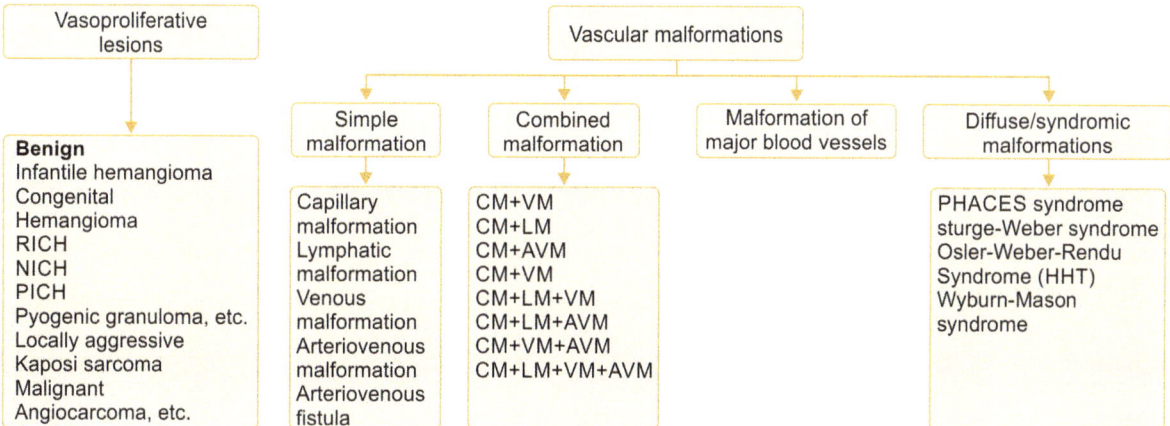

Flowchart 7: International Society for the Study of Vascular Anomalies (ISSVA) classification of ocular anomalies.

(HHT: hereditary hemorrhagic telangiectasia; NICH: noninvoluting congenital hemangioma; PICH: partially involuting congenital hemangioma; RICH: rapidly involuting congenital hemangioma)

12. Define carotid cavernous fistula (CCF).

Definition

An abnormal communication between the arteries and veins within the cavernous sinus (CS) which may be direct or dural (indirect) is known as carotid cavernous fistula.

Types and Etiology

Direct CCF: Direct connection from internal carotid artery (ICA) to CS. It can be due to trauma, rupture of aneurysm of ICA, Ehlers-Danlos Syndrome, or iatrogenic.

Dural CCF: Indirect connection between cavernous arterial branches and CS. Causes include hypertension, fibromuscular dysplasia, and Ehlers-Danlos type IV.

Clinical Features

Carotid cavernous fistula is more marked in direct than dural fistulas and depend on the flow within the fistula (high flow or low flow).

Symptoms:
- Bruit
- Diplopia
- Tearing
- Red eye
- Foreign body sensation
- Blurred vision
- Headache, confusion, aphasia

Signs:
- Congestion
- Cork screwing of conjunctival vessels (arterialization of venules)
- Chemosis
- Limitation of motility
- Bruit
- *Features of raised orbital pressure:* Pulsatile mires on applanation and venous stasis retinopathy
- Retinal vein occlusions
- *Optic neuropathy:* Glaucomatous or nonglaucomatous
- Sixth nerve palsy is most often seen; other cranial nerves (III, IV) may also be affected.

Evaluation

Ultrasound or Doppler can show an enlarged superior ophthalmic vein (SOV).
Computed tomography or MR angiography can identify the enlarged and detailed CS pathology.
    Gold standard: Digital subtraction angiography which identifies the site of fistula

Management

Direct CCF: Endovascular intervention is the treatment preferred; coils, liquid embolic agents, or a combination may be used.

Dural CCFs often resolve spontaneously: They can be managed conservatively in mild cases. Endovascular intervention is indicated if progression is noted.

 13. Define dacryops.

Definition

Dacryops refers to lacrimal ductal cysts of the primary or accessory lacrimal glands **(Flowchart 8)**.

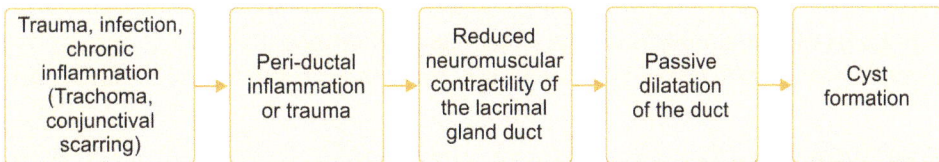

Flowchart 8: Etiopathogenesis of dacryops.

Classification (Bullock)

- Palpebral lobe cysts (simple dacryops)
- Orbital lobe cysts
- Accessory lacrimal gland cysts of Krause and Wolfring
- Ectopic lacrimal gland cysts

Clinical Features (Table 13)

Symptoms: Painless mass or translucent cyst, mechanical ptosis, and foreign body sensation.

Differential Diagnosis

- Tumors
- Foreign body granulomas
- Sarcoidosis
- Tuberculosis
- Dermoid or epidermoid cysts
- Other cystic lesions: Inclusion cyst, lymphatic cysts

Investigations

Ultrasound: Single-walled cyst with low internal echoes

Computed tomography: Well-defined cystic lesion with fluid densities and normal address in bone

Magnetic resonance imaging: Helps identify an ectopic lacrimal gland cyst

Management

- Can be observed if small
- If symptomatic, surgery is the primary modality of treatment.
- Complete excision is preferred over incomplete excision or aspiration to avoid recurrence.
- Depending on the location, conjunctival or cutaneous approaches may be chosen.
- Achieving in excision of intact cyst is preferred to avoid recurrence.

TABLE 13: Clinical features of dacryops based on location.

Type	Signs
Palpebral lobe cysts (simple dacryops)	• Variable sized nontender bluish gray cyst in superotemporal quadrant • Inflammatory signs can be present in presence of infection
Orbital lobe cysts	*Present with mass effect:* Proptosis, eyelid edema, globe dystopia
Accessory lacrimal gland cysts of Krause and Wolfring	• Cyst arising from Krause glands involved superior–inferior fornices • Wolfring gland dacryops occur over upper border of tarsus and can cause ptosis from levator disinsertion or mechanical effect
Ectopic lacrimal gland cysts	Can occur in the caruncle, bulbar conjunctiva, eyelids, or within the orbit. Inflammation, proptosis, ptosis, limitation of ocular motility, and vision loss can result

Complications

Infection is rare and presents with inflammation mimicking orbital cellulitis or abscess.

Computed tomography scan or MRI can help delineate the lesion and excision biopsy confirms the diagnosis.

 14. Discuss mucocele.

The etiopathogenesis of mucocele is shown in **Flowchart 9**.

Causes of obstruction of sinus ostium include fractures, sinonasal surgery, osteomas, polyps, and congenital anomalies.

Clinical Features (Table 14)

Mucocele commonly occurs in adults and can present early in children with cystic fibrosis.

Ocular and orbital symptoms arise when the mucocele extends into the orbit. Symptoms depend on the sinus involved.

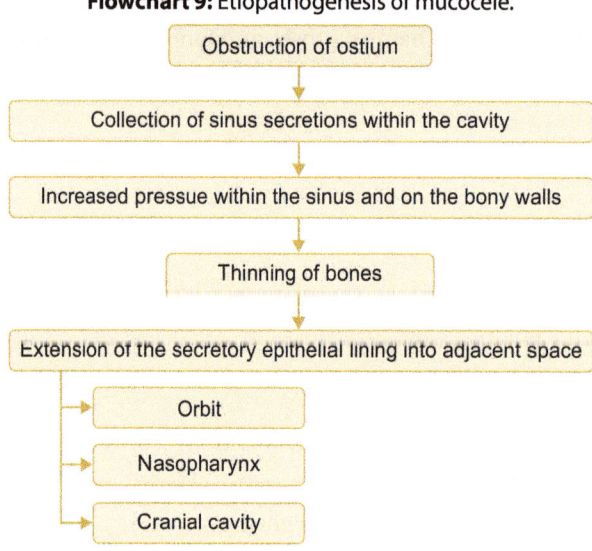

Flowchart 9: Etiopathogenesis of mucocele.

TABLE 14: Clinical features of mucocele.

Frontoethmoidal mucocele	Maxillary mucocele	Sphenoid and posterior ethmoidal mucocele
• Inferior or inferolateral globe dystopia • Proptosis • Hypertelorism (more common with bilateral mucoceles) • Epiphora	• Proptosis • Sometimes enophthalmos due to erosion of orbital floor	• Proptosis • Vision loss

Diagnosis

Computed tomography scan orbits and peripheral nervous system (PNS): Well-defined isodense homogenous mass with epicenter within any of the sinuses. Thinning and displacement of bony walls may be seen with extension into the orbit, brain, or nasopharynx.

Treatment of Mucocele

The management of mucocele is shown in **Flowchart 10**.

Globe dystopia and proptosis usually improve with surgical correction.

Flowchart 10: Management of mucocele.

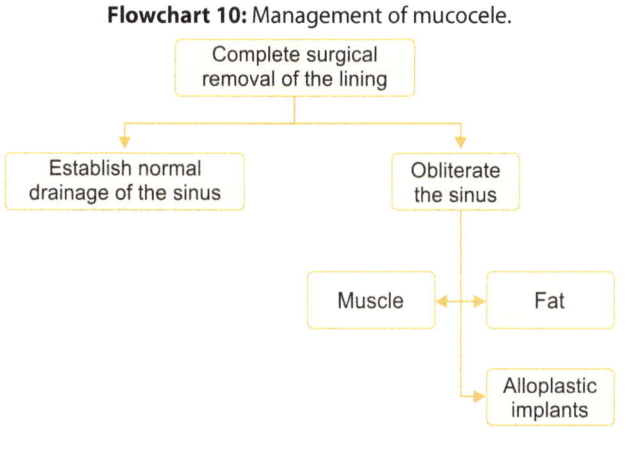

TABLE 15: Types of encephalocele.

Term	Location
Occipital	Occiput
Encephalocele of cranial vault	• Interfrontal • Anterior fontanelle • Interparietal • Posterior fontanelle • Temporal
Frontoethmoidal	• *Nasal* • *Naso-orbital** • *Nasoethomidal*
Basal	• Transethmoidal • Sphenoethmoidal • Transsphenoidal • Frontosphenoidal/spheno-orbital

*Subgroup with ophthalmic manifestations.

 15. Define encephalocele. Mention the types, evaluation, and principles of its management.

Definition

Cephalocele refers to herniation of intracranial contents through a defect in the skull and depending on the contents, they are termed meningocele, meningoencephalocele, encephalocele, or ventriculocele **(Table 15)**.

Clinical Features

Naso-orbital encephaloceles:
- Proptosis
- Globe dystopia is usually lateral as the encephaloceles usually occupy from the medial aspect of the orbit through a defect in the lacrimal and ethmoidal bones.
- Sometimes, the lesion may result from dysplastic orbital roof and cause inferior globe dystopia.
Occipital encephaloceles may affect visual function.

Evaluation

Neurological Examination
- Associated systemic anomalies to be looked for are dextrocardia, pulmonary hypoplasia and laryngomalacia, renal agenesis, and myelomeningocele.
- Arhinencephaly and anophthalmia in anterior encephaloceles
- Neurologic examination is of utmost importance.

Magnetic resonance imaging: To visualize the amount of brain structures herniated

Computed tomography: To assess bony defects

Angiography: To exclude the presence of major vessels in herniated contents

Differential Diagnosis

These lesions need to be distinguished from nasal glioma, nasal polyp, and dermoid cyst and can also present as a medial canthal mass.

Treatment

- *Frontoethmoidal encephaloceles* can be operated electively and in the presence of hydrocephalus.
- *Basic principles of surgery*

- Removal of unnecessary herniated contents into the sac
- Watertight closure of the dura
- Repair of bone defect
- Closure of skin
- Acceptable cosmesis
- Avoid further damage to the sac which can precipitate infection and herniation.
- Hydrocephalus when present can be addressed in same sitting.

Suggested Reading

1. Abdolrahimzadeh B, Piraino DC, Albanese G, Cruciani F, Rahimi S. Neurofibromatosis: an update of ophthalmic characteristics and applications of optical coherence tomography. Clin Ophthalmol. 2016;10:851-60.
2. Abou-Al-Shaar H, Krisht KM, Cohen MA, Abunimer AM, Neil JA, Karsy M, et al. Cranio-orbital and orbitocranial approaches to orbital and intracranial disease: eye-opening approaches for neurosurgeons. Front Surg. 2020;7:1.
3. Albert DM, Miller J, Azar DT, Young LH (Eds). Albert & Jakobiec's Principles and Practice of Ophthalmology. Philadelphia: Saunders/Elsevier; 2008.
4. Alvarez H, Orning J, Castillo M. Orbital vascular lesions: a review of clinical and imaging findings. Exp Rev Ophthalmol. 2013; 8(2):151-66.
5. Andrew NH, Coupland SE, Pirbhai A, Selva D. Lymphoid hyperplasia of the orbit and ocular adnexa: a clinical pathologic review. Surv Ophthalmol. 2016;61(6):778-90.
6. Avery RA. Orbital/periorbital plexiform neurofibromas in children with neurofibromatosis type 1: multidisciplinary recommendations for care. Ophthalmology. 2017;124(1):123-32.
7. Bicer T, Soylemez H. Epibulbar osseous choristoma. Case Rep Ophthalmol Med. 2014;2014:292619.
8. Binning MJ, Liu JK, Kestle JRW, Brockmeyer DL, Walker ML. Optic pathway gliomas: a review. Neurosurg Focus. 2007;23(5):E2.
9. Biswas A. Eyelid Tumours: Clinical Evaluation and Reconstruction Techniques. Berlin: Springer; 2014.
10. Calandriello L, Grimaldi G, Petrone G, Rigante M, Petroni S, Riso M, et al. Cavernous venous malformation (cavernous hemangioma) of the orbit: current concepts and a review of the literature. Surv Ophthalmol. 2017;62(4):393-403.
11. Cauduro RS, Ferraz Cdo A, Morales MS, Garcia PN, Lopes YC, Souza PH, et al. Application of anterior segment optical coherence tomography in pediatric ophthalmology. J Ophthalmol. 2012;2012:313120.
12. Chaudhry IA, Elkhamry SM, Al-Rashed W, Bosley TM. Carotid cavernous fistula: ophthalmological implications. Middle East Afr J Ophthalmol. 2009;16(2):57-63.
13. Delfini R, Missori P, Iannetti G, Ciappetta G, Cantore G. Mucoceles of the paranasal sinuses with intracranial and intraorbital extension: report of 28 cases. Neurosurgery. 1993;32:901-6.
14. Esmaeli B. Ophthalmic Oncology. New York, Dordrecht, Heidelberg, London: Springer; 2011.
15. Galindo-Ferreiro A, Alkatan HM, Muinos-Diaz Y, Akaishi PM, Galvez-Ruiz A, Cruz AV. Accessory lacrimal gland duct cyst: 23 years of experience in the Saudi population. Ann Saudi Med. 2015;35(5):394-9.
16. Gorlin RJ, Goltz RW. Multiple nevoid basal-cell epithelioma, jaw cysts and bifid rib. A syndrome. N Engl J Med. 1960;262:908-12.
17. Grossniklaus HE, Eberhart CG, Kivela TT (Eds). WHO Classification of Tumors of the Eye, 4th edition. Lyon: IARC; 2018.
18. Henderson AD, Miller NR. Carotid-cavernous fistula: current concepts in aetiology, investigation, and management. Eye (Lond). 2018; 32(2):164-72.
19. Kalangu KKN. Management of encephaloceles. In: Sindou M (Ed). Practical Handbook of Neurosurgery. Vienna: Springer; 2009.
20. Katowitz JA, Katowitz WR. Pediatric oculoplastic surgery, 2nd edition. New York: Springer; 2017.
21. *Klippel-Feil syndrome. Genetics Home Reference. US National Library of Medicine.* [online] Available from https://ghr.nlm.nih.gov/condition/klippel-feil-syndrome. [Last accessed April, 2023].
22. Kurup SP, Lissner GS. Characterization of dacryops infections. Ophthalmic Plast Reconstr Surg. 2015;31(1):58-62.
23. Lee AG. Neuroophthalmological management of optic pathway gliomas. Neurosurg Focus. 2007;23(5):E1.
24. Mauriello JA, Flanagan JC. Surgical approaches to the orbit. In: Mauriello JA, Flanagan JC (Eds). Management of Orbital and Ocular Adnexal Tumors and Inflammations. Berlin: Springer; 1990.
25. Mombaerts I. The many facets of dacryoadenitis. Curr Opin Ophthalmol. 2015;26(5):399-407.
26. Naffziger HC. Exophthalmos; some principles of surgical management from the neurosurgical aspect. Am J Surg. 1948;75(1):25-41.
27. Osguthorpe JD, Saunders RA, Adkins WY. Evaluation of and access to posterior orbital tumors. Laryngoscope. 1983;93(6):766-71.
28. Perry JD, Singh AD. Clinical Ophthalmic Oncology: Orbital Tumors, 2nd edition. Berlin: Springer-Verlag; 2014.
29. Shields JA, Shields CL, Eagle Jr RC, Arevalo F, De Potter P. Ophthalmic features of the organoid nevus syndrome. Trans Am Ophthalmol Soc. 1996;94:65-86.
30. Shields JA, Shields CL. Eyelid, Conjunctival, and Orbital Tumors, 3rd edition. China: Wolters Kluwer; 2016.
31. Stallard HB. A plea for lateral orbitotomy (Krönlein's operation). Br Med J. 1947;1(4499):408.
32. Sundar G. Vascular lesions of the orbit: conceptual approach and recent advances. Indian J Ophthalmol. 2018;66:3-6.
33. Tanaboonyawat S, Idowu OO, Copperman TS, Vagefi MR, Kersten RC. Dacryops—a review. Orbit. 2020;39(2):128-34.
34. Topilow NJ, Tran AQ, Koo EB, Alabiad CR. Etiologies of proptosis: a review. Intern Med Rev (Wash D C). 2020;6(3).
35. van der Meulen J. Orbital neurofibromatosis. Clin Plast Surg. 1987;14(1):123-35.
36. Yanoff M, Duker JS. Ophthalmology, 4th edition. Amsterdam: Elsevier; 2014.

1.25 Socket

Richa Dharap Wagh, Tarjani Dave

Q 1. Discuss definition, etiology, clinical features, morphologic types, assessment, and management of contracted socket with special notes on anophthalmic socket in a child.

Definition: Contracted socket is *defined as* shrinkage and shortening of all or a part of socket tissues leading to a decrease in depth of fornices and/or orbital volume, ultimately leading to an inability in retaining prosthesis. Simply put, there is inadequate space, with tissue loss.

An ideal anophthalmic socket has the following features **(Figs. 1A to D)**:
- Well-centered appropriately sized orbital implant
- Healthy overlying conjunctival lining
- Adequate depth of fornices
- Socket is able to hold an appropriately sized prosthesis that mimics the appearance of the contralateral eye, being cosmetically pleasing and symmetric.
- Eyelid is in position, symmetric in appearance to the contralateral eye, providing complete eye closure and enabling uniform wetting of the ocular surface and prosthesis.

Etiology

Preoperative	Intraoperative	Postoperative
• Trauma-related eye loss • Mechanical • *Burns:* Chemical, thermal	*Excessive tissue manipulation:* Conjunctiva or Tenon's capsule handling	Poorly fitting prosthesis and long-term use of stock eye
Chronic infection-related eye loss	Inappropriate size of implant	Socket postradiation therapy
Cicatrizing conjunctival disease [e.g., Stevens–Johnson syndrome (SJS), pemphigoid]	Excess use of cautery	Socket infection
Previous socket surgery, predisposing to excessive scarring	Excessive tissue sacrifice	Chronic inflammation
		Frequent handling of prosthesis
		Failure to maintain regular polishing and prosthesis health

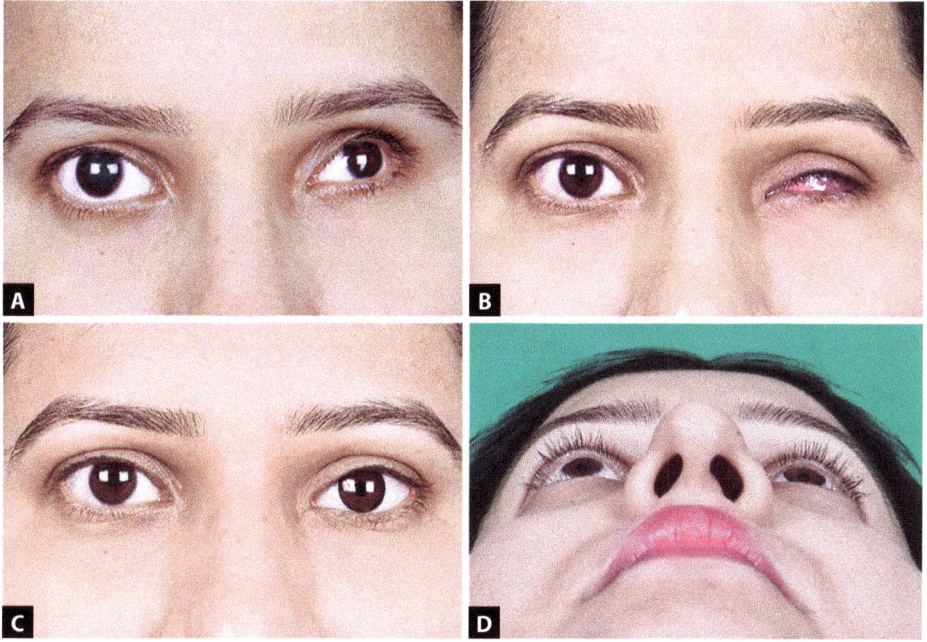

Figs. 1A to D: Ideal anophthalmic socket. (A) Left eye with phthisis bulbi; (B) Following evisceration with a 20 mm implant; (C) Following placement of a custom ocular prosthesis with a good aesthetic outcome; (D) Minimal enophthalmos with the ocular prosthesis.

Clinical Features

Complaints of pain, redness or discharge from socket, ocular discomfort, instability with frequent falling of prosthesis, poor movement of the ocular prosthesis, inability to close the eyes with the prosthesis on, and hollowed out appearance of periorbital tissues. The details of the primary eye removal surgery including indication, date of surgery, implant type, previous eye surgery or history of trauma, and prior radiation therapy should be obtained.

Examination

The examination of any socket consists of three parts as follows (**Figs. 2A to D**):
1. Examination with the prosthesis
2. Examination without the prosthesis
3. Examination of the prosthesis.

Examination with the Prosthesis

It is imperative to perform a preliminary examination with the ocular prosthesis in place. External appearance and facial symmetry, eyelid position and evaluation for ptosis or eyelid malpositions such as entropion, and lower eyelid retraction are performed. Eyelid closure is assessed for any lagophthalmos, and assessment of prosthesis movement is done. In addition, features of postenucleation socket syndrome (PESS), such as enophthalmos, superior sulcus deformity, ptosis or eyelid retraction with relevant measurements, lower eyelid sagging indicating laxity of the lower eyelid, and backward tilt of the ocular prosthesis, are noted. The above examination gives an estimate of the *volume and surface deficit*.

Examination Without the Prosthesis

The prosthesis is then removed. Socket inflammation, discharge from the socket, presence of an implant, and whether the implant is well covered and central are assessed. Next, the socket and the conjunctival fornices are examined carefully for *surface loss*. The socket is gently palpated over a closed eyelid or with a gloved finger to confirm the presence and location of the orbital implant. The degree of movement of the socket is assessed and documented by asking the patient to look in all directions of gaze. Any discharge, bleeding, conjunctival inflammation, implant exposure, granulomas, cysts, adhesion bands, or fornix contracture are noted. Papillae need to be ruled out by everting the upper eyelid. Depth of fornices can be measured using a lens spatula, which is then held over a graduated scale. The quality of socket, whether dry or moist, gives

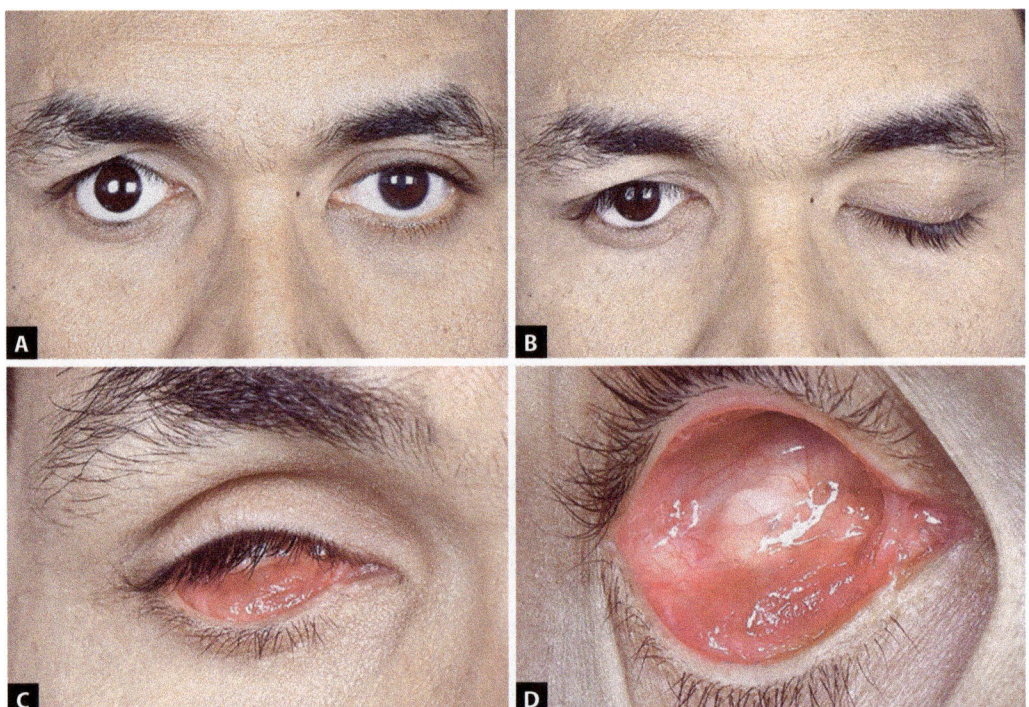

Figs. 2A to D: Examination of a case of contracted socket. (A) Right contracted socket with a prosthesis. There is evidence of superior sulcus deformity and lower eyelid laxity. (B) Right contracted socket with lagophthalmos. (C) Right contracted socket without prosthesis. (D) Right contracted socket with shallow inferior fornix and medial symblepharon.

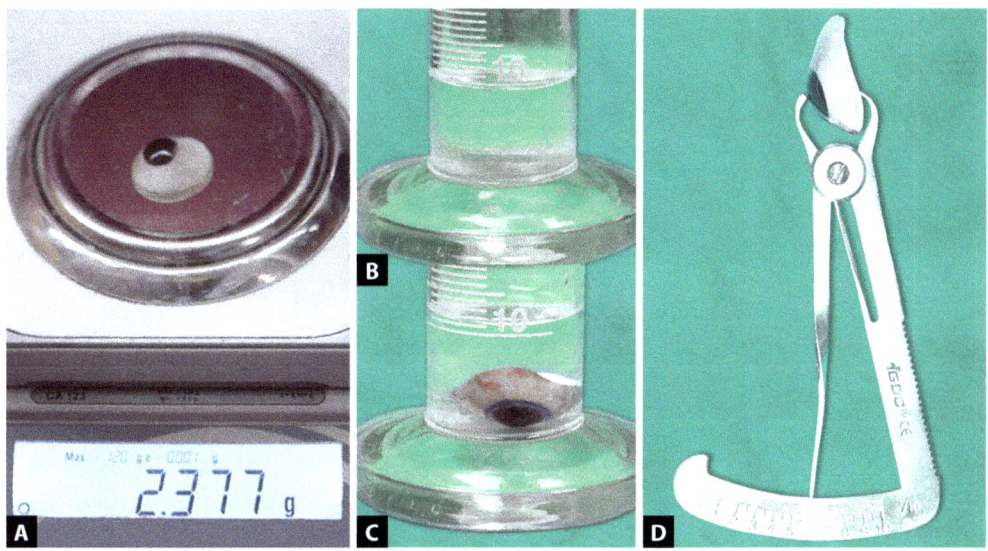

Figs. 3A to D: Examination of the prosthesis. (A) Weight of the prosthesis; (B and C) Volume of the prosthesis being measured with a water column; (D) Thickness of the prosthesis.

a clue to its vascularity and residual viable tissue. Patency of the lacrimal drainage system must be assessed in presence of any watering or discharge.

Examination of the Prosthesis

Its thickness, weight, and volume are documented. It is also examined for scratches, surface irregularities, or deposits **(Figs. 3A to D)**.

Clinical photographs with and without prosthesis in place, including the positive clinical findings, as well as photographic documentation of the prosthesis with its dimensions are good habits to maintain.

Summary of history and examination findings in a case of contracted socket	
History	• Present symptoms • Past history of previous eye removal surgery • Identification of any predisposing factors for contracture from history
Examination	• External examination with prosthesis in place: Volume • Socket examination after removal of prosthesis: Surface • Examination of prosthesis

Classification

There are several classification systems for contracted socket:
- Based on onset
- Based on bony and soft-tissue contracture
- Based on clinical signs of soft-tissue contracture
- Based on surface and volume loss.

Classification Based on Onset (Figs. 4A and B)

Congenital contracted socket	Acquired contracted socket
Congenital contracted socket associated with congenital clinical anophthalmos	Acquired contracted socket following trauma
Congenital contracted socket associated with severe microphthalmos	• Acquired contracted socket following infection • Acquired contracted socket following iatrogenic tissue loss • Acquired contracted socket following cicatrizing conjunctivitis • Acquired contracted socket following poor prosthesis fitting • Acquired contracted socket following radiation

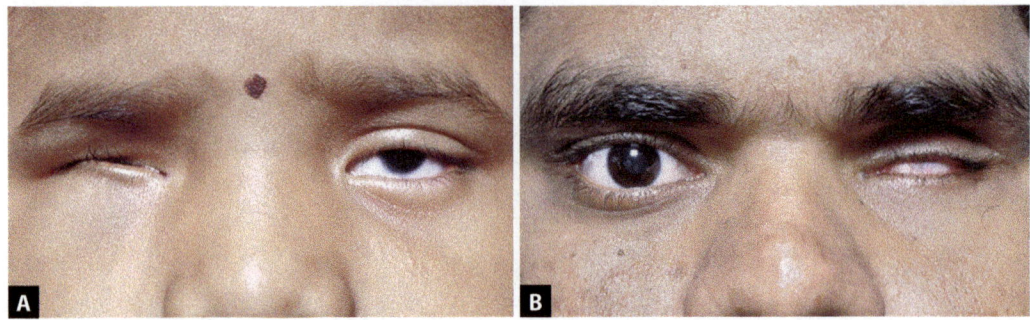

Figs. 4A and B: (A) Congenital contracted socket with right orbitopalpebral cyst and (B) left acquired contracted socket.

Classification Based on Bony and Soft-Tissue Contracture

Soft-tissue contracture	Bony contracture	Combined bony and soft-tissue contracture
• Shelving of lower fornix • Loss of verical fornices • Loss of horizontal fornices • Loss of all fornices	• Micro-orbitism	• Micro-orbitism with varying degrees of contracted socket

Classification Based On Soft-Tissue Contracture (Gopal Krishna classification) into Five Grades as Follows

Grade	Description
0	Socket lined by healthy conjunctiva, having deep well formed fornices
1	Inferior fornix shallowing or shelving, forming a downward slope, pushing lower eyelid down and out, preventing retention of prosthesis (*inferior fornix*)
2	Loss of upper and lower fornices (*vertical fornices*)
3	Loss of upper and lower, medial and lateral fornices (all *four fornices*)
4	Loss of all four fornices with shortening of the horizontal and vertical palpebral apertures (*global loss*)
5	Recurrent contracted socket after repeated attempted socket reconstruction

Note: Mnemonic: IVF Gynec Research.

It is important to note that the above classification outlines only the surface loss.

Classification Based on Surface and Volume Loss

Surface loss	Volume loss	Combined surface and volume loss
• Shelving of lower fornix • Loss of verical fornices • Loss of horizontal fornices • Loss of all fornices	• Absence of orbital implant • Inadequately sized orbital implant	• Congenital • Acquired

This classification system gives a practical approach to the management of contracted socket.

Management

Goal of treatment: Achieve a healthy socket with fair volume lined by adequate epithelial lining to house an acceptable prosthesis with satisfactory cosmesis.

As we are aware, the first step of any treatment is *primary prevention*. It is important to recognize and avoid any factors that might predispose to formation of contracted socket.

- Meticulous history to identify preexisting risk factors, for example, history of trauma, chemical injury, chronic infections, cicatrizing disease.
- Appropriate surgical steps include careful handling of tissues during dissection, preservation of conjunctiva and Tenon's, tension-free closure over the implant, and avoiding excessive cautery. Mandatory use of conformer post operatively to maintain the surface area. This should be used till it is replaced by permanent prosthesis.
- Fabrication of an appropriately sized prosthesis with smooth edges
- Prosthesis care such as using adequate lubrication to prevent friction
- Prosthesis maintenance: Regular six monthly polishing and five yearly replacement of new prosthesis.

Management of contracted socket can be summarized as follows:

Parameters	Shallow fornix	Surface loss	Volume loss	Management
1	Yes	No	No	Prosthetic management Fornix formation sutures
2	Yes	+ (mild) ++ (moderate) +++ (severe)	No No No	Fornix formation with AMG Fornix formation with MMG Fornix formation with MMG
3	Yes	No	+ (mild) ++ (moderate) +++ (severe)	Hyaluronic acid gel filler injection Autologous fat transfer Autologous fat transfer Porex wedge implant Implant exchange Secondary implant
4	Yes	Yes	Yes	Dermis fat graft Secondary implant + FFS + MMG
5	Yes	Dry	Severe	Orbital prosthesis

(AMG: amniotic membrane graft; FFS: fornix formation suture; MMG: mucous membrane graft)

Adjunctive treatment:

	Correction of surface loss	
Mild	**Moderate**	**Severe**
Intralesional injections: Steroid or 5-FU	Addressing anterior lamellar shortening: Skin grafting	Extensive MMG (labial + buccal mucosal grafting) Wrapped conformer technique
• Addressing eyelid malposition: • Anterior lamellar repositioning • Tarsal fracture	Addressing posterior lamellar shortening: • Tarsal fracture • Retractor recession • Application of spacer • Hard palate and auricular cartilage	Deep socket reconstruction with special conformers
Pressure conformers to deepen fornices	Pressure conformers to deepen fornices	Extensive skin grafting in case of dry sockets
		Oculofacial prosthesis/exenteration prosthesis/osseo-integrated prosthesis

(FU: fluorouracil; MMG: mucous membrane graft)

- *Acquired causes of anophthalmic socket in a child:*
  Acquired anophthalmia in a 3-year-old child could be following eye removal surgery:
  - The most common cause is enucleation for advanced retinoblastoma.
  - Another advanced intraocular tumor in a child could be medulloepithelioma.
  - Enucleation might also have been performed for a painful blind eye following advanced Coats disease or diffuse retinal capillary hemangioma.
  - Evisceration might have been performed following severe trauma to the eye or in advanced buphthalmos with nil visual potential or developmental anomalies such as a large corneal dermoid with disorganized anterior segment or a painful blind eye in a child.
- *Congenital clinical anophthalmos:*
  History should elicit the following points:
  - *Onset of anophthalmia:* Congenital clinical anophthalmos is the term used for the absence of the eyeball since birth. Congenital absence of the eye will cause a small bony orbit, a constricted mucosal socket, short eyelids, and reduced palpebral fissure and malar prominence. Anophthalmia in a 3-year-old child can also be acquired following eye removal surgery such as evisceration and enucleation.
  - *History of possible etiologies for anophthalmic socket:* Genetic mutations, chromosomal abnormalities, and prenatal environment can all cause anophthalmia. Anophthalmia is an extremely rare disease and is mostly rooted in genetic abnormalities. The following genes are commonly implicated:
    - *Role of SOX2:* The commonly associated genetic mutation is in the *SOX2* gene. Sox2 anophthalmia syndrome is an autosomal dominant inheritance, but the majority of patients who suffer from Sox2 anophthalmia are the first in

their family history to have this mutation due to germline mosaicism. Some of these gene mutations will cause the Sox2 protein not to be formed, while other mutations will yield a nonfunctional version of this protein. Without this Sox2 protein, the activity of genes that is important for the development of the eye is disrupted.
- *Role of RBP4 (retinol-binding protein):* The *RBP4* gene has recently been linked to autosomal dominant form of anophthalmia. This form of anophthalmia has variable penetrance and a maternal inheritance such that the disease occurs only when a mother and fetus both carry an RBP4 mutation. This mutation predisposes the fetus to vitamin A deficiency, which in the initial months of pregnancy, when the eye is developing, may lead to anophthalmia. This form of anophthalmia is the first that may be intervened upon with vitamin A supplementation of retinyl esters during the initial months of pregnancy.
- *Environmental influences:* Children who have had gestational-acquired infections, especially toxoplasma, rubella, and influenza infections, may develop anophthalmia. Other environmental factors are maternal vitamin A deficiency, exposure to X-rays during gestation, solvent abuse, and exposure to thalidomide.

- *History of associated syndromes:*
There are several syndromic associations of anophthalmia. These include:
  - *SOX2 and variant genes:* Anophthalmia–esophageal–genital (AEG) syndrome
  - Pituitary abnormalities and OTX2 variants: Although there is no syndromic eponym, defects in OTX2 and variant genes include pituitary anomalies with anophthalmia and microphthalmia.
  - PAX6-associated mutations include eye and brain defects
  - *Retinoic acid synthesis pathway members:* STRA6 and Matthew–Wood syndrome
  - SHH signaling: Curry–Jones syndrome
  - *Genes involved in BMP signaling:* Waardenburg anophthalmia syndrome (WAS)
  - *Genes of the mitochondrial respiratory complex:* Microphthalmia with linear skin defects syndrome (MLS; also known as microphthalmia, dermal aplasia, and sclerocornea or MIDAS) is recognizable due to characteristic manifestations of anophthalmia or microphthalmia, sclerocornea and corneal opacities, and patchy, erythrodermatous skin lesions.
  - Bosma arhinia microphthalmia syndrome and deleterious variant in SMCHD1
  - Gorlin–Chaudhry–Moss syndrome
  - Warburg Micro syndrome, Martsolf syndrome, and RAB18 deficiency
  - Anophthalmia, rhizomelic skeletal dysplasia, and MAB21L2 variants

- History of prior ocular surgeries and conservative management for congenital anophthalmia
  - *When:* Treatment for congenital anophthalmia ideally begins at birth.
  - *Why:* Conformer expansion should be initiated promptly to aid expansion of the horizontal palpebral fissures (HPF) and the fornices.
  - *How:* Conformers act by giving an omnidirectional vector of expansion. This expansion is better achieved with the help of customized conformers that are made by taking an impression of the eye socket. Conformers need to be changed every 3 weeks for adequate expansion. Hydrogel conformers work on the principle of imbibing fluid and expanding two to three times the original size within a short period of time.

Types of conformers:
- *Graduated stem conformers:* These are readily available in standard sizes.
- *Custom conformers:* These are customized to patient's socket.
- *Hydrogel conformers:* These are available in standard sizes with a fixed expansion rate.
- *Three-dimensional (3D) printed conformers:* These are fabricated by scanning the patient socket and 3D printing the conformer.
  - History of prior use of ocular prosthesis and its regimen for care of ocular prosthesis
    - *Evaluation of congenital anophthalmia in a 3-year-old child:* The evaluation should include assessment of the HPF, the fornix depth, and the socket volume. Presence of an associated orbitopalpebral cysts needs to be evaluated. A high-riding lower eyelid is suggestive of an associated inferior orbitopalpebral cyst. These parameters are measured after every visit of socket expansion. The presence of bony contracture needs to be assessed.
    - *Management of congenital anophthalmia in a 3-year-old child:* The management aims at equalizing the HPF in both eyes in unilateral cases and expanding the socket area and the HPF to normal for age in bilateral cases by conformer expansion followed by orbital volume expansion. Management details are highlighted in **Figures 5 and 6**. Orbital volume expansion can be achieved by enucleation with implant if there is no bony contracture. Alternately, a dermis fat graft or an orbital tissue expander can be placed for orbital volume expansion.

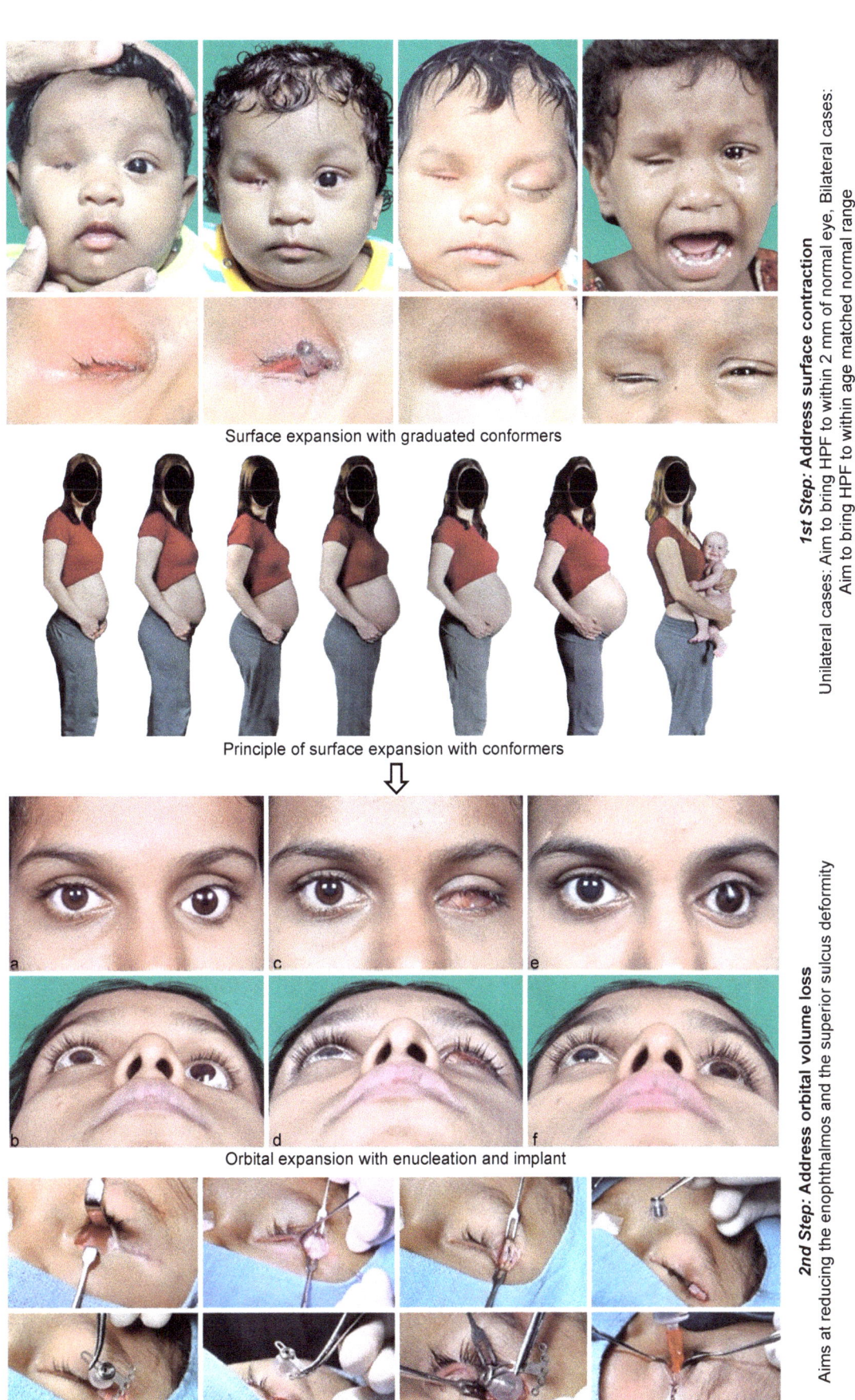

Fig. 5: Management protocol for congenital clinical anophthalmia. (HPF: horizontal palpebral fissure)

Management Protocol: Co-existent orbito-palpebral cyst
It the cyst produces inability to retain conformer, cyst aspiration + sclerotheraphy is performed
(ethanolamine oleate/sodium tetradecyl sulfate)

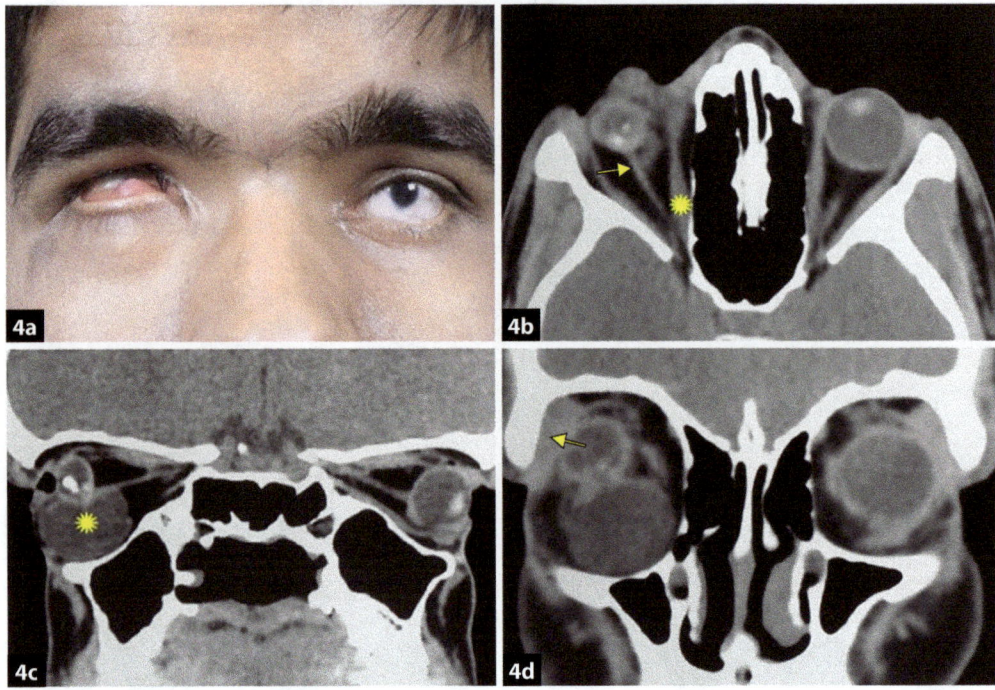

Clincial examination of an orbitopalpebral cyst:
4a: A high riding lower eyelid indicating a cyst
4b: Axial CT: rudimentary eyeball, intact extraocular muscles and optic nerve
4c: Saggital reconstruction CT: inferior orbitopalebral cyst
4d: Coronal CT: orbital volume expansion on right side

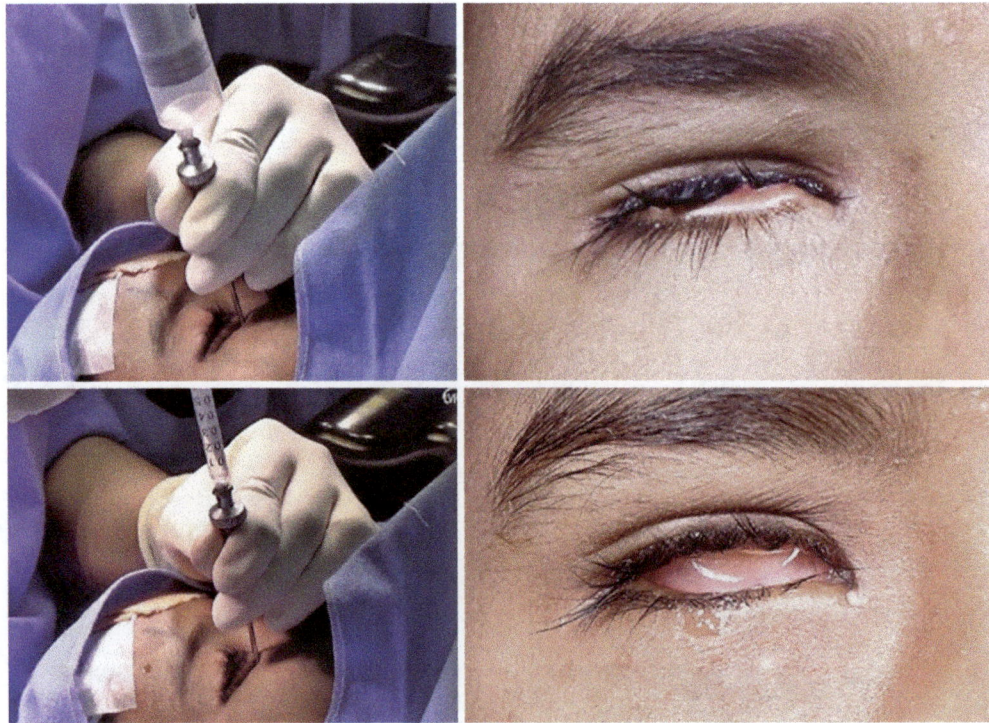

- Cyst aspiration
- Visual potential assessed
- Sclerotherapy performed if no visual potential deemed

- Precyst aspiration
- Postcyst aspiration + Sclerotherapy with central conformer

Fig. 6: Highlights in the management of orbitopalpebral cysts. (CT: computed tomography)

For patients with an associated orbitopalpebral cyst, the cyst aids in orbital expansion and hence should be retained till 2–3 years of age. If the cyst hinders conformer placement, cyst aspiration and sclerotherapy are performed, followed by conformer expansion as discussed above.

Counseling

- Thorough counseling of the patient should be done, explaining the primary problem and the final prognosis.
- Need for multiple surgeries, not only of the socket but also of the eyelid, and need for frequent modification or change of prosthesis with the incurring costs and clinic visits must be emphasized.
- Possibility of suboptimal cosmetic outcome should always be explained.
- Patient must be informed about the need to use other body tissues, such as oral mucosa, for ocular reconstruction.
- Surgical reconstruction should be considered when the eye is quiet.

 2. Discuss indications and techniques of evisceration and enucleation.

Evisceration

Introduction

Evisceration is a surgical technique by which all intraocular contents are removed while preserving the remaining scleral shell, extraocular muscle attachments, and surrounding orbital adnexa. The surgery often includes placement of an implant into the evisceration cavity to maintain the orbital volume.

Indications

- Endophthalmitis
- Penetrating ocular trauma
- Painful blind eye.

Contraindications

- Known or suspected intraocular malignancy
- Phthisis bulbi and microphthalmia (relative).

Surgical Technique

- Careful preoperative evaluation should be performed to ensure that there is no intraocular malignancy in the operative eye when planning an evisceration.
- If there is no view of the posterior pole, B-scan or computed tomography (CT) scan should be used to rule out malignancy.
- Correct laterality of the evisceration must be carefully confirmed prior to initiation of the surgery, and utmost detail must be paid to the surgical checklist.
- Evisceration may be performed under general anesthesia or, in some cases, local anesthesia with intravenous, monitored sedation. Retrobulbar administration of anesthetic with epinephrine is often given to reduce intraoperative bleeding and postoperative pain. The volume of block given should be minimal to avoid a tense orbit that might hinder implant placement.
- The patient is appropriately prepared and draped in a sterile manner and an eyelid speculum is placed.
- Local anesthetic may be injected into the subconjunctival space to demarcate available conjunctiva and Tenon's capsule and aid in hemostasis. Alternatively, several drops of 10% topical phenylephrine can be applied to the ocular surface before the procedure to provide hemostasis.
- A 360° conjunctival peritomy is then made at the limbus. The Tenons capsule is dissected from the sclera using blunt dissection with Steven's scissors in the four oblique quadrants between the recti muscles. This dissection helps in the step of sclerotomies.
- A full-thickness incision is then made at the limbus so that scissors may be introduced to excise the cornea in a circumferential manner.
- All intraocular contents, including uveal tract, crystalline lens, vitreous humor, and retina, are removed. Techniques for removing the intraocular contents include use of a periosteum elevator, evisceration spoon, spatula, or other instruments. These contents are sent for histopathologic examination.

- Hemostasis at the posterior pole and vortex veins may then be achieved with cautery and direct pressure.
- Absolute or 70% alcohol may then be instilled to denature and remove all remaining uveal material and microorganisms from the scleral shell. Care must be taken to keep the alcohol within the sclera and not contact the conjunctiva since alcohol produces severe inflammation.
- The alcohol is washed out with normal saline.
- The next step involves performing sclerotomies to allow placement of an adequately sized implant. A good sized orbital implant helps to decrease the superior sulcus hollowing and anophthalmic ptosis, which ultimately results in a better cosmetic result. This is particularly helpful in globes that are phthisical and would potentially limit the size of an implant if placed within the scleral shell only.
- The techniques of sclerotomy are as described below:

Technique	Description
Two-flap (petal) sclerotomy	The sclera is divided from the limbal end to the optic nerve in two oblique quadrants between the extraocular muscles. This divides the sclera into two flaps both the flaps are disinserted from the optic nerve by a circumferential incision 3 mm from the optic nerve. Each flap is suspended by two recti muscles
Four-flap (petal) sclerotomy	The sclera is divided from the limbal end to the optic nerve in four oblique quadrants between the extraocular muscles. This divides the sclera into four flaps. All the four flaps are disinserted from the optic nerve by a circumferential incision 3 mm from the optic nerve. Each flap is suspended by a rectus muscle
Circumferential equatorial sclerotomy	A circumferential incision is made at the equator of the scleral shell to divide the shell into an anterior and a posterior component. The anterior component allows a tension-free closure
Anterior relaxing sclerotomy	Relaxing anterior sclerotomies can be performed in the oblique quadrants to increase the aperture of the scleral shell through which an implant is inserted
Posterior radial sclerotomy	Radial sclerotomies are initiated in the posterior half of the scleral rims from beyond the vortex veins to the optic nerve. These sclerotomies are performed in the four oblique quadrants
Anterior relaxing with posterior sclerotomies	The abovementioned sclerotomies are performed simultaneously
Evisceration with retained corneal button	The corneal button is retained and a T-shaped incision is made at the limbus with the vertical limb of the T extending posteriorly toward the optic nerve in an oblique quadrant. This incision is used to scoop out the intraocular contents as well as to insert an implant

- Implant material is surgeon dependent and includes spherical implant choices of acrylic, polymethyl methacrylate (PMMA), silicone, hydroxyapatite (HA), porous polyethylene, and aluminum oxide. The implant may be placed directly into the scleral shell or may be first wrapped in donor sclera, mesh, or other materials.
- Closure is performed in three layers, i.e., the sclera, anterior tenons, and conjunctiva. A conformer is placed and a temporary tarsorrhaphy may be performed to help retain the conformer.
- Perioperative antibiotics are often administered and are especially important in cases of evisceration in the setting of endophthalmitis. The duration of antibiotic therapy has been reported to range from 5 days to several weeks, depending on the nature of the infection.
- Postoperative pain can be managed by injection of retrobulbar anesthetic or ethanol prior to patching. A pressure patch is applied and removed after 1 day. The suture tarsorrhaphy is removed after 1 week. The patient may visit an ocularist for prosthesis fitting 6–8 weeks following surgery (**Figs. 7A to L**).

Enucleation

Introduction

Enucleation is the surgical procedure that involves removal of the entire globe and its intraocular contents, with preservation of all other periorbital and orbital structures.

Indications

- Intraocular malignancy or high suspicion for intraocular malignancy (most commonly uveal melanoma and retinoblastoma)
- Trauma
- Blind, painful eye
- Sympathetic ophthalmia
- Microphthalmos.

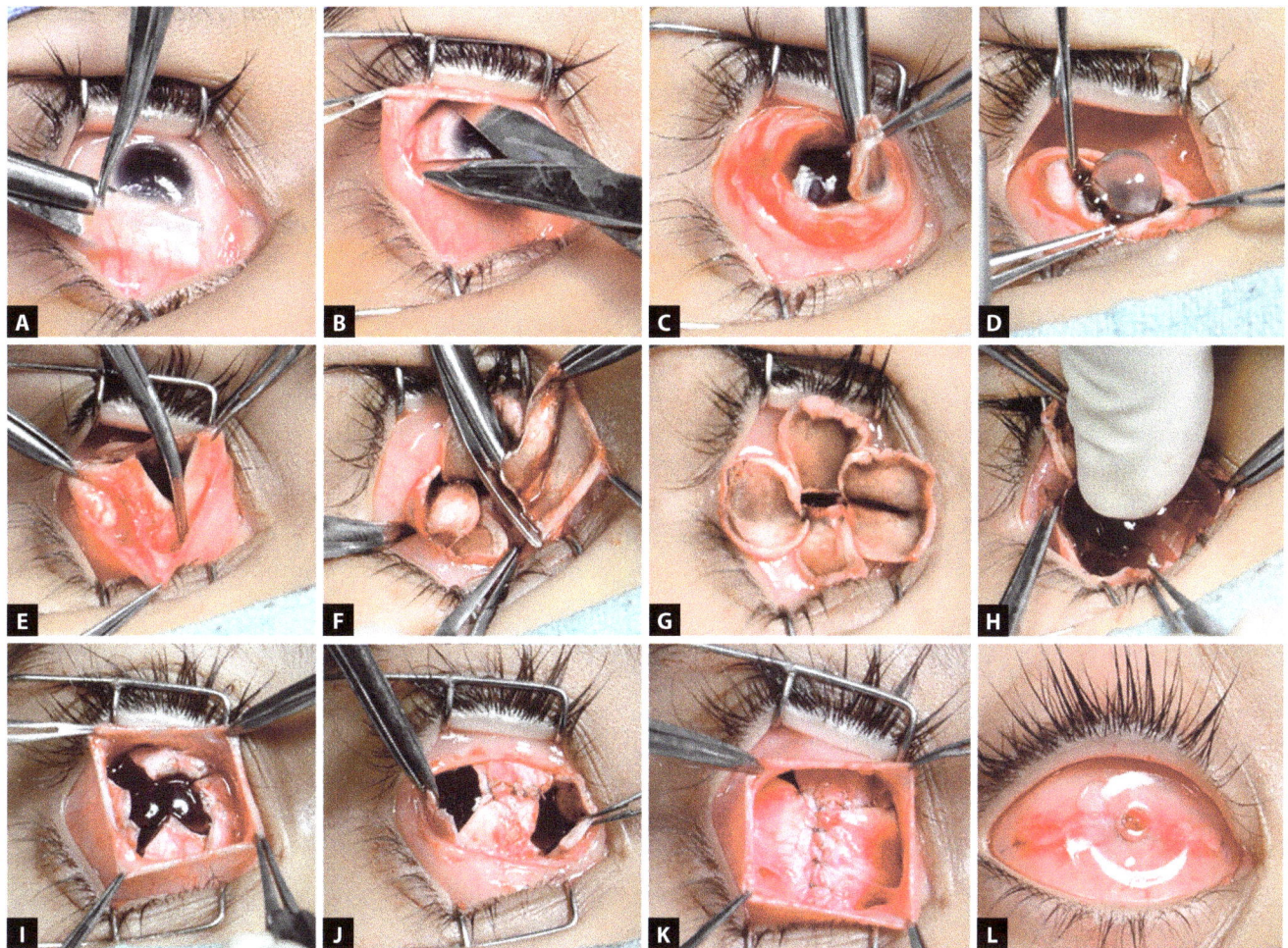

Figs. 7A to L: From top left: Peritomy (A), Tenon's capsule dissection (B), excision of corneal button (C), scooping out of intraocular contents (D), sclerotomy to make four flaps (E), posterior sclerotomy to disinsert the petals from the optic nerve (F & G), insertion of polymethyl methacrylate (PMMA) implant (H), view after implant insertion (I), closure of vertical flaps (J), closure of horizontal flaps (K), and after conformer placement (L).

Surgical Technique

- Enucleation is performed under general anesthesia.
- After a time-out is performed to confirm the correct operative eye with the entire operating room team, the face is prepared and draped in sterile fashion.
- A limbal conjunctival peritomy is performed with Wescott scissors for 360°. Blunt dissection in the sub-Tenon's plane is then carried out in each of the oblique quadrants with Stevens scissors.
- Each rectus muscle is then identified, isolated with a muscle hook, secured with suture, and cut at the insertion to the globe.
- The superior and inferior oblique muscles are isolated and transected.
- Once the globe is determined to rotate freely, the optic nerve is identified, strummed, and cut with enucleation scissors or an enucleation snare wire.
- Some surgeons prefer to first clamp the optic nerve with a curved hemostat prior to transection to encourage further hemostasis.
- An attempt should be made to cut a long segment of the optic nerve, particularly in situations of intraocular malignancy where histologic examination of the optic nerve is crucial.
- Additional hemostasis is then achieved with direct pressure in the intraconal space and cautery of the optic nerve if needed.
- An implant is then placed in the intraconal space to replace volume lost by the enucleated globe, achieve cosmetic symmetry with the fellow socket, and allow for motility of the prosthesis.
- In certain circumstances, including severe infection, a surgeon may choose not to place an implant at the time of enucleation and elect to place an implant in a second surgery.

- A three-layered closure is then carried out, i.e., posterior tenons, anterior tenons, and the conjunctiva with absorbable sutures.
- Antibiotic drops are instilled and a clear plastic conformer is placed over the closed conjunctiva. A suture tarsorrhaphy is performed to retain the conformer.
- Perioperative antibiotics are often administered. The duration of antibiotic therapy has been reported to range from 5 days to several weeks, depending on the nature of the infection.[5]
- Postoperative pain can be managed by injection of retrobulbar anesthetic or ethanol prior to patching. A pressure patch is applied and removed after 1 day. The suture tarsorrhaphy is removed after 1 week. The patient may visit an ocularist for prosthesis fitting 6–8 weeks following surgery.

Myoconjunctival Technique of Enucleation with Implant

This is a technique of enucleation where the motility of the extraocular muscles can be translated to the respective fornices where the prosthesis rests. This helps in improving the prosthesis motility. In this technique, each rectus muscle is hooked, and two sets of sutures are passed through the muscle. A 4.0 silk suture is passed close to the muscle insertion as performed in a standard enucleation technique. These sutures help in providing traction to the globe while transecting the optic nerve. A second 6.0 Vicryl suture is placed 6–8 mm from the first suture. The muscle is transected between the two sutures. After the globe is enucleated and implant placed, the Vicryl suture is exteriorized into the respective fornix. This helps in translating the contractions generated within the extraocular muscles to the prosthesis and hence improved motility **(Figs. 8A to P)**.

Choice of Immediate Versus Delayed Implant

Some surgeons choose to place the implant in a secondary staged procedure days to weeks after the initial evisceration, particularly in the setting of acute infection, believing that the rates of implant extrusion may be higher with primary implantation at the time of evisceration.

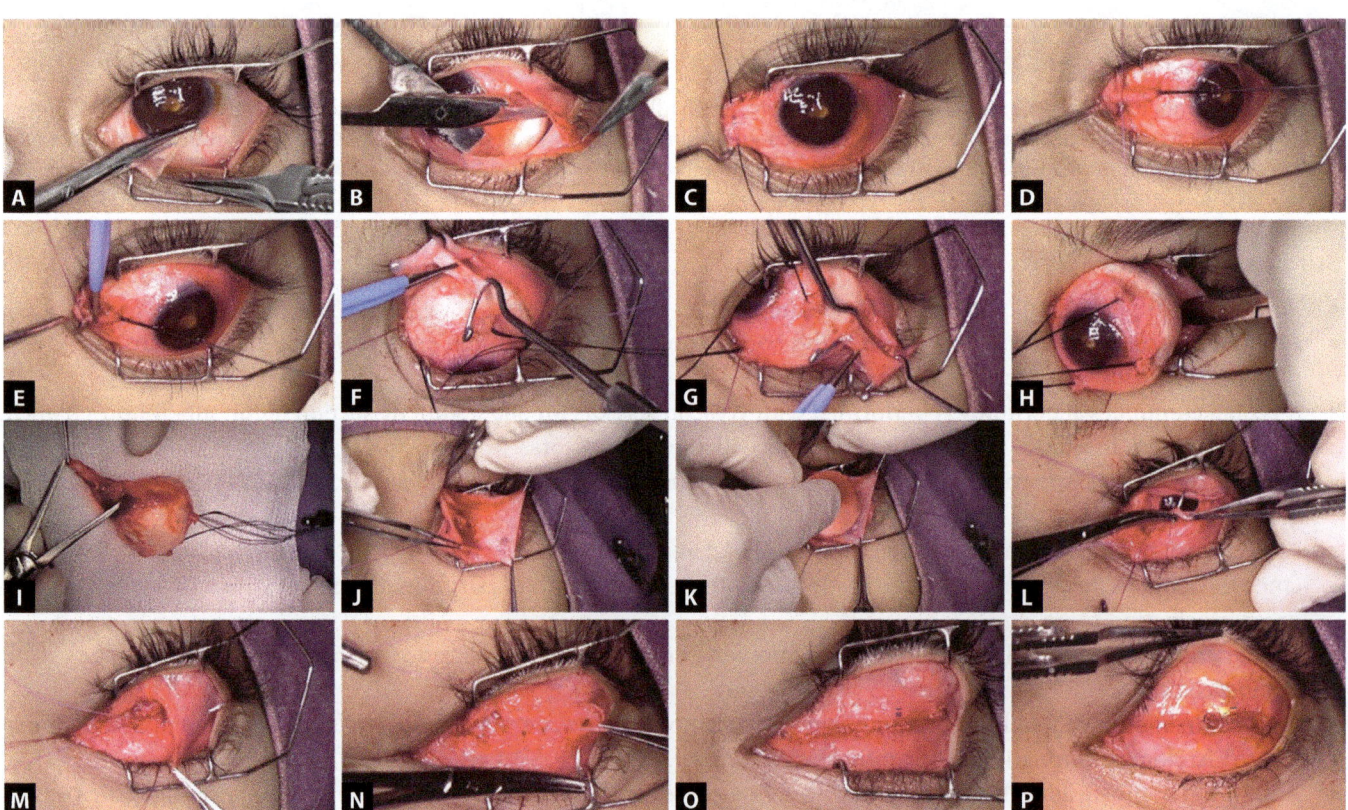

Figs. 8A to P: From top left: (A) Peritomy, (B) Tenon's capsule dissection, (C) tagging of medial rectus with 4.0 silk, (D) myoconjunctival suture passed 6 mm from the silk suture with 6.0 Vicryl, (E) muscle cut between the two sutures, (F) superior oblique cut, (G) inferior oblique cut, (H) optic nerve cut, (I) length of the optic nerve cut section measured, (J) intraconal space exposed, (K) implant placed, (L) posterior Tenon's capsule closed with interrupted sutures, (M) myoconjunctival sutures exteriorized to the respective fornices, (N) anterior Tenon's capsule closed with 6.0 Vicryl interrupted sutures, (O) conjunctiva closed with 6.0 Vicryl continuous sutures, and (P) conformer placed.

Evisceration Versus Enucleation

Advantages of evisceration over enucleation:
- Shorter operative time
- Less complex surgery
- More cost efficient
- Less disruption of orbital tissues
- Improved motility
- Less chance of spread to nervous system in cases of infection
- Less painful.

Disadvantages of evisceration over enucleation:
- Risk of sympathetic ophthalmia
- Risk of dissemination of intraocular tumors.

Q 3. Discuss indications, techniques, surgical steps, and complications of exenteration. Discuss the methods of rehabilitation.

Introduction

Exenteration is a surgical procedure involving removal of the entire globe and its surrounding structures including muscles, fat, nerves, eyelids, and sometimes the bony orbit and surrounding paranasal sinuses (extent determined by disease being treated) **(Figs. 9 and 10)**.

Indications

- Ill-defined orbital tumors where resection with a tumor-free margin improved survival
- Adnexal tumors such as squamous cell carcinoma, basal cell carcinoma, and sebaceous gland carcinoma with orbital extension
- Conjunctival melanoma and ocular surface squamous neoplasia with orbital extension

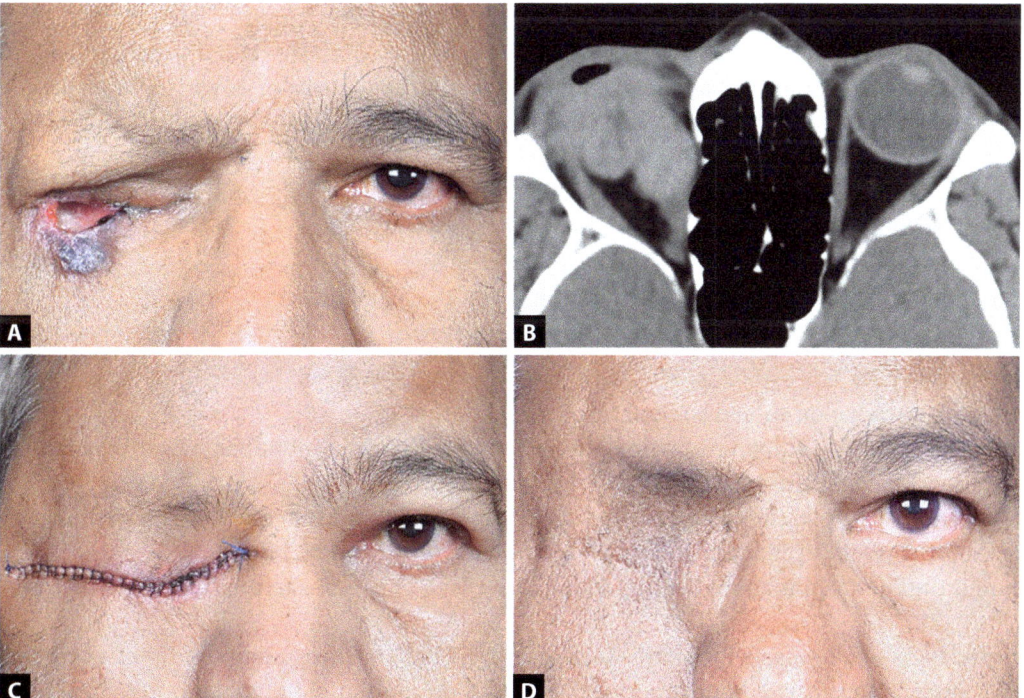

Figs. 9A to D: Right eye (RE) basal cell carcinoma with orbital extension treated with anterior orbital exenteration. (A) RE lower eyelid basal cell carcinoma with loss of eyeball contour; (B) Ct orbit demonstrating loss of globe contour and orbital extension of the lesion; (C) Day 1 postoperative following RE eyelid sparing anterior orbital exenteration; (D) 6 weeks postsurgery following anterior orbital exenteration.

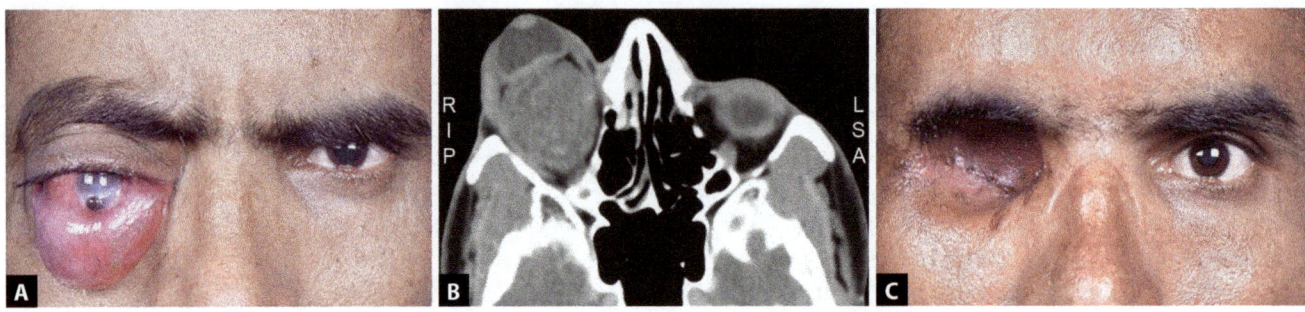

Figs. 10A to C: Right eye (RE) orbital mucormycosis treated with anterior orbital exenteration. (A) RE proptosis; (B) RE orbital mucormycosis (microbiology proven); (C) post-total exenteration.

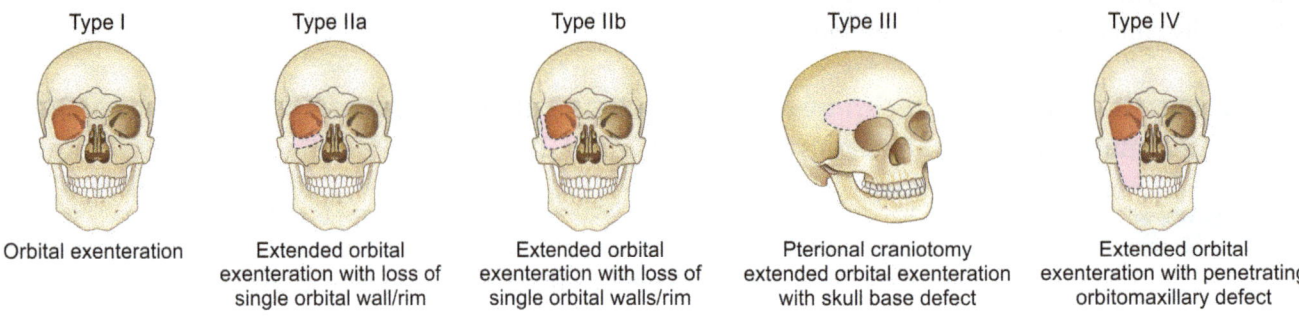

Fig. 11: Types of extended orbital exenteration.

- Uveal melanoma and retinoblastoma with orbital extension
- Lacrimal gland adenoid cystic carcinoma localized to the orbit
- Life-threatening infections such as mucormycosis where debulking the infected tissues reduces mortality.

Types of Exenteration

- Subtotal or anterior exenteration sparing the eyelids
- Total exenteration involving removal of the eyelids and complete orbital structures
- Extended or radical exenteration involving removal of the eyelids and complete orbital structures with the periorbita

Widespread orbital and periorbital tumors or infections may require exenteration of surrounding paranasal sinuses and parts of the cranial cavity. In such situations, extended orbital exenteration may be classified as follows **(Fig. 11)**.

- *Type I:* Orbital exenteration
- *Type IIa:* Extended orbital exenteration with loss of single orbital wall
- *Type IIb:* Extended orbital exenteration with loss of several orbital walls
- *Type III:* Extended orbital exenteration with skull base defect
- *Type IV:* Extended orbital exenteration with penetrating orbito-maxillary defect.

Surgical Technique

- Careful preoperative evaluation should be performed.
- General anesthesia should be employed. In exceptional situations, local retrobulbar, infraorbital, and periorbital nerve blocks may be used if general anesthesia is absolutely contraindicated.
- A 4-0 black silk suture is passed through the skin, orbicularis muscle, and superficial tarsus of the upper and lower lids and tied together to close the eyelids and to provide traction during the procedure.
- A skin incision is outlined 4 mm above the upper and lower lash line and extended at the canthi to meet in an ellipse **(Fig. 12A)**.
- A skin and orbicularis oculi muscle incision is placed with a blade or the monopolar tip of a radiofrequency device. Suborbicularis dissection is carried out superiorly and inferiorly until the periosteum just outside the orbital rim is exposed for 360° **(Figs. 12B to D)**.
- An incision is then made through the periosteum for 360° about 4 mm outside of the orbital rim to expose the underlying bone **(Fig. 12E)**. The superomedial neurovascular bundles are cauterized.

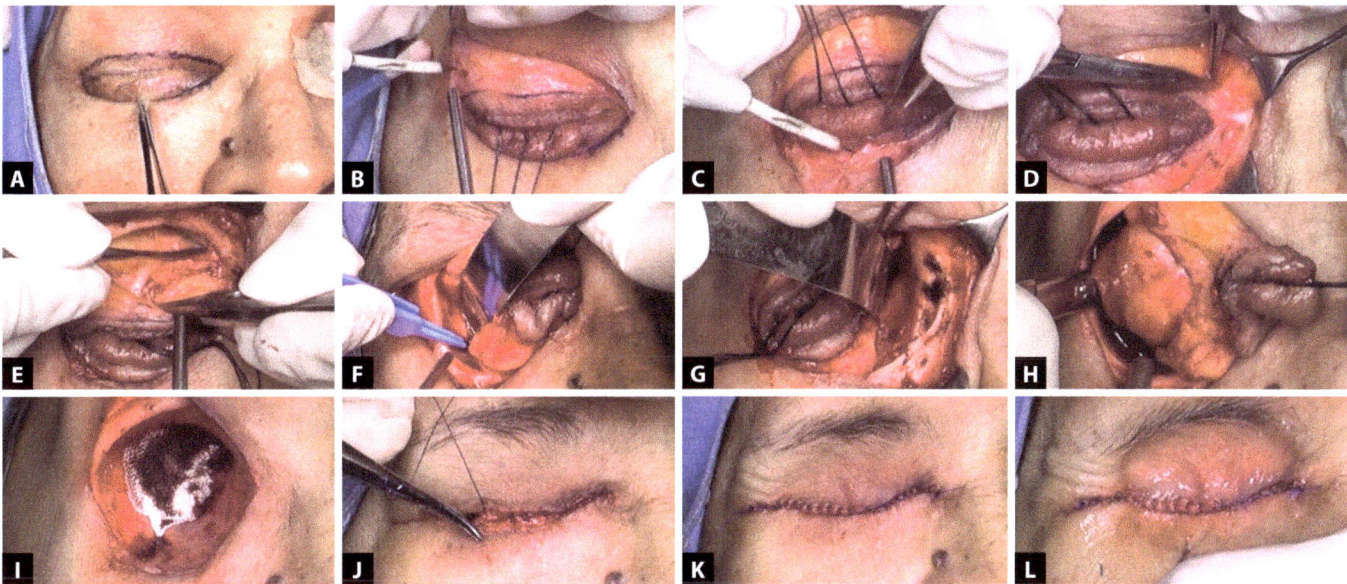

Figs. 12A to L: From top left: (A) Skin marking 4 mm from the eye margin; (B) Skin incision taken with the monopolar tip of a radiofrequency machine; (C) Suborbicularis dissection done; (D) Medial canthal tendon incised close to the orbital rim; (E) Orbital rim exposed all 360°; (F) Neurovascular bundles cauterized; (G) Nasolacrimal duct cut; (H) Enucleation scissors used to dissect orbital contents out at the posterior orbit; (I) Hemostasis achieved; (J) Orbicularis closed with 6.0 Vicryl; (K) skin closed with 4-0 Prolene; (L) Air from the socket aspirated.

- Medially, the medial canthal tendon is dis-inserted from the orbital rim.
- A periosteal elevator is used to free the periosteum for 360° around the bony orbital margin and into the orbital cavity **(Figs. 12E and F)**. The medial orbit is approached in the end since it is highly vascular. Care must be taken when using the periosteal elevator nasally to prevent fracturing the thin lamina papyracea of the ethmoid bone. The infraorbital, zygomaticofacial, zygomaticotemporal, and ethmoid neurovascular bundles are cauterized **(Fig. 12F)**. The nasolacrimal duct is cut at the junction of the sac and the duct in the lacrimal sac fossa **(Fig. 12G)**.
- When the periosteum is free posteriorly, the enucleation scissors are inserted between the periosteum and bone inferotemporally and gently advanced to the orbital apex **(Fig. 12H)**.
- The tissues are then cut as close to the orbital apex as possible, and the orbital contents are removed by continued traction on the silk sutures in the eyelids while cutting the residual adhesions in the posterior orbit.
- The socket is immediately packed with a gauze, and indirect pressure is applied to achieve hemostasis. The gauze is then removed, and the orbital apex is inspected. Residual soft tissue at the orbital apex is removed piecemeal, and bipolar cautery and repeat packing are used until there is no further bleeding. Absorbable gelatin sponges dipped in tramadol or an absorbable hemostat such as *Surgicel* may be used to control hemostasis **(Fig. 12I)**.
- A rubber drain may be placed in the socket after complete hemostasis, and the skin of the upper and lower eyelids are sutured together in two layers. The orbicularis is sutured with 6.0 Vicryl and the skin is sutured with 4-0 Prolene continuous interlocking sutures **(Figs. 12J and K)**.
- This leaves the residual orbital cavity filled with air that is aspirated with syringe prior to patching the socket **(Fig. 12L)**. One skin suture is tied to the drain if placed and the drain is removed after a week. Alternately, the exenterated socket is aspirated daily for collection of blood within the socket until the aspirate is <4 cm^3 in volume. An orbital prosthesis can be fabricated and dispensed after 6 weeks.

Complications (Figs. 13A to C)

- Extensive bleeding necessitating a blood transfusion
- Communication between the orbit and nasal cavity due to fracture of the thin ethmoid bones during surgery
- Cerebrospinal fluid (CSF) leak
- Postoperative infection
- Discharging fistula
- Wound gape.

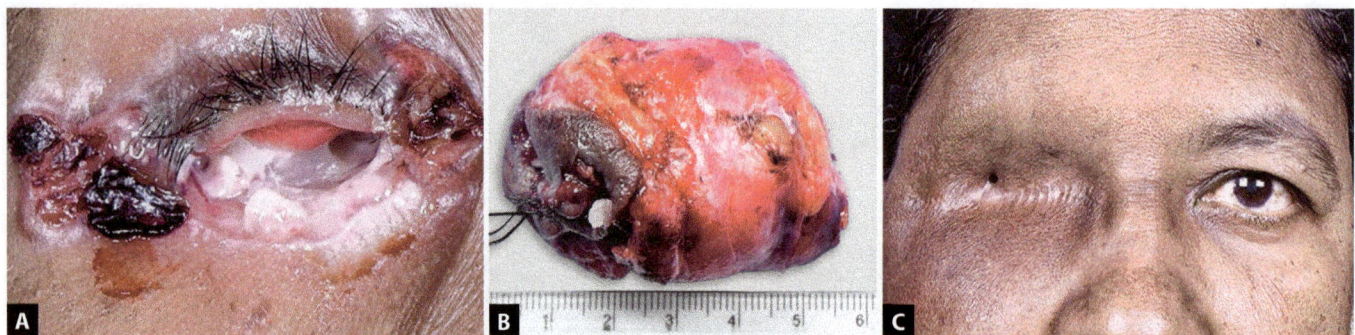

Figs. 13A to C: Right eye (RE) discharging anterior fistula following anterior exenteration. (A) RE adnexal and anterior orbital basal cell carcinoma; (B) RE anterior exenteration; (C) Discharging anterior fistula.

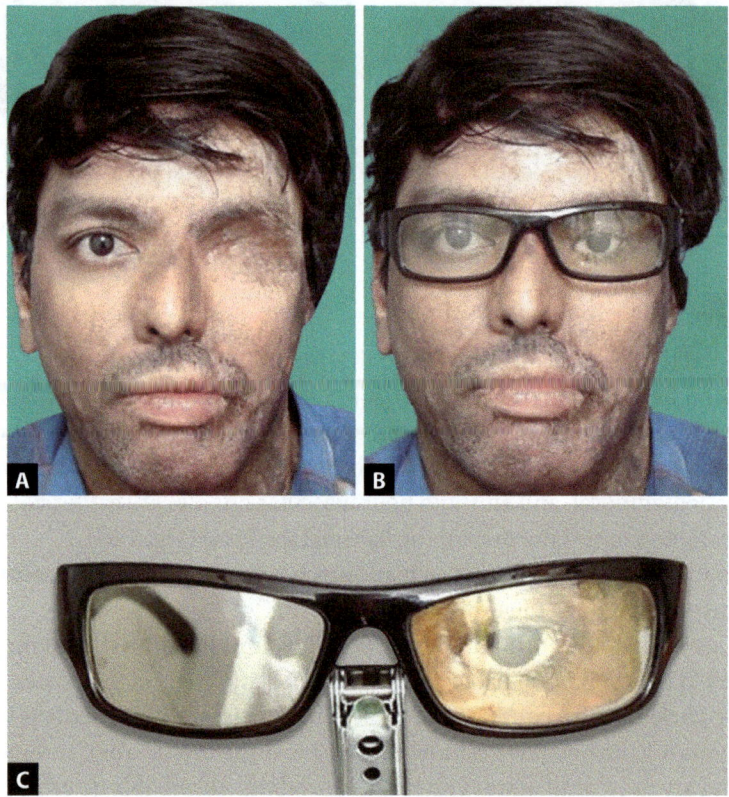

Figs. 14A to C: A spectacle-retained acrylic prosthesis.

Postoperative Rehabilitation of the Orbital Cavity

Following exenteration of the orbit, the empty socket can be rehabilitated by an orbital prosthesis. An orbital prosthesis should be aesthetic, durable, light weight, and economical. Choice of material depends upon the size and depth of the orbital defect, patient aesthetic demands, size and type of defect, type of lifestyle, and the financial condition. Most commonly used materials for fabrication of facial prosthesis are acrylic and silicone elastomers. Acrylic offers advantages such as adequate longevity, remarkable aging properties, low cost, easy to process, better adherence of prosthesis to spectacle frame, and minimal maintenance. Silicone materials are preferred nowadays, as they provide better marginal adaptation and more lifelike appearance than acrylic. But they are expensive and lack the ability of chemical or mechanical bonding with a spectacle frame.

There are three kinds of orbital prosthesis:
1. Spectacle-retained acrylic prosthesis **(Figs. 14A to C)**
2. Adhesive-retained silicone prosthesis **(Figs. 15A to C)**
3. Osseo-integrated prosthesis retained with the help of magnetic implants **(Figs. 16A to C)**

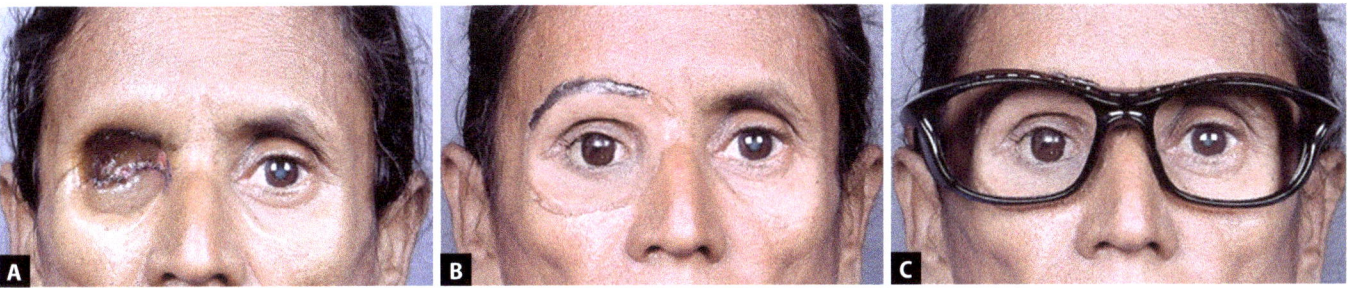

Figs. 15A to C: Adhesive retention silicone prosthesis. (A) Post-right eye (RE) eyelid sparing exenteration; (B) With adhesive retention silicone prosthesis; (C) With a spectacle frame to hide the brow discrepancy.

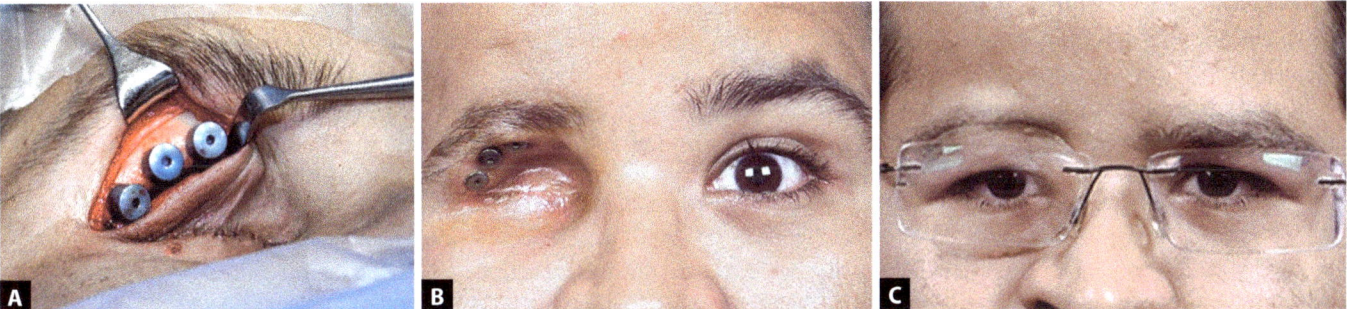

Figs. 16A to C: Osseo-integrated orbital prosthesis. (A) Right eye (RE) magnetic orbital implants placed in the superolateral rim; (B) Postoperative healing over the implants; (C) Magnet-retained right silicone prosthesis.

 4. What are orbital implants and their indications? Enumerate different materials for orbital implants. What are the advantages and complications of orbital implants?

Definition: An *implant* is any material inserted into the body to replace a missing biological structure, support a damaged biological structure, or enhance an existing biological structure. Orbital implants are used after enucleation or evisceration surgery to replace the lost ocular volume and provide an adequate support for the external prosthesis.

Need for Placement

Why	When	What	How

• Volume replacement	• Indications:
	  – Primary
	  – Secondary
		• Classification
		• Advantages
		• Disadvantages
			• Surgical procedure

WHY: Volume Replacement

The orbital volume is 30 mL and the globe contributes to 7 mL of this volume. This 7 mL needs to be replaced after any destructive eye surgery. In an ideal situation, 70% of this volume is contributed by orbital implant, and 30% by an external ocular prosthesis. An 18 mm orbital implant can replace an average deficit of only 3.1 mL, which will subsequently warrant the use of a larger prosthesis. Hence, accurate implant sizing prior to placement is extremely important for a satisfactory postoperative aesthetic outcome.

The number on size of the implant represents the diameter of the implant in millimeters, and sizes range from 12 to 23 mm. Mathematically, a 20–22 mm implant fills a volume of 4.2–5.6 mL. Implant sizing can be done by using one of the following methods:

- *Axial length of the fellow eye:* Kaltreider formula

    Size = (axial length – 2) mm

- *Age of the patient:* 18 mm in children, 20 mm in adults
- Use of intraoperative sizer after removal of globe or eye contents
- *Empiric size selection:* The largest implant that provides tension-free closure

- Calculation of volume loss using graduated cylinder to measure the removed contents

$$V_{implant} = V_{tissue\ loss} - V_{tissue\ wrap} - V_{prosthesis}$$

where $V_{implant}$ is the volume of required implant, $V_{tissue\ loss}$ is the total tissue loss after removal of contents, $V_{tissue\ wrap}$ is the volume of the wrapping material (applicable if wrapping is to be done), and $V_{prosthesis}$ is the volume of the prosthesis, which is ideally taken as 2 mL.

WHEN: Indications

Implant placement is indicated after all evisceration and enucleation surgeries for adequate volume replacement, but the time of placement can differ according to individual case. In practice, most implants are placed primarily, i.e., at the time of enucleation or evisceration. Exceptions to this are in cases of severe ocular or orbital trauma, where there is extensive tissue loss and loss of tissue planes. It is important to note that all endophthalmitis and panophthalmitis cases undergoing evisceration are not contraindications to implant placement, and decision needs to be individualized on a case-to-case basis. Decision to defer implant placement may be taken in case sclera or surrounding tissues appear unhealthy because such cases are prone to implant exposure and extrusion.

Secondary implant placement is done as a subsequent surgery after resolution of residual inflammation and infection. But as tissue healing occurs, fibrosis also sets in; hence, secondary implant surgeries are more challenging to perform.

Primary implant	Placed during the time of evisceration or enucleation surgery, except in cases of severe ocular trauma or infections
Secondary implant	Placed at a later date following the original enucleation or evisceration procedure. An implant exchange procedure is also included in a secondary implant surgery.

WHAT: Types of Implants

Characteristics of an ideal implant are:
- Biocompatible and nondegradable
- Simple to implant
- Adequate volume replacement of the lost globe
- Good motility and support transmitted to the overlying ocular prosthesis
- Low rate of complications
- Economical.

Biomaterials: Historically, materials such as wool, clay, sponge, rubber, paraffin, ivory, cork, cartilage, fat, bone, and metals such as gold, silver, platinum, aluminum, or vitallium have been used as implants in anophthalmic sockets. Early implants had high rates of exposure and extrusion in addition to poor motility and cosmesis. Hence, the advent of different types of materials and designs of implants surfaced. A brief summary of different materials used in the present times as orbital implants is shown.

Synthetic	Polymers	Polymethyl methacrylate (PMMA), silicon, polyethene, polytetrafluoroethane (PTFE)
	Ceramics	Glass, hydroxyapatite (HA), aluminum oxide
	Composites	Teflon-carbon, HA-silicon, HA-alumina
Biogenic	Autologous	Dermis fat graft
	Allografts	Implants wrapped with sclera/dermis/pericardium
	Xenografts	Cancellous bone

Orbital implants can be classified as porous or nonporous.

Nonporous implants: As the name suggests, these are made up of nonporous material and hence cannot interact with the surrounding orbital tissues. Silicon spheres and PMMA spheres are examples of nonporous implants. These are the implants of choice in children and elderly age groups or in case of placement of a temporary implant. These are also the first choice in case of tumor or infection, where any fibrovascular growth needs to be avoided.
- *Silicon:* Available as a solid sphere
- *PMMA:* Available as a solid sphere, hollow sphere, and in hemisphere shapes. PMMA has also been used to manufacture the quasi-integrated design of implants. Baseball implant, a PMMA implant wrapped in donor sclera, has been a popular implant used in the past. A hollow acrylic implant was manufactured to address increasing rates of migration attributed to the increased weight of the implant.

Advantages of nonporous implants:
- Time tested materials
- Easy availability
- Smooth external surface
- Cheap.

Porous implants: These implants are composed of porous matrix that allows the fibrovascular tissue to permeate throughout the implant's core architecture. The purpose of this biointegration was to reduce the rates of migration and extrusion. Porous polyethylene (Medpor), HA (Bio-Eye), and aluminum oxide (Bioceramic) are the most commonly used porous implants.

- *Hydroxyapatite* belongs to a class of calcium orthophosphates. It has a structure very similar to apatites present in the mammalian bone, hence providing good strength at the same time inciting minimal tissue reaction, although HA is known to cause giant cell reaction. Originally derived from corals, HA is now synthetically manufactured. The microarchitecture is identical to cancellous bone and lends the material its porous nature. Vascular ingrowth starts slowly and is completed by 6–7 months. As compared to the original bovine cancellous bone-derived implant, HA has a lower porosity that gives it more strength. This property is useful to withstand the pressure of drilling during pegging. The original Bio-Eye has a rough external surface and hence mandates wrapping. This abrasive surface is associated with conjunctival thinning with increased potential for exposure, infection, and pyogenic granuloma formation. Newer generations of synthetic HA, for example, coated Bio-Eye, have a smoother surface, which allows direct suturing of the muscles to these implants.
- *Porous polyethylene* is made by polymerization of ethylene molecules. It is a cheap and easily available material. Although less biocompatible than HA, it has a smooth nonabrasive external surface, with a soft nonbrittle core, that allows easy insertion and direct suturing of muscles, obviating the need for wrapping of the implant. It is said to cause less inflammation than HA. Newer improved designs provide porous anterior surface with increased fibrovascular ingrowth, with prefabricated tunnels and suture holes.
- *Alumina* is the cheapest of the three implants. It has a smoother surface than HA. Fibroblasts proliferate more rapidly on alumina than HA. A protein coating is formed around the implant after insertion, causing least inflammatory reaction.

Advantages of porous implants:
- The risk of migration of the implant within the orbit is reduced.
- It has a reduced risk of extrusion after complete fibrovascular ingrowth.
- The implant permits better movement of the ocular prosthesis since it allows for pegging.
- The motility peg allows the weight of the ocular prosthesis to be borne by the implant rather than by the lower eyelid.
- The implant has a low complication rate in the hands of an experienced surgeon.

Disadvantages of porous implants:
- Expensive
- Additional surgical time for wrapping, etc.
- Additional surgical procedure if pegging is considered
- Implant exchange and removal is challenging due to fibrovascular ingrowth
- Needs removal in case of suspected infection, as its porous nature provides a surface area for biofilm of the organisms to grow.

What is Wrapping and Pegging?

Wrapping is done to facilitate insertion of implants with a rough surface. Additional advantages of wrapping include providing an added layer of protective barrier to prevent exposure, adding volume to the implant, and enabling attachment of extraocular muscles in case of nonintegrated implants. When used, an additional 2 mm must be subtracted to calculate the implant size.

Materials used:

Autogenous tissue	Synthetic
Donor sclera, pericardium, fascia lata, temporalis fascia, acellular dermis, periosteum	Polyglactin (Vicryl) mesh, polyester urethane, polyglycolic acid, polytetrafluoroethane (PTFE) sheet

Traditional wrapping involves covering the implant completely with the wrapping material. If sclera is being used, the edges of the sclera are sutured after placing implant in the scleral pocket, and four small windows are cut out for attachment of recti muscles. Vicryl mesh is used to cover the surface completely, as fibrovascular ingrowth can take place through the mesh.

A modified technique of providing additional protective cover is anterior scleral capping. A scleral cap is sutured to the anterior one-third of the implant to provide an extra layer over it.

Disadvantages:
- Adds expense and surgical time
- Additional second site surgery with increased morbidity
- Theoretical risk of disease transmission using autogenous tissue.

Pegging is a method to establish direct coupling between the implant and the prosthesis, which translates into enhanced prosthesis movements and hence improved cosmesis. It can be done in case of porous implants after completion of fibrovascular ingrowth, usually around 6 months. Vascularity should be confirmed on contrast-enhanced magnetic resonance imaging (MRI) prior to peg placement. A motility peg, made up of PMMA or titanium, is inserted within a sleeve that is drilled on the anterior surface of the buried orbital implant.

Practical considerations for pegging:
- It is an optional procedure for those who desire improved motility and cosmesis.
- Use of the pegging system has declined over the years due to complications such as foreign body granulomas, recurrent inflammation, and discharge associated with it.
- It also leads to increased chances of exposure and thus extrusion.

Depending upon how the implants are linked to the surrounding orbital structures and overlying prosthesis, they can be nonintegrated, quasi-integrated, or integrated (mechanically or biologically, or magnetically coupled) **(Table 1)**.

TABLE 1: Types of implants with their advantages and disadvantages.

Type	Description	Examples	Advantages	Disadvantages
Nonintegrated	• Nonporous, no attachment to surrounding orbital tissues • Do not allow fibrovascular in-growth • Uninterrupted conjunctival lining over the implant, without any attachment with the prosthesis	• Silicon spheres • Polymethyl methacrylate (PMMA) spheres	• Smooth external surface • Can be used in case of tumor or infection • Cheap and easily available • Useful as temporary implant when implant exchange is anticipated	• Poor motility if not wrapped • Increased chances of migration as they do not integrate
Quasi- or semi-integrated (buried integrated)	• Nonporous, but have specific apparatus for attachment to the extraocular muscles • Uninterrupted conjunctival lining with indirect contact between orbital implant and ocular prosthesis • Irregular anterior surface allows the translation of movement to custom shaped prosthesis	• Cutler implant I • Allen implant • Iowa implants I and II • Universal implant	• Good motility because of tunnels provided for muscle attachment • Made up of easily available cheap material	• Anterior irregular surface causes chronic pinching of conjunctiva and Tenon's tissue • Discomfort and high rate of erosion with subsequent exposure and extrusion • Require specialized prosthesis to fit shape
Integrated, mechanical (exposed integrated)	• Specific apparatus for attachment to the extraocular muscles • Conjunctival lining is interrupted in order to allow direct coupling of the implant to the ocular prosthesis (with or without a peg)	Cutler implant II	• Theoretically, good prosthesis motility	• High rates of complications such as exposure and extrusion • Chronically inflamed conjunctival surface with redness and discharge
Bio-integrated	• Porous material implants • Direct biological integration of implant with surrounding orbital structures • Can be integrated with prosthesis with pegging system	• Porous polyethylene (Medpor) • Hydroxyapatite (Bio-Eye) • Aluminum oxide (Bioceramic)	• Provides the best motility • Reduced risk of migration and extrusion • Cosmesis can be enhanced using the pegging system	• Need for additional procedure such as peg placement • Requires implant removal in case of infection, without attempting conservative measures • Less economical, with higher cost of the implant, expense of the second-stage procedure and the required modifications to the ocular prosthesis

Implant Complications

The most common complications are those involving volume deficits and eyelid malpositions. These are related to the use of implants of inappropriate size and, subsequently, a heavy prosthesis. Conjunctival thinning, discharge, and pyogenic granuloma can occur. Complications associated with orbital implants can be classified as (1) complications directly attributable to implant placement **(Figs. 17A to F)** and (2) complications due to socket surgery **(Figs. 18A to J)**.

	Treatment
Complication due to the implant	
Socket/orbital infection	*Mild:* Antibiotics and anti-inflammatory agents *Severe:* Implant removal and healing with secondary intention, secondary implant at a later date
Implant exposure	*Limited:* Conservative with antibiotics and lubricants *Extensive:* Covering with conjunctival flap/patch graft/implant exchange
Implant extrusion	Secondary implant
Implant migration	*Mild:* Modify prosthesis *Moderate to severe inferotemporal:* Customized floor implant *Any other quadrant:* Implant removal with dermis fat graft
Complications due to socket surgery	
Volume deficit	*Nonsurgical:* Hyaluronic acid gel filler injections *Surgical:* Autologous fat transfer, implant exchange, subperiosteal floor implant, dermis fat graft
Conjunctival retention cysts	• Cyst aspiration with sclerotherapy • Cyst excision
Lower eyelid laxity	Lateral tarsal strip
Upper eyelid blepharoptosis	*Mild:* Prosthesis modification *Moderate to severe:* Ptosis correction
Entropion	*Mild:* Prosthesis modification *Moderate to severe:* Posterior lamellar grafts and anterior lamellar repositioning

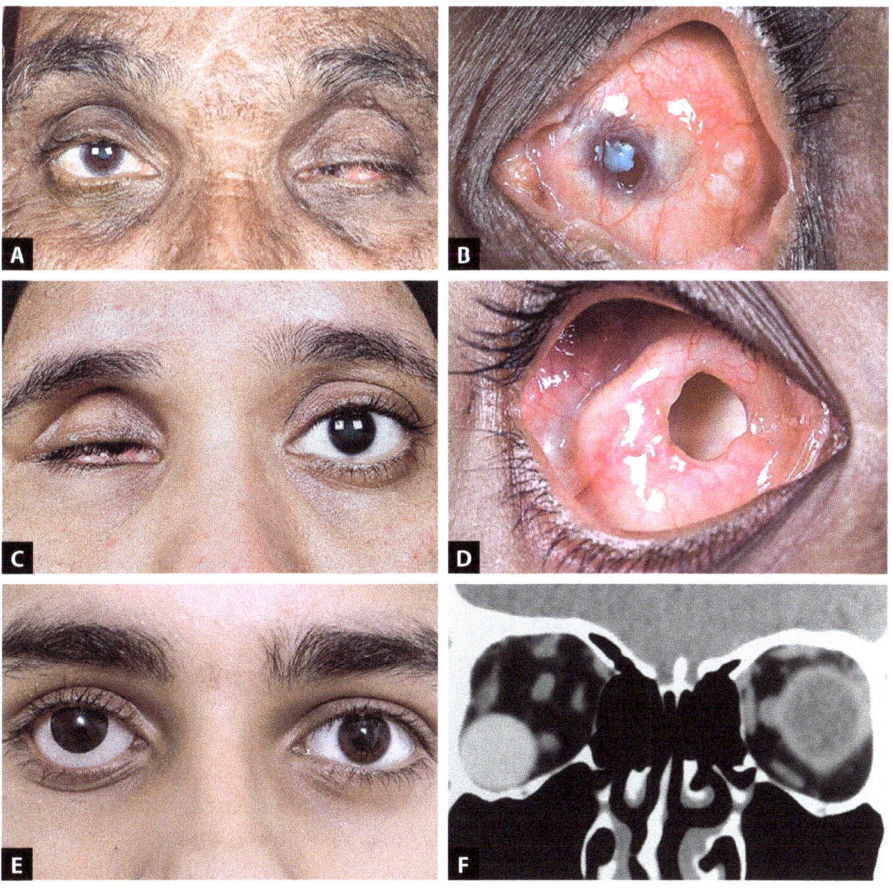

Figs. 17A to F: Implant complications. (A and B) Implant exposure; (C and D) Implant extrusion; and (E and F) Implant migration.

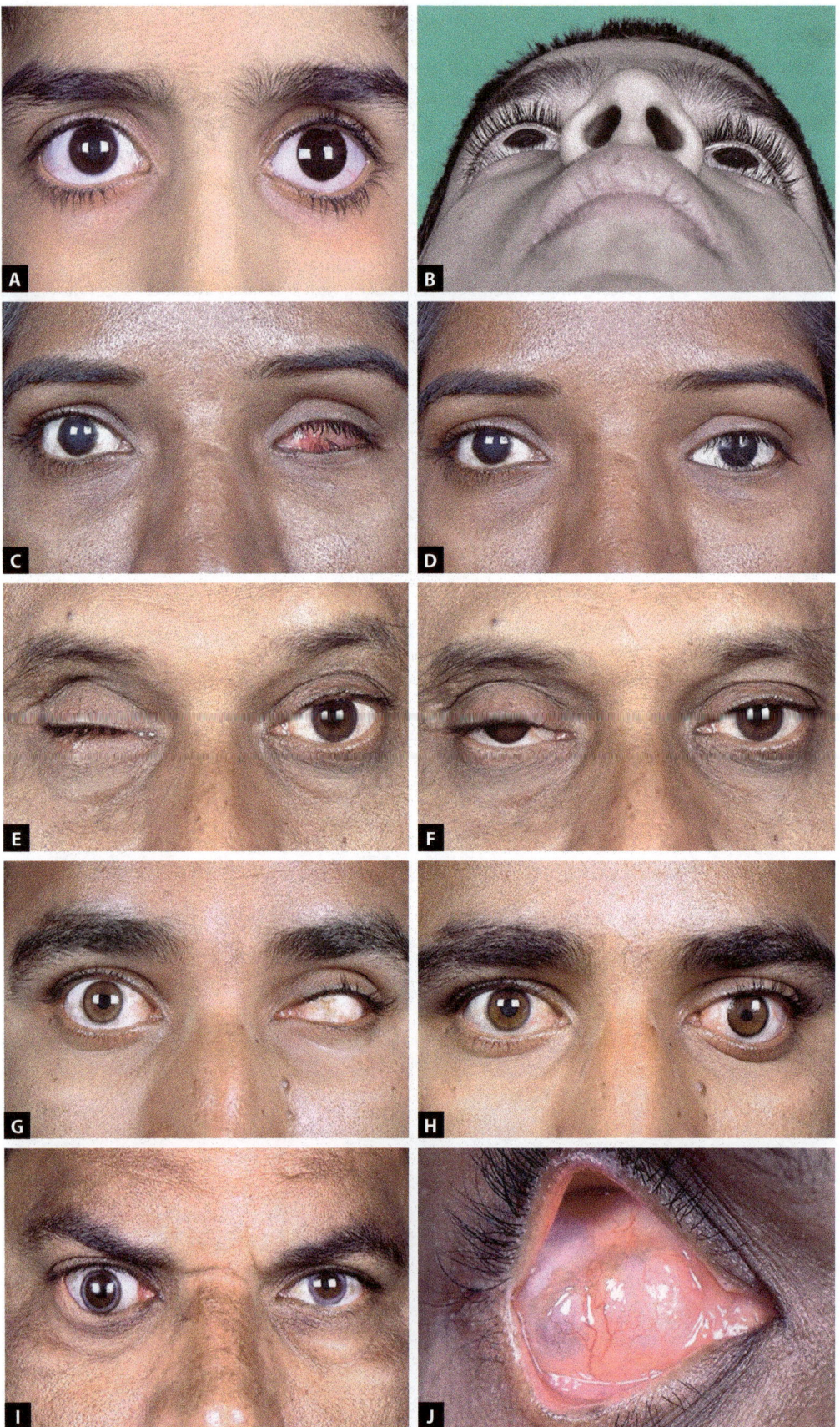

Figs. 18A to J: Socket surgery complications. (A and B) Volume loss with left superior sulcus deformity and enophthalmos due to a small implant; (C and D) Left upper and lower eyelid entropion; (E and F) right upper eyelid blepharoptosis; (G and H) Left lower eyelid retraction; (I and J) Right conjunctival retention cyst.

In spite of multiple studies on different implants, there are no standard guidelines established for their use. At present, implant choice is governed by patient factors, surgeon experience and preference, ease of use, and cost.

Suggested Reading

1. Allen R. Exenteration with placement of a full thickness skin graft. Oculoplastics Surgery Techniques. University of Iowa Health Care. Ophthalmology and Visual Sciences Video Library.
2. Baino F, Perero S, Ferraris S, Miola M, Balagna C, Verné E, et al. Biomaterials for orbital implants and ocular prostheses: overview and future prospects. Acta Biomater. 2014;10(3):1064-87.
3. Ben Simon GJ, Schwarcz RM, Douglas R, Fiaschetti D, McCann JD, Goldberg RA. Orbital exenteration: one size does not fit all. Am J Ophthalmol. 2005;139:11-7.
4. Dave T. Outcomes of volume replacement after evisceration and enucleation with implant. AIOS Proc. 2017.
5. Fay A, Dolman PJ. Diseases and Disorders of the Orbit and Ocular Adnexa E-Book: Expert Consult. Elsevier Health Sciences; 2016.
6. Johnson TE. Management of the contracted socket. Anophthalmia. Cham: Springer; 2020. pp. 193-208.
7. Jordan DR, Klapper SR. Evaluation and management of the anophthalmic socket and socket reconstruction. Smith and Nesi's Ophthalmic Plastic and Reconstructive Surgery, 3rd edition. Berlin: Springer; 2012. pp. 1131-73.
8. Kaltreider SA, Lucarelli MJ. A simple algorithm for selection of implant size for enucleation and evisceration: a prospective study. Ophthalmic Plast Reconstr Surg. 2002;18(5):336-41.
9. Krishna G. Contracted sockets—I (aetiology and types). Indian J Ophthalmol. 1980;28(3):117-20.
10. Leatherbarrow B. Oculoplastic Surgery, 3rd edition. New York: Thieme Medical Publishers; 2019.
11. Nagendran ST, Lee NG, Fay A, Lefebvre DR, Sutula FC, Freitag SK. Orbital exenteration: the 10-year Massachusetts eye and ear infirmary experience. Orbit. 2016;35:199-206.
12. Rong AJ, Johnson TE. Orbital implants and wrapping materials. Anophthalmia. Cham: Springer; 2020. pp. 93-106.
13. Spiegel JH, Varvares MA. Prevention of postexenteration complications by obliteration of the orbital cavity. Skull Base. 2007;17: 197-203.
14. Tripathy D, Rath S. Evisceration with primary orbital implant in fulminant endophthalmitis/panophthalmitis. Orbit. 2015;34(5): 279-83.
15. Tyers AG. Orbital exenteration for invasive skin tumours. Eye (Lond). 2006;20:1165-70.

1.26 Conjunctival Epithelial Tumors and OSSN

Nupur Goel, Anasua G Kapoor

Q 1. Enumerate/classify all the conjunctival tumors/tumors of the ocular surface.

Introduction

Tumors of the ocular surface have a wide clinical spectrum and include several forms of epithelial, stromal, caruncular, and secondary tumors.

Tumors affecting the conjunctiva and cornea include benign and malignant neoplasms arising from the conjunctival epithelium, conjunctival stroma, and structures within the stroma including the blood vessels, nerves, fat, and lymphoid tissue. Corneal tumors can arise specifically from the corneal epithelium and rarely does the stroma promote a tumor. Most corneal tumors are secondary to extension from an adjacent conjunctival tumor. Conjunctival tumors are relatively infrequent.[1]

Conjunctival tumors	Benign	Malignant
Epithelial tumors		
Nonmelanocytic	• Papilloma • Keratoacanthoma • Reactive hyperplasia • Inverted follicular keratosis • Keratotic plaque • Hereditary benign intraepithelial dyskeratosis • Oncocytoma • Dacryoadenoma	• Conjunctival intraepithelial neoplasia (CIN) • Invasive squamous cell carcinoma (SCC)

Contd...

Contd...

Conjunctival tumors	Benign	Malignant
Melanocytic	• Nevus • Ocular melanocytosis • Complexion-associated melanosis • Primary acquired melanosis	Malignant melanoma
Stromal tumors		
Vascular	• Pyogenic granuloma • Lymphangiectasia and lymphangioma • Varix • Cavernous hemangioma • Capillary hemangioma • Hemangiopericytoma • Glomus tumor	Kaposi sarcoma
Fibrous	Fibrous histiocytoma	
Neural	• Neuroma and neurofibroma • Schwannoma	
Histiocytic		
Myogenic/myxomatous	Myxoma	
Lipomatous	Lipoma	
Lymphoproliferative	Benign reactive lymphoid hyperplasia	• Lymphoid and plasmacytic tumors • Leukemia
Choristomas	• Dermoid • Dermolipoma • Simple and complex choristomas	
Xanthomatous	Juvenile xanthogranuloma	
Caruncular tumors	• Papilloma • Nevus • Lipoma • Sebaceous hyperplasia and adenoma • Oncocytoma	• SCC • Melanoma • Sebaceous carcinoma • Lymphoma • Kaposi sarcoma
Metastatic tumors		Tumors metastasizing from primary tumors located in the breast, lungs, cutaneous melanoma, etc.
Secondary tumors		Tumors extending from the eyelid, orbit, intraocular structures, and paranasal sinuses

 2. Enumerate the epithelial tumors of the conjunctiva.

Epithelial tumors of the conjunctiva[1,2]

	Benign	Malignant
Nonmelanocytic	• Papilloma • Keratoacanthoma • Reactive hyperplasia • Inverted follicular keratosis • Keratotic plaque • Hereditary benign intraepithelial dyskeratosis • Oncocytoma • Dacryoadenoma	• Conjunctival intraepithelial neoplasia (CIN) • Invasive squamous cell carcinoma (SCC)
Melanocytic	• Nevus • Ocular melanocytosis • Complexion-associated melanosis • Primary acquired melanosis	Malignant melanoma

 3. Discuss the nonmelanocytic benign epithelial tumors of the conjunctiva.

Nonmelanocytic benign epithelial tumors of conjunctiva[1,3]

Tumor		Pathogenesis	Morphology	Malignant potential	HPE	Treatment
Squamous papilloma	Children	Infection of the conjunctival epithelium with human papillomavirus (HPV) 6, 11, or 16 Virus is acquired through transfer from the mother's vagina to the newborn's conjunctiva as the child passes through the mother's birth canal	• Solitary or multiple • Sessile or pedunculated • Becomes confluent in extreme cases to form massive papillomatosis • Appears most often as a pink or red mass with fleshy frond or finger-like projections in the inferior fornix, most common medially • Also seen in bulbar conjunctiva but rarely in the cornea	Low malignant potential	Numerous vascularized papillary fronds lined by acanthotic epithelium	Small sessile: Periodic observation Larger or more pedunculated lesions (generally symptomatic with foreign body sensation, chronic mucous production, hemorrhagic tears, incomplete eyelid closure, and poor cosmetic appearance): Surgical excision by the "no-touch technique" followed by cryotherapy
	Adults	May be associated with HPV infection and immunocompromised status	• Unilateral and solitary • Seen at the limbus, encroaching the cornea as it grows • Can also arise in the caruncle	Low malignant potential	Numerous vascularized papillary fronds lined by acanthotic epithelium	Surgical excision by the "no-touch technique" followed by cryotherapy is the treatment of choice Other reported treatment modalities include laser, dinitrochlorobenzene immunotherapy, interferon alpha 2b (IFN α-2b), and topical mitomycin C (MMC) drops
Inverted papilloma		Papilloma may invaginate inward into the underlying conjunctiva and substantia propria to	• Presents as a mixed inverted exophytic papilloma • Rarely, it appears as solid or cystic solitary nodule at the limbus, plica semilunaris, and tarsal conjunctiva	Tendency towards malignant transformation into transitional cell carcinoma, SCC, or mucoepidermoid carcinoma		Treatment is by local excision

Contd...

Contd...

Tumor	Pathogenesis	Morphology	Malignant potential	HPE	Treatment
Conjunctival pseudo-epitheliomatous hyperplasia	• Reactive inflammatory proliferation of the epithelial cells, which simulates carcinoma clinically and histopathologically • Conjunctival lesion secondary to irritation by concurrent or preexisting stromal inflammation such as pterygium, pinguecula, allergic conjunctivitis, and foreign body	Elevated leukoplakic pink lesion in the limbal area	Benign	Massive acanthosis, hyperkeratosis, and parakeratosis of the conjunctival epithelium	Complete excision and additional cryotherapy would constitute optimal management, as difficulty prevails in clinically and histologically differentiating the lesion from low-grade SCC
Keratoacanthoma	Variant of conjunctival pseudoepitheliomatous hyperplasia	• An elevated mass with hyperkeratosis or leukoplakia is the usual presentation • Onset as well as the progression is rapid	Benign	Massive acanthosis, hyperkeratosis, and parakeratosis	Complete excision and cryotherapy
Dacryoadenoma	Rare condition affecting children and young adults	Translucent and fleshy pink lesion in the bulbar, forniceal, or palpebral conjunctiva	Benign	Appears to originate from the surface epithelium and proliferate into the stroma, forming glandular lobules similar to the lacrimal gland	Complete excision
Conjunctival epithelial cyst	Two subtypes—inclusion cysts and ductal cysts. Inclusion cysts are further classified as spontaneous or posttraumatic	• Smooth translucent lesions containing clear fluid. The contents may be turbid, containing epithelial debris seen layered like pseudohypopyon • May remain stable and asymptomatic and rarely undergo spontaneous resolution	Benign	Ductal cysts are lined by two layers of the epithelium and may contain secretory material	Excision is the treatment of choice for a cyst that enlarges or becomes symptomatic

Contd...

Contd...

Tumor	Pathogenesis	Morphology	Malignant potential	HPE	Treatment
Hereditary benign intraepithelial dyskeratosis	• Specifically seen among the inbred Caucasians, African-Americans, and Native Americans known as Haliwa Indians but is also seen in the population of other descent • Generally presents in the first decade of life	Rare autosomal dominant condition of the conjunctiva and other mucous membranes	• Elevated hyperemic and fleshy V-shaped plaque on the nasal and temporal bulbar conjunctiva and limbus • It may be asymptomatic or can cause redness and discomfort. Severe form can lead to corneal vascularization, opacification, and loss of vision	• No risk of malignancy, but recurrence is common. • Hence, complete excision with clear margins is warranted.	Marked acanthosis and hyperkeratosis of the conjunctival epithelium with prominent dyskeratosis	Smaller symptomatic lesions are treated conservatively with lubricants and topical steroids, while larger lesions undergo local resection with ocular surface reconstruction
Keratotic plaque	Thickening and keratinization of conjunctival epithelium	Leukoplakic lesion that may develop in the bulbar conjunctiva is usually in the interpalpebral region	Little or no malignant potential	Acanthosis, hyperkeratosis, and parakeratosis. Dyskeratosis is always absent.	
Actinic keratosis	Clinically, it may often be indistinguishable from conjunctival intraepithelial neoplasia (CIN). Rose bengal staining of the surface of the lesion tips the clinical suspicion in favor of CIN	• Focal leukoplakic lesion occurring at the interpalpebral area presenting as flat, white plaque sometimes with a frothy covering • Usually located over a chronically inflamed pingueculum or pterygium	Progresses very gradually and shows no tendency toward aggressive growth	Proliferation of surface epithelium with keratosis	• Actinic keratosis is a relative indication for surgical excision and supplemental cryotherapy • Close observation of the lesion, until progression is documented, is a reasonable option

(HPE: histopathological examinations; SCC: squamous cell carcinoma)

4. Describe the pathogenesis and clinical features of OSSN.

Introduction

Ocular surface squamous neoplasia (OSSN) is a term given by Lee and Hirst[2] in 1995 to denote a spectrum of neoplasm that originates from squamous epithelium ranging from simple dysplasia to invasive squamous cell carcinoma (SCC), involving the conjunctiva, the limbus, and the cornea.[4] *"Ocular surface"* denotes the involvement of the conjunctiva or cornea, *"squamous"* excludes other epithelial cells such as basal cells and melanocytes, and *"neoplasia"* includes both dysplastic and carcinomatous lesions.

Epidemiology

Ocular surface squamous neoplasia is the most common nonpigmented malignancy of the ocular surface, with an incidence that ranges from 0.03–1.9 per 100,000/year in the Caucasian population to 3–3.4 per 100,000/year in African ethnicity populations.[5]

Pathogenesis and Risk Factors[1,5]

Primary risk factor	*Nonmodifiable risk factors*	*Modifiable risk factors*	*Putative risk factors*	*Systemic associations*
UVB radiation, with people chronically exposed to direct solar light and those involved in outdoor occupations being at the most risk	• Male gender • Age	• Cigarette smoking • Vitamin A or retinol deficiency • Chronic trauma or inflammation • Exposure to petroleum products • Use of topical voriconazole	• HIV-1 and 2 • HPV-16 and 18 • Hepatitis B and C	• Xeroderma pigmentosum • Papillon–Lefèvre syndrome

(HIV: human immunodeficiency virus; HPV: human papillomavirus; UV: ultraviolet)

The *"limbal transition zone theory"* of OSSN proposed by Lee and Hirst is based on the long-living and high proliferation rate of the limbal stem cells. The limbal stem cells have the responsibility for corneal epithelial replacement. Any alteration here may lead to abnormal epithelial maturation which may result in metaplasia.[6]

It is thought that the breakdown of the human body's immune surveillance against the tumor creates a "permissive environment" for other risk factors to trigger malignant transformation of the epithelial cells. For example, HPV infection, which is associated with HPV-induced inhibition of the tumor-suppressor protein retinoblastoma (Rb), may interact synergistically with sunlight exposure, which can cause ultraviolet (UV) radiation-related DNA damage, including the formation of pyrimidine dimers (CC-TT) and epigenetic changes in the p16 gene promoter and lead to triggering of the neoplastic transformation of the cell lineage.[5]

Clinical Features[1]

- Mostly unilateral; rarely, it is bilateral in immunosuppressed patients.
- In middle aged and older patients
- Usually starts in interpalpebral conjunctiva and then grows and straddles the limbus and then may or may not involve the cornea
- Fleshy or nodular, sessile minimally elevated lesion
- Surface keratin, feeder vessels, and secondary inflammation
- In dark-skinned people, the mass is commonly pigmented.
- Human immunodeficiency virus (HIV)-related lesions are often larger, with forniceal extension, and feature more areas of leukoplakia with pronounced feeder vessels.
- Most common signs and symptoms are a red eye, ocular irritation, and the appearance of a new mass in the eye.
- Vision is usually unaffected unless it encroaches the center of the cornea.
- In very advanced cases, necrotizing scleritis, associated with severe pain and visual loss, has been described.

Oculoplasty and Tumors

Morphological Classification[6]

Conjunctival

Placoid
- Gelatinous
- Papilliform
- Velvety
- Leukoplakic

Nodular

Diffuse: Can masquerade as chronic conjunctivitis. It is also important to examine the tarsal conjunctiva after everting the eyelid of patients with OSSN to detect contiguous or multifocal involvement of the tarsal conjunctiva

Nodulo-ulcerative: Recently described nodulo-ulcerative pattern of OSSN, which is characterized by ulceration/necrosis of the conjunctiva and sclera surrounded by indurated and thickened conjunctiva and sclera with associated feeder vessels and keratin

Corneal

- Primary corneal ocular surface squamous neoplasia (OSSN) or encroachment from conjunctival OSSN
- When the involvement is limited to the corneal epithelium with only minimal limbal involvement, it is called primary corneal dysplasia[4]
- OSSN arising from the cornea alone is uncommon
- Appear as a subtle wavy, advancing, gray, superficial opacity that may be relatively avascular or may have fine blood vessels
- Sharply defined fimbriated borders, the convex leading edge spreads in an arc away from the limbus, and often white dots are present over the grey epithelium
- Potentially more aggressive than the conjunctival variant[6]

Grades/microscopic appearance of OSSN: The first case of OSSN was described in 1860 by Von Graefe.[2] The initial cases of squamous neoplasms described in the literature were cases of SCC. Subsequently, it has been recognized that both invasive and noninvasive subtypes of squamous neoplasms occur.[2]

Dysplasia
Dysplastic cells in the basal layers of epithelium

↓

Preinvasive OSSN
Carcinoma in situ (CIS)/Corneal –Conjunctival Intraepithelial Neoplasia (CCIN)
No longer normal surface cells

↓

Invasive Squamous cell carcinoma
Final stage of this tumor where dysplastic epithelial cells invade beyond the basement membrane to the conjunctival substantia propria or corneal stroma

- *Mild:* Less than a third thickness occupied by atypical cells
- *Moderate:* Three-quarter thickness occupied by atypical cells
- *Severe:* Nearly full thickness occupied by atypical cells

Most of these lesions have a relatively benign course, but malignant behaviors have been reported

Generally, it is a slow-growing tumor that rarely metastasizes (<1%), but is capable of causing extensive local tissue destruction.

Local invasion is the most prevalent mechanism of tumor spread. Advanced cases can infiltrate the cornea and sclera to have the intraocular extension. Intraocular invasion may be associated with iritis, glaucoma, retinal detachment, or rupture of the globe. Rarely, the tumor may extend into the orbit causing proptosis.[1] Metastases are rare, and the first site of extraocular involvement is regional lymph nodes. Nodal development has been noted to precede the development of systemic dissemination; thus, regular neck examination is recommended so potential curative radical neck dissection may be undertaken before the onset of distal metastases.

Aggressive variants:
- Spindle cell SCC
- Mucoepidermoid SCC
- Adenoid SCC

Differentiating Features between Conjunctival Intraepithelial Neoplasia and Invasive Squamous Cell Carcinoma

Conjunctival intraepithelial neoplasia (CIN)	Invasive squamous cell carcinoma (SCC)
CIN accounts for 39% of all premalignant and malignant lesions of the conjunctiva and for 4% of all conjunctival lesions	Incidence of invasive SCC is of much lesser frequency, varying from 0.02 to 3.5/100,000 population
Precancerous and no potential to metastasize	Invasive generally has a low potential for metastasis
Leukoplakia is absent/minimal	• Extensive leukoplakia • Presence of feeder vessels and intrinsic vascularity favors SCC • Nodular lesion causes suspicion of invasive SCC

There are no consistent clinical criteria for distinguishing CIN from invasive SCC. However, there are some changes suggestive of malignant transformation.[5]

- A diffuse or multifocal configuration
- Brown pigmentation
- Median basal diameter of >10 mm
- Thickness of >1 mm.

Diagnosis

The diagnosis of OSSN is usually made clinically. Vital dye staining with rose bengal, toluidine blue, or lissamine green can help determine the diagnosis as well as to outline the borders of the tumors.

Histopathological evaluation using incisional and excisional biopsy	• Gold standard for diagnosis[5] • An incisional biopsy to establish the diagnosis is not usually indicated unless the tumor is large and diffuse. In such instances, map biopsies, similar to those used for conjunctival involvement of sebaceous carcinoma, may be advisable[2]
Impression cytology/exfoliative cytology	• Can be used to identify superficial dysplastic lesions • But they cannot assess the potential invasive growth of these lesions • Require a dedicated preparation and immediate analysis after tissue sampling
In vitro confocal microscopy (IVCM)	• Reveals such ocular surface squamous neoplasia (OSSN) features as pleomorphic epithelial cells, hyperreflectivity of the epithelium, demarcation line between normal and neoplastic area, enlarged nuclei with prominent nucleoli in the basal epithelium ("starry sky" appearance), and loss of limbal dendritic cells
High-resolution or ultra-high-resolution anterior segment optical coherence tomography (HR-OCT)/AS-OCT	• OSSN has a classic appearance on OCT with three characteristic features: (1) Hyperreflective, (2) thickened epithelium with (3) an abrupt transition point between normal and abnormal epithelium • Advantage of OCT is that images are easily and quickly obtained in a noncontact manner • HR-OCT can also play a role in the ongoing surveillance of OSSN, especially in identifying residual subclinical disease despite apparent clinical resolution • However, the diagnostic sensibility of this latter imaging modality is dependent on the training level of the users and ranges from 94 to 100%, with a specificity of up to 100% • HR-OCT also allows for the detection of treatment response and subclinical recurrence • Limitations of the technology are that the region of scanning is manually determined by the technician and as such, without automated scanning technology of the entire ocular surface, areas of subclinical disease may not be captured • Shadowing can obscure the depth of penetration, especially in thick tumors • The main limitation of HR-OCT is the impossibility to perceive deep invasion of the tumor or the histologic grade
Ultrasonic biomicroscopy (UBM)	• Examination using UBM reveals a hyperechoic tumor surface with a generally hypoechoic tumor stroma; this pattern differs from the hyperechoic orbital tissues and is easily identifiable in cases of orbital invasion • Advantage: Detecting the infiltration of adjacent structures due to its higher penetration and capability to achieve a better resolution of the posterior margin of the lesions • Limitation: Time-consuming and highly operator-dependent, and requires direct contact with the eye

Differential Diagnoses[7]

Ocular surface squamous neoplasia mimics the following conditions: Pterygium, pinguecula, hyperkeratotic plaque, Bitot spot, chronic conjunctivitis, episcleritis, and necrotizing scleritis

Other tumors: Epibulbar choristoma, pagetoid sebaceous gland carcinoma, amelanotic and melanotic nevi, and melanoma

 5. Discuss and describe the management options of OSSN.

Management options for OSSN.

	Surgical excision	*Topical chemo/immunotherapy*
Advantages	• Smaller lesions (<4 mm) • Diagnostic and therapeutic • Frequent follow-ups avoided	• Treating entire ocular surface, corneal lesions • Multifocal and extensive lesions
Disadvantages	• High recurrence rate (30–56%) • Limbal stem cell deficiency (LSCD), symblepharon, conjunctival scarring	• Higher cost • Frequent follow-up • Adverse effects • Compliance • Longer time for resolution

- *Surgical excision*: Surgical removal of conjunctival lesions is carried out following the Shields' "no touch" technique to avoid the potential risk of seeding. The steps of surgical excision include the following:[1]

1	*Complete excision with 4 mm margin clearance:* Conjunctival incision is made approximately 4 mm outside the clinically determined tumor margin. The incision incorporates full-thickness conjunctiva and Tenon's fascia. Dissection is carried out in the episcleral plane (if there is no episcleral adhesion) to reach the limbus
2	*Lamellar sclerectomy (0.2–0.3 mm depth):* Thin lamellae of the tumor-free sclera, 0.2 mm in depth including 2.0 mm outside the adherent conjunctival mass is removed if scleral fixity is noted
3	*Alchohol keratoepitheliectomy (AKE) with 2 mm margin:* Absolute alcohol is applied with cotton-tipped applicator to the involved cornea to allow for controlled corneal epitheliectomy 2 mm outside the corneal component. The corneal epithelium is scrolled off to the limbus using a controlled sweeping motion with a beaver blade
4	The *entire tumor is removed in one piece* without touching the tumor by excising it along the limbus
5	*Base cryotherapy:* Cryotherapy, double freeze–thaw cycle, is applied to the edge of the remaining bulbar conjunctiva and the scleral base if there was episcleral adhesion. Limbal cryotherapy should be limited to 6 clock hours
6	*Closure of conjunctival defect* • Direct • Amniotic membrane graft • Dissection duration of >6 clock hours: Limbal stem cell deficiency (LSCD) can be prevented with intraoperative limbal epithelial transplantation

The reported recurrence rate of OSSN is 15–52%. Lee and Hirst reported a 17% recurrence after excision of conjunctival dysplasia, 40% after excision of CIN, and 30% for SCC of the conjunctiva. With adjunctive cryotherapy, the recurrent rate appears to be reduced from 28.5 and 50% after simple excision to 7.7 and 16.6% after excision with cryotherapy in primary and recurrence OSSN. Cryotherapy is known to decrease the recurrence rate by destruction of any residual tumor tissue beyond the horizontal or deep surgical margin of the wound. It has the advantage of reaching both tumor cell islands and deeply infiltrated cells, thus obviating the need for radical surgery.[6] It acts by directly destroying the tumor cells initially by lowering the temperature and later by obliteration of the microcirculation resulting in ischemic necrosis.[6] Cryotherapy may also act via an immunologic response to liberated tumor antigens, which may play a late role in ongoing policing of residual or recurrent tumor cells at a cellular level.[6] With the protocol-based technique as described above, the recurrence rate can be limited to <5%.[1]

Alternatively, to minimize the amount of tissue removed, a modified Mohs technique with intraoperative control of surgical margins has also been suggested.[5]

Enucleation or orbital exenteration is reserved for cases with intraocular or periocular invasion, respectively.

- *Topical chemo/immunotherapy:* Due to the relatively high rate of recurrence after surgical excision, various topical treatments have been advocated as a sole therapy for OSSN. Topical therapy offers a nonsurgical method for treating the entire ocular surface with less dependence on defining the tumor margin, potentially eliminating subclinical lesions. Topical treatment can offer a high drug concentration, avoiding systemic side effects. Furthermore, the increased stress, pain, and trauma associated with surgical procedures are avoided.

Indications for topical chemo-/immunotherapy in noninvasive OSSN:[1]
- >2 quadrants of conjunctival involvement
- >180° of limbal involvement
- Clear corneal extension encroaching the papillary axis
- Positive margin after excision
- Patient not fit for surgery

Commonly used topical chemotherapeutic agents:
- Mitomycin C (MMC)
- 5-Fluorouracil (5-FU)
- Interferons [recombinant human interferon alpha-2b (IFN-α2b)].

These agents can be used as primary treatment or with the adjunction of surgical resection—before (chemoreduction), intraoperatively, or after (chemopreventive) the procedure—to reduce the risk of recurrence.

Chemo/immunotherapeutic agents in OSSN:[1,8]

Drugs	Type	Mechanism of action	Formulation	Dosage	Adverse effects	Comments
MMC	Alkylating agent	Under aerobic condition generates free radicals Cytotoxicity → Lipid peroxidation → →Inhibition of DNA and protein synthesis →Inhibits cell migration and production of extracellular matrix	Topical: 0.02–0.04% drops	Four times a day for 1 week followed by 2–3 weeks off until the eye is quiet. Usually three to four cycles until resolution (alternative: 7–14 day cycles)	• Conjunctival hyperemia • Blepharospasm • Corneal punctate erosion • Punctal stenosis • Limbal stem cell deficiency	• Due to the risk of punctal stenosis, punctal plugs should be inserted prior to initiating topical MMC • The 2–3-week medication holiday in each cycle helps with patient comfort and compliance
5-FU	Pyrimidine analog	Inhibits thymidylate synthetase Inhibits production and incorporation of thymidine into DNA Inhibits RNA synthesis	Topical: 1% drops	Four times a day for 1 week with 3 weeks off (alternative: Four times daily for 2 days to 4 weeks)	• Eyelid erythema • Conjunctival hyperemia • Corneal punctate erosion	• To reduce symptoms, topical corticosteroids are used in conjunction with preservative free artificial tears • Punctal or canalicular stenosis can occur with systemic 5-FU treatment but not with topical 5-FU use
IFN α-2b	Type 1 IFN	Immune-mediated suppression of IL-10 stimulates IL-2 and IFN-γ m RNA Antiproliferative Antiviral • Immunotherapy: Widely used as a primary modality for unresectable extensive tumors • Immunoreduction: Helps in reducing the tumor size, ideally followed by complete excision of the residual tumor. Immunomodulation: The long-term use of topical IFN helps to prevent recurrence	Topical: 1 MIU/mL (alternative: 2–3 MIU/mL) Subconjunctival injections 1 million IU/mL 3 million IU/mL 10 million IU/mL (alternative: 10 MIU/month)	Topical: Four times a day drops continuously Subconjunctival: Weekly injections until resolution (typically 4–5 weeks)	Hyperemia and follicular conjunctivitis have infrequently been reported along with formation of epithelial microcysts • Flu-like malaise with injections • To lessen the severity of the side effects, 1 g of oral acetaminophen is administered at the time of the injection and then as needed until symptoms resolve	• Ease of use • Minimal side effects • More side effects (e.g., flu-like symptoms) • Benefits of decreased out-of-pocket costs (because the medication is usually covered by insurers) • Quicker resolution • No need for compounding • Assured compliance
Cidofovir	Antiviral agent with activity against double-stranded DNA viruses	Incorporation of the molecule into replicating DNA, where it causes direct DNA damage and promotes cellular apoptosis	2.5 mg/mL topical			Encouraging efficacy as secondary treatment in multirefractory OSSN

(DNA: deoxyribonucleic acid; 5-FU: 5-fluorouracil; IFN α-2b: interferon alpha-2b; IL-10: interleukin 10; MMC: mitomycin C; OSSN: ocular surface squamous neoplasia; RNA: ribonucleic acid)

Comparison of commonly used chemo/immunotherapeutic drugs in OSSN.

	Interferon alpha-2B	5-FU	MMC	Result
Complete resolution	95% (75–100%)	91% (82–100)	90%	Similar
Recurrence	4–20%	0–28%	Average 20%	Similar
Adverse effects	15%	42%	76%	MMC > 5-FU > IFN
Time to resolution	3.5–4 months	1.25 months	4 months	MMC = IFN >5-FU
Cost per cycle	500$	37$	300$	IFN > MMC >5-FU

(5-FU: 5-fluorouracil; IFN: interferon; MMC: mitomycin C)

Radiotherapy[1,3]

Two forms of radiotherapy are employed for conjunctival tumors, namely external beam radiotherapy and custom-designed plaque radiotherapy. External beam radiotherapy to a total dose of 3,000–4,000 cGy is used to treat conjunctival lymphoma and metastatic carcinoma when they are too large or diffuse to excise locally. Side effects of dry eye, punctate epithelial abnormalities, and cataract should be anticipated.

Custom-designed plaque radiotherapy to a dose of 3,000–4,000 cGy can be used to treat conjunctival lymphoma or metastasis. A higher dose of 6,000–8,000 cGy can be employed to treat the more radiation-resistant melanoma and SCC. In general, plaque radiotherapy is reserved for those patients who have diffuse tumors that are incompletely resected and for those who display multiple recurrences. The two designs for conjunctival custom plaque radiotherapy include a conformer plaque technique with six fractionated treatment sessions as an outpatient or a reverse plaque technique with the device sutured onto the episcleral as an inpatient.

Plaque brachytherapy (ruthenium-106) is used to control gross or microscopic residual tumors where deep sclerocorneal invasion precludes complete excision. In such cases of invasive disease, brachytherapy or proton beam radiotherapy can be used in the attempt to salvage the eyeball.

6. Discuss the tumor, node, metastasis (TNM) staging of OSSN.

Tumor staging is assessed using the TNM definitions, as stated in the American Joint Committee on Cancer (AJCC) recommendations, with T describing features of the primary tumor, N describing involvement of the regional nodes, and M describing the spread of distant metastasis.

The eighth edition of the AJCC classification has been recently released, and the definitions for T1 and T2 differ from those in the seventh edition. In the seventh edition, the definition of T1 and T2 was based solely on the tumor size, whereas in the eighth edition T classification is based both on the tumor size (≤5 or >5 mm) and the invasiveness of the basement membrane and adjacent structures, namely fornix, plica semilunaris, caruncle, eyelid lamellae, orbit, sinuses bone, and brain.[5]

TNM staging	Definition
Primary tumor (T)	
TX	Cannot assess the primary tumor
T0	No evidence of primary tumor
Tis	Carcinoma in situ
T1	Tumor (<5 mm in greatest dimension) invades through the basement membrane without invasion of adjacent structures*
T2	Tumor (<5 mm in greatest dimension) invades through the basement membrane with invasion of adjacent structures*
T3	Tumor invades adjacent structures excluding the orbit
T4	Tumor invades orbit with or without further extension
T4a	Tumor invades orbital soft tissues without bone invasion
T4b	Tumor invades the bone
T4c	Tumor invades adjacent paranasal sinuses
T4d	Tumor invades the brain

Contd...

Contd...

Lymph node (N)	
NX	Regional lymph nodes cannot be assessed
N0	Regional lymph node metastasis absent
N1	Regional lymph node metastasis present
Systemic metastasis (M)	
M0	No distant metastasis
M1	Distant metastasis
Histopathologic grade (G)	
GX	Grade cannot be assessed
G1	Well differentiated
G2	Moderately differentiated
G3	Poorly differentiated
G4	Undifferentiated

*Adjacent structures in all cases include the cornea, forniceal/palpebral/tarsal conjunctiva, intraocular chambers, caruncle and plica semilunaris, lacrimal puncta and canaliculi, anterior/posterior eyelid lamellae, and eyelid margin.

 7. Discuss the drawbacks of TNM classification and enumerate a new proposed clinical classification of OSSN/Discuss stage-based protocol management of OSSN.

More recent statistics based on either the seventh or the eighth edition have revealed that only a few lesions presented as in situ, while the majority of the cases fell cumulatively in the T3 or T4 category. This can be explained by the fact that OSSN often grows with limbus involvement, shifting the lesion directly to the T3 category, notwithstanding a small dimension. Another limitation of the TNM classification is the inclusion of those lesions with intraocular extension into the T3 category, even though they require enucleation for tumor control, rather than local excision. To overcome these drawbacks of the TNM classification, a new clinical-based classification scheme has been proposed which provides general advice for tumor management.

New clinical classification proposed for ocular surface squamous neoplasia.[5]

Grade	Limbal involvement (clock hours)	Maximal basal diameter (mm)	Treatment
Grade I: Ocular surface squamous neoplasia (OSSN) with no invasion into ocular coats clinically and on imaging*			
A (small)	≤3	≤5	Surgical excision with margin control
B (large)	>3 to <6	>5 to <15	Immunotherapy or immunoreduction
C (diffuse)	≥6	≥15	Immunoreduction
Grade II: OSSN with invasion into ocular coats (sclera/corneal stroma) on imaging*			
	Any	Any	Excision with lamellar sclerectomy or keratectomy + cryotherapy of margins and base with plaque brachytherapy
Grade III: OSSN with intraocular invasion			
	Any	Any	Enucleation
Grade IV: OSSN with intraorbital extension†			
	Any	Any	Exenteration

*Imaging in grades I and II relies on ultrasound biomicroscopy.
†Confirmed by computed tomography or magnetic resonance imaging.

Clinical Course and Prognosis of Ocular Surface Squamous Neoplasia

Carcinoma of the ocular surface is generally regarded as low-grade malignancy. Overall, OSSN has a good/fair prognosis, with little tendency to metastasize and a low mortality rate. Recurrences take place most frequently within the first 6 months after resection. Recurrent lesions tend to be of the same histologic grade as the primary tumor and generally do not demonstrate progressive malignant change.

Recurrence rate is closely dependent on:
- Involvement of surgical margins
- Presence of feeder vessels
- HIV infection status
- Histopathologic grade
- Availability of adjunctive therapies, such as cryotherapy, immunotherapy, or chemotherapy
- Irritation as a presenting symptom as well as corneal location was also identified as risk factors for recurrence.

Recently, the overexpression of the tumor-suppressor gene *p16INK4a* has been identified as a biomarker of diffuse growth pattern, early age of presentation <50 years, and metastasization in late T stages.

References

1. Honavar SG, Manjandavida FP. Tumors of the ocular surface: a review. Indian J Ophthalmol. 2015;63(3):187.
2. Gupta S, Sinha R, Sharma N, Titiyal JS. Ocular surface squamous neoplasia. Off Sci J Delhi Ophthalmol Soc. 2012;23(2):89-96.
3. Shields CL, Shields JA. Tumors of the conjunctiva and cornea. Surv Ophthalmol. 2004;49(1):3-24.
4. Tananuvat N, Lertprasertsuke N. Ocular surface squamous neoplasia. Intraepithelial Neoplasia. London: InTech; 2012. pp. 35-62.
5. Cicinelli MV, Marchese A, Bandello F, Modorati G. Clinical management of ocular surface squamous neoplasia: a review of the current evidence. Ophthalmol Ther. 2018;7(2):247-62.
6. Lee GA, Hirst LW. Ocular surface squamous neoplasia. Surv Ophthalmol. 1995;39(6):429-50.
7. Bhadduri A. AIOS Ready Reckoner, 2nd edition, Ocular Surface Squamous Neoplasia. p. 15.
8. Al Bayyat G, Arreaza-Kaufman D, Venkateswaran N, Galor A, Karp CL. Update on pharmacotherapy for ocular surface squamous neoplasia. Eye Vision. 2019;6(1):1-2.

Neuro-ophthalmology

2.1 Cranial Nerve Palsy

Gunjan Saluja

 1. Discuss third cranial nerve (CN) palsy—etiology, clinical feature, and management.

Etiology

The common etiologies of third nerve palsy include vascular ischemia, trauma, intracranial neoplasm, hemorrhage, and idiopathic. Ischemic changes arising from a microvascular disorder such as diabetes mellitus and hypertension are the most common systemic causes of acquired third nerve palsy. However, the etiology and presentation of acquired third nerve palsy vary at different levels (*See* **Figure 9** of Section 2.3.1 *Anatomy and Physiology*).

- *Supranuclear lesions:* Lesions at the level of the cerebral cortex or the supranuclear pathway cause conjugate paresis of both the eyes.
- *Nuclear lesions and fascicular lesions:* Vascular diseases, demyelination, and tumors are the main cause of third nerve palsy at this level.
- *Basilar portion:* The primary causes of isolated palsy in this level chiefly include aneurysms, diabetes mellitus, and extradural hematoma. Aneurysms arising from the posterior communicating artery, posterior cerebral artery, or superior cerebellar artery can cause compression of the third nerve. Extradural hematoma results in a tentorial pressure cone and herniation of the temporal lobe. The third nerve gets compressed by the herniation as it passes over the tentorial edge, leading to third nerve palsy.
- *Intracavernous portion:* A large number of CNs lie in the vicinity of the third nerve in the cavernous sinus, hence pathologies of the cavernous sinus in diabetes, pituitary apoplexy, aneurysm, or carotid cavernous fistula result in multiple nerve palsies of the CN IV, CN VI, and the first division of CN V.
- *Intraorbital portion:* Trauma, tumors, and Tolosa-Hunt syndrome are the main causes of intraorbital third nerve palsy.

Third nerve palsy in children: Most cases of third nerve palsy in children are congenital, other causes of third nerve palsy besides this include local inflammation, trauma, aneurysm, and ophthalmoplegic migraine.

Clinical Features

Symptoms

Patients with third nerve palsy present with complaints of:
- *Diplopia:* Patients present with symptoms of acute onset diplopia along with drooping of eyelids, which can be horizontal or vertical. However, sometimes patients may not appreciate diplopia due to severe ptosis. Fixed dilated pupil due to the involvement of efferent fibers of the pupillary pathway can lead to glare.
- *Headache:* The presence of severe headache and orbital pain is usually associated with aneurysm and inflammation.
- *Other associated features:* Although rare, the patient may complain of difficulty in reading, protrusion of the eye, chemosis, headache, pain, and vomiting. Other accompanying neurological features can be present which include contralateral hemiparesis in Weber's syndrome, contralateral tremors in Benedict syndrome, and ipsilateral ataxia in Nothnagel syndrome **(Fig. 1)**.

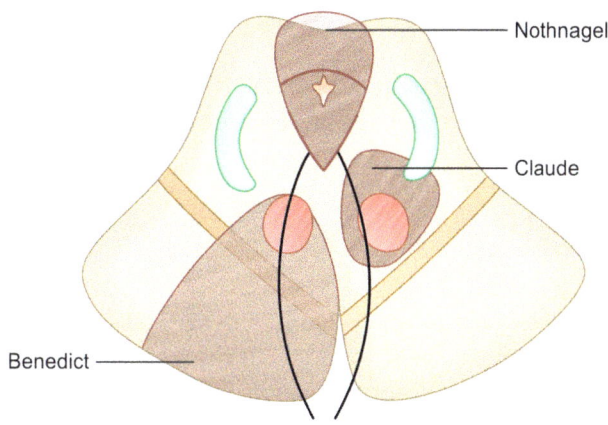

Fig. 1: Benedikt's syndrome, Weber syndrome, and Nothnagel syndrome.

Systemic History

It is important to rule out the systemic history of coronary artery disease, hypertension, and diabetes mellitus. History of trauma and history of central nervous tumor, radiation should be ruled out. Recurrent episodes of oculomotor nerve palsy can be noted in patients of diabetes mellitus and ophthalmoplegic migraine.

Signs

Ocular Examination

- *Visual acuity:* Visual acuity, especially for near, can be reduced due to the involvement of the pupil.
- *Ptosis:* Ptosis in third nerve palsy occurs due to the involvement of levator palpebrae superioris (LPS) and is usually severe.
- *Extraocular movements:* The eyes are fixed in a down and out position. This occurs due to palsy of the medial rectus (MR), superior rectus (SR), inferior rectus (IR), and inferior oblique (IO). It is due to the unopposed action of superior oblique (SO) and lateral rectus (LR) that the eyes are fixed in a down and out position.
- *Pupil:* The pupil must be carefully examined in a case of third nerve palsy as it gives an insight into the etiology. Accordingly, third nerve palsy can be broadly classified as pupil involving or pupil sparing. Pupil involving third nerve palsy usually is seen in patients with aneurysm and intracranial space-occupying lesions, as the pupilomotor fibers are present on the outer surface of the oculomotor nerve, on the contrary, microvascular ischemic causes result in pupil-sparing third nerve palsy, due to involvement of the vasa nervorum.
- *Aberrant regeneration in third nerve palsy:* Change in the actions of muscles supplied by the third nerve can occur due to regrowth of damaged nerve fibers following complete or severe third nerve palsy. It is more likely to occur when the endoneurial sheath has been breached by trauma, tumor, or an aneurysm. It may occur from weeks to months after the onset of the third nerve paresis.
  - *Pseudo-Von Graefe's sign:* Elevation of the upper eyelid on downward gaze or adduction
  - Adduction of the eye on attempted upward or downward gaze
  - Limitation of elevation and depression of the eye with retraction of the globe on attempted vertical movement
  - *"Pseudo-Argyll Robertson pupil":* Greater constriction of the pupil to convergence than to light and gaze-evoked pupillary constriction
- *Binocular function:* Binocular function can be assessed with Worth's four dot test and Bagolini's striated glass test after neutralization of deviation. The binocular function is usually absent in congenital and early age onset third CN palsy with a large angle of deviation. Those with late-onset and in partial third CN palsy binocular function are usually intact.
- *Diplopia charting:* Diplopia charting can be done using red–green glasses by projecting a streak of light on the testing screen at 1 meter. It measures horizontal, vertical, and torsional misalignments simultaneously and is valuable in determining the surgical approach by assessing the different contributions in the cardinal positions of gaze.
- *Hess chart:* The affected eye shows a markedly constricted field whereas the contralateral eye demonstrates overaction of its muscles.
- *Forced duction test:* Forced duction test (FDT) is a clinical test, which should be done preoperatively to reveal any restriction, and is thus vital for surgical planning. The test is typically performed under topical anesthesia, the conjunctiva

is held at limbus with Pierce Hoskin forceps or globe-holding forceps, and the patient is asked to look in the opposite direction of testing muscle to relax the concerned muscle.
- *Active force generation test:* Active force generation test (AFGT) is done under topical anesthesia by asking the patient to look in the direction of the muscle being tested; the presence of a tug is suggestive of residual action in the paralytic muscle.

Investigations

Neuroimaging

Imaging is indicated in all cases with age <50 years and patients with age >50 years, without any comorbidities, in patients with associated symptoms such as headache, nausea, vomiting, in cases of pupil involving third nerve palsy, ocular pain, proptosis, papilledema, loss of corneal sensation, history of trauma and nonresolving or worsening of palsy. A wide range of life-threatening causes (e.g., aneurysm) can be there hence a low threshold should be adopted for neuroimaging. Computed tomography (CT) angiography is usually the preferred modality by most physicians and helps to rule out an aneurysm. Newer modalities such as magnetic resonance imaging (MRI) brain and orbits with venography can provide additional information.

Blood Investigations

Erythrocyte sedimentation rate (ESR), C-reactive protein (CRP), complete blood count (CBC), blood sugar, lipid profile, blood pressure, and homocysteine levels help in the assessment of vascular risk factors assessment.

Lumbar Puncture

Lumbar puncture may be required after ruling out space-occupying lesion if a rare etiology such as infection (e.g., syphilis, Lyme disease) or vasculitis (including giant cell arteritis) is suspected.

Management

Observation

- Simple observation is appropriate in presumed microvascular cases, and a majority of the cases show signs of recovery at 2 weeks and recover by 3–6 months.
- During the observation period to avoid diplopia, temporary prisms can be useful if the angle of deviation is small. Uniocular occlusion with an eye patch or opaque contact lens may be necessary to avoid diplopia if the ptosis component is partial or recovering.
- Young children should be treated with alternate patching to prevent amblyopia.
- Systemic control of diabetes and hypertension is essential to prevent further worsening.

Surgical Treatment

Surgical treatment of the ocular motility element and ptosis should be contemplated only after the spontaneous improvement has ceased, usually not earlier than 6–12 months from onset.

For the surgical purpose, it can be divided into three groups.
1. Complete third CN palsy supramaximal LR recession, periosteal fixation of LR, transposition of LR to MR, Scott procedure, Peter's procedure (SO to MR).
2. Partial third CN palsy MR resection and LR recession (adjustable procedure for the co-operative patient), vertical transposition of SR and IR to MR, surgeries on SR, and IR for correction of vertical deviation.
3. Aberrant regeneration to LPS to do surgery on the normal eye which takes the advantage of fixation duress for correction of ptosis, and same side surgery may worsen the same.

Botulinum toxin: The role of botulinum toxin in the management of acute or chronic third-nerve paresis has not been adequately investigated. Toxin injection into the uninvolved LR muscle is sometimes used to prevent its contracture when recovery time is prolonged.

Flowchart 1 summarizes the management algorithm of third nerve palsy.

Q 2. Discuss clinical features and management of third nerve palsy.

Same as the above Answer.

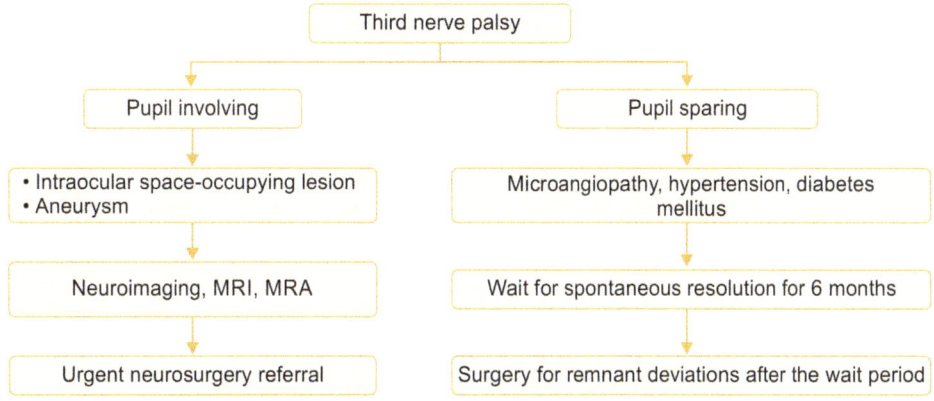

Flowchart 1: The management algorithm of third nerve palsy.

(MRA: magnetic resonance angiography; MRI: magnetic resonance imaging)

Q 3. Discuss anatomy of third, fourth, sixth cranial nerve, and enumerate the lesions of each nucleus.

Refer to the anatomy Chapter.

Q 4. Explain causes, investigations, and management of acute onset third nerve palsy.

Same as the above Answer.

Q 5. Fourth cranial nerve palsy—

- A 27-year-old driver developed left eye hypertropia following an accident. How will you diagnose and manage him?
- Describe pathway of the fourth cranial nerve. Enumerate the causes of fourth nerve palsy (acquired) with respect to the site of affections.

Etiology of Fourth Nerve Palsy

- *Congenital:* Idiopathic lesions are common, and many of these remain asymptomatic until decompensation occurs in adult life due to reduced fusional ability.
- Acquired
- *Trauma:* Closed head trauma usually results in bilateral fourth nerve palsy.
- Microvascular ischemic causes such as diabetes hypertension can also lead to fourth nerve palsy. Tumor and aneurysm are other relatively less common causes of fourth nerve palsy.

Clinical Features

Symptoms

- The patients usually present with complaints of sudden onset hypertropia associated with vertical diplopia which is worse in downgaze and head posture.
- The age of onset helps to differentiate between congenital and acquired fourth nerve palsy, past photographs can be useful for documentation of head posture.

- Birth history should be thoroughly taken to rule out birth trauma.
- Amblyopia in the congenital cases is rarely seen due to the presence of a head posture.
- History of trauma and systemic illness such as diabetes mellitus and hypertension must be ruled out (*See* **Figure 10** of Section 2.3.1 *Anatomy and Physiology*).

Signs

- *Ocular examination:*
  - *Visual acuity:* Vision may be reduced in congenital cases due to amblyopia.
  - *Facial asymmetry and abnormal head posture:* A compensatory head posture is adapted by the patients to avoid diplopia. The functions of SO muscle include intorsion, depression, and abduction, therefore, to compensate for each of these, there is a characteristic head posture. For example, in a case of right superior oblique paresis (SOP), the held tilt would be toward the left shoulder to compensate for in torsion, chin depression is present to compensate for depression action and there will be face turn to the same side to compensate for abduction. In bilateral cases since intorsion and abduction of both the eyes is affected there is no head tilt or face turn unless the involvement is asymmetrical.
- *Facial asymmetry:* Persistent abnormal head posture in cases of congenital IV nerve palsy can lead to facial asymmetry. Facial asymmetry arising due to premature fusion of the coronal axis (plagiocephaly) on one side results in the retro placement of trochlea, making the SO muscle more parallel to the coronal than the sagittal axis (de-sagittalization) and causes laxity of the SO tendon thus reducing all of its action.
- *Extraocular movements:* A limitation of depression in adduction is noted, and can be associated with IO overaction (over-elevation in adduction).
- *Cover test:* The strabismus examination should be performed after correcting the compensatory head posture. The affected eye shows a hyperdeviation and an associated esodeviation. There will be hypertropia of the affected eye which increases on opposite gaze and same side head tilt, also known as Park's three-step test.
- *Park's three step test:* The test is illustrated with the example of right SOP. The test helps to identify the paralyzed cyclovertical muscle.

  Step 1: To assess which eye is hypertrophic in the primary gaze, in case of right hypertropia, the following muscles could be involved:
  - Depressors of the right eye, i.e., SO and IR causing hypertropia of the right eye.
  - Elevators of the left eye, i.e., SR or IO causing hypotropia of the left eye.

  Step 2: To assess which lateral direction worsens hypertropia—If the right hypertropia increases on the left, gaze implicates a right SO or left SR involvement. An increase in the hypertropia in the right gaze implicates that either the right IR or left IO is involved. In this case, the deviation will be worse in opposite gaze, so now from four muscles, we have zeroed down to two muscles left SO or right SR deviation.

  Step 3: Bielschowsky's head tilt test—The head-tilt test is performed with the patient fixating at a straight ahead target at 3 meters.

  On head-tilt test, the hypertropia worsens on right tilt due to overaction of right SR muscle. On the tilting, the head the eye toward the shoulder intorts and elevates, as the SO is paralyzed the SR needs to overact to bring about the desired intorsion, which is accompanied by elevation. Thus, worsening the hypertropia on the same side head tilt.

  In patients with bilateral SO palsy, there is alternate hypertropia in adduction.

  Other features of bilateral SO palsy:
  - Right hypertropia in left gaze and left hypertropia in right gaze, though orthophoria may be present in primary position with more than 10° of cyclodeviation (measured using double Maddox rods or by synoptophore)
  - "V" pattern esotropia is often present.
  - Bilaterally positive Bielschowsky's head tilt test
  - Chin down position.
- *Hess charting:* The affected eye will show a markedly constricted field whereas the other eye demonstrates overaction of the yoke muscles. In a patient of recently acquired left fourth nerve palsy would have the following abnormalities, the chart of the left eye with right eye fixing will be smaller than the right, with a left chart showing underaction of the SO and overaction of the IO.

- *Evaluation of torsion:* Unilateral fourth nerve palsy is characterized by <8° of cyclodeviation while bilateral cases may have >10° of cyclodeviation.

    Torsion can be measured objectively and subjectively. Objectively the torsion can be measured by fundus photography and indirect ophthalmoscopy.

    Subjectively torsion can be measured by synaptophore, Bagolini's striated glasses, and double Maddox rod test.
- *Fundus photography and indirect ophthalmoscopy:* Normally, the fovea is located between the two horizontal lines, one passing through the center of the disc and the other cutting the lower pole of the disc tangentially. The usual location is in the middle of these two horizontal lines, in cases of SO palsy because of extorsion there is downward displacement.
- *Maddox rod:*
    - *Double Maddox rod test:* Maddox rods contain a series of horizontal cylinders, and are placed one in front of either eye. Each eye will therefore perceive the vertical line of light. In the presence of cyclodeviation, the line perceived by the paretic eye will be tilted and, therefore, distinct from that of the other eye. One Maddox rod is then rotated until till both lines become parallel to each other. The amount of rotation can be measured in degrees and indicates the amount of cyclodeviation.
- *Field charting:* Vertical displacement of blind spot suggests torsion.
- *Forced duction test:* Exaggerated FDT, described by Guyton, is done to look for laxity on the SO tendon. The globe is grasped with Pierce Hoskin's forceps in the superior temporal and inferonasal quadrant. The globe is retracted inside the orbit and the eye is elevated and adducted. The globe is rocked in the intorsion and extorsion movement. A normal taut SO tendon will cause the globe to pop up during this maneuver and a click is felt by the examiner. It is always imperative to compare it with another eye to differentiate between the normal and lax tendons. To test tension in the IO muscle—the globe is grasped inferotemporal and superonasal quadrant and is then retracted, depressed, and adducted.
- *Checking fourth cranial nerve function in the third palsy:* A limbal or conjunctival landmark is noted and the patient is asked to look down, but due to the palsy of IR, the patient will not be able to look down in abduction, however, as the SO is functioning, intortion will be present, which can be noted from the conjunctival landmark, suggesting that the fourth CN is intact.

Investigations

- Blood investigations to rule out risk factors such as diabetes, hypertension, and other cause of microangiopathy should be done.
- Neuroimaging is required only when it is associated with other neurological signs.

Management

Observation

Congenital decompensated and presumed microvascular palsies commonly resolve spontaneously. All patients are seen every 1–2 months while being monitored for stability/recovery. Unilateral cases of vascular origin usually recover within 6 months. Small-unrecovered deviations with vertical/horizontal diplopia can be managed long-term by incorporating prisms into spectacles.

Surgical Management

The surgical management of SO palsy depends upon the following factors:
- Laxity of SO tendon
- Presence of IO overaction
- Amount of deviation in primary position
- The gaze of maximum deviation.

    The algorithm for the management of SO palsy has been summarized in **Flowchart 2**.

6. Discuss management of unilateral and bilateral fourth nerve palsy.

Flowchart 2: Management of superior oblique palsy.

```
Vertical diplopia
      ↓
Park's three step test (maximum hypertropia on contralateral head tilt)
      ↓
Head posture in previous childhood pictures
      ├──────── Absent ────────┬──────── Present ────────┐
      ↓                                                   ↓
Low vertical fusional vergence              High vertical fusional vergence
      ↓                                                   ↓
Acquired superior oblique palsy             Congenital superior oblique palsy
      ↓                                                   ↓
                                            Management by Knapp's classification
      ↓                                                   ↓
Age <40 years                               Age >40 years
      ↓                                                   ↓
Imaging to rule out space-occupying lesion  Risk factors of mononeuropathy
                                              ├── Present ──┬── Absent ──┐
                                              ↓                          ↓
                                            Observe                   Imaging
```

	Hypertropia worse on adduction and upgaze	Right inferior oblique weakening
	Hypertropia worse on adduction and downgaze	Right superior oblique strengthening (tuck)
	Hypertropia worse on abduction	• Tuck superior oblique, if RHT <25 PD • Tuck superior oblique, with inferior oblique weakening, if RHT >25 PD
	Hypertropia worse on abduction and downgaze	• First procedure, tuck right superior oblique, with inferior oblique weakening • Second procedure, strengthen right inferior rectus
	Hypertropia worse on downgaze, abduction and adduction	Tuck right superior oblique, or weaken left inferior rectus
	Bilateral superior oblique palsy	Bilateral superior oblique tuck
	Traumatic palsy, Brown's plus syndrome	

For right superior oblique palsy
(PD: prism diopter; RHT: right hypertropia)

7. Discuss sixth cranial nerve palsy—management options in a case of lateral rectus palsy with visually disabling diplopia.

Etiology

The four most common causes are idiopathic (26%), hypertension (19%), coexistent diabetes and hypertension (12%), and trauma (12%).

The etiologies of sixth nerve palsy can be broadly classified into congenital and acquired causes:
- *Congenital:*
  - Following birth trauma
  - Hereditary
  - Infection (maternal)
  - Failure of LR development
  - Mobius syndrome (sixth nerve palsy with accompanying seventh nerve palsy)
- *Acquired:* The common acquired causes are:
  - Trauma
  - Space-occupying lesions
  - Infections, bacterial, or viral
  - Raised intracranial pressure
  - Postviral inflammation
  - Multiple sclerosis
  - Diabetes
  - Ophthalmoplegic migraine

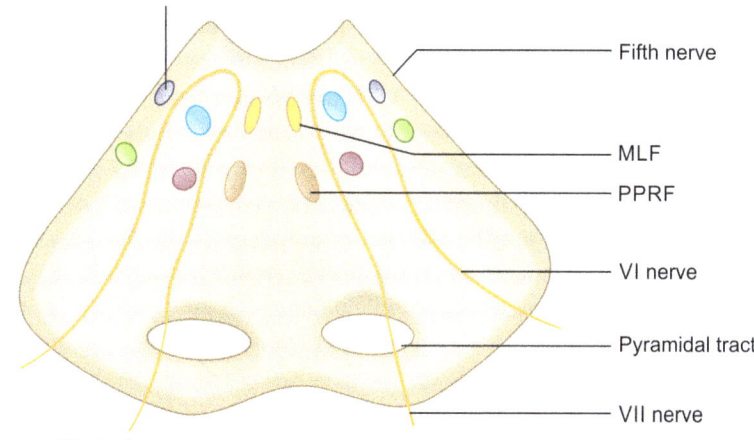

Fig. 2: Millard–Gubler and Foville syndrome. (CN: cranial nerve; MLF: median longitudinal fasciculus; PPRF: posterior pontine reticular formation; SOF: superior orbital fissure)

- In older adults, vascular lesions such as diabetes, hypertension, space-occupying lesions, and senile LR weakness can lead to sixth nerve palsy.
- *False localizing signs:* Raised intracranial pressure can cause stretching one or both sixth nerves due to their long intracranial course or the compression against the petrous tip resulting in sixth nerve palsy.
- *Foville syndrome (Fig. 2):* Foville (inferior medial pontine) syndrome results from vascular disease or tumors involving the dorsal pons and is characterized by the sixth nerve paresis, horizontal conjugate gaze palsy, ipsilateral V, VII, VIII CN palsy, and ipsilateral Horner's syndrome.
- *Millard–Gubler syndrome (MGS) (ventral pontine syndrome):* MGS most frequently is caused by vascular diseases, tumors, or demyelination. In addition to ipsilateral sixth nerve palsy, there is contralateral hemiplegia and often an ipsilateral lower motor neuron (LMN) facial nerve palsy.

Symptoms

In acquired cases, the patient presents with acute onset horizontal diplopia.
History of diabetes mellitus, hypertension, viral infections, immunization, and neurosurgery must be noted, as they help to find the underlying cause.

Ocular Examination

- *Head posture:* The patient with sixth nerve palsy typically acquires a face turn on the ipsilateral side. Face turn in congenital cases may prevent amblyopia and maintain binocular single vision and can be confirmed by looking at the previous pictures.
- *Extraocular movements:* Ocular motility examination reveals the presence of severe limitation of abduction.
- *Fundus examination:* Besides the anterior segment examination, it is essential to carry a fundus examination to look for papilledema.
- *Past pointing:* Past pointing indicates recent onset. It can be tested by asking the patient to point with his finger the object viewed by the paretic eye (hand-eye coordination) with a septum not allowing him to have visual feedback to correct the coordination due to paresis. In the presence of paresis, extra innervation is required for a movement in the direction of

the field of action of the paretic muscle which is perceived by the brain as if the object is located farther than it is, giving extra-innervation to the hand for pointing. This causes past pointing.
- *Diplopia charting:* The subjective deviation is recorded by asking the subject to quantify the separation between the double images, which are dissociated by red-green glasses. This is repeated in all the nine diagnostic positions. In paralytic strabismus, the separation is maximal in the field of action of the paretic muscle.
- *Hess and Lee's chart:* Hess and Lee's chart also reveals the presence of limitation of abduction and a smaller square of the affected eye.
- *Forced duction test:* The FDT is done to look in mechanical restriction due to MR. Under the topical anesthesia, the examiner passively moves the patient's eye in the direction opposite to that in which mechanical restriction is suspected. For example, in a case of right LR limitation, there may be a contracture of the right MR. After the topical anesthesia, the medial limbal conjunctiva is grasped firmly with a toothed forceps and the globe is lifted from the orbit. The patient is asked to look in abduction so that the MR is relaxed. The examiner then tries to passively move the eye in the abduction.

    Care must be taken not to abrade the cornea. If the examiner can successfully manage to move the eye until the lateral limbus touches the lateral canthus that means that there is no mechanical restriction and, the motility defect is caused by paralysis of the LR muscle. If resistance is encountered, it means that the FDT is positive, mechanical restrictions do exist medially which may be due to contracture of the MR muscle, conjunctiva, or Tenon's capsule.

    Important causes for MR contracture include thyroid eye disease, entrapment of medial contents after fracture, myositis, and cysticercosis. Some patients initially have pure nerve palsy, but contracture of the antagonist muscle results in secondary mechanical restriction of movement. FDT can be falsely negative if the globe is not lifted out of the orbit while performing the test for recti muscle and if not depressed inside the orbit while performing the test for oblique muscles.
- *Active force generation test:* Active force generation test is used to evaluate the ability of a muscle to move the eye against a resisting force. After topical anesthesia, the paralytic muscle is held with the fixation forceps and the patient is asked to look in the direction of the limited duction; the amount of force generated by the muscle is felt as a tug by the examiner. The test should be repeated in the other eye for the comparison of the forces.

Investigations

Neuroimaging

Neuroimaging is essential in patients with acute onset sixth nerve palsy, without any underlying systemic disorder and in patients with papilledema, to rule out intracranial space-occupying lesion.

Management

Conservative Management

- Conservative management and observation form the first line of management and include systemic control of diabetes and hypertension.
- Use of a patch, or an opaque-colored cosmetic contact lens to avoid diplopia
- Prisms can be advised in the management of patients with a small angle of deviation, up to 14 prism diopter (PD).

Surgical Management

Surgical management is indicated in patients with no signs of recovery even after 6 months.

The management depends upon FDT and AFGT.

The algorithm has been summarized in **Flowchart 3**.

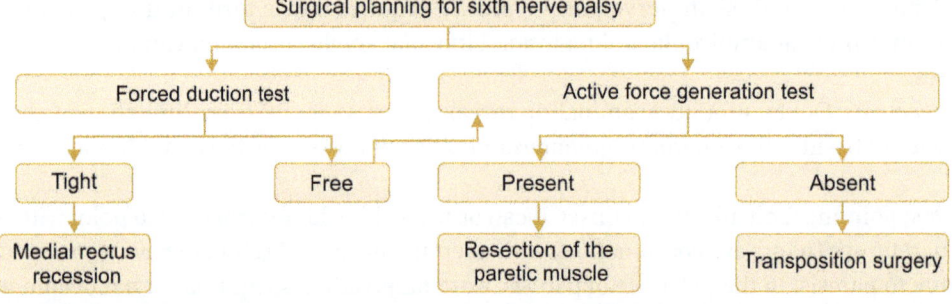

Flowchart 3: Surgical management algorithm for sixth nerve palsy.

2.2 Ocular Myopathies

Gunjan Saluja

Q 1. Discuss clinical features and diagnostic tests of ocular myasthenia, important differential diagnosis and points to differentiate, or etiology, types, clinical picture, differential diagnosis, and management of myasthenia gravis.

Introduction

A neuromuscular junction abnormality arises from the antibody-mediated autoimmune reaction on postsynaptic acetylcholine (Ach) receptors or altered release of presynaptic Ach **(Fig. 1)**.

The various neuromuscular junction abnormalities include:
- Myasthenia gravis
- Lambert–Eaton syndrome
- Botulism
- Organophosphate toxicity.

Of all the neuromuscular junction abnormalities stated above, myasthenia gravis is the most common and results from the formation of autoantibodies against the postsynaptic Ach receptors, ophthalmic manifestations of myasthenia gravis include ptosis and diplopia and are characterized by diurnal variation, with symptoms improving at rest and worsening on long hours of work.

Etiopathogenesis

The disease dates back to 1879 when Erb gave the first detailed description of the disease.

Myasthenia gravis has two peaks, the first peak occurs in second to the third decade, and the second peak occurs in sixth to the seventh decade, the disease most commonly affects females. It is frequently thymic hyperplasia, which is thought to be the source of autoantibodies, HLA-B7 and HLA-DR2 have a positive association with myasthenia.

Physiology of Neuromuscular Junction

The neuromuscular junction consists of a large myelinated nerve fiber ending to a skeletal muscle fiber, the nerve fiber forms a complex of branching nerve terminals, which invaginates into the surface of muscle fiber and lies outside the muscle fiber plasma membrane, the entire structure is called motor end plate and the space between the nerve terminal and muscle fiber membrane is called the synaptic cleft.

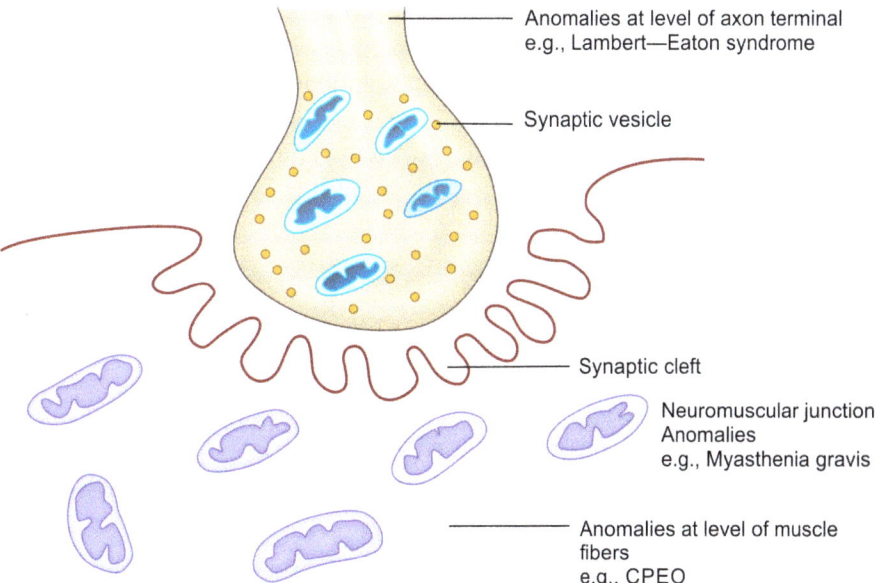

Fig. 1: Neuromuscular junction and the anomalies. (CPEO: chronic progressive external ophthalmoplegia)

The axon terminal end has mitochondria which is the main source of adenosine triphosphate (ATP), which is needed for the synthesis of Ach; Ach is synthesized in the axonal cytoplasm and is absorbed rapidly into the vesicles. When a nerve impulse reaches the neuromuscular junction, Ach is released in the synaptic space, which then binds with Ach receptors, which in turn causes a conformational change in the Ach-gated channels, allowing the sodium ions to enter the muscle fiber and to cause contraction of the muscle.

Pathogenesis

In myasthenia gravis, there is the formation of antibodies against Ach receptors in the neuromuscular junction, so that Ach fails to bind with its receptor resulting in the failure to initiate the opening of voltage-gated sodium channels, and muscle depolarization does not occur. A pure ocular form of the disease can exist, the characteristic features of extraocular muscles, such as rapid contraction and high-firing frequency of twitch fibers, make them vulnerable to the disease, besides extraocular muscle, muscles of mastication, and breathing are affected commonly.

Clinical Features

Symptoms

- Diplopia and ptosis are usually the first symptoms of the disease.
- The initial symptoms may be triggered after an emotional upset or upper respiratory tract infections or after pregnancy.
- The characteristic features of the disease are its diurnal variation, with the symptoms improving on waking up and worsening on fatigue and during evening hours.
- The generalized form of myasthenia gravis usually involves proximal muscles of the upper and lower limbs, as a result, the patient gives a typical history of difficulty in lifting heavy weights, combing hair, climbing stairs, and squatting.
- Other features of generalized myasthenia which involve 75% of patients include facial weakness, jaw weakness dysarthria, dysphagia, and erector spinae involvement that results in difficulty in maintaining an erect posture.

Signs

Ocular signs result from the involvement of mainly orbicularis oculi, levator palpebrae superioris, and extraocular muscles. Signs have been summarized in **Table 1**.

Systemic History

Myasthenia gravis, being an autoimmune disease, can be associated with other autoimmune diseases such as thyroid disease, systemic lupus erythematosus, neuromyelitis optic spectrum disorders, and pernicious anemia, which are found with increased frequency in patients with myasthenia gravis.

Investigations

- *Ach receptor antibody:* The test is 80% sensitive and is positive in only 50% of patients of ocular myasthenia, these patients with positive Ach receptor antibody are likely to have thymoma.
- *Antimuscle-specific kinase (anti-MuSK) antibody:* Anti-MuSK antibody can be positive in patients with negative Ach receptor antibody.
- Thoracic imaging (MR and CT) can be done to look for thymoma and also to rule out lung tumor if Lambert–Eaton syndrome is suspected.

TABLE 1: Signs for ocular myasthenia gravis.

Signs due to levator palpebrae superioris	• Ptosis • Cogan's lid twitch • Lid hopping
Signs due to orbicularis oculi involvement	• Peek sign • Weakness on forced closure
Signs due to extraocular muscle weakness	• Paresis of 3rd, 4th, and 6th nerve paresis (not following any particular pattern) • Gaze palsy • Complete ophthalmoplegia • End gaze nystagmus • Pseudo-internuclear ophthalmoplegia

- *Ice pack test:* A lower temperature inhibits the breakdown of Ach by acetylcholinesterase, as a result of which Ach concentration increases in the neuromuscular junction, as a result, it replaces the Ach receptor antibody and binds with the Ach receptors, thus improving the symptoms.

   In ice pack test, the ice pack is placed over the ptotic lid, for 2 minutes, clinical pictures are taken before and after the test, an improvement in the ptosis after 2 minutes indicates a positive ice pack test, which is around 75% sensitive.

- *Sleep test:* The sleep test is based on the principle of improvement of clinical signs of myasthenia after rest. The patient is asked to take rest for 30 minutes in a dark, silent room, clinical pictures of ptosis and extraocular movements are taken before and after 30 minutes, an improvement in clinical signs indicates a positive test.

- *Fatigue test:* The patient in this test is asked to look toward the wall for sometime, the worsening of clinical signs indicates a positive test.

- *Edrophonium test:* Edrophonium is a preferred agent for the diagnosis of myasthenia gravis, because its action is reversible and the drug is short-acting. An intravenous test dose of 0.2 mL (2 mg) edrophonium hydrochloride is given, if any allergic reaction or adverse reaction of the drug is noted, then the test is immediately terminated. If no adverse reaction is noted then the remaining 0.8 mL of the drug is injected after 60 seconds, heart rate and electrocardiogram of the patient must be continuously monitored.

   A second syringe containing 0.5–1 mg of atropine must be readily available to counteract the adverse reactions of edrophonium.

   Uncommon potential side effects include bradycardia and death; hence, resuscitation facilities must be available in case of emergency.

   Pre- and post-test deviation measurements and Hess charting can increase the sensitivity of this test.

- *Thyroid function test:* As myasthenia gravis can be associated with autoimmune thyroid disease, thyroid function tests must be done.

- *Repetitive nerve stimulation test:* The test shows a decrease in compound muscle action potential by 10% in the 4th or 5th response to a train of nerve stimuli.

- *Electromyography:* Electromyography (EMG) is performed over the deltoid muscle in generalized myasthenia and over orbicularis oculi, levator palpebrae superioris muscle in ocular myasthenia cases, EMG in myasthenia shows a characteristic decremental response.

- Single fiber electromyography (SFEMG) demonstrates "jitter", which indicates the variability of propagation time to individual muscle fibers supplied by the same motor neuron. The sensitivity of SFEMG is approximately 90%. In particular, SFEMG of the superior rectus and levator palpebrae superioris muscle is extremely sensitive for the detection of ocular myasthenia gravis.

Management

The main therapies for myasthenia gravis include:
- Acetylcholinesterase inhibitors
- Corticosteroids
- Immunosuppressants.

Acetylcholinesterase Inhibitors

Mechanism of action: Acetylcholinesterase inhibitors prevent the degradation of Ach, increasing its concentration in the neuromuscular junction thus increasing the transmission across the synapse. These agents form the first line of management because of their ability to provide immediate symptomatic improvement in muscle weakness and the absence of long-term side effects.

Pyridostigmine is the most common agent prescribed and has a duration of action of 2–8 hours, with starting dose being 30–60 mg every 4 hours, a dose over 120 mg can result in cholinergic crisis.

Adverse effects: The common adverse effects arising from these agents are due to increased concentration of Ach and include:
- Gastrointestinal disturbances (nausea, diarrhea, and abdominal cramps)
- Muscle twitching
- Bradycardia.

   Overdosage results in sialorrhea, blurred vision, and worsening of weakness (cholinergic crisis).

   Diplopia often does not improve with pyridostigmine and may be treated with an immunosuppressive agent.

Corticosteroids

Corticosteroids having anti-inflammatory action are beneficial in myasthenia patients not responding to pyridostigmine.

If treatment with corticosteroids is planned, diabetes and tuberculosis should be excluded.

Immunosuppressants

Azathioprine, cyclosporine, and mycophenolate mofetil are utilized for the long-term management of myasthenia gravis and may be used in combination with prednisone and pyridostigmine. Blood counts, liver function, and renal function must be monitored.

Rituximab is usually reserved for patients with severe disease.

Plasmapheresis

It effectively reduces circulating autoantibodies and is typically reserved for patients with the myasthenic crisis or is used preoperatively for patients undergoing thymectomy, improvement is rapid but transient.

Intravenous Immune Globulin

Like plasmapheresis, intravenous immune globulin produces rapid improvement.

Systemic Management

Patients with myasthenic crisis require aggressive pulmonary treatment, often need intubation and mechanical ventilation.

Crutch Glasses

Crutch glasses can be used in patients with ptosis and poor Bell's phenomenon.

Strabismus Surgery in Myasthenia

Diplopia is more refractory to medical management. Strabismus surgery has been reported to relieve diplopia in such patients, strabismus surgery has been indicated in patients with stable deviations for >6 months. Favorable surgical results can be obtained in the form of binocular single vision in primary position, conventional recession resection of affected muscles according to deviation can help to achieve good results.

Thymectomy

Thymectomy is indicated for all patients who have a thymoma. Thymectomy results in complete remission in 35–45% of patients and the benefits of thymectomy may appear after 2–3 years, yet some patients respond almost immediately after surgery. It is usually recommended for patients under the age of 55 years who have a generalized disease. Ectopic rests of active thymic tissue result into a poorer prognosis. A trans-sternal approach is preferable to allow adequate visualization of the thoracic cavity and total thymus removal.

Lambert–Eaton Myasthenic Syndrome

Lambert–Eaton myasthenic syndrome (LEMS) is a triad of muscle weakness, autonomic dysfunction, and hyporeflexia. The disorder unlike myasthenia, which affects neuromuscular junction, is a presynaptic disorder affecting the calcium-gated voltage channels, thus resulting in Ach release failure.

The syndrome is associated with small cell lung carcinoma, and the non-neoplastic form is associated with pernicious anemia, thyroid disease, Sjögren's syndrome, and other autoimmune disorders.

Clinical Features

Patients usually present with dry eye and are associated with keratoconjunctivitis sicca-like features. The onset of the disease is rapid in the neoplastic form of the disease, whereas the non-neoplastic form remains stable. Ptosis, intermittent diplopia, sluggishly reacting pupil, and tonic pupil may also be present.

Slowed saccadic velocities can normalize after exercise.

TABLE 2: Differentiating points between myasthenia gravis and Lambert–Eaton syndrome.

Features	Ocular myasthenia	Lambert–Eaton syndrome
Pathophysiology	Antibodies against acetylcholine receptor	Antibodies against voltage-gated calcium channels
Location of defect	Postsynaptic	Presynaptic
Progression	• Craniocaudal • Ocular features appear first	From limbs to face
Effect of exercise	Worsens the symptoms	Improves the symptoms
Deep reflexes	Intact	Brisk
Autonomic disturbances	Absent	Present
Electromyographic response	Decremental response	Incremental response

Autonomic involvement is present in 50% of cases, which results in dry mouth, constipation, hypohidrosis, impotence, orthostatic hypotension, and urinary retention. Unlike myasthenia gravis, muscle strength improves following voluntary contraction or repetitive testing.

Investigations

- *Electromyography:* Electrophysiological studies confirm the diagnosis. Low rates of nerve stimulation (2–3 Hz) produce a decremental response, but high rates (20–50 Hz) cause an increase in the compound action potential. SFEMG shows changes similar to those found in myasthenia gravis.
- Anti-Ach receptor antibodies are not present.
- Voltage-gated calcium channel (VGCC) antibodies have been found in about 50% of patients.
- Chest imaging (CT and MRI) can be helpful to rule out associated lung carcinoma.
Differences between ocular myasthenia have been summarized in **Table 2**.

2. Discuss the tests for malingering.

Introduction

Intentionally counterfeiting a disease with benefit instinct is malingering. If the subject believes that he/she is ill, then it is called "conversion reaction" or "hysteria". In the case of conversion, the subject really lives his/her symptoms and cannot control them or even know that they are psychogenic in origin.

Malingering can be broadly classified into four types. The feigning of a nonexistent disease is *simulation*. The pretence that a certain condition is worse than it actually is *exaggeration*. Assignment to a disease or injury of an origin other than the real one is *false attribution* and pretence that a disease does not exist is *dissimulation*, thus dissimulation is a form of reverse malingering and is found in candidates for insurance or entry into service.

The individual may malinger to have defective vision, due to total blindness in one eye, partial blindness in one eye, and total or partial blindness in both eyes.

In hysteria, the patient is malingering on a subconscious level, whereas a malingerer is malingering on a conscious level. Malingering can be approached either by a psychological assessment of the patient or by trapping the patient with various tests.

Psychological Approach

This is based on the knowledge of an individual and his behavior. The reaction of the patient during examination such as disgruntled aggressive behavior and overplaying his part should be noted.

Various tests have been devised for malingering and the choice of tests depends upon the presenting symptoms of the patient, the following tests can be done in patients presenting with total blindness in one eye.

Total Blindness in One Eye

- *Binocular alignment:* Both eyes move equally in all directions when testing for extraocular movements and both eyes keep their fixation on the target. An eye with severely limited vision will fail to follow the parallel movement.

- *Objective prism test:* A high base-out prism when placed in front of an eye, it moves the eye inward involuntarily, to fuse two images, but a blind eye will not make any movement.
- *Double prism test:* A base-to-base double prism is properly aligned in front of the good eye and an opaque disc is put before the "blind" eye. A card with a horizontal line is shown to him. Even with one eye, an individual should see two lines, but a malingerer to prove his blindness in one eye will pretend to see one line.
- *Pinhole test:* A pinhole disc is placed in front of a good eye while the "blind" eye is left uncovered, the trial frame is tilted slightly so that the pinhole gets out of the visual axis. If the individual continues to read then he is doing so with the "blind" eye.
- *Plus 10 reading test:* A plus 10D lens is placed in front of the good eye. A reading card with fine print is then gradually moved away if the individual continues to read then he is doing so with the "blind" eye.
- *Friend test:* The patient is asked to wear red and green goggles and is asked to read the "Friend". The red glass is placed in front of the right eye and green in front of the left eye, if the person reads all the letters of the word, then it is suggestive that he is using both the eyes.
- *Synoptophore test:* A pair of fusion pictures in the synoptophore, i.e., rabbits, is shown if the individual sees both the controls, he clearly has good vision in each eye.
- *Tests for stereopsis:* Stereopsis is the highest level of binocularity if the individual can read the stereopsis charts correctly than he is using both his eyes.
- *Perimetry:*
  - Malingering could be easily diagnosed in Goldmann perimetry. Complex procedures of Goldmann perimetry confuse simulator, but an experienced simulator could overcome Goldmann perimetry.
  - Crossed or spiraling isopters defects are common in Goldmann and appear like generalized contraction in automated perimetry and are diagnosed as a functional loss. The field is tested continuously in the clockwise and anticlockwise direction starting with stimulus I4e, as larger stimuli are involved III4e and V4e, there is often further constriction.
- *Tangent screening:* In tangent screening, patient is tested at a distance of 1 meter with a 9-mm stimulus size, the patient is then moved back to 2 meter and the response is marked with 18-mm stimulus size, causing the field to expand twice, failure of the field to expand indicates a nonorganic component.
- *Pupillary reflex:* The pupillary examination would be helpful in discrimination of simulation in visual field loss. In cases of asymmetric visual acuity or visual field loss, the problem must be of either intraocular (retinal) or the optic nerve, and optic nerve lesion must cause relative afferent pupillary defect (RAPD). So, in cases of unilateral visual acuity or field loss cases if a clinical ocular examination is normal and no afferent pupillary defect presents, then it is a simulation case.
- *Laboratory tests:* In cases related to optic nerve dysfunction, laboratory tests are significant. In cases with a suspect of pre- and retrochiasmal lesions, computerized tomography and magnetic resonance imaging with contrast matter are necessary. No lesion in imaging increases suspicion of malingering. Visual Evoked Potential (VEP) recording with normal latency and amplitudes strengthens the probability of malingering.

Tests for Partial Blindness in One Eye

- *Jackson's convex and concave cylinder test:* A plus 6.00 cylinder and a minus 6.00 cylinder are placed with their axes superimposed in front of the good eye so that one lens neutralizes the other. While the patient is reading the distant chart, the front cylinder is gradually rotated until its axis is perpendicular to that of the other, so that if the patient is still able to read, he is doing so with the poor eye.
- *Special test cards:* Malinger usually tends to read only the first line on the vision chart, i.e., a vision of 6/60, therefore if the top letter is made of the size of the 6/24 line, and if he reads this, he has a vision of 6/24 line.
- *Amblyoscopic test:* The tubes of this instrument are so arranged that images are crossed when looking through them, if the patient claims his right eye to be blind, he will see the picture only on the left side thinking that he is seeing with his left eye. The test thus is a proof of deception, either conscious or subconscious.
- *Cycloplegia test:* A cycloplegic drug is used in the normal eye and normal saline is used in the eye with low vision and the patient is asked to read. Since the normal eye cannot read because of paralyzed accommodation, the ability to read gives a proof of malingering.

The tests described above for complete blindness in one eye above may also be used for partial blindness.

Tests for Malingering with Total or Partial Blindness in Both Eyes

It is rare for a malinger to claim loss of sight in both eyes, hysterical patients usually come with bilateral defective vision. The following tests are used for feigned total or partial blindness in both eyes.

- *Menace reflex:* A sudden surprise movement of the examiner's hand toward the face of the patient often causes the patient to blink. Even if a person learns to suppress a blink, he will have an increase in pulse rate.
- *Prism test:* A base-in-prism is placed in front of one eye if vision is present, the eye will move outward and then inward when the prism is removed.
- *Opticokinetic nystagmus test:* When a patient is asked to look at a rotating drum marked with vertical stripes, he will develop nystagmus, with fast and slow components.

Examination of Pupil and Accommodation for Malingering

Accommodation Paralysis

Accommodation paralysis causes blurring of near vision, making the subjects dependent on hypermetropic lenses. The far vision is normal. After a few hours of cycloplegia when pupils get back to normal, subjects feel comfortable. Failure of the patient to read despite correct near correction raises the possibility of the nonorganic lesion.

Convergence and Blinking

Some people can easily imitate convergence when the subject converges his/her eyes, and if miosis is observed, it is malingering.

Fixed, Dilated Pupil

A fixed dilated pupil can be associated with oculomotor nerve palsy, pharmacologic blockade, and Adie's pupil. A pharmacologic blockade may occur due to inadvertent or purposeful application of mydriatic or cycloplegic eye drops. The pilocarpine test can help to distinguish pharmacologic blockade with Adie's pupil, 1% pilocarpine cannot overcome receptor blockade and the pupil remains large, whereas in Adie's pupil diluted concentration of 0.125% pilocarpine can cause constriction of the pupil.

Eyelid Position and Function Malingering

Ptosis

A person with true ptosis will always try to elevate his lids and brow is usually elevated. Patients who feign ptosis do not make any effort to elevate the lid and maintain a drooping eyelid and with upgaze, ptosis resolves usually.

Blepharospasm

Nonorganic blepharospasm may be unilateral or bilateral and typically affects children and young adults; it can also be triggered by an emotionally traumatic event and may cause nonorganic ptosis.

Management

The suspicion of malingering must be raised in patients with vision loss, without any pathologies of the anterior and posterior segment.

Patients with nonorganic visual complaints are best managed with an understanding approach and words of encouragement; it is important to allow patients a graceful way out of the situation and reassuring that their problem will resolve over time. The symptoms often resolve in 1–2 follow-up visits. A consultation with a psychiatrist must be warranted in patients with underlying psychological illness.

2.3 Anatomy and Physiology

Gunjan Saluja

 1. Discuss anatomical subdivision of optic nerve.

The optic nerve takes its origin from the ganglion cells of retina; both the X and Y ganglion cells join together as they leave the globe and form the optic nerve. The optic nerve head, or the papilla, is a flat disc with a depression at the center known as optic cup; retinal ganglion cells exit from the papilla.

Neuro-ophthalmology

The optic nerve is 50–60 mm long and has four main anatomical subdivisions. They are:
1. Intraocular
2. Intraorbital
3. Intracanalicular
4. Intracranial.

Intraocular: The intraocular portion of the optic nerve is around 1 mm in length. The axons of the nerve traverse the sclera through the lamina cribrosa which contains 200–300 sieve-like channels. Just behind the sclera, the optic nerve acquires dural sheath and arachnoid membrane. The dural sheath is contagious with the periorbital dural sheath of the optic canal, and the arachnoid membrane is the continuation of the arachnoid in the intracranial space. Just behind the sclera, the optic nerve also acquires the myelin coating.

Thus, due to the addition of myelin, the diameter of the optic nerve increases from 1.5 mm at the optic disc to 3 mm **(Figs. 1A and B)**.

Intraorbital: The intraorbital portion of the optic nerve is about 25–30 mm in length. The central retinal artery and central retinal vein travel anteriorly within 10–15 mm of the optic nerve.

Intracanalicular: The length of this portion of the optic nerve is about 10 mm; as the nerve enters in the optic canal, the dural sheath of the nerve fuses with the periorbita. The optic canal lies in the sphenoid bone. Within the optic canal, the optic nerve lies with ophthalmic artery and sympathetic plexus. The nerve is separated from the superior orbital fissure by the lateral wall of the lesser wing of sphenoid. The canal runs superiorly and medially.

Intracranial: The intracranial portion of the nerve measures about 20 mm; the optic nerve in the brain lies under the falciform ligament of dura mater, which may compress the nerve, if the lesions are arising from the sella or sphenoid bone. The intracranial portion of the nerve ends in the optic chiasma.

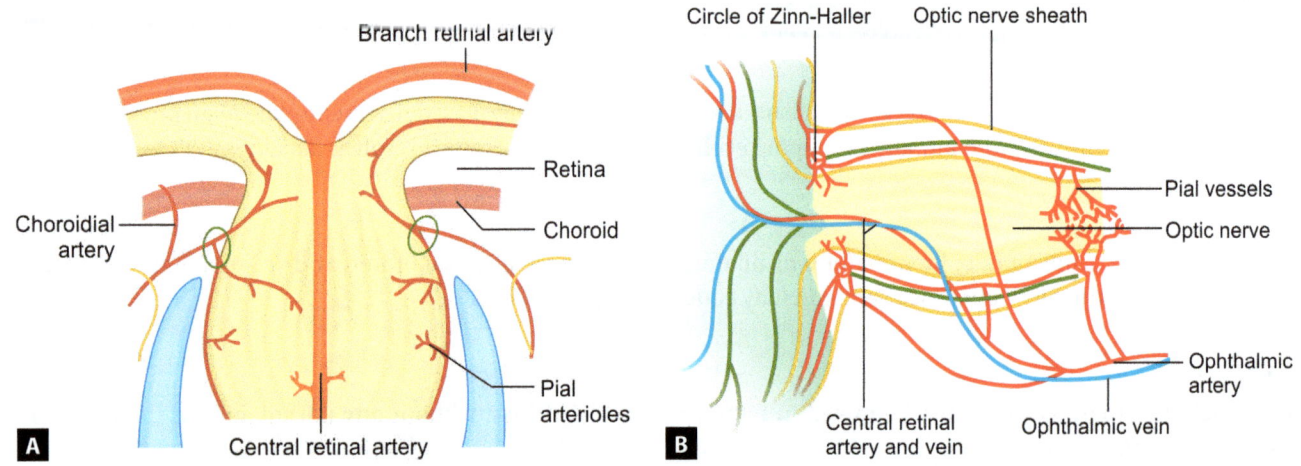

Figs. 1A and B: Blood supply of (A) intraocular portion of optic nerve and (B) intraorbital portion of optic nerve.

Clinical Implication

Anatomical subdivision	Length (mm)	Diseases common
Intraocular	1	• Ischemic optic neuropathy • Demyelinating disorders
Intraorbital	25	• Traumatic optic neuropathy
Intracanalicular	10	• Traumatic optic neuropathy
Intracranial	20	• Ischemic optic neuropathy • Demyelinating disorder • Compressive optic neuropathy

Q 2. Describe the vascular supply of the optic nerve head and its clinical importance (with a well-labeled diagram).

The blood supply of the optic nerve can be classified according to the portion of the optic nerve.

Intraocular Portion (Optic Nerve Head) (Figs. 1A and B)

The intraocular portion of the optic nerve can further be divided into prelaminar, laminar, and retrolaminar regions:
- *Prelaminar:* The prelaminar region of the optic nerve receives its blood supply by branches of short posterior ciliary arteries.
- *Laminar:* The region of lamina cribrosa is supplied by the branches of short posterior ciliary artery and arterial circle of Zinn–Haller.
- *Retrolaminar region:* The retrolaminar region of the optic nerve is supplied by recurrent pial vessels, and the central retinal artery provides branches to the optic nerve from pial plexus.

Intraorbital Portion (Fig. 1B)

The intraorbital portion of the optic nerve is supplied by preaxial and axial systems.

Preaxial system: It is derived from ophthalmic artery, long posterior ciliary artery, short posterior ciliary artery, lacrimal artery, and central retinal artery.

Axial system: It is derived from intraneural branches of the central retinal artery, central collateral arteries, and central artery of the optic nerve.

Intracanalicular Portion

The intracanalicular portion is supplied by ophthalmic artery, long posterior ciliary artery, short posterior ciliary artery, lacrimal artery, and central retinal artery.

Intracranial Portion

The intracranial portion receives its blood supply from the branches of the internal carotid artery, anterior cerebral artery, small recurrent branches from the ophthalmic artery, and twigs from the anterior communicating artery.

Clinical Implication

A reduction in the blood supply of the optic nerve head due to occlusion of the posterior ciliary arteries, hypotension, or excessive blood loss results in ischemic optic neuropathy. Similarly, occlusion of the retrobulbar region of the optic nerve will result in posterior ischemic optic neuropathy.

Q 3. Discuss the anatomy of optic chiasma.

The optic chiasm (derived from a Greek word whose literal meaning is "to mark with an X") or optic chiasma is an X-shaped space, which lies on the undersurface of the brain, above the pituitary gland, directly in front of the hypothalamus. It is formed by the decussating nerve fibers (axons) of the two optic nerves, one from each eye.

Anatomical Location and Relations

The optic chiasm is a flattened structure, which is 3.5 mm in height and 15 mm in width and is situated about 10 mm above the pituitary gland, thus making it susceptible to damage secondary to pituitary pathologies. The pituitary gland rests in the sella turcica portion of the sphenoid bone and the chiasma is separated from the pituitary gland by a space called inferior chiasmatic cistern. The chiasma is in continuation contiguous with the anterior–inferior floor of the third ventricle at the base of the brain.

Chiasma usually hangs directly over the pituitary fossa of the sphenoid bone; however, due to variations in the lengths of the optic nerves, the chiasm can be:
- Prefixed chiasma, i.e., lying above the chiasmatic sulcus or the tuberculum sellae
- Postfixed chiasma, i.e., lying above the dorsum sellae (**Figs. 2A and B**).

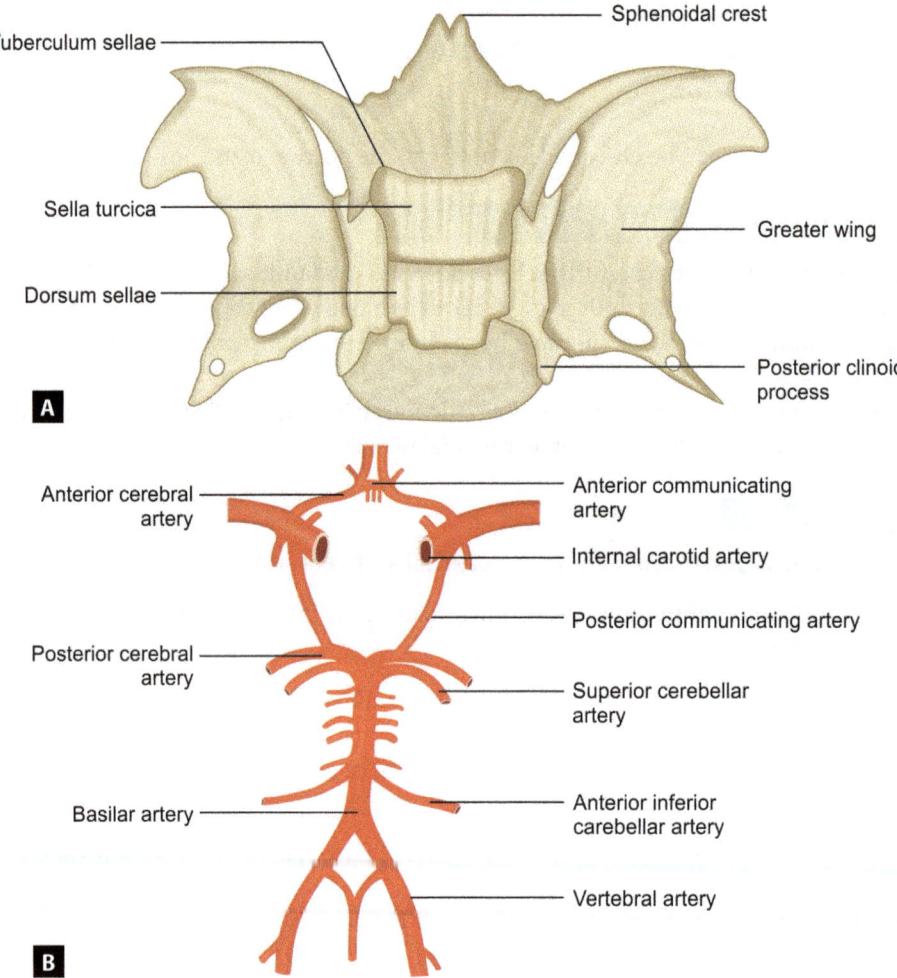

Figs. 2A and B: (A) Anatomy of sella; (B) Circle of Wills.

Laterally, chiasma is related to the supraclinoid segments of the carotid arteries. Inferolaterally, it is related to the cavernous sinuses.

Formation of Optic Chiasma

The optic nerve passes through the optic canal present in the lesser wing of the sphenoid, and decussates within chiasma at a ratio of 60:40, that is, 60% of the nasal fibers cross over to the opposite side and the remaining temporal fibers remain uncrossed.

Beyond the chiasma, in the optic tract also the temporal fibers remain uncrossed. The optic tract fibers then synapse in one of the six layers of the lateral geniculate body (LGB). Superior nasal quadrant retinal fibers remain superior and cross more posteriorly in the chiasm and macular fibers cross through the chiasm in its central and posterior portions.

Arterial Supply

Circle of Willis encircles optic chiasma; hence, its blood supply is derived from the arteries constituting the circle of Willis which are **(Fig. 2B)**:
- Left and right anterior cerebral arteries
- Left and right internal carotid arteries
- Left and right posterior cerebral arteries
- Left and right posterior communicating arteries.

The arterial supply of the chiasm is derived from the anterior cerebral and communicating arteries from above and the posterior communicating, posterior cerebral, and basilar arteries from below.

Neuro-ophthalmology

Q 4. Describe the anatomy of visual pathway with diagram.

Refer to **Figure 3**.

Q 5. Discuss the anatomy of lateral geniculate body and visual cortex.

Lateral Geniculate Body

Lateral geniculate body is a projection nucleus of thalamus and plays an important role in visual processing. The lateral geniculate nucleus has broad connections and receives input from the extrastriate cortex as well as from the midbrain and the hindbrain. LGB acts as a relay point for transferring the visual information from the optic tract to optic radiation. There is a 1:1 ratio of the axons entering the LGB and exiting it.

Location: LGB is located in the posteroventral region of the thalamic nuclei, immediately abutting the pulvinar and posterior to the inferior choroidal point of the choroid plexus.

The name has been derived due to its location, which is relatively lateral to the medial geniculate nucleus and geniculum (meaning joint) from the sharp bend of its fibers.

Structure: LGB is structurally divided into six layers/laminae of gray matter with intervening white matter composed of axons and dendrites. The gray matter laminae consist of six layers of irregularly stacked cones, numbering one ventrally to six dorsally.

The layers 1 and 2 lying ventrally consist of loosely arranged magnocellular cells and the four layers lying dorsally (3, 4, 5, and 6) consist of small- and medium-sized, parvocellular cells. The retinal ganglion signals from the ipsilateral eye synapse on layers 2, 3, and 5, and signals from the contralateral eye synapse on layers 1, 4, and 6. M cells in the LGN receive input from the large-field, motion-sensitive Y-type retinal ganglion cells, while P cells receive input from the small-field, color-sensitive X-type retinal ganglion cells. Koniocellular cells project into regions ventral to each of the P and M laminae.

Lateral geniculate body is also the point of origin for the optic radiations, which project via the internal capsule to the primary visual cortex (V1) **(Fig. 4)**.

Intergeniculate leaflet (IGL) is a distinct area lying in between the dorsal and ventral layers of the lateral geniculate nucleus which projects to the suprachiasmatic nuclei of hypothalamus via the geniculohypothalamic tract and to the pineal gland via the geniculopineal tract, implicating the LGB in the modulation of circadian/diurnal rhythms.

Visual fibers' representation in LGB: Macular fibers coming in the optic tract occupy two third of LGB, upper retinal fibers occupy the anterior one third of LGB, and lower retinal fibers occupy lateral half of the anterior one third of LGB.

Blood supply: LGB receives its blood supply from the branches of the posterior cerebral artery, the lateral posterior choroidal branch, and the internal carotid artery from its anterior choroidal branch.

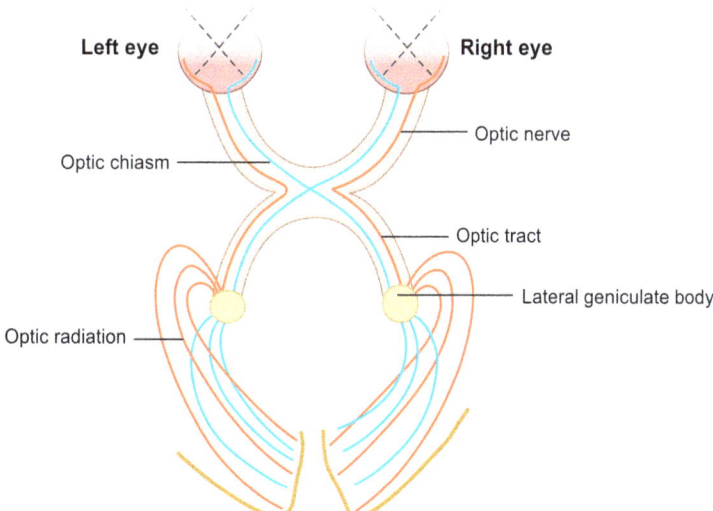

Fig. 3: Visual pathway.

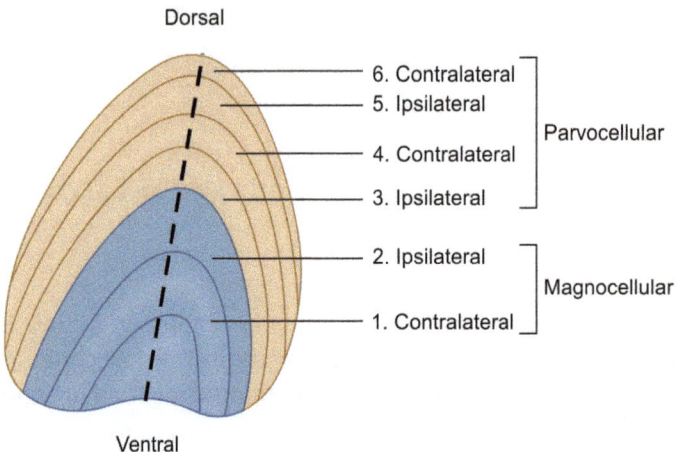

Fig. 4: Anatomy of lateral geniculate body.

Lesions in the lateral geniculate nucleus can result in contralateral homonymous hemianopias and quadrantanopia; due to projections to the suprachiasmatic nucleus, lesions of LGB can also disrupt the effects of stimuli that generally modulate circadian rhythm.

Visual Cortex

The occipital lobe is the smallest of the four lobes of the cerebral hemisphere. It is present posterior to the parietal and temporal lobes, forming the caudal part of the brain, with its posterior-most part being the occipital pole, and is primarily responsible for visual processing. It contains the primary and association visual cortex. The occipital lobe is separated from the parietal and temporal lobes on the medial surface by the parieto-occipital sulcus and on the lateral surface by an imaginary line that extends from the parieto-occipital sulcus to the preoccipital notch. The medial surface of the occipital lobe has a characteristic calcarine sulcus (calcarine fissure) extending from the parieto-occipital sulcus to the occipital pole.

The upper and lower banks of calcarine sulcus house the primary visual cortex receiving visual information from the contralateral half. The primary visual cortex, also known as V1 or Brodmann area 17, surrounds the calcarine sulcus on the occipital lobe's medial aspect. The secondary visual cortex, also known as V2, V3, V4, V5, or Brodmann areas 18 and 19, surrounds the primary cortex and receives information from it **(Figs. 5A to D)**.

Types of Cells in Occipital Cortex
- *Simple cells:* They are side-by-side, arranged, excitatory and inhibitory receptive fields. Simple cells are arranged side by side with excitatory and inhibitory receptive fields. These cells that respond the best to a light source in a specific orientation are mainly found in the V1 layer of the occipital cortex.
- *Complex cells:* They are found in V1–V3 and respond to the summation of several receptive fields that become integrated from many simple cells. Complex cells respond the most to a moving stimulus across the cell's receptive field and to movement in a particular direction.
- *End-stopped cells:* These cells respond the best to moving lines of specific lengths, corners, and edges.
  Collectively all the cells—simple, complex, and end-stopped cells—are critical for processing specific features to a stimulus.

Layers of Occipital Cortex

The occipital cortex has been divided into six layers by Brodmann:
1. *V1, Brodmann area 17 (V1, primary, calcarine, or striate cortex):* The primary visual cortex V1 is the first to receive the signals from the optic radiations and is divided into six distinct layers, each comprising different cell types and functions. Layer 4 consists of mainly simple cells and receives the information from the lateral geniculate nucleus. The macular fibers terminate more posteriorly. Layers 2, 3, and 6 of V1 mainly consist of complex cells.
2. *V2, Brodmann area 18:* V2 receives integrated information from V1, resulting in an increased level of complexity and response patterns to objects. The cells in V2 respond to differences in color, spatial frequency, moderately complex patterns, and object orientation. V2 has feed-forward connections with V3–V5 and feedback connection with V1.

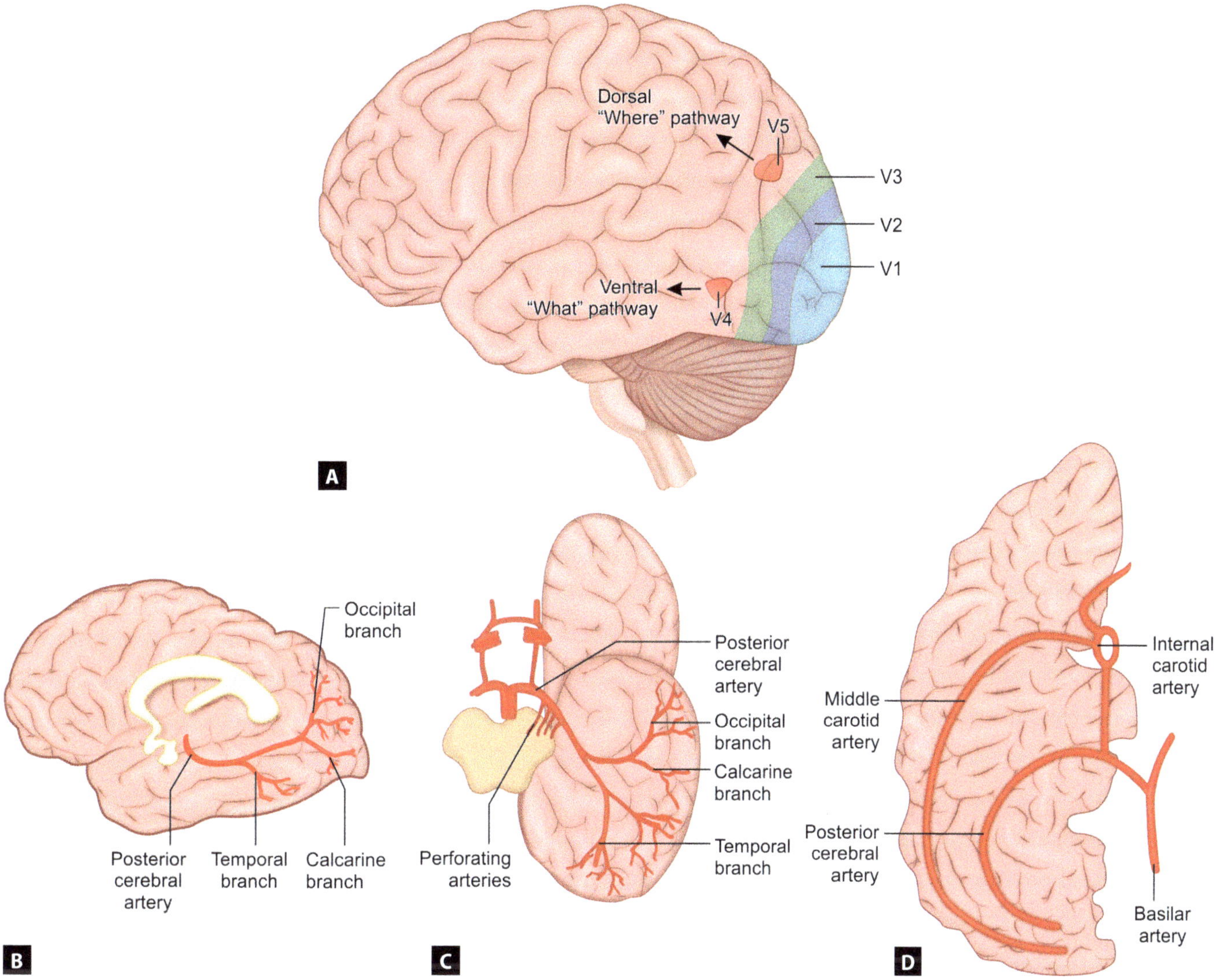

Figs. 5A to D: (A) Anatomy of visual cortex; (B to D) Blood supply to occipital cortex.

3. *V3:* This lies in the posterior parietal lobe and receives signals from V1 and V2. V3 further sends the efferent signals to the basal ganglia and midbrain.
4. *V4:* This is located within the lingual and fusiform gyri and is sensitive to color.
5. *V5:* This is located posterior and within the superior temporal sulcus and gyrus subangularis, sensitive to movement and direction, V5 is very sensitive to movement and direction. V5 corresponds to the medial temporal visual region, receiving inputs from ipsilateral V1.
6. *V6:* The dorsomedial area (DM) also known as V6, appears to respond to visual stimuli associated with self-motion and wide-field stimulation. Although its existence in new world monkeys is described, in humans its existence is controversial. Few authors believe V6 is nothing but area V5 only.

6. Discuss the supranuclear control of ocular movements.

Supranuclear pathways involve the pathways lying above the cranial nerve nucleus, i.e., relay information from the cortex to the cranial nerve nucleus, whereas the infranuclear pathways arise from the cranial nerve nucleus to the extraocular muscles. These are comparable to the upper motor neuron and lower motor neuron (LMN) of the motor system, where the upper motor neurons comprise the pathways originating from the motor cortex to the anterior horn and LMN comprises the pathways arising from the anterior horn of the spinal cord to the peripheral muscles.

The various eye movements include the following:
- Saccades
- Pursuit

- Vergence
- Vestibular eye movements
- Positional movements.

Pathways for Various Eye Movements

The impulse for intentional saccades originates from the contralateral frontal eye field area, whereas the impulse for reflexive saccades originates from the parietal eye field area, located in the posterior parietal cortex. The impulse further passes to posterior pontine reticular formation (PPRF), located in the pons.

Posterior pontine reticular formation plays an important role in controlling ocular movements and has deep connections with the superior colliculus, PPRF supplies the ipsilateral sixth nerve nucleus after which the impulse passes to the contralateral third nerve nucleus through the median longitudinal fasciculus (MLF) to supply medial rectus. The path is therefore known as the frontomesencephalic pathway **(Figs. 6A to C)**.

Vertical Saccades

The fibers from the cortex project to the rostral interstitial nucleus of the MLF of Cajal, located in the rostral midbrain. These fibers further project bilaterally to the oculomotor and trochlear nuclei, after passing through the posterior commissure.

Pursuit (Fig. 7)

Pursuit movements are smooth following ocular movements, required to maintain the foveation and stabilize the retinal image.

The neural pathway for pursuit originates in the primary visual cortex, specifically from the peristriate cortex of the occipital motor area, Brodmann's area 19, or area V1. Projections are then sent to the extrastriate V5, which includes the middle temporal (MT) and medial superior temporal (MST) areas which lie in the superior temporal sulcus. The pursuit movement is initiated from MT and is maintained by MST. The signals from MST are then sent to the frontal eye fields, which signals the generation for pursuit movements.

The fibers, for both horizontal and vertical pursuits, then descend through the internal capsule, and just above the level of the sixth nerve nuclei, they cross over to the opposite side of brain stem and eventually end in "pontine center" for lateral gaze in the dorsolateral pontine nucleus.

Velocity signals are projected from here to the floccular region and to the vermis lobules of the cerebellum. The flocculus maintains pursuit during steady constant tracking.

The role of cerebellum is to sort out eye and head rotations in the tracking process and to sort out the ocular pursuit signal from visual and eye–head motor inputs; the signals are then transmitted to the medial longitudinal fasciculus to the third, fourth, and sixth cranial nerve nuclei and finally to the relevant extraocular muscles via the respective cranial nerves.

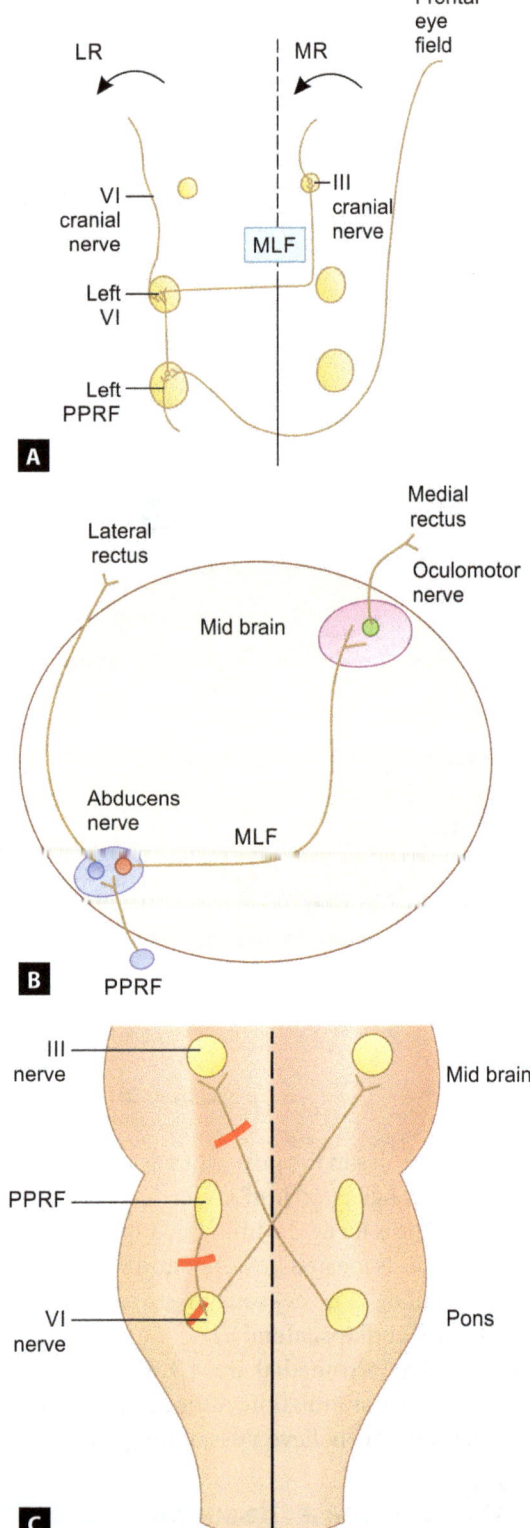

Figs. 6A to C: (A) Supranuclear pathway of saccade; (B) Internuclear ophthalmoplegia; (C) One-and-a-half syndrome. (LR: lateral rectus; MLF: median longitudinal fasciculus; MR: medial rectus; PPRF: posterior pontine reticular formation)

Vestibulo-ocular Reflex (Fig. 8)

The vestibulo-ocular reflex (VOR) is mediated with the help of a peripheral sensory apparatus consisting of semicircular canals and saccule and utricle, a central processing mechanism, and motor output through extraocular muscles.

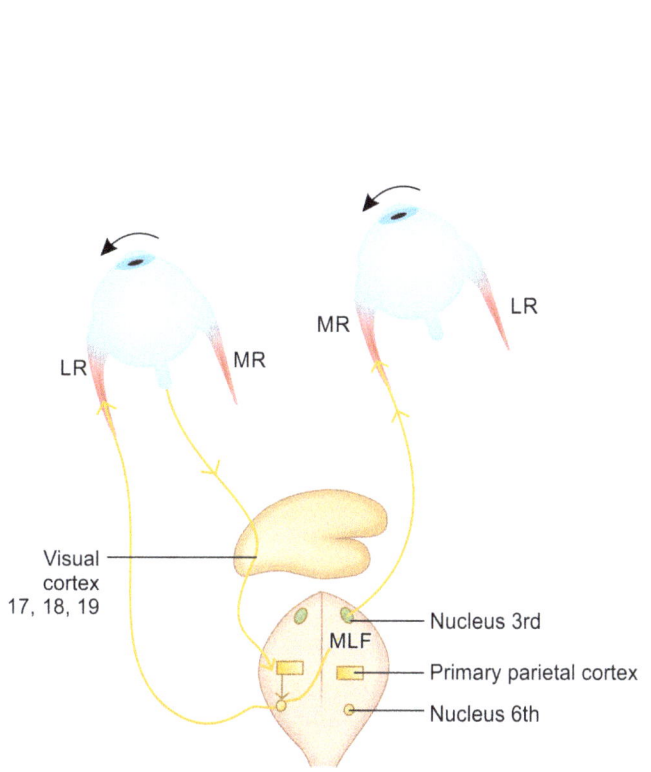

Fig. 7: Pursuit pathway. (LR: lateral rectus; MLF: median longitudinal fasciculus; MR: medial rectus)

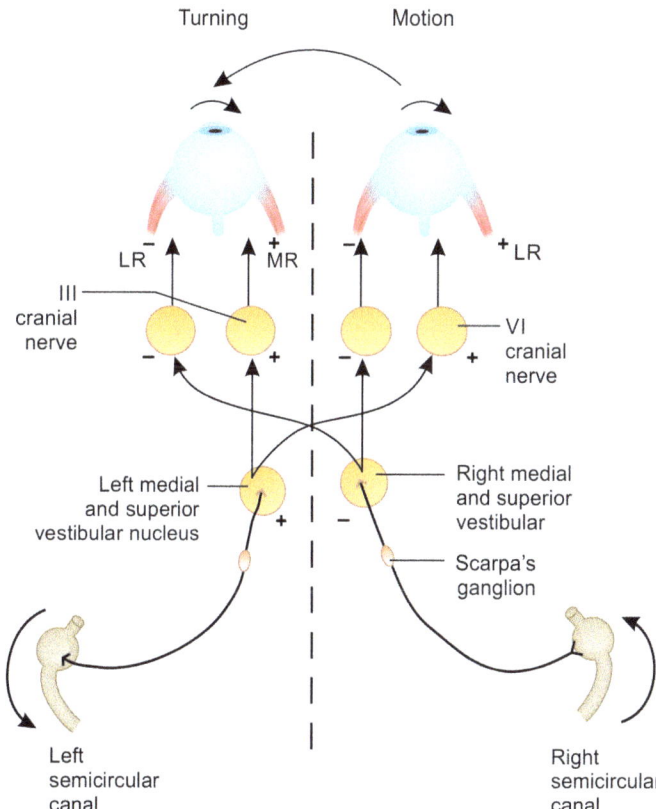

Fig. 8: Vestibulo-ocular pathway. (LR: lateral rectus; MR: medial rectus)

The function of VOR is to maintain the foveation with head movements; as a result, whenever the head moves, the eyes move in the opposite direction by the same amount to maintain the clear image.

Semicircular Canals

There are six bony semicircular canals arranged in three planes: anterior, posterior, and horizontal on both sides, with each plane having a pair of canals. Semicircular canals are sensitive to angular acceleration and detect head rotation. The dilated portion of the semicircular canal is called the ampulla, which has hair cells.

These hair cells are embedded in a fluid and gelatin-like structure. The hair cells are known as crista ampullaris and the gelatinous cup-like material above it is known as cupula.

In between the bony semicircular canal and the membranous portion, perilymph is present and endolymph is present on the inner side.

With rotation of the head, the endolymph will move in the opposite direction causing the movement of gelatinous material, and further causing bending of the hair cells and their depolarization. These signals from semicircular canals are further transmitted to the median and superior vestibular nuclei located in the vestibular nerve.

Otolith Organs

Otolith organs are sensitive to linear acceleration and help in detection of the head position relative to gravity and head translation. The utricle lies in the posterior part of bony vestibule and receives openings of semicircular ducts; the saccule lies anterior to the vestibule. The sensory epithelium of saccule and utricle is macula.

The macula consists of a membrane made of gelatinous mass and on top consists of crystals of calcium carbonate called otoliths. The cilia of hair cells project in the gelatinous layer. Linear movements cause the displacement of otolithic membrane, stimulating it, and further transmitting the information through the vestibular nerve to the inferior and median vestibular nuclei. From the vestibular nuclei, the information is further transmitted to the nuclei of the third and sixth cranial nerves through the medial longitudinal fasciculus.

The vestibular system also sends the information via the inferior cerebellar peduncle to the cerebellum to modulate the VOR. The flocculonodular lobe and fastigial nuclei are responsible for fine-tuning.

7. Discuss internuclear ophthalmoplegia (INO).

See Answer of Q8.

 8. Discuss one-and-a-half syndrome, its cause, and clinical features.

The etiologies of INO include:
- Demyelinating lesions such as multiple sclerosis
- Vascular causes—infarction and hemorrhage in the brain stem
- Tumors of brain stem and 4th ventricle
- Chiari malformation
- Wernicke encephalopathy
- *Metabolic disorders:* Hepatic encephalopathy, abetalipoproteinemia, Fabry disease
- Hydrocephalus due to subdural hematoma
- Bacterial and viral meningoencephalitis
- Syphilis
- Progressive supranuclear palsy
- Intoxications by drugs such as tricyclic antidepressants, toluene, propranolol, phenothiazine, D-penicillamine
- Brain stem trauma due to cervical hyperextension.

Lesions of the MLF produce INO. In unilateral lesions, INO is characterized by weakness of adduction ipsilateral to the side of the lesion that can vary from a complete loss of adduction beyond the midline to a mild decrease in the velocity of adduction, and nystagmus can be observed in the contralateral eye on abduction. The abduction nystagmus is characteristic of INO.

Vestibular slow phases, pursuit and optokinetic following movements, and saccades and quick phases of nystagmus are all affected by the MLF lesion.

Convergence is intact, despite the absence of voluntary adduction.

Lesions that damage the MLF may also damage the abducens nucleus, fascicle, or both on either side of the brain stem. Lesions that damage the MLF on one side and the ipsilateral abducens nucleus produce the one-and-a-half syndrome. The only preserved horizontal eye movement is the abduction of the contralateral eye.

Investigations

Neuroimaging aids in evaluating the exact site of lesion and the nature of lesion.

Management

Management depends upon the underlying etiology.

 9. Discuss anatomy, nerve supply, and action of third, fourth, and sixth cranial nerves.

The extraocular movements are chiefly governed by third, fourth, and sixth cranial nerves.

Third Cranial Nerve/Oculomotor Nerve

The third cranial nerve originates in the midbrain at the level of superior colliculus. The main motor nucleus of the third cranial nerve consists of the subnuclei, which supply the ipsilateral medial rectus, inferior rectus, and inferior oblique and contralateral superior rectus; besides this, the central nucleus supplies the levator palpebrae superioris (LPS).

An accessory parasympathetic nucleus supplies the Edinger–Westphal nucleus, which sends the preganglionic parasympathetic fibers, along with oculomotor fibers.

Course of the Nerve

After originating, the fasciculus which consists of efferent fibers passes through the red nucleus, and after emerging from the midbrain the fibers pass through the interpeduncular space.

The nerve in the interpeduncular space passes between the superior cerebellar and posterior cerebral arteries and enters the cavernous sinus. In the cavernous sinus, the nerve lies in the lateral wall of the sinus, above the trochlear nerve.

In the anterior part of the cavernous sinus, the nerve divides into superior and inferior divisions and enters the orbit through the superior orbital fissures passing within the annulus of Zinn.

The superior division of the nerve then supplies the superior rectus and LPS. On the contrary, the inferior division of the nerve supplies the inferior rectus, inferior oblique, and medial rectus **(Fig. 9)**.

Clinical Significance

As there is one single central nucleus of LPS, the nuclear lesions will cause bilateral ptosis. Similarly, as the main motor nucleus supplies the contralateral superior rectus, a lesion will cause contralateral superior rectus palsy.

Interpeduncular Portion

The nerve here lies in close proximity with the posterior cerebral and superior cerebellar arteries; hence, it can be easily compressed by the aneurysms arising from them. The pupillomotor fibers lie in the outer portion of the nerve and are supplied by pial vessels; therefore, they are the first to be involved in case of a compressive lesion.

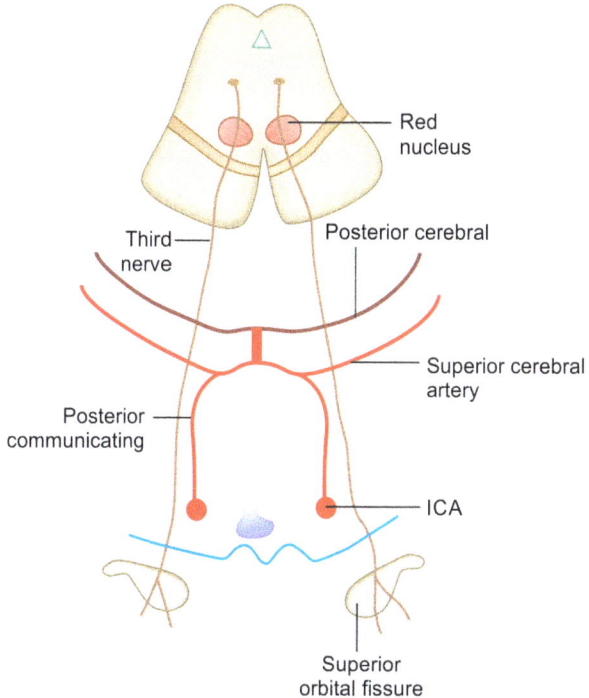

Fig. 9: Course of third nerve. (ICA: internal carotid artery)

Anatomy of Fourth Cranial Nerve

The fourth cranial nerve is an entirely motor nerve and is different from other cranial nerves, as it is the only one to arise from the dorsal aspect and to cross completely on the opposite side. The nucleus of the fourth cranial nerve lies in midbrain at the level of inferior colliculus.

The nerve fibers leaving the nucleus turn posteriorly and decussate completely in the medullary velum. The nerve then runs between the posterior cerebral and superior cerebellar arteries, like the third nerve. It pierces the dura of the roof of cavernous sinus and lies in the lateral wall of cavernous sinus, beneath the oculomotor nerve and above the ophthalmic division of the trigeminal nerve. The nerve passes through the superior orbital fissure and lies outside the annulus of Zinn. The nerve enters the orbit to supply the superior oblique muscle **(Fig. 10)**.

Anatomy of Sixth Cranial Nerve

The sixth cranial nerve, abducens, is the most commonly involved cranial nerve. Its long, tortuous course predisposes it to be easily involved. Abducens is also the first cranial nerve to be involved in cases of cavernous sinus thrombosis and in cases of elevated intracranial pressure.

The nucleus of the sixth cranial nerve lies at the level of pons, ventral to the floor of the 4th ventricle; the fibers leave the brain stem ventrally at the pontomedullary junction.

The fibers of the seventh cranial nerve wrap around the sixth nerve nucleus; as a result of this, ipsilateral LMN facial nerve palsy is also common along with sixth nerve palsy. The nerve then enters the prepontine basilar cistern and passes

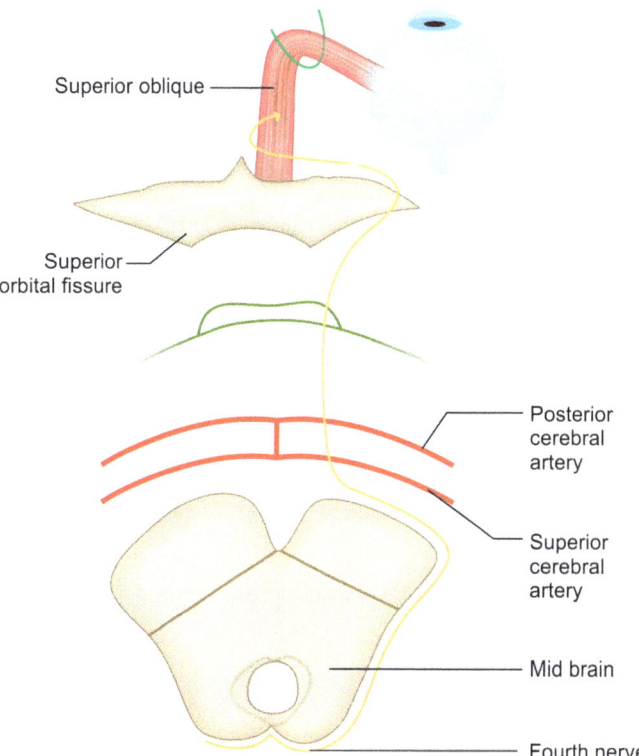

Fig. 10: Anatomy of fourth cranial nerve.

upward close to the base of the skull where it is crossed by the anterior inferior cerebellar artery. The nerve then pierces the dura below the posterior clinoids and angles forward over the tip of the petrous bone, passing through the inferior petrosal sinus, underneath the petroclinoid ligament to enter the cavernous sinus. In the cavernous sinus, the sixth nerve is situated in the medial wall and lies in close relation to the internal carotid artery. The nerve then enters the orbit through the superior orbital fissure within the annulus of Zinn to innervate the lateral rectus **(Fig. 11)**.

 10. Describe the anatomy of the cavernous sinus and its communications.

Cavernous sinus is located in the middle cranial fossa, on either side of the body of sphenoid. Anteriorly, the sinus extends to the superior orbital fissure and posteriorly extends up to the apex of petrous bone.

Fig. 11: Anatomy of the 6th cranial nerve. (SOF: superior orbital fissure)

Relations of the Cavernous Sinus

Superiorly, the cavernous sinus is related to optic tract, internal carotid artery, and anterior perforated substance. Foramen lacerum, junction of body and greater wing of sphenoid, is inferiorly related to the sinus. Medially, the sinus is related to hypophysis cerebri and sphenoid sinus and is related to temporal lobe with uncus laterally.

Structures within the Cavernous Sinus

The lateral wall of the cavernous sinus consists of the following cranial nerves (from up to down):
- Oculomotor nerve
- Trochlear nerve
- First two divisions of trigeminal nerve, which are ophthalmic and maxillary
  The medial wall consists of:
  - Internal carotid artery
  - *Abducens nerve:* Lies inferior to internal carotid artery **(Fig. 12)**.

Communications of Cavernous Sinus (Fig. 13)

The incoming channels of cavernous sinus *from orbit* include:
- Superior ophthalmic vein
- Central retinal vein, which may drain into the superior ophthalmic vein and then drain into cavernous sinus; the vein can also directly drain to cavernous sinus

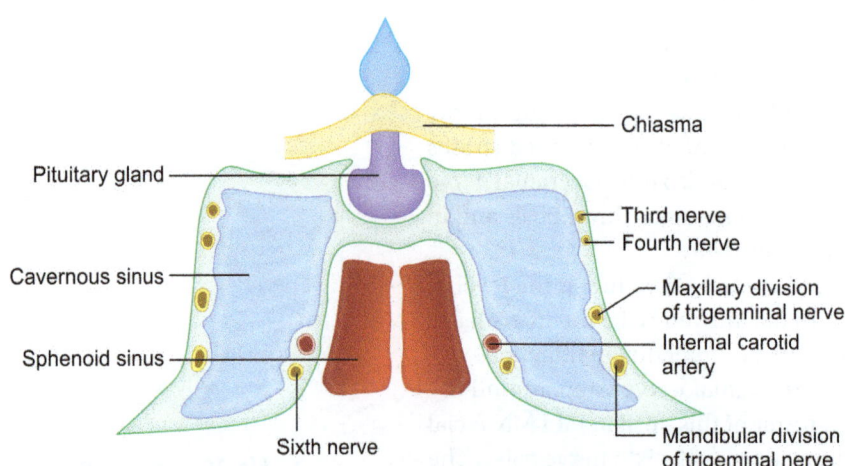

Fig. 12: Anatomy of cavernous sinus.

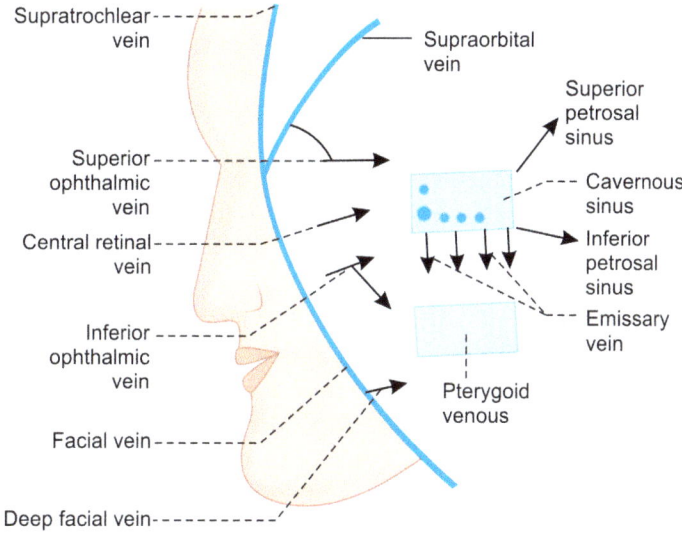

Fig. 13: Communication of cavernous sinus.

- Inferior ophthalmic vein
- Medial ophthalmic vein.

Tributaries from Brain
Superficial middle cerebral vein and inferior cerebral vein from the temporal lobe are the tributaries that arise from the brain.

Tributaries from Meninges
Sphenoparietal sinus and frontal trunk of the middle meningeal vein are the tributaries that arise from meninges.

Cavernous sinus drains into:
- Transverse sinus through superior petrosal sinus
- Internal jugular vein through inferior petrosal sinus
- Pterygoid plexus through emissary veins.

Clinical Implication
Cavernous sinus thrombosis.

2.4 Optic Nerve

Gunjan Saluja

 1. Explain signs of optic nerve dysfunction or various investigations available to assess the optic nerve function or how would you evaluate the integrity of visual pathways? Discuss briefly about localization of their lesions in the context of neurological disorder.

Optic nerve function tests: It consists of following as described here.

Color Vision
Color vision is defined as the ability of the human eye to differentiate between various colors excited by different wavelength of light. Color is created by utilizing two properties of light, energy, and frequency of vibration or wavelength.

Theories of color vision: There are various theories given for explaining the concept of color vision.

These mainly include:

- *Trichromatic theory:* Trichromatic theory of color vision was developed, in the later half of the 19th century, based on the work of Maxwell, Young, and Helmholtz. According to this theory, there are three types of cone receptors, sensitive to red—570 nm (L cone), green—535 nm (M cone), and blue regions—445 nm (S cone) of the spectrum, respectively.

    Red, green, and blue were considered three primary colors and all other colors are seen by combination of these colors, but contrary to this theory three "color separation" images are not transmitted directly to the brain.

    It has been found that gene for blue sensitive cones is located in chromosome number 7, and genes for red and green sensitive cones are located in X chromosome.

- *Herring's opponent theory:* Herring proposed an opponent colors theory of color vision based on various subjective observations, which included appearance of hues, simultaneous contrast, after-images, and color vision deficiencies. Herring also noted that certain hues were perceived together. For example, a color perception is not described as reddish-green or yellowish-blue, while combinations of red and yellow, red and blue, green and yellow, and green and blue are readily perceived. This suggested to Herring that there was something fundamental about red-green and yellow-blue pairs causing them to oppose one another. Thus, our visual system interprets color in antagonistic way.

    Herring proposed that there were three types of receptors, but these receptors had bipolar responses to light-dark, red-green, and yellow-blue.

- *Dominant modulator theory:* Granit (1947) proposed a dominator/modular theory of color vision according to which there were "modulators", which responded to only a narrow part of visible spectrum and another group was of "dominators" which responds to a broad band of spectrum.

- *Modern theory of opponent colors:* Retinal neurons encode color into opponent signals, outputs of all three cone types are summed (L + M + S) to produce an achromatic response that matches the Commission Internationale de l'Eclairage (CIE) V(λ) curve as long as the summation is taken in proportion to the relative populations of the three cone types. Differencing of the cone signals allows construction of red-green (L – M + S) and yellow-blue (L + M – S) opponent signals. The transformation from LMS signals to the opponent signals serves to decorrelate the color information carried in the three channels, thus allowing more efficient signal transmission.

Physiology of Color Vision

The process of perceiving colors begins from the cone receptors, which have a sharp onset, and offset, further the action potential generated in the cones is transmitted by electronic conduction to other cells of retina across the synapses. The horizontal cells have been seen to show two different types of response, luminosity response, and chromatic response, both of which are hyperpolarizing for a part of spectrum and depolarizing for the other part.

The bipolar cells show a center surround response, with one spectrum of wavelength causing hyperpolarization and depolarization by the other spectrum. The exact role of amacrine cells is not known but is believed to act as color control.

There exist two types of color-opponent ganglion cells, the red-green color cells which utilize the signals from red/green cones to detect their contrast and blue-yellow opponent color cells which obtain a summated output from red-green cones and is contrasted with the blue cones.

Following this color information is transmitted by the parvocellular pathway of lateral geniculate body to the layer IVc of the visual cortex, from where the information is transmitted to the blobs in layers II and III and center-surround cells.

Color Attributes

Color has three attributes, which include hue, saturation, and lightness.

1. *Hue:* Hue is determined by the wavelength of a particular color, at the wavelength of 480 and 590 nm of the visible spectrum, this ability to differentiate between two colors is maximum.
2. *Saturation:* Saturation defines the brilliance and intensity of color and is estimated by the amount of wavelength of light added before it is distinguishable.
3. *Lightness:* Lightness depends on the luminosity. The luminosity function varies between photopic vision and scotopic vision, this shift is known Purkinje shift.

Tests for Color Vision

- *Pseudoisochromatic chart test:* Pseudoisochromatic charts have been named so, as the symbol appears to be of the same color as that of background for the affected individual and the subject is required to identify the symbol, which is embedded in the background. There are various pseudoisochromatic plates present such as Ishihara's plate and Hardy–Rand–Rittler plates.

These test plates consist of a series of cards on which colored dots of discs of various sizes are printed to form a multicolored figure against a multicolored background. The figure is some easily identifiable letter, Arabic numeral, or geometric configuration. The difference between figure and background dots is in color. Size, lightness, and saturation of the dots may be different so that identification of the intended figure by cues other than hue is less likely.

- *Arrangement tests:* Observer is required to arrange color samples by similarity in a sequential color series.

  These colors are mounted in caps, which are numbered on the back and can be moved about freely during performance. Arrangement tests may be designed for evaluation of fine hue discrimination and for evaluation of color confusion.

  Arrangement tests are easy to administer. Such tests require manual dexterity, patience, concentration, and the understanding of abstract ordering. Hence, they are less suitable for young children. The Farnsworth Panel D-15 has 15 caps and FM 100-hue test has 100 caps; 100-hue test is more time consuming, but is a sensitive indicator of aptitude for hue discrimination D-15 and 100-hue tests differentiate among protan, deutan, and tritan defects.

  Order of the caps arranged by the observer is plotted directly on the score sheet on a diagram that shows correct cap positions; extending in a circle from the reference cap. Errors occur when caps are misplaced from the correct order. The scorer draws lines connecting the caps in their actual order, when in correct order; the lines retrace the hue circle. Subjects with normal color vision may make at most one or two minor errors. Dichromats and extreme anomalous trichromats make multiple (6–12) crossovers, forming a nearly parallel series of lines. The axis of the crossover lines is characteristic of the type of defect; the axes corresponding to protan, deutan, and tritan defects are indicated on the scoring sheet.

- *Edridge-green lantern test:* The Edridge-green lantern is designed to produce a range of colors and tints; in addition to the seven-colored lanterns, it also contains seven modifying glass filters, and seven aperture sizes. The colored filters represent signal colors; modifying filters represent smoke, fog, and rain, and various aperture sizes represent color judgments made at different distances.

  Test is performed in a dark room at a distance of 20 feet. The lights are presented in random order, and the observer names the colors of lights. Administration is complicated for the examiner because of the five rotating discs (containing the colored filters, the modifying filters, and the apertures), the lantern can be rotated singly or jointly, making hundreds of combinations possible.

- *Holmgren wool test:* The Holmgren wool test was one of the original tests, which was designed to screen red–green color defects. The test consists of 75 small strands and 3 large strands of colored wools. The large strands serve as test colors, and the smaller strands act as matching colors. The skeins are placed in a heap. The subject is asked to select skeins from the heap that nearly matches the test skein in color. There is no exact match; similarly colored skeins, or skeins of lighter or darker shades of the same color, may be selected.

- *Nagel's anomaloscope:* Nagel's anomaloscope is based on principle of mixing of two colors to produce another color.

  The instrument is designed to present a circular split field. In the lower half, a spectral yellow (589 nm) appears. Turning a knob can continuously vary the luminance of the yellow half. Upper half of the field is filled with a mixture of spectral yellow–green (545 nm) and spectral red (670 nm). A knob can continuously adjust relative proportions of green and red, from all green through any mixture to all red. Patient adjusts red and green ratio (0–73) till it matches the hue of lower yellow, normal is 45.

Anomalies of Color Vision (Flowchart 1)

Congenital Color Vision Defects

The congenital color vision defects are genetically inherited; most common are red–green defects which are inherited as X-linked recessive disorder. The congenital color vision defects can be broadly classified as achromatopsia or dyschromatopsia.

Dyschromatopsia: It can be classified into anomalous trichromacy and dichromacy.
- *Anomalous trichromacy:* It is a common congenital color vision defect, which occurs when one of three cone pigments are altered in its spectral sensitivity and can be of three types—protanomaly, deuteranomaly, and tritanomaly.
  - *Protanomaly:* Protanomaly is a color vision defect, in which photopic sensitivity for red light is low and is a hereditary X-linked disorder.
  - *Deuteranomaly:* It is the most common color vision defect, affecting photopic sensitivity for green light, hence as compared to normal individuals, the deuteranomalous individual will require more green light, and is a hereditary X-linked disorder.

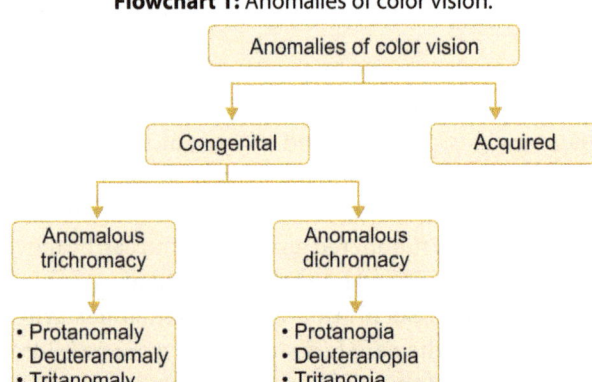

Flowchart 1: Anomalies of color vision.

- *Tritanomaly:* It is a rare color vision deficiency, causing deficiency of blue sensitive retinal pigment and these patients require more blue light as compared to normal control.
- *Dichromacy:* Dichromacy is a moderately severe color vision defect in which one of the three basic color vision mechanisms is absent or nonfunctioning.
  - *Protanopia:* Color vision deficiency, characterized by complete absence of red cones
  - *Deuteranopia:* Color vision defect, characterized by absence of green cones and is inherited as X-linked disorder
  - *Tritanopia:* Tritanopia is characterized by absence of blue cones.

Achromatopsia: Achromatopsia is characterized by complete cone deficiency, and occurs when two or all three cone pigments are missing. Achromatopsia can be complete or incomplete.

Acquired Color Defects

A change in color vision may be caused due to serious ocular and systemic conditions, which changes in severity and type. The severity of defect may be greater in one eye and does not have any gender predisposition. Acquired color defects may occur secondary to damage to macula or optic nerve.

Blue–yellow color vision defect is usually seen in patients with chronic serous chorioretinopathy, macular edema, and shallow retinal detachment.

Red–green color vision defects are usually seen in patients with optic nerve dysfunction such as optic neuritis, Leber's optic atrophy.

Acquired blue color defect can be due to age-related nuclear sclerosis.

Contrast Sensitivity

Contrast sensitivity implies the ability of observer to perceive differences between an object and its background and to be able to discriminate it from the same. According to Michelson's formula and Weber's definition, contrast sensitivity is defined as a measure of the difference in luminance and amount of reflected light from two adjacent surfaces, which are lighter and darker with respect to each other and can be expressed as a percentage, with the maximum being 100%. Thus, if the lighter surface is white, it will ideally reflect all light and if the darker surface is black and it will reflect no light, the contrast ratio is 1 and if converted into percentage, measures 100%. Self-illuminated Snellen visual acuity charts are high-contrast charts, approximately 100%, this means we are measuring visual acuity in Snellen chart in 100% contrast, and this scenario of 100% contrast is rarely encountered in day-to-day life and most tasks are performed under low-contrast conditions, therefore contrast sensitivity measurements form an integral part of current ophthalmic practice.

Types: There are two major types of contrast sensitivity, which can be assessed:
1. *Spatial:* Spatial contrast sensitivity refers to the detection of striped patterns at various levels of contrast and spatial frequencies. Width of the stripes is defined as the spatial frequency that expresses the number of pairs of light and dark bands subtending an angle of one degree at the eye. Thus, in high spatial frequencies, the bands are narrower and in low spatial frequencies, the bands are wider.
2. *Temporal:* Temporal contrast sensitivity refers to the time-related processing in the visual system. Human contrast system is most sensitive in detecting contrast differences occurring at about four cycles per degree, i.e., at this spatial frequency, the normal human eye will detect lower contrast differences than at any other frequency. The higher frequency cut-off

is related to the optical limits of the human visual system's ability to resolve details and is about 60 cycles per degree. The low frequency drop-off is due to lateral inhibition within the retinal ganglion cells (RGCs).

Contrast sensitivity tests: Tests for contrast sensitivity can be grating contrast tests such as Arden's, Regan's, and Cambridge low-contrast grating test or letter contrast tests such as Pelli Robson's and Bailey–Lovie low-contrast visual acuity chart.

- *Grating contrast test:*
  - *Arden gratings:* Arden introduced a booklet with seven plates, the contrast changes from top to bottom, with increasing spatial frequency and covers a range of 1.76 log units, plates are studied at a distance of 57 cm, each plate is assigned a score of 1–20, a score of 82 with sum of scores of all plates is considered normal.
  - *Cambridge low-contrast gratings:* The test consists of a set of 10 plates and is performed at a distance of 6 m. The pages of this booklet are presented in pair, with one page in each pair being blank and the other having gratings. The pages are shown in decreasing contrast and are stopped when first error is made.
- *Letter contrast test:*
  - *Pelli–Robson contrast sensitivity chart:* The Pelli–Robson Chart, designed by Denis Pelli and John Robson, consists of letters of decreasing contrast, arranged in a pair of three, with two triplets in one row. The contrast decreases from one triplet to another by 0.15 log units, 2.25 log units being the best.

    To perform the test, the chart is hung at a distance of 1 metre, such that the center of chart is approximately at level of subject's eye. The chart is illuminated uniformly and subject is made to read the chart horizontally beginning from the upper left corner. The test is concluded when subject names two of the three letters of the chart incorrectly.

    The test should be performed after giving proper refractive correction under appropriate lighting conditions and should be avoided after any contact procedures.
  - *Functional acuity contrast test (FACT) chart:* FACT chart, developed by Dr Arthur Ginsberg, offers a sensitive and comprehensive measure of functional visual acuity. This chart effectively evaluates the patient's vision over a wide range of size and contrast, closely simulating the normal visual environment.

Factors affecting contrast sensitivity:
- Age, contrast sensitivity decreases with increasing age and is believed to decrease by about 10% for each decade.
- *High-refractive errors decrease the contrast sensitivity:* Postrefractive surgery, also there is a reduction in the contrast sensitivity, one of the reasons for reduced contrast sensitivity after refractive surgery is the increased high-order aberrations induced by the procedure.
- Amblyopia causes lower contrasts for all grating sizes than the fellow eye. A linear relation exists between contrast sensitivity function and visual acuity in the amblyopic eye. As visual acuity decreases, the contrast sensitivity function also decreases and peak sensitivity shifted to lower spatial frequencies.
- Glaucoma decreases contrast sensitivity over all grating sizes and affects both parvocellular and magnocellular pathways.
- Cataract affects lower frequencies. It affects lower contrast sensitivity at some or all grating sizes. Symptoms of glare may exacerbate the results.
- Patients with macular degenerations and diabetic retinopathy demonstrate greater contrast sensitivity loss for all grating sizes with increased degeneration.
- Multiple sclerosis (MS) and optic neuropathy due to pituitary adenomas affect middle grating sizes.
- Drugs such as ibuprofen have been reported to cause loss of contrast over all grating sizes, which can be due to transient multifocal lesions of the visual pathway, scotoma and color vision changes are other deleterious effects of the drug.

Visual Evoked Potential (VEP)

The most common electrophysiological test done in neuro-ophthalmic disorders is the visual-evoked response. The VEP, as the name suggests, is the record of electric potential generated in the occipital cortex when a stimulus is shown to the patient.

Electrodes: The electrodes are placed on the occipital cortex, and the response generated is recorded. The electrodes are placed such that both hemispheres are equally recorded. The inion electrode is placed near the area of visual cortex, and is called the active electrode. Reference electrode is placed over the nonvisual cortex at the vertex and detects minimal activity in response to visual stimulation. The ground electrode is placed over the forehead.

Stimuli: The stimuli can be either in the form of a flash of light (diffuse light spot) or in the form of a pattern, depending on the stimuli shown VEP can be flash or pattern VEP.

In flash VEP, the stimuli are presented repetitively randomly or regularly within a short period of time. The electrical activity thus generated is recorded graphically by an x-y plotter on the contrary in pattern VEP a checkerboard pattern is shown to the patient; hence, a proper refractive error correction should be given to avoid any variations in the result during pattern VEP.

Response generated: The standard flash VEP is characterized by two negative waves and two positive waves in the sequence N1, P1, N2, and P2, the amplitude and implicit times depend on check size, contrast and alteration frequencies of the stimulus. The wave most often used for clinical studies is, however, P100, which is the first positive wave, recorded at 100 ms. The amplitude of this response is defined as the height of potential measured from pack to trough.

Indications:
- *Demyelinating lesion:* A delay in the generation of the P wave is suggestive of increase in the latency and is a characteristic feature of demyelinating diseases.
- *Ischemic toxic and compressive optic neuropathy:* A decrease in the amplitude of P wave is present in ischemic, toxic, and compressive optic neuropathies.
- *Optic atrophy:* VEP helps in measurement of optic nerve function and is also helpful in monitoring hydrocephalus and idiopathic intracranial hypertension (IIH).
- *Visual acuity:* Sweep VEP can be used to determine the visual acuity in preverbal children. Sweep VEP gives two types of visual acuity minimum discriminable angle.
- *Nonorganic vision loss:* VEP also helps to diagnose nonorganic vision loss, a person denying vision, but having a response on VEP is likely to have nonorganic vision loss.
- *Visual fields assessment:* VEP can also help to localize the optic pathway lesions, asymmetric amplitudes recorded over both the hemispheres is suggestive of hemianopic visual field loss, similarly in chiasmal lesions with bitemporal hemianopia, a decreased amplitude of VEP can be recorded over contralateral hemisphere when each eye is separately stimulated.

Visual Fields

Visual field analysis plays an important role in the management of the various neuro-ophthalmic disorders. It helps in exact localization of the visual pathway defect, and in monitoring the disease course. Normal visual field in each eye is approximately, 60° superiorly, 70–75° inferiorly, 60° nasally, and 100–110° temporally. The optic disc forms the physiological blind spot and is located 15° temporally in each eye.

Evaluation of the visual field: Most of the tests to evaluate visual fields are subjective and are based on the patient's ability to appreciate the target. The common tests used to evaluate visual fields are Goldmann perimetry and automated static perimetry using Humphrey visual fields.
- *Goldmann perimetry:* Goldmann perimetry is an example of kinetic perimetry, which is performed using a moving target, such that the target moves from an area of nonvisibility to the visible area.
  Patient's head is placed on the chin rest and one eye of the patient is patched. He is then asked to fixate on a central point and stimuli in the form of white light dots are projected in the inner surface of bowl. The stimulus is moved from the unseen periphery to the patient's field of view.
  The test can be easily performed in elderly patients and in patients with low visual acuity.
- *Humphrey's visual field:* Humphrey's visual field uses the principle of automated perimetry, it is more sensitive, but is more time consuming and require good patient co-operation. Patient's head is placed on the chin rest and one eye of patient is covered, patient is then asked to fixate at the central spot. The white light dot stimuli are projected in the inner surface of bowl, randomly. Patient is given a buzzer in one hand and is asked to press the buzzer whenever he sees the stimulus. The size of stimulus remains the same but its intensity varies. This test helps to test central 10, 24, and 30°.

Humphrey's visual field-testing strategies: Swedish interactive threshold algorithm (SITA) and SITA standard are most commonly used. The test is completed in 3 minutes (each eye) with SITA fast technique and in 6 minutes (each eye) with SITA standard technique.

Interpretation of various visual field defects is summarized in **Table 1**.

Optical Coherence Tomography

Optical coherence tomography (OCT) can detect subtle anatomical variations, and helps in assessment of optic nerve head abnormality. Hence, it is useful in patients with congenital optic disc abnormalities such as disc pit, disc coloboma, optic

TABLE 1: Interpretation of various visual field defects.

Visual field defects caused by lesions in visual pathway

• Retina	
• Macular pathologies	• Central and paracentral defects
• Degenerative retinopathy	• Progressive constriction of peripheral visual fields
Optic nerve	• Central, paracentral defects, centrocecal scotoma (optic neuritis, hereditary optic neuropathy, and toxic optic neuropathy)
	• Altitudinal defects (ischemic neuropathy)
Chiasma	Bitemporal hemianopia
Retrochiasmal lesion	Homonymous hemianopia
Occipital lobe (PCA infarct)	Homonymous hemianopia with macular sparing
Parietal lobe lesion (Superior fibers of optic radiation)	Pie in the floor
Temporal lobe lesion	Pie in the sky

(PCA: posterior cerebral artery)

disc atrophy, and disc hypoplasia. It will also be useful in conditions with progressive structural alteration such as in cases of disc edema, ischemic optic neuropathies, and systemic disorders.

Optical coherence tomography uses the principle of laser interferometry, the OCT system profile combines them in 2-dimensional line scans (B scan) and further to 3-dimensional scans thus producing depth resolved tissue image.

Currently available OCT uses spectrometer to analyze the backscattered light from the tissue interfaces simultaneously, thus increasing the resolution of images and reducing the acquisition time.

Peripapillary retinal fiber layer imaging measures the thickness of retinal nerve fiber layer (RNFL) in a concentric circle around optic disc, and displays thickness measurements in superior, inferior, nasal, and temporal quadrants and smaller segments. These measurements are reproducible and thus are helpful in regular monitoring of the progression. Although RNFL thickness is the most common parameter measured, ganglion cell layer (GCL) is a better indicator of visual function.

The line scan provides a cross-sectional image of the desired area and can be oriented horizontally or obliquely through optic disc or through papillomacular bundle, and will be helpful in the diagnosis of structural abnormalities of optic nerve head.

Indications:

Multiple sclerosis: MS is characterized by the progressive demyelination of axons. RNFL continues as optic nerve and is unique as it lacks myelin sheath, but is an ideal structure to visualize the process of neurodegeneration, neuroprotection, and neurorestoration. RNFL thickness and macular volumes are reduced in patients with MS.

Axonal loss of RNFL is the most severe in those cases of MS, which have significant cerebral demyelination. Moreover, the disorganization of the RNFL can be demonstrated even when there was no history of an episode of optic neuritis.

Optical coherence tomography can also help in understanding the pathogenesis of MS and can also help in progressive monitoring of the disease process.

Optical coherence tomography in ischemic optic neuropathies: OCT in ischemic optic neuropathies helps to monitor disc edema resolution and RNFL loss over time thus, providing a good correlation with the Humphrey's visual field.

Optical coherence tomography in toxic optic neuropathy (TON): TONs are associated with the loss of RNFL. OCT shows considerable loss of the nerve fibers.

In methyl alcohol toxicity on the contrary, initially in the acute, there is peripapillary nerve fiber swelling due to accumulation of intraretinal fluid; however, with the progression in the chronic phase the retinal nerve fiber thickness is diffusely reduced.

Optical coherence tomography in papilledema: Papilledema is traditionally monitored using stereoscopic fundoscopy and photography. OCT in papilledema reveals an increase in the RNFL thickness, which eventually normalizes with eventual thinning as the edema resolves. The optic nerve head in papilledema is elevated with smooth internal contour and subretinal hyporeflective space (SHYPS) and a recumbent "lazy V" pattern. OCT is also helpful in diagnosis of subtle disc edema.

2. Discuss the evaluation and management of disc edema.

Approach to the patient of disc edema depends upon whether the patient has unilateral or bilateral disc edema. The investigations and management of a case of disc edema should be tailored according to the underlying etiology.

Unilateral Disc Edema

Unilateral disc edema usually results from papillitis, neuroretinitis, and ischemic optic neuropathies. Acute stages of Leber's hereditary optic neuropathy (LHON) can present with unilateral disc edema with telangiectasia being the characteristic feature. The common feature in each of these is the sudden onset profound vision loss, hence the investigations must be advised taking in considerations age, gender, and presenting feature of each of the etiology when suspecting them to be the underlying cause.

Bilateral Disc Edema

Pseudopapilledema

It is mandatory to first rule out pseudopapilledema to avoid any nonessential investigations. Common causes of pseudopapilledema include optic nerve head drusen and hypermetropia. The differentiating features of true and pseudo disc edema have been summarized in **Flowchart 1**. Ultrasound B scan helps to rule out optic nerve head drusen and shows the presence of a high amplitude spike at the level of disc.

True Disc Edema

Papilledema: Bilateral disc edema associated with increased intracranial pressure (ICP) is termed as papilledema.

Etiology: The common causes include—
- Grade 5 hypertensive retinopathy (Keith–Wegner–Beker classification)
- Intracranial space-occupying lesion
- Spinal cord tumors
- Cerebral venous thrombosis.
  If disc edema cannot be explained by the above-mentioned etiology, then diagnosis of IIH should be considered.

Pathogenesis of papilledema: Papilledema results from the translaminar elevation of cerebrospinal fluid (CSF) pressure gradient which is further transmitted down the optic nerve sheath from the intracranial cavity and produces axoplasmic flow stasis and resultant intraneuronal ischemia, further causing vision loss.

Symptoms: Patients usually present with complaints of headache with no to mild blurring of vision. Some patients may also complain of diplopia in lateral gazes, resulting from sixth nerve palsy.

Signs:
- *Visual acuity:* Visual acuity is usually good in the initial stages of papilledema, until the late stages when optic atrophy ensues in.
- *Pupil:* Relative afferent pupillary defect (RAPD) cannot be elicited in patients with bilateral involvement and will have sluggishly reacting pupil.
- *Extraocular movements:* Extraocular movements must be examined to look for any limitation of abduction and sixth nerve palsy which can result from stretching of nerve due to increased intracranial tension and causes a false localizing sign.
- *Color vision:* Color vision is reduced and can be established simply by using a red object to check for red color desaturation.
- *Fundus examination:* Fundus examination reveals the presence of an elevated disc with blurred margins and surrounding flame-shaped hemorrhages, exudates and presence of Paton's lines (Paton's lines result from displacement of retina due to underlying edema; throwing the peripapillary retina into a series of folds running concentrically with the edge of disc).
- Spontaneous venous pulsation (SVP) results from the variation in the pressure gradient along the retinal vein as it traverses the lamina cribrosa. When the ICP rises, the intracranial pulse pressure also rises to equal the intraocular pulse pressure and the SVP ceases.
- *Grading:* Frisen's grading of papilledema helps to determine progression of the papilledema.
  - *Grade 1:* Blurring of nasal disc margin with normal temporal margins
  - *Grade 2:* Blurring of 360° of disc margin with few flame-shaped hemorrhages

- *Grade 3:* Blurring of disc margin with surrounding hemorrhages and exudates
- *Grade 4:* Optic atrophy.

Spontaneous venous pulsation results from the variation in the pressure gradient along the retinal vein as it traverses the lamina cribrosa. When the ICP rises, the intracranial pulse pressure also rises to equal the intraocular pulse pressure and the SVP ceases.

Investigation:

30° test: Increase in the ICP causes an increase in the optic nerve sheath diameter. The difference in the optic nerve sheath diameter (ONSD) in primary position as compared to an eccentric 30° gaze is a useful test to detect papilledema. Optic nerve sheath diameter can be measured with the help of ultrasound B scan, 3 mm behind the globe from inner edge to inner edge of optic nerve. The site 3 mm behind the globe is recommended as it is believed to be the site with maximum pressure changes along the optic nerve. When the eye rotates to 30° eccentric gaze position, the CSF within the sheath redistributes itself posteriorly, reducing the ONSD. Usually, a reduction of ONSD of more than 10% from primary position to 30° from fixation is considered positive for fluid in the sheath and a marker of potential increased ICP.

- *Visual fields:* Visual field examination reveals the presence of enlarged blind spot.
- *Fundus fluorescein angiography:* Fundus fluorescein angiography reveals the presence of disc leakage in true optic disc edema as opposed to disc staining without leakage in pseudo papilledema.
- *Optical coherence tomography:* OCT in papilledema reveals an increase in the RNFL, which eventually normalizes with eventual thinning as the edema resolves. The optic nerve head in papilledema is elevated with smooth internal contour and subretinal hyporeflective space and a recumbent "lazy V" pattern. OCT is also helpful in diagnosis of subtle disc edema.
- *Magnetic resonance imaging (MRI) brain:* MRI brain must be the initial investigation advised (after ruling out pseudopapilledema) to exclude the diagnosis of space-occupying lesion.
- *Magnetic resonance venography (MRV):* MRV helps to rule out cerebral venous thrombosis. Cerebral venous thrombosis can be further attributed to a large number of causes, which include Behcet's disease, septic, and tumor emboli, autoimmune diseases such as systemic lupus erythematosus (SLE) and primary coagulopathy. Hence, once cerebral venous thrombosis is detected on MRV, investigations to diagnose the underlying pathology must be done.
- *Lumbar puncture:* After excluding the space-occupying lesion, lumbar puncture should be done, and increased opening pressure, should warrant further investigation.

Management:

The management depends upon the underlying etiology.

Flowchart 2 summarizes the approach to a patient with disc edema.

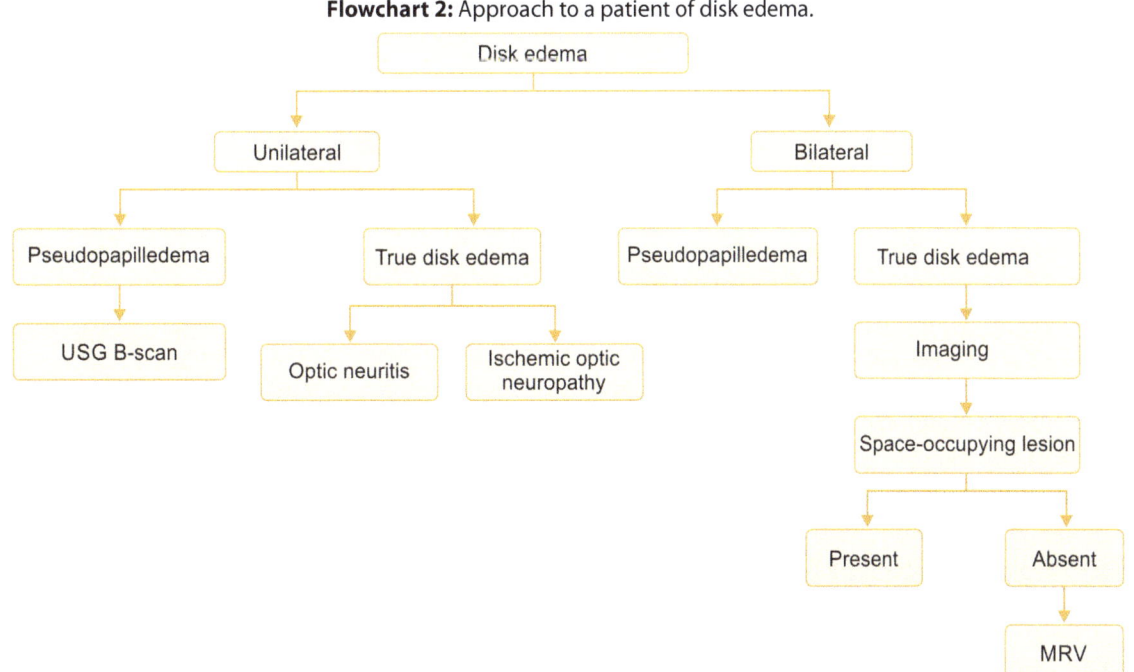

Flowchart 2: Approach to a patient of disk edema.

(MRV: magnetic resonance venography; USG: ultrasonography)

3. Explain differential diagnosis, evaluation, and management of unilateral disc edema.

See above Answer.

4. Discuss etiopathogenesis, differential diagnosis, and management of unilateral swelling of on head.

See Answer to the above Question.

5. Discuss traumatic optic neuropathy.

Traumatic optic neuropathy may occur directly or indirectly after cranio-orbital trauma. Optic nerve damage can be caused due to direct transection, avulsion, ischemia, or orbital hemorrhage.

Direct optic nerve injuries can result from penetrating trauma, especially associated with orbital fractures; whereas indirect optic nerve injury is caused by the transmission of forces to optic nerve from a distant site, without any overt damage to the surrounding tissue structures.

Etiopathogenesis

Traumatic optic neuropathy occurs in 0.5–2% of patients who suffer closed head trauma.

The intracanalicular portion of optic nerve is more susceptible to injury due to its compact space. The nerve may be damaged by shearing and avulsion of its nutrient vessels, or by pressure transmitted along bone to optic canal as the nerve lies in a close compacted space in the optic canal, the canalicular portion of optic nerve becomes more susceptible to injury, the next most common site is intracranial portion of the optic nerve, as it lies in close proximity to the falciform dural fold, making it susceptible for damage.

The optic nerve injuries can be caused by primary or secondary mechanism.
- *Primary mechanism:* The primary mechanism is due to immediate mechanical shearing of RGC axons, an irreversible process that results in neuronal loss.
- *Secondary mechanism:* Following the primary mechanism, optic nerve swelling develops and as the nerve lies within the tight canal, it results in compartment syndrome and ischemia, thus compromising blood supply to the RGCs and causing the cell death by apoptosis.

Clinical Features

Symptoms

The strong clinical suspicion of traumatic optic neuropathy arises when there is loss of vision after a history of blunt or penetrating trauma especially in the region of forehead, brow or to face. The most common mechanism of injury as stated in IONT study was motor vehicle accident, bike accident, fall, and assault.

Signs
- *Visual acuity:* Visual acuity is invariably reduced significantly in all the patients of traumatic optic neuropathy.
- *Pupil:* RAPD can be elicited in patients with unilateral traumatic optic neuropathy, but in patients with bilateral traumatic optic neuropathy, both the pupils will be sluggishly reacting and show light near dissociation.
- *Anterior segment:* Anterior segment must be examined to look for other signs of blunt trauma.
- *Fundus:* Fundus examination must be done to look for retinal dialysis, breaks. Optic nerve findings may vary, and depend upon the site of trauma.

Anterior injuries may cause optic nerve avulsion, appearing a ring of hemorrhage, compromised retinal vascular supply can lead to retinal infarction or central retinal artery occlusion and with more posterior injuries, which are more common, fundus can look entirely normal. Disc pallor develops usually about 6 weeks following the initial injury.

Investigations
- *Color vision and contrast sensitivity:* Color vision and contrast sensitivity will be affected, as such as in other pathologies affecting the optic nerve.

- *Visual fields:* Visual field examination requires sufficient level of vision and may help to localize the lesion. Moreover, there are no pathognomonic visual field features associated with traumatic optic neuropathy.
- *Optical coherence tomography in traumatic optic neuropathy:* A few case reports and clinical studies have demonstrated the role of OCT in traumatic optic neuropathy, and it had been found that there is progressive loss of RNFL thickness as the disc pallor ensues. Besides, another study has demonstrated an increased choroidal thickness in patients with traumatic optic neuropathy, which can be explained due to impaired blood circulation and vascular remodeling of the optic nerve head and choroid.
- *Visual evoked response (VER):* VER can be helpful in cases, where assessment of pupillary response is difficult, as in bilateral cases.
- *Neuroimaging:* High-resolution computed tomography (HRCT) is the diagnostic procedure of choice as it can delineate bony fractures better than MRI. Orbital and optic canal fractures as well as optic nerve sheath hemorrhages can be better detected on CT scan. MRI is superior for imaging soft tissue and assessing chiasmal damage.

Management

Medical and surgical management of traumatic optic neuropathy is needed for the following reasons:
- To reduce edema
- To make more space for the edematous nerve
- To use neuroprotective agents to reduce the damage cascade which is set up at the moment of injury.

Surgical Management

Indications of immediate surgical management include:
- Orbital hemorrhage compromising optic nerve that can be relieved by lateral canthotomy and cantholysis.
- Patients with impacted bony fragment impinging on optic nerve, other school of thought on the contrary states that optic canal fracture is a poor prognostic factor for visual recovery, as an impinged bony fragment can transect the optic nerve causing loss of a large proportion of ganglion cell axons, which are less likely to recover.

Surgery: Intra- and extracranial surgical techniques have been used to achieve optic nerve decompression in TON, minimally invasive extracranial approaches using transethmoidal, endonasal, or sublabial routes are preferred.

Complications of surgery are CSF leak, meningitis, and exacerbation of traumatic optic neuropathy.

Medical Management

The use of steroids in traumatic optic neuropathy is controversial. Some of the studies have shown that patients of traumatic optic neuropathy, treated with corticosteroids, have a faster recovery while there are studies, which have shown no effect of steroids in management of traumatic optic neuropathy.

The proponents of steroid therapy believe that the anti-inflammatory properties of steroids can reduce edema and thus decrease the loss of ganglion cells due to compression; moreover, steroids in high doses have antioxidant and free radical scavenger property, as used in optic neuritis, can also help in neuroprotection.

The first evidence of utilization of steroids in the management of traumatic optic neuropathy was suggested by National Acute Spinal Cord Injury Study-II (NACS-II).

The NACS-II was a multicenter clinical trial, which evaluated the role of mega dose of steroids in patients of acute brain and spinal cord injury and found that patients who presented within 8 hours of trauma. The study concluded that mega dose of steroids, 30 mg/kg loading dose, followed by 5.4 mg/kg for next 24 hours, showed a significant improvement in the visual outcomes. This led to a widespread use of steroids in traumatic optic neuropathy.

But other studies had contradictory results, corticosteroid randomization after significant head injury (CRASH) trial evaluated the role of mega dose of steroids in traumatic brain injury, but the study had to be stopped early due to increased number of deaths in the treatment group.

 6. Discuss the clinical features, differential diagnosis, and management of optic neuritis.

Optic neuritis is defined as the inflammation of optic nerve and its sheath, if the optic nerve head (optic disc) is edematous, the term papillitis is used and on the other hand, if the optic nerve head is normal and shows no signs of inflammation, the term retrobulbar neuritis is used.

TABLE 2: McDonald's criteria for multiple sclerosis (MS).

Number of attacks	Lesion	Criteria for diagnosis
0 (progression from onset)	—	1 year of disease progression, and 2 of 3 criteria Dissemination in space in brain* Dissemination in space in spinal cord* Positive CSF
1	• 1 • 2	• Dissemination in space and time • Dissemination in time
2 or more	• 1 • 2 or more	• Dissemination in space • None

*Dissemination in space: one or more T2 lesion in MS typical regions which are juxtacortical, periventricular, spinal cord, infratentorial. Dissemination in time: simultaneous asymptomatic contrast-enhancing and nonenhancing lesions at any time or a new T2 or contrast-enhancing lesion on follow-up MRI irrespective of the timing.
(CSF: cerebrospinal fluid; MRI: magnetic resonance imaging)

Types

Optic neuritis can be classified according to the etiology and the appearance of the optic disc.

Etiological Classification

- *Demyelinating:* Optic neuritis can occur as a forme fruste form of MS, and can also be associated with other demyelinating disorders such as Devic's disease [neuromyelitis optica (NMO)] which forming a separate spectrum of disorders. Devic's disease is characterized by necrotizing demyelinating lesions of bilateral optic nerves and spinal cord and occurs due to formation of serum antibody, NMO-IgG, which targets the autoantigen aquaporin-4, a useful marker for the diagnosis. The spinal lesions extend contiguously over three of more vertebral segments. MS and optic neuritis: The incidence of optic neuritis has been recorded as 1–5 cases/100,000/year, with the incidence being higher at the higher latitudes. 15–20% of patients with MS can have acute demyelinating optic neuritis as the presenting feature; 50% of patients of MS can develop optic neuritis in the due course of disease. Similarly optic neuritis can be the first presenting feature of MS, as noted in 38% of patients in optic neuritis treatment trial (ONTT).
- *McDonald diagnostic criteria for MS:* Significant clinical history and presentation along with neuroimaging abnormalities with or without CSF abnormalities or abnormal VEP response is sufficient for diagnosis of MS; however, only recurrent optic neuritis in the absence of other clinical or laboratory manifestations is not sufficient for diagnosis. **Table 2** summarizes McDonald criteria.
- *Parainfectious:* Usually occurs following a viral infection or immunization.
- *Infectious:* Occurs due to sinus infections or in association with cat scratch fever, syphilis, Lyme disease, cryptococcal meningitis in patients with acquired immunodeficiency syndrome (AIDS), and herpes zoster.
- *Autoimmune:* Occurs in association with systemic causes such as sarcoidosis, SLE, polyarteritis nodosa, and other forms of vasculitis.

Morphological Classification

- *Papillitis:* In papillitis, optic nerve head is affected, fundus examination shows the presence of a hyperemic and edematous disc, which can be associated with peripapillary flame-shaped hemorrhages.
- *Neuroretinitis:* Neuroretinitis is associated with papillitis along with macular star. Macular star results from exudation in peripapillary retina, and penetrates the outer plexiform layer resulting into typical appearance of macular star. Macular star appears after 2 weeks; hence, it becomes essential to re-examine the patient of papillitis after 2 weeks. Neuroretinitis is more commonly associated with infectious etiologies such as syphilis and cat scratch disease.
- *Retrobulbar neuritis:* Optic nerve head is not involved and appears to be normal in acute stages, till in the chronic stage optic atrophy ensues in.

Clinical Features

The average age of onset is typically in the 30s, with common age group being 20–50 years and it predominantly affecting females.

TABLE 3: Distinguishing features between typical and atypical optic neuritis.

	Typical	Atypical
Age	Young adult	Pediatric cases, older age
Laterality	Unilateral	Bilateral
Clinical course	Mild-to-moderate loss of vision followed by spontaneous improvement after 2 weeks	Severe vision loss progressing for >2 weeks; no spontaneous improvement noted for longer duration
Pain on eye movements	Mild-to-moderate periocular pain worsening on eye movements	Severe periocular pain
Fundus	Normal or edematous disk	Severe disk edema, macular star, and retinal exudates
Other findings	Uthoff's phenomenon, Pulfrich effect	Family history and neoplastic history

Symptoms

The patients typically present with complaints of sudden onset blurring of vision, and can be associated with pain on extraocular movements, especially upgaze which can be explained by the attachment of some fibers of superior rectus to dura mater. The maximum severity of pain is seen by 24–36 hours which subsides within 48–72 hours. Both eyes can be simultaneously involved in 10% or in rapid succession, bilateral cases are more common in children (12–15 years) **(Table 3)**.

Signs

- Relative afferent papillary defect can be noted.
- Color vision and contrast sensitivity are reduced. Abnormal color vision was noted in 94% of the involved eyes using Fransworth–Munsell 100 hue test in ONTT.
- *Uthoff's phenomenon:* Temporary loss of vision with exercise in patients of optic neuritis. Exercise increases body temperature, due to which the nerve impulses are blocked or slowed down in a demyelinated nerve. Uthoff's phenomenon is associated with MS. Blockade of ion channels, heat shock proteins, circulatory changes, effects of serum calcium, and unidentified humoral substance have been hypothesized and investigated as a cause of Uhthoff's phenomenon in MS.
- *Pulfrich's phenomenon:* The phenomenon was first described by Pulfrich in 1922, wherein lateral motion of an object in the field of view is interpreted by the brain as having a depth component. Patient is shown a pendulum, a person with demyelinating disorder can appreciate a three-dimensional movement of the pendulum, which can be explained due to a relative difference in signal timings between the two eyes in demyelinating disorders. Pulfrich's phenomenon causes difficulties with tasks involving judgement of moving objects, such as playing certain sports, crossing roads, or driving.
- *Lhermitte's sign:* Lhermitte's sign is described by the patients as an electric shock such as pain that runs from the head down to the back, through the arms and legs and is due to demyelination of dorsal columns of cervical spine.

Investigations

- *Visual field:* Central/centrocecal scotoma is typically noted in optic neuritis; however, in ONTT, all types of visual field defect were noted. Visual field defect typically resolves at 1 year in 56% patients and in 76% patients at 10 years.
- *Visual evoked response:* VER is not specific, and shows a delay in P100 latency indicating a slow conduction along the optic nerve, VER also helps to detect subclinical disease in the fellow eye. VER abnormalities persist even after complete recovery, and 80–90% of patients will have an abnormal VER at the end of 1 year and 35% will return to normal in 2 years.
- *Optical coherence tomography:* OCT shows RNFL thinning which is evident after edema resolves.
- *Optical coherence tomography-angiography (OCT-A):* OCT-A measurements in MS patients can help to detect retinal vascular impairment. The optic nerve head flow index (ONH-FI) is measured by OCT-A and allows for visualization of the density and caliber of retinal vessels and flow velocity. A significant decrease in ONH-FI in MS patients with a history of optic neuritis as compared to healthy controls has been observed in various studies. Optic nerve damage in MS patients with optic neuritis can be detected most accurately when ONH-FI and structural OCT parameters are considered in combination. These findings have demonstrated the usefulness of OCT-A in studying vascular abnormalities associated with MS.
- *Imaging:* Contrast-enhanced fat suppressed MRI of orbit and brain is the imaging protocol of choice and shows the enhancement of inflamed optic nerve. Periventricular demyelinating plaques are a characteristic of MS. MRI also helps to estimate the cumulative probability for developing MS as suggested by ONTT. A negative MRI at baseline indicated the risk of MS to be 25%, on the other hand, presence of a single lesion doubled the 15-year risk to 50%, while three or more lesions caused a threefold increase in the risk, viz., to 78%.

- *Blood investigations:* Blood investigations should be advised when suspecting infections, autoimmune diseases, in cases of recurrent optic neuritis, atypical cases, cases with bilateral simultaneous involvement, in pediatric patients (age <15 years) and before initiating steroids. Blood investigations include:
  - Complete blood count
  - Erythrocyte sedimentation rate (ESR)
  - C-reactive protein (CRP) levels
  - Chest X-ray and Mantoux test should be advised to rule out tuberculosis.
  - Venereal disease research laboratory test (VDRL), fluorescent treponemal antibody absorption (FTA-ABS), and TORCH profile are advised besides the above-mentioned investigations in cases of neuroretinitis.
  - *Cerebrospinal fluid analysis:* CSF analysis shows nonspecific abnormalities such as increased lymphocytes (10–100) and elevated protein. Presence of oligoclonal bands predicts the progression to MS.

Management

Routine treatment of demyelinating optic neuritis is not advised and eventually resolves by itself.

Treatment is considered only for the patients who:
- Require faster recovery
- Have severe bilateral visual loss
- In patients with poor vision in the fellow eye.

Steroids in optic neuritis: Steroids in optic neuritis are used for acute exacerbations.

Regimen: Intravenous (IV) methylprednisolone 1 g daily for 3 days followed by oral prednisolone (1 mg/kg/day) for 11 days and then tapered over 3 days. Oral corticosteroids alone were associated with an increased risk of recurrence of optic neuritis in ONTT hence this form of therapy should be avoided.

Optic neuritis treatment trial.
- *Objective:* ONTT was a prospective interventional trial conducted with an objective to evaluate the efficacy of steroids in the management of optic neuritis and to establish relation between optic neuritis and MS.
- *Methods:* Patients were randomized into three arms: placebo, oral (low-dose) prednisone (1 mg/kg/day for 14 days), and high-dose IV methylprednisolone (250 mg four times daily for 3 days), followed by oral prednisone (1 mg/kg/day for 11 days).
- *Results:* At 6 months, color vision and contrast sensitivity and visual fields were found to be significantly better in the methylprednisolone arm; however, after 1 year, there was no significant difference between treated and untreated patients in any of the functional outcome. Intravenous methylprednisolone was found to accelerate the rate of visual recovery over the first 15 days. By day 30, nearly complete recovery occurred in all patients. No significant difference was found between oral prednisolone and placebo in any of the parameter. At 12 months, all three groups were similar in terms of visual functions. In a subsequent analysis, patients randomized to receive treatment with high-dose IV methylprednisolone in conjunction with 11-day low-dose oral prednisone taper exhibited a significantly reduced risk of developing clinically definite MS (defined by the development of new neurologic symptoms attributable to demyelination other than optic neuritis in either eye occurring at least 4 weeks after the study entry and lasting >24 hours with abnormality documented on neurological examination) over the subsequent 2 years. Beyond 2 years, no significant disease-modifying effects of steroids were seen.

Other Options

- Longer-acting agents (delay the development of CDMS):
  - *Disease-modifying drugs:* Interferon β-1a and -1b, glatiramer acetate. The results of trials on various disease-modifying drugs have been summarized in **Table 4**.
  - *Immunosuppressive:* Mitoxantrone, natalizumab, and fingolimod
- *Intravenous immunoglobulins (IVIGs):* IVIGs have been tried for acute optic neuritis but with no long-term effects on visual function or on the latency of VEP responses after AON.
- *Plasma exchange (PLEX):* PLEX has demonstrated efficacy in the treatment of refractory AON and in AON associated with NMO. The addition of PLEX to IV methylprednisolone in the acute treatment of NMO-associated AON has showed significant improvement in high-contrast acuity, visual fields, and temporal RNFL thickness, but not low-contrast letter scores or color vision. The early, first-line use of PLEX in the treatment of AON is yet to be evaluated. PLEX is presumed to mediate a therapeutic effect, at least in part, through the removal of pathogenic humoral and plasma factors.

TABLE 4: Studies for various management options of optic neuritis.

Study	Objective	Inclusion	Results
• Controlled high-risk subjects avonex multiple sclerosis prevention study • CHAMPS	IM weekly INF-β1a vs. placebo	Two white matter lesions in MRI >3 mm	Weekly INF-β1a IM decreased 3-year probability of developing clinically definite multiple sclerosis (CDMS)
Controlled high-risk subjects avonex multiple sclerosis prevention surveillance CHAMPION	5-year continuation of CHAMPS	Compared those who received Avonex from the starting of CHAMPS vs. those who were switched from placebo after 30 months	Those who were started on Avonex from the beginning of the study had fewer relapses
ETOMS	Subcutaneous INF-β1a (Rebif) 22 µg weekly vs. placebo within 3 months of presentation	>4 T2-weighted lesions in MRI	Weekly subcutaneous INF-β1a within 3 months of initial presentation decreased probability of developing CDMS
• Betaferon in newly emerging multiple sclerosis for initial treatment • BENEFIT	INF-β1b 250 µg Betaseron vs. placebo	>2 T2-weighted MRI lesions >3 mm in size within 2 months	INF-β1b 250 µg every alternate day decreased 2-year probability of developing CDMS
• Early glatiramer acetate treatment in delaying conversion to clinically definite multiple sclerosis of subjects presenting with clinically isolated syndrome • PreCISe	Glatiramer acetate 20 mg every day subcutaneously vs. placebo	>2 T2-weighted MRI lesions >6 mm	Glatiramer acetate 20 mg every day subcutaneously for 3 years, reduced risk of developing CDMS
• Prevention of relapses and disability by interferon (IFN) β-1a subcutaneously in multiple sclerosis • PRISMS	IFN-β1a 22 µg and 44 µg SC vs. placebo in relapsing-remitting multiple sclerosis		Both treatment groups had fewer relapses

(IM: intramuscular; MRI: magnetic resonance imaging)

- *Erythropoietin:* Systemic infusion of erythropoietin with and without methylprednisolone has demonstrated beneficial effects on RGC function and survival in a rat model of experimental autoimmune encephalomyelitis. Erythropoietin administration increases protein levels of various antiapoptotic factors such as phospho-Akt, phospho-MAPK 1 and 2, and Bcl-2 which help to limit the apoptosis of RGCs after AON. Erythropoietin administration has shown partial recovery of pattern reversal VEPs and improvement in flash electroretinograms and significant improvement in the thickness of peripapillary RNFL. A recent trial showed 33,000 IU erythropoietin is effective in managing optic neuritis as an adjuvant to methylprednisolone.
- *Teriflunomide:* Teriflunomide selectively and reversibly inhibits dihydro-orotate dehydrogenase, an important enzyme in the pyrimidine synthesis pathway, leading to a reduction in proliferation of activated T and B lymphocytes. In MS, it reduces lymphocyte infiltration in the central nervous system (CNS), reduced axonal loss, and improves the neurological functioning.
- *Adrenocorticotropic hormone:* Adrenocorticotropic hormone reduces the inflammatory axonal loss following optic neuritis.
- *Dimethyl fumarate (DMF):* DMF has been approved for the use of relapsing remitting type of MS; DMF has also shown beneficial effect in optic neuritis associated with MS. DMF is believed to act by targeting the lymphocytes.
- *Antibody against LINGO1 (anti-LINGO):* Leucine-rich repeat and immunoglobulin-like domain-containing protein (LINGO1) is a CNS protein that acts as a negative regulator of oligodendrocyte precursor, and delays their differentiation to promote CNS remyelination. Hence, anti-LINGO1 antibodies will promote remyelination.

 7. Discuss toxic amblyopia/etiology, clinical feature, and management of toxic optic neuropathy.

Toxic optic neuropathy is characterized by the visual impairment resulting from damage to the visual pathway by the toxins; the term toxic amblyopia used previously is a misnomer as it is an optic neuropathy rather than amblyopia.

The anterior visual pathway is susceptible to be damaged by a large number of toxins, which can be in the form of medications or due to exposure to a toxin in the workplace. Thus, TON can be defined as damage caused to the papillomacular bundle resulting in a central or centrocecal field defect, and is attributed to its peculiar blood supply.

Etiopathogenesis

Toxic optic neuropathy can result from exposure to toxins, ingestion of toxins, and from elevated serum levels of certain drugs. The various etiologies have been summarized in **Flowchart 1**. The common among them are tobacco, methyl alcohol ingestion, chronic alcoholism, antitubercular drugs, and antibiotics such as linezolid and chloramphenicol.

Unusual configuration of vascular supply of the optic nerve head may predispose it to the accumulation of toxic agents, although the underlying pathogenesis of TON by most of the agents remains obscure, and is believed to be due to mitochondrial injury and imbalance of intracellular and extracellular free radical homoeostasis.

Pathogenesis of a few common agents has been described below.

- *Methyl alcohol:* Methyl alcohol poisoning still remains an important cause of toxic optic neuropathy and especially amongst the low socioeconomic class. Methyl alcohol is metabolized in the liver by the enzyme alcohol dehydrogenase, leading to the formation of formaldehyde, following which formic acid is formed. Toxicity develops from a combined effect of the metabolic acidosis (H^+ production) and an intrinsic toxicity of the formate ion itself, which inhibits the mitochondrial electron transport chain.
- *Tobacco and chronic alcoholism leading to toxic optic neuropathy:* The underlying pathogenesis of toxic optic neuropathy in tobacco and chronic alcoholism is chiefly due to deficiency of vitamin B complex, chronic exposure of tobacco leads to accumulation cyanide, which inhibits the electron transport chain, thus leading to disruption of ATP production and ultimately impairing the axonal transport system.
- *Ethambutol:* Ethambutol is a bacteriostatic agent, and is the first-line drug used in antitubercular treatment (ATT) regimen. The drug is a chelating agent, which disrupts one of the several metal-containing enzyme systems in the nucleic acid structures of mycobacteria. Chelating properties of ethambutol remain the main cause of neurotoxicity, and it causes calcium flux into mitochondria. Toxicity is classically described as dose- and duration-related and is reversible on discontinuation of therapy. The toxicity appears unpredictable, and, therefore, the drug should be used cautiously. The toxicity is seen in 1–5% of patients taking antituberculosis treatment regimen and symptoms usually start 2–8 months after the drug is started.

    Dosage of 25 mg/kg/day in intensive phase and 15 mg/kg/day in maintenance phase is considered safe as well as effective, although toxicity has been reported below this dosage too.
- *Isoniazid:* Isoniazid is another first-line antitubercular drug, given concurrently with ethambutol. Vision improves when administration of the drug is ceased. Pyridoxine 25–100 mg/day may help to stabilize or even reverse isoniazid-induced toxic neuropathy.

    Physicians should remember that if a patient on ATT develops toxic optic neuropathy and does not improve on stopping ethambutol then isoniazid should also be stopped.

    A baseline ophthalmologic examination should be done before treatment with either ethambutol or isoniazid is started and should include fundus examination, color vision, contrast sensitivity, and visual fields.
- *Amiodarone:* Amiodarone is a commonly used antiarrhythmic drug, and has been associated with a large number of ocular side effects, including corneal verticillata, or vortex keratopathy, anterior subcapsular cataract and nonarteritic anterior ischemic optic neuropathy (NAION). However, NAION is usually unilateral, but amiodarone-induced toxicity is usually bilateral. The mechanism remains unclear and is believed that it may relate to a lipidosis that is induced by the drug, which has been supported by histopathologic studies of the optic nerve in these patients.
- *Linezolid:* Linezolid belongs to oxazolidinone group of antibiotics and shows activity against methicillin-resistant Staphylococcus species, penicillin-resistant Streptococcus species, and vancomycin-resistant enterococci; the drug is usually well tolerated, with few side effects, but toxic optic neuropathy can result from its prolonged use of 5–10 months, and is hypothesized to be caused by mitochondrial dysfunction.
- *Vigabatrin:* An antiepileptic medication is used in the management of infantile spasms and refractory seizures. Vigabatrin causes constriction of visual field; the field defects start as bilateral nasal defects and progress to concentric bilateral field constriction with preservation of central vision.

    Visual field monitoring hence must be done at every 6 months, as vigabatrin-associated visual field defects are irreversible and are due to combined effects of retinal and optic nerve head toxicity. Taurine deficiency is believed to cause retinal phototoxicity.

Clinical Features

Symptoms

Patient complains of painless diminution of vision, which is gradually progressive and is associated with color vision disturbances.

Systemic History

History of tuberculosis, intake of ethambutol, chronic alcoholism or methyl alcohol intake, chronic alcoholism, and smoking must be obtained.

Signs

- *Visual acuity:* Visual acuity varies from minimal reduction of visual acuity to no light perception (NLP) in rare cases (e.g., methanol ingestion).
- *Pupil:* Relative afferent papillary defect present.
- *Optic disc:* The optic disc can be normal or hyperemic in early stages and can develop disc pallor in later stages.

Investigations

Systemic Investigations

- Complete hemogram, total and differential blood counts, and urine analysis must be done.
- Liver function tests can be deranged in case of chronic alcoholism.
- Serum vitamin B_{12} levels and serum folate levels must be monitored, to rule out any nutritional deficiency.

Ophthalmic Investigations

- *Color vision and contrast sensitivity:* Dyschromatopsia is the earliest sign of toxic optic neuropathy and hence color vision and contrast sensitivity tests can be used for early diagnosis of drug-induced toxicity.
- *Visual field examination:* Static (Humphrey) or kinetic (Goldmann) visual field examination is essential in the evaluation of a patient suspected of having toxic/nutritional optic neuropathy. Central or cecocentral scotoma with preservation of the peripheral field is characteristic of toxic optic neuropathy and most frequently found in them. Centrocecal defect results from the involvement of papillomacular bundle, which is most frequently involved.
- *Neuroimaging in toxic optic neuropathy:* Neuroimaging usually is normal in optic nerve-induced toxic optic neuropathy; they are usually indicated to rule out other causes and to confirm the diagnosis.
- *Electrophysiological test:* VER reveals reduced amplitude of P100 wave, with near normal latency, differentiating it from demyelinating causes.
- *Optical coherence tomography:* OCT is a useful tool for the early diagnosis of toxic optic neuropathy, and can quantify loss of RNFL as an early sign of drug-induced toxicity, and thus can also be used for monitoring.

Differential Diagnosis

Differential diagnosis of toxic optic neuropathy includes other causes of gradual progressive optic neuropathy, which can be due to compressive optic neuropathy, infiltrative optic neuropathy, or hereditary optic neuropathy.

Treatment

The foremost step in managing toxic optic neuropathy, as with any toxic process, is to remove the offending agent, which may also cause reversal of the process.

Medical therapy includes multivitamin supplementation, needed in many patients with toxic neuropathy.

Patients with toxic/nutritional optic neuropathy should be observed initially every 4–6 weeks and then every 6–12 months depending on their recovery. Visual acuity, pupils, optic nerves, color vision, and visual fields should be assessed at each visit. Vision may gradually recover to normal over several weeks, and may take months for full restoration, though there is always the risk of permanent residual vision deficit.

Management of a Few Common Specific Toxic Optic Neuropathies

- Methyl alcohol toxicity

- Definitive diagnosis of methanol toxicity requires a confirmed increase in the serum methanol level with gas chromatography (>20 mg/dL), where peak levels are achieved 60–90 minutes after ingestion. A low arterial pH (<7.2) correlates the best with formate levels.
- Supportive therapy includes airway management, correction of electrolyte disturbances, and providing adequate hydration. To correct metabolic acidosis, buffer such as sodium bicarbonate can be used.
- Antidote therapy is directed toward delaying methanol metabolism and can be achieved by the use of either ethanol or fomepizole.
- Ethanol is also metabolized by the enzyme aldehyde dehydrogenase, such as methanol, and the enzyme has 10–20 times more affinity for ethanol as compared to methanol. Fomepizole is also metabolized by the same enzyme, but unlike ethyl alcohol does not cause CNS depression.
- Ethanol however is more commonly used due to its easier cost effectiveness and better availability, and is given IV as a 10% solution in 5% dextrose. A loading dose of 0.6 g/kg is given followed by an IV infusion of 0.07–0.16 g/kg/h.
- Intravenous pulse steroids have been proven to be effective in saving vision in patients of toxic optic neuropathy, and is probably due to anti-inflammatory effects of steroids.
- *Tobacco and ethyl alcohol-induced toxic optic neuropathy:* Nutritional depletion is an important cause of vision detonation in alcohol and tobacco-induced optic neuropathy, and visual improvement in these patients seems to be related to improved nutrition. Therefore, it should be overemphasized to patients that stopping smoking or reducing the consumption of alcohol is critical to their recovery and abstinence from alcohol and tobacco combined with an improved diet and vitamin supplementation remains the mainstay of therapy. Injections of hydroxocobalamin have also been successful in treating patients with tobacco-induced TON. Hydroxycobalamin converts free cyanide generated to cyanocobalamin, an analog of vitamin B12, thus reducing its toxicity.
- *Isoniazid toxicity:* Isoniazid toxicity may be associated with bilateral optic disc swelling. Another atypical feature is that the visual fields often take the appearance of bitemporal hemianopic scotomas. Vision improves when administration of the drug is ceased. Pyridoxine 25–100 mg/day may help to stabilize or even reverse isoniazid-induced toxic neuropathy. Although it has been used to reverse the toxicity of isoniazid, vision may improve simply by stopping the drug

Thus, a baseline ophthalmologic examination should be done before treatment is instituted with any drug associated with optic nerve toxicity. It should include fundus examination, color vision, contrast sensitivity, and visual fields. All these parameters should be monitored periodically as long as they are on the drug to detect any optic nerve toxicity as soon as possible, for this reason physicians must also be aware about the various toxic drugs.

 8. Discuss the optic disc anomalies.

Following are the different optic disc anomalies seen in clinical practice.

Optic Disc Pit

It is a round oval gray, crater-like depression in the optic disc, first described by Wiethe in 1882.

Etiopathogenesis

The exact etiology underlying the development of optic disc pit (ODP) remains obscure.

Congenital pits are believed to be due to imperfect closure of superior edge of embryonic fissure. Histologically, pit is the herniation of rudimentary neuroectodermal tissue into a pocket-like depression within the nerve substance. Its pathogenesis is unknown.

Various theories have been put forward; it is hypothesized that incomplete closure of the fissure results in microcommunication between the pit and subarachnoid space, others believe that pit arises due to coloboma, but contrary to coloboma, pits are usually unilateral and are rarely associated with iris or fundal coloboma. Absence of lamina cribrosa is noted at the site of pit. ODP is often complicated by the serous macular detachments, source of subretinal fluid (SRF) causing serous macular detachment remains controversial; some believe that SRF originates most likely from vitreous cavity, while other school of thought states that fluid arises from the subarachnoid space that surrounds the optic nerve. A lamellar macular hole may develop later.

Acquired ODPs on the contrary are associated with glaucoma and presents as localized region of susceptibility to the elevated intraocular pressure.

Clinical Features

Symptoms

Optic disc pits are usually asymptomatic, unless complicated by serous macular detachment. In the presence of serous detachment, patients may complain of metamorphopsia, micropsia, and blurred vision.

Signs

Optic disc pit is usually an incidental finding. It commonly involves temporal optic disc but may be situated in any sector. It is often associated with adjacent peripapillary retinal pigment epithelium changes in unilateral cases; the involved disc is slightly larger than the normal disc.

Diagnosis

- *Visual field:* Visual field defects are variable; the most common defect appears to be a paracentral arcuate scotoma and enlarged blind spot. Serous macular detachment causes enlarged blind spot.
- *Optical coherence tomography:* OCT in case of ODP can demonstrate trace amounts of subretinal fluid if present, and may also show schisis such as separation between inner and outer retina.

Management

- *Laser photocoagulation:* Laser spots are applied temporally to the optic disc produce laser scars which act as a barrier between the ODP and the subretinal space, preventing the entrance of fluid into the macula.
- *Pars plana vitrectomy (PPV):* PPV combined with laser application or internal limiting membrane peeling and/or gas tamponade remains the treatment of choice in cases with foveoschisis. The rationale for using PPV is based on the theory about vitreous participation and especially the vitreous traction on the macula, both of which contribute in the appearance of ODP maculopathy. The induction of posterior vitreous detachment (PVD) by PPV and the release of the vitreous traction at the macula are the factors that facilitate the absorption of the subretinal fluid.
- *Macular buckling:* In macular buckling surgery, a scleral sponge is fixed at the posterior pole corresponding to the macula at 6–12 O'clock position without application of additional gas, laser, or cryotherapy. The buckle provides compression ab externo and acts as a barrier, preventing the flow of the fluid from the ODP to the macula. The procedure is not widely practiced due to the prolonged learning curve and a difficult technique.
- *Fibrin glue application:* Fibrin glue application in the optic nerve head along with PPV fluid air exchange, drainage of subretinal fluid, and temporal peripapillary laser has been successfully tried for the management of ODP with serous macular detachment.

Optic Disc Coloboma

Etiopathogenesis

Optic disc coloboma (ODC) is inherited as sporadic or an autosomal dominant disorder and is associated with mutation in *PAX6* gene. Coloboma results from incomplete opposition of embryonic fissure, and is usually present inferiorly.

Optic disc coloboma can occur in isolation or in association with choroidal and retinal coloboma.

Clinical Features

Patient usually presents with decreased visual acuity, which can be due to coloboma or secondary to serous retinal detachment. Vision loss is variable and is difficult to predict, fundus features include well-demarcated excavation lying within enlarged disc, excavation is off centered and lies inferiorly.

Neuroretinal rim (NRR) is thin or absent inferiorly, superior NRR may be spared. Coloboma can be differentiated from morning glory syndrome by absence of abnormal vasculature and glial tuft. ODC can be associated with multisystem disorders such as charge syndrome, Walker–Warberg syndrome, Aicardi syndrome, and Goldenhar syndrome.

Morning Glory Syndrome

Morning glory syndrome also occurs due to failure of closure of embryonic fissure and is associated with abnormal retinal vasculature, glial proliferation, and pigmentary changes.

Clinical features: Visual acuity is usually poor, varies from 20/200 to FCCF, and has myopic refractive error.

Disc in morning glory syndrome is funnel shaped with peripapillary excavation and glial proliferation, which occurs over the center of disc; vessels are large and tortuous with S-shaped loop. Retinal folds, subretinal neovascularization, and serous retinal detachment are other fundus features.

Management

Imaging of brain should be done to rule out any other associated CNS and midline anomaly in patients with ODC, other systemic anomalies should also be ruled out.

Tilted Optic Disc

Etiopathogenesis

Tilted optic disc is a coloboma, which varies in appearance depending on degree of mal closure of embryonic fissure. Incomplete closure of embryonic closure also results in coloboma of retina, RPE, choroid, and disc, as the fissure closes at the end from inferior to inferonasal end, most colobomas arise in this region.

Clinical Features

Both males and females are equally affected. Vision is rarely affected and is not associated with significant systemic and neurological features. Fundus examination reveals tilting of optic disc without actual rotation, superotemporal aspect of the disc is elevated, and inferonasal portion of the disc, long axis of the disc, is obliquely oriented. Congenital absence of inferonasal tissue gives appearance of rotation of disc pole. Other features may result from complications of staphyloma resulting in excessive stretching of Bruch's membrane, causing Lacquer cracks and CNVM formation. Medullated nerve fibers can also be associated with the tilted optic disc. Tilted optic can be associated with situs inversus and suprasellar tumors.

Investigations

Visual field most commonly shows presence of superotemporal deficit, which is due to lack of axons in the inferonasal part.

Electrophysiological investigations: VER is suggestive of delayed latency.
   Electroretinogram is suggestive of reduced amplitude of both photopic and scotopic waves.
   Electrooculogram is associated with reduced amplitude.

Myelinated Nerve Fibers

Myelinated nerve fibers occur in 0.5–1% of the population, appearing as well-demarcated patches with feathery borders, and obscure the underlying retinal vessels. Although most cases are asymptomatic, visual function can be affected due to myopia, amblyopia, and strabismus.

Etiopathogenesis

The process of myelination of optic pathways begins at 5 months of gestation. It progresses in a retrograde pattern; from lateral geniculate body to optic tracts, optic chiasma and at last, myelination of optic nerve takes place at 8 months of gestation. Anomalous myelination occurs, when myelination extends beyond the posterior portion of lamina cribrosa to reach the disc and peripheral retina.

The exact pathogenesis is not clear. Oligodendrocytes are the main supporting cells and are responsible for myelination of long axons of the central nervous system. Besides, the optic pathways, during development lamina cribrosa, act as a barrier and prevent the progenitor oligodendrocytes to enter the developing eye, thus myelination stops at the lamina cribrosa and the fibers anterior to lamina remain unmyelinated. Myelinated retinal nerve fibers thus can occur due to the damage to lamina cribrosa, or can result if the oligodendrocyte progenitors migrate to the retina before the development of lamina cribrosa.

Clinical Features

The anomaly equally affects both males and females, and is inherited as autosomal dominant disorder.
   Patients are usually asymptomatic, and myelinated nerve fibers are just an incidental finding.
   Myelinated nerve fibers are unilateral in 80% of patients and patients with sufficient number of myelinated fibers may present with amblyopia, high myopia, nystagmus, and strabismus.

On fundus examination, myelinated areas have a whitish, feathery appearance, continuous with the disc at upper and lower poles.

Visual field: Relative scotomas may develop depending on the location of myelinated RNFL. Optic disc involvement can cause enlarged bind spot while isolated involvement of peripheral retina will result in isolated peripheral scotoma.

Fundus autofluorescence: Myelin blocks florescence and appears dark on autofluorescence.

Optical coherence tomography: OCT shows thick retinal nerve fiber, causing hyper-reflectivity with backscattering of light resulting in decrease visibility of retinal layers behind myelination.

Systemic associations with myelinated retinal fibers:

The anomaly can be associated with:
- Gorlin syndrome (basal cell nevi syndrome)
- Autosomal dominant vitreoretinopathy and limb deformities
- Epilepsy
- Craniosynostosis
- Turner syndrome
- Down syndrome.

Management

There is no treatment for myelinated nerve fibers, but the other associated pathologies must be taken care of, such as myopia must be corrected, amblyopia if present should be managed accordingly by advising patching, and strabismus must be corrected surgically.

 9. Describe the clinical features, diagnosis, and management of idiopathic intracranial hypertension.

Idiopathic intracranial hypertension, also known as pseudotumor cerebri, usually affects obese female of childbearing age. The term pseudotumor cerebri is preferred, as many cases, which were previously thought to be idiopathic, may have an identifiable cause. Pseudotumor cerebri is characterized by signs and symptoms of isolated raised ICP, and normal imaging and CSF studies.

Etiopathogenesis

The exact etiopathogenesis of the disease still remains obscure, various risk factors associated with IIH are obesity, tetracycline, oral contraceptives, vitamin A toxicity, iron deficiency anemia, hypothyroidism, and Adison's syndrome.

The optic nerve is formed by around 1.2 million axons, which must maintain their orthograde (optic nerve to brain) and retrograde flow (brain to optic nerve). Any obstruction of the axonal transport mechanism can result into disc edema, also as optic nerve sheath is continuous with the subarachnoid space containing CSF, an increase in the CSF pressure can cause compression of the optic nerve.

Risk Factors

Isolated increase in CSF pressure not related to any mass can be due to increased production of CSF or due to impaired absorption of CSF by arachnoid villi. Weight gain, endocrine changes, hypercoagulable states, and obstructive sleep apnea are the commonly associated risk factors for IIH. Role of vitamin A in IIH remains obscure and can be suggested due to impaired CSF absorption by excessive retinol and retinol-binding protein.

Obesity considered associated with IIH can be due to release of adipose tissue-derived retinol-binding protein from adipose tissue. Increased intra-abdominal, visceral fat, as in polycystic ovarian diseases, is also associated with elevated levels of adipose tissue-derived retinol-binding protein. Another theory which was put forward, explaining the relation of obesity with IIH, was associated with increased intra-abdominal pressure, causing increased cardiac filling pressure, thus impeding venous return from brain and subsequently leading to an increased intracranial venous pressure and IIH, but this theory fails to explain IIH in nonobese patients.

Clinical Features

Symptoms

The typical profile of a patient of IIH usually is of an obese female in the childbearing age.

Patients of IIH usually present with complaints of headache, decreased visual acuity, transient obscuration of vision, and pulsatile tinnitus.

Diplopia can result secondary to sixth cranial nerve palsy, which is a nonspecific sign of increased ICP.

History of use of drugs such as tetracycline, oral contraceptives, corticosteroids, nalidixic acid, and cyclosporine must be obtained.

Signs

- *Visual acuity:* The visual acuity can be normal or reduced.
- *Extraocular movements:* Involvement of sixth cranial nerve can result to limitation of abduction.
- *Fundus examination:* Bilateral and symmetric papilledema is the hallmark sign of IIH, but papilledema can also be unilateral or asymmetrical. The Frisen scale may be used to grade severity of the papilledema.

Dandy's diagnostic criteria for IIH:
- Papilledema
- Normal neurological examination except for cranial nerve abnormalities
- *Neuroimaging:* Normal brain parenchyma without hydrocephalus, mass or structural lesion and no abnormal meningeal enhancement or venous sinus thrombosis on MRI and MR venography; if MRI is unavailable or contraindicated, contrast-enhanced CT may be used.
- Normal CSF composition
- Elevated CSF opening pressure (≥25 cmH$_2$O) in a properly performed lumbar puncture.

A diagnosis of IIH is definite in patients fulfilling A–E; the diagnosis is probable if A–D are met but the CSF pressure is lower than specified.

Investigations

- *Contrast sensitivity:* Contrast sensitivity is usually low in patients of IIH.
- *Visual fields:* Visual field examination is mandatory in patients of IIH and helps in diagnosis as well as for follow-up. The fields usually are associated with enlarged blind spot.
- *Neuroimaging:* Neuroimaging is needed to exclude secondary causes of intracranial hypertension. MRI, including MR venography, is the imaging of choice. The imaging findings in IIH include:
  - Flattening of the posterior pole
  - Distension of perioptic subarachnoid space
  - Enhancement (with gadolinium) of the prelaminar optic nerve
  - Empty sella
  - Intraocular protrusion of the prelaminar optic nerve
  - Vertical tortuosity of the orbital optic nerve
  - Stenosis of one or both transverse cerebral venous sinuses
- *Lumbar puncture:* IIH is associated with elevated CSF opening pressure. Pressure is usually >25 cm water, taken with patient lying in lateral decubitus position. CSF analysis must also be done to rule out inflammation, tumor cells, and infection.
- *Optical coherence tomography:* OCT shows increased thickness of peripapillary RNFL and can be used for monitoring of IIH.

Management

Goal of treatment in IIH is preservation of vision and reduction of symptoms (usually headache). Hence, the management must be tailored according to the severity of symptoms and urgency of treatment.

First step in management of IIH is to identify and ameliorate conditions such as obesity, sleep apnea, causative medications, and venous sinus thrombosis. Poor visual prognosis is associated with high-grade papilledema, severe and rapidly progressive vision loss, macular edema, venous sinus thrombosis, and systemic hypertension that requires a more aggressive treatment.

Conservative Management

Observation without medical or surgical intervention is indicated in an asymptomatic patient who presents with papilledema. The precise relationship between weight gain or obesity and raised ICP is not clear, but the benefits of weight reduction have been demonstrated repeatedly. Studies have demonstrated that loss of approximately 6% of body weight is associated with a reduction in papilledema and discontinuation of systemic treatment. Diet control and exercise are one of the most effective ways to assist a patient in weight loss. If weight loss through diet and exercise fails, bariatric surgery has been shown to positively benefit IIH, but it carries risks of anastomotic leaks, small bowel obstruction, malabsorption, and gastrointestinal bleeding.

Medical Management

In a patient with good visual acuity and with primary complaints of headache, medical management is indicated.

Carbonic Anhydrase Inhibitors

Carbonic anhydrase inhibitors (CAIs), such as acetazolamide, are the treatment of choice. The IIH Treatment Trial (IIHTT) is a multicenter, double-blind, placebo-controlled, North American clinical trial that reported the results of use of acetazolamide with a low-sodium weight-reduction diet compared with diet alone. Use of acetazolamide resulted in modest improvement in visual field function in patients with mild visual loss. The trial also reported improved quality of life outcomes at 6 months with acetazolamide.

Mechanism of action: CAIs such as acetazolamide and methazolamide present in the choroid plexus, decrease CSF production, and also act as mild diuretics.

Dose: Acetazolamide in adult patients is usually started at 1 g daily (250 mg QID or 500 mg BID), with a maximum recommended daily dose of 4 g.

Adverse effects: Adverse effects of acetazolamide include paresthesias, lethargy, and altered taste. Hypokalemia is an important adverse effect and hence electrolytes must be monitored.

Topiramate

Topiramate is an antiepileptic drug; it inhibits carbonic anhydrase and can suppress appetite. It has proven to have similar effects such as acetazolamide in terms of papilledema and headache. The dose of topiramate in IIH is from 25 to 50 mg BD. The drug has side effects such as depression, cognitive slowing, and has potential teratogenic risks.

Nonsteroidal Anti-inflammatory Drugs

Nonsteroidal anti-inflammatory drugs (NSAIDs) such as paracetamol may be started in the first few weeks following diagnosis. Indomethacin may have some advantage due to its effect of reducing ICP.

Surgical Management

In acute or rapidly progressive disease, cases of treatment failure are the indications of surgical management.
- *Cerebrospinal fluid diversion procedures:* The commonly performed surgical procedures include CSF diversion using ventriculoperitoneal, ventriculoatrial, or lumboperitoneal shunt and optic nerve sheath decompression. CSF shunting is the most widely performed surgical treatment for IIH. Shunting results in rapid normalization of the ICP, resolution of papilledema, and improvement of vision. All shunt procedures have a high long-term failure rate and often need revision because of obstruction or failure.
- *Optic nerve sheath decompression:* It is an effective treatment in patients with papilledema and severe visual loss but does not improve headache. ONSD rapidly reduces papilledema and bilateral improvement in visual function is seen in many cases. The procedure has little effect on ICP, but symptomatic improvement is due to local reduction in pressure on the nerve by lowering the intrasheath pressure. In long run, it results in fibrous scar formation between the dura and the optic nerve, thus protecting the anterior optic nerve from ICP. Patients with improvement or apparent remission after ONSD should remain under close follow-up, as long-term visual decline may still occur.
Venous sinus stenting can also be tried in patients with IIH, as stenosis of distal transverse sinus is related to IIH.

10. Describe the typical and atypical clinical features, evaluation, and management arteritic AION (anterior ischemic optic neuropathy).

See Answer to Question 11.

 11. Describe the approach to a 73-year-old male patient who complains of a profound unilateral loss of vision in one eye, followed by a similar loss on the other after 8 weeks. What are the diagnosis, clinical features, investigations, and management of such a case?

Arteritic-anterior ischemic optic neuropathy (A-AION) is an acute, often painful optic neuropathy that occurs predominantly in elderly patients and can result to permanent vision loss. Thus, A-AION is an ophthalmic emergency.

Etiopathogenesis

Arteritic-anterior ischemic optic neuropathy is most commonly associated with giant cell arteritis (GCA).

Giant cell arteritis, also known as temporal arteritis, is a systemic autoimmune disease primarily affecting the elderly. It is characterized by granulomatous inflammation of large- and medium-sized arteries. GCA in eye has a special predilection to involve the posterior ciliary artery, resulting in its thrombotic occlusion. Since, posterior ciliary artery is the main source of blood supply to optic nerve head; its occlusion results in infarction of a segment or the entire ONH, depending upon the area of ONH supplied by occluded PCA. This results in development of A-AION, leading to massive visual loss in one or both eyes. Other rare causes include other types of vasculitis, such as polyarteritis nodosa, SLE, and herpes zoster.

Clinical Features

Symptoms

- GCA is the most common associated cause of A-AION, which is a disease of middle-aged and elderly patients.
- Females are more commonly affected than males.
- Patient may have amaurosis fugax, which is one of the earliest symptoms.
- Patients typically complaint of rapid onset unilateral visual loss accompanied by decreased visual acuity, which is typically severe: <20/200. Other less common ocular features include diplopia and eye pain.
- Other systemic manifestations include headache and tenderness of temporal arteries, jaw claudication, malaise, loss of appetite, anorexia and weight loss, fever, joint and muscle pain, and ear pain.

Signs

- A relative afferent pupillary abnormality is present in unilateral optic neuropathies.
- *Fundoscopy:* Ophthalmoscopic examination reveals, chalky-white pallor of optic disc with edema, which may be severe, and is the hallmark of A-AION.
- The disc most often is diffusely swollen, but a segment of more prominent involvement may be present with flame-shaped hemorrhages located adjacent to the disc. The peripapillary retinal arterioles are frequently narrowed. Other ophthalmic manifestations include cotton-wool spots, central retinal artery occlusion, cilioretinal artery occlusion (which is erroneously diagnosed as "branch retinal artery occlusion"), choroidal ischemic lesions, and rarely ocular ischemia.
- Up to 20% patients may have occult GCA, without overt systemic symptoms.
- Other uncommon presentations include hearing loss, vertigo, facial pain, lingual paralysis, and carotid bruits.

Diagnosis

Laboratory Studies

The A-AION is associated with an increase in the inflammatory markers, characterized by an elevated ESR (up to 70–120 mm/min) and/or serum CRP may aid in diagnosis. Elevation of both ESR and CRP has 97% specificity for temporal arteritis. GCA is also associated with thrombocytosis, the platelet counts can be increased in the acute AION.

Visual Field Examination

Visual field examination shows altitudinal field defects.

Biopsy

Diagnosis of temporal arteritis is made by superficial temporal artery biopsy (TAB), which is recommended in cases of AION with clinical suspicion of arteritis. Biopsy findings of intimal thickening, internal limiting lamina fragmentation, and chronic inflammatory infiltrate with giant cells are confirmatory for GCA. GCA is characterized by skip lesions, hence a negative biopsy does not rule out arteritis, if initial biopsy is found to be negative and suspicion for GCA is high, a biopsy of the contralateral temporal artery should be considered.

Imaging

Acute GCA, in ultrasonography, displays a noncompressible, hypoechoic lesion commonly seen as concentric arterial wall thickening described as "halo sign." Ultrasonography is easily available, safe, and has a high resolution of 0.1 mm. Using a 15 MHz transducers, a temporal artery halo is usually detectable in stenotic segments. Ultrasound is more sensitive than TAB as TAB evaluates only a limited anatomical region. High positive predictive value of arteritis on color duplex ultrasound has indicated that TAB may be unnecessary in cases of suspected GCA. Color duplex ultrasonography of the temporal artery has 100% sensitivity and 91% specificity.

OCT, FA, and OCT-A

Fundus fluorescein angiography is associated with delayed choroid filling, normal choroid filling is completed in 3–5 seconds.

Optical coherence tomography helps in assessing sectoral disc edema, RNFL thickness, and also helps to document the resolution to a normal or an atrophic optic disc.

Optical coherence tomography-A clearly identifies the boundary of the ischemic area at the level of the optic nerve head, which is comparable to optic disc filling defects detected by FA.

Differential Diagnosis

The main differential diagnoses of A-AION can include—NAION, atypical optic neuritis, infiltrative optic neuropathies, anterior orbital lesions with optic nerve compression, and diabetic papillopathy.

Treatment

- *Corticosteroids:* A-AION is associated with GCA; hence, steroids form the mainstay of management, and to prevent any further visual loss. In cases with high index of suspicion, high-dose corticosteroids must be started immediately as an emergency measure, "every minute counts".
    1 g IV methylprednisolone must be started initially for 3 days followed by high dose of oral steroids, as high as 100 mg/day.
    High-dose steroid therapy must be maintained till both ESR and CRP settle down to a stable, low level, which usually takes 2–3 weeks. CRP usually settles much earlier than the ESR, following which gradual tapering of steroids must be done.
- *Steroid-sparing agents:* The potential adverse effects of corticosteroids include—osteoporosis, diabetes, cataract formation, hence in these subset of patients, steroid sparing agents such as methotrexate must be considered.
- *Tocilizumab:* Tocilizumab is a monoclonal antibody, which binds to alpha chain of human interleukin-6 (IL-6) receptor, thus downregulates acute phase reactions and is effective against corticosteroid-resistant A-AION.
- *Leflunomide:* Leflunomide is also a steroid-sparing agents which acts by inhibiting dendritic cell maturation, monocyte, and lymphocyte activation, by inhibiting the production of several cytokines, including tumor necrosis factor alpha, ILs—IL-2, IL-6, and IL-12 and metalloproteinases (MMP1, MMP3, and MMP9), which have been implicated in pathogenesis of GCA.

 12. Describe etiopathogenesis, clinical features, and management of AION.

See Answer to Question 13.

13. Discuss ischemic optic neuropathy—diagnosis and management.

Ischemia of optic nerve can occur at different locations and most frequently occurs in optic nerve head; the ischemic optic neuropathies can be classified according to the site and etiology.

The most common site is the anterior 1 mm of optic nerve head, which results in optic nerve head edema and is associated with visible disc edema. AION can result from arteritic or nonarteritic causes. Similarly, posterior ischemic optic neuropathy involves the retrobulbar portion of optic nerve and can result from either arteritic or nonarteritic causes.

Etiopathogenesis

Nonarteritic anterior ischemic optic neuropathy is the most common cause of acute optic neuropathy in patients over the age of 50 years.

A large number of etiologies have been suggested for the NAION, which includes:
- Diabetes mellitus
- Hypertension
- Hypercholesterolemia
- Hyperhomocystinemia
- Sleep apnea.

Nonarteritic anterior ischemic optic neuropathy is mainly associated with laminar and retrolaminar infarction, as reported in various histopathological studies and commonly involves the short posterior ciliary artery and its distal branches. The most commonly proposed pathogenic theory for NAION states that insufficiency of the optic disc circulation is exacerbated by structural crowding of nerve fibers which eventually causes inadequate oxygenation and results to ischemia, leading to acute optic disc swelling (ODS) and SRF accumulation. ODS can result to compartment syndrome and subsequent axonal degeneration and loss of RGCs by apoptosis.

Clinical Features

Symptoms

The patient is typically a 50-year-old patient, with complains of sudden onset diminution of vision, frequently visual impairment is reported after awakening, which can be due to nocturnal hypotension.

Systemic History

Patient usually is a known case of diabetes mellitus, hypertension, or hypercholesterolemia.

Signs
- *Pupil:* Relative afferent papillary defect can be demonstrated in patients with a normal fellow eye.
- *Fundus:* Optic disc edema in NAION may be diffuse or segmental.

The disc is usually small hyperemic unlike in A-AION which is associated with pallid disc edema. A focal region of more severe swelling is often seen and typically displays an altitudinal distribution.

Diffuse or focal telangiectasia of the edematous disc can also be present. The finding represents the development of microvascular shunts, from ischemic to nonischemic region of optic nerve head, "luxury perfusion".

The disc at risk is the one which has smaller diameter and demonstrates a small or absent physiological cup, thus resulting in structural crowding of the axons at the level of cribriform plate. Hard and soft exudates can be present in up to 7% of patients.

Investigations

Systemic Investigations

Systemic investigations include complete blood count, CRP, and ESR, to rule out A-AION and other autoimmune and infective etiologies.

Color Vision and Contrast Sensitivity

As like any other optic nerve pathology, color vision and contrast sensitivity are affected, and there loss is proportional to vision loss.

Visual Field

Visual fields in patients of NAION show a typical inferior altitudinal field defect.

Visual Evoked Response

Visual evoked response shows a reduced amplitude, with normal latency.

Optical Coherence Tomography

Optical coherence tomography is a useful tool in diagnosis of NAION, the findings vary according to the disease activity, in the initial stages when there is optic disc edema, OCT studies show an increase thickness of peripapillary RNFL with a hyporeflective subretinal space. Later, when optic disc atrophy develops, the RNFL becomes thinner, corresponding to the areas of visual field defect. RNFL can even be affected in the sectors corresponding to a relatively unaffected hemifield in visual field.

Fluorescein Fundus Angiography

Fluorescein angiographic studies in NAION are suggestive of impaired optic disc perfusion, with delayed peripapillary choroidal filling and delayed disc filling, thus suggesting that impaired flow to the optic nerve head in NAION is distal to short posterior ciliary arteries, and possibly occurs at the level of the paraoptic branches that supply the optic nerve head directly.

Optical Coherence Tomography-Angiography

Optical coherence tomography-angiography in patients of NAION demonstrates the loss of peripapillary capillaries and flow impairment in retinal peripapillary capillaries which correspond to structural OCT deficits of RNFL, GCL, and automated visual field deficits.

A potential clinical application of OCT-A in NAION can be for monitoring the recovery, as studies have revealed partial recovery of peripapillary vascular flow with improvement in visual function.

Management

Nonarteritic anterior ischemic optic neuropathy management options include medical and surgical management, but controversies exist in the choice of treatment.

Medical Management

Steroids

Use of steroids in NAION still remain controversial as earlier studies had shown a beneficial effect of steroid in NAION, but controversies arose when other group of studies showed no beneficial effect of steroids, intravitreal steroid implants have also been tried and have shown beneficial effects.

The rationales given by Hayreh et al. for the use of steroid in NAION are:
- Steroids possibly decrease capillary permeability.
- Reduces edema in optic nerve and retina.
- Faster resolution of optic disc swelling reduces the compression of capillaries in the optic nerve head.
- Improves blood flow.
- Restores function and survival of ganglion cells.

Role of Antiplatelet Agents in NAION

There are a very few case reports and studies suggesting the use of aspirin and other antiplatelet drugs in the management of acute NAION, in one of retrospective study done in 23 patients for the use of aspirin, no significant difference was present between the two groups in terms of visual acuity and mean deviation on automated perimetry.

Newer modalities in the management of NAION are now targeting the enzymes such as capsase-2 an important enzyme in the apoptotic pathway, so as to limit the ganglion cell loss.

Surgical Management

Optic nerve sheath decompression has been tried to overcome the compartment syndrome. The ischemic optic neuropathy decompression trial (IONDT) was a randomized, multicenter trial, done to find the efficacy of optic nerve sheath decompression in patients of NAION, and compared Optic nerve sheath decompression surgery in 119 patients with no treatment in 125 controls. The study revealed no significant benefit of ONSD, instead ONSD can be associated with several adverse effects and recommended that ONSD should not be performed for NAION.

Disease Course and Visual Outcome

Vision can worsen in the initial 2 weeks of presentation and stabilizes by 2 months.

According to Hayreh et al., approximately 50% of patients of NAION had a visual acuity of 20/30 or better and nearly one-quarter had visual acuity of 20/200 or worse, of which 41% of patients with visual acuity of 20/70 or worse at presentation showed improvement at 6 months. Recurrence can be seen in 3–8% of the patients. Involvement of the fellow eye ranges from 15% to 24% over 5 years.

Arteritic Anterior Ischemic Optic Neuropathy
See above Answer

14. Describe optic nerve head drusen.

Optic nerve drusen is a calcified hyaline deposit present within optic nerve head, the incidence is 3.4 per 1,000 individuals and can be as high as 10–20 per 1,000 as reported in autopsy studies. Optic nerve drusen buried within the optic disc can mimic papilledema, misdiagnosing it as true disc edema may lead to invasive and unnecessary workup. These concretions can enlarge throughout life, they are mostly asymptomatic, but may lead to significant visual field loss through acute vascular events and slowly progressive mechanisms.

Etiopathogenesis

The underlying etiology and pathogenesis of optic nerve drusen are not known. Optic nerve drusen can result from disturbance in axonal metabolism, associated with reduced axoplasmic flow, congenitally dysplastic discs with a propensity for drusen formation, or a small scleral canal causing physical compression of the optic nerve, resulting in ganglion cell death, with extrusion and calcification of mitochondria. Retinitis pigmentosa and angioid streaks are commonly associated with optic nerve drusen.

Optic nerve drusen can present in 9% of patients of retinitis pigmentosa, and is believed to be due to RGC axonal degeneration. Degenerating axons extrude mitochondria, which become calcified and form drusen. Optic disc drusen have been associated more commonly with a few subtypes of retinitis pigmentosa including Usher syndrome, in which it results from mutation of *m*embrane-type *F*rizzled-*r*elated *p*rotein (*MFRP*) gene and the syndrome of nanophthalmos-retinitis pigmentosa–foveoschisis–optic disc drusen, associated with mutation in the crumbs homolog 1 (*CRB1*) gene. Other common association of optic nerve drusen is with angioid streaks; the incidence reported can be as high as in 25%, and has been hypothesized due to deposition of polyanions in the abnormal elastin fibrils; resulting in elastin mineralization of lamina cribrosa. Calcium binds to these polyanions, resulting in formation of macromolecules, which further disrupt axonal transport and lead to the formation of drusen.

Clinical Features

Symptoms

Optic nerve drusen is typically asymptomatic, and is often diagnosed incidentally, few patients may complain of transient visual obscuration (TVO), which probably is secondary to transient disc ischemia.

Signs

Disc drusen can be buried or exposed:
- Buried drusen may cause only subtle elevation of the disc and obscuration of the physiologic cup, giving appearance of a crowded disc.
- Exposed drusen are usually larger, appear as multilobular yellowish-white nodule, which are best seen with retroillumination and glow with semitranslucent appearance. Occasionally, hemorrhages or neovascularization appear

in the optic disc and extend into the peripapillary region. Bilateral findings are seen in 75% of patients, the excrescences are commonly seen in the nasal half of the disc.

Investigations

- *Visual field defects:* Visual field defects are more common in superficial drusen as compared to buried drusen, and, therefore, visual field defects tend to increase in frequency with increasing age. The common visual fields associated with disc drusen include—nasal inferior arcuate scotoma (32%), unspecified nasal defect (21%), constricted visual field (21%), and enlarged blind spot (18%).
- *B-scan ultrasonography:* Ultrasonography (USG) B-scan is considered to be the gold standard imaging modality to detect optic disc drusen. Drusen characteristically appear hyperechoic with posterior shadowing. The B-scan is able to scan the entire area of the optic disc using sweeping movements of the ultrasound probe.
- *Fundus autofluorescence:* Optic disc drusen display autofluorescence, which can be detected on preinjection control photography, but it is not useful in patients with buried drusen.
- *Orbital computed tomography:* Orbital CT detects calcification of drusen, but has the risk of radiation exposure.
- *Optical coherence tomography:* OCT shows the presence of a hyper-reflective lumpy bumpy deposit in layer and thinning of RNFL, on the contrary, RNFL thickness is increased in papilledema. Other features seen in OCT helpful in differentiating papilledema from pseudopapilledema are lazy V pattern with smooth internal contour of optic nerve head and SHYPS thickest near the optic nerve head with gradual tapering away from the optic nerve in true papilledema and a "lumpy bumpy" internal contour with abrupt decline in SHYPS observed in optic nerve drusen causing pseudopapilledema.
- *Optical coherence tomography-angiography:* OCT-A of the optic nerve head in patients of optic nerve drusen reveals the presence of capillary narrowing in the superficial capillary plexus layer, areas of capillary dropout, and decreased vascular density. OCT-A also helps in early prediction of axonal damage, supporting the hypothesis that enlarged drusen can compress the surrounding vessels causing acute or chronic ischemia.

Complications

The prognosis of optic nerve head drusen is usually good; however, optic nerve head drusen can cause complications such as NAION, choroidal neovascularization, and central retinal artery, and vein occlusion.

15. Discuss the ocular aspects of multiple sclerosis.

Refer to Question 9.

16. Discuss drug-induced optic neuropathies.

Refer to Question 7.

17. Describe the clinical features, diagnosis, and management of a case of methyl alcohol poisoning.

Refer to Question 7.

2.5 Pupil

Gunjan Saluja

1. Discuss examination of the pupil and its significance.

The pupillary light reflex represents the sum of the entire neuronal input beginning from the photoreceptors, bipolar cells, ganglion cells, and axons of ganglion cells. Therefore, damage anywhere along this portion of the visual pathway reduces the amplitude of pupil movement in response to a light stimulus. Observation of the difference in pupil movements between the two eyes in response to alternating the light back and forth between the two eyes is the basis for the alternating light test, or "swinging flashlight" test, used to assess the relative afferent pupillary defect (RAPD).

Swinging Flashlight Test

In a normal individual, on showing a bright flash of light, the pupil of that eye should constrict, and the pupil of the contralateral eye must also constrict due to consensual reflex.

Procedure
- The test should be done in a dimly illuminated room, with the patient fixed at a distant target to avoid miosis.
- A bright stimulus is used to elicit pupil constriction, and the light is directed from below the level of the patient's eyes.
- The light source is then briskly and rhythmically moved from one eye to another several times.

Quantification of Relative Afferent Pupillary Defect

Quantification of RAPD can be done using neutral density filters. The neutral density filter is placed in front of the normal eye, and the density of the filter is increased till the afferent pupillary defect appears in the normal eye. Accurate quantification of RAPD is accomplished by determination of log unit difference needed to balance the pupil reaction between the two eyes.

Interpretation

The RAPD is a sensitive indicator of the afferent pupillary pathway defect.

Retina

Unilateral large retinal lesions such as retinal detachment, central retinal artery occlusion, and central retinal vein occlusion (ischemic) can lead to clear RAPD.

On the contrary, dense cataracts and corneal opacities do not produce relative afferent papillary defects, which can be explained to be due to:
- Dark-adapted retina behind the cataract
- Beam of light coming through the pupil can be diffused by cataract or the corneal opacity to cover a broader area of the retina than normal.

Optic Nerve

Optic nerve damage will always produce RAPD, with the largest RAPD occurring due to unilateral optic nerve disorders. In cases of resolved optic neuritis, though visual acuity may be regained, optic disc pallor and RAPD still exist.

Optic Chiasma

Compressive lesions of optic chiasma can also produce asymmetric visual loss; however, in patients with bitemporal hemianopia, RAPD may not be present due to symmetrical involvement.

Optic Tract

A complete lesion of the optic tract produces contralateral homonymous hemianopia and causes RAPD in the contralateral eye, i.e., in the eye with temporal field visual loss. This is because the number of fibers crossing to the opposite side outnumbers the uncrossed fibers in chiasma.

Pretectal Nucleus

A unilateral lesion in the pretectal nucleus will cause damage to the pupillary fibers coming from the ipsilateral optic tract, causing contralateral RAPD. Lesions involving the lateral geniculate body and the proximal portion of the retro-geniculate body may cause RAPD not due to lesion of the pathway but due to the involvement of intercalated neurons between visual pathways and pupillomotor pathways of pretectum.

 2. Describe the pupillary pathways in detail with diagram.

The afferent pupillary pathway begins in the retina, which consists of approximately 60 million rods, 3 million cones, and a minority (<5%) of retinal ganglion cells that are intrinsically photosensitive, with each of them having a distinct contribution to the pupillary light reflex. The rods and cones are responsible for rapid modulation in pupillary size with changes in ambient light sensitivity; on the contrary, intrinsically photosensitive retinal ganglion cells mediate a slower but more sustained pupillary response to light.

The signals are further transmitted through the ipsilateral optic nerve, consisting of fibers from the nasal and temporal retina.

The temporal retinal fibers (nasal visual field), whereas fibers from the nasal retina (temporal visual field) decussate in the chiasma and contribute to the contralateral optic tract.

The pupillary fibers, unlike the fibers of visual pathways, do not synapse in the lateral geniculate nucleus; instead, the pupillary fibers enter the dorsal midbrain through the brachium of the superior colliculus and synapse in the olivary pretectal nucleus. Half of the fibers synapse with the ipsilateral Edinger–Westphal (EW) nucleus and the other half of the fibers decussate in the posterior commissure to reach the contralateral EW.

Edinger–Westphal nuclei are paired structures present in the dorsal rostral midbrain. The neurons of the EW nucleus form the parasympathetic fibers of the oculomotor nerve. After exiting the midbrain, the subarachnoid space, the pupillomotor fibers lie on the mediodorsal aspect of the third nerve, in proximity to the posterior communicating artery.

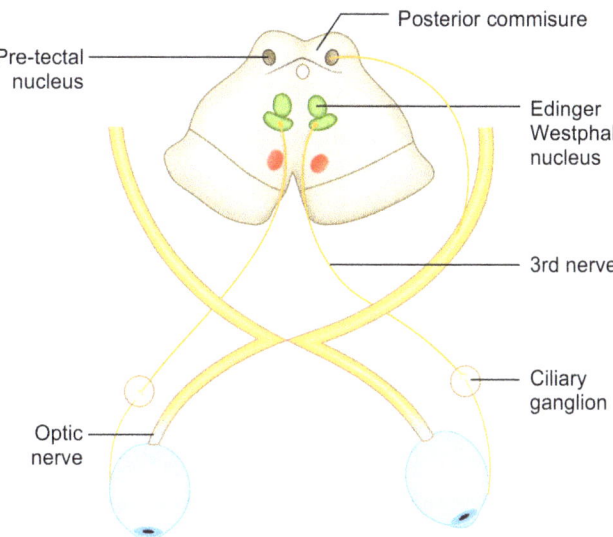

Fig. 1: Pupillary pathway.

The pupillomotor fibers then enter the cavernous sinus along with the third cranial nerve.

In the anterior cavernous sinus, the nerve divides into a superior and inferior division with the pupillomotor fibers exclusively lying along with the inferior division of the oculomotor nerve, which also innervates the inferior rectus, inferior oblique, and medial rectus.

The pupillary fibers further synapse in the ciliary ganglion.

The axons of ciliary ganglion innervate the pupillary constrictors as well as the ciliary muscles allowing accommodation. Thus, through this path, bilateral pupils are supplied **(Fig. 1)**.

The normal pupil is circular and 3–4 mm in size and is placed centrally. Pupils are relatively small at birth, largest during adolescence, and further tend to grow smaller with increasing age.

Pupillary contraction to light is an important neuronal reflex because it gives information about the integrity of both the afferent visual system and the efferent neuronal outflow to each pupil. The pupils are controlled by two muscles of ectodermal origin: Sphincter pupillae and dilator pupillae. When maximally contracted, the size of the pupil may be <1 mm; when maximally dilated, it may be >9 mm.

 3. Discuss the physiological basis and causes of light-near dissociation.

Pupils under normal conditions constrict on exposure to light and constrict as a part of the near triad, which includes miosis and convergence. In light-near dissociation, pupillary constriction with near reflex is preserved, but pupillary constriction with light reflex is absent.

Argyll Robertson Pupil

Argyll Robertson pupils are characterized by the presence of accommodation reflex, but light reflex is absent. The pupils are typically small and dilate poorly in the dark. The site of lesion in Argyll Robertson pupil is in the region of the Sylvian aqueduct in the rostral midbrain. The fibers responsible for accommodation reflex enter the EW nucleus ventrally; hence, they are spared. However, the light reflex fibers lie dorsally and are involved.

Argyll Robertson syndrome is a pathognomonic feature of neurosyphilis.

Other causes include diabetes, encephalitis, multiple sclerosis, age-related degenerative diseases of the central nervous system, and systemic inflammatory disorders such as sarcoidosis.

Parinaud's Syndrome

Parinaud's syndrome is characterized by the classic triad of limitation of upgaze, with lid retraction on attempted upgaze (Collier's sign) and light-near dissociation.

The rostral interstitial nucleus of medial longitudinal fasciculus (riMLF) and interstitial nucleus of Cajal (INC) regulate the vertical gaze pathways. Both INC and riMLF decussate in the posterior commissure and are present near the cerebral aqueduct; thus, dorsal midbrain lesions affect the vertical gaze.

Pupils are large and fail to respond to light reflex; however, the near reflex is preserved.

The causes of Parinaud's syndrome include tumors of the pineal gland compressing the dorsal midbrain and hydrocephalus, and in cases with aqueductal stenosis, it can be the first sign.

Aberrant Regeneration of Third Nerve

The light reflex can be restored by aberrant regeneration after the damage to the preganglionic oculomotor nerve. Oculomotor nerve fibers for extraocular muscles can be misdirected toward the iris sphincter. These pupils usually have features of the tonic pupil, with absent slow sustained contraction to near effort.

Q 4. Describe the sympathetic nervous system of the eye with the help of a diagram. Also, describe the various pharmacological tests to diagnose the abnormalities of the sympathetic nervous system.

The sympathetic innervation in the eye innervates the retractors of the upper eyelid (Muller's muscle) and lower eyelid, pupillary dilator muscle, and vasomotor control and consists of first-order, second-order, and third-order neurons **(Fig. 2)**.

First-Order Neuron

The first-order neuron begins from the ipsilateral hypothalamus and extends up to the ciliospinal center of Budge and Waller at the level of C8–T1.

Second Order Neuron

The second-order neurons arise from the ciliospinal center of Budge and pass to the pulmonary apex, which then passes through the stellate ganglion and goes up to the carotid sheath to the superior cervical ganglion near the bifurcation of the common carotid artery.

Third-Order Neuron

The postganglionic, third-order neuron arises from the superior cervical ganglion behind the angle of the mandible and up along with the course of the carotid artery. Within the cavernous sinus, sympathetic fibers leave the internal carotid artery and enter the orbit along with the nasociliary branch of the trigeminal nerve.

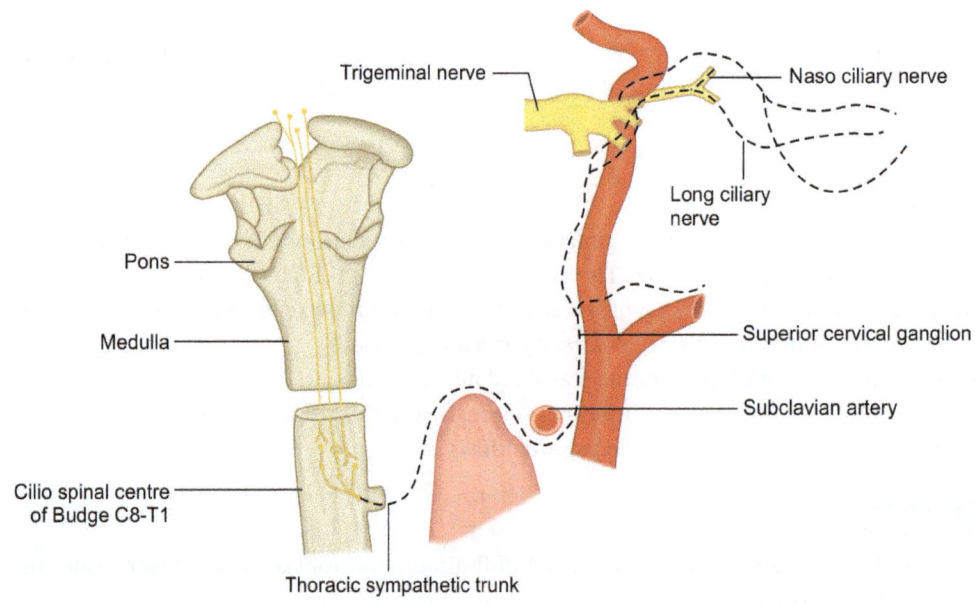

Fig. 2: Horner's syndrome.

Pharmacological Tests for Localization of the Lesion

Ten Percent Cocaine Test
Cocaine blocks the reuptake of norepinephrine at the sympathetic nerve endings. 10% percent cocaine in normal individuals causes dilation of the pupil to 8 mm within 4–5 minutes, but patients with Horner's syndrome will not respond.

Apraclonidine Test
Apraclonidine is a direct alpha receptor agonist. It has no effect on eyes with intact sympathetic innervation. 0.5 or 1% Apraclonidine after 45 minutes of instillation in Horner's syndrome causes dilation of Horner's pupil due to denervation hypersensitivity, and ptosis improves.

One Percent Hydroxyamphetamine Test
One percent hydroxyamphetamine can be used to distinguish preganglionic and postganglionic Horner's syndrome and is performed after 24–48 hours of cocaine test.

Mechanism of action of hydroxyamphetamine
Hydroxyamphetamine promotes the release of noradrenaline from the intact nerve endings.

Procedure
One percent hydroxyamphetamine is instilled in the cul-de-sac and the pupil diameter is measured after 45 minutes.

In postganglionic lesions, the nerve endings are destroyed due to anterograde degeneration destroying the noradrenaline stores, causing no mydriatic effect.

A false-negative response can be produced if the test is performed within 7 days as the norepinephrine stores are not depleted.

 5. What is anisocoria, indications for its investigation, and management?

Physiological anisocoria is present in 10% of the population in room light and 20% of the population in dim light, with a difference of 0.4 mm pupil diameter. Anisocoria causes less amount of light to enter the retina of the eye with a smaller pupil and causes a false impression of RAPD.

Etiology

Structural Defects
Structural defects of iris due to congenital defects such as aniridia, iris coloboma, congenital ectopic pupils, polycoria, persistent pupillary membrane, iridocorneal endothelial syndrome, and other developmental anomalies can lead to anisocoria.

Acquired conditions such as neovascularization of iris, sphincter atrophy, trauma to iris, surgical trauma, posterior synechiae, and angle-closure glaucoma can also lead to anisocoria.

More Anisocoria in Dim Light

Horner's Syndrome
Horner's syndrome results from the interruption of sympathetic innervations to the eye. The sympathetic innervation in the eye innervates the retractors of the upper eyelid (Muller's muscle) and lower eyelid, pupillary dilator muscle, and vasomotor control, thus resulting in the classic triad of ptosis, miosis, and anhidrosis. The ptosis is mild to moderate, and involvement of lower lid retractor leads to apparent enophthalmos and narrowing of the palpebral fissure **(Fig. 2)**. The first-order neuron begins from the ipsilateral hypothalamus, extends up to the ciliospinal center of Budge and Waller at the level of C8–T1, and stays lateral in the brainstem and cervical cord, causing unilateral Horner's syndrome. Central Horner's syndrome is associated with contralateral hemiparesis, hypesthesia, and Wallenberg syndrome.

Preganglionic Horner's Syndrome

The second-order neurons arise from the ciliospinal center of Budge and pass to the pulmonary apex, which then passes through the stellate ganglion and goes up to the carotid sheath to the superior cervical ganglion near the bifurcation of the common carotid artery. Common causes of preganglionic Horner's syndrome are malignancy, lung and breast cancer, and accidental or surgical trauma to cervical vertebrae.

Postganglionic Horner's Syndrome

The postganglionic, third-order neuron arises from the superior cervical ganglion behind the angle of the mandible and up along with the course of the carotid artery. Within the cavernous sinus, sympathetic fibers leave the internal carotid artery and enter the orbit along with nasociliary branch of the trigeminal nerve. Trauma, tumor, inflammatory lesions, and metastatic lesions can also involve the third-order neurons.

Congenital Horner's Syndrome

Congenital Horner's syndrome can be caused secondary to brachial plexus injury during birth, congenital tumor, and viral infections. Patients with congenital Horner's syndrome may have associated heterochromia iridis.

Congenital Horner's syndrome can be associated with a hemifacial flush when crying, which is seen on the opposite side, due to failure of vasodilation on the side of congenital Horner's syndrome.

Pharmacological Tests for Localization of the Lesion

Ten Percent Cocaine Test

Cocaine blocks the reuptake of norepinephrine at the sympathetic nerve endings. Ten percent cocaine in normal individuals causes dilation of the pupil to 8 mm within 4–5 minutes, but patients with Horner's syndrome will not respond.

Apraclonidine Test

Apraclonidine is a direct alpha receptor agonist. It has no effect on eyes with intact sympathetic innervation. 0.5 or 1% Apraclonidine after 45 minutes of instillation in Horner's syndrome causes dilation of Horner's pupil due to denervation hypersensitivity, and ptosis improves.

Hydroxyamphetamine Test

One percent hydroxyamphetamine can be used to distinguish preganglionic and postganglionic Horner's syndrome and is performed after 24–48 hours of cocaine test.

Mechanism of action of Hydroxyamphetamine

Hydroxyamphetamine promotes the release of noradrenaline from the intact nerve endings.

Procedure

One percent hydroxyamphetamine is instilled in the cul-de-sac and the pupil diameter is measured after 45 minutes.

In postganglionic lesions, the nerve endings are destroyed due to anterograde degeneration destroying the noradrenaline stores, causing no mydriatic effect.

A false-negative response can be produced if the test is performed within 7 days as the norepinephrine stores are not depleted.

- Palsy of the iris dilator muscle causes miosis and failure of dilation of the pupil in dim light; as a result, anisocoria increases in dim light.
- *Pharmacologic stimulation of iris sphincter:* Stimulation of the iris sphincter causes the pupil to be nonreactive and is worse during dim light as the pupil will not dilate and remain constricted.

More Anisocoria in Light

- *Damage to parasympathetic outflow to the iris sphincter:* The parasympathetic pathway is responsible for the constriction of the pupil; hence, damage to the parasympathetic outflow will result in persistent dilation of pupil and failure of constriction in bright light, thus increasing anisocoria in bright light.

A final common pathway for the pupillary reaction to light and near begins in mesencephalon with oculomotor nuclei to ciliary ganglion and through the short ciliary nerve to iris sphincter.

Lesions anywhere in this pathway can cause absolute paralysis of pupillary constrictor.
- *EW nucleus damage:* Most lesions in the EW nucleus cause papillary abnormalities along with oculomotor nucleus involvement.
- *Damage to pupillomotor fibers in oculomotor nerve fascicle:* Damage to oculomotor nerve fascicles due to inflammation, ischemia, and infection can lead to complete or incomplete isolated 3rd nerve palsy.
- *Damage to pupillomotor fibers in the subarachnoid portion of the oculomotor nerve:* As the oculomotor nerve passes between the posterior cerebral artery and the superior cerebellar artery, the pupillary fibers here are superficial and are prone to be compressed by the aneurysm and space-occupying lesion.
- *Damage to ciliary ganglion and iris root:* Damage to postganglionic parasympathetic innervation of intraocular muscles will lead to poor pupillary dilation. Poor pupillary reaction to light can result from regional palsy of the iris sphincter, paresis of accommodation, and supersensitivity of denervated muscle.

Slow tonic redilation after constriction of nerve stimuli results in the tonic pupil.

Etiologies of Tonic Pupil

Local Causes

Inflammation, tumors, infiltrative disorders, and infections such as herpes zoster, measles, syphilis, diphtheria, influenza, and rheumatoid arthritis can lead to damage to the ciliary ganglion.

Neuropathic Tonic Pupil

Generalized widespread, peripheral, or autonomic neuropathy in cases of syphilis, diabetes mellitus, and spinocerebellar ataxia can lead to damage to the ciliary ganglion or short ciliary nerves.

Adie's Tonic Pupil

The etiology of Adie's tonic pupil is obscured in many cases but can be associated with secondary viral or bacterial infection causing inflammation and damage to neurons in the ciliary ganglion.

In Adie's syndrome, deep tendon reflexes may be reduced.

Clinical Features

Patients with Adie's tonic pupil are usually asymptomatic, but can also present with the following:
- Mydriasis
- Difficult in near vision and glare
- Initially, the patients may have only loss of deep tendon reflexes.
- With time, resting pupil size may be smaller; however, the normal tone of the pupil never returns. The tonic pupil may become smaller over time, known as "Little old Adie's pupil".
- Excessive sweating may be noted on one side. The triad of excessive sweating, reduced deep tendon reflex, and Adie's pupil is known as Ross's syndrome.

On examination, the anisocoria increases in bright light. Direct light reflex is absent, but the near reflex is present or tonic due to aberrant reinnervation of the sphincter. The slit-lamp examination further shows the presence of sectoral vermiform movements due to segmental denervation in most of the cases. Instillation of 0.125% pilocarpine constricts the pupil due to cholinergic denervation supersensitivity. A normal pupil does not respond to this diluted concentration of pilocarpine.

Management

Adie's syndrome is managed by prescribing 0.125% reconstituted pilocarpine three times a day. Reading glasses can be prescribed to improve the near vision.

In patients with no improvement with pilocarpine and glasses, thoracic sympathectomy can be done as a definitive treatment for hyperhidrosis.
- *Pharmacologic stimulation of iris dilator:* Cocaine, oxymetazoline, and phenylephrine dilate the pupil, leaving the sphincter intact.

- *Sympathetic hyperactivity:* Tadpole pupil is an intermittent and benign phenomenon in which the pupil of one eye becomes distorted for a minute or two. The pupil of one eye is pulled in one direction like the tail of a tadpole and is thought to be due to repeated bursts of sympathetic innervations. Whiplash injury due to low cervical or thoracic spinal cord causes episodes of irritation of sympathetic ganglion, resulting in episodes of dilation of pupil and sweating.

Q 6. Describe Horner's syndrome, its etiology, clinical features, diagnosis, and differential diagnosis.

It is discussed in detail in Question 5.

2.6 Chiasmal and Retrochiasmal Lesion

Gunjan Saluja

Q 7. Discuss the anatomy of optic chiasma. Briefly discuss the various lesions affecting visual fields (role in health and disease).

Q 8. Discuss pituitary lesions for ophthalmologist.

Q 9. Discuss chiasmal syndromes.

See Answer of Question 10 for Question 7, 8, 9.

Q 10. Describe the causes and ocular manifestations of chiasmal lesions.

Anatomy of Chiasma

Refer to the anatomy Question.

Chiasmal Lesions

Etiology

The chiasmal lesions include:
- Pituitary adenoma
- Pituitary apoplexy
- Meningioma
- Glioma
- Craniopharyngioma
- Other less common chiasmal syndromes
- Chordoma, germinoma, endodermal sinus tumor, leukemia, and Hodgkin's and non-Hodgkin's lymphoma
- Nasopharyngeal carcinoma and metastatic carcinomas
- Nonneoplastic lesions compressing chiasma
- Sphenoid sinus mucocele, arachnoid cyst, Rathke's cleft cyst, epidermoid cyst, fibrous dysplasia, histiocytosis X, dolichoectasia of the internal carotid artery, and aneurysm of large vessels of the circle of Willis
- Cavernous hemangiomas, arteriovenous malformations, aneurysms, and venous angiomas may compress the chiasma
- Toxins
- Trauma.

Pituitary Adenoma

Pituitary adenoma is the most common etiology of chiasmal dysfunction and can affect patients of any age group.

Pituitary tumors can be classified as:
- *Benign adenomas*, the most frequent pituitary tumor
- *Invasive adenomas* invade adjacent skull base structures and its meningeal coverings
- *Pituitary carcinomas*.

The benign adenomas usually remain asymptomatic, and the increased risk of chiasmal involvement is associated with macroadenomas of >10 mm.

Pituitary Apoplexy

Pituitary apoplexy is the sudden enlargement of a pituitary gland as a result of hemorrhage or infarction (most commonly hemorrhagic infarction) of a pituitary adenoma.

Predisposing factors for pituitary apoplexy include pregnancy, estrogen therapy, obstetrical hemorrhage (Sheehan's syndrome), diabetes mellitus, bleeding disorders, long-term anticoagulation, blood dyscrasias, radiation therapy, trauma, angiography, atheromatous emboli, cardiac surgery, coughing, positive-pressure ventilation, and vasoactive agents.

The presentation of acute pituitary apoplexy is variable and its course is unpredictable.

Meningioma

Chiasma can be compressed from below by the suprasellar meningiomas of the sphenoid planum or tuberculum sellae. Compression can also be caused by meningiomas arising from the diaphragm sellae, medial sphenoid ridge, and olfactory groove. It is typically seen in patients of middle and late age groups.

Craniopharyngioma

The anterior lobe of the pituitary forms embryologically from Rathke's pouch, an embryological structure connected to the pharynx. In children and young adults, embryonic vestigial epithelial remnants of Rathke's pouch between the anterior and posterior lobes of the pituitary may develop into a benign, frequently cystic tumor called craniopharyngioma.

The extension of the craniopharyngioma in the third ventricle can lead to hydrocephalus.

Optic Glioma

Gliomas, also called pilocytic astrocytomas, are not uncommon in the perichiasmal region; gliomas infiltrating the chiasm also involve the hypothalamus and usually affect children.

Inflammation

Inflammation due to sarcoidosis, syphilis, granulomatous diseases, arachnoiditis, abscess, demyelinating disease, and lymphoid hypophysitis can also compress the chiasma due to edema.

Toxins

Direct damage to the chiasma can be caused by drugs such as chloramphenicol, ethambutol, isoniazid, and vincristine.

Traumatic Chiasmal Syndrome

The traumatic chiasmal syndrome usually results from penetrating head trauma, road traffic accidents, falls from height, assaults, stab wounds, and gunshot wounds. Direct injury can result from orbital or cerebral trauma disrupting the anatomic and functional integrity of the optic nerve.

Indirect injury to chiasma can result from blunt trauma to the forehead and further transmission of force through the cranium to the intracanalicular portion of the optic nerve.

Ocular Features

- Patients with chiasmal lesions can complain of difficulties related to unrecognized loss of their peripheral field or may complain of unilateral or bilateral central or peripheral vision loss. Patients with bitemporal hemianopia can experience loss of depth perception at near. Pituitary adenomas, craniopharyngiomas, and aneurysms can also cause gradual onset progressive and fluctuating vision loss, which is associated with loss of color vision and red dyschromatopsia in the temporal hemifield.
- Lesions arising from the cavernous sinus and causing the compression of optic chiasma can also be associated with multiple cranial nerve palsies leading to ophthalmoplegia, facial pain, numbness, and difficulty in near vision.

- Para sellar tumors can also be associated with typical see-saw nystagmus characterized by elevation and intorsion of one eye and simultaneous depression and extorsion of the other eye. This typical nystagmus has been postulated to be the result of compression of intestinal nucleus of the Cajal or inferior olivary nucleus.

Systemic Features

Patients with space-occupying lesions frequently complain of frontal headache. Pituitary endocrine dysfunction can lead to a variety of symptoms and signs due to the specific hormone produced. Increased secretion of growth hormone leads to features of acromegaly, which include thick lips, enlarged eyebrows, increased size of hands and feet, and metabolic changes, including diabetes mellitus and hypertension.

Increased levels of prolactin lead to the amenorrhea–galactorrhea syndrome in women and impotence in men.

Increased levels of adrenocorticotropic hormone (ACTH) lead to changes in body habitus, full-moon face, and centripetal obesity. Hypothalamic dysfunction may also manifest as urinary frequency as a result of diabetes insipidus, heat or cold intolerance caused by a disturbance of temperature regulation, behavioral changes, lethargy, decreased libido, and decreased or increased appetite.

Investigations

Visual Field Testing

Visual field tests help in localization of the lesion in the chiasma and hence should be carefully performed. The chiasmal disorders typically follow a vertical midline defect and have a typical vertical step, although early chiasmal compression often lacks a clear vertical step.

Chiasmal diseases should be tested either with a single central isopter or static threshold sensitivity within the central 15–20° from fixation.

The type of defect helps in exact localization of the lesion, compression of the anterior angle of chiasma caused by sphenoidal meningioma, typically leads to junctional scotoma, which is characterized by scotoma in one eye and temporal field loss in the other.

Similarly, direct compression of the chiasma from below by the pituitary adenoma causes bitemporal superior quadrantanopia or bitemporal hemianopia.

Bitemporal inferior quadrantanopia can occur with compression of the body of the chiasm from above by craniopharyngioma.

Hemifield Slide Phenomenon

Loss of normal partial overlap of the temporal field of one eye and nasal field of the other eye leads to a lack of physiological linkage between two remaining hemifields, causing difficulty in reading and diplopia.

Neuroimaging

Neuroimaging with the help of magnetic resonance imaging (MRI) is an absolute indication for patients who have symptoms or signs referable to the chiasm or parachiasmal region.

Computed tomography (CT) with fine cuts (1.5–3 mm) of axial and coronal views is an acceptable alternative. MRI helps in better definition of the anatomical relationships of chiasma to the surrounding structures and the absence of artifacts from the bone. CT, on the contrary, helps in the detection of tumoral calcifications and bony erosion and destruction by meningiomas and craniopharyngiomas.

Systemic Investigations

A complete endocrinological workup must be done to detect the lesions involving the pituitary hypothalamic axis.

 11. Discuss cortical blindness.

The ability to recognize visually presented objects and words depends on the integrity not only of the visual pathways and primary visual area of the cerebral cortex (area 17 of Brodmann) but also of those cortical areas that lie just anterior to area 17, that is, areas 18 and 19 of the occipital lobe and area 39, which is the angular gyrus of the dominant hemisphere (visual association areas). Hence, impairment to any of these areas can lead to cortical blindness.

Etiology

The etiology of cortical blindness can be classified according to the underlying cause, which can be acute vision loss, chronic vision loss, or brief visual impairment.

Acute Vision Loss

Acute-onset cerebral vision loss can arise due to vascular causes such as infarction in the territory of a posterior cerebral artery, sagittal sinus thrombosis, bacterial meningitis, and trauma.

Infarction typically arises due to thromboembolic events located in the heart of the vertebrobasilar system. Occlusion of the basilar artery results in ischemia along with the distribution of the cerebral artery.

Thus, along with vision loss, other features might also be noted, such as memory deficits, vertical gaze palsy, and quadriparesis.

Chronic Vision Loss

Chronic cortical blindness can result from a large number of causes, which include:
- Intracranial space-occupying lesions
- Brain abscess
- Adrenoleukodystrophy
- Subacute sclerosing panencephalitis
- Creutzfeldt-Jakob disease
- Demyelinating disorders
- Chronic mercury poisoning.

Brief Visual Impairment

Brief visual impairment of cerebral origin can be associated with migraine, presyncope attacks due to postural hypotension, vasovagal attacks, and cardiac arrhythmia that can lead to short episodes of bilateral vision dimming. This can be associated with feelings of giddiness, lightheadedness, paresthesia, or excessive sweating.

Features of Cortical Blindness

Information from the retina is transmitted to the primary visual cortex (V1, also known as the striate cortex or Brodmann area 17). From here, visual information is transmitted to the (V2) prestriate cortex, from where the information is processed and further transmitted to V3 and extrastriate cortex. The areas in the extrastriate cortex can be broadly organized in two interconnected pathways, which include the ventral ("what?") and the dorsal ("where?") pathways.

The ventral pathway runs inferiorly along the occipital and temporal lobes and plays an important role in the recognition of objects; hence, damage to these pathways can lead to an inability to recognize the objects. The dorsal pathway runs superiorly from the occipital to the parietal lobe and helps in the localization of objects. The characteristic features of cortical blindness include loss of all visual sensations with normal fundoscopic examination, preservation of light and accommodation papillary reflexes, and loss of menace reflex.

Disorders of Recognition

Cerebral Achromatopsia

The term indicates deficient color perception, and patients are unable to name colors. This feature results from bilateral impairment of fusiform and lingual gyri (ventral occipital cortex).

Visual Agnosia

Visual agnosia implies an inability to recognize an object or a particular aspect of an object using vision alone, although the basic visual pathways are preserved and function normally. Visual agnosia usually results from a lesion of ventral pathways.

Impaired visual recognition could occur at two levels: Apperceptive (i.e., impairment in basic visual processing) and associative (i.e., impairment in accessing stored visual memories or access to meaning).

Prosopagnosia

Prosopagnosia is the inability to recognize familiar faces, and the patient may also have associated defects in recognition of other specific objects. Prosopagnosia results from the damage to bilateral occipital lobes or damage to the right inferior occipital lobe.

Akinetopsia

Patients with lesions of the dorsal pathway V5 experience loss of perception of visual motion with the intact perception of color and texture.

Alexia Without Agraphia

Alexia without agraphia or pure alexia is an inability to read the letters while maintaining the ability to write. The patients thereby may be able to write a dictation but would not be able to read it. The severity may vary, ranging from global alexia to "letter-by-letter reading", in which patients recognize letters but have difficulty assembling them to form words, with longer words being progressively more difficult.

The condition typically results from the damage to the fibers originating from the left occipital lobe to the splenium of the corpus callosum.

Disorders of Visual–Spatial Relation

Simultanagnosia

Simultanagnosia refers to a failure to generate a global percept of a complex visual scene despite an intact ability to perceive the individual elements that make up that scene. It represents a restricted window of attention. Patients are usually very symptomatic, often rendered functionally blind. It is most commonly seen in the context of stroke affecting the parietal lobes, but the frontal lobes may be involved.

When testing with Ishihara's pseudo-isochromatic plate, the patient correctly identifies the colors but will not be able to identify the numbers.

Balint Syndrome

Balint syndrome commonly results from ischemic infarctions in bilateral parietal and occipital areas. Balint syndrome is associated with difficulties in visual and spatial coordination and is characterized by optic ataxia, oculomotor apraxia, and simultanagnosia. Optic ataxia results in a lack of coordination between visual input and hand movements, which means that patients are unable to complete a visually guided task. Oculomotor apraxia is the inability to voluntarily shift gaze despite the intact function of extraocular muscles.

Visual Allesthesia

Allesthesia is a condition in which a stimulus is perceived at a location remote from its application and is usually associated with somatic stimuli.

Disorders of Vision Awareness

Anton Syndrome

Anton–Babinski syndrome is the denial of vision loss, which is associated with the emergence of memories of events and experiences that never took place along with vision loss and cortical blindness. Anton syndrome can result from the damage to either the primary occipital cortex area 17, secondary occipital cortex areas 18 and 19, or angular gyrus.

Riddoch Phenomenon

Riddoch phenomenon is also known as stereostatic dissociation, which is the dissociation between the static stimuli and kinetic stimuli. It is characterized by the ability of the patient to visualize only the moving objects in the blind hemifield, resulting in normal kinetic perimetry; on the contrary, the static perimetry will be abnormal.

Hemispatial Neglect

Hemispatial neglect results from the damage to the contralateral parietal lobe and is characterized by the inability to perceive and process stimuli on one side of the body or environment.

Visual Hallucinations

Temporal lobe lesions may lead to olfactory gustatory hallucinations, and the visual phenomenon in this area is usually complex and is associated with formed hallucinations.

Parietal lobe lesions may lead to formed or unformed hallucinations; on the contrary, the occipital lobe lesions characteristically lead to unformed hallucinations associated with white or colored flashes of light, kaleidoscopic colors, moving discs, and flickering or hexagonal arrays.

Hallucinations are usually described in hemianopia or quadrantanopia.

Palinopsia

Palinopsia is a cortical phenomenon seen with disorders of the parieto-occipital area and is characterized by the presence of afterimages even after the removal of the original stimulus. The afterimages may also be associated with hemifield defects, with pallinoptic images appearing in the blind hemifield.

2.7 Miscellaneous

Gunjan Saluja

 1. Describe superior orbital fissure syndrome, its clinical presentation, and management.

Orbital Apex Syndrome

The term superior orbital fissure syndrome (SOFS) or Rochon–Duvigneaud syndrome is applied to lesions located immediately anterior to the orbital apex, including the structures exiting through the superior orbital fissure, thus resulting in multiple cranial nerve palsies, which include oculomotor nerve (III), trochlear nerve (IV), abducens nerve (VI), and the ophthalmic branch of the trigeminal nerve (V1) in the absence of optic nerve pathology. Orbital apex syndrome, besides the above-mentioned features, will also include the features of optic nerve involvement.

Etiology

- *Trauma:* It is the most common cause of SOFS. The syndrome is commonly associated with motorcycle accidents, zygomatic fractures, and orbital fractures.
- *Neoplasms:* Burkitt's lymphoma, leukemia, rhabdomyosarcoma, metastases from breast carcinoma, lung carcinoma, and renal carcinoma
- *Infections:* Meningitis, syphilis, sinusitis, herpes zoster
- *Autoimmune etiologies:* Systemic lupus erythematosus (SLE), sarcoidosis, Tolosa–Hunt syndrome, microscopic polyangiitis, Churg-Strauss syndrome, nonspecific orbital inflammation
- *Iatrogenic:* Postorbital and sinonasal surgeries
- *Vascular:* Cavernous sinus thrombosis, carotid-cavernous fistula, carotid artery aneurysm
- *Other causes:* Neurofibromatosis, mucocele, fibrous dysplasia.

Pathogenesis

The structures passing through the superior orbital fissure can be compressed by bony fragments or mass or by edema of the surrounding tissues as in cases of inflammation due to infectious and autoimmune etiologies. Moreover, the orbital muscle cone is a narrow space, which is bounded by the intermuscular membrane and Tenon's capsule; hence, any edema or masses in this area compromise delicate neural structures.

The sixth nerve passes through the annulus of Zinn and lies in close proximity to the greater wing of the sphenoid, making it the most vulnerable. On the contrary, the trochlear nerve is the least commonly involved as it lies outside the common tendinous ring of Zinn where it is well protected.

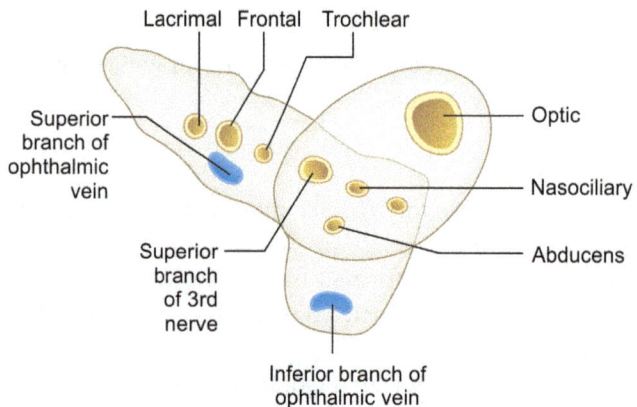

Fig. 1: Superior orbital fissure.

Clinical Features

The important structures passing through the superior orbital fissure are the third nerve (superior and inferior divisions), sixth nerve, and nasociliary nerve. The trochlear nerve, along with the frontal and lacrimal nerves, passes outside the annulus of Zinn. Hence, the clinical features arising will collaborate with the involvement of the structures mentioned **(Fig. 1)**.

Third nerve: The involvement of the superior division of the oculomotor nerve leads to ptosis and elevation deficit in abduction (superior rectus). The involvement of the inferior division of the oculomotor nerve will lead to defective depression in abduction (inferior rectus), elevation in adduction (inferior oblique), adduction (medial rectus), and loss of sympathetic supply of pupillomotor fibers, leading to the fixed pupil.

Simultaneous involvement of the sixth nerve leads to defective abduction.

Fourth nerve palsy results in limitation of depression in adduction (superior oblique).

Nasociliary nerve: Loss of corneal sensation.

Lacrimal hyposecretion and eyelid or forehead anesthesia: Due to damage to branches of the ophthalmic division of the trigeminal nerve.

Vision loss along with the above-mentioned features will be suggestive of *optic nerve involvement*, leading to a diagnosis of the orbital apex syndrome.

Investigations

Imaging

Localization of the etiology is of utmost importance in which imaging plays an important role; gadolinium contrast-enhanced magnetic resonance imaging is the investigation of choice in patients with suspected inflammatory disorders, vasculitis, sarcoidosis, and nonspecific inflammatory disorders. The enlarged dilated tortuous superior ophthalmic vein is an important feature of carotid-cavernous fistula, which can be further supported by computed tomography angiography with venous sequences.

Fat suppression helps to visualize the lesions of the cavernous sinus and orbital apex.

Computed tomography is useful in patients with fractures involving the base of the skull and in those where the zygomaticomaxillary or nasoethmoidal regions are involved.

Blood Investigations

Total leukocyte count, differential leukocyte count, and erythrocyte sedimentation rate are helpful in patients with suspected underlying infectious etiology.

Peripheral smear and bone marrow biopsy can be helpful in patients with suspected lymphoma or leukemia. In patients with suspected vasculitis as the underlying cause, cytoplasmic antineutrophil cytoplasmic antibody (c-ANCA) and perinuclear antineutrophil cytoplasmic antibody (p-ANCA) can be advised. Similarly, in patients with suspected sarcoidosis, serum angiotensin-converting enzyme (ACE) and serum calcium levels can be helpful.

It is important to differentiate between the infectious (fungal) and inflammatory etiology as initiating steroids in those patients can further worsen the disease.

Management

Management depends upon the underlying etiology.

 2. Discuss the clinical features and management of migraine.

Migraine is a common cause of primary headache, which is disabling due to its severity and repetitive bouts. It is more common in females as compared to males. Family history is usually present. Primary dysfunction involves afferent sensory neurons of the trigeminal nerve; the activation of trigeminal nucleus caudalis causes the release of vasoactive chemokines at vascular endings of the trigeminal nerve; and these neuropeptides cause dilation of pial arteries, increase vascular permeability, and induce an inflammatory response, thus activating trigeminal afferent fibers within the walls of the blood vessels.

Clinical Features

Attacks are episodic, start at puberty, and reduce as the age advances and can be associated with variable degrees of remission. Headache in typical cases is unilateral and is of throbbing nature.

Headache is usually unilateral and can be associated with or without aura.

Other associations include vomiting, photophobia, allodynia, and nausea.

The attacks can be predisposed by:
- *Hormonal factors:* Migraine is linked to the hormonal changes during puberty, young adulthood, and menopause. The attacks may be exaggerated during pregnancy and menstruation.
- Emotional stress, sleep deprivation, or excess sleep and hunger can lead to migraine.
- Certain food items such as chocolate, cheese, wine, alcohol, citrus fruits, food additives, exercise, vasodilators, and contraceptive pills can predispose migraine.

Clinical Variants

Migraine with Aura

- The classic migraine/migraine with aura begins from a small scotoma, which gradually expands and is bounded by a shimmering, zigzag, and silvery pattern of image which moves temporally into periphery and later disappears.
- Loss of vision may be present, which expands into periphery and later breaks.
- Typically, they are hemianopic and perceived by patient as monocular. Imagery builds over minutes with positive phenomenon typically having movement.
- Aura lasts for 60 minutes and is typically followed by a throbbing headache on the contralateral side, which is associated with photophobia.
- The attacks last for 4–72 hours.

Basilar Migraine

Basilar migraine results from transient ischemia along distribution of basilar artery, and can be accompanied with diplopia, vertigo, ataxia, dysarthria, and loss of consciousness, which may be a part of the aura and is transient.

Migraine Aura without Headache

- Migraine aura may be present without associated headache and must be differentiated from transient ischemic attacks. Symptoms include scintillating scotoma, transient homonymous hemianopia, peripheral visual field constriction causing tunnel vision, and episodic diplopia.
- Symptoms typically last for 60 minutes and are transient.
- A residual field defect suggests underlying cerebrovascular pathology.

Migraine without Aura

Migraine without aura is the most common migraine and has no associated preceding neurologic symptoms.

Hemiplegic Migraine

Hemiplegic migraine is the prolonged headache lasting for hours or days followed by hemiparesis, which recovers slowly over days.

Management

Drugs in Acute Migraine

The treatment should be initiated with nonsteroidal anti-inflammatory drugs (NSAIDs). In case there is no response with NSAIDs, triptan should be tried. Opioid use must be avoided in acute migraine.

Triptans

- Triptans are 5HT1B/1D receptor agonists, which inhibit the release of calcitonin gene-related peptide (CGRP) and inflammatory peptide in the meninges, thus preventing the pain signal from returning from periphery to trigeminal nucleus caudalis. 5HT1B receptors constrict the blood vessels and are contraindicated in patients with vascular disease.
- Commonly used triptans are almotriptan, rizatriptan, sumatriptan, and zolmitriptan.
- Side effects of triptan include tingling, flushing, sensation of warmth, heaviness, pressure, shortness of breath, and palpitations.

Prophylaxis of Migraine

Indications

- Recurring migraine interfering with patients' quality of life
- Four or more attacks in 1 month
- Long duration of aura

Drugs used for prophylaxis include:
- Propranolol
- Amitriptyline
- Gabapentin
- Valproate
- Topiramate.

3. Discuss the clinical features and management of essential blepharospasm.

Benign essential blepharospasm (BEB) is characterized by bilateral episodic contraction of orbicularis oculi and has no underlying etiology. The exact pathogenesis of blepharospasm is not known but can be caused by basal ganglia dysfunction.

Clinical Features

- The diagnosis of BEB is made clinically.
- The age of onset is between 40 and 60 years with females being affected more. Family history of dystonia or postural tremor increases the risk of blepharospasm.
- The spasms initially are mild and infrequent but can progress to interfere with daily activities of the patient. Patients typically describe an initial period of awareness of increased blink rate. The spasms further progress to constant progressive repetitive forceful eyelid closure, with or without apraxia of eyelid opening. Stress, fatigue, bright lights, driving, and social interactions can exacerbate blepharospasm and are usually associated with anxiety disorders. Singing, walking, driving, and placing pressure on brow may suppress symptoms.
- Blepharospasm can be associated with facial grimacing, cogwheeling in neck and extremities, and Meige syndrome. Other causes of blepharospasm such as dry eye, blepharitis, meibomitis, keratoconjunctivitis sicca, intraocular inflammation, narrow-angle glaucoma, aniridia, and meningeal irritation must be ruled out. History of prior neuroleptic use must be elucidated, which can cause tardive dyskinesia.

Investigations

Magnetic resonance imaging is unnecessary unless other neurologic abnormalities are suspected such as lower pontine mass, thalamic infarct, putaminal hemorrhage, and frontal cortical infarct which can cause blepharospasm.

Management

Supportive Care

Supportive care can be given in the form of artificial tears and chromatic lenses.

Oral Medications

A large number of medications have been used to manage blepharospasm, which are muscle relaxants such as baclofen and benzodiazepines, analgesics, antidepressants, antihistamines, anticholinergics, and antiepileptics such as phenytoin, carbamazepine, and serotonin antagonist (cyproheptadine). The oral medications can be tried in patients not willing for botulinum toxin injection.

Botulinum Toxin

The anaerobic bacillus *Clostridium botulinum* produces six antigenically distinct types of neurotoxin, of which botulinum toxin A has been approved by the Food and Drug Administration (FDA) for the treatment of blepharospasm. Botulinum toxin binds to the receptors present at the neuromuscular junction, enters the axons, and inhibits the release of acetylcholine.

Botulinum toxin is a large protein of high molecular weight, which is stabilized to a nontoxic protein and stabilizers. The toxin is supplied as a lyophilized powder, which needs to be reconstituted with sterile saline. Shaking the vial prior to its injection must be avoided to prevent the shearing of protein. The concentration of botulinum toxin used for blepharospasm is 2.5 units/0.1 mL; the total dose delivered in the eyelid is 12.5–15.0 units. The amount of toxin injected is gradually increased if the spasms recur before 10–12 weeks.

Sites of Injection

Two in the upper eyelid, one in the lower eyelid, with additional injections into corrugator supercilii in patients with brow contraction are administered with a 30-gauge needle. The upper eyelid injections must be avoided in central part to prevent ptosis.

It takes several days to achieve the effect of toxin, with the response lasting for 10–12 weeks.

With each subsequent injection, the effect of toxin reduces and has a variable response.

Local side effects of botulinum toxin include pain, hematoma, ptosis, diplopia, and lagophthalmos. All these side effects of the toxin are self-limited, with minimum systemic absorption.

CHAPTER 3

Strabismus

Priyanka Ramesh, Gunjan Saluja

Anatomy and Physiology

Q 1. Discuss muscle pulley.

Extraocular muscle pulleys are sheets of tissue made up of collagen, elastin, and smooth muscle that encircle the extraocular muscles and also attach to the walls of the orbit and adjacent connective tissue. The existence of pulleys was proposed by Demer and Miller and now has been confirmed by high-definition magnetic resonance imaging (MRI) of the orbit. They are located in a coronal plane, around 5-6 mm behind the equator. They encase the posterior part of the muscle and prevent the movement of the muscle belly during ocular movements. They are richly innervated and they also change their positions depending on different gazes. The orbital fibers of the extraocular muscles are attached to the pulley whereas the global fibers traverse anteriorly and attach to the sclera. These pulleys act like a functional origin of the extraocular muscles.

Abnormal location of pulley or any pathology in the pulley has been proposed as a mechanism of ocular motility disorders.

- Heterotopia of the muscle pulley is one of the theories for pattern strabismus. There is vertical displacement of the lateral rectus (LR) pulley. Inferior displacement will give rise to V pattern strabismus with upshoots and less depression in adduction and conversely the superior displacement of the pulley leads to A pattern with elevation of the abducting and depression of the adducting eye. There can be abnormalities of the pulley in certain disorders such as craniosynostosis syndromes and connective tissue disorders such as Marfan's syndrome and Ehler-Danlos syndrome. It can also be damaged in acquired conditions such as trauma or age-related degeneration of the pulley fibers.
- Globe size and pulley disparity can also lead to "strabismus fixus" in high myopes **(Figs. 1 and 2)**.

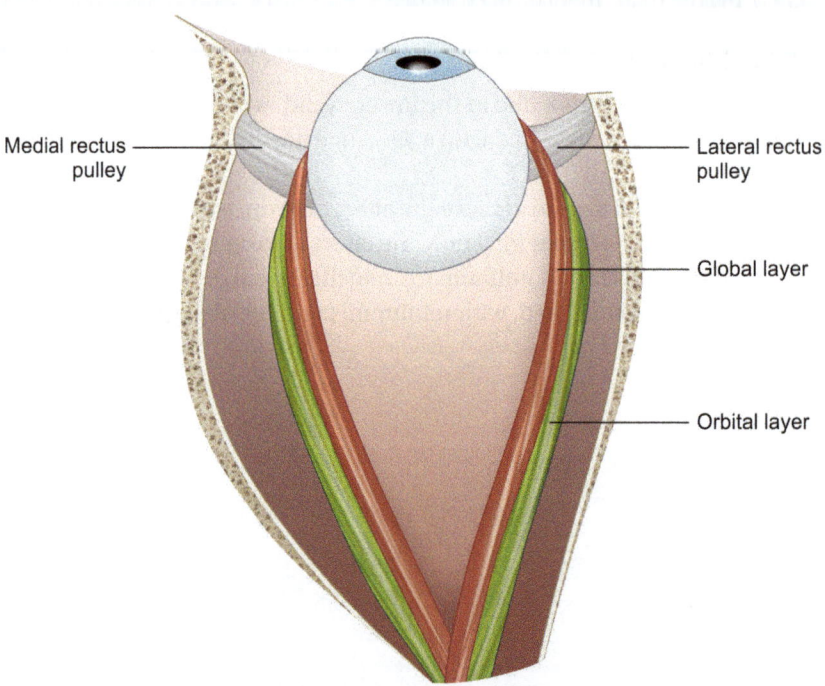

Fig. 1: Pulleys of medial recti and lateral recti.

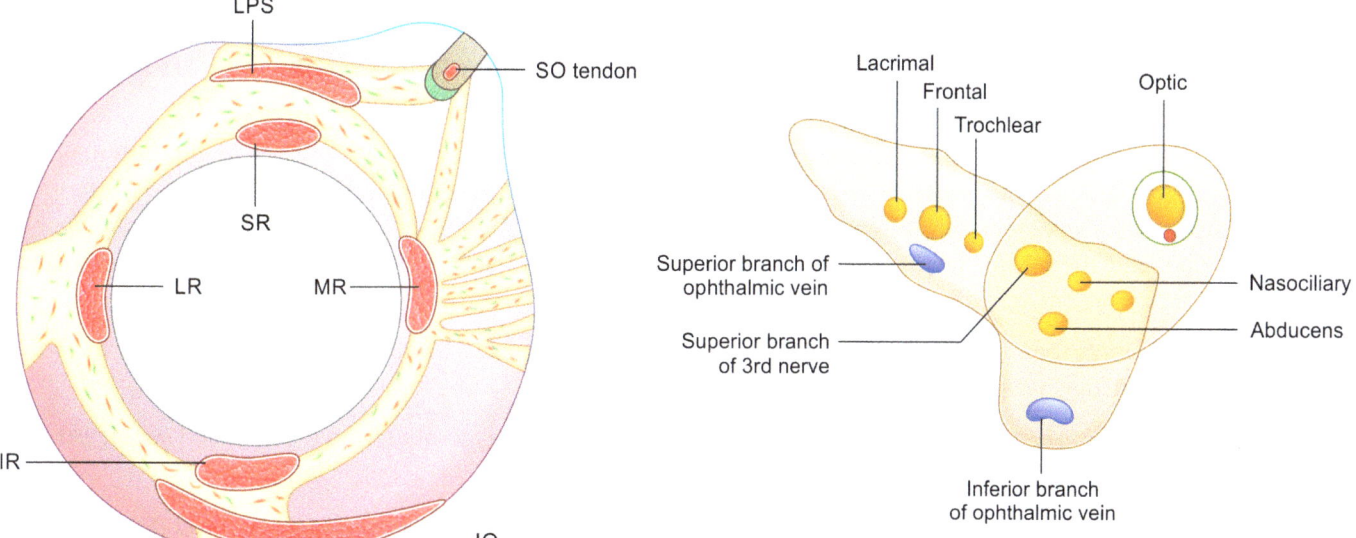

Fig. 2: Extraocular muscle (EOM) pulley system.
(IO: inferior oblique; IR: inferior rectus; LPS: levator palpebrae superioris; LR: lateral rectus; MR: medial rectus; SO: superior oblique; SR: superior rectus)

Fig. 3: The superior orbital fissure, the annulus of Zinn, and the structures passing through the various areas.

 2. Describe annulus of Zinn.

The annulus of Zinn is a common tendinous ring of origin of the recti muscles situated at the apex of the orbit. It lies on the lesser and greater wing of sphenoid. It is elliptical in shape and it encloses the optic canal and also divides the superior orbital fissure into three parts.

The superior part of the annulus of Zinn gives origin to the superior rectus (SR), the medial part to the medial rectus (MR), the inferior part to the inferior rectus (IR), and the lateral part to the LR. The superior orbital fissure is divided into the upper, middle, and lower part by the annulus.

Structures passing through the upper part are:
- Lacrimal nerve
- Frontal nerve
- Trochlear nerve
- Superior ophthalmic vein and recurrent branch of the ophthalmic artery

Structures passing within the tendinous ring are:
- Two divisions of the third cranial nerve, the superior and inferior
- Nasociliary nerve
- Abducens nerve

Structure passing through the lower part is:

Inferior ophthalmic vein.

The optic canal is enclosed in the annulus of Zinn. It contains the optic nerve and the ophthalmic artery **(Fig. 3)**.

 3. Discuss the origin, insertion, function, nerve, and blood supply of extraocular muscles, with a note on their development.

There are six extraocular muscles that bring about the ocular movements. The MR, LR, SR, IR, and two oblique muscles—the superior and inferior oblique (IO).

Superior Rectus

Origin: It arises from the common tendinous origin of the upper part of the annulus of Zinn. The origin is superolateral to the optic foramen. The origin of the levator palpebrae superioris (LPS) is present above the origin of the SR.

Course in the orbit: The SR travels anterolaterally through the orbit making an angle of 23° with the long axis of the globe. Above the SR is the LPS and the frontal nerve. Inferiorly, it is separated by the ophthalmic artery, nasociliary artery, and nerves by orbital fat. The tendon of the superior oblique (SO) after getting reflected by the trochlea is present beneath the muscle. Laterally, there is the lacrimal artery and nerve and medially there is the ophthalmic artery and nasociliary nerve.

Insertion: The SR pierces the Tenon's capsule and attaches on the sclera around 7.7 mm away from the limbus in an oblique fashion. The length of the insertion is around 10.8 mm.

Blood and nerve supply: The SR is supplied by the superior division of the oculomotor nerve. The blood supply is by the lateral muscular branch of the ophthalmic artery.

Actions: The primary action of the SR is elevation and the elevation action is maximum in abducted position of the globe because of the angulation of the SR fibers to the long axis of the globe. The secondary actions are adduction and intorsion.

Inferior Rectus

Origin: It is the shortest extraocular muscle. It originates from the inferior part of the annulus below the optic foramen.

Course in the orbit: The muscle moves anteriorly making an angle of around 23° with the anteroposterior axis of the globe. Above it is the optic nerve and inferior division of the oculomotor nerve. Laterally, it is related to the IO. Inferiorly, it is related to the floor of the orbit and the infraorbital nerve and vessel. Inferiorly, it is also related to the IO as it crosses and the sheaths unite.

Insertion: It attaches on the sclera around 6.5 mm from the limbus. The insertion is around 9.8 mm long in an oblique fashion. Its fascial sheath is also attached to the lower lid.

Nerve and blood supply: Blood supply is by the medial muscular branch of the ophthalmic artery and nerve supply is by the inferior division of the oculomotor nerve.

Actions: The primary action is depression which acts best when globe is abducted because of the angulation of the fibers. The secondary actions are adduction and extorsion.

Medial Rectus

Origin: It is the largest extraocular muscle. It takes origin from the medial part of the annulus of Zinn. It arises both from superior and inferior area of the optic canal and also from the dura of the optic sheath.

Course in the orbit: It passes along the medial wall of the orbit. It is related superiorly to the SO, ophthalmic artery, ethmoidal branch, and the infratrochlear and ethmoidal nerves. Inferiorly is the floor of the orbit, medially the medial orbital wall, and laterally the optic nerve and fat.

Insertion: It is inserted on the sclera around 5.5 mm from the limbus. The insertion is a straight line around 10.3 mm.

Nerve and blood supply: Nerve supply is by the inferior division of the oculomotor nerve. The blood supply is by the medial muscular branch of the ophthalmic artery.

Action: It acts as a pure adductor in the primary position.

Lateral Rectus

Origin: It is originated from the lateral part of the annulus of Zinn where it crosses the superior orbital fissure. The origin is in the shape of a U and it has two heads—an upper head and a lower head.

Course in the orbit: It travels anteriorly along the lateral orbital wall. Superiorly is the lacrimal artery and nerve. Inferiorly is the floor of the orbit and the tendon of IO passes the LR inferiorly and then medially. Medially it is related to the optic nerve, the abducens nerve, ciliary ganglion, and the ophthalmic artery. Laterally in the anterior part of the globe, it is related to the lacrimal gland.

Insertion: It pierces the Tenon's capsule and attaches on the sclera around 6.9 mm from the limbus. The attachment is vertical measuring around 9.2 mm.

Nerve and blood supply: It is supplied by the abducens nerve and blood supply by the lacrimal artery and lateral muscular branch of ophthalmic artery.

Actions: It is a pure abductor when the eye is in primary position.

Superior Oblique

It is the longest and thinnest extraocular muscle.

Origin: Arises from the body of sphenoid above and medial to the optic foramen. The insertion overlaps the insertion of the LPS.

Course and insertion: It travels anteriorly between the superior and medial wall of the orbit to reach the trochlea which is a cartilaginous pulley attached to the spina trochlearis on the frontal bone. From here, the muscle gets reflected posterolaterally to form a tendon 10 mm behind the trochlea and finally gets inserted. The insertion is a fan-shaped insertion with a width of about 11 mm. It is curved with concave part facing the trochlea. The anterior end of the insertion is about 13.8 mm from the limbus and 3–4.5 mm behind the insertion of the SR. The posterior end is about 18.8 mm behind the limbus and 13.6 mm behind the insertion of the SR. The direct part of the muscle is around 40 mm and reflected tendon is around 19.5 mm.

Actions: The SO-reflected tendon makes 55° angle with the axis of the globe. It acts as a depressor in adducted position. The primary action of SO is intorsion and the subsidiary actions are abduction and depression.

Blood and nerve supply: Nerve supply is by the trochlear nerve and blood supply is by the superior muscular branch of the ophthalmic artery.

Inferior Oblique

Origin: It originates by a rounded tendon on the medial part of the orbital floor lateral to the opening of the nasolacrimal duct. Few fibers also arise from the lacrimal fascia. It is the only muscle originating from the front of the orbit and has the shortest tendon.

Course in the orbit: It passes laterally and backward making an angle of around 45° with the long axis of the globe. Inferiorly, it is related to the periosteum.

Insertion: It is attached to the inferolateral part of the sclera behind the equator with a curved incision. The width of the incision is around 9 mm, anterior end is around 10 mm behind the LR, and the posterior end is about 1 mm behind and 2 mm in front of the anatomical location of the fovea.

Actions: The primary action is extorsion. The secondary actions are abduction and elevation. Since the muscle makes an angle of 45° with the long axis, it acts as a pure elevator in adduction.

Blood and nerve supply: Nerve supply is by the inferior division of the oculomotor nerve. Blood supply is by the infraorbital and medial muscular branches of the ophthalmic artery **(Figs. 4 to 6) (Table 1)**.

Development of the Extraocular Muscle

The extraocular muscles are mesenchymal in origin. All the muscles originate from a mesenchymal mass of tissue beginning posteriorly at the apex of the orbit around the optic nerve and progress anteriorly. The tendons fuse with the sclera at the end of 3 months. The LR, the SR, and the LPS develop first at 5th week followed by the MR and SO at 6 weeks and finally the IR and IO. The muscles innervated by the 3rd cranial nerve develop from premandibular condensations and the LR and SO develop from the maxillomandibular mesoderm.

4. Describe briefly origins, insertions, and action of extraocular muscles.

Refer to Answer 3.

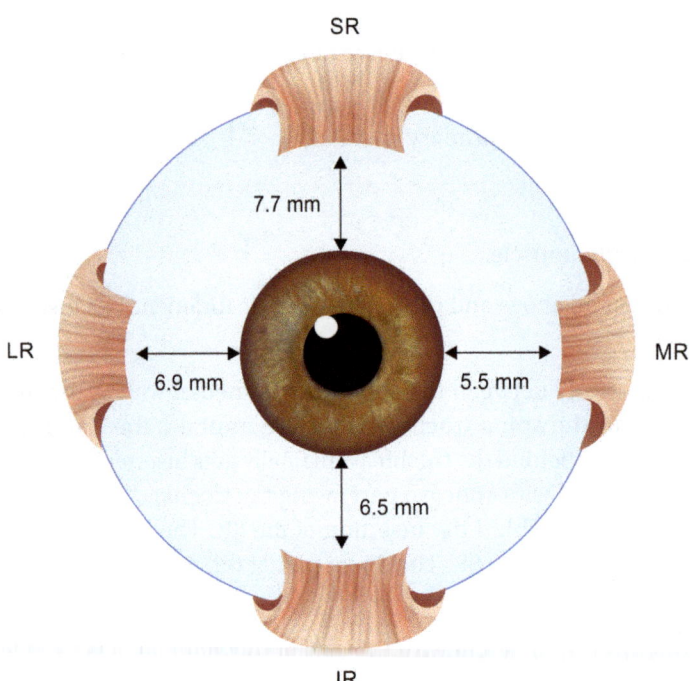

Fig. 4: Insertions of recti muscles.
(IR: inferior rectus; LR: lateral rectus; MR: medial rectus; SR: superior rectus)

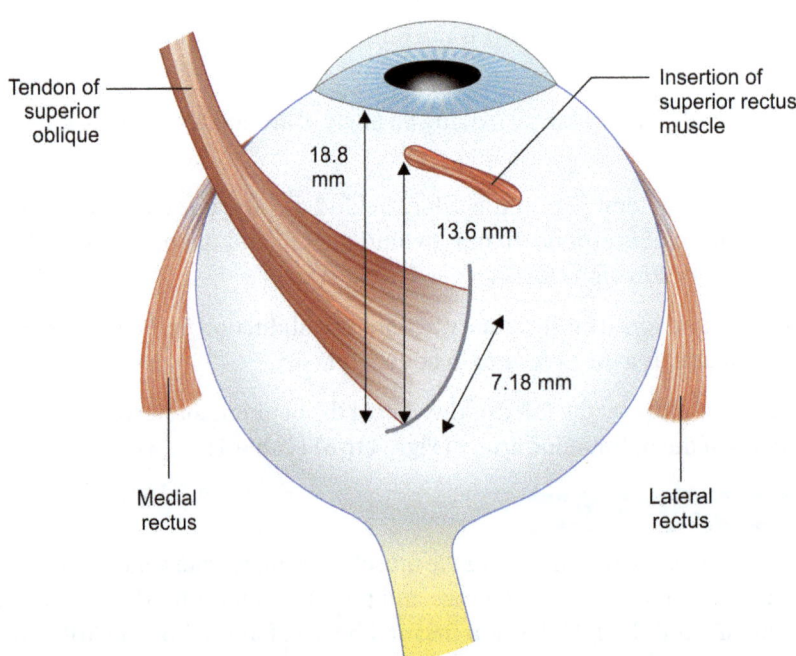

Fig. 5: Insertion of superior oblique tendon.

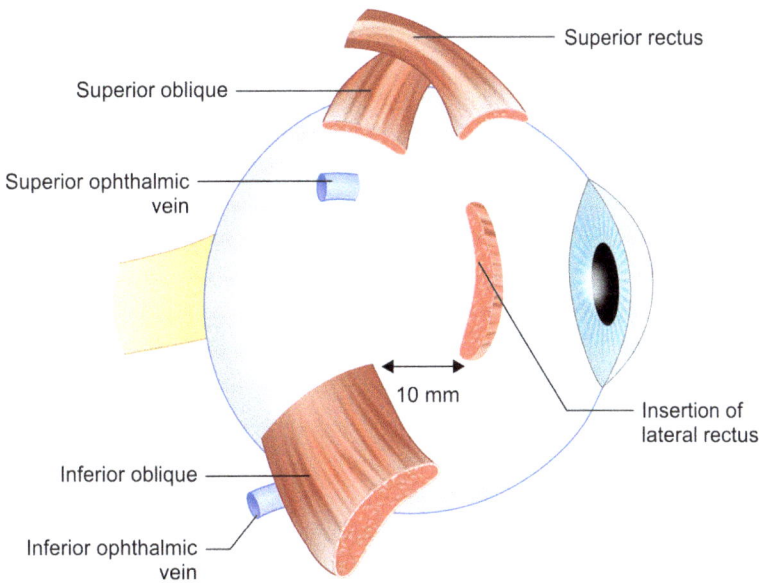

Fig. 6: Insertion of inferior oblique tendon.

TABLE 1: The actions of the extraocular muscles.

Muscle	Main action	Subsidiary action
Medial rectus	Adduction	–
Lateral rectus	Abduction	–
Superior rectus	Elevation	Intorsion and adduction
Inferior rectus	Depression	Extorsion and adduction
Superior oblique	Intorsion	Depression and abduction
Inferior oblique	Extorsion	Elevation and abduction

 5. Describe anatomy of superior oblique muscle. Discuss mechanism of its muscle action in various direction of gaze.

It is the longest and the thinnest extraocular muscle.

Origin: It arises from the body of sphenoid above and medial to the optic foramen. The insertion overlaps the insertion of the LPS.

Course and insertion: It travels anteriorly between the superior and medial wall of the orbit to reach the trochlea, which is a fibrocartilaginous loop attached to the spina trochlearis on the inferior surface of the frontal bone. The SO passes through the loop and the trochlea acts like a pulley. It is surrounded by the synovial sheath at this point **(Fig. 7)**.

From here, the muscle gets reflected posterolaterally to form a tendon 10 mm behind the trochlea and finally gets inserted. The insertion is a fan-shaped insertion with a width of about 11 mm. It is curved with concave part facing the trochlea. The anterior end of the insertion is about 13.8 mm from the limbus and 3–4.5 mm behind the insertion of the SR. The posterior end is about 18.8 mm behind the limbus and 13.6 mm behind the insertion of the SR. The direct part of the muscle is around 40 mm and reflected tendon is around 19.5 mm.

Actions: The SO reflected tendon makes 55° angle with the axis of the globe. It acts as a depressor in adducted position. The primary action of SO is intorsion and the subsidiary actions are abduction and depression.

Blood and nerve supply: Nerve supply is by the trochlear nerve and blood supply is by the superior muscular branch of the ophthalmic artery.

6. Discuss the various laws governing the ocular movement. Discuss the clinical implication.

There are four laws governing the ocular motility:
1. Hering's law of equal innervation
2. Sherrington's law of reciprocal innervation
3. Donder's law
4. Listing's law.

Hering's law of equal innervation: This law states that corresponding or "yoke" muscles get equal and simultaneous innervation to being about motor coordination between the two eyes and binocular movement. This is seen both in versions and vergences. For example, for levoversion, the left LR and the right MR receive simultaneous and equal innervation.

Sherrington's law of reciprocal innervation: This law states that during binocular movement, the direct antagonist receives equal and simultaneous inhibition of innervation. This allows the opposing muscle to relax and hence bring out ocular movement. For example, in levoversion, the left LR gets excitatory stimulus and the left MR gets simultaneous and equal inhibitory stimulus.

Donder's law: This law states that to each position of the line of sight belongs a definite orientation of the horizontal and vertical meridians relative to the coordinates of space. The orientation of the retinal meridians depends on the amount of elevation, depression, or horizontal eye movement and out of the three degrees of freedom of rotation of the eyeball, the rotation around the anteroposterior axis is restricted. Hence, there is no cyclorotation that happens. The orientation of the meridians is same irrespective of the path taken to reach there.

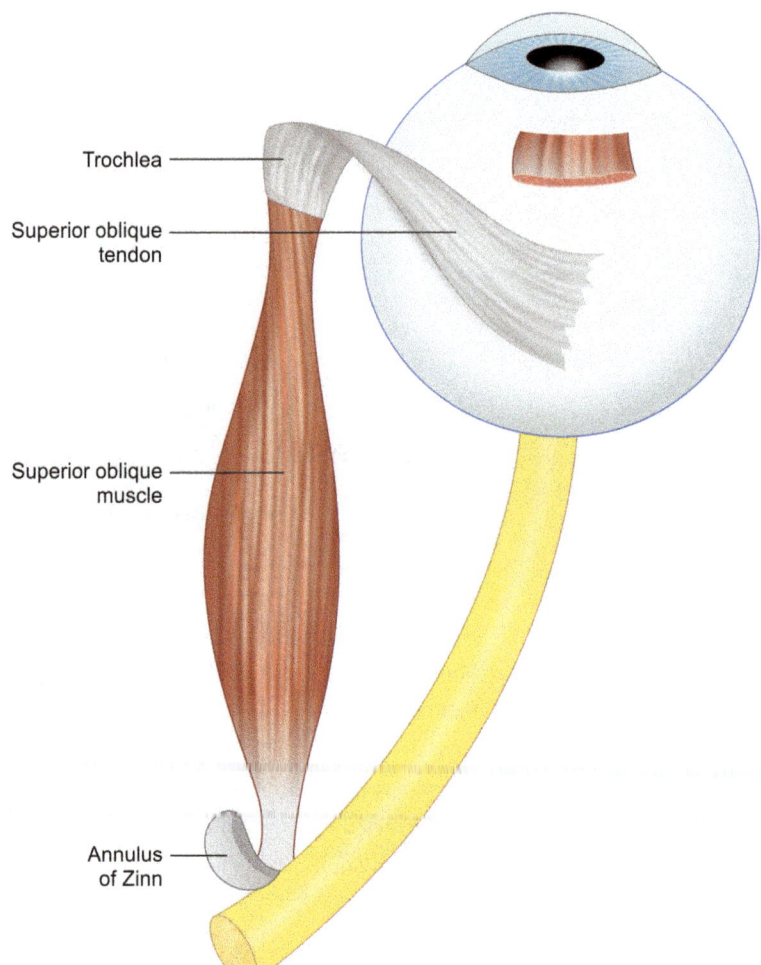

Fig. 7: Course of superior oblique tendon and its insertion.

Listing's law: This is similar to the Donder's law. All ocular movements from the primary position occur due to rotation along a single plane called the Listing's plane which is in the equatorial plane. It implies that all ocular movements are true to the meridian and no torsion occurs.

Clinical Implications of the Laws of Ocular Motility

- *Hering's law:* Hering's law is responsible for the binocular ocular motility. It is responsible for versions and vergences. It is responsible for symmetric convergence and also in cases of asymmetric convergence. In asymmetric convergence, there is combined convergence as well as lateral version. This law explains the primary and secondary deviations in case of paralytic strabismus. The paralytic muscle receives extra innervation when the paralytic muscle is the fixing eye, and hence according to Hering's law, the yoke muscle also receives extra innervation resulting in more amount of deviation in the normal eye making the secondary deviation more than the primary deviation.

  Dissociated vertical deviations (DVDs) defy Hering's law of equal innervation. In DVD, the undercover eye is hypertropic and there is excycloduction. When the fixation is changed and the fixing eye is kept undercover, the hypertropic eye will move down to take up fixation. By the virtue of Hering's law, the covered eye should have moved down or become hypotropic. Instead, it becomes hypertropic under cover.

- *Sherrington's law:* According to this law, the direct antagonistic muscle relaxes equally when an extraocular muscle contracts hence preventing co-contraction of the muscles. In Duane's retraction syndrome (DRS), this law is not followed. There is simultaneous innervation to both the medial and the LR resulting in limitations of adduction and abduction along with retraction of the globe.

7. Describe various types of eye movements and various neuroanatomic pathways controlling eye movements.

The different types of ocular movements include:
- *Rapid eye movements:* Voluntary and spontaneous saccades, fast phase of vestibular and optokinetic nystagmus
- *Slow eye movements:* Voluntary pursuit, vergence movements, and slow phase of vestibular and optokinetic nystagmus

Saccades: This is a rapid eye movement to bring the object of interest on the fovea. The amount of movement that occurs depends on the distance of the object from the fovea. It is controlled by the prefrontal cortex or the ipsilateral paramedian pontine reticular formation (PPRF) for horizontal and riMLF (rostral interstitial medial longitudinal fasciculus) for vertical eye movement. It has a latency of 200 ms and velocity of 300–700 m/s. The retinal blurring during the saccade is not appreciated due to increase in the visual threshold.

Smooth pursuit: It is a tracking movement to follow a regularly moving object. It maintains the object on the fovea throughout the movement. It is controlled by the ipsilateral parieto-occipital cortex (higher center), pretectal nuclei of the midbrain, brainstem reticular formation, and cerebellar flocculi. It has a latency of 125 ms and velocity of 30–60 m/s.

Vergences: These movements help in alignment of the eyes with respect to each other so that the image falls on corresponding points of the retina in both eyes thereby achieving fusion. Thus, the stimulus for this is binasal or bitemporal disparity in the image. Fusional vergence is also associated with accommodation and miosis. It has a latency of 160 ms and velocity of 20 m/s. It is mediated by the temporoparietal cortex and the pretectal midbrain.

Vestibular reflex: These include movements to counteract the movements of the neck and head to keep the object of regard on the fovea. The stimulation of the semicircular canals, otoliths, or neck receptors gives rise to these movements. The latency is 100 ms and velocity is 300 m/s. The controlling pathway is in the contralateral vestibular nucleus and the PPRF.

Neuroanatomic Pathways Controlling Eye Movements

The central nervous system pathways controlling the ocular movements can be divided into the supranuclear pathway and the nuclear and infranuclear pathways.

The supranuclear pathway involves the cortical network and the network in the brainstem area.
- *Cortical area:* The saccades are controlled by the frontal cortex, the smooth pursuit by the parieto-occipital and the vergence eye movement by the temporoparietal cortex.
- Pontine paramedian reticular formation and median longitudinal fasciculus—control the horizontal eye movement. The PPRF receives connections from the cortex and vestibular system and helps in direct stimulation of the abducens nucleus to bring about lateral eye movement. The PPRF is also connected to the medial longitudinal fasciculus (MLF) which in turn is connected to the oculomotor nerve.
- Mesencephalic reticular formation, rostral interstitial nucleus of median longitudinal fasciculus, and posterior commissure are the areas which control the vertical eye movements. They receive the commands from the cortex.
- Vestibular nucleus gives the commands for the reflex eye movements. The vestibular nucleus supplies the PPRF or the MRF and bring about either the vertical or horizontal eye movement.

The nuclear and the infranuclear pathways consist of the cranial nerve nuclei and their connections and the cranial nerves.
- The oculomotor nucleus is present in the midbrain in the periaqueductal gray matter. It has subnuclei for supplying the extraocular muscles including the LPS and it also has the Edinger-Westphal nucleus which supplies the parasympathetic fibers to the ciliary muscles and the sphincter pupillae. All the muscles are supplied by the ipsilateral nuclei except the SR which is supplied by the contralateral nuclei and the LPS where bilateral LPS is supplied by a

single nucleus. Hence, in case of nuclear 3rd nerve palsy, there is bilateral ptosis and opposite side SR involvement. Since the Edinger-Westphal also supplies bilaterally, in nuclear lesion, there is loss of pupillary constriction in both eyes.
- The trochlear nucleus gives rise to the trochlear nerve which supplies the SO. It is situated in the midbrain at the level of the inferior colliculus. The nerve decussates dorsally when it exits from the midbrain. Hence, in nuclear lesions, the contralateral SO is involved.
- Abducens nucleus supplies the LR and it is present in the pons close to the nucleus of the facial nerve such that the nerve curves around the facial nerve nucleus when in exits from the pons. It is present near the floor of the fourth ventricle and it is closely related to the PPRF.
- *Internuclear connections between the abducens and the oculomotor nucleus:* The abducens nucleus is connected to the oculomotor nucleus by the internuclear neurons in the MLF. The LR of one side is connected to the MR of the contralateral side which helps in bringing about horizontal gaze movement **(Fig. 8)**.

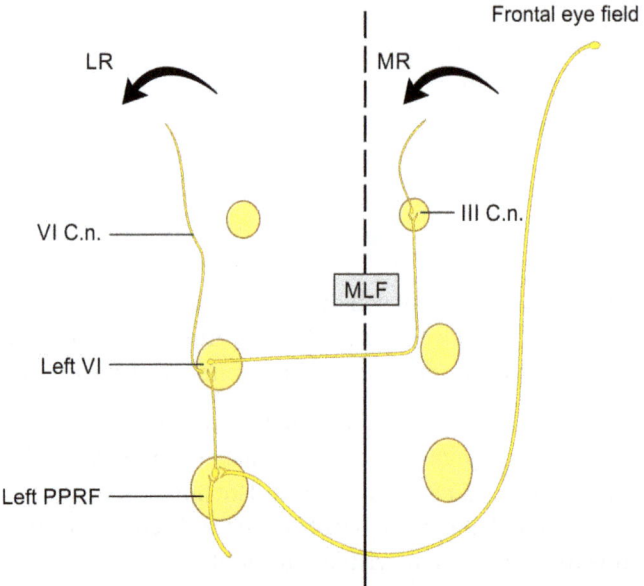

Fig. 8: Connections between the abducens nucleus and the oculomotor nucleus. (C.n: cranial nerve; LR: lateral rectus; MR: medial rectus; MLF: medial longitudinal fasciculus; PPRF: paramedian pontine reticular formation)

Binocular Vision

Q 8. Describe binocular vision—evolution, development, grades, and tests for assessment of binocular single vision.

Binocular vision is the phenomenon by which objects seen separately by the two eyes are perceived as a single object. Any object imaged on the two primary visual directions seem to be superimposed and as if in the same area in space even though they are separated.

Images falling on the fovea of both eyes will be perceived to be in front of the person, that is in front of the imaginary cyclopean eye. Images falling on the corresponding points of the retina will appear as a single image and other points are called as disparate points.

Evolution and Development of Binocular Vision

Hubel and Weisel's experiments helped in understanding the development of binocular vision. The layer 4-c of the visual cortex contains the ocular dominance columns. In all humans, at birth, the cortical cells are connected equally to both eyes. 10% of the cells are connected to right eye and 10% to the left eye. 80% are connected binocularly where central 20% have equal connections with both eyes and the rest have a predominance to any one eye. The inputs to the ocular dominance columns start segregating at the last weeks of intrauterine life and is almost complete by 4-6 weeks. The visual development continues till 0–5 years up to 9 years. In case there is deprivation of stimulus to any one eye, the ocular dominance column cells from that eye start representing the other eye thereby developing amblyopia in the affected eye. This process is reversible till the age of cortical plasticity.

Correspondence and Disparity Theory for Binocularity

When images fall on the corresponding points of the retina, they are perceived as a single image. When disparate points are stimulated, diplopia occurs. However, if there is horizontal disparity and it falls within the Panum's area, the images are fused and due to the horizontal disparity, there is perception of depth or stereopsis which increases as the disparity increases and with further increase diplopia ensues.

Grades of binocular vision: There are three grades of binocular vision.
1. *Simultaneous macular perception:* The ability of the visual cortex to perceive two images which stimulate corresponding area or fovea of both the eyes.

2. *Fusion:* This is a phenomenon by which two objects which are slightly dissimilar are perceived as a single image when they stimulate corresponding points of the retina.
3. *Stereopsis:* This is the highest form of binocular vision and it is the perception of depth.

Tests for binocular vision:
- After image test
- Synoptophore
- Worth forth dot test
- Maddox rod test
- Bagolini striated glasses.

These tests help in detection of abnormalities in binocular vision such as suppression or anomalous retinal correspondence (ARC).

- *After image test:* This is based on the principle of after image. The foveae of both eyes are stimulated with straight line, horizontal for right eye and vertical for left eye with the central portion being black to provide fixation as well as to protect the fovea. The patient then visualizes the after image in a darkroom or with eyes closed and the response is recorded **(Fig. 9)**.
  - *Symmetrical cross-response:* This is seen normally in the absence of squint. And in the presence of squint, it signifies normal bifoveal fixation. Irrespective of the type of deviation, symmetrical cross is seen with normal retinal correspondence (NRC).
  - *Asymmetrical crossing:* This is seen in cases of ARC. The amount of separation between the two lines gives the subjective angle of deviation.
  - If any one line is absent, then it suggests suppression of that eye.
- *Synoptophore:* This is based on the principle of haploscope. Both eyes are given separate stimulus with the help of two separate tubes with eye piece, prisms, and illumination system. Different slides can be presented to the patients and responses can be recorded. Simultaneous macular perception, fusion as well as stereopsis can be checked. Subjective deviation can be checked which can confirm the presence of ARC and also check the angle of anomaly **(Fig. 10)**.
- *Worth four dot test:* This uses red green glasses for dissociation of the two eyes. It is done at a distance of 6 m. The chart consists of four colored dots. Two green on either side, one red on top and, white below **(Figs. 11A to D)**. The patient is made to wear the red glass before right eye and green glass before the left eye. The following responses can be seen.

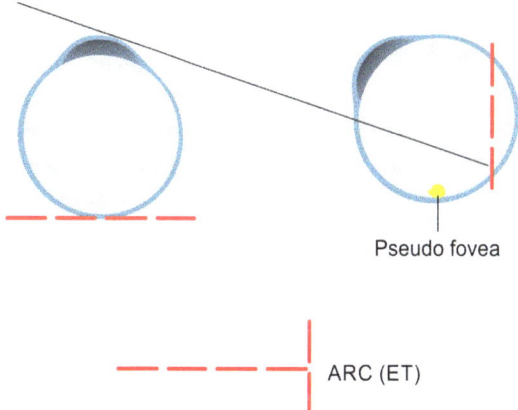

Fig. 9: Response obtained from after image test in a patient with esotropia and ARC. (ARC: anomalous retinal correspondence; ET: Esotropia)

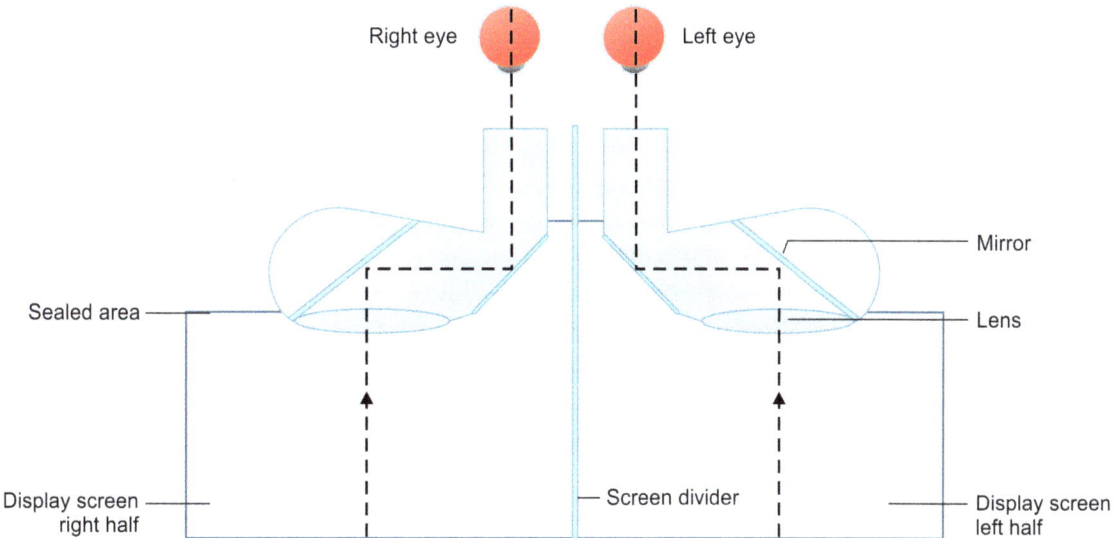

Fig. 10: Schematic diagram of synoptophore.

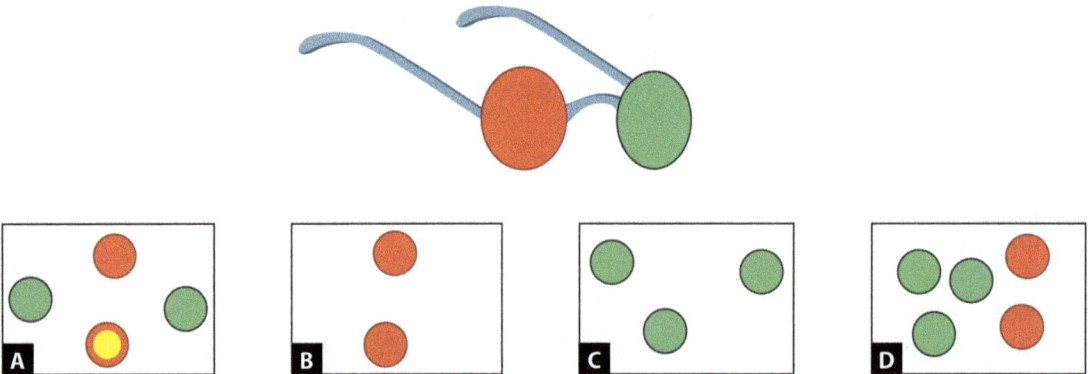

Figs. 11A to D: *Different responses of Worth four dot test:* (A) Normal response; (B) Left suppression; (C) Right suppression; (D) Diplopia response.

- *Four dots:* In normal binocular response without squint, all four dots are seen. This response is also seen in harmonious ARC in the presence of manifest deviation.
- *Five dots:* Here, the patient sees two red dots and three green dots. This is seen in manifest deviation with NRC without suppression. In the presence of esotropia, there is uncrossed diplopia and in exotropia there is crossed diplopia.
- *Presence of either two red dots or three green dots:* In this depending on which eye is suppressed, patients with right eye suppression see three green dots and with left eye suppression see two red dots.

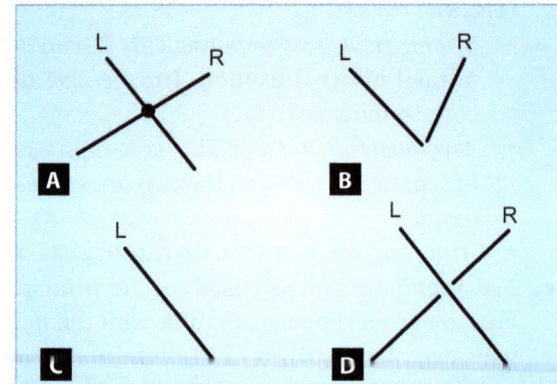

Figs. 12A to D: Different responses In Bagolini striated glass test; orthophoria with NRC and strabismus with harmonious ARC (A); Diplopia response (B); Right eye suppression (C); Central suppression scotoma (D). (ARC: anomalous retinal correspondence; NRC: normal retinal correspondence)

- *Bagolini striated glasses:* It is the most physiological test for binocularity. The striated glasses have striations which convert a point source of light into a straight light. The striations are right angle to each other in the two eyes **(Figs. 12A to D)**.
  - *Symmetrical cross response:* This is seen normally in the absence of manifest squint with and in ARC in presence of manifest squint.
- Diplopia response is seen in case of manifest squint without suppression.
- Absence of any one slant line is seen in case of suppression.
- A central scotoma can be seen in case of fixation point scotoma in manifest squint with ARC.
- Double Maddox rod test is similar to the Bagolini's test. Here, Maddox rod, which has multiple cylinders to convert a point source of light to a straight line, is used. One eye it can be oriented to create a vertical line and another to create a horizontal line.

Measurement of Suppression Scotoma

Extent of suppression: The extent of suppression can be charted under binocular conditions. Patient is asked to fixate with one eye and other eye is tested.

Various methods of measuring suppression scotoma are:
Prism: Prism is used to displace the central object peripherally till it can be visualized in different directions. Patient recognizes diplopia when the image falls outside the scotoma.

Binocular perimetry: The arrangement of testing apparatus is such that fixation target is common to both eyes but test object is seen only by one eye.
- *Lee's screen:* One eye is charted while the other eye fixates through mirror.
- Two Bjerrum screens at 90° to each other
- *Polaroid scotometer:* Using polaroid dissociation, one eye fixates and field of the other eye is charted.
  Depending on the test used, different responses can be obtained.

- When more dissociating tests are used such as prisms or Lee's screen a single large scotoma is seen.
- With less dissociating test such as phase difference haploscope or polaroid scotometer two discrete scotomas are seen.

 9. Discuss anatomical and physiological basis of binocular vision.

Refer to Answer 8.

 10. Describe sensory adaptation to strabismus. What is fusional vergence?

Manifest deviation results in stimulation of noncorresponding points of the retina resulting significant distress in the form of diplopia and confusion. The cortex adapts to this to eliminate the diplopia in children due to plasticity of the cortex. They can be motor adaptations or sensory adaptations. The sensory adaptations are suppression, ARC, and eccentric fixation.

- *Suppression:* This is a cortical mechanism in which the image from the deviating eye is ignored. This requires a long-standing constant large angle deviation. The suppression can be facultative, where the images from one eye are ignored only in binocular conditions but when the other eye is closed, the images from the earlier suppressed eye are processed normally. When the suppression is present even in monocular conditions, then it is called as obligatory suppression and this leads to the development of amblyopia. The presence of suppression can be diagnosed by testing the sensory status of the eye with the help of after image test, Bagolini striated glasses, synoptophore, or Worth four dot test.
- *Anomalous retinal correspondence:* In the presence of small angle deviation, instead of the fovea getting stimulated in the deviating eye an extrafoveal point gets stimulated. As an adaption to avoid diplopia, the fovea of the deviating eye loses its primary visual direction and fovea of one eye and extrafoveal point of the other eye share common subjective visual direction. During monocular conditions, the fovea still remains dominant over the extrafoveal point and fovea regains its straight-ahead gaze. This adaptation results in preservation of binocularity even in the presence of manifest squint. The ARC can be harmonious or unharmonious. In harmonious ARC, the amount of ARC completely compensates for the amount of deviation. Hence, the subjective angle is zero. In case of unharmonious ARC, the amount of ARC is not full, hence there is some amount of subjective deviation as well. The difference between the objective and subjective deviation gives the angle of anomaly. ARC can be detected using Bagolini's glasses, synoptophore, and the after-image test.
- *Eccentric fixation:* When the fovea loses its primary visual direction even in monocular conditions and the extrafoveal point starts assuming the straight-ahead gaze.

Fusional Vergence

Vergences are the ocular movements that occur in opposite directions also known as disjunctive movements. It occurs to maintain binocular vision, fixation, and fusion. The different vergence movements are:
- *Convergence:* Inward movement of both eyes
- *Divergence:* Outward movement of both eyes
- *Sursumvergence or deorsumvergences:* This is the vertical fusional vergences
- *Cyclovergence:* Torsional vergence movement

Stimulus for fusional vergence: The retinal disparity is the stimulus for fusional vergence. When an object comes closer to the eye, noncorresponding points of the retina are stimulated, this results in correctional movement to bring the image on the corresponding points of the retina. The disparity should be beyond the Panum's fusional area. There is an upper limit for the fusional vergence, beyond which the eyes cannot fuse and diplopia ensues.

The controlling center for vergence movement is said to be in the temporoparietal cortex/pretectal midbrain. The convergence center is thought to be in the nucleus of Perlia. It has a latency of 160 ms and velocity of 20 m/s. There is a continuous feedback loop.

Convergence: It can be voluntary or involuntary. There are four types of involuntary convergence:
1. *Tonic convergence:* This is the resting tone in the muscles which keep the eyes aligned. It is absent in deep sleep and general anesthesia and hence eyes are divergent in these cases. The tone is very high in children.
2. *Proximal convergence:* This is the convergence that occurs due to the psychological feeling that the image is close to the eyes.
3. *Accommodative convergence:* This is the convergence that occurs along with accommodation as a synkinetic movement along with pupillary constriction.

4. *Fusional convergence:* This is the convergence that occurs in response to retinal disparity in an attempt to restore fusion and binocular vision.

Measurement of Vergences

- *Using prism bars:* Prism bars can be used to induce retinal disparity and check for the fusional effort by the patient. The strength of the prism can be increased till the patient develops diplopia, this is called as the break point and then the prisms can be reduced till the patient starts appreciating binocular single vision and this is called as the recover point. This can be done for convergence using base-out prism, divergence using base in prisms, and also for base-up prisms in deorsumvergence and base down in sursumvergence.
- *Using synoptophore:* Synoptophore can be used for the measurement of horizontal vergences by moving the arms of the synoptophore and also for vertical and torsional fusion by moving the image.
  - Normal ranges for distance
  - *Convergence:* 20 prism diopter (PD)
  - *Divergence:* 6-8 PD
  - *Vertical vergences:* 3-4 PD
  - *Torsional vergences:* 8-22°.

11. Describe stereopsis.

Stereopsis is defined as relative ordering of visual objects in depth, that is, in the third dimension. It is the ability of the brain to perceive relative depth. It is considered as the highest level of binocularity.

Physiological basis of stereopsis: Because of the lateral displacement of the two eyes, the images formed on the corresponding points of the two eyes are not exactly alike but have a slight disparity. This disparity is perceived as depth. Horizontal disparity between the images falling on the corresponding points of the retina results in stereopsis when the images are fused by the cortex. The disparity should be within the Panum's area of fusion for this to occur. If the amount of horizontal disparity is more than what can be fused by the cortex, diplopia occurs. Vertical disparity does not result in stereopsis.

Development of stereopsis: Stereopsis is absent in infants <3 months of age. It rapidly develops and reaches normal level by 6 months.

Tests for stereopsis: The different mechanisms of stereopsis testing are:
- *Haploscopic principle:* Here, the two eyes are dissociated with the help of two tubes with angled mirrors such that different stimuli can be given to the two eyes. For example, synoptophore.
- *Anaglyph principle:* Here, the dissociation is brought about by using conjugate colors, red and green. The test consists of stereo-paired images in red and green and the patient performs the test using red–green glasses. For example, the Netherlands organization (TNO) test..
- *Vectographic principle:* This uses the principle of polarized light. Two stereo-paired images are present such that one light passing through one is polarized in one direction and the light passing through the other is polarized in a different direction and the patient performs the test using polarized filter glasses. For example, Titmus fly test and Randot.
- *Panographic principle:* This is a real-depth stereogram where there are a grid of cylinders with random dot pattern which will cause slightly different images to fall on the two eyes resulting in real depth perception. Glasses are not required for this test. For example, Lang stereotest.
- *Real depth:* Here, there is an actual difference in the placement of the objects. No glasses are required. For example, Frisby–Davis distance and near test.

1. *The Netherlands organization test:* It has seven plates which have to be read using red–green glasses. It is done at a distance of 40 cm. It can be used in children above 3 years, tests 15–480 seconds of arc.
2. Titmus stereo test is based on vectographic principle. It has a stereofly card and polaroid glasses. It tests near stereopsis and can be done in children from 3 years onward. The fly tests 3,500 arc seconds. Graded testing from 40 to 800 arc seconds also present. Stereo butterfly test is based on the same principle. It has the image of a butterfly instead of a fly.
3. *Randot test:* This is also based on vectographic principle with random dot stereogram. It requires polaroid glasses. There is a distant stereoacuity testing variant as well. It can be done in children >3 years. Tests 400–20 seconds of arc.
4. *Frisby–Davis test:* They have both near and distance. Near Frisby–Davis consists of glass plates with images and patient has to identify which image is in the front. The distance stereoacuity test consists of a background illuminated box with

different symbols attached to transparent rods giving the appearance that they are free floating. The patient is asked to tell which symbol is in the front. Distance test is done at 6 m and measures between 5 and 50 seconds of arc.
5. *Synoptophore:* This is based on the haploscopic principle. The two eyes receive separate stimuli by two tubes with angled mirrors and illuminating lamp. There are specific slides for stereopsis. Slides which have similar images but have slight horizontal disparity give the illusion of depth.
6. *Lang's two-pencil test:* This is a test which can be done bedside without the need for expensive equipment and measures only gross stereopsis. The patient is made to touch the tip of a pencil held by the examiner with another pencil. If patient is unable to perform, then we can conclude that gross stereopsis is absent.

 12. Define abnormal retinal correspondence. Explain its development and methods of diagnosis.

In the presence of small angle deviation, instead of the fovea getting stimulated in the deviating eye, an extrafoveal point gets stimulated. As an adaption to avoid diplopia, the fovea of the deviating eye loses its primary visual direction because of suppression of the foveal image and fovea of one eye and extrafoveal point of the other eye share common subjective visual direction. During monocular conditions, the fovea still remains dominant over the extrafoveal point and fovea regains its straight-ahead gaze. This adaptation results in preservation of binocularity even in the presence of manifest squint. The ARC can be harmonious or unharmonious. In harmonious ARC, the amount of ARC completely compensates for the amount of deviation. Hence, the subjective angle is zero. In case of unharmonious ARC, the amount of ARC is not full, hence there is some amount of subjective deviation as well. The difference between the objective and subjective deviation gives the angle of anomaly.

The different tests for ARC are:
- *After-image test:* In this, both the eyes are stimulated by a bright line vertical in one and horizontal in the other successively after closing the other eye. The center of the line is covered by a black dot to provide fixation and to protect the fovea from the bright light. Since the eyes are stimulated monocularly and patient is made to fix at the central black dot, the foveae of both the eyes are stimulated. Now, the patient is made to sit in a dark room to get a positive after image or in a bright light to get a negative after image. Since the foveae of both eyes are stimulated, in orthophoria as well as in the presence of manifest deviation with NRC, a symmetrical cross-response is seen. In case of ARC, an asymmetrical cross-response is seen as the visual direction of the fovea becomes eccentric. It is crossed in case of esotropia and uncrossed in case of exotropia **(Fig. 9)**.
- *Bagolini striated glasses:* These are plano glasses with striations at 90° to each other in the two eyes. One eye has striations at 35° and the other at 145°. The striations convert a point source of light into an oblique line. Both eyes are stimulated simultaneously. In case of orthophoria, a cross-response is seen. In cases of manifest deviation, if cross-response is seen, it indicates ARC **(Figs. 12A to D)**.
- *Synoptophore:* It uses tubes and angled mirrors to dissociate the two eyes. Stimulus is given to the fovea of both eyes separately. In the presence of manifest squint, if the patient sees a superimposed images, then there is NRC. If there is a diplopia response, then there is ARC. The objective and subjective angle of deviation can also be calculated. If the objective angle is equal to the subjective angle, then there is NRC. If the subjective angle is zero, then there is complete sensory adaptation for the squint and the angle of anomaly is equal to the objective deviation and the ARC is harmonious. If the subjective angle is not zero, but is lesser than the objective deviation, the ARC is said to be unharmonious **(Fig. 10)**.

 13. What are the methods of measurement of stereopsis? Discuss the sensory and motor adaptations to strabismus?

Tests for stereopsis: The different mechanisms of stereopsis testing are:
- *Haploscopic principle:* Here, the two eyes are dissociated with the help of two tubes with angled mirrors such that different stimuli can be given to the two eyes. For example, synoptophore.
- *Anaglyph principle:* Here, the dissociation is brought about by using conjugate colors, red and green. The test consists of stereo-paired images in red and green and the patient performs the test using red–green glasses. For example, TNO test.
- *Vectographic principle:* This uses the principle of polarized light. Two stereo-paired images are present such that one light passing through one is polarized in one direction and the light passing through the other is polarized in a different direction and the patient performs the test using polarized filter glasses. For example, Titmus fly test and Randot.

- *Panographic principle:* This is a real-depth stereogram where there are a grid of cylinders with random dot pattern which will cause slightly different images to fall on the two eyes resulting in real-depth perception. Glasses are not required for this test. For example, Lang stereotest.
- *Real depth:* Here, there is an actual difference in the placement of the objects. No glasses are required. For example, Frisby–Davis distance and near test.

1. *The Netherlands organization test:* It has seven plates which have to be read using red–green glasses. It is done at a distance of 40 cm. It can be used in children >3 years, tests 15–480 seconds of arc.
2. *Titmus stereo test* is based on vectographic principle. It has a stereofly card and polaroid glasses. It tests near stereopsis and can be done in children from 3 years onward. The fly tests 3500 arc seconds. Graded testing from 40 to 800 arc seconds also present. Stereo butterfly test is based on the same principle. It has the image of a butterfly instead of a fly.
3. *Randot test:* This is also based on vectographic principle with random dot stereogram. It requires polaroid glasses. There is a distant stereoacuity testing variant as well. It can be done in children >3 years. Tests 400–20 seconds of arc
4. *Frisby–Davis test:* They have both near and distance. Near Frisby–Davis consists of glass plates with images and patient has to identify which image is in the front. The distance stereoacuity test consists of a background illuminated box with different symbols attached to transparent rods giving the appearance that they are free floating. The patient is asked to tell which symbol is in the front. Distance test is done at 6 m and measures between 5 and 50 seconds of arc.
5. *Synoptophore:* This is based on the haploscopic principle. The two eyes receive separate stimuli by two tubes with angled mirrors and illuminating lamp. There are specific slides for stereopsis. Slides which have similar images but have slight horizontal disparity give the illusion of depth.
6. *Lang's two-pencil test:* This is a test which can be done bedside without the need for expensive equipment and measures only gross stereopsis. The patient is made to touch the tip of a pencil held by the examiner with another pencil. If patient is unable to perform, then we can conclude that gross stereopsis is absent.

Sensory and Motor Adaptations of Strabismus

Strabismus results in noncorresponding points of the retina getting stimulated resulting in diplopia and confusion with the absence of binocularity. Confusion is controlled by strong foveal rivalry and for diplopia, there are certain sensory and motor mechanisms.

The sensory adaptations are suppression, ARC, and eccentric fixation.

- *Suppression:* This is a cortical mechanism in which the image from the deviating eye is ignored. This requires a long-standing constant large angle deviation. The suppression can be facultative, where the images from one eye is ignored only in binocular conditions but when the other eye is closed, the images from the earlier suppressed eye are processed normally. When the suppression is present even in monocular conditions, then it is called as obligatory suppression and this leads to the development of amblyopia. The presence of suppression can be diagnosed by testing the sensory status of the eye with the help of after-image test, Bagolini striated glasses, synoptophore, or Worth four dot test.
- *Anomalous retinal correspondence:* In the presence of small angle deviation, instead of the fovea getting stimulated in the deviating eye an extrafoveal point gets stimulated. As an adaption to avoid diplopia, the fovea of the deviating eye loses its primary visual direction and fovea of one eye and extrafoveal point of the other eye share common subjective visual direction. During monocular conditions, the fovea still remains dominant over the extrafoveal point and fovea regains its straight-ahead gaze. This adaptation results in preservation of binocularity even in the presence of manifest squint. The ARC can be harmonious or unharmonious. In harmonious ARC, the amount of ARC completely compensates for the amount of deviation. Hence, the subjective angle is zero. In case of unharmonious ARC, the amount of ARC is not full, hence there is some amount of subjective deviation as well. The difference between the objective and subjective deviation gives the angle of anomaly. ARC can be detected using Bagolini's glasses, synoptophore, and the after-image test.
- *Eccentric fixation:* When the fovea loses its primary visual direction even in monocular conditions and the extrafoveal point starts assuming the straight-ahead gaze.

The motor mechanisms are fusion, head posture, and blind spot mechanism:
- *Fusion:* These involve controlling the deviation by fusional vergences. Exodeviation is controlled by fusional convergence and esodeviation by fusional divergence. It results in latent squint. Fusional convergence is stronger than fusional divergence. Fusional effort can lead to asthenopia in the patient.
- *Head posture:* This is seen mostly in incomitant strabismus where the amount of deviation is not equal in all gazes. The patient assumes a head posture such that gaze is fixed in the direction of least deviation or no deviation. For example, in case of right LR palsy, patient assumes a right face turn. Sometimes, the head posture can be in such a way that maximum deviation occurs and the diplopia image can be ignored.

- *Blind spot mechanism:* An esotropia of around 15° results in the image falling on the blind spot and hence avoiding diplopia. This mechanism is used in incomitant squints, where the fixing eye is chosen depending on whether the image of the other eye falls on the blind spot.

 14. What are the sensory adaptations in strabismus and their clinical significance?

Sensory and motor adaptations of strabismus: Strabismus results in noncorresponding points of the retina getting stimulated resulting in diplopia and confusion with the absence of binocularity. Confusion is controlled by strong foveal rivalry and for diplopia, there are certain sensory and motor mechanisms.

The sensory adaptations are suppression, ARC, and eccentric fixation.
- *Suppression:* This is a cortical mechanism in which the image from the deviating eye is ignored. This requires a long-standing constant large angle deviation. The suppression can be facultative, where the images from one eye is ignored only in binocular conditions but when the other eye is closed, the images from the earlier suppressed eye are processed normally. When the suppression is present even in monocular conditions, then it is called as obligatory suppression and this leads to the development of amblyopia. The presence of suppression can be diagnosed by testing the sensory status of the eye with the help of after-image test, Bagolini striated glasses, synoptophore, or Worth four dot test. *Clinical significance:* Absolute suppression can become amblyopia which results in reduced visual acuity which is reversible only if identified early.
- *Anomalous retinal correspondence:* In the presence of small angle deviation, instead of the fovea getting stimulated in the deviating eye, an extrafoveal point gets stimulated. As an adaption to avoid diplopia, the fovea of the deviating eye loses its primary visual direction and fovea of one eye and extrafoveal point of the other eye share common subjective visual direction. During monocular conditions, the fovea still remains dominant over the extrafoveal point and fovea regains its straight-ahead gaze. This adaptation results in preservation of binocularity even in the presence of manifest squint. The ARC can be harmonious or unharmonious. In harmonious ARC, the amount of ARC completely compensates for the amount of deviation. Hence, the subjective angle is zero. In case of unharmonious ARC, the amount of ARC is not full, hence there is some amount of subjective deviation as well. The difference between the objective and subjective deviation gives the angle of anomaly. ARC can be detected using Bagolini's glasses, synoptophore, and the after-image test.
- *Eccentric fixation:* When the fovea loses its primary visual direction even in monocular conditions and the extrafoveal point starts assuming the straight-ahead gaze
  Clinical significance: The measurement of squint using prism bar cover test (PBCT) is unreliable in these conditions due to eccentric point of fixation.

 15. Discuss anomalous retinal correspondence.

Refer to Answer 12.

 16. Describe Worth four dot test.

This is a test used to check the binocular status of the patient. It has to be performed using a red–green glass for the dissociation between the two eyes. It can be done for distance at 6 m and also at near at 33 cm. The test object consists of four lights: two green lights next to each other, one red light above, and one white light below. The patient has to look at these lights with the red glass in front of right eye and green glass in front of the left eye. Normally, the patient should see two green lights, one red, and one white light. In case of manifest deviation with NRC, he will see five lights, three green and two red lights which are crossed in case of exotropia and uncrossed in case of esotropia. If there are suppressions, the images from the eye which is suppressed will not be seen. So, the patient will see either two reds or three green dots. In case of abnormal retinal correspondence, the patient will still be able to see four dots even in the presence of manifest deviation **(Figs. 11A to D)**.

 17. Discuss method and significance of Bagolini striated glasses test.

Bagolini striated glasses are used for the testing of binocularity in a patient. It consists of plano glasses which have striations at right angle to each other. That is at 45° in one eye and 135° in the other. The glasses do not have any refractive power and do not stimulate accommodation. It converts a point source light into an oblique streak of light depending on the striations. There is dissociation between the two eyes as each eye sees a streak of light which are right angle to each other. It is the least dissociative and most physiological. The patient is made to wear the glasses over his preexisting refractive correction and light is shone on it. Normally in the absence of manifest deviation, the patient sees a symmetrical cross-response. In case of manifest squint with ARC, the patient still sees a symmetrical cross-response. In case of suppression, only one line is seen depending on the eye which is fixating. In case of the presence of a central scotoma, the central part of the crossing of the lines is not seen. In case of manifest squint recent onset especially in adults, where patient has diplopia, the patient sees two separate lines (**Figs. 12A to D**).

 18. What is the difference between a Horopter and Panum's area? Describe sensory and motor adaptations to strabismus.

Horopter

Horopter is an imaginary plane joining the corresponding retinal points in space. It is a plane in which the objects present will appear to be equidistant from the observer. The horopter is not constant and it depends on the position of the observer as well as the gaze. The horopter can be charted using vertical sticks and it appears as the longitudes of earth and hence it is also called as the "Longitudinal Horopter" and it is a flattened dome (**Fig. 13**). When a circle is drawn joining all the corresponding points of the retina, it is called as the theoretical or the geometric horopter and it does not coincide with the actual horopter. This theoretical horopter is called as the Vieth-Müller circle and the deviation of the actual horopter from the Vieth-Müller circle is called as Hering–Hillebrand deviation.

Panum's Area

All images falling on the corresponding points of the retina are seen as a binocular single image. Hence, any image falling in the plane of the horopter is seen as a single image, but there are small areas around the corresponding points where the images can still be fused to create a single image and this is called as Panum's area of binocular fusion (**Fig. 13**). This area is also responsible for the perception of depth. The cortical effort for the fusion because of slight disparity in the images falling on the two eyes gives the perception of depth.

Sensory and motor adaptations of strabismus: Strabismus results in noncorresponding points of the retina getting stimulated resulting in diplopia and confusion with the absence of binocularity. Confusion is controlled by strong foveal rivalry and for diplopia, there are certain sensory and motor mechanisms.

The sensory adaptations are suppression, ARC, and eccentric fixation.
- *Suppression:* This is a cortical mechanism in which the image from the deviating eye is ignored. This requires a long-standing constant large angle deviation. The suppression can be facultative, where the images from one eye is ignored

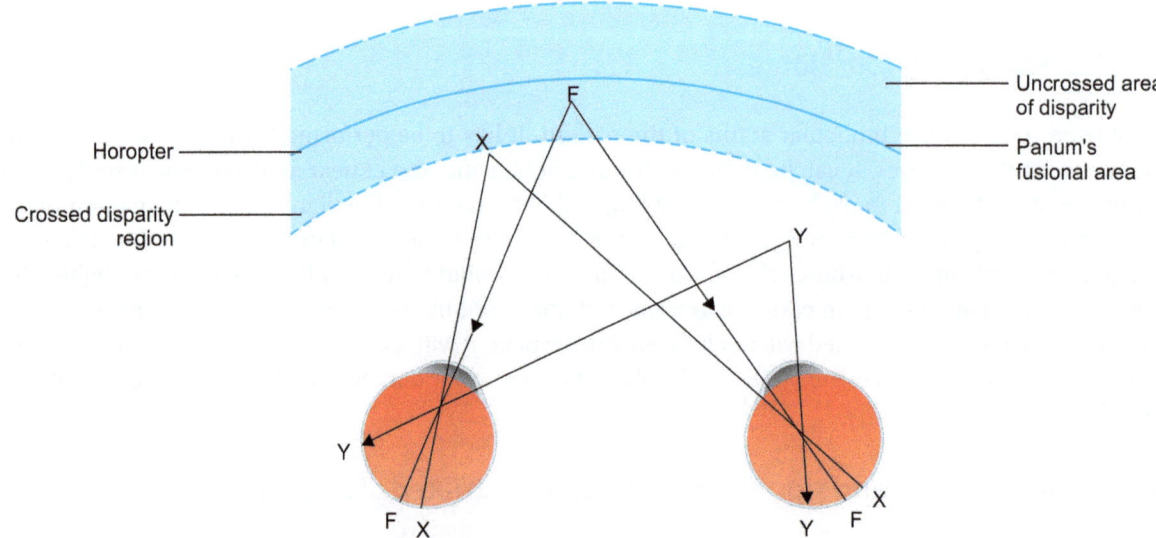

Fig. 13: Horopter and Panum's area of fusion.

only in binocular conditions but when the other eye is closed, the images from the earlier suppressed eye are processed normally. When the suppression is present even in monocular conditions, then it is called as obligatory suppression and this leads to the development of amblyopia. The presence of suppression can be diagnosed by testing the sensory status of the eye with the help of after image test, Bagolini striated glasses, synoptophore, or Worth four dot test.

- *Anomalous retinal correspondence:* In the presence of small angle deviation, instead of the fovea getting stimulated in the deviating eye, an extrafoveal point gets stimulated. As an adaption to avoid diplopia, the fovea of the deviating eye loses its primary visual direction and fovea of one eye and extrafoveal point of the other eye share common subjective visual direction. During monocular conditions, the fovea still remains dominant over the extrafoveal point and fovea regains its straight-ahead gaze. This adaptation results in preservation of binocularity even in the presence of manifest squint. The ARC can be harmonious or unharmonious. In harmonious ARC, the amount of ARC completely compensates for the amount of deviation. Hence, the subjective angle is zero. In case of unharmonious ARC, the amount of ARC is not full, hence there is some amount of subjective deviation as well. The difference between the objective and subjective deviation gives the angle of anomaly. ARC can be detected using Bagolini's glasses, synoptophore, and the after-image test.
- *Eccentric fixation:* When the fovea loses its primary visual direction even in monocular conditions and the extrafoveal point starts assuming the straight-ahead gaze

The motor mechanisms are fusion, head posture, and blind spot mechanism:

Fusion: These involve controlling the deviation by fusional vergences. Exophoria is controlled by fusional convergence and esophoria by fusional divergence. It results in latent squint. Fusional convergence is stronger than fusional divergence. Fusional effort can lead to asthenopia in the patient.

Head posture: This is seen mostly in incomitant strabismus where the amount of deviation is not equal in all gazes. The patient assumes a head posture such that gaze is fixed in the direction of least deviation or no deviation. For example, in case of right LR palsy, patient assumes a right face turn. Sometimes, the head posture can be in such a way that maximum deviation occurs and the diplopia image can be ignored.

Blind spot mechanism: An esotropia of around 15° results in the image falling on the blind spot and hence avoiding diplopia. This mechanism is used in incomitant squints, where the fixing eye is chosen depending on whether the image of the other eye falls on the blind spot.

Esotropia

 19. Define esotropia. Describe classification and management of esotropia in children.

Esotropia is the inward deviation of either eyes.

Classification of esodeviations:
- *Comitant esodeviation:*
  - *Accommodative esotropia:*
    - Refractive accommodative
    - Nonrefractive accommodative
    - Hypoaccommodative
    - Partially accommodative
  - *Nonaccommodative esotropia:*
    - Infantile esotropia
    - Nonaccommodative convergence excess
    - Acquired (basic) esotropia
    - Acute onset esotropia
    - Divergence insufficiency/paralysis
    - Cyclic esotropia
    - Recurrent esotropia
  - *Microtropia:*
    - Nystagmus blockage syndrome

- *Incomitant esotropia:*
  - Paralytic
  - *Nonparalytic:*
    - A-V pattern esotropia
    - Retraction syndrome
    - Mechanical restrictive esodeviations—congenital fibrosis of the extraocular muscles (CFEOM), thyroid ophthalmopathy, and orbital wall fracture
- Secondary esodeviations—sensory and consecutive.

Management of Esotropia In Children

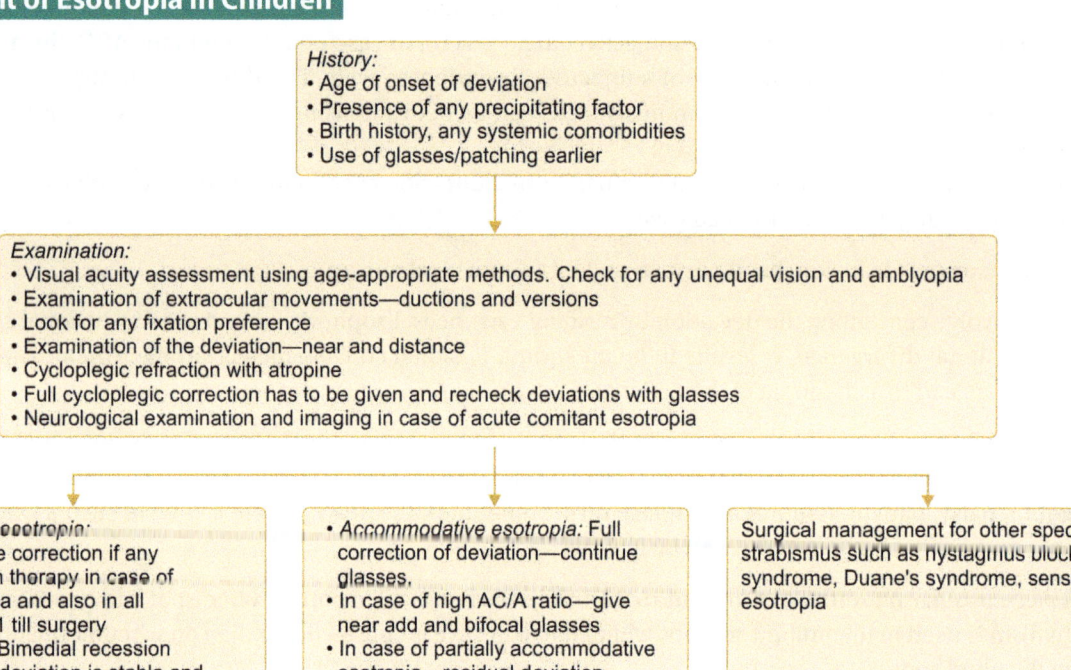

 20. Describe investigation and management of esotropia in 1-year-old child.

Investigations of Esotropia in a 1-Year-Old

- *History:* A good history by the parents is essential. History regarding the onset of squint, the duration if it is constant or intermittent as well as the eye which deviates should be asked. History regarding the visual status such as fixation, presence of eye contact, recognition of mother and following and playing with toys should be asked. History of noticing any head posture should be asked.
- General examination by a pediatrician to rule out any developmental delay or other systemic involvement
- *Visual status assessment:* Different methods of assessment of the visual acuity are present for infants. A rough method in the OPD is to look for fixation of either eyes, if it is central steady and maintained, to check if the child follows light and object. Check if the child has a fixation preference to any one eye in case of esotropia which suggests that visual acuity may be better in that eye. Check if the child resists occlusion of either eyes.

Other formal methods of visual acuity testing are:
- Catford drum test
- Preferential looking test
- Teller acuity chart
- Visual Evoked Response (VER)
- Boeck Candy test

- Worth's ivory ball test
- Sheridan ball test
- Anterior segment as well as a dilated fundus evaluation is a must to rule out any intraocular pathology that could be causing low vision in any eye resulting in deviation.
- *Refraction:* This is the most important step in any case of strabismus. Uncorrected refractive errors especially hypermetropia has to be addressed in any case of esotropia. In a 1-year-old child, refraction has to be done with atropine. Ointment atropine is given thrice a day for 3 days and then refraction is done. Full cycloplegic refraction is given.

Evaluation of the Squint

- *Head posture:* Presence of head posture has to be looked when the child walks into the clinic before the child is made aware of our examination. Head posture such as face turn toward the fixing eye is seen in Ciancia syndrome or can be seen in nystagmus to achieve null position.
- Hirschberg test will allow to check for the presence of squint. Children can be given colorful fixation targets, toys to maintain fixation. Cover test is done to confirm the presence of squint and rule out pseudoesotropia which can be seen in the presence of epicanthal folds. Uncover test will help in latent squints. One can check if the squint is freely alternating or there is a fixation preference at this stage. We should also check for the presence of cross-fixation. Presence of nystagmus should be checked and if the amplitude increases on covering one eye (manifest-latent).
- The ductions and versions have to be checked. All nine gazes have to be checked. Most importantly abduction has to be checked for any limitation. Comitant esotropias do not have abduction limitation. Abduction limitation is seen in congenital 6th nerve palsy or in Duane's syndrome. Reflex eye movements when the head is moved can be used to confirm limitation. In cases with cross-fixation or in case inhibitional or habitual palsy, the eye can be patched for a long time and then the duction can be checked in the other eye. Presence of either inferior or SO overactions, A–V patterns and DVD have to be checked.
- Performing PBCT in children with esotropia is difficult. Approximate amount of squint can be quantified using the Hirschberg test. If the pupillary reflex falls on the pupillary margin, it is 15°, midway between the pupil and the limbus is around 30° and at the limbus is around 45°. Krimsky's method of quantification of the squint where the prism is kept on the deviating eye and the pupillary reflex is centralized.
- Optokinetic nystagmus has to be checked. Infantile esotropia will have asymmetric optokinetic nystagmus. Here, there is asymmetry in the smooth pursuit. The temporal to nasal pursuit is normal but the nasal to temporal movement has cogwheel pattern. Pursuit asymmetry is normally present in infants up to the age of 5 months.

However, any insult caused during this period of development can lead to the persistence of this asymmetry. Pursuit asymmetry remains a tell-tale sign of infantile esotropia, and persists even after surgery if surgery is not done in infancy.

Management of Esotropia in a 1-year-old Child

The management depends on the type of esotropia. The main differential diagnosis includes:
- Infantile esotropia
- Congenital abducens nerve palsy
- Duane's retraction syndrome
- Nystagmus blockage syndrome

1. The main step initially is to give the appropriate refractive correction. Complete cycloplegic refractive correction. In the presence of amblyopia, or if there is a fixation preference, then occlusion therapy has to be advised. In a child of 1 year, conventional full-time occlusion for 2 days of the dominant eye has to be done. Even in cases where there is free alternation, it is suggested to do 1:1 occlusion of the eyes.
2. Amblyopia therapy has to be completed prior to any surgical intervention.
3. Surgical intervention is advisable only after correction of amblyopia, once the squint is freely alternating, there is a large angle of deviation which is confirmed on repeated evaluation and it is constant.
4. Surgical planning in children has to be careful as the small globe will result in larger amount of correction as compared to adults. MR recessions are the preferred surgery.

 21. Discuss management of congenital esotropia.

Refer to Answer 20 for the investigation and evaluation of esotropia.

Management of Esotropia

- Refractive error should be checked. Refraction should be done under ointment atropine as children have very strong accommodation. Full cycloplegic refraction has to be given.
- If there is presence of fixation preference and unequal visual acuity, amblyopia therapy has to be completed prior to surgical intervention. Full-time occlusion depends on the age. Up to 2 years, 2:1 is advised and subsequently one day is increased for every year such as 3:1, 4:1, and 5:1. And >6 years, it is maintained as 6:1. Even in the absence of fixation preference, 1:1 alternate patching is advised till surgery to correct temporonasal bias.
- Surgical intervention should be planned when there is a stable and large angle deviation which has been seen in subsequent visits. Any accommodative component has to be ruled out or corrected. The squint must be freely alternating and the child should allow enough examination to check for inferior or SO overactions and presence of A-V patterns.
- *Surgery:* MR recessions or combined MR recession and LR resection can be planned. 3–4.5 PD is corrected per 1 mm surgery of MR and 2–3 PD is corrected per mm surgery on LR. IO weakening procedures should be added in patients with associated IO overaction.
  - Similarly, if SO overaction with A pattern is present, a SO weakening procedure must be done, as MR recession alone without SO weakening procedure will lead to worsening of A pattern.
- Chemodenervation with botulinum toxin has been tried. Botox injection to the MR results in weakening of the muscle and reduction squint. It is not the mainstay.

Surgical Outcomes

- Optimal goal—is the presence of orthophoria, normal visual acuity, NRC, reduced stereopsis, and stable alignment.
- Desirable goal—is the presence of microtropia, very small angle esotropia or ecotropia with abnormal retinal correspondence with central or parafoveal fixation, mild amblyopia, and reduced or absent stereopsis.
- Acceptable goal—having eso- or exotropia of 10–20 PD. Good cosmetic outcome. May have ARC but suppression or amblyopia is seen. Less stable alignment.
- Unacceptable goal—having large angle residual esotropia or consecutive exotropia. Poor cosmetic outcome, presence of amblyopia, and suppression with unstable angle of deviation. Will require resurgery.

 22. Discuss infantile esotropia—clinical features, evaluation, indications for intervention, and management. Also write a note on postoperative complications.

Infantile esotropia is a manifest esodeviation that has an onset between birth and 6 months of age. It is also called essential infantile esotropia or congenital esotropia.

Clinical Features

- The age of onset is between birth and 6 months.
- The esotropia is of large angle usually >30°.
- The angle is stable and it usually increases with time.
- Initially, the esotropia is freely alternating but later they develop a fixation preference. Sometimes, there can be early fixation preference. Cross-fixation is present when freely alternating.
- Children do not have any neurological abnormalities.
- On refraction, these children usually do not have a significant refractive error. They may have mild-to-moderate hypermetropia.
- Amblyopia is seen in 30–40% of children.
- There may be associated IO overaction, dissociative vertical deviation, manifest latent nystagmus or rarely manifest nystagmus. There can be A or V patterns. Limitation of abduction can be seen.
- Asymmetric optokinetic nystagmus is seen. There is asymmetry in the smooth pursuit. The temporal to nasal pursuit is smooth but the nasal to temporal has a cogwheel pattern.

There are two variants of infantile esotropia:
1. *Ciancia syndrome:* This consists of infantile esotropia with bilateral abduction limitation with manifest latent nystagmus which increases in abduction and reduces in adduction. Hence, the fixing eye is kept in adduction and the patient has a face turn toward the fixing eye.

2. *Lang's syndrome:* Early onset esotropia with dissociative vertical deviation, nystagmus, and excyclotorsion of the nonfixing eye.

Refer to Answers 20 and 21 for investigations and management of infantile esotropia.

Postoperative Complications

- *Overcorrections or undercorrections:* Exact measurement of the squint in children is difficult and the amount of correction in children is also more than in adults due to smaller eyeballs. Also, in children <6 months, due to poorly developed posterior segment, the results are unpredictable.
- *Slippage of the muscle tendon:* The recessed or resected muscle can slip resulting in limitation of movement and deviation.
- *Vomiting:* This is seen in children following strabismus surgery due to handling of the muscles as well as anesthetic drugs.
- *Infections:* Usually rare, there can be suture abscess or cellulitis.
- *Suture granuloma and reactions:* Less common with Vicryl sutures
- *Tenon's prolapse and conjunctival cysts:* This occurs due to improper closure of the conjunctiva and prolapse of the Tenon's capsule. Improper apposition of the conjunctiva leads to the conjunctival cells to be imbedded leading to conjunctival cyst.
- Dellen formation can occur due to disturbance in the tear film.
- Anterior segment ischemia is rare and happens when three or more adjacent recti are operated upon. There is corneal edema, thinning, segmental iris atrophy, keratic precipitates and anterior chamber flare and late onset cataract.

23. What is AC/A ratio. What are the methods of measuring it? Briefly discuss the disorders resulting from altered AC:A ratio.

Accommodation and convergence are synkinetic movements. When a near object has to be viewed, there occurs an accommodation and corresponding to that, there is a convergence that happens. The amount of convergence per unit of stimulus of accommodation can be expressed as AC/A ratio with the unit prism Diopter/Diopter. The AC/A ratio is not constant and it depends on the individual.

The methods of measuring AC/A ration are:
- *Heterophoria method:* In this method, the ocular deviation is first measured at distance fixation with the appropriate refractive correction with accommodation at rest and next at 33 cm when the accommodation is acting. The method also takes into account the interpupillary distance (IPD). The AC/A ratio is then calculated by the formula IPD + near deviation – distance deviation/fixation distance at near in diopters. For the deviation, esotropia has a + sign and exotropia has a – sign.
- *Gradient method:* Here, the distance for fixation is fixed, but the patient is given lenses to either stimulate or relax accommodation. If it is done with fixation at 6 m, concave lenses are given to stimulate accommodation and if it is done at 33 cm, convex lenses are given to relax accommodation. It is done after wearing appropriate refractive correction and deviation is measured with accommodation relaxed and stimulated. Esodeviations are considered with + sign and exodeviations with – sign. The formula is, near deviation – distance deviation/power of the lens in diopters. Gradient method gives lesser AC/A ratio compared to the heterophoria method and it gives a more true estimate.
- *Fixation disparity method:* Here, the changes in the fixation disparity when there is forced convergence with the help of base out prisms and the fixation disparity when accommodation is stimulated with lenses are compared. And the AC/A ratio is calculated by seeing what stimulus of accommodation and convergence produces the same amount of fixation disparity. This is not used much practically.
- *Haploscopic method:* This again a laboratory method using two tubes that separate the two eyes, i.e., using a haploscope.

Disorders of AC/A

- Children with accommodative esotropia can have abnormality in the AC/A ratio and the management depends on this. In refractive accommodative esotropia, there can be either high or normal AC/A ratio. In children with normal AC/A ratio, the difference between near and distance deviation is <15 PD. In case of high AC/A ratio, the children have more deviation for near. This is due to excessive convergence per unit of accommodation. In high AC/A ratio, in order to relax accommodation, children will require near add, bifocals in addition to the hypermetropic refractive correction. Miotics can be used to reduce the accommodation effort but they are less precise than spectacle correction and have adverse effects such as headache. In nonrefractive esotropia, there is high AC/A ratio, children have no significant esotropia for distance but >15 PD esodeviation for near. They also require near addition for relaxing accommodation.

Accommodative esotropia depending on the AC/A ratio can be classified as:
- Refractive normoaccommodative and refractive hyperaccommodative esotropia, or nonrefractive hyperaccommodative and nonrefractive hypoaccommodative esotropia.
- Abnormal AC/A ratio can also be seen in intermittent exotropia in simulated divergence excess type. Here, the distance deviation is more than the near deviation and it is not a true excess, but there is an apparent reduction in the near deviation due to the increased convergence during accommodation. This can be confirmed by giving the patient a near addition of +3D to relax the accommodation and then measuring the deviation.
- In children with intermittent exotropia, giving over minus glasses may be of benefit in children with high AC/A ratio.

 24. Describe different protocols for management of congenital esotropia.

Refer to Answer 21.

 25. Discuss the management of esotropia in a 5-year-old child.

The main differential diagnoses of a 5-year-old child with esotropia include:
- Accommodative esotropia—refractive, nonrefractive, hypoaccommodative, or partially accommodative esotropias
- Nonaccommodative—late onset essential esotropia, acute comitant, microtropia, cyclic esotropia, sensory esotropia, and nystagmus blockage syndrome
- Paralytic or restrictive causes—6th nerve paralysis, DRS

Accommodative esotropia is the most common cause of esotropia in this age group.

Evaluation of a 5-year-old child with esotropia:
- *History:* A good history by the parents is essential. History regarding the onset of squint, the duration if it is constant or intermittent as well as the eye which deviates should be asked. History of any increase in deviation during near work and history of use of glasses should be asked. History of noticing any head posture should be asked. Accommodative esotropia starts usually around second year of life.
- General examination by a pediatrician to rule out any developmental delay or other systemic involvement.
- *Visual status assessment:* Visual acuity of both eyes has to be tested. Tumbling E chart, Landolt's C chart, Sheridan letter chart, HOTV chart, or picture identification charts can be used.
- Anterior segment as well as a dilated fundus evaluation is a must to rule out any intraocular pathology that could be causing low vision in any eye resulting in deviation.
- *Refraction:* This is the most important step in any case of strabismus. Uncorrected refractive errors especially hypermetropia has to be addressed in any case of esotropia. In this case of a 5-year-old child, atropine is the recommended cycloplegic of choice. Ointment atropine is given thrice a day for 3 days and then refraction is done. Full cycloplegic refraction is given. If the child is not accepting the glasses, mild cycloplegic drops can be given for a few weeks.

Evaluation of the Squint

- *Head posture:* Presence of head posture has to be looked when the child walks into the clinic before the child is made aware of our examination. Head posture can be present in cases of 6th nerve palsy and in DRS.
- Hirschberg test will allow to check for the presence of squint. Children can be given colorful fixation targets, toys to maintain fixation. Cover test is done to confirm the presence of squint. Uncover test will help in latent squints. One can check if the squint is freely alternating or there is a fixation preference.
- The ductions and versions have to be checked. All nine gazes have to be checked. Most importantly abduction has to be checked for any limitation. Comitant esotropias do not have abduction limitation. Abduction limitation is seen in 6th nerve palsy or in Duane's syndrome. Presence of either inferior or SO overactions, A-V patterns, and DVD have to be checked.
- Prism bar cover test has to be performed for quantification of the squint. Deviations should be measured for distance as well as near and also with and without glasses. This is because in some types of accommodative esotropia, there can be high AC/A ratio leading to increased deviation for near. If there is increased deviation for near, the deviation has to be rechecked with +3D lens in place to relax accommodation.

- AC/A ratio has to be calculated either using gradient or heterophoria method.
- Sensory status has to be checked to look for the presence of suppression, abnormal retinal correspondence, and also for the presence of stereopsis. If the child is cooperative, binocular status can be checked by Bagolini striated glasses or Worth four dot test. Stereopsis can be checked with any of the distance and near stereoacuity tests.

Management of Esotropia in a 5-year–old Child

The management will depend on the type of esotropia.
- *Management of accommodative esotropia:*
  - Refraction is essential and should be done under ointment atropine and full cycloplegic refraction has to be prescribed without correcting for the cycloplegic effect.
  - In cases of accommodative esotropia, the deviation gets corrected fully on use of glasses. If the near deviation is more than the distance deviation, then the child will have high AC/A ratio and will require bifocals to relax the accommodation and prevent accommodative convergence.
  - In cases of partially accommodative esotropia, some amount of deviation will remain even after refractive correction. In these cases, if the deviation is significant, surgical intervention can be planned.
  - In case of nonrefractive accommodative esotropia, there is no significant deviation for distance, but there is deviation for near due to high AC/A ratio, these patients benefit from near addition.
  - Miotics can be used in place of glasses but are not preferred as they do not give a precise correction of the refractive error and are associated with adverse effects such as brow ache, nausea, iris cysts, lens opacity, angle closure glaucoma, and retinal detachment. Echothiophate iodide 0.03% is used for this.
  - For small residual deviation after glasses, prisms can be used. For more significant deviation, surgery in the form of MR recessions can be done. Posterior fixation or Faden of the MR can be combined with recession.
  - In case of nonaccommodative convergence excess esotropia, bifocals and miotics are ineffective. It requires surgical management which is unconventional large recessions.
  - In cases of acute onset esotropia, neurological causes should be ruled out by a through neurological work-up and imaging.

26. Describe evaluation and management of accommodative esotropia.

Refer to Answer 25.

27. Classify esotropia. How would you plan the management of convergence excess esotropia in a 5-year-old child? Describe the choice of procedure and surgical planning in detail.

Refer to Answer 19 for classification of esotropia.

Management of Convergence Excess Esotropia

Investigations:
- A good history about the age of onset of deviation, any history of use of glasses and if the deviation increases on near work or reduces with the use of glasses.
- Visual acuity assessment has to be done for the patient. Age-appropriate methods of visual acuity assessment have to be done.
- Refraction under atropine has to be performed for detection of hypermetropia. Full cycloplegic refraction has to be prescribed in cases of esotropia.
- Squint work-up has to be done with the Hirschberg test, cover and uncover test. Deviations have to be measured both for near and distance and also with and without glasses. In convergence excess type of accommodative esotropia, the near deviation is more than the distance deviation by around >15 PD. The near deviation should be remeasured with +3D for the relaxation of the accommodative convergence.
- AC/A ratio has to be calculated for these children.
- Sensory evaluation to detect suppression, ARC, and the amount of stereopsis

Management:
- After the appropriate correction of the hypermetropia, if there is an accommodative esotropia, the distance correction will be completely corrected with glasses.
- For the near deviation, bifocal glasses should be given to relax the accommodation. Executive type bifocals are preferred in children.
- Miotics have been proposed as a treatment option in these cases, but are not preferred because glasses give a more accurate correction of the refractive error and the miotics are associated with adverse reactions such as brow ache, iris cysts, retinal detachment, shallow anterior chamber, and also lens opacities.
- If there is a partially accommodative esotropia, where there is distance deviation even after correction with glasses, prisms can be prescribed for small angle deviation or surgery can be planned for larger deviations. MR recession is planned depending on the amount of deviation. This can be combined with posterior fixation suture or Faden of the MR for further weakening.

Exotropia

28. Discuss intermittent divergent squint (IDS) management, prognostic factors, and controversies.

Intermittent exotropia is the most common form of exotropia and is intermittent in presentation which gradually progresses.

Management of IDS

- A good history has to be taken from the parents regarding the onset of the deviation, any precipitating factors, and the progression of the amount of deviation. History regarding the time duration for which the squint is more apparent has to be asked.
- Initial investigations must be done as any case of squint. Visual acuity assessment and refraction under cycloplegia should be done. Cover test, uncover test, and alternate cover test should be done. Duction and versions have to be checked. Any oblique overactions have to be checked. Measurements of the deviation using PBCT should be done with glasses for both distance as well as near. Deviations at distance longer than 6 m have to be checked. In case the near deviation is less than the distance deviation, then Scobee and Burian occlusion test has to be done in cases of simulated divergence excess and then the deviation has to be assessed to neutralize the tenacious proximal fusion. If the deviation is still high after this, +3D should be used to relax the accommodation and then the deviation has to be measured. AC/A ratio has to be calculated in these patients. Evaluation has to be done at multiple times and at multiple visits to ensure the full deviation has manifested and measured.

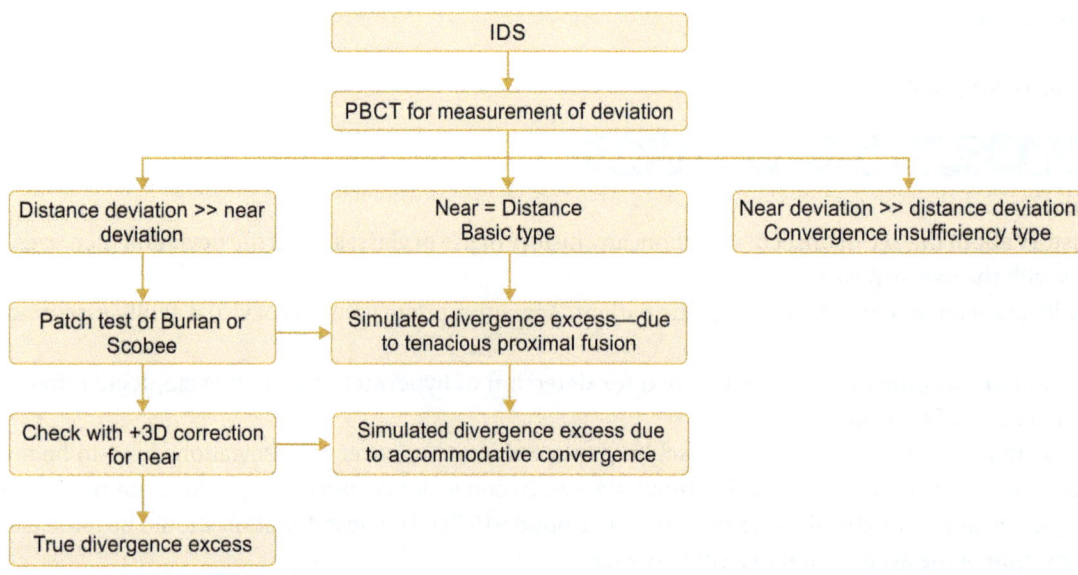

- Sensory evaluation should be done using Bagolini striated glasses, Worth four dot test, after image test and synoptophore. Both near and distance stereoacuity testings have to be done.

TABLE 2: The revised New Castle scoring.

	Score
Home control	
XT or monocular eye closure seen:	
Circle appropriate score	
Never	0
<50% of time fixing in distance	1
>50% of time fixing in distance	2
>50% of time fixing in distance + seen at near	3
Clinic control	
Circle appropriate score near and distance	
Near	
Immediate realignment after dissociation	0
Realignment with aid of blink or re-fixation	1
Remains manifest after dissociation/prolonged fixation	2
Manifest spontaneously	3
Distance	
Immediate realignment after dissociation	0
Realignment with aid of blink or re-fixation	1
Remains manifest after dissociation/prolonged fixation	2
Manifest spontaneously	3
Total NCS: (Home + Near + Distance) =	

- New castle score has to be calculated. Home control + clinic control >3 suggests need for surgical management **(Table 2)**. Calhounz staging also has to be determined. Any progression from stage 2 to 3 requires surgical intervention.

Management of IDS

- *Nonsurgical management:*
  - Correction of the existing refractive error will result in improvement of the visual acuity and the fusional capacity of the child. In myopia, full correction has to be given to promote accommodative convergence. In case of hypermetropia, <+2.00D is not corrected except in older patients where it has to be corrected to give relief from asthenopia.
  - *Using of over minus glasses:* This is useful only in patients with high AC/A ratio, such that the over minus will stimulate accommodation resulting in accommodative convergence. This is more accepted in younger children. Older patients develop asthenopic symptoms.
  - *Use of prisms:* Base-in prisms can be used to ensure binocular vision. We can undercorrect the prism correction to stimulate fusion.
  - *Orthoptics:* This helps in increasing the fusional control and helps in controlling the exodeviation. It can help in converting tropia into phoria. It can be done in the clinic using synoptophore or can be done at home using pencil push up exercise or simple home orthoptic trainer. Physiological diplopia should be appreciated by the patient.
- *Surgical management:*
  Indications:
  - Constant large angle deviation which is observed >50% of the times by parents
  - Progression from Calhoun stage 2 to stage 3, i.e., exotropia for distance and intermittent exotropia for near with suppression scotoma for distance.
  - New Castle score of ≥3
  - Deterioration of distance stereopsis, increasing deviation. Patient has to be observed at multiple sittings with repeated measurements of deviation prior to planning surgery.

Surgical options: In the presence of divergence excess exotropia symmetrical lateral recession of both eyes can be done. In case of A or V pattern, with oblique overactions, the obliques can be tackled or shifts of the LR can be planned. In cases of convergence insufficiency, bimedial resections have been proposed. Unilateral recession resections have also been done.

Prognostic Factors of IDS

- *Timing of the surgery:* Long-standing deviation present since childhood indicates poor prognosis for the return of normal binocular vision postsurgery. Ideal surgery should be done prior to the development of suppression scotoma.

- *Calhoun staging:* Calhoun divided the clinical presentation into four stages:
  1. Exophoria at distance, orthophoria for near. Asymptomatic
  2. Intermittent exotropia for distance, orthophoria/exophoria for near. Symptomatic for distance but no suppression scotoma
  3. Exotropia for distance and exotropia or intermittent exotropia for near, suppression scotoma for distance
  4. Exotropia for near and distance. No binocularity.

From this, we can see that stage 3 and 4 have poorer prognosis due to development of suppression scotoma. Ideally, surgery has to be done when there is progression from stage 2 to 3. Stage 4 suggests loss of binocularity and poor prognosis.

Stereopsis: These patients develop abnormalities in stereopsis earlier for distance as compared to near. Singh et al. suggested monitoring of distance stereopsis by FD2 test to decide on timing of surgery. A distance stereoacuity worse than 20 seconds of arc-needed surgery. A stereoacuity of >70 seconds of arc suggested poor prognosis.

Controversy in IDS

- *Timing of surgery:* Knapp advised early surgery to avoid the sensory adaptations of squint and to preserve binocularity, but others such as Jampolsky advice to wait till the child is older so that better examination and accurate diagnosis is possible to prevent consecutive esotropia. Newcastle score gives an objective method to decide on the timing of surgery, but it is better to have a case-to-case decision.
- *The choice of surgery:* Some surgeons advise bilateral LR recessions while some suggest unilateral recession and resection. For convergence insufficiency type, some suggest bimedial resections while some suggest slanting recession of the LR. For cases with high AC/A ratio, bilateral LR recession with posterior fixation suture for the MR has been suggested.

 29. Discuss intermittent divergent squint management, prognostic factors, and controversies.

Refer to Answer 28.

 30. Classify exotropia in children. Discuss its management.

Classification of exotropia:
- Comitant:
  - *Primary:*
    - Infantile exotropia
    - Intermittent exotropia
  - *Secondary:*
    - Sensory exotropia
    - Consecutive exotropia
- Incomitant:
  - Paralytic
  - Restrictive
  - Musculofascial anomalies
  - Dissociated horizontal deviation.

Management of Exotropia

Refer to Answer 28 for evaluation of exotropia and management of IDS.

Vertical Deviation

 31. Describe etiology, diagnosis, and management of superior oblique overaction.

Superior oblique overaction results in depression in adduction. This depression in adduction can be because of primary or secondary causes.

- *Primary causes:* Primary SO overaction is obscure. Certain factors can result in apparent overaction of the SO muscle.
  - Craniofacial abnormalities such as hydrocephalus which result in anterior placement of the trochlea and sagittalization of the SO resulting in stronger action.
  - *Muscle pulley:* Heterotopia of the muscle pulleys can result in apparent overactions of the SO.
- *Secondary causes:*
  - Paralysis of the IO
  - Paralysis of the contralateral IR
  - Contracture of contralateral SR due to contralateral SO palsy.

Diagnosis of Superior Oblique Overactions

- There is A pattern of strabismus on examination. Deviation has to be measured in 25° upgaze and 35° downgaze. A 10 PD difference is considered as significant.
- The oblique overactions have to be checked in versions. The oblique overaction can be divided into mild, moderate, or severe depending upon whether the hypotropia is seen in primary gaze, when the eye is adducted or only in the direction of action of the SO.
- Examination has to be done to rule out secondary causes such as IO paralysis, contralateral SO paralysis with SR contracture.
- The presence of any cyclodeviations can be subjectively measured by using a Maddox wing, double Maddox rod, diplopia charting using red green glass with a horizontal target, synoptophore, and blind spot charting. Objectively, the presence of torsion can be confirmed by examination of the fundus. Normally, the fovea is present between the lines passing through the center of the disc and the line passing through the lower end of the disc.

Management of Superior Oblique Overaction

Superior oblique overaction can be managed by weakening procedure of the SO. The various weakening procedures are:
- *Tenotomy:* This involves the disinsertion of the entire muscle after hooking and identifying it. It is unpredictable and causes weakening of all the actions including intorsion.
- *Posterior tenectomy of the SO:* This involves hooking the muscle and its identification. Only the posterior fibers responsible for depression are cut. The anterior 1–2 mm of fibers responsible for intorsion are spared.
- Recession of the entire muscle by disinserting and reinserting 4 mm nasal to the SR.
- Prieto–Diaz technique is also a full thickness recession and inserting the tendon 12 mm from the limbus 6 mm from the nasal end of the SR. This prevents the limitation of depression in abduction.
- Recession of only the anterior fibers
- Lengthening of the SO tendon can be done by placing silicone expanders, splitting the tendon longitudinally and joining the cut ends, z-technique of lengthening can be used.

 32. Describe management of vertical diplopia.

Refer to Answer 33.

 33. A 45-year-old patient presents with sudden onset vertical diplopia. What is the differential diagnosis? Discuss evaluation and management of acute-onset vertical diplopia.

Differential diagnoses of sudden onset vertical diplopia are:
- Superior oblique palsy
- Oculomotor nerve palsy
- Myasthenia gravis
- Dysthyroid ophthalmopathy
- Orbital floor fracture with IR entrapment
- Heavy eye syndrome.

Evaluation of Vertical Diplopia

- A thorough history has to be taken regarding the onset of diplopia. History of road traffic accident, history of head injury, has to be asked for both 3rd and 4th nerve palsy. History of vomiting and headache for raised intracranial pressure has to

be asked. History of any direct trauma to the globe leading to floor fracture should be asked. History of diurnal variation of the diplopia which suggests myasthenia gravis has to be asked.
- *Examination:* Head posture has to be checked. There can be face turn or head tilt. Face turn to right side can be seen in defective right SR, right IR, left IO or left SO, and vice versa. Head tilt is an important finding. SO palsy patients have opposite side head tilt. And in case of bilateral SO palsy, there may be chin down position.
- *Ocular deviation:* Hirschberg test and cover–uncover test has to be performed to confirm the presence of squint. Ductions and versions have to be performed to look for any limitation of movement. Deviation can be measured using a PBCT. Presence of torsional component can be checked subjectively using Maddox wing, synoptophore, double Maddox rod, and blind spot charting. Objectively, it can be assessed by fundus evaluation to look for torsion.
- Park's 3-step test has to be performed to confirm the muscle involved in case of hypertropia. SO palsy shows improvement in hypertropia on same side gaze and opposite side head tilt. This test will be unreliable in the presence of contracture/entrapment or fibrosis of a vertical rectus, in restrictive strabismus, in case of myasthenia gravis or in case of thyroid ophthalmopathy.
- Diplopia charting with red green glasses with horizontal target and Hess or Lees charting has to be done. Forced duction test for the vertical recti and exaggerated forced duction test for the oblique muscles has to be done.
- Fundus examination to rule out papilledema
- *Investigations:* SO palsy and oculomotor palsy patients should undergo MRI brain with contrast to look for any intracranial space-occupying lesions. CT orbits has to be done in cases of suspected orbital floor fracture. Systemic work-up is done to rule out ischemic 4th nerve palsy if MRI is normal. Thyroid profile test is also done in cases of suspected thyroid eye disease. Tensilon test and neurology work-up in cases of myasthenia gravis have to be done.

Management of Vertical Diplopia

Management depends on the cause of diplopia:
- *Superior oblique palsy:* In acute SO palsy, any life-threatening causes such as intracranial space-occupying lesions have to be tackled first. For the diplopia, patients can be advised to patch the affected eye to avoid diplopia. Initially, the patients are followed up regularly to check for worsening or improvement in the diplopia. In case of ischemic palsy, systemic work-up and control of the systemic comorbidities is advised. Once the causative factor is removed, the patient is observed for at least 6 months for signs of improvement. Patient can be given prismatic correction for the diplopia. If there is significant diplopia with hypertropia, surgical management can be done. Surgical options include IO weakening, SO tuck, and Harada–Ito procedure.
- In case of thyroid ophthalmopathy, systemic medications for the thyroid disease have to be started. The patient has to be followed up to check for stability of the deviation. Prisms can be given in the meantime.
- In case of myasthenia gravis, neurology work-up has to be done and medical management planned.
- Orbital floor fracture can be treated with floor fracture repair with release of the entrapped muscle and plating. Residual hypotropia after the surgery due to damage and fibrosis of the IR can be treated with surgery or prism.

34. Discuss dissociated vertical deviation.

This condition was described by Bielschowsky. This condition is characterized by elevation and excycloduction of the occluded eye with slow depression and incycloduction when the cover is removed and the eye takes fixation again. It is usually bilateral but can be asymmetric. It can be associated with exotropia or esotropia including infantile esotropia. The condition does not follow Herring's law.

Mechanism

The mechanism of DVD is not fully known. The possible theories are:
- *Spielmann's theory—binocular stimulation imbalance:* Failure to develop binocularity can lead to persistent immature monocular circuits. These can be either visual or vestibular. Vertical pursuit asymmetry can be noted in DVD patients with better pursuits directed when down to up than vice-versa. Variability of DVD with postural changes suggests involvement of vestibular or otolithic pathways. In a patient with strabismus, where binocularity is disturbed, these biases become manifest.
- *Bielschowsky's theory:* Alternate and intermittent excitation of subcortical centers governing vertical divergence can give rise to DVD.

- *Brodsky's theory:* According to Brodsky's theory, DVD is a manifestation of primitive dorsal light reflex, when light stimulus falls from one side of fish, it misregisters it as its subjective vertical meridian with a counterclockwise tilt. Therefore occurs a clockwise tilt for equal binocular stimulation. This righting reflex causes vertical divergence of eyes to prevent the corrective body tilt. Therefore downward movement of ipsilateral eye and upward contralateral eye occurs.

Other theories proposed for DVD are:
- Manifestation of atavistic oculomotor reflexes present in birds and fishes
- More elasticity of the elevators compared to the depressor muscles. Bilateral paresis of the depressors or imbalance between the innervation of the elevators and depressor
- Oblique muscle induced cycloversion
- Nystagmus-dampening mechanism (Guyton's theory).

Clinical Features

- There is spontaneous elevation and excycloduction of either eye when fusion is interrupted either by cover or when patient is day dreaming or fatigued. When the elevated eye refixates, the movement is slow and there is incycloduction which can be appreciated by seeing the limbal vessels.
- When red filter is placed on any eye, the red image is always lower as the eye with the filter placed is elevated.
- *Bielschowsky's phenomenon:* When a neutral density filter is placed on the fixing eye, and the density is gradually increased, the occluded eye starts to move down and the fixing eye starts elevating. If it is increased further, the occluded eye can be depressed as well.
- There can be head posture-head tilt opposite to the side with more vertical deviation. Chin depression also has been described.
- The elevation is present both in adduction and abduction.
- When head is tilted backward in asymmetric cases, the amount of deviation reverses.
- Measurement can be done by prism bar uncover test. The prism is kept base down on the occluded eye. The cover is shifted to the fixing eye and the refixation is noticed. The prisms are increased till the eye does not move down to take up fixation.

Differences between DVD and inferior oblique overaction (IOOA):

Clinical features	DVD	IOOA
Elevation	Seen in primary, adduction and abduction	Maximum in adduction. Absent in abduction
Superior oblique overaction	May coexist	Usually there is underaction of SO
V pattern	Absent	Present
Pseudoparesis of SR of the other eye	Absent	Present
Intorsion on refixation	Present	Absent
Speed of refixation	Slow refixation	Fast refixation
Bielschowsky phenomenon	Present	Absent
Latent nystagmus	Often present	Absent

Management of DVD

The different surgical procedures described for DVD are:
- Superior rectus recession with IR resection
- Posterior fixation suture for the SR
- Supramaximal SR recession
- Inferior oblique weakening with anterior positioning.

 35. What are dissociated vertical deviations (DVDs)? How do you differentiate a DVD from an inferior oblique overaction? What is the management of DVDs?

Refer to the Answer 34.

Q 36. Discuss double elevator palsy.

Double elevator palsy is a condition in which there is limitation in elevation both from primary position, in adduction as well as abduction. The affected eye is hypotropic and it can be associated with ptosis. Since elevation is limited in all the three positions, it was called as double elevator palsy thinking both SR and IO are affected. Since the pathology can be restriction in IR as well, it was renamed "monocular elevation deficit (MED)".

Causes of MED

- *Congenital:* Due to supranuclear defects, primary SR paresis or IR restriction
- *Acquired:* Cerebrovascular accidents associated with hypertension, thromboembolism, or vasculitis. Sarcoidosis, intracranial space-occupying lesions, infectious etiology such as syphilis and cysticercosis.

Clinical Features

- There is hypotropia of the affected eye when the normal eye is fixing. Rarely, the affected eye might be preferred for fixation, in that case the normal eye will be hypotropic. There may be associated horizontal squint.
- There is limitation of elevation both in adduction and abduction. There is associated ptosis and pseudoptosis components. Ptosis is seen in the hypotropic eye because of the fascial attachments between the LPS and the SR. Pseudoptosis is the ptosis that disappears when the hypotropic eye takes upfixation.
- Head posture—chin elevation can be seen
- Bell's phenomenon can be affected depending upon the type of MED. It is normal in supranuclear type and affected in IR restriction and SR paresis types.
- *Diplopia:* This is absent in case of congenital MED but will be seen in cases of acquired MED.
- Upward saccade is affected depending upon the type of MED.
- *Forced duction test (FDT):* It will be tight if there is IR restriction. Active force generation test will show SR paresis if present.

Types of MED—given by Ziffer et al.:

- *Primary IR restriction or fibrosis:* FDT shows tight IR. Upward saccades are normal till the IR restriction comes into play. Bell's phenomenon is poor.
- *Primary SR palsy:* FDT is free. The upward saccade is slow both below and above midline. Bell's phenomenon is poor.
- *Supranuclear type:* It is usually congenital. Vertical saccade is mildly affected or normal below midline but absent above midline.

Differential diagnosis: Brown's syndrome, CFEOM, and congenital third nerve palsy for congenital

Acquired: Thyroid ophthalmopathy, orbital floor fracture with IR entrapment, and myasthenia gravis

Management (Flowchart 1)

- Complete work-up with squint work-up along with FDT and evaluation of saccades.
- Surgical correction:

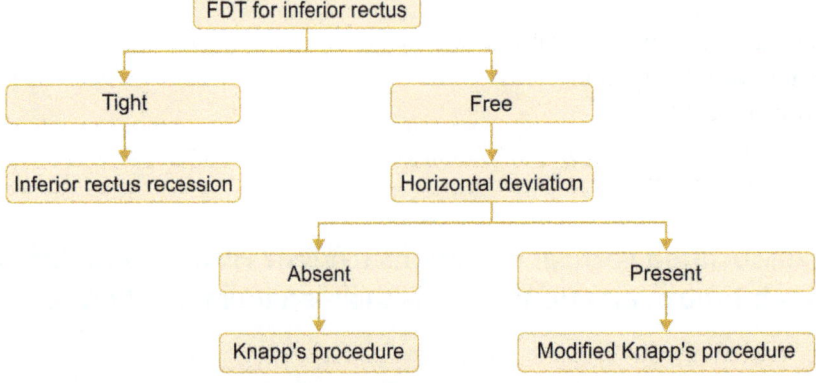

Flowchart 1: The management of double elevator palsy.

(FDT: forced duction test)

- *Knapp's procedure:* This is a transposition procedure where the medial and LR are transposed to the SR.
- *Augmented Knapp's procedure:* Where along with the Knapp's procedure, posterior fixation sutures are placed to give more action.
- *Modified Knapp's procedure:* Here, not the full tendon, but a partial tendon of medial and LR is transposed.
- Inferior rectus recession—done in case FDT is tight for IR

37. Describe surgical management of monocular elevation deficit.

Refer to the Answer 36.

38. Discuss management of vertical diplopia.

Refer to Answer 33.

Restrictive Strabismus

39. What are congenital cranial dysinnervation disorders (CCDDs)? Give classification for CCDDs.

Congenital cranial dysinnervation disorders are a group of congenital, nonprogressive abnormalities of cranial musculature due to developmental anomalies of one or more cranial nerves with primary or secondary dysinnervation. There may be absent normal innervation for the muscles or there can be aberrant muscle innervation. It may be associated with secondary muscle pathology and orbital or bony abnormalities.

The conditions included under CCDDs are:

Disorder	Cranial nerve involved	Genetic abnormality
Duane's syndrome	6th CN	HOXA1, CHN1 gene (DRS gene)
Congenital fibrosis of the extraocular muscles (CFEOM)	3rd and 4th cranial nerves	KIF21A, PHOX2A TUBB3, TUBB2B
Mobius syndrome	6th and 7th nerve	
Horizontal gaze palsy with progressive scoliosis	6th nerve	ROBO3
Brown's syndrome	4th nerve	

It is also said to include congenital 3rd nerve and 4th nerve palsy and also Marcus Gunn jaw-winking ptosis.

Neuroimaging Features of CCDDs

Routine MRI will miss the features of CCDDs. It requires high-resolution MRI which shows the hypoplasia or absence of the involved cranial nerve nucleus, hypoplasia of the extraocular muscles, and orbital or bony abnormality.

40. Discuss the etiopathogenesis and clinico-investigative approach to restrictive strabismus.

Restrictive strabismus is a kind of incomitant strabismus causes either due to abnormality in the muscle structure or innervation which prevents the relaxation of the muscles leading to restriction.

Etiology and Pathogenesis of Restrictive Strabismus

- *Congenital restrictive strabismus:*
  - *Duane's retraction syndrome:* The restriction is due to abnormal innervation of the LR which results in co-contraction of the medial and LR.
  - *Brown's syndrome:* There is restriction in the SO tendon due to abnormalities in the tendon, its sheath, or the trochlea. It can be congenital or acquired.

- *Congenital fibrosis of extraocular muscles:* It is the congenital fibrosis by the extraocular muscles and associated adhesions between the extraocular muscles, Tenon's capsule, and the sclera.

However, all these pathologies are now believed to be due to innervational disorders which further leads to secondary effects of restriction.

- *Acquired restrictive strabismus:*
  - *Thyroid ophthalmopathy:* This is a condition characterized by autoimmune response characterized by accumulation of glycosaminoglycans and fibroblasts in the orbit and associated thickening of the extraocular muscles results in limitation of movement.
  - *Orbital myositis, myocysticercosis, and pseudotumor of the orbit:* This is an inflammatory pathology where there is thickening of the extraocular muscles and tendon resulting in limitation of movement.
  - *Orbital fracture with muscle entrapment:* Blow-out fractures of the orbit after blunt trauma can lead to entrapment of the muscles most commonly the IR in floor fractures which result in fibrosis of the muscle and limitation.
  - *Muscle fibrosis secondary to trauma or surgery:* Surgeries such as retinal detachment surgeries with band and buckle, previous strabismus surgery, and glaucoma implant surgeries can lead to injury of the muscles and adhesions which can cause restrictive strabismus.
  - *Acquired Brown's syndrome:* Inflammatory pathology in the SO tendon or sheath such as juvenile rheumatoid arthritis, rheumatoid arthritis, systemic lupus erythematosus can lead to fibrosis of the tendon resulting in Brown's syndrome.

Clinico-investigative Approach to Restrictive Strabismus

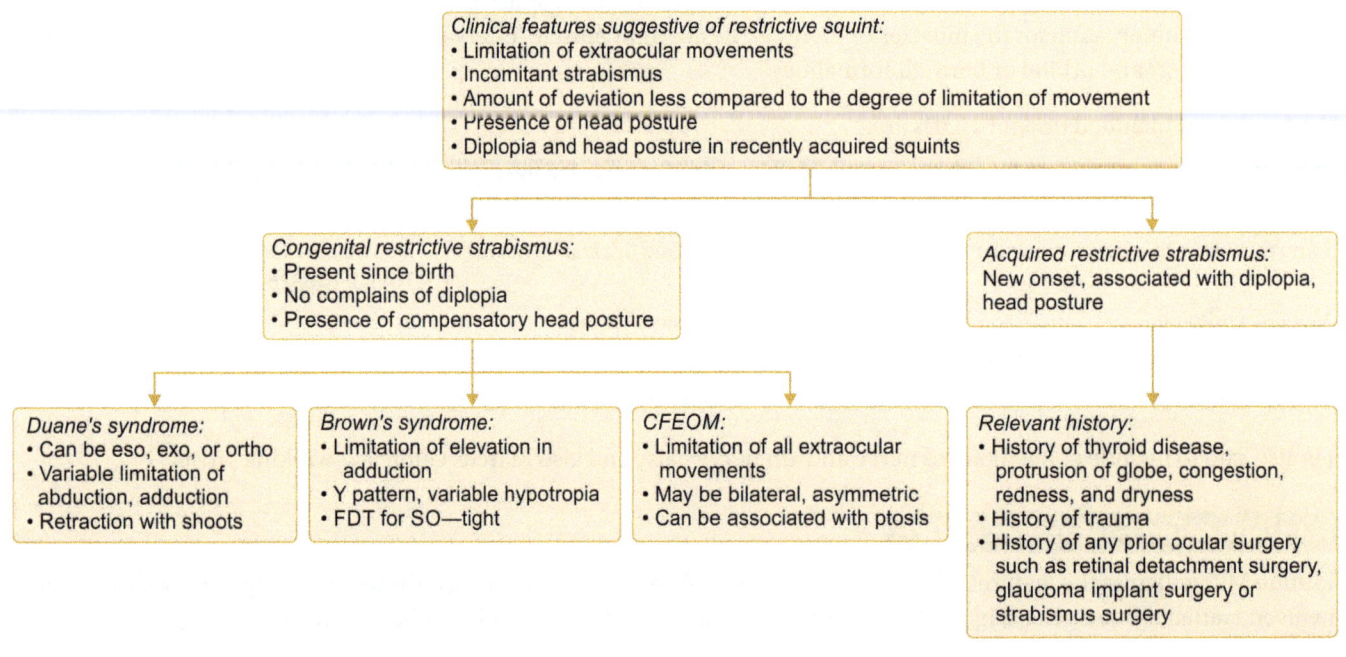

(ANA: antinuclear antibody; CBC: complete blood count; CFEOM: congenital fibrosis of the extraocular muscle; CRP: C-reactive protein; ESR: erythrocyte sedimentation rate; IGG4: immunoglobulin-G4)

41. What is Brown's syndrome?

Brown's syndrome is a type of restrictive strabismus where there is limitation of elevation in adduction due to abnormality in the SO tendon or sheath.

The clinical features are:
- Limitation of elevation in adduction with normal elevation in adduction.
- FDT shows severe restriction for elevation of the eye in adducted position but free in abducted position. Positive exaggerated FDT for SO
- Divergence in upgaze—Y pattern
- Other variable features are—limitation of elevation in primary position, widening of lid aperture, downshoot in adduction, hypotropia, and head posture

The causes described for Brown's syndrome are:
- Anomalies of the tendon sheath—the Tenon's capsule around the SO tendon forms the sheath which encloses it. The presence of abnormality or tightness in the sheath which gets relieved on removal of the sheath has been demonstrated in many cases.
- Tight tendon of the SO can result in restriction of elevation.
- Impaired slippage of the tendon through the trochlea which can be congenital or acquired. Acquired cases are seen post-traumatic and also inflammation of the trochlea such as tenosynovitis.
- Congenital abnormalities of the trochlea or the SO tendon.
- Acquired abnormality of the SO tendon or muscle such as metastasis, trauma to the trochlear region resulting in fibrosis
- Abnormalities of the IO and its adjacent structures are seen in orbital blow out fracture or secondary to paralysis of the IO.
- Idiopathic—after SO tucking surgery

Grades of Brown's Syndrome

- Mild—restricted elevation in adduction. No downshoot and no hypotropia in primary position
- Moderate—restriction in elevation in adduction with downshoot. No hypotropia in primary position
- Severe—restriction in elevation with downshoot and hypotropia in primary position
  Brown's plus is associated with SO overaction.
  Canine tooth syndrome where there is trauma at the region of the SO. It is associated with SO palsy so there is limitation in depression and elevation in adduction.

Management

- Complete tenectomy of the SO or its sheath has been tried. Some surgeons combine it with IO weakening.
- Superior oblique tendon lengthening procedure using silicone expanders, chicken sutures, or loop sutures
- In acquired Brown's syndrome, investigations such as MRI brain and orbits should be done to detect any pathology in the SO tendon or trochlea. Blood investigations such as complete blood count (CBC), erythrocyte sedimentation rate (ESR), C-reactive protein (CRP), and antinuclear antibody (ANA) profile have to be done. Trial of systemic or perilesional steroids can be given. Nonsteroidal anti-inflammatory drugs (NSAIDs) have also been tried. It is usually self-limiting and immediate surgical intervention is not indicated.

42. What is Duane's retraction syndrome? Enumerate the types and describe the clinical features. Describe management of a case of Duane's retraction syndrome with abnormal head posture.

Duane's retraction syndrome is a condition that comes under congenital cranial dysinnervation disorder. It is also known as Stilling–Turk–Duane syndrome. It is characterized by limitation of abduction and/or adduction, retraction of the globe on attempted adduction, and variable upshoot or downshoot.

Pathogenesis

Initially, it was thought to be because of an inelastic band in the place of LR.

Later, it has been proposed to be due to innervational abnormalities of the LR. There is abnormal and paradoxical innervation to the LR on abduction and adduction.

Recent high-resolution MRI has demonstrated abnormality in the development of the 6th cranial nerve and the condition has been classified as a congenital cranial dysinnervation disorder.

Classification of DRS

Huber's classification based on the innervation to the LR and the MR:

Types	Innervation	Clinical presentation
1	LR innervation absent in abduction LR innervation present in adduction	Limitation of abduction and adduction with retraction during adduction
2	LR innervation present during adduction and abduction	Variable abduction Adduction limitation with retraction
3	Both LR and MR innervation present in adduction and abduction	Limitation of adduction and abduction with retraction

Based on the type of deviation in primary position, it can be classified as:
- Eso-DRS
- Exo-DRS
- Ortho-DRS.

Clinical Features

- There is variable limitation of both adduction and abduction depending upon the pattern of innervation.
- There can be esodeviation, exodeviation, or no obvious deviation in the primary position.
- There is presence of globe retraction associated with narrowing of the palpebral aperture. This is seen because of co-contraction of the MR and the LR or can be due to tight inelastic muscle.
- There can be upshoots or downshoots occurring due to "Bridle effect" or "Leash effect" due to the tight LR. The globe slips during adduction because of the tight muscle which leads to the upshoot or downshoot.
- There can be abnormal head posture in the way of face turn with face turn usually toward the side of DRS seen more with eso-Duane. Even in ortho Duane, the face turn can be present to avoid upshoots or downshoots
- The condition can be bilateral as well.
- *Associations:* There are many ocular and systemic conditions associated with DRS such as:
  - Goldenhar syndrome—oculo-auriculo-vertebral dysplasia. There is presence of preauricular tag, sinus, and epibulbar dermoid.
  - Klippel–Feil syndrome—short neck, vertebral anomalies such as cervical fusion, low posterior hair line
  - Wildervanck syndrome—has deafness along with features of Klippel–Feil syndrome.
  - Ocular anomalies—coloboma, persistent hyaloid arteries, iris dysplasia, pupillary anomalies, microphthalmos, and gustolacrimal reflex.

Management of DRS

A detailed anterior and posterior segment evaluation along with visual acuity testing and refraction has to be done to look for any low vision and its cause including amblyopia.

Detailed motor and sensory examination along with measurement of the head posture has to be done.

The indications of surgical management are:
- Obvious deviation of the eye in primary position
- Significant head posture
- Presence of significant retraction or shoots.

Management of Esotropic DRS

Flowchart 2 depicts the management of esotropic DRS.

Management of Exotropic DRS

Flowchart 3 depicts the management of exotropic DRS.

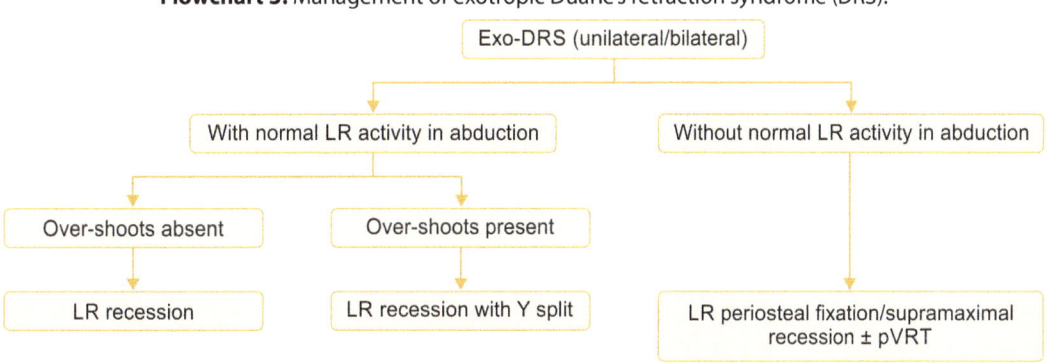

Flowchart 2: Management of esotropic Duane's retraction syndrome (DRS).

(FDT: forced duction test; LR: lateral rectus; MR: medial rectus; PD: prism diopter; pVRT: partial vertical rectus transposition; SRT: superior rectus transposition)

Flowchart 3: Management of exotropic Duane's retraction syndrome (DRS).

(LR: lateral rectus; pVRT: partial vertical rectus transposition)

Source: Adapted from Gaur N, Sharma P. Management of Duane retraction syndrome: a simplified approach. Indian J Ophthalmol. 2019;67(1):16-22.

Management of Ortho DRS

Here, the indication of surgery is the presence of significant upshoot, downshoot, or retraction. Variable recession of both MR and LR with Y splitting of the LR can be done for this.

 43. Describe classification and principles in the management of Duane retraction syndrome.

Refer to the Answer 42.

Strabismus Surgeries

 44. Describe inferior oblique weakening procedures.

Indications of IO weakening procedures:
- Presence of V pattern with associated IO overaction
- Superior oblique palsy
- Dissociated vertical deviations
- Double elevator palsy where the contralateral IO is weakened
- DRS with upshoots

- Torsional Kestenbaum
- Other paralytic/restrictive strabismus

Contraindications of IO weakening procedures:
- V pattern without any IO overaction
- Presence of intorsion of the globe. It will worsen with weakening of the IO.

Approach and Technique of IO Weakening

Conjunctival approach either by limbal, paralimbal, or fornix-based incision depends on the surgeon's preference.

The conjunctival incision is made in the inferotemporal quadrant. The LR is first identified and hooked. The globe is retracted superonasally and the border if the IO is identified in the fornix. A smooth tipped blunt hook is inserted and the IO is lifted. Once it is confirmed that the entire muscle is hooked, the intermuscular septum and attachments are dissected and the muscle is cut using a tenotomy scissors. The cut end is secured using 6-0 Vicryl sutures.

Methods of IO Weakening

- *Fink's method:* This is a method of recession without changing the course of the muscle. The IO is reinserted at a point 6 mm inferior and 6 mm posterior to the inferior end of the LR. This gives 8 mm of recession. For 10 mm recession, a point 2 mm posterior to this is taken and for 6 mm recession, a point 2 mm anterior is taken.
- *Park's method of recession:* The IO is inserted 2 mm lateral and 3 mm posterior to the lateral end of the insertion of the IO. This gives 10 mm of recession along with anterior positioning.
- *Elliot and Nankin method:* This is a method of recession with anterior positioning. The one end of the IO is placed at the lateral end of the insertion of the IR and the other end posterior to this point. It can be augmented by inserting one end 1 or 2 mm anterior to the lateral end of the insertion of IR.
- Anterior and nasal transposition by Stager-IO is inserted 2 mm nasal to the insertion of the IR.
- *Pure anteropositioning:* This is a method of anterior positioning without any recession. It does not affect torsion. It gives recession equal to Fink's recession. The IO is inserted next to the inferior end of the LR insertion.
- *Total anteropositioning:* This completely weakens the elevator action. Here, the IO is placed anterior to the IR.
- *Myectomy:* It is not predictable and it will not give graded recessions. It is no longer preferred. Here, the IO is isolated and cut using tenotomy scissors.
- *Denervation and extirpation:* Here, the nerve to the IO is identified and cut to make the IO lax. The muscle is then disinserted from the origin and completely cut and removed. This is done only in cases where there is persistent IO overaction even after recession or myectomy.
- *Recession of anterior fibers:* Here, there is selective weakening of the extorsion. Only the anterior fibers are separated from the rest of the muscle and recessed.

Complications of IO Weakening Surgery

- *Fat adherence syndrome:* It occurs if more of adipose tissue is dissected during isolation of the IO. There will be bleeding and subsequent scarring in the inferotemporal quadrant.
- *Damage to the LR:* The LR can be caught in the hook while trying to isolate the IO. This is more common if the LR has already been recessed.
- *Pupil dilation:* Permanent or temporary mydriasis can occur due to damage to the nerve to the ciliary ganglion. It occurs due to excessive trauma or traction to the IO muscle.
- *Hemorrhage from the IO muscle:* This occurs as the IO is highly vascular. Hemorrhage can lead to ecchymosis, subconjunctival hemorrhage, or rare cases bleed into the orbit.
- There can be under- or overcorrections.
- *Pseudo-IO overaction:* This happens after anterior placement of the IO more than 1 mm from the IR. This results in limitation of elevation in abduction and increasing elevation in adduction.

 45. Discuss nonsurgical management of esotropia.

Nonsurgical management has a role to play in the management of accommodative esotropias and also in infantile esotropia till surgical intervention is planned.

Nonsurgical management in infantile esotropia:
- The first step is cycloplegic refraction and giving full refractive correction. Atropine is the preferred cycloplegic agent. It is given for three times a day for 3 days and refraction is done on the fourth day.
- If there is presence of amblyopia, then patching should be advised. Conventional full-time occlusion of the better eye is done. Till the age of 2 years, it is done as 2:1 and subsequently 3:1, 4:1, 5:1 for 3, 4, and 5 years. 6 years onward, it is done as 6:1.
- Even in the absence of amblyopia, 1:1 occlusion is done to prevent contracture of the MR and prevent developing fixation preference.
- Botulinum toxin injection into the MR results in temporary weakening of the MR and alignment of the eyes. This is a temporary procedure.

Nonsurgical management of accommodative esotropia: Accommodative esotropias are associated with abnormality in the accommodative convergence mechanism.
- The first step is the correction of underlying hypermetropia. Cycloplegic refraction under atropine is preferred and full cycloplegic refraction should be given. In cases of refractive normo-accommodative esotropia, the deviation responds well to refraction.
- If there is high AC/A ratio, then the deviation is more for near than for distance. In these cases, bifocals are prescribed to reduce the accommodative effort for near. Bifocals are also the treatment of choice in nonrefractive hyperaccommodative type of esotropia with high AC/A ratio and also in hypoaccommodative type where the near point of accommodation is receded and there is a weak accommodation.
- The bifocals should be executive type of bifocals and it should bisect the pupils. Progressive glasses are not prescribed in children.
- Miotics therapy can be given instead of glasses. They are not preferred as they are not as precise as glasses. They can be used as a temporary measure.
- Prisms can be prescribed for small residual deviation. Base-out prisms are given.

46. Discuss Faden operation.

Faden operation was a technique first described by Cuppers. It is also called as posterior fixation suture or retroequatorial myopexy. The term Faden means thread or suture in German.

Faden operation is a procedure in which the muscle belly is suture to the sclera at a point behind the equator of the globe such that the functional insertion of the muscle changes making it weaker. The mechanisms of action of Faden operation are:
- It shifts the functional insertion of the muscle hence reducing the maximum ocular rotation. It acts as a weakening procedure but mainly in the direction of the action of the muscle and there is no effect in primary or the normal resting position.
- Since it is a weakening procedure, increased innervation will be supplied to the muscle and also the yoke muscle of the fellow eye. This is useful in nerve palsies where the Faden can be placed on the yoke muscle of the paralyzed muscle in the contralateral eye thereby increasing innervation to the paralyzed muscle.
- Because of the presence of suture, the effective contraction of the muscle fibers also reduces leading to weakening of the muscle.

Indications of Faden procedure are:
- Incomitant strabismus such as LR or IR paresis, restrictive strabismus such as thyroid myopathy
- Duane's retraction syndrome, double elevator palsy
- Accommodative esotropia with deviation being more for near
- Nystagmus blockage syndrome
- Dissociated vertical deviation
- Nystagmus with cross fixation.

Surgical Procedure

The conjunctival incision can be limbal or fornix base. After a good exposure, suture is passed through the muscle belly and into the sclera at premeasured distance from the muscle insertion.
- *Medial rectus:* 12–14 mm
- *Inferior rectus:* 14–16 mm

- *Lateral rectus:* 16–20 mm
- *Superior rectus:* 14–16 mm.

 47. What are adjustable sutures in squint surgery?

Adjustable recession surgery is a technique where the amount of recession can be modified to give more precise outcomes. It was described originally by Jampolsky.

Indications of Adjustable Recessions

- In paralytic or incomitant squint where patient has diplopia and accurate correction is needed.
- In case of large angle deviation where results may be inconsistent.
- In case of resurgery or previously injured muscle where results are more unpredictable.
- In case of thyroid eye disease with severe restriction and aberrant innervation in nerve palsy.

Surgical Procedure

Limbal incision is the preferred route of surgery. After hooking and separating the muscle from the attachments, recession is done. The sutures are passed through a scleral tunnel and secured using "one and a half knot." The conjunctiva is sutured leaving some bare sclera. In the postoperative period, the one and a half knot is loosened and the amount of recession is varied and sutures are secured. Another technique is the sliding noose technique. 6-0 Vicryl or nonabsorbable sutures are used.

The readjustment has to be done within 24 hours and can be done either with topical or local anesthesia. Globe is held by using fixation forceps or bucket handle sutures. The adjustment is made asking the patient is fixate at a distance and a cover-uncover test can also be performed. The sutures are tied and ends are trimmed.

 48. Evaluate various transposition surgeries in strabismus.

Transposition surgeries are those procedures, where a weak or paralytic muscle is strengthened by attaching an adjacent muscle to strengthen it. It is mainly done in paralytic strabismus, slipped or lost muscle, DRS, and double elevator palsy.

The broad indications of transposition procedures are:
- To improve the rotation of the globe
- To expand the binocular diplopia-free field
- Shift residual binocular field into the primary position.

The prerequisites for transposition surgery are that the FDT should be free and no restrictive component should be present. The duction should be short of midline and saccadic velocity should be <100°/s.

The different transposition procedures are:
- *Transpositions for abduction limitation:*
  - Full tendon transposition where the full tendon of the superior and the inferior recti is transposed to the LR. Care should be taken to avoid anterior segment ischemia. In crossed transposition, the SR is inserted to the inferior border of the LR and IR is inserted to the superior border.
  - *Hummelsheim procedure:* This is a partial tendon transfer. The SR and IR are split and the lateral halves are inserted to the LR.
  - *Jensen's procedure:* This is a partial tendon transfer where the SR and IR are split but not disinserted. The split halves are inserted to the split halves of the LR. This minimizes the risk of anterior segment ischemia as the muscle is not disinserted.
  - *Nishida's procedure:* This is also a partial tendon transfer but utilizes sutures to shift the force vectors. The IR and SR are split up to 15 mm from the insertion. Then at around 8–10 mm from insertion, sutures are passed through the IR and SR and then passed through the sclera 8 mm posterior to the LR insertion above and below the muscle. A modification of this method involves not splitting the muscle but only uses sutures. A suture is passed around 8–10 mm behind the insertion of the SR and IR and then it is passed through the superotemporal and inferotemporal quadrant of the sclera around 10–12 mm behind the limbus.
  - O'Connor's is a full tendon transposition procedure with cinching of the LR.

- *Superior or IR transpositions:* This involves transposition of only the superior or IR. It improves abduction limitation. It prevents anterior segment ischemia.
- *Procedures for vertical muscle palsy:*
  - *Knapp's procedure:* It is done in cases of MED. The lateral and medial recti are transposed superiorly. A modification is where the muscle tendons are split and then transposed. Augmentation of Knapp's can be done by putting posterior fixation sutures.
  - *Inverse Knapp's palsy:* Similar to Knapp's done for double depressor palsy
- *Procedures for third nerve palsy:*
  - *Superior oblique tendon transfer:* This is done to treat adduction limitation in third nerve palsy due to weak MR. The SO tendon is isolated and disinserted. The tendon is brought near the MR and attached at the superior end of the MR insertion.
  - *Lateral rectus to MR:* Here, the LR is isolated, separated from all the attachments and attached near the MR. The muscle is brought to the other side using the superior route. If there is hypertropia, then it can be brought through the inferior route to cause hypotropia. Y splitting of the LR such that one arm is above and one arm is below the MR insertion has also been described.

Complications of transpositions:
- Improper testing of the muscle functions can lead to erroneous outcomes. If the LR is not fully paralyzed, the transpositions may lead to exotropia. If the muscles used for transpositions are also paralyzed, then the transpositions will be ineffective. Improper testing of FDT for the fibrosis of the antagonistic muscle will lead to poor results.
- There can be undercorrections or late overcorrections.
- Induced vertical deviations can occur with vertical rectus transpositions.
- Anterior segment ischemia.

49. Describe IO weakening procedures.

Refer to Answer 44.

50. What is anterior segment ischemia?

The blood supply to the anterior segment of the eye is mainly by the anterior ciliary vessels. They are branches of the ophthalmic artery and are around 7 in number. The arteries originate posteriorly and traverse anteriorly long with the recti muscles. Hence, conventional, full tendon squint surgeries can result in disruption of the anterior ciliary vessels leading to anterior segment ischemia.

The risk factors for anterior segment ischemia are:
- Strabismus surgery to three or four recti muscles
- Advancing age
- Associated orbital or systemic diseases such as diabetes mellitus, hypercoagulability, leukemia, hypertension, atherosclerosis, thyroid eye disease, prior uveitis, carotid-cavernous fistula
- Other ocular surgeries such as scleral buckle, cryotherapy, and diathermy.

Clinical Features

Mild cases have iritis. Severe cases have severe iritis, iris atrophy, corectopia, corneal edema or clouding, nonreactive pupils, cataract, glaucoma, hypotony, and eventually phthisis bulbi.

Management

In acute cases, it can be treated with cycloplegics and corticosteroids.

Steps to prevent anterior segment ischemia:
- Limit the number of rectus muscles operated in a single sitting
- Space out the surgical procedures. Have a gap of 6 months to 1 year
- Limbal incisions disrupts the perilimbal conjunctival–episcleral collateral network hence fornix incision is preferred.
- Opt for partial tendon or vessel-sparing transposition procedures to reduce risk of anterior segment ischemia.

51. Discuss nonsurgical management of strabismus.

Management of strabismus is a mixture of surgical and nonsurgical management. Nonsurgical management is usually initiated prior to the surgical management and may need to be continued in the postoperative period as well. The aim of the nonsurgical management includes:
- Correction of refractive error
- Treatment of amblyopia, suppression, and abnormal retinal correspondence
- Utilizing glasses to manage deviations, e.g., accommodative esotropia and IDS
- Use of prisms in small angle deviations
- Management of convergence insufficiency.

The various methods of nonsurgical management are:
- *Optical therapy:*
    - Use of proper refraction with appropriate cycloplegia. In esotropia, full cycloplegic refraction has to be given. Atropine is the preferred cycloplegic of choice in cases of esotropia and children <8 years of age. Proper refraction and appropriate refraction are the treatment of choice in refractive accommodative esotropia.
    - Cases of accommodative esotropia with high AC/A ratio will need bifocals to reduce the deviation for near. Bifocals are also given for nonrefractive hyperaccommodative or hypoaccommodative esotropia.
    - Overminus glasses are given in intermittent exotropia as a method to stimulate accommodation and reduce the exodeviation. It is a good option in cases with high AC/A ratio. This is not a permanent treatment but a temporary measure.
    - *Prisms:* Small deviations can be corrected using prisms. It can be given for small residual or consecutive deviations. It can be given for incomitance squints with small amount of deviation and diplopia. Around 7–8 PD is accepted per eye and with Fresnel prisms 25–30 PD is accepted. It is usually not preferred, as it reduces the quality of vision, induces optical aberrations, and makes glasses heavier and cosmetically unacceptable. Prisms can be used for convergence insufficiency. Base-in prisms are used for this. It has to be undercorrected so that some effort has to be used by the patient. Prisms are also used in abnormal retinal correspondence.
- *Orthoptic treatment:* This involves the treatment of abnormal retinal correspondence, suppression, improving fusional vergences, and treatment of amblyopia.
    - *Suppression treatment:* The principle of treatment is to preferentially stimulate the suppressed eye or differential stimulation favoring the suppressed eye. There are different techniques for this include using red filter over the dominant eye and doing tasks in red which is visible only in the suppressed eye, using cheiroscope or Pigeon-Cantonnet stereoscope. The method most commonly used is synoptophore which uses different slides which stimulate both eyes individually with alternate or simultaneous flashing.
    - *Abnormal retinal correspondence treatment:* Small cosmetically acceptable deviation with ARC is acceptable. Occlusion therapy and binocular stimulation are used to treat ARC.
    - *Amblyopia management:* Amblyopia is managed by preferential stimulation of the amblyopic eye. It can be done by occlusion, penalization using drugs such as cycloplegics, partial occlusion using scotch tape, active vision therapy, pleoptics, and dichoptics. Medical drug therapy such as levodopa-carbidopa and even citicoline has been used in amblyopia therapy.
    - *Therapy for convergence insufficiency:* It can be done with pencil push-ups, home orthoptic trainer or can be done in the clinic using synoptophore.
- *Medical therapy:*
    - *Miotics:* Miotics can be used in accommodative esotropia to help accommodation. Echothiophate 0.03%, 0.06%, and 0.123% solution is available. This therapy is not preferred, as it is not as accurate as bifocals and the drugs can have adverse reactions such as nausea, vomiting, abdominal cramps, frequent micturition.
    - Cycloplegics can be used in accommodative esotropia for refraction and also to relax accommodation to make children accept glasses.
    - *Newer drugs:* Levodopa-carbidopa has been studied as a treatment option in amblyopia. Recently, citicoline has also been explored as an option in amblyopia therapy.
- *Botulinum toxin injection:* Botulinum toxin is a neurotoxic agent produced by the bacteria *Clostridium botulinum*. It inhibits the release of acetylcholine from the motor end plate hence inhibiting motor response to a stimulus. When injected in the muscle, it results in temporary paralysis of the muscle. It is used in paralytic squints as an immediate

treatment prior to surgical management where it is injected into the antagonist of the paralyzed muscle. It is also used in infantile esotropia where it is injected into the MR. This will reduce the deviation and help in alignment of the eye. It is usually not preferred as it is temporary and needs repeated injection.

Miscellaneous

 52. Describe classification of amblyopia/discuss amblyopia, and recent trends in management.

Amblyopia is defined as unilateral or bilateral reduction in visual acuity due to vision deprivation or abnormal binocular interaction which cannot be explained by any organic cause and is reversible by therapy in appropriate cases.

Classification of Amblyopia

- *Strabismic amblyopia:* This is due to presence of strabismus which leads to abnormal binocular interaction. It is more common with esotropia than exotropia as exotropia is usually intermittent to begin with and in esotropia, the fovea of the deviating eye has to compete against the temporal field of the other eye which is stronger than the nasal hemifield.
- *Anisometropic amblyopia:* This is due to high-refractive error in any one eye. It can be anisomyopic or anisohyperopic. Amblyopia develops with lower amounts of hyperopia than myopia as near vision is preserved in myopia.
- Stimulus deprivation amblyopia, e.g., due to congenital cataract, ptosis covering the pupil, and corneal opacity.
- *Ametropic amblyopia:* This is due to bilateral high-uncorrected refractive error.
- Amblyopia associated with nystagmus.
- Organic amblyopia—where there are subtle organic causes.

Clinical Features

- *Reduction in visual acuity:* A two-line reduction of visual acuity is considered as significant. Recognition visual acuity such as Snellen's chart is more affected than resolution visual acuity such as Teller's acuity chart. In strabismic amblyopia, recognition visual acuity is more affected. Whereas in anisometropic amblyopia, both grating and recognition visual acuity
- Poor stereopsis and decreased contrast sensitivity
- Strabismic amblyopia is not degraded by neutral density filters and may show better visual acuity with neutral density filter. This is not seen with anisometropic amblyopia which shows same degradation of visual acuity in the normal and amblyopic eye.
- Crowding phenomenon is seen in amblyopia where visual acuity is better with single optotypes than line acuity due to abnormal contour interaction.
- Fixation abnormalities such as poor fixation and eccentric fixation can be seen.
- Smooth pursuit and saccade abnormality.

Management of Amblyopia

- Removing the amblyopiogenic factor—correction of refractive error, correction of deviation, cataract surgery, and ptosis surgery
- Refraction with appropriate cycloplegic
- Occlusion therapy—occlusion of the normal eye can be done to preferentially stimulate the affected eye. Occlusion can be done with patch of the normal eye. Full-time occlusion was advocated earlier. The amblyopia treatment study has shown good results with even part-time occlusion for 6 hours and 2 hours. The number of days is decided on the age of the child 2 days till 2 years, number of days equal to the age till 6 years and then 6 days a week. Follow-up is done every 6 weeks. Two follow-ups are needed to say that there has been no improvement.
- Penalization can be tried where worse eye is given optical advantage either by optical method where high plus glasses are given, pharmacological method where cycloplegics are given or partial occlusion where one spectacle glass is made partially opaque with tape or nail varnish.
- *CAM vision stimulator:* It is a method where the amblyopic eye is preferentially stimulated with high-contrast grating patterns.

- *Pleoptics:* Here, the fovea of the amblyopic eye is preferentially stimulated. Bangerter used to dazzle the rest of the retina and then stimulate only the fovea whereas, Cuppers used after images to stimulate the fovea.

Recent Advances in Amblyopia Therapy

- *Perceptual learning:* In this, the patient is made to repeatedly do visual tasks such as letter detection, Vernier acuity, contrast detection, and positional discrimination either binocularly or uniocularly.
- *Binocular treatment:* It focusses on dissociated stimulation of both the eyes so as to improve amblyopia and also to develop binocularity and stereopsis. This includes dichoptics where red–green dissociation is used to separately stimulate the two eyes. They come as games on tablets or smartphone which the child plays with both eyes open. Now, virtual reality goggles-based games are also being studied.
- *Pharmacotherapy:*
  - *Levodopa:* This is a drug used in parkinsonism and has been found to be of benefit in increasing visual acuity in the amblyopic eye by increasing dopaminergic synapse transmission which is present in visual processing.
  - *Citicoline:* This drug acts in the central nervous system to increase cerebral metabolism and dopaminergic neurons. It also acts as a neuroprotectant and has been tried in addition to patching with good results.

53. Discuss classification and management of amblyopia.

Refer to Answer 52.

54. Describe classification, management, and strategies for prevention of amblyopia.

For classification and management, refer to Answer 52.

Prevention of Amblyopia

- Risk of amblyopia development is maximum in the critical period (0–5 years) when the synapses are still malleable and the best results of amblyopia therapy is also in the same period (up to around 12 years).
- *Strabismic amblyopia:* Esotropia has higher chances of development of amblyopia. Any child with esotropia must be checked for fixation preference or resistance to occlusion of either eye. Visual acuity assessment with age-appropriate methods should be checked wherever possible. Occlusion therapy has to be started at diagnosis and continued till vision is equalized in both eyes and fixation preference is lost. Surgical management should be done only after management of amblyopia. In case there is no amblyopia, 1:1 occlusion can be started to prevent amblyopia till surgery and immediate surgical intervention has to be planned.
- *Anisometropic and ametropic amblyopia:* Early detection of refractive error and its appropriate refractive correction
- *Stimulus deprivation amblyopia:* Early detection of cataract, severe ptosis, corneal opacity, and early surgery. Risk of amblyopia is more in unilateral cases and hence early surgery in unilateral cases is a must.

55. Describe microtropia.

Microtropia is a condition where there is small amount of deviation which may not be picked up by routine examination.

Clinical Features

- Small-sized deviation around 5–8°.
- Fixation can be foveal or nonfoveal with relative scotoma on the fixation spot.
- Amblyopia, subnormal stereoacuity, and ARC
- Normal or near normal fusional amplitudes
- Positive and negative cover test
- *Positive four PD test:* A 4 PD base-out prism is kept in front of the right eye. If there was any microtropia in the right eye, there is no movement due to foveal scotoma. If the left eye has microtropia, then there is no inward movement of the left eye for fusional adduction.

Classification of Microtropia

- *Park's monofixation syndrome:* There is presence of macular scotoma with peripheral fusion and presence of gross stereopsis.
- *Lang's microtropia*—has three types:
  - *Type 1:* Characterized by central fixation
  - *Type 2:* Characterized by eccentric fixation without identity that is the angle of anomaly and is not equal to the amount of eccentricity of fixation
  - *Type 3:* Characterized by eccentric fixation with identity where the angle of anomaly is equal to the amount of eccentric fixation, hence there is no movement in cover–uncover test.

It can also be classified as:
- Primary
- *Secondary:* After surgery for deviation.

Management of Microtropia

- Detection of refractive error and amblyopia
- Management of amblyopia with occlusion.

 56. Describe etiology, clinical feature, and management of AV pattern deviations.

AV pattern deviations are horizontal deviations which have vertical incompetence. They can be:
- A esotropia—the amount of deviation is more in upgaze
- A exotropia—amount of deviation is more in downgaze
- V esotropia—amount of deviation is more in downgaze
- V exotropia—amount of deviation is more in upgaze
- Y pattern—where there is exotropia in upgaze only. Seen in Brown's syndrome
- Diamond pattern—seen in esotropia, where amount of deviation is more in both upgaze and downgaze
- X pattern—seen in exotropia where amount of deviation is more in upgaze and downgaze

Etiology: There are many schools of thoughts about the causes for patterns:
- Horizontal school of thought—medial and LR overaction or underaction can lead to patterns. In V esotropia, there is MR overaction which leads to increased adduction in downgaze. V exotropia can occur due to LR overaction which causes increased abduction in upgaze. Similarly, A exotropia occurs due to MR underaction and A esotropia there is underaction of LR.
- *Vertical school of thought:* This suggests that the vertical recti lead to the patterns. SR underaction will lead to less adduction in upgaze and V pattern. SR underaction will lead to secondary IO overaction as well as SO underaction. Hence, the vertical and obliques actions are interconnected.
- *Oblique school of thought:* This is now the most widely accepted theory for the AV patterns. V pattern occurs due to IO overaction and A pattern occurs due to SO overaction.
- *Orbital structural factors:* These occur due to variation in the facial features such as mongoloid slant is associated with A esotropia and V exotropia.
  Variations in the structures of the skull which alters the position of the trochlea can lead to patterns. Desagittalization where the oblique tendon becomes more parallel to coronal plane is seen in plagiocephaly and results in weakening of the SO leading to V pattern and in sagittalization, where the SO lies more in the sagittal plane due to hydrocephalus can give A pattern.
- *Anomalous muscle insertions:* Abnormal insertion of the recti will give rise to vertical vectors which can cause patterns. In V patterns, the MR is inserted higher and LR lower.
- *Heterotopia of the muscle pulleys:* With the description of muscle pulleys by Demers et al., it has been found that altered position of the muscle pulleys can lead to patterns. Inferior displacement of the LR pulley leads to V pattern and upshoot in adduction.

Clinical Features

- *Head posture:* Children can present with chin up or down head posture. V exotropia presents with chin up position and A exotropia presents with chin down position.

- All horizontal deviations must be checked for presence of oblique muscle overactions and presence of patterns.
- Deviation is measured in upgaze of 25° and downgaze 35°. A difference of 15 PD is significant in V pattern and 10 PD difference is significant in A pattern.

Management of AV Patterns

- Horizontal rectus recession and resection are done for the horizontal deviation.
- If associated with oblique overactions—if the patterns are associated with oblique muscle overactions, then oblique muscle weakening should be done. In case of V patterns, IO weakening procedure can be done. Depending on the amount of overaction, Parks or Fink recession for mild and Elliot and Nankin's recession with anterior positioning can be done for more severe overaction. Posterior tenectomy of the SO is preferred for SO overaction.
- If there is no oblique overaction, then the horizontal recti shifting is done. In V pattern, the MR is shifted down and the LR is shifted up. In A pattern, the MR is shifted up and the LR is shifted down.
- Slanting recession of the horizontal recti can be done. In V esotropia pattern, MR is recessed more inferiorly and in A esotropia, it is recessed more superiorly.

57. A 14-year-old boy is brought by his parents with occasional deviation of the eyes. Discuss differential diagnosis, evaluation, and management of such a case.

Differential diagnoses of occasional deviation of the eyes are:
- Intermittent exotropia
- Intermittent esotropia.

Refer to Question 25 and Question 28 for evaluation and management.

58. Describe the role of botulinum toxin in strabismus.

Botulinum toxin is a neurotoxic agent produced by the bacteria *C. botulinum*. Infection by this bacterium resulted in paralysis of bulbar and skeletal muscles. Its use in weakening of extraocular muscles was first described by Alan Scott.

Mechanism of Action

The botulinum toxin A is 150 kDa. It acts on the nerve endings which stimulate the motor end plate. The toxin attaches to the gangliosides on the surface membrane of the nerve ending using the carboxy terminus. Next the toxin is entered into the cell with the process of endocytosis which occurs through the amino-terminus. This toxin then inhibits the release of acetylcholine from the vesicles hence preventing the end plate potential. The effect lasts for 2–4 months.

Method of Injection

The dose of botulinum toxin used is 2.5 units per muscle. It is injected into the muscle with the help of electromyography (EMG). It is done under local anesthesia in adults and in ketamine anesthesia in children. The muscle is identified and the EMG is connected which shows continuous activity. The toxin is injected at the junction of anterior two-thirds and posterior one-third. The activity on the EMG stops soon after the injection. Care must be taken to avoid perforation of the globe and extravasation of the toxin to other muscles.

Indications

- In paralytic muscle especially in LR palsy, it is injected in the MR to weaken the MR. This allows alignment of the eyes and improved diplopia-free fields.
- In thyroid eye disease, it is useful if done before the fibrosis of the muscle occurs.
- In congenital esotropia, it is injected in the MR to paralyze the MR and allow alignment of the eyes. It has a longer lasting effect in children.
- In poststrabismus surgery over- or undercorrection
- Apart from strabismus surgery, it is also used in the treatment of essential blepharospasm and also in hemifacial spasms.

Adverse Effect

It can cause ptosis, paralysis, or weakness of the adjacent extraocular muscles. It can also cause pupillary dilation and accommodation weakness. It can cause dry eye, reduced lacrimation, foreign body sensation, and retrobulbar hemorrhage.

 59. Describe methods of testing visual acuity in children/pediatric vision assessment.

Visual acuity assessment in children is a challenge due to inability to read the normal Snellen's chart.

Visual assessment in children <1 year:
- *Catford drum test:* This consists of optotypes of various sizes which is present on an oscillating drum. The smallest optotype which elicits a pendular movement of the eyes is considered as the visual acuity. It is done at a distance of 60 cm.
- *Preferential looking tests:* These include tests which have a pattern which the infant will prefer to fix at a pattern than a plain area and depending on the visual acuity, patterns of a particular resolution can be seen by the child.
    - *Teller acuity card:* It contains grating patterns which is shown to the child. In <6 months, it is done at a distance of 38 cm and in 7 months to 3 years, it is done at a distance of 84 cm. It measures resolution visual acuity. It measures near acuity and can miss conditions such as myopia and also it can overestimate the visual acuity.
    - *Cardiff acuity cards:* This is based on vanishing optotypes principle. They consist of a series of cards with picture optotypes drawn in white lines present at one end and blank space at the other. These optotypes are visible only at a particular distance. The child is shown the cards and rotated to see if the child fixes on the optotype and changes fixation according to the movement of the card.
- *OKNOVIS:* This is based on the principle of arrestovisography. These consist of optotypes of different sizes which are shown to the child to arrest the optokinetic nystagmus. The smallest optotype which can arrest the optokinetic nystagmus suggests the visual acuity.
- *Visually evoked response:* It is recording of the cortical electrical activity after a visual stimulation. The visual stimulation can be flash or pattern (checker board or stripe) type. Pattern reversal is the preferred method. The P100 latency and amplitude are checked.
- *Indirect methods of assessment of visual acuity:* These include certain observations or examinations that can be done in the OPD setting which give clues regarding low vision.
    - *Reflexes:* Such as blink response to light, pupillary reactions and menace reflex can be elicited.
    - *Fixation pattern:* Both eyes should be checked for central, steady, and maintained fixation, presence of fixation preference, and resistance to occlusion of either eye. Presence of any nystagmus, eccentric fixation. In the absence of squint, deviation can be induced by a prism and checked, if any particular eye is preferred for taking up fixation.
    - Ability of the child to follow objects can be checked. The pattern of smooth pursuit, any jerky motion, any nasotemporal asymmetry can be checked.

Visual Assessment in Children Between 1 and 2 Years

- Cardiff acuity and Teller's acuity can be performed in this age group.
- *Boeck candy test:* This consists of using small edible candies to assess visual acuity. The ability of the child to pick up the candy and eat. It can be done uniocularly to check difference between the two eyes.
- *Worth's ivory ball test:* Here, balls of different diameters 0.5–1.5″ are shown to the child and rolled on the floor asking the child to bring the ball back to the examiner. The smallest size which the child can retrieve gives the visual acuity.
- *Sheridan's ball test:* These consist of Styrofoam balls which can be rolled on the floor similar to the previous test or are mounted on a black wall and fixation pattern is assessed.

Visual Assessment in Children Between 2 and 3 Years

- *Miniature toy test:* This test is done at a distance of 10 feet. The child is asked to identify pairs of toys from many toys.
- *Coin test:* This consists of coins of various sizes and the child has to differentiate between the coins from different distances.
- *Dot visual acuity test:* This consists of an illuminated light box with dots of different sizes progressively becoming small. The smallest size which the child can identify gives the visual acuity.

Visual Assessment in Children between 3 and 5 Years

- *E chart:* This consists of the letter E of various sizes with the arms pointing in different directions which the child has to identify and show. It is done at a distance of 6 m. The child can be taught by the mother to help in the testing. It can be used for screening purpose.
- *C chart by Landolt:* It is similar to the E chart, where the letter C is used and the child has to point where the opening of the letter C is.
- *Sjögren hand and arrow chart:* Where the child has to show the direction of the arrows.
- *Sheridan's letter chart:* It uses alphabets which child has to recognize. It is done at a distance of 3 m. They come as 5 letter sets, 7 letter sets, or 9 letter sets.
- *Lippman's HOTV test:* It is similar to the Sheridan's test using only 4 letters done at a distance of 3 m.
- *Lea's symbol chart:* Here, different shapes in Snellen's equivalent are shown to child and key cards are provided. The child has to identify the symbols and show them in the key cards.
- Snellen's visual acuity chart can be used where children are made to read the letters from a distance of 6 m.

Suggested Reading

1. Bosley TM, Abu-Amero KK, Oystreck DT. Congenital cranial dysinnervation disorders: a concept in evolution. Curr Opin Ophthalmol. 2013;24(5):398-406.
2. Bron A, Tripathi R, Tripathi B. Wolff's Anatomy of the Eye and Orbit, 8th edition. Germany: Taylor & Francis; 1997.
3. Burke J. Inverse Knapp procedure. Eye (Lond). 2001;15(Pt 1):5.
4. Clark RA. The role of extraocular muscle pulleys in incomitant non-paralytic strabismus. Middle East Afr J Ophthalmol. 2015;22(3):279-85.
5. Flanders M. Restrictive strabismus: diagnosis and management. Am Orthopt J. 2014;64:54-63.
6. Gaur N, Sharma P. Management of Duane retraction syndrome: a simplified approach. Indian J Ophthalmol. 2019;67(1):16-22.
7. Goray A, Kamlesh, Dhiman S, Thacker P, Goel Y, Babita, et al. Monocular elevation deficit—simplified. DJO. 2015;26:7-13.
8. Ishida Y, Hayashi O, Oda S, Kakinoki M, Miyake T, Inoki Y, et al. A simple muscle transposition procedure for abducens palsy without tenotomy or splitting muscles. Jpn J Ophthalmol. 2005;49:179-80.
9. Knapp P. The surgical treatment of double elevator paralysis. Trans Am Ophthalmol Soc. 1969;67:304-2.
10. Kraus CL, Culican SM. New advances in amblyopia therapy I: binocular therapies and pharmacologic augmentation. Brit J Ophthalmol. 2018;102:1492-6.
11. Levi DM, Li RW. Perceptual learning as a potential treatment for amblyopia: a mini-review. Vision Res. 2009;49(21):2535-49.
12. Porciatti V, Schiavi C, Benedetti P, Baldi A, Campos EC. Cytidine-5¢-diphosphocholine improves visual acuity, contrast sensitivity and visually-evoked potentials of amblyopic subjects. Curr Eye Res. 1998;17(2):141-8.
13. Rosenbaum AL, Santiago AP. Clinical Strabismus Management: Principles and Surgical Techniques. United Kingdom: Saunders; 1999.
14. Saxena R, Sharma M, Singh D, Sharma P. Full tendon medial transposition of lateral rectus with augmentation sutures in cases of complete third nerve palsy. Br J Ophthalmol. 2018;102(6):715-7.
15. Sharma P (Eds). Strabismus Simplified, 2nd edition. New Delhi: CBS Publishers and Distributers; 2013.
16. Sharma P, Gaur N, Phuljhele S, Saxena R. What's new for us in strabismus? Indian J Ophthalmol. 2017;65(3):184-90.
17. Singh A, Nagpal R, Mittal SK, Bahuguna C, Kumar P. Pharmacological therapy for amblyopia. Taiwan J Ophthalmol. 2017;7(2):62-9.
18. Taylor JN. Surgical management of oculomotor nerve palsy with lateral rectus transplantation to the medial side of the globe. Aust N ZJ Ophthalmol. 1989;17:27-31.
19. von Noorden GK, Campos EC. Binocular Vision and Ocular Motility: Theory and Management of Strabismus. United Kingdom: Mosby; 2002.

Sclera

Aditi Dubey

Q 1. Classify scleral inflammation.

Scleral inflammation gives rise to a spectrum of conditions, ranging from a trivial self-limiting episode to a vision-threatening necrotizing process. Clinical classification of episcleral and scleral inflammation is important not only for diagnosis but also to know the prognosis.[1]

Episcleritis: The episclera is the thin densely vascularized layer of connective tissue overlying the sclera and situated below the Tenon's capsule. In simple terms, it is inflammation of episcleral tissues. It can be:
- Simple
- Nodular.

Scleritis: Sclera is an opaque, elastic, and resilient tissue of the eye.[2] It can be compared to an incomplete shell comprising approximately 90% (five-sixths) of the outer coat of the eye. Scleritis is a severe inflammation of the scleral tissue. This painful inflammatory condition can be classified as:
- *Anterior scleritis:*
  - Diffuse scleritis
  - Nodular scleritis
  - *Necrotizing scleritis:* It consists of two varieties:
    - With inflammation
    - Without inflammation (scleromalacia perforans)
- *Posterior scleritis.*

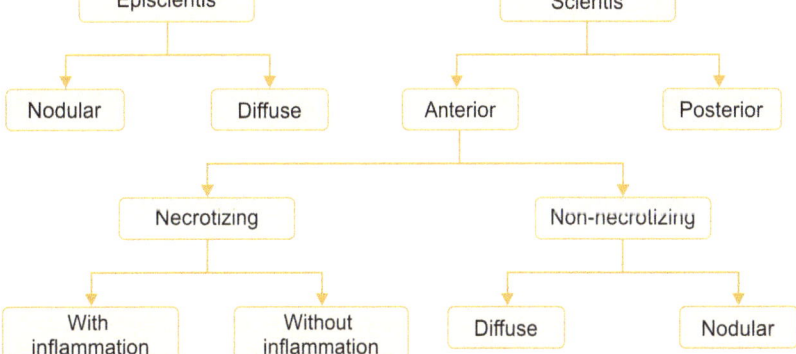

Flowchart 1: Classification of scleral inflammation.

This classification system proposed by Watson and Hayreh is widely accepted **(Flowchart 1)**.[3]

Q 2. Discuss classification of scleritis its clinical features, investigation, and management of scleritis.

Classification of Scleritis

Refer to Answer 1.

Clinical features of scleral inflammation:
- Most common in the fourth to sixth decades
- Recurrences and remissions are common
- Unilateral or bilateral involvement simultaneous or at various times.

Anterior Scleritis

Symptoms
- Pain—insidious in the onset, severe in intensity, penetrating in character, localized to the eye, radiates to the forehead, jaws, and the sinuses, and is only temporarily relieved by analgesics.
- Redness—gradual in the onset, progressive, bluish-red tinge in appearance, sectoral, or diffuse depending on the type.
- Translucent (blue–gray) sclera—in recurrent attacks of scleral inflammation
- Photophobia.

Signs
- Scleral and episcleral edema on slit-lamp examination with red-free light
- Deep episcleral vessels are more congested than the superficial episcleral vessels
- No conjunctival congestion
- Miosis
- Transient myopia
- Reduced visual acuity due to complications, e.g., keratitis, uveitis, glaucoma, cataract, exudative retinal detachment, and macular edema.

Posterior Scleritis

Inflammation of the sclera posterior to the ora serrata may spread to choroid, retina, and optic nerve. On fundus examination:
- Fundus mass—subretinal in nature
- Choroidal folds—a series of alternating light and dark lines confined to the posterior pole, often temporal, and rarely extending beyond the equator, arranged in a horizontal and parallel pattern, surrounding a subretinal mass
- Retinal striae
- Choroidal or retinal detachments
- Disc or macular edema
- Diplopia
- Flashes of light (photopsia)
- Tenderness
- Proptosis
- Lid swelling, lid retraction, and limitation of ocular movements
- Reduction in vision due to transient hyperopia, choroidal or retinal detachments, distortion of the macula, cystoid macular edema, and optic neuritis.

Grading of Scleritis

McCluskey and Wakefield proposed a scoring system for the extent and severity of the disease. Another grading system was given by Sen et al. based on their cross-sectional interobserver agreement study on National Eye Institute's digital photo archive. The high-resolution photographs were taken after application of 10% phenylephrine and scleral inflammation was graded as shown in **Table 1**.[4]

TABLE 1: Grading of scleritis.

Grade	Grading description
0	No scleral inflammation with complete blanching of vessels
0.5	Trace inflammation with minimally dilated deep episcleral vessels
1	Mild scleral inflammation with diffuse mild dilatation of deep episcleral vessels
2	Moderate scleral inflammation with tortuous and engorged deep episcleral vessels
3	Severe scleral inflammation with diffuse significant redness of sclera and obscuration of deep episcleral vessels with edema and erythema
4	Necrotizing scleritis with or without uveal show

Scleritis and episcleritis is commonly associated with various connective tissue disorders. **Table 2** Shows the systemic association of episcleritis and scleritis.

Clinically the episcleral and scleral inflammation can be differentiated. **Table 3** Shows the differential features of episcleritis and scleritis.

TABLE 2: Diseases associated with episcleritis and scleritis.	
Noninfectious	• Connective tissue diseases and other inflammatory conditions • Rheumatoid arthritis • Systemic lupus erythematosus • Ankylosing spondylitis • Reactive arthritis • Psoriatic arthritis • Arthritis and inflammatory bowel disease • Relapsing polychondritis
Vasculitic diseases	• Polyarteritis nodosa • Allergic granulomatous angiitis (Churg–Strauss syndrome) • Granulomatosis with polyangiitis (Wegener) • Behçet's disease • Giant-cell arteritis • Cogan's syndrome • Vasculitic diseases associated with connective tissue diseases and other inflammatory conditions
Miscellaneous	• Atopy • Rosacea • Gout • Foreign body granuloma • Chemical injury
Infectious	• Bacterial • Fungal • Viral • Parasitical

S. no.	Clinical characteristics	Episcleritis	Scleritis
		TABLE 3: Differentiating features of episcleritis and scleritis.	
1.	Presenting symptom	• Redness • Irritation	• Severe excruciating pain (deteriorates at night) • Redness
2.	Tenderness	Nil or minimal	Moderate to severe
3.	Color of vessels	Bright red in color	Purple red in color
4.	Movement of congested vessels	Moved easily with the help of cotton bud	Cannot be moved easily with cotton bud
5.	10% phenylephrine test	Blanching of vessels occurs	Blanching of vessels does not occur
6.	Inflammation site	Episcleral congestion	Congestion of deeper episcleral vessels; Scleral edema

Investigating a Case of Scleritis

Scleritis should undergo a thorough systemic examination and serological investigation to rule out the presence of any systemic disease. Many a time scleral inflammation can be the initial manifestation of these systemic diseases and many of them can be life-threatening, the systemic evaluation in such patients can be rewarding. Following investigations should be done:

- Routine blood investigations such as complete blood count (CBC) and erythrocyte sedimentation rate (ESR) should be advised in all patients with scleritis. Liver function tests (LFT), renal function tests, and blood glucose levels are usually done to establish baseline normal levels and to monitor response to steroid or immunosuppressive treatment.
- Rheumatoid factor is an autoantibody directed against the Fc region of immunoglobulin G (IgG). The classic Rose–Waaler test is a hemagglutination test for rheumatoid factor in the serum. The latex agglutination test is also widely available. Enzyme-linked immunosorbent assay (ELISA) can measure IgG, IgA, and IgM rheumatoid factors. Oligoarticular rheumatoid arthritis (RA) may be associated with a negative test for IgM rheumatoid factor but a positive test for IgG rheumatoid factor.
- The antineutrophil cytoplasmic antibody (ANCA) test has been very helpful in the diagnosis of Wegener's granulomatosis (WG). Cytoplasmic antineutrophil cytoplasmic antibody (cANCA) is found to be more specific for WG than perinuclear antineutrophil cytoplasmic antibody (pANCA).
- Antinuclear antibodies (ANAs) are done in clinical suspicion of systemic rheumatic diseases or collagen vascular diseases such as systemic lupus erythematous (SLE).
- *Tests for SLE:* Antiribosomal antibodies, antibodies to double-stranded deoxyribonucleic acid (dsDNA), and Anti-Sm (Smith) antibodies are specific for SLE.
- *Tests for tuberculosis (TB):* If suspected clinically, tuberculin skin test or Mantoux test for the diagnosis of latent TB. Cross-reactivity of the antigen used in the test with bacillus Calmette–Guérin (BCG) and environmental nontuberculous mycobacteria, booster effect on repeated injection of purified protein derivative (PPD) leading to false-positive results is a major concern. Interferon-gamma release assay (IGRA) is more specific than the tuberculin skin test. Chest X-ray and high-resolution computerized tomography (HRCT) have been found in diagnosis of TB.
- *Test for sarcoidosis:* Serum angiotensin-converting enzyme (ACE) and serum lysozyme. These tests are not fully specific for the disease and may be raised in various other systemic conditions. Definitive diagnosis of sarcoidosis is made by solid-tissue biopsy showing classic noncaseating granulomas. Radiological evidence of bilateral hilar lymphadenopathy is considered as pathognomonic of this clinical entity.
- *Syphilis:* Various tests are available for the diagnosis of syphilis. Dark-field microscopy provides direct identification of Treponema pallidum. Serological tests include nontreponemal tests such as venereal disease research laboratory (VDRL) tests and rapid plasma reagin (RPR) tests, and treponemal tests such as fluorescent treponemal antibody absorption (FTA-ABS) and microhemagglutination assay for T. pallidum (MHA-TP) assays detect antibodies against T. pallidum.
- *Laboratory diagnosis of infectious scleritis:* The sample obtained is microscopically examined, using Gram's and Giemsa staining methods and potassium hydroxide (KOH) 10% or calcofluor white preparation. These tests give useful information for initial antimicrobial treatment in infectious scleritis. Culture is done in fresh blood agar, chocolate agar, Sabouraud dextrose agar, non-nutrient agar with an overlay of Escherichia coli, thioglycolate broth and brain heart infusion broth, etc.

Treatment of Scleritis

The primary aim of the treatment of scleral inflammation is to control the inflammatory process to relieve the symptoms and thereby reduce the damage to the eye.

Good visual outcome if adequate treatment is initiated shortly after its onset. The main modality of treatment is medical, although some conditions may require surgical treatment also.

- *Medical management of scleritis:* The mainstay of treatment:

First line of treatment	— Oral nonsteroidal anti-inflammatory drug (NSAID) and topical steroid	
(Non-necrotizing scleritis)	↓ Not responding	
Second line	Systemic steroids	
	↓ Not responding	
Third line	Immunosuppressive	First line (necrotizing scleritis)

TABLE 4: List of nonsteroidal anti-inflammatory drugs for scleral inflammation.		
i.	Diflunisal	500 mg bid
ii.	Naproxen	250–500 mg bid
iii.	Ibuprofen	800 mg tid
iv.	Fenoprofen	600 mg tid
v.	Ketoprofen	100 mg tid
vi.	Flurbiprofen	100 mg tid
vii.	Indomethacin	75 mg SR bid
viii.	Diclofenac	75 mg SR bid
ix.	Piroxicam	20 mg qid
x.	Mobic Meloxicam	7.5–15 mg qid

(SR: sustained-release)

- *Systemic NSAIDs:* Systemic NSAID therapy cyclooxygenase (COX) inhibitor is almost invariably effective. There are various agents that are used given in **Table 4** along with dose. Although indomethacin sustained-release 75 mg BD is considered as first choice, if available. However, long-term NSAIDs should be avoided in the view of systemic side effects.
- *Corticosteroids:* Topical steroids are given as adjuvant to the oral NSAID; the agents widely used are loteprednol 0.5%, prednisolone acetate 1%, etc.

    Oral corticosteroids are indicated in cases which are nonresponsive to first line of therapy or with posterior or necrotizing disease. The starting dose is 1 mg/kg/day, the weekly reduction by 10 mg/week and once 40 mg/day is reached the further reduction to maintenance dose of 5 mg/day is dependent in clinical response.

    Intravenous corticosteroids are for cases where aggressive management of the scleral inflammation is required like threatened scleral or corneal perforation in necrotizing scleritis. Pulse therapy of intravenous (IV) methyl-prednisolone is given 500 mg-1 g for 3 days. It is followed by high dose of oral steroid or immunosuppressive agents.

    As corticosteroids can have serious side effects on long-term use so steroid treatment should be initiated and maintained after systemic work up. Special caution must be taken in diabetics and hypertensive cases.

    The role of periocular steroids is still controversial in scleritis and not widely used.
- *Immunosuppressive agents are indicated in cases of:*
    - Anterior necrotizing scleritis
    - Posterior scleritis not responding to steroid or requiring long-term steroids
    - Scleritis associated with a systemic autoimmune disease or collagen vascular disease.

    Various immunosuppressants have been tried for treatment of scleritis and these include antimetabolites (methotrexate, azathioprine, and mycophenolate mofetil), alkylating agents (chlorambucil and cyclophosphamide), and T-cell inhibitors (cyclosporine and tacrolimus). Most commonly and widely used is methotrexate with or without a short course of oral steroid in tapering dosage. Dosage of methotrexate is 0.1–0.5 mg/kg/week; low-dose therapy is started at a dose of 7.5 mg/week and it can be increased up to 25 mg/week. It is given orally once a week along with folic acid analog. As it causes hepatotoxicity and bone marrow suppression, CBC and LFT monitoring are essential.

    Azathioprine and cyclophosphamides are next-line drugs.
- *Surgical management of scleritis:* Tectonic surgical procedures rarely may be required to preserve the integrity of the globe. Patch grafts might need to be performed along with systemic immunosuppression in cases of extensive scleral melts and uveal show. Donor sclera (fresh, glycerine preserved, or frozen) is most commonly used. Other options such as fascia lata, periosteum, aortic tissue, polytetrafluoroethylene, dura mater, split thickness dermis, processed pericardium, and Conjunctiva–Muller muscle flap have also been tried.

 3. Discuss etiopathogenesis, clinical features, evaluation, and management of necrotizing scleritis.

Anterior scleritis can also be of necrotizing variety with inflammation and necrotizing without inflammation (scleromalacia perforans).

Necrotizing Scleritis without Inflammation

It is the most severe form with bilateral involvement and potentially vision-threatening condition. The most common association is with RA.

Pathophysiology

Due to vasculitis secondary to immune complex deposition in autoimmune diseases like RA there is vascular shutdown of the episcleral bed, resulting in avascular necrosis and the ectasia of the sclera. In advance cases, the necrotizing scleritis may spread to the equator and circumferentially and can involve the entire globe.

Clinical Features

Severe pain and tenderness, white, avascular areas of localized scleral edema and congestion, and the edges of these lesions are more inflamed than the center. In advance cases, underlying uveal tissue becomes visible as the sclera becomes thin and translucent.

Necrotizing Anterior Scleritis without Inflammation (Scleromalacia Perforans)

As the name suggests, it has no minimal signs of inflammatory pathology. It is a rare entity but vision threatening.

Pathophysiology

It occurs predominantly in patients with long-standing RA.

Clinical Features

No minimal signs of inflammation, no pain or tenderness, and blurred vision. In advance cases, the sclera progressively thins and the underlying dark uveal tissue is visible. Staphylomas, peripheral corneal thinning, and spontaneous perforation are rare but are prone to rupture with minimal trauma.

Other ocular problems include conjunctivitis and the complications of uveitis and/or scleritis, such as cataract, seclusion of the pupil, iris bombe, secondary glaucoma, or macular edema depending on the other structures involved.

Systemic manifestations of RA in form of malaise, fatigue, and weight loss can also be present along with articular and extra-articular manifestations in cases of necrotizing scleritis.

Evaluation and treatment are discussed in Answer 2.

4. Discuss clinical features and types of anterior and posterior scleritis.

Refer to Answer 1 and Answer 2.

5. How will you investigate a case of scleritis?

Refer to Answer 2.

6. Discuss management of necrotizing scleritis.

Refer to Answer 3.

References

1. Majumder PD, Biswas J. Scleral Inflammations: An Update. AIOS CME Series no. 29; 2013.
2. De la Maza MS, Tauber J, Foster CS. The Sclera, 2nd edition. New York Dordrecht Heidelberg London: Springer; 2012.
3. Carlos EP, Fabio M. Systemic disorders associated with episcleritis and scleritis. Curr Opin Ophthalmol. 2001;12:471-8.
4. Sen HN, Sangave AA, Goldstein DA, Suhler EB, Cunningham D, Vitale S, et al. A standardized grading system for scleritis. Ophthalmology. 2011;118:768-71.

Retina

5.1 Common Retinal Disorders and Surgery

Mahesh Kumar MH, Navneet Sidhu, Monika Kapoor

Q 1. Discuss the development of eye and retinal disorders related to development of eye.

Development of Eye and Retinal Disorders Related to Development of Eye

The development of the eye commences at day 22 of embryonic life which has eight pairs of somites and is 2 mm in length. The eyeball is formed from these primordial structures:
- Optic vesicle—from prosencephalon
- Lens placode
- Mesenchyme
- Visceral mesoderm.

Formation of Optic Vesicles

The earliest sign of eye development is the formation of the lens placodes, which are small surface ectoderm thickenings on both sides of the developing head. At the same time, the neural ectoderm forms two optic pits that fill up to form pouches on either side of the midline; these pouches are termed the optic vesicles which are derived from prosencephalon. The narrow neck of these vesicles called the optic stalk directly connects the optic vesicle and the developing forebrain.

Formation of Optic Cup

Once the optic vesicle touches the inner aspect of the surface ectoderm, the vesicle invaginates to form a bilayered optic cup; the inner layer forms the neural retina, whereas the outer layer forms the retinal pigment epithelium (RPE). As the optic cup forms, two processes take place:
1. First, the surface ectoderm begins to invaginate to form the lens.
2. Second, the area between the cup and the surface ectoderm fills with a combination of mesodermal and neural crest-derived cells—the ectomesenchyme that will form much of the anterior segment of the eye. The invagination of the optic cup occurs asymmetrically with a ventral fissure that facilitates entry of mesodermal and neural crest cells. The fissure closes at its center first and then "zips" both anteriorly and posteriorly.

Formation of Lens Vesicle

Around day 27 of embryonic development, the surface ectoderm overlying the optic vesicle begins to thicken and form the lens placode. It gradually deepens and forms a lens vesicle which is separated from the surface ectoderm on day 33 of embryonic development **(Table 1)**.

Retinal Disorders Related to Development of Eye

- *Retinal coloboma:* It is due to incomplete closure of the optic fissure. It may involve the sensory retina and RPE. The choroid is also involved in such cases, since differentiation of the choroid depends on intact RPE.

TABLE 1: Chronology of embryonic and fetal development of the eye.

Time	Events
22 days	Optic primordium appears in neural folds (1.5–3.0 mm)
25 days	Optic vesicle evaginates. Neural crest cells migrate to surround vesicle
28 days	Vesicle induces lens placode
Second month	• Invagination of optic and lens vesicles • Hyaloid artery fills embryonic fissure • Closure of embryonic fissure begins • Pigment granules appear in retinal pigment epithelium • Primordia of lateral rectus and superior oblique muscles grow anteriorly • Eyelid folds appear • Retinal differentiation begins with nuclear and marginal zones • Migration of retinal cells begins • Neural crest cells of corneal endothelium migrate centrally. Corneal stroma follows • Cavity of lens vesicle is obliterated • Secondary vitreous surrounds hyaloid system • Choroidal vasculature develops • Axons from ganglion cells migrate to optic nerve • Glial laminal cribrosa forms • Bruch membrane appears
Third month	• Precursors of rods and cones differentiate • Anterior rim of optic vesicle grows forward, and ciliary body starts to develop • Sclera condenses • Vortex veins pierce sclera • Eyelid folds meet and fuse
Fourth month	• Retinal vessels grow into nerve fiber layer near optic disc • Folds of ciliary processes appear • Iris sphincter develops • Descemet membrane forms • Schlemm canal appears • Hyaloid system starts to regress • Glands and cilia develop
Fifth month	• Photoreceptors develop inner segments • Choroidal vessels form layers • Iris stroma is vascularized • Eyelids begin to separate
Sixth month	• Ganglion cells thicken in macula • Recurrent arterial branches join the choroidal vessels • Dilator muscle of iris forms
Seventh month	• Outer segments of photoreceptors differentiate • Central fovea starts to thin • Fibrous lamina cribrosa forms • Choroidal melanocytes produce pigment • Circular muscle forms in ciliary body
Eighth month	• Chamber angle completes formation • Hyaloid system disappears
Ninth month	• Retinal vessels reach the periphery • Myelination of fibers of optic nerve is complete to lamina cribrosa • Pupillary membrane disappears

- *Ocular albinism:* It is due to absence of melanocytes from the RPE. The fovea is not developed. There is a decreased number of rods. Also, there is abnormal optic nerve projection to the lateral geniculate nucleus with more crossed fibers as compared to normal. This causes low vision.

 2. Describe the embryological evolution of the retina.

Embryological Evolution of the Retina

The retina forms two overlapping layers:
1. The neural retina forms from the inner surface of the optic cup, whereas
2. The RPE forms from the outer surface.

Neurosensory Retina

- Forms during 4–5th week of gestation.
- Consists of two zones—Outer primitive zone and inner marginal zone (layer of His)
- Neuroepithelial cells divide by 6–7th week of gestation to form inner and outer neuroblastic layers.
- Subsequently various layers of the retina develop, whose differentiation starts during 6th week of gestation and is completed by 5.5 months of embryonic life. However, macula develops completely by 8th month of gestation.

Retinal Pigment Epithelium

Outer wall of the optic cup has cells which become pigmented around 6th week of gestation. The posterior layer forms the RPE and the anterior part continues forward as pigment epithelium of the ciliary body and iris.

Retinal Vessels

- Mesenchyme in the optic stalk differentiates to form the hyaloid artery.
- The posterior part of the hyaloid artery forms the central retinal artery and the anterior part closes, which in some cases may persist as a persistent fetal vasculature (PFV).
- A branch of the primitive maxillary vein within the optic stalk forms the central retinal vein.
- The retinal vasculature continues to develop till 3 months after birth, nasal periphery before the temporal periphery. Thus, premature infants are at a higher risk of developing retinopathy of prematurity (ROP).
- The vitreous is likely formed by both mesodermal and ectodermal components: neural ectoderm cells of the inner optic cup probably contribute the primary vitreous connective fibers, and the mesoderm forms the hyaloid vasculature.
- The primary vitreous forms a central conical structure that contains the hyaloid vasculature and is surrounded by secondary vitreous, which eventually replaces the primary vitreous by the 6th fetal month. Retinal development occurs concentrically, beginning in the center of the optic cup and extending peripherally. Lamination of the neural retina occurs at approximately 8–12 weeks of gestation.
- Ganglion cells appear to be the first to differentiate; they proliferate rapidly early in the second trimester.
- The internal and external limiting membranes form when cells cease to proliferate and begin to differentiate.
- The optic nerve develops from the optic stalk, which is the narrow stalk that connects the optic vesicle with the forebrain. The optic stalk is highly active in regulating cell migration into and around the developing eye, mostly through the release of ligands and expression of growth factor receptors.
- The stalk initially forms from neuroectodermal cells surrounded by neural crest cells. In the 6th week of gestation, neuroectodermal cells begin to vacuolate and degenerate, providing space for axons from the ganglion cells of the inner retina. The surrounding neural crest cells form meninges, whereas neuroectodermal cells form surrounding oligodendrocytes (to make myelin sheaths). Peripheral nerves, including most cranial nerves, are surrounded by myelin supplied by Schwann cells. The exception is the optic nerve, which is surrounded by oligodendrocytes. This difference is an important reason the optic nerve is susceptible to optic neuritis.

 3. Discuss anatomy and blood supply of retina.

Anatomy of Retina

- Retina extends from the optic disc to the ora serrata. The total surface area is about 266 mm^2.
- The retina can be divided into the optic disc, macula lutea, and the periphery.
- *Optic disc:* It measures 1.5 mm in diameter. Here all the retinal layers terminate except the nerve fiber layer (NFL) which continues into the optic nerve.
- *Macula lutea/area centralis:* It is the yellow area, measuring 5.5 mm in diameter, located temporal to the optic disc. It corresponds to 15° of visual field.
- *Fovea centralis:* It is the central depressed part of the macula. It is 1.5 mm in diameter and corresponds to 5° of visual field. It is the most sensitive part of the retina.
- *Foveola:* Forms the center of the fovea. It is 0.15 mm thick.
- *Ora serrata:* The peripheral part which forms the junction of the retina and the ciliary body.
  - *Dentate processes:* These are the tooth-like extensions of the retina on the pars plana.

Microscopic Structure

There are 10 layers from outside to inward:
1. RPE
2. Layer of rods and cones
3. External limiting membrane
4. Outer nuclear layer (ONL)
5. Outer plexiform layer (OPL)
6. Inner nuclear layer (INL)
7. Inner plexiform layer (IPL)
8. Ganglion cell layer (GCL)
9. NFL
10. Internal limiting membrane (ILM).

Blood Supply of Retina

The retina receives its nutrition from two discrete circulatory systems:
1. Retinal blood vessels
2. Choroidal blood vessels.
   Both are derived from the ophthalmic artery, which is the first branch of the internal carotid artery.

The major branches of the ophthalmic artery are:
- Central retinal artery
- Posterior ciliary arteries
- Muscular branches.

The retinal blood vessels provide nourishment for the inner retinal layers and carry off waste products from them. The outer retinal layers are avascular and are supplied by diffusion from the choriocapillaris.

- The central retinal artery is an end artery. In the area of the lamina cribrosa, its lumen measures about 170 μm in diameter. Typically, just before its exit from the optic nerve the central retinal artery divides into the superior and inferior papillary arteries, which in turn divide into nasal and temporal quadratic branches.
- The anatomic division of the retinal arteries into superior and inferior halves is usually maintained throughout the retina because normal retinal vessels rarely cross the horizontal raphe.
- The major branch arteries are about 110 μm in diameter as they cross the disc margin. They course within the NFL and GCL of the retina.
- Usually, after the first branch, the retinal arteries contain no elastic fibers and no internal elastic membrane, which are criteria for arteries, and thus the term arterioles is more appropriate.
- No nerve fibers have been found in the media or adventitia of human retinal vessels. Although the ophthalmic artery contains sympathetic nerve fiber endings and therefore is under the control of the autonomic nervous system, apparently no central regulation of the blood flow occurs in the retina itself.
- The retinal arteries and arterioles remain in the inner retina, and only capillaries are found as deep as the INL. The retinal venous drainage of the retina generally follows the arterial supply. The retinal veins (mainly venules) are present in the inner retina, where they occasionally interdigitate with their associated arteries.
- When two vessels cross, the artery usually lies anterior (vitriad) to the vein, and the two vessels share a common adventitial coat. Many more arteriovenous crossings occur temporally than nasally because the nasal vessels assume a much straighter course. The crossings are important because they represent the most common site of branch retinal vein obstructions. The retinal veins drain into the central retinal vein, which also acts as the major efferent channel for the vessels of the optic nerve.
- Near the disc, the retinal veins are approximately 150 μm in diameter.
- In the retina, the capillaries are arranged in laminar meshworks. Depending on the thickness of the retina, the laminar meshwork can vary from three layers at the posterior pole to one layer in the periphery. Like capillary networks elsewhere in the body, the retinal capillaries assume a meshwork configuration to ensure adequate perfusion to all retinal cells.
- The deeper layer has a mesh diameter of about 50 μm (15–130 μm) and the more superficial layer has a slightly larger meshwork of about 65 μm (16–150 μm) diameter. Besides the laminar characteristic of the retinal capillaries, they also show other variations.

- A capillary-free zone is present around each of the larger retinal arteries and veins, but it is more prominent around arteries, where it measures up to 100 µm in diameter.
- In the fovea and the far retinal periphery, retinal capillaries are absent. The foveal avascular area is 400–500 µm in diameter.

 4. Describe anatomy and histology of macula.

Anatomy of Macula

The central area of the retina, or macula, measures approximately 5.5 mm in diameter and is centered between the optic nerve head (ONH) and the temporal vascular arcades. On histologic examination, this area features two or more layers of ganglion cells, accounting for half of all the ganglion cells in the retina. Oxygenated carotenoids, in particular lutein and zeaxanthin, accumulate within the central macula and contribute to its yellow color **(Table 2)**.

- The central 1.5 mm of the macula, which is called the fovea (or fovea centralis), is specialized for high spatial acuity and color vision.
- The fovea has a margin, a downward slope, and a floor known as the foveola, a 0.35-mm diameter region where cones are slender, elongated, and densely packed. At the very center of the foveola is a small depression, 150–200 mm in diameter, known as the umbo.
- Within the fovea is a region devoid of retinal vessels known as the foveal avascular zone (FAZ). The geometric center of the FAZ is often taken to be the center of the macula and thus the point of fixation; it is an important landmark in fluorescein angiography (FA).
- Surrounding the fovea is the parafovea, a ring 0.5 mm in width where the GCL, INL, and OPL (also known as Henle fiber layer) are thickest. Surrounding this zone is the perifovea, a ring approximately 1.5 mm wide. Thus, the umbo forms the center of the macula, and the periphery of the perifovea forms its margin, which is sometimes referred to as the area centralis.

Histology of Macula

- In foveal region, there are no rods, cones are larger and more in number.
- Rest of the layers are thinner.
- Foveola consists of cones exclusively. The rest of the retinal layers are absent in this layer.
- In the region surrounding the foveola, cones are arranged obliquely (Henle's layer).
- The GCL is 2–6 layers thick.

TABLE 2: Anatomical terminology of the macula (area centralis).

Term	Synonym	Histologic definition	Clinical observation (size)
Macula	Area centralis	Contains two or more ganglion cell layers	Area between vascular arcades 5.5 mm in diameter centered 3.0 mm temporal and 0.8 mm inferior to the center of the optic disc
Fovea	Fovea centralis	A depression in the inner retina, has a margin, slope, and floor, the photoreceptor layer of which is entirely cones	A concave central retinal depression seen on slit lamp examination 1.5 mm in diameter (about 1 disc diameter, or 5°)
Foveola		The floor of the fovea features cones only, arranged in the shape of a cake (gateau nucleaire), where the inner nuclear layer and ganglion cell layers are laterally displaced	0.35 mm in diameter, usually smaller than the foveal avascular zone
Umbo	Fixation light reflex	Small (150–200 µm) center of the floor of the foveola; features elongated cones forming a bouquet of cones	Observed point corresponding to the normal light reflex but not solely responsible for this light reflex
Parafovea		Margin, where the ganglion cell layer, inner nuclear layer, and Henle layer is thickest (i.e., the retina is thickest)	Ring 0.5 mm in width surrounding the fovea
Perifovea		From the outermost limit of the parafovea to the outer limit of the macula	Ring 1.5 mm in width surrounding the parafovea

5. Discuss the anatomy and development of the macula. Describe different zones of macula and their clinical importance.

Kindly refer **Table 2**.

6. Discuss the importance of IS/OS (inner segment/outer segment) junction.

Inner Segment/Outer Segment Junction

- The IS of each photoreceptor is comprised of IS myoid and IS ellipsoid (IS el).
- The IS el is the distal-most portion of the IS and adjacent to the IS/OS junction.
- About 75% of the content of the IS el is tightly packed with mitochondria (long, thin, and bundled parallel in a healthy retina).
- The IS and OS are connected by a cilium, measuring approximately 0.25 µm by 1 µm, which is composed of microtubules.
- A narrow gap can be seen (50–200 nm) on electron microscopy imaging and separates the IS from the OS.
- The passage, which includes the connecting cilium is called IS/OS junction.
- The ovoid mitochondria with multiple internal membranes (cristae) were thought to contribute to a high refractive index in this region and optically serve as microlenses.
- The optical coherence tomography (OCT) back reflection from the IS/OS junction seems to arise from the abrupt change in the optical index of refraction at the IS/OS junction, and the IS el mitochondria (lipid-rich) are thought to contribute to the high refractive index of the IS.
- Advances in the OCT technology-enabled details of retinal microstructural changes associated with various retinal disorders, in particular the integrity of photoreceptor layers as visualized using OCT has been demonstrated to have a more robust correlation with visual acuity (VA) than retinal thickness measurements alone.
- It has drawn attention to the continuity of these layers as possible predictive indicators of VA in various conditions that affect macula.
- Currently available spectral domain OCT has an axial resolution between 4 and 7 µm. And transverse resolution of approximately 15 µm. It enables delineation of four hyper-reflective bands in outer macula.
- The term "ZONE" defines anatomic regions without recognized histopathological correlation to a specific retinal layer.
- The ellipsoid zone (EZ) was previously referred to as IS/OS junction and it is now thought to be formed mainly by mitochondria within ellipsoid layer of outer portion of IS of photoreceptors.
- Outer retinal bands (ORL) from innermost to outermost include ELM, EZ, interdigitation zone (IZ), and RPE band.

Importance

- Attenuation, discontinuity, and disruption of these bands have been reported as likely hallmarks of photoreceptor dysfunction or damage in a variety of retinal diseases.
- *In dry age-related macular degeneration (AMD):* Disruption of EZ has been associated with VA impairment and may occur with progression of drusen or regression of subretinal drusenoid deposits.
- *In neovascular AMD:* Integrity of EZ at baseline was reported as a positive prognostic factor for visual outcome following three monthly injections of anti-vascular endothelial growth factor (VEGF).
- *In diabetic macular edema (DME):* EZ disruption at fovea was reported as an important predictor of VA and progression of DR.
- *In full-thickness macular holes (FTMH):* After vitrectomy for FTMH, outer foveal photoreceptors disruptions are typically apparent on OCT and are associated with cystic spaces in outer retinal layers of the fovea.
- *In epiretinal membrane (ERM):* Preoperative disruptions of EZ were associated with poorer VA results postoperatively.

7. Discuss foveal avascular zone.

Anatomy and Development

Foveal avascular zone is located inside the fovea and varies from 600 to 1,000 µm.
- Surrounding the fovea are parafoveal and perifoveal areas about 0.5 mm and 1.5 mm in diameter. In the parafoveal region, the GCL, INL, and OPL are the thickest.

- The FAZ is defined when the superior temporal and inferior temporal quadrantic arteries (above and below, respectively) meet along the raphe in temporal retina sometime between 25 and 28D, approximately.
- FAZ forms at 37 weeks of gestation and continues to undergo remodeling up to approximately 15 months after birth.
- Small or absent FAZ was found in all preterm infants who had a gestational age of ≤30 weeks, and a normal FAZ was found in all infants who had a gestational age of ≥36 weeks.
- The macular pigment appears at about 17 weeks of gestational age and is believed to drive the formation of the FAZ. Its spatial distribution is correlated with the size of the FAZ.
- The fovea is made up of the cone photoreceptors and Müller cells, and the rod photoreceptors are absent from the central fovea.
- The Müller cells inhibit the migration of astrocytes into the central fovea so that an astrocyte-free zone is formed.
- The astrocyte-free zone plays an important role in forming the FAZ because astrocytes induce the migration of retinal vessel cells across the retina.

Detection

Foveal avascular zone is visible on:
- Fundus fluorescein angiography (FFA)
- Optical coherence tomography angiography (OCTA)

Fundus fluorescein angiography could only highlight the superficial FAZ not deeper vascular layers.

Optical coherence tomography angiography provided with noninvasive, dyeless, and in-depth evaluation of FAZ. OCTA could assess not only the superficial capillary plexus (SCP) and FAZ but also the deep capillary plexus (DCP) and its FAZ. OCTA enables us to measure and define FAZ characteristics across the three superficial (SCP), middle (MCP), and deep (DCP) capillary plexuses.

- The SCP had its upper boundary located 3 μm below the ILM and lower boundary located 15 μm below the IPL. Meanwhile, DCP had its upper boundary 15 μm below IPL and its lower boundary located 70 μm below IPL.
- In superficial retinal plexus, the border of the FAZ is well-delineated, and vascular network distribution is coarse and related to retinal blood vessel distribution. Meanwhile, the border of FAZ in deep retinal plexus is indistinct with fine and compact distribution of its vascular network.
- The OCTA is believed to be more accurate than the FA to demarcate and measure the FAZ, as it is not obscured by leakages, pooling, or staining from fluorescein. However, shadows from hemorrhage and macular edema may affect the FAZ measurements by the OCTA.
- *Gender distribution of FAZ:* It is reported that females have larger vertical and horizontal diameters in both superficial and deep FAZ except horizontal diameter in deep FAZ.
- Because the FAZ is avascular, it is more deformable and more elastic than the rest of the vascularized retina.
- The FAZ appears to be specified by local expression of the antiangiogenic pigment epithelium-derived factor (PEDF) by ganglion cells at the incipient fovea and in the emerging fovea during its formation.

Function and Clinical Implication

- The intact microvascular structure of the FAZ is critical for providing a satisfactory visual function.
- Macular ischemia is often diagnosed by disruption and irregularities of FAZ.
- Visual impairment resulting from ischemic maculopathy secondary to diabetic retinopathy (DR) or retinal venous occlusions is clearly associated with disruption of the FAZ architecture.
- *Normal FAZ:* FAZ in normal individual was described in the OCTA as an intact well-demarcated round or oval area of reduced capillary density with a border without gaps, holes, or interruption of the capillary network in both superficial and deep plexuses. Its normal longest diameter is located either on vertical or horizontal axis. The FAZ diameters in normal individuals are similar in SCP, MCP, and DCP.
- *Foveal hypoplasia:* Conditions associated with foveal hypoplasia are albinism, aniridia, ROP, and achromatopsia.
- ROP has smaller foveal pits coupled with a smaller or even an absent FAZ.
- Albinism is known to lack a FAZ and to have pronounced foveal hypoplasia.
- FAZ enlargement can be used as an index of nonperfusion, which could be translated to ischemia of central retina. The FAZ shape is identical in the OCTA and FA, and the FAZ size was correlated in both.
- In diabetics, the FAZ is enlarged due to vasculature disintegrity.
- The FAZ often appeared to be asymmetrical due to gaps, holes, or interruption of the capillary networks which form an irregular circle with hyporeflection that demarcates the enlarged FAZ.

- Maximum diameter of the FAZ was usually neither on the horizontal nor on the vertical axis. Additionally, the FAZ diameters are not the same in SCP, MCP, and DCP.
- Furthermore, the FAZ is enlarged in diabetics not only before developing apparent DR but even before systemic diagnosis of diabetes mellitus (DM), so it could also be used as a predictor for whom may need closer follow-up.
- DME patients with larger FAZ were reported to be nonresponders to laser therapy, who may benefit more from anti-VEGF treatment.

8. Write short note on contrast sensitivity.

Contrast sensitivity is the ability to perceive slight changes in luminance between regions which are not separated by definite borders.

Types of Contrast Sensitivity

- *Spatial contrast sensitivity:* Spatial contrast is a physical dimension, optical parameter referring to the light-dark transition of a border or an edge in an image that delineates the existence of a pattern or an object.

  As visual activity is ability to resolve fine detail in well-illuminated, high-contrast black and white patterns. A contrast sensitivity function is derived by measuring the lowest detectable contrast across a range of spatial frequencies.

  Contrast = $I_{max} - I_{min}/I_{max} + I_{min}$

  Where, I_{max} = Brightness of background; I_{min} = Brightness of object.

  Thus, for perfectly black letters (100% nonreflecting) on perfectly white paper (100% reflecting) → contrast is equal to 100% as seen in Snellen's visual activity charting.
- *Temporal contrast sensitivity:* The contrast sensitivity function is generated for time-related (temporal) processing in the visual system by showing a uniform target field modulated sinusoidal in time rather than a function of spatial position.

Common Contrast Sensitivity Tests

- *Sine wave gratings:*
  - Functional acuity contrast test (FACT)
  - Visitech VCTS chart
  - CSV1000
  - Sine wave grating tests in chart form
- *Low contrast optotype tests:*
  - Lea test
  - Pelli Robson letter chart
  - Melbourne edge test
  - Mars letter contrast sensitivity test
  - Cambridge low contrast gratings.

Procedure

Should employ:
- Criterion-free procedure
- Uniform progression of contrast
- Adequate number of trials at each contrast
- Reliable sensitivity estimate.

Sine wave greetings tend to be less reliable as they provide limited number of trials at several spatial frequencies. Accurate measurement requires hundreds of trials and >1 hour.

Newer modalities → 50–100 trials (duration 5–10 minutes); and based on Bayesian adaptive test procedure uses adaptive Bayesian statistics to select optimum spatial frequencies and contrast to fit the free parameters.

Factors Affecting Contrast Sensitivity

- Refractive errors—higher frequencies affected
- Age—decreases with age
- Lenticular changes—reduces low spatial frequencies

- Ocular and systemic diseases—decreased in retinal, optic nerve, visual pathway diseases, glaucoma, ocular hypertension, multiple sclerosis, DM, and amblyopia.

 9. Write short note on retinal pigment epithelium.

Anatomy

- The RPE is a monolayer of hexagonal cells extending from the margin of the optic disc to the ora serrata, where it is continuous with the pigmented epithelium of the pars plana of the ciliary body.
- The RPE cells are cuboidal in cross-section and joined near their apical margins by junctional complexes that include maculae and zonulae adherents (intermediate spot and belt junctions, respectively), as well as zonulae occludentes (tight belt junctions).
- In the zonulae occludentes between adjacent RPE cells, the plasma membranes are fused and are impermeable to water and ions. These continuous belts of tight junctions constitute the outer blood–retinal barrier, which blocks extracellular movement of water, ions, and macromolecules between the choriocapillaris and the subretinal space.
- The RPE cells are essential for photoreceptor health and have several other functions, including vitamin A metabolism and regeneration in the visual cycle, phagocytosis and degradation of shed OS tips, light absorption by melanin granules, heat exchange, secretion of the matrix surrounding the photoreceptor IS and OS, and active transport of materials between the choriocapillaris and the subretinal space.
- The RPE cells are smaller (approximately 10–14 μm diameter) and contain more melanin in the macula, and are flatter and wider (up to 60 μm diameter) with less pigment in the periphery. Photoreceptor density also varies across the retina, but a relatively constant ratio of 45 photoreceptors per RPE cell is found in all retinal regions.
- Each RPE cell is polarized with an apical part adjacent to the subretinal space and a basal portion facing Bruch's membrane (BM). The apical surface has numerous long microvilli that envelop the photoreceptor OS and are involved in phagocytosis of shed OS tips.
- The apical portion also contains numerous cytoplasmic filaments, microtubules, and football-shaped melanin granules. The melanin is thought to absorb stray light, decreasing light scatter within the eye.
- The midportion of the RPE cell contains the nucleus, cytoplasmic organelles for protein synthesis (ribosomes, rough endoplasmic reticulum, and Golgi apparatus), smooth endoplasmic reticulum, phagosomes containing OS tips undergoing digestion by lysosomal enzymes, and lipofuscin granules.
- The lipofuscin granules, which increase in number with normal aging, represent residual OS lipids incompletely digested by lysosomal activity. The lipofuscin granules are autofluorescent and are relatively sparse in the RPE of children. RPE cells in older eyes are engorged with lipofuscin granules, which also contain incompletely digested melanin granules. The highest density of RPE lipofuscin is found in the macula; this high concentration of lipofuscin granules may compromise RPE functions and has been suggested to cause macular degeneration.
- The lateral and basal surfaces of the RPE cells are highly specialized, containing a variety of different receptors and ion channels. The RPE basal surfaces are infolded, increasing the area of the RPE surface membrane. The basal RPE surface rests on a basal lamina that forms the innermost layer of BM. The other layers of BM are the inner collagenous, elastin, outer collagenous, and the basal lamina.

Physiology

The RPE cells have electrogenic sodium–potassium pumps in the apical membrane and chloride bicarbonate exchange transporters in the basal membrane. The net effect of the pumps, transport systems, and passive ion channels is movement of water across the RPE in a retina-to-choroid direction, promoting adhesion of the neurosensory retina to the RPE.

Functions of Retinal Pigment Epithelium

- *Cellular junction and cytoskeleton:* Actin (7 nm), microtubules (25 nm), and intermediate filaments (10 nm)
- *Bruch's membrane synthesis and remodeling:* BM nutrition and excretion from retina. Collagen XVIII → Endostatin → inhibits choroidal neovascular membrane (CNVM)
- *Light absorption:* Melanin absorbs stray photons, sharpens vision, and inhibits photo-oxidative stress
- *Phagocytosis of OS receptor:* Receptor mediated recognition → attachment → internalize → degradation. Cathepsin D and S

- Roll in visual cycle
- Protection from oxidative stress
- *Maintains avascular outer retina:* PEDF, COL XVIII.
- Immune privilege and immune response
- Nutrients ion and water transport
- Secretion of cytokines and growth factors.

Growth Factors by Retinal Pigment Epithelium

- *PEDF:* Neuroprotection neurogenesis and antiangiogenesis
- *VEGF:* Angiogenesis, endothelial cell survival factor, and maintenance of choriocapillaries fenestrations
- *NGF (nerve growth factor):* Survival and maintenance of sympathetic and sensory neurons ocular immune response
- *BDNF (brain-derived neurotrophic factor):* Survival and growth of neurons
- *NT-3 (neurotrophin-3):* Neurogenesis stimulus
- *IGF-1 (insulin-like growth factor):* Myelination, neuroprotection, and synaptogenesis
- NPD 1 (neuroprotectin-1)
- TGF (transforming growth factor)-beta
- GM-CSF (granulocyte-macrophage colony-stimulating factor)
- *MCP-1 (monocyte chemotactic protein-1):* Monocyte chemoattractant
- FGF (fibroblast growth factor) and HGF (hepatocyte growth factor)
- Interleukin-6 and 8.

 10. Discuss macular pigments in health and disease.

Macular Pigments

Macular pigment is a generic term used to describe the yellow pigment composed principally of three isomeric carotenoids:
1. Lutein
2. Zeaxanthin
3. Meso-zeaxanthin (MZ)

Highest levels of MP: Henle's fibers at fovea, INL at parafovea.

Main Function
- Optical filter for blue light
- Antioxidant protection by decreased peroxidation of long-chain polyunsaturated fatty acid (PUFA)
- Veiling luminance.

Dominance in Normal Population
- Lutein (L)—peripheral macula
- Zeaxanthin (Z)—mid peripheral macula
- MZ—epicenter of macula
  At fovea L:Z ratio is 1:2.4. (Serum L:Z is 3:1).
  Hydroxyl (-OH) in carotenoids can pass blood–brain barriers (BBB) and ocular barriers.
  Stereo isomeric forms: Lutein = 8 and Zeaxanthin = 3.
  Z and MZ: More capable of eliminating reactive oxygen species (ROS). But L:Z:MZ—1:1:1, 1 is essential.

Antioxidative Properties
- Quenching singlet oxygen
- Triplet state photosensitizers
- Decreased peroxidation of membrane phospholipids
- Scavenging ROS
- Decrease the lipofuscin formation.

Optical Properties
- Filtration of blue light (400–500 nm)
- *Reduces chromatic aberration:* Enhances visual equity and contrast sensitivity.
- Reduces discomfort with glare.
- Improves photo stress recovery time.
- Improves macular function and neural processing speed.

Clinical Measurement
- *Psychophysical methods:*
  - Heterochromatic flicker photometry
  - Motion photometry
- *Optical methods:*
  - Autofluorescence spectrometry
  - Imaging reflectometry
  - Raman spectrometry.

Macular Pigmentary Changes in Diseases

- *AMD:* Low-grade inflammation and hypoxia in outer retina → oxidative stress → AMD. Inverse relationship between dietary intake of L and Z and risk of AMD. Age-related eye disease studies (AREDS), Rotterdam study. Taurine, omega-3 fatty acids, zinc, antioxidant, lutein (TOZAL) study.
- *ROP:* level of oxygen → Production of hypoxia inducible factor, and VEGF.
  Trials have shown 50% reduction in progression of early to threshold ROP with L, Z supplementation.
- *DR:* Prolonged hyperglycemia → oxidative stress.
  L and Z can block pathways by quenching oxygen radicals.
  Neuroprotective activities of Lutein prevent neuronal losses.
  Hu et al. L/Z supplementation in DR → increased macular pigment optical density (MPOD), better visual equity, and improved macular edema.
- *Cataract:* Trials have shown delayed progression of cataract following L/Z supplementation.

 11. Write short note on phosphenes.

Glowing visual sensations evoked by stimuli other than luminance changes are called phosphenes.

It can be spontaneous or provoked.
- Gentle pressure on eyelids
- Electric/magnetic stimulation
- Stimulation of cortex.
  Prolonged visual deprivation → increased cortical excitability to incoming visual input.
  Various forms of patterns: Sparks, glowing circles or part of it, spiral moving in concentric circles.
  Retinal phosphenes include self-illumination, pressure or mechanical phosphenes, electrical phosphenes, radiation phosphenes, and light energy induced phosphenes.

Conditions Associated with Phosphenes

- *Optic neuritis:* Mechanical aggravation of a damaged or inflamed optic nerve. An early sign of optic nerve demyelination in multiple sclerosis.
- *Severe myopia:* Changes in eye pressure and vitreous traction → stimulates visual cells mechanically leading to phosphenes. Preluding retinal detachment.
- *Migraine:* Prominent symptom—Phosphenes + Aura
- Associated with retrochiasmal disorders
- Associated with pharmacological agents. For example, ivabradine (narcotic-induced anesthesia).
- *Leber's and vitamin-A deficiency:* Inappropriate and constant activation of opsin
- *Electric stimulation of visual cortex:* Both in blind and seeing subjects. Transcranial magnetic stimulation (TMS)

12. Write short note on color vision theories.

The different theories of color vision are:
- *The trichromatic theory:* Thomas Young and Hermann Van Helmholtz
- Granit's dominator and modulator theory
- Herring's opponent color theory.

Trichromatic Theory

Suggested by Young and modified by Helmholtz. So, it is also called Young–Helmholtz theory. According to this theory, there are three types of cones with different pigments:
1. Erythrolabe (Porphyropsin = red)—maximum absorption at 565 nm
2. Chlorolabe (Lodopsin = green)—maximum absorption at 535 nm
3. Cyanolabe (Cyanopsin = blue)—maximum absorption at 440 nm

According to the theory, any color consists of a mixture of the three primary colors in varying proportions. So, the identification of each color is by the relative frequency of impulse from each cone.
- Fails to explain the black sensation as black is considered a color too.
- Fails to explain how peripheral color-blind zones perceive yellow–white or gray sensations.

Granit's Dominator and Modulator Theory

With help of microelectrodes into ganglion cells.
- *Dominators:* (Y ganglion cells) detects the intensity of light (not frequency, color). Response to whole visual spectrum
- *Modulators:* (X ganglion cells)
  - Blue 450–470 nm
  - Green 520–540 nm
  - Red-yellow.

Herring's Opponent Color Theory

Extension of trichromatic theory: According to this theory, some colors are "mutually exclusive."
- *Four primary colors:* Red, yellow, blue, and green.
- *Stimulus (light):* One sensation on breakdown and one sensation on resynthesis.
- Complementary colors become antagonistic to their respective primary color.

Methods to Check Color Vision

- ISHIHARA pseudoisochromatic plates—16, 24, 38 plates
  Red-green color deficiency:
  - 1st plate—demonstration/malingerers
  - Transformation (2–9th)—appears different to color deficient subject
  - Vanishing (10–17th)—not seen by color deficit
  - Hidden digit (18–21st)—ony individual with colour vision could recognise figure, Normal person cannot
  - Diagnostic (22–25th)—seen by normal
- American Optical Company (Hardy, Rand Rittler)
- City university test
- The standard pseudo-isochromatic plates
- *Anomaloscope:* Gold standard
  The subject is asked to mix red and green colors in adequate proportion to match the yellow color disc.
- *Farnsworth Munsell D-15 test:* Patient is asked to arrange 15 colored discs in sequential order.
- *F-M 100 Hue test:* 85–88 movable color in four boxes and 22 colors
- Holmgren's wool test
- Eldridge Green Lantern.

13. Describe the mechanism of dark adaptation with respect to anatomy and physiology involved.

- Dark adaptation refers to the ability of the visual system (both rods and cones mechanisms) to recover sensitivity to the decreasing surrounding background light.
- The time taken to see in dim illumination is called "dark adaptation time". The rods are much more sensitive to illumination than cones.
- Dark adaptometry can be performed by instruments called photometers or adaptometers, which can control and vary the amount of light entering the eye to a definite and known extent.
- *Procedure:* The retina is exposed to an intense light for a time sufficient to bleach 25% or more of rhodopsin (1,500 mLb) → following this, the normal rods become insensitive to light → cones only respond to very bright stimuli → subsequent recovery of light sensitivity can be monitored by placing the subject in the dark and periodically exposing them to spots of light of varying intensity in the visual field and asking if they are perceived.
- The intensity of the flashes can be controlled by neutral density filters. The readings are repeated till no further rise in sensitivity is noted and the results are plotted in log units of brightness against time.

Dark Adaptation Curve

- Normal curves indicating central retinal field are biphasic with:
  - Initial rapid segment of cone function (cone adaptation)
  - Second slower segment of rod function (rod adaptation)
- The kink on the curve is called the rod-cone break (alpha point).
- Dark adaptation takes 15–30 minutes. The alpha point occurs after 7–10 minutes of dark adaptation.

Mechanisms of Dark Adaptation

- *Neutral adaptation:* It is fast, and represents reversal of neutral light adaptation of photoreceptors and other retinal cells.
- *Photochemical adaptation:* It is slow, and involves pigment regeneration.
  The process of adaptation is primarily based on changes in visual pigment.

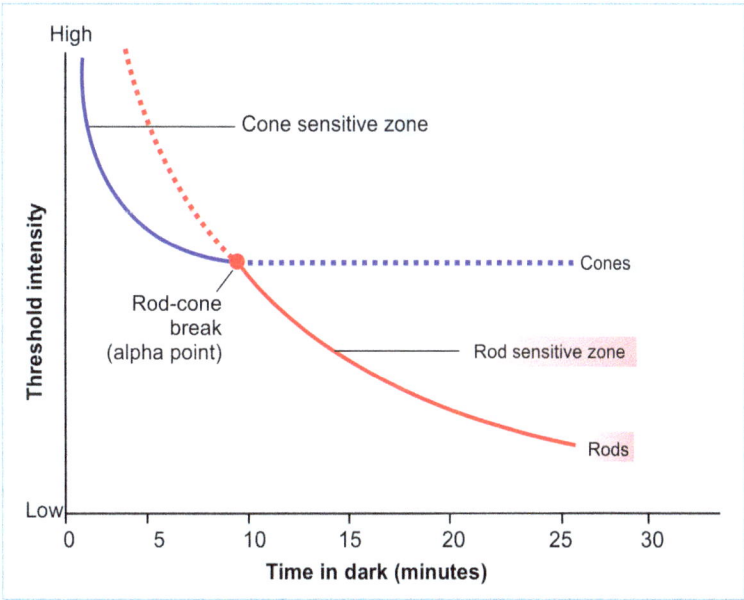

- *Photoreceptor behavior to light:*
  - In the steady state of equilibrium, a high density of Na-K$^+$ pumps enables the photoreceptor to maintain a constant intracellular concentration of Na$^+$ and K$^+$.
  - An outward K$^+$ current through nongated K$^+$ selective channels, tends to hyperpolarize the photoreceptors at about –70 mV.
  - An inward Na$^+$ current carried by cyclic guanosine monophosphate (cGMP) gated sodium channels, called "dark current" depolarizes the cell to around –40 mV.

- Changes in the relative polarization of the photoreceptor cells, results in adaptations to different background illuminance.
- In the dark, cGMP levels are high and keep Na^+ channels open allowing a steady inward current called dark current.
- The dark current keeps the cell depolarized → depolarization opens the voltage-gated calcium channels → increased intracellular Ca^{+2} causes vesicles of glutamate to merge with cell membrane and release it into synaptic cleft.
- Photoreceptor cells are depolarized in the dark and this relative switching off activates the next cell.
- Light stimulation of photoreceptor brings about a cascade of reactions at molecular level, conversion of 11-cis-retinaldehyde to All- trans configuration.
- Light-activated rhodopsin now interacts with transducin → promotes release of phosphodiesterase (inhibitory) → breaks down cGMP to 5-cGMP → lowered cGMP concentration leads to closure of Na^+ channels → hyperpolarization of the cells. → decrease in release of excitatory neurotransmitter glutamate from the channel.

- *The absolute threshold values of dark adaptation depend on:*
  - State of adaptation
  - Stimulus variables
  - Methodological variables
  - Variability of sensitivity of retina depending on retinal location.

14. Describe iridofundal coloboma.

Introduction

- Ocular colobomata are caused by defective embryogenesis.
- Coloboma generally results from a failure of the fetal or choroidal fissure to close during the 5-7th week of fetal life, at the 7-14 mm stage.
- This is the period between the invagination of the optic vesicle and the closure of the fetal fissure. Almost any ocular structure may be involved, including the cornea, iris, ciliary body, zonule (lens), choroid, retina, optic disc, and/or optic nerve.
- Failure of a portion of the fetal fissure to close results in the defect we recognize as an ocular coloboma; disc coloboma results from nonclosure of the most anterior portion of the optic stalk.

Clinical Features

Typical/Atypical

- The "typical" coloboma is in the inferonasal quadrant, caused by defective closure of the fetal fissure. It is the most frequent.
- Coloboma located anywhere other than the inferonasal quadrant of the globe is termed "atypical".

Complete/Incomplete

- A complete iris coloboma is a full-thickness defect, involving both the pigment epithelium and the iris stroma. It may be:
  - Total, extending to the iris root and giving rise to the "keyhole pupil", or
  - Partial, involving only the pupillary margin and causing a slightly oval pupil.
- An incomplete iris coloboma is usually partial thickness, involving either the pigment epithelium or the iris stroma. It tends to be wedge-shaped and is best demonstrated by iris transillumination.

Posterior Segment Coloboma

- The inner layers of the fetal fissure, comprising progenitor neuroretinal cells, are approximated at its margins, normally closing during the 5th or 6th week of gestation. The neuroretinal cells then completely cover the inside of the globe. Failure of simultaneous fusion of the outer layers—the future RPE—leads to coloboma involving both the RPE and the neurosensory retina.
- *Coloboma of choroid* is infrequent, occurring in only 0.14%. Histological findings include absence of the RPE. The overlying retina is hypoplastic and gliotic, and sometimes has rosettes. Where retinal tissue is recognizable, the retinal layers are reversed, with the rods and cones facing inward and the NFL adjacent to the sclera. The underlying

choroid is either hypoplastic or absent altogether. Whereas, the RPE at the edge of the defect is hyperplastic. The thin sclera may have cystic spaces filled with glial proliferation, sometimes exuberant enough to resemble a neoplasm.
- *Macular coloboma* is usually bilateral, symmetrical, circumscribed, and excavated defects that involve both the choroid and retina.
  They have been classified into three main types:
  1. Pigmented macular coloboma
  2. Nonpigmented macular coloboma
  3. Macular coloboma associated with abnormal vessels
- The visual prognosis depends primarily on the involvement of the optic nerve, macula, and papillomacular bundle.
- Retinochoroidal colobomata induce absolute scotomata if they are severe. Macular colobomata are associated with loss of central vision.
- *Coloboma of optic nerve:* Retinochoroidal colobomata can involve both the macula and the optic nerve to varying degrees. Isolated optic disc colobomata present as enlarged, white, sharply delineated, bowl-shaped excavations of the disc, 2–8 D in depth.
- Optic disc involvement has been classified into six types, increasing in severity from a normal disc outside the chorioretinal coloboma as the mildest form to a nonidentifiable disc shape with blood vessels emerging from the superior border of a large chorioretinal coloboma.

Complications

- Retinal detachment and cataract are the most common complications associated with retinochoroidal coloboma.
- Rhegmatogenous retinal detachments (RRDs) have been reported in 4–40% of cases, usually because of breaks within or adjacent to the coloboma. Histologic sections indicate that a central break in the inner layer of the retina and a break in the outer layer at the margin of the coloboma are both necessary to produce rhegmatogenous detachment.
- Non-RRD occurs, usually after infancy, in two-thirds of individuals with autosomal dominant, isolated optic nerve coloboma.
- A variety of cataracts have been associated with coloboma, including isolated pigment clumping on the lens capsule at the equator, subcapsular and cortical opacification, anterior and posterior polar cataracts, and total opacification. Lens subluxation occurs infrequently.
- Secondary glaucoma (and related angle abnormalities), amblyopia, anisometropia, and sensory strabismus may occur.

Evaluation and Treatment

Iris Coloboma

- Because the iris defects themselves impose no visual defect; treatment is indicated only for cosmesis. One useful approach is to fit a cosmetic contact lens that resembles a normal iris and is designed to match the fellow eye in appearance. Such lenses can be optically corrective. Cosmetic contact lenses also are useful for microcornea associated with coloboma and microphthalmia.
- Surgical repair is not generally performed unless other intraocular surgery is indicated. After implantation, the coloboma may be repaired with nonabsorbable sutures.
- Repair of iris coloboma is helpful to provide a stable platform for anterior chamber (AC) lens implantation and may prevent progressive synechia formation and secondary angle closure.

Retinochoroidal Coloboma (Table 3)

- In patients under 30 years of age, coloboma-associated retinal detachments are more common in males.
- Prophylactic laser treatment applied posteriorly along the edge of the coloboma and cryopexy anteriorly has been recommended.
- In cases requiring surgery, the preferred initial treatment is laser photocoagulation (LPC). Vitrectomy and air-fluid exchange with a buckle may be indicated subsequently, and are more successful than scleral buckling alone.
- Cases with associated severe microphthalmia, treatment during infancy with cosmetic scleral shells may be helpful.

Differential Diagnosis

- Iris abnormalities in aniridia, heterochromia irides, iris nevi, iris trauma, iris atrophy, and Rieger syndrome can mimic a coloboma.

TABLE 3: Classification of retinochoroidal coloboma.

Ida Mann classification	
Type 1	Coloboma extending above the anatomic disc
Type 2	Coloboma extending up to the superior border of the disc
Type 3	Coloboma extending below the lower border of the disc
Type 4	Coloboma involving the disc only
Type 5	Coloboma below the disc with normal retina between
Type 6	Pigmented lesion in periphery
Type 7	Coloboma in extreme periphery
Lingam Gopal classification	
Type 1	Normal optic disc located outside the coloboma
Type 2	Abnormal optic disc located outside the coloboma
Type 3	Colobomatous disc located outside the coloboma
Type 4	Normal disc located within the coloboma
Type 5	Colobomatous disc located within the coloboma
Type 6	No recogizable disc within the coloboma

- Retinochoroidal colobomata are easily differentiated from inflammatory lesions and all the other causes of leukocoria.
- Congenital optic pits and optic nerve staphylomata can also be confused with optic nerve colobomata.

 15. Write short note on optic nerve head drusen.

- Optic disc drusen are a form of calcific degeneration in some of the axons of the optic nerve.
- *Pattern of inheritance:*
  - Genetically, optic disc drusen have an autosomal dominant pattern of inheritance.
  - Inheritance of small optic disc size is thought to be a risk factor in drusen formation. They appear more often in whites and rarely in blacks.
  - Small inherited optic disc size and mesodermal dysplasia resulting in vascular dysplasia are factors that may influence the development of optic disc drusen.

Clinical Symptoms and Signs

- Most patients with optic disc drusen are asymptomatic. Up to 8.6% have reported transient visual obscurations.
- *Visual field defects:*
  - Appear in nearly 90% of cases.
  - Majority are peripheral in nature.
  - If progressive and severe, the loss of field can lead to blindness, even in young adults.
  - Progressive central vision loss is rare.
  - Can first appear during childhood; even before drusen appear on the disc.
  - Become more numerous and worsen in degree of severity.
  - The pattern is most commonly an arcuate NFL defect.
- When visible, optic disc drusen look-like yellow crystals within the substance of the ONH. The margins are often indistinct. Papilledema is what optic disc drusen mimic.
- Optic disc drusen, over time, appear as elevated, lumpy irregularities on the anterior-most portion of the disc.
- The nasal optic disc is the usual place exposed drusen are noted. These lesions are bilateral in >85% of cases, buried or visible.
- Cilioretinal arteries are associated with optic disc drusen. Often the scleral canal is small. The optic nerve that contains drusen is anomalous by nature.
- The pathogenesis of optic disc drusen is thought to be due to slowed axoplasmic flow, thus forming calcific excrescences.

- The field defects could arise from pressure on the NFL resulting from a combination of the presence of the optic disc drusen and vascular compromise.

Diagnosis

- Fundoscopic evaluation with direct and indirect ophthalmoscopy
- Visual field testing
- B-scan ultrasonography can expose calcium deposits even if they are invisible ophthalmoscopically. The use of high gain helps to isolate optic disc drusen.
- FA is also useful. In the preinjection phase optic disc drusen demonstrate autofluorescence. In the late phase, staining is observed.
- Computed tomography (CT) and even facial X-rays can show the presence of calcium in the optic nerve, but small lesions can be missed.
- Electroretinograms are useful when NFL and VA are subnormal.
- Visual evoked potentials (VEPs) are abnormal in >95% of cases due to peripapillary NFL malfunction, P100 latency is prolonged.
- *Newer technologies:* OCT, GDx (scanning laser polarimetry), and Heidelberg retinal tomography (HRT) are commercially available. These tests examine NFL thickness. NFL loss is a pathologic finding observed with optic disc drusen.

Complications of Optic Nerve Head Drusen

- Pathologic vascular abnormalities occur in a variety of ways in association with optic disc drusen.
- Optociliary shunts are collateral networks that form between the retinal venous system and the choroidal network as a result of increased central retinal venous pressure. As optic disc drusen enlarge with age shunt vessels become more apparent.
- Vascular occlusions can occur due to the structural abnormality of the nerve head. Anterior ischemic optic neuropathy (AION) is the most common cause of visual loss in patients with optic disc drusen.
- Central retinal artery occlusion (CRAO) and central retinal vein occlusion (CRVO) may occur in conjunction with optic disc drusen.
- Peripapillary subretinal neovascularization secondary to optic disc drusen has been reported.
- Other hemorrhages include superficial flame-shaped hemorrhages and deep peripapillary hemorrhages.
- Deeper hemorrhages can appear encircling the disc in the subretinal or subretinal pigment epithelial spaces. The hemorrhages may be due to occult neovascularization, direct venous compression, or vascular wall erosion by sharp-edged drusen.

Systemic diseases associated with drusen:
- Retinitis pigmentosa
- Pseudoxanthoma elasticum
- Angioid streaks.

Treatment of Optic Nerve Head Drusen

- In the presence of visual field loss and optic disc drusen enlargement—intraocular pressure (IOP) lowering medications.
- In case of glaucoma and disc drusen—careful follow-up with serial visual fields, nerve fiber analysis, and repeated IOP testing. Surgical treatment consisting of optic nerve sheath fenestration is controversial.
- LPC of subretinal neovascular membranes should be considered only if central acuity is threatened.

 16. Discuss the role of indocyanine green (ICG) dye in ophthalmology.

Dyes are chemical compounds that bind to various substances in nature to induce color. When dyes color living tissues or cells, they are called vital dyes.

Biochemistry

- Indocyanine green is a tricarbocyanine anionic vital dye with a mass of 775 Da.
- It has amphiphilic properties that allow it to bind to both cellular and acellular elements in living tissues.

- The hydrophilic dye is delivered as a sterile powder, and in 1959 it was approved by the Food and Drug Administration (FDA) for indicator dilution studies and liver function testing.
- Both the absorption and fluorescence maximums of ICG are within the near-infrared range.
- ICG is useful in retinal angiography, because it improves the visualization of choroidal tissues. In ocular surgery, its use remains off-label despite widespread popularity.
- The dye is commercially provided as a powder to achieve final concentrations of 0.05–0.5%.
- It is recommended that the green dye initially be diluted in distilled water before further dilution in saline solution, because of a higher risk of precipitation in saline.

Uses of Indocyanine Green Dye in Ophthalmology

- *In corneal surgery:* ICG was used for assessment of endothelial cell viability. The green dye did not compromise cell integrity, as determined by electron microscopy, when rabbit and human corneal endothelia were exposed to 0.5% ICG for 3 minutes.
- *ICG in keratoplasty [deep lamellar endothelial keratoplasty (DLEK)]:* After dissection and excision of the host posterior stromal disc, including DM and endothelial cells, ICG is used to stain corneal stroma of the donor disc transplanted to the host AC. After being placed by an air bubble, ICG staining allowed visualization of the tissue interface through the host corneal stroma. After 24 hours the ICG disappears from the cornea, with no signs of inflammation.
- *For identification of conjunctival cysts:* ICG can be injected through a 27-gauge needle into the conjunctival cyst. Following the flushing of residual ICG solution, the cyst becomes clearly visible as a green-stained structure.
- *For anterior capsule:* ICG staining for capsule visualization in conditions with poor or no red reflex has been reported since the end of the 1990s, using concentrations ranging from 0.125% to 0.5%.
- *For ILM staining:*
    - ICG adheres well to the extracellular matrix components of the ILM, such as collagen type 4, laminin, and fibronectin.
    - Clinical data showed that macular closure rate may be achieved in 74–100% of patients using ICG-guided ILM peeling.
    - The potential toxic effects of ICG on the retina are:
        - ICG may persist after MH surgery for up to 36 months.
        - Complications of ICG-assisted chromovitrectomy include RPE changes, visual field defects, and optic nerve atrophy, migrating to subretinal space through the MH, causing retinal damage.
    - This high rate of RPE abnormalities may be related to the ICG concentration, technique of application, ICG exposure to light, or a combination of factors. Recent studies have utilized ICG in a concentration of 0.05% and osmolarity around 290 mOsm with few or no signs of RPE toxicity.
    - ICG has been also used to facilitate ILM peeling in other diseases for persistent macular edema from causes such as CRVO, DME, Irvine–Gass syndrome, and vitreomacular traction syndrome. Significant improvement in VA was observed only in patients with DME.
- *For ERMs:*
    - ICG allows better visualization of ERMs in vitrectomy for proliferative diabetic vitreoretinopathy (PDVR), idiopathic ERMs, and proliferative vitreoretinopathy (PVR).

Dye-induced Retinal Toxicity

- The subretinal injection of dyes may be associated with a greater risk of toxicity than intravitreal injection.
- This might be because the presence of Muller glial cells and their basement membrane (ILM) between the vitreous dyes and the neural cells has a blocking effect.
- Visual field defects as a complication after vitrectomy for MH surgery vary in different clinical series from 1% up to 70%.
- Proposed mechanisms include mechanical trauma to the ONH, disturbance of the chorioretinal circulation, and dehydration injury of the NFL during fluid–gas exchange.
- The iodine present in the ICG solution may be responsible for the observed retinal toxicity. Iodine and its derivative compounds such as sodium iodate are highly toxic and a single injection leads to necrosis of practically the complete RPE.
- Cellular damage at the vitreoretinal interface, including nonspecific shrinkage and disruption of the cellular architecture caused by induction of osmotic levels of >500 mOsm.
- The presence of sodium iodine in the ICG solution requires dilution in water, thereby resulting in a hypotonic solution of 248–275 mmol/kg.

- *Light-mediated damage:* The overlap of ICG absorption spectra with different types of endoillumination for vitreoretinal surgery may pose the risk of phototoxicity to the retina.
- Intravitreous ICG along the ILM may enhance light absorption and increase the local temperature on the retina, the so-called photo-oxidation type I. Indeed, photo-oxidation type I with ICG has been reported in the treatment of choroidal neovascularization using photodiode laser.
- First, every vital dye injected intravitreally has a dose-dependent toxicity to the retinal tissue. ICG or IfCG should be injected in concentrations below 0.05%.
- Very low amount of dye injection onto the preretinal membrane, avoidance of long macular exposure to endoillumination, and removal of sodium and iodine from staining solutions by applying IfCG instead of ICG and diluting the dye in glucose 5%

17. Discuss cherry red spot.

A cherry red spot (CRS) is a clinical sign seen in the context of thickening and loss of transparency of posterior pole of the retina.

It is an ophthalmoscopic evidence of pathology that may involve the peripheral layers of the retina and multiple systems of the human body.

Mechanism

- Diseases associated with accumulation of storage material (such as glycolipids or sphingolipids) in the retinal cellular layers result in swelling and loss of transparency of the multilayered ganglion cells giving it a white appearance.
- The foveola, the thinnest part of the retina being almost devoid of ganglion cells, retains its relative transparency allowing the normal choroidal vasculature to be seen through it.
- These histological features result in the appearance of the central red area (normal foveola) that is surrounded by dull halo resulting from attenuation of transparency of the surrounding area.
- Later in the course of the disease, ganglion cell death makes the spot less prominent. Atrophy of retinal NFL and optic atrophy may also follow.
- Occlusion of the central retinal artery is also associated with CRS.
- CRS seen in methanol poisoning is due to macular cystoid edema and in quinine poisoning due to retinal edema.

Clinical Features

It is a fundoscopy finding, visualized on direct ophthalmoscopy or slit lamp biomicroscopy.
- The CRS is visualized as a bright to dull red spot at the center of macula, surrounded and accentuated by a grayish white or yellowish halo. Its color is due to the pigment epithelium and choroid, and therefore may demonstrate color variability according to the race.

Causes of Cherry Red Spot

- CRS is associated with inherited metabolic conditions, CRAO, orbital contusion, and orbital ischemia due to vasospasm.
- In metabolic disorders, it is seen more consistently in certain conditions such as Tay-Sachs disease, Sandhoff's disease, and Sialidosis (evident in most cases by the time psychomotor retardation and mental deterioration set in).
- It may be seen in many cases of Infantile Niemann-Pick disease type IA and GM1 gangliosidosis and occasionally in metachromatic leukodystrophy.
- Other conditions associated with CRS include Farber's disease, Goldberg's disease, Gaucher's disease (infantile form), Hurlers syndrome, mucopolysaccharidosis VII, Hallervorden-Spatz syndrome, cryoglobulinemia, and Leber's congenital amaurosis.
- The CRS varies in its appearance which reflects the differing amounts of substrate and the toxicity of the deposited material.
  - Opaquely white in Tay-Sachs disease and Sandhoff's disease,
  - Faintly gray in Farber's disease, metachromatic leukodystrophy, and
  - More diffuse in Niemann-Pick disease.
- The opacity correlates with the severity of the visual loss in Tay-Sachs and Sandhoff's disease, in contrast to the normal vision in Farber's disease.
- However, late in the course of the disease, the loss of CRS coincides with optic atrophy.

Causes of Cherry Red Spot-like Lesions and Pseudo-Cherry Red Spot

Cherry Red Spot-like Lesion
- Adult Niemann–Pick disease (ring of perifoveal crystalloid deposits)
- Gaucher's disease (atypical macular CRS)
- Lactosylceramidosis (increasing redness of macula)
- Sea blue histiocyte syndrome (perifoveal yellowish-white scintillating granules in doughnut-shaped pattern).

Pseudo-Cherry Red Spot

Conditions such as macular hemorrhage (MH) with retinal detachment could be considered as pseudo-CRS, because the abnormality is in the foveola rather than the parafoveal area.

Management

- *Cherry red spot is seen bilaterally:* In metabolic disorders, quinine and other drug toxicity and, Leber's congenital amaurosis.
- *CRS is seen unilaterally:* In CRAO orbital contusions, MH with retinal detachment, or MH.
- CRS is more commonly associated with CRAO in adults. The age, health of patient, history of trauma or vascular disease, and unilaterality of lesion may help to distinguish it from the metabolic disorders.
- Early diagnosis allows for appropriate counseling and prenatal diagnosis (for example, determination of levels of hexosaminidase A and B levels in Sandhoff's disease).
- CRAO, an ophthalmic emergency, should be treated within 24 hours: treatment options include:
  - Medical and surgical lowering of IOP
  - Carbon dioxide rebreathing, steroids (in vasculitis)
  - Vasodilator drugs
  - Hyperbaric oxygen
  - Antifibrinolytic drugs
  - Barbiturate coma
  - Free radical scavengers, and antioxidants.

 18. Discuss ocular manifestations of leukemia.

- Leukemia is a malignant proliferative disorder of leukopoietic bone marrow stem cells and widespread infiltration of other organs, tissues, and peripheral blood by immature neoplastic leukocytes.
- Ocular disorders have been reported in 30–90% of cases of leukemia.
- *Ophthalmic involvement can be classified into:*
  - *Primary or direct:* Anterior segment, uveal infiltration, orbital infiltration, cranial nerve palsies, and papilledema
  - *Secondary or indirect:* Retinal or vitreous hemorrhage, infections, and vascular occlusions
- Ophthalmic involvement in leukemia is associated with significant ocular morbidity and vision loss.
- Myeloid leukemias were more commonly observed to have ocular manifestations (56%) as compared to lymphoid leukemias (46%).
- Ophthalmic signs in patients suffering from leukemia were described as "leukemic retinopathy".

Primary Manifestations

Orbit and Eyelids

Leukemic cells may infiltrate the soft tissues, extraocular muscles, or lacrimal glands. It is more common in acute lymphoblastic leukemias (ALLs). Eyelids involvement can present with edema, inflammation, chemosis, and pain.

Conjunctiva

Hyperemia and edematization of the lower palpebral conjunction can be unusual sign of ALL.

Sclera

Scleral infiltration is common during ALL, around episcleral vessels.

Cornea

It is hardly ever affected by direct infiltration because cornea is an avascular structure.

Anterior Chamber and Iridocorneal Angle

In ALL, hypopyon has been estimated at 2.5-18% of relapsed cases depending on the stage of the disease. AC involvement in cases of ALL is typically bilateral. The mechanism by which the cells migrate into AC is not clear.
- In children, spontaneous hyphema is also a presentation of leukemia.
- Radiotherapy is warranted in infiltration of AC.

Retina

It is involved in leukemia very commonly. Up to 70% of all patients with leukemia show fundus changes.
- Early manifestations are venous dilatation and tortuosity.
- Other manifestations include retinal vascular sheathing, superficial retinal or intraretinal hemorrhages, and cotton-wool spots comprising "leukemic retinopathy".
- *Retinal hemorrhages:* These may occur in all levels of retina with focal destruction, usually at posterior pole, maybe round or flame-shaped hemorrhages with a white component in the center (consists of leukemic cells and debris, platelet-fibrin aggregates and septic emboli).
- Large leukemic infiltrates can cause total retinal detachment.
- Smaller infiltrates tend to be perivascular.
- Subretinal infiltrates are referred to as subretinal hypopyon.
- Cotton-wool spots are probably due to ischemia from anemia, hyperviscosity, or leukemic infiltration.
- Less frequent manifestations—microaneurysms which tend to be peripheral.
- ILM generally acts as an effective barrier to leukemic cell infiltration.
- Serous retinal detachment may develop as a result of choroidal involvement by leukemic cells or due to incompetence of the outer blood retinal barrier including pigment epithelial changes.

Choroid

It is the most frequently involved ocular tissue in leukemia, but is not clinically apparent.
- Leukemic cell infiltration causes partial occlusion of choriocapillaries and delay of choroidal circulation.
- It can be diffuse or perivascular involvement.
- Overlying retina shows photoreceptor damage, RPE atrophy, and serous retinal detachment (RD), usually affecting posterior pole.

Optic Nerve

- It is usually involved in CNS leukemia (13–18%).
- Symptoms include lethargy, blurred vision, loss of VA, or diplopia when cranial nerves 3, 4, and 6 are affected.
- Papilledema is the most frequent sign of optic nerve involvement. It can be due to direct infiltration of the nerve by leukemic cells, increased IOP, or swelling because of retrolaminar leukemic invasion.
- Optic nerve can also be affected without the presence of papilledema.
- It can also be the first sign of ALL or of extramedullary relapse after remission.
- Involvement carries a poor prognosis.
- Treatment options include intrathecal chemotherapy and radiotherapy.

Secondary Manifestations

Orbit and Eyelids

- These are affected after remission, or secondary to chemotherapy, radiotherapy, or graft-versus-host reaction.
- Lacrimal glands are frequently affected → either by direct infiltration by leukemic cells, graft-versus-host reaction, or radiation causing a tear dysfunction or dry eye.

Conjunctiva

- Hyperviscosity can produce vascular anomalies in conjunctiva, which is more frequent in chronic leukemias.

- Most common involvement of conjunctiva comes from conjunctivitis, secondary to dry eye after a graft-versus-host reaction.
- Dysfunction of the meibomian glands is another common manifestation of chronic graft against host disease.
- Direct toxicity of methotrexate is associated with appearance of keratoconjunctivitis sicca.

Sclera

Occasionally immunocompromised patients suffer opportunistic infectious scleritis.

Cornea

- Drugs used in chemotherapy such as cytarabine produces corneal toxicity by interfering with epitheliums synthesis of deoxyribonucleic acid (DNA).
- Patients with secondary immunosuppression present with infections with herpes and fungi.

Anterior Chamber

- Extramedullary relapse of acute leukemias may masquerade as hypopyon uveitis.
- Ischemia of anterior segment may occur secondary to anemia or hyperviscosity.
- Cataract may develop due to steroids, chemotherapy drugs use, or radiotherapy.

Retina

- Life-threatening opportunistic infections by cytomegalovirus (CMV), herpes, protozoal, and fungal infections are noted.
- CMV is the most common viral infection noted in immunocompromised states. The virus invades the retina causing necrosis, vascular sheathing, hemorrhage, and combined exudative and RRD.
- Other viruses (herpes simplex, varicella zoster, and mumps) can cause necrotizing retinitis.
- Candida typically appears as focal, deep white lesions that may be singular or multiple. It may extend into vitreous causing uveitis and retinitis with characteristic cotton balls in the vitreous.
- Aspergillus is also a common cause of infection in leukemia.

Choroid

Choroid secondary affection is much less common than primary. Retinochoroidal infarction can be seen during the treatment of ALL.

Optic Nerve

- Secondary involvement of optic nerve includes toxicity of chemotherapy, antibiotics, or radiotherapy, ischemia after anemia, opportunistic infections in immunocompromised infections.
  - The treatment of ocular manifestations is difficult because the effect of chemotherapy in the eye is limited. Radiotherapy is frequently used for treatment.

 19. Discuss micropulse retinal laser.

- *Laser interaction with human tissue depends on:*
  - Laser wavelength
  - Pulse duration
  - Irradiance (energy per area)
- *Laser photocoagulation (LPC):* The main laser tissue is a thermal effect due to an increase in the temperature of retinal tissue by 10°C.
  - *First theory:* Photoreceptors require vast amounts of oxygen for normal function → LPC destroys these cells → reduces oxygen consumption by retina and improves oxygenation of the remaining part → consequently, production of VEGF significantly diminishes.
  - *Second theory:* Insertion of laser power on RPE → results in tissue scarring, production of "heat shock proteins" by surrounding laser spot surviving tissue → results in immunomodulation of cell function, normalizes production of certain cytokines → reduces chronic inflammation.
- *Micropulse laser therapy (MPLT):*
  - The micropulse mode is an additional feature of commercially available lasers of different wavelengths: 532 nm, 577 nm, or 810 nm.

- The micropulse laser mode delivers energy in succeeding train of very short pulses, with alternative "on" and "off" times with a duty cycle concept.
- The duty cycle is defined as the length of the time of "power on" divided by the total time laser is used (e.g., 5% duty cycle means that each micropulse of energy is "on" for 100 µs followed by 1,900 µs in the "off" mode).
- This cycle is repeated multiple times within one laser shot, i.e., 100 times with a 5% duty cycle.
- Micropulse laser treatment has been extensively used for selected retinal diseases.
- The idea of subthreshold laser therapy is not to leave any marks on the retina.

- *Laser power settings:*
  - Maximum permissible exposure (MPE)—one-tenth of the laser exposure—is good to produce biological effect.
  - Power level of subthreshold micropulse laser therapy (SMPLT)—two therapeutic approaches exist:
    1. *Laser power titration:* It is recommended to be performed on the border of edematous and healthy retina. The titration method itself bears the risk of overtreatment → resulting in thermal coagulation of retinal tissue.
    2. Setting power to fixed low values (200–300 mW for yellow laser).

- *Clinical applications of SMPLT:*
  - Central serous chorioretinopathy (CSCR)
  - DME
  - Proliferative diabetic retinopathy (PDR)
  - Macular edema secondary to vein occlusion

- *SMPLT in CSCR:* CSCR represents an accumulation of serous fluid under neurosensory retina. It is sometimes accompanied by RPE detachments and alterations of RPE (atrophy or hypertrophy) is characteristic in the chronic form of CSCR.
  - LPC was used in treating chronic cases of CSCR persisting for >4 months or recurrent CSCR.
  - SMPLT improves cell function → thus improving pumping efficacy of RPE. And it also reduces inflammatory processes by reducing the production of cytokines.
  - It was noted that SMPLT was efficacious in improving retinal morphology in chronic CSCR. Complete resolution of SRF is achieved in 60–80% of cases.

- *SMPLT in DME:*
  - Laser photocoagulation for DME is now being used rarely because of side effects of visual field scotomas and secondary choroidal neovascularization.
  - SMPLT is used now as a nondamaging retinal therapy for DME.
  - The possible suggested mechanism of action: Stimulation of retina by SMPLT reduces VEGF levels → consequently most potent proedema factor is compromised.
  - As RPE cell function is improved, the elimination of intraretinal and subretinal fluid is also more efficient.
  - SMPLT is much cheaper, so it would be economically rational to include it in the process of treating DME.

Indications

- Patients reluctant to receive intravitreal injections
- Noncompliant patients
- Patients with contraindicated anti-VEGF therapy due to systemic reasons
- Financial restrictions
- Group of patients with small diabetic edema of short duration and good VA.
- *SMPLT for severe nonproliferative diabetic retinopathy (NPDR) or PDR:* SMPLT PRP works similar to anti-VEGF injections preserving retinal sensitivity.
- *SMPLT in ME secondary to retinal vein occlusion (RVO):* SMPLT is tried as an alternative to LPC and anti-VEGF in macular edema secondary to venous occlusion.
  - It seems to be superior to LPC in improving best-corrected visual acuity (BCVA), as it leaves retinal cells intact.
  - The latest studies do not favor intravitreal ranibizumab against SMPLT in the treatment of ME.
- Therapy by micropulse laser is cheap and safe, highly efficacious in resolving fluid in CSCR.
- The position of laser in DME and ME secondary to RVO is yet to be determined.
- Pan-retinal photocoagulation with SMPLT is currently a form of experimental therapy and its efficacy needs to be confirmed.

20. Write a short note on choroidal effusions (ciliochoroidal effusion, ciliochoroidal detachment, and choroidal detachment).

An abnormal accumulation of fluid in the suprachoroidal space: Hypotony is the main cause of fluid accumulation in the suprachoroidal space after surgery, although inflammation and venous congestion may also be contributing factors. Choroidal effusion further exacerbates hypotony by reducing aqueous humor production and, possibly, by increasing uveoscleral outflow.
- Serous choroidal effusion
- Hemorrhagic choroidal effusion
- Idiopathic ciliochoroidal effusion/uveal effusion syndrome.

Etiological Classification

- *Ocular disorders (specific):*
  - *Tumors:* Primary, metastatic
  - Nanophthalmos
- *Ocular inflammations:*
  - Scleritis
  - Vogt–Koyanagi–Harada (VKH)
- *Ocular trauma:*
  - Nonsurgical
  - *Postsurgical:*
    - Cataract surgery
    - Glaucoma surgery
    - Retina surgery
- *Systemic/nonocular diseases:*
  - *Severe hypertension (HTN):* Malignant HTN, eclampsia
  - Disseminated supravascular coagulopathy
  - Carotid-cavernous fistula.

Pathophysiology

In a normal eye, the suprachoroidal space is essentially nonexistent because of close apposition of the choroid to the sclera. In pathologic conditions that disrupt the normal ocular fluid dynamics and hydrostatic and oncotic pressure gradients, fluid accumulates in this potential space.

Choroidal effusions represent tissue edema and are best understood through Starling's law, which elucidates the balance of hydrostatic and osmotic gradients between the choroidal capillaries and interstitial space of the eye. These mechanisms suggest that choroidal effusions form either as a result of increased transudation through the choroidal capillary walls or from a drop in IOP caused by an increase in uveoscleral outflow of aqueous humor. Choroidal effusions may also be a precursor of suprachoroidal hemorrhage.

Risk Factors

- Low IOP
- Glaucoma surgery in the setting of over filtration or a bleb leak
- Medications—perioperative antimetabolites: Mitomycin C (MMC)—during trabeculectomy
- Aqueous suppressants—timolol or dorzolamide
- Glaucoma drainage device implantation
- Late choroidal effusions—latanoprost use in eyes with prior cataract extraction
- Systemic medications—sulfonamides, tetracycline, diuretics, and selective serotonin reuptake inhibitor (SSRIs).
- Iridotomy
- Pre-existing conditions—nanophthalmos and Sturge-Weber syndrome.

Clinical Features

- *Serous:* Small, peripheral effusions may be asymptomatic, with minimal to no shallowing of the AC. Large effusions may cause refractive changes from anterior displacement of the lens-iris diaphragm and resultant myopia. Patients may experience an absolute scotoma at the site of effusion.
- *Hemorrhagic:* Unlike serous choroidal effusions, which typically develop painlessly, hemorrhagic choroidals generally have an abrupt onset with severe pain and marked reduction in VA. When hemorrhagic choroidals are associated with high IOP, hyperosmotic agents and aqueous suppressants are recommended. The visual outcomes and overall prognosis are worse with hemorrhagic choroidals.

Diagnosis

- Choroidal effusions are diagnosed clinically and usually appear elevated, may appear in a four-lobed presentation because of firm attachments of the choroid to the vortex veins.
- Ultrasonography offers a method for detecting a small accumulation of fluid in the supraciliary-choroidal space not readily apparent on clinical examination. B-scan echography helps to differentiate choroidal effusions from retinal detachments. On echography, effusions are notable for their anterior angle and extension to the ora serrata.
- Low-lying choroidals may be seen with the use of sulfa-derivative medications, such as topiramate, as the mechanism of secondary angle closure in these cases does not involve a pupillary block mechanism, and laser peripheral iridotomy is ineffective in breaking the acute attack.
- *Acute intraoperative effusions:* In some cases, choroidal effusions may occur during intraocular surgery and can precede an expulsive hemorrhage. An early sign of this phenomenon is loss of the normal red reflex. Proper treatment in this scenario involves immediate closure of the incision. The closure is often followed by a rapid rise in IOP to 80 mm Hg or greater with a subsequent normalization of IOP within 15–30 minutes, leaving a localized area of effusion.

21. Discuss amaurosis fugax.

Introduction

- The term amaurosis fugax is often used to describe transient monocular visual loss mainly associated with vascular thromboembolic events arising from the internal carotid arterial system.
- The condition is not common in children and more likely to have a benign cause.
- In adults, the cause is mainly atherosclerotic emboli from the carotid artery bifurcation.

Epidemiology

Over the age of 50 years who have other vascular risk factors which include hypertension, hypercholesterolemia, smoking, previous episodes of transient ischemic attacks (TIAs), and claudication.

Other risk factors:
- Diabetes
- Heart disease
- Cocaine use.

Pathophysiology

Thromboembolism originating from the carotid circulation, as well as hypoperfusion caused by the stenosis of this circulation, are the underlying mechanisms. Hollenhorst plaque and the cholesterol particle appear refractile, yellow, and bright.

Other factors:
- Vasospasm
- Elevated plasma viscosity, for example with leukemia, multiple myeloma
- Atherosclerotic cerebrovascular disease.
  Loss of vision is usually unilateral, painless, and transient.
  In most cases, the vision loss may vary from a few seconds to a few minutes.

Symptoms

- Complaint of sudden monocular vision loss that can last between 2 and 30 minutes.
- Can involve the entire visual field or can be partial.
- Patients often describe it as a "curtain coming down" in front of their eye or as a generalized darkening or shadow.
- Episodes spontaneously resolve.
    In anyone over the age of 60 years experiencing multiple episodes, giant cell arteritis should be suspected, and further investigations should be undertaken.
- Cholesterol plaques (Hollenhorst plaques) → retinal ischemia → CRAO or branch retinal artery occlusion can develop. In some patients, particularly those with the ocular ischemic syndrome, exposure to bright lights can provoke the episodes, as vascular insufficiency of the retinal photoreceptors combined with increased metabolic demand leads to blurred or decreased vision. Vision usually returns to normal once the photoreceptors have completely hyperpolarized.

Investigations

- Evaluation of hypertension, DM, and hyperlipidemia
- *Blood investigations:* Complete blood count, prothrombin time and partial thromboplastin time, erythrocyte sedimentation rate, and C-reactive protein
- Carotid Doppler, magnetic resonance angiography, and CT angiography.
- Electrocardiogram, Holter monitoring, and transesophageal echocardiography.

Treatment/Management

- Controlling and treating the underlying vascular risk factors.
- Endarterectomy in symptomatic patients who have carotid stenosis >70% reduces future risks of stroke.
- Carotid stenting has been found comparable to endarterectomy.
- Treatment of ocular ischemic syndrome involves panretinal photocoagulation or anti-VEGF.

Prognosis

If amaurosis fugax with significant carotid artery plaques is not treated, the patient risks a major stroke within 12 months. Those who undergo carotid endarterectomy have a good prognosis but the risk of adverse cardiac events still remains.

Retinal Arterial Microaneurysm

- An acquired focal aneurysmal dilation of an arteriole, usually within the first three orders of the retinal arterial system. Retinal arterial microaneurysm (RAM) typically occurs along the temporal branches, often at points of bifurcation or arteriovenous crossing.
- Visual loss may occur secondary to macular edema, exudate, hemorrhage and neurosensory retinal detachment, and photocoagulation may expedite visual recovery.

Pathology

Thickening of the arteriolar vessel wall → focal areas of ischemia, remodeling of the greater intimal collagen → dilation of the vessel diameter. Breaks within the arteriolar wall result in a fusiform dilation of the wall, increasing the risk of exudation and rupture.

Signs and Symptoms

- Patients with retinal arterial macroaneurysms may be visually asymptomatic, and the abnormality may be found only on routine funduscopic examination.
- The onset of RAM is often insidious, but patients occasionally present with acute, severe visual loss. It has three clinical forms:
    1. Quiescent
    2. Hemorrhagic
    3. Exudative

Quiescent RAM: This is an incidental finding and seldom results in visual symptoms.

Hemorrhagic RAM: Present acutely, with rapid visual deterioration. On examination, a saccular or fusiform dilation along the first or second-order arteriole is seen. A characteristic multilayered hemorrhage involving the vitreous, as well as the preretinal, intraretinal, and subretinal spaces.

Exudative RAM: More gradual, indolent course, presence of lipid deposition in a circinate pattern surrounding the lesion, as well as intraretinal edema and accumulation of subretinal fluid.
- The classic appearance provides an easy diagnosis; however, variable presentations such as subretinal hemorrhage, macular exudate, and ERMs can make the diagnosis difficult.
- Aneurysmal changes are also seen with von Hippel, Leber's, Coat's DR, RVO, retinal arteritis, Eales disease, CMV retinitis, radiation retinopathy, sickle cell retinopathy, Takayasu's disease, and the hyperviscosity and aortic arch syndromes.

Clinical Evaluation
- A complete assessment of RAM requires a combination of clinical examination and imaging studies, such as B-scan ultrasonography, FFA, indocyanine green angiography (ICGA), and OCT. B-scan to exclude conditions such as retinal tears, detachments, and breakthrough hemorrhage from polypoidal choroidal vasculopathies.
- FFA to diagnose and delineate the suspected lesion. The typical RAM fills up uniformly in the early phase, revealing a fusiform dilation of the arteriole with late leakage. The presence of a thrombus may result in filling defects.
- *ICGA:* If significant hemorrhage renders FFA inconclusive, ICGA allows deeper penetration through the areas of hemorrhage.
- *OCT:* Spectral-domain OCT (SD-OCT) enables visualization of the lesion as well as associated complications. The macroaneurysm will appear as a round or oval hyper-reflective lesion in the inner retinal layers. Demarcate the extent of lipid deposition and accumulation of intraretinal and/or subretinal fluid.

Treatment
- Optimize blood pressure control
- Management of the ocular manifestations of RAM depends on the VA in the affected eye, as well as the location of the lesion and associated consequences.

Observation: Good VA, with the RAM located inferiorly or nasally, and minimal exudation or hemorrhage. Often, RAM with associated retinal or breakthrough vitreous hemorrhage will thrombose and subsequently regress without further intervention.

Argon laser photocoagulation:
- Significant hemorrhage or exudation threatening the macula, especially when the RAM is located superotemporally, early retinal argon photocoagulation is recommended.
- RAMs complicated by subfoveal hemorrhage → disorganization of the retinal inner layers and associated neurosensory detachment → Subsequent fibrosis and atrophy may result in permanent central vision loss.
  Anti-vascular endothelial growth factor can be administered in such cases.

Yttrium aluminum garnet (YAG) laser hyaloidotomy: Large, nonresolving premacular hemorrhage promotes dispersion of the blood into the vitreous, where it may be more readily absorbed.

Intravitreal gas: Prolonged submacular hemorrhage (SMH) may be toxic to the underlying photoreceptor and retinal pigment epithelial cells. Displacement of the hemorrhage may be achieved by injection of expansile intravitreal gas, with or without the aid of adjunctive tissue plasminogen activator with pars plana vitrectomy.

 22. Write short note on Terson syndrome.

It was discovered by French ophthalmologist, Albert Terson in 1990.
- Characterized by intraocular hemorrhages, such as vitreous, subhyaloid, or intraretinal/sub-ILM hemorrhage, associated with subarachnoid hemorrhage (SAH) within the same admission period as first SAH diagnosis, or within 3 months of that diagnosis.
- Higher incidence in patients under 40 years old.
- Vitreous hemorrhage is an indicator of poor prognosis in patients with subarachnoid hemorrhage higher frequency in patients with consciousness disturbance, lower Glasgow Coma Scale (GCS) score, and higher Hunt–Hess grade.
- Mild retinal hemorrhages were associated with a better prognosis than large preretinal hemorrhages or vitreous hemorrhages.
- Retinal hemorrhage in a patient who has temporarily lost consciousness is very suggestive of aneurysmal rupture especially of the internal carotid and anterior communication.

Pathogenesis of Vitreous Hemorrhage

- Increased intracranial pressure forces blood into the subarachnoid space and along the optic nerve sheath into the preretinal space, or
- Sudden rise in intracranial pressure lead to decrease in venous return to the cavernous sinus or obstruct the retinochoroidal anastomoses and central retinal vein, leading to venous stasis and hemorrhage.

Treatment

- Timely surgical intervention with 23G vitrectomy for the treatment of intraocular hemorrhage is associated with better visual prognosis.
- In Terson syndrome with bilateral visual loss, it is reasonable to consider early vitrectomy in one eye and observe the other both approaches resulted in the same visual outcome.

 23. Write short note on dyes used in ILM peeling.

- Chromovitrectomy refers to the usage of vital dyes in vitreoretinal surgery to aid in the visualization of ocular tissues and anatomic planes, especially ILM, vitreous and ERMs.
- The ILM is a fine, multilaminar, semitransparent membrane 2.5-μm thick, it acts as a basal membrane for the Mueller cells, and plays a main role in the pathogenesis of various vitreoretinal interface diseases, especially in the macular area.
- ILM has a main role in the development and treatment resistance of diffuse DME, as it thickens almost three times its normal size.
- Surgical removal of the ILM in these conditions has proven to be effective in anatomic and functional improvements. The main technical difficulty is to remove and peel the membrane completely because it is transparent and multilaminar, making visualization challenging.

Brilliant Blue G Dye

- Most frequently used
- Introduced by Enaida et al. in 2006
- It is anionic amino triarylmethane.
- 280 mOsm osmolarity molecular weight—854 and 7.4 pH
- It is safe, no dose-dependent or time-dependent toxicity.
- As it has a great affinity for the ILM, it is easy to use at low concentrations and obviates the need for fluid-air exchange.
- 0.25 mg/mL brilliant blue G in balanced salt iso-osmolar solution. After injecting, wait for 30–45 seconds, extract the dye by active aspiration and proceed to peel the ILM, using ILM forceps.
- The edge in the temporal foveal area is held, and in a concentric movement pulling inward we perform the maculorrhexis, pulling the ILM flap very carefully without exceeding the vascular arcade, and it is important to try to perform the peeling in only one maneuver.

Trypan Blue

- Blue hydrophilic anionic azo dye is used to stain ERMs.
- Weakly stain the vitreous and ILM.
- Unable to cross cell membranes in living cells, only able to stain dead cells with compromised cell membranes.
- ERM contains a relatively high number of dead glial cells, and thus has a high affinity for trypan blue.
- Due to its hydrophilicity, trypan blue also has a weak affinity for the ILM and vitreous. Fluid-air exchange should first be performed to ensure that the dye localizes to the macula.
- Used in 0.15% concentration or a 3:1 mixture of 0.15% trypan blue to 10% glucose dense solution that does not require fluid-air exchange before injection.
- New indication for the use of trypan blue was to stain the edges of an open retinal tear on subretinal administration facilitating its identification during vitrectomy.

Bromophenol Blue

- Chemically, it is tetrabromophenosulfonaphthalein, has a molecular weight of 670 Da, and a chemical formula $C_{19}H_{10}Br_4O_5S$.
- Blue triarylmethane dye that has high affinity for the ILM and ERMs. Bromophenol blue is used at a concentration of 0.13–0.2% and does not require fluid-gas exchange.
- In vitro studies have demonstrated low toxicity to the retina with significantly less toxic effects than ICG.

Patent Blue

- Blue anionic triarylmethane dye stain for ERMs.
- Chemical formula of $C_{27}H_{31}N_2NaO_6S_2$ and a molecular weight of 582 Da.
- Moderate affinity for ERMs and a low affinity for the ILM.
- Used as an iso-osmolar solution at 0.25% concentration or diluted in 0.25% glucose. Similar safety profile to trypan blue when used in the vitreous space and low toxicity when injected subretinally.
- Surgical case reports have not reported any postoperative visual field defects or grossly visible RPE changes.
- Its use in vitreoretinal surgery is off-label, and it does not yet have FDA approval.

Indocyanine Green and Infracyanine Green

- Tricarbocyanine anionic dye with a molecular formula of $C_{43}H_{47}N_2NaO_6S_2$ and a molecular weight of 775 Da.
- Green dye with amphiphilic properties.
- ICG demonstrates greatest affinity to the extracellular matrix components of the ILM, thereby exhibiting an ability to selectivity stain the ILM.
- ICG is a green anionic cyanine dye useful for ILM staining. High affinity for components of the extracellular matrix presents in the ILM such as collagen type IV and laminin.
- ICG requires initial dilution in distilled water (if diluted in saline, the dye can precipitate), then be subsequently diluted in a balanced saline solution to create a less hypo-osmolar solution.
- ICG's toxicity when used intraocularly, shown to be toxic to chorioretinal cells when exposed to moderate-to-high concentrations.
- Proposed to cause toxicity when applied and exposed to light through a photochemical mechanism.
- Infracyanine green (IFCG) is another green anionic cyanine dye that is very chemically and pharmacologically similar to ICG.
- Its main difference is that it does not contain sodium iodide unlike ICG (ICG contains 4–5% iodine in part as a byproduct of its synthesis and in part due to the presence of an iodine moiety on the molecule).
- Advantage of not requiring initial dilution in distilled water to avoid precipitation. It also avoids exposure of the retina to toxic iodide.

Triamcinolone Acetonide

- Synthetic nonsoluble corticosteroid is used to stain the cortical vitreous or ILM. It is composed of white crystals in an aqueous suspension. These crystals are responsible for their staining ability, as they bind avidly to acellular tissues such as vitreous and also deposit on the ILM.
- The duration that triamcinolone acetonide remains in the eye depends on the specific formulation; crystals can remain in the vitreous cavity for up to 40 days after instillation.
- The half-life is around 18 days in nonvitrectomized eyes and 3 days in vitrectomized eyes.
- Application consists of injecting 0.1–0.3 mL with a concentration of 40 mg/mL.
- Triamcinolone acetonide has been shown to be more effective in highlighting vitreous than trypan blue, IFCG, and fluorescein.
- It has anti-inflammatory properties, and intravitreal injections are approved for the treatment of macular edema and uveitis with added benefit of decreasing postoperative inflammation and vitreoretinopathy.
- It is nontoxic to the retina and remains a relatively safe option.
- Slightly increased risk in the development of cataracts and increased IOP with intravitreal triamcinolone use.

24. Write short note on micro-incision vitrectomy surgery.

Introduction

The evolution of vitrectomy surgery has come a long way from open sky vitrectomy to sutureless micro-incision vitrectomy surgery (MIVS). It is also known as transconjunctival sutureless vitrectomy (TSV). In 2002, Fuji et al. introduced 25G vitrectomy, followed by 23G vitrectomy in 2005 by Eckdart and Stanley Chang. 23G has combined benefit of both 25G and 20G. 27G vitrectomy has been introduced by Oshiwara in 2010.

Indications

- *23G:* It can be used in any case but is more suitable in cases of rhegmatogenous retinal detachment surgery and for diabetic vitrectomies. It can be used in the case of trauma especially foreign body removal and endophthalmitis.
- *25G and 27G:* Mainly macular surgery (ERM, macular hole, macular pucker). Simple cases of vitreous hemorrhage can be managed. Pediatric cases can be managed with it.

Advantages

- Sutureless—better patient comfort
- Less conjunctival scarring—helpful in patients undergoing multiple surgeries and in ocular surface disorders
- Reduced surgically induced inflammation
- Less surgery-induced astigmatism
- Safety—less chances of inadvertent retinal breaks because of high cut rate and smaller port aperture
- Easy dissectibility.

Disadvantages

- Prolong surgery timings
- Higher infusion pressure can cause optic nerve damage
- Deformability (bending or breakage)
- Limitation of maximum flow across the port
- Retinal injury in case where it is displaced anteriorly because of long blades.
- Not useful in cases of nucleus drop
- Not suitable in cases where extensive dissection is needed such as tractional retinal detachment.

Instrumentation

It is sutureless surgery. Three microcannulas are inserted through the conjunctiva and sclera in pars plana through two-step incision. The different cannulas and their diameters include:
- Inner diameter of conventional 20G cannula was 0.9 mm
- Inner diameter of 25G is 0.57 mm
- Inner diameter of 23G is 0.65 mm
- Inner diameter of 27G is 0.40 mm

  Comparative to 20G cannula MIVS cutter port is smaller and closer to the tip helping in safely doing vitrectomy closer to detached retina, membrane segmentation or delamination and vitreous base shaving. Cutting rate can be 5,000–8,000 cpm.

Illumination

There is 35% reduction in amount of illumination with 20% reduction in light pipe diameter. New generation Xenon and Mercury vapor illumination sources greatly improved illumination in MIVS surgery.

Rigidity

It is very flexible which can cause bending or breakage of instruments. It is difficult to maneuver globe with these instruments. This problem is more with 25 and 27G. To overcome it 25+ and 27+ has been introduced by adding 5 mm supporting sleeve near proximal end to make it stiffer and less malleable. But it reduces the effective working length.

Aspiration and Flow Rates

Flow through a tube is proportional to the fourth power of the radius of the tube A/C to Poiseuille law. Because of the reduction in diameter in MIVS higher infusion and aspiration rates are necessary to optimize flow and vitreous removal.

Complications

- *Wound leakage:* Biplanar incision, proper wound construction, and oblique/angled entry reduce this complication.
- *Postoperative endophthalmitis:* Variable results of different studies. Most of them suggest less chances than conventional 20G vitrectomy surgery.

25. Discuss ocular phototoxicity.

Introduction

The eyes are very sensitive to sunlight. Light transmission through eye is required for its basic biological functions but at the same time, intense sunlight exposure causes hazards to ocular structures. Low or high altitude, outdoor employment are particular risk factors.

Factors Causing Ocular Phototoxicity

- *Intensity of light:* It is directly proportional to ocular phototoxicity. Greater the intensity of light, more damage to ocular structure. The eye can be damaged by exposure to reflective sunlight from snow which is known as snow blindness. Staring at the sun during an eclipse can also damage eyes. Less intense light for a prolonged duration causes slowly age-related damage.
- *Wavelength of light:* As the wavelength of light decreases energy of light increases which causes more damage to eye. Longer wavelengths are less energetic but at the same time penetrate the eyes more deeply. The human eye has unique filtering characteristics which determine in which area of the eye particular wavelength of light will be absorbed. The human cornea absorbs light below 295 nm, so most energetic light [most of ultraviolet B (UV-B) and all UV-C] do not reach up to lens. The lens absorbs most of UV-B and all UV-A. Only visible spectrum (400–700 nm) reaches the retina. In younger age lens can transmit small part of UV-B, but elderly lens filters out much of blue visible light.
- *Oxygen tension:* Tissue with greater oxygen content is more prone to oxidative and photo-oxidative damage. Cornea is highly oxygenated tissue hence more prone to damage. Oxygen supply in retina is through blood which varies in different layers of retina. So, it has varying sensitivity.

Site of Damage

- *Cornea:* Temporary damage to epithelial and endothelial cells (as they have a high potential for regeneration) causes keratitis.
- *Uvea:* Mainly protected because of iris pigmentation.
- *Lens:* Epithelial cells which are in direct contact with aqueous humor are more prone to phototoxic damage. Inner fiber membrane can also be damaged through damage to the lipids and intrinsic membrane proteins. Phototoxicity damage can lead to modification of DNA and certain amino acids. Covalently bound chromophores may act as endogenous sensitizers. All these can lead to change in the refractive index of the lens material leading to aggregation and ultimately opacification.
- *Retina:* It can damage retinal pigment epithelial tissues choroid and the photoreceptors. Extensive damage can lead to permanent blindness.

Defence Systems

As the age progresses, age defence materials decreases. Antioxidant enzymes (superoxide dismutases and catalases) and antioxidants (Vitamin E, C, lutein, zeaxanthin, lycopene, glutathione, and melanin) are the defense system of eye.

Mechanisms

Mechanism of damage can be inflammatory or photo-oxidative. In inflammatory process, initial insult to tissue causes a cascade of events that results in wider damage to the tissue. In photo-oxidation reaction, sensitized compound absorbs light and excited to a singlet, then triplet, and then produces free radicals and ROS which in turn damage the ocular tissues.

Repair

Lens damage is irreversible. The cornea and retina has sufficient repair systems.

Chromophores

It absorbs light. It can be endogenous or exogenous. For ocular phototoxicity, its presence is mandatory. Endogenous chromophores are DNA and proteins in cornea, proteins, and melanin in uvea, yellow chromophores in lens and lipofuscin in retina. Exogenous can be herbal medication or diagnostic dye. Any compound which has a tricyclic, heterocyclic, or porphyrin ring structure is a potential ocular chromophore.

Ocular Clinical Features

- *Cornea:* Because UV-B causes photo-keratitis, pinguecula and pterygium.
- *Uvea:* Uveal melanoma is the most common malignant tumor of eye. Ultraviolet light is a known risk factor.
- *Lens:* Cataracts
- *Retina:* Macular degeneration, the leading cause of irreversible blindness in the increasing age population.

 26. Write short note on perfluorocarbon liquid (PFCL).

Introduction

Perfluorocarbon liquids (PFCLs) are fluorochemicals in which all the oxygen atoms are replaced by fluorine. It is industrially produced by methods such as electrochemical fluorination, oligomerization, and telomerization, since it has low surface tension and viscosity and specific gravity ranging from 1.76 to 2.00. It is an ideal intraoperative tool in vitreoretinal surgery.

Types

- Perfluorooctane (PFO)
- Perfluoroperhydrophenanthrene (Vitreon)
- Perfluorodecalin (PFD)
- Perfluorotributylamine (PFTB)
- Perfluoro-octyl bromide (PFOB).

Indications in Vitreoretinal Surgery

- *Retinal detachment with severe PVR:* The application of PFCL in PVR surgery has changed its surgical management. Before PFCL era during this surgery, anterior PVR dissection has to be done before proceeding posteriorly. But now posterior dissection of PVR is possible because of PFCL. The injection of PFCLs after initial dissection helps in opening the funnel and hence better visualization of proliferative membranes and decreases the incidence of postoperative surgery reproliferation.
- *Giant retinal tears:* The mobility of the detached retina is high in this case causes difficulty in manipulation. PFCL stabilizes the detached retina during vitrectomy and displaces subretinal fluids. Its use in giant retinal tears with no severe PVR, helps in preserving lens during surgery.
- *Diabetics retinopathy:* It helps to flatten shrunken retina. It also helps in detachments that appeared during removal of tight vitreoretinal adhesions. It helps in doing LPC using low energy.
- *Relocating and stabilizing detached retina for further maneuvers:* Its specific gravity is twice than perfusion solution, so during vitrectomy. PFCLs generate a force against the interface downward. It helps in stabilizing detached retina and helps in maneuvering. When slowly injected it also causes drainage of subretinal fluid through retinal breaks hence avoiding posterior retinotomy. Sometimes it helps in identifying unseen breaks when subretinal fluid is coming through it.
- *Dislocated crystalline lens or intraocular lens (IOL) in vitreous cavity:* Since their gravity is less than PFCL, it floats up when injecting into vitreous cavity, hence helpful in removal as well as improving the safety of the process. The injection is stopped once the lens has reached the iris plane. Once it comes in AC phaco can be done. It provides support underneath the nucleus.

- *Retinopathy of prematurity and other complex pediatric retinal detachment:* Perfluorooctane has a vital role here. Since posterior proliferative changes are mainly inferior, silicon oil and gas are less effective. PFCL can be used as a temporary postoperative tamponade.
- *Intraocular foreign body removal:* Use of PFCL helps in lifting it away from retina and hence helps in removal safely.
- *Penetrating trauma with posterior foreign body:* Penetrating trauma can be associated with lens injury vitreous hemorrhage and retinal detachment. PFCL plays a vital role in surgery.
- *Protecting macula:* Agents or drugs which can cause toxicity to macula, small amount of PFCL can be injected before to form a bubble covering macular area.
- *Suprachoroidal hemorrhage:* It may be useful in expressing suprachoroidal hemorrhage from sclerotomies.

Complications

- Perfluro Octane (PFO) impart damage mechanically. Short-term use is safer. Intraretinal macrophages and foam cells are observed after 1–2 weeks of intravitreal placement. As duration increases, narrowing of the OPL and degenerative thinning of outer nuclear layer is noted.
- Clinical observation—significant pigment epithelial atrophy seen in subretinal PFCL areas. Younger patients are more prone to inflammation.
- Role in sticky silicone oil formation.
- Secondary membrane formation.

Recent Developments

Hydrogenated hydrofluorocarbons liquids (HFCLs): It is a modification to reduce specific gravity and increase lipophilic properties so that it can be tolerated better as long-term vitreous tamponade.

Perfluorocarbon Perfused Vitrectomy

It helps in PFCL perfusion instead of balanced salt solution during vitrectomy. Oxygenated or nonoxygenated PFCL is used in the recycling or nonrecycling process respectively. In severe DR, oxygenated PFCL can be an advantage for the circulation compromised retina. It also helps in hemostasis.

27. Discuss intravitreal implants and uses.

- An intravitreal implant is a drug delivery system, injected or surgically implanted in the vitreous of the eye, for sustained release of pharmacologic agent to the posterior and intermediate segments of the eye.
- They deliver a continuous concentration of the drug over a prolonged period of time.
- Corticosteroid implants are being studied for conditions that lead to macular edema due to uveitis, DR, and retinal venous occlusions.
- Goal of therapy—to reduce the inflammation in the eye while minimizing the adverse effects of the drug.
- *Four intravitreal corticosteroid implants are:*
  - *Fluocinolone acetonide 0.19 mg (iluvien):*
    - Rod-shaped device made of polymide and polyvinyl alcohol
    - Can be inserted with a 25G needle
    - Sustains up to 3 years
    - Medically indicated for treatment of DME patients who have been treated previously with a course of steroids and did not have clinically significant rise in IOP.
  - *Fluocinolone acetonide 0.59 mg (retisert):*
    - Sterile implant consisting of a tablet. The tablet is encased in a silicone elastomer cup with a release orifice and membrane, the entire elastomer cup assembly is attached to a suture tab.
    - It is implanted via pars plana incision and suturing.
    - It is released at a rate of 0.3–0.4 µg/day over a period of approximately 2.5 years.
    - Medically indicated for the treatment of chronic, noninfectious intermediate, posterior, or panuveitis.
  - *Fluocinolone acetonide 0.18 mg (yutiq):*
    - Nonbiodegradable injectable implant
    - It has a 36-month sustained release.

- It is released at a rate of 0.25 μg/day.
- Indicated for chronic noninfectious uveitis affecting the posterior segment of the eye.
- *Dexamethasone 0.7 mg (ozurdex):*
  - It is composed of a biodegradable copolymer of lactic acid and glycolic acid with micronized dexamethasone.
  - It is implanted in vitreous cavity through pars plana using a 22G applicator.
  - Provides dexamethasone for up to 6 months.
  - *Medically indicated for the treatment of:*
    - Noninfectious ocular inflammation or uveitis, affecting the intermediate, or posterior segment of the eye.
    - Macular edema following CRVO or branch retinal vein occlusion (BRVO)
    - DME
- Fluocinolone acetonide—nonerodible, delivers drugs up to 30–36 months.
- Dexamethasone—bioerodible, lasts up to 6 months.

Uses

- Uveitis
- Macular edema after venous occlusion
- Diabetic macular edema
- Age-related macular degeneration.

Regulatory Status

- Ozurdex was approved by US FDA in 2009 for the treatment of macular edema following BRVO or CRVO. Approved in 2010 for noninfectious uveitis affecting posterior segment of the eye. Approved in 2014 for DME.
- Iluvien was FDA approved in 2014 for DME in patients previously treated with a course of corticosteroids.
- Retisert was approved by FDA in 2014 and Yutiq was approved by FDA in 2018 for the treatment of chronic noninfectious uveitis affecting the posterior segment of the eye.

 28. Discuss intravitreal steroids and uses.

Intravitreal injections have provided a logical method to bypass the blood retinal barrier so as to provide clinically effective doses of therapeutic agents to the ocular target tissue.

Mechanism of Action

- Steroids have an inhibitory effect on angiogenesis and inflammatory reactions by reducing the migration and activation of inflammatory cells.
- Has a direct angiostatic effect by upregulation of extracellular matrix protein plasminogen activator inhibitor-1.
- Inhibit the production of vascular endothelial growth factors.
- Inhibitory effect on plasmin → stabilizes endothelial and basement membranes and reduces vascular permeability and leakage.
- Downregulate intracellular adhesion molecule expression, which is an important stimulus for the development of neovascular membranes and an inflammatory mediator released by photodynamic therapy (PDT).
- So, steroids work for a number of retinal conditions characterized by inflammation, vascular leakage, and new blood vessel growth.

Uses of Intravitreal Triamcinolone Acetonide

- *In diabetic macular edema:*
  - Intravitreal triamcinolone acetonide (IVTA) is a promising therapy for DME (diffuse type) refractory to laser therapy.
  - IVTA has helped in decreasing the macular thickness, absorption of hard exudates, and a resultant improvement in VA. Positive effects reach its peak by 1–3 months.
- *In retinal vein occlusions:* IVTA has been effective in macular edema secondary to CRVO and BRVO (SCORE study).
- *Macular edema due to other causes:* IVTA has also been widely used in treating pseudophakic cystoid macular edema, uveitic cystoid macular edema, and macular edema in retinitis pigmentosa with variable results.

- *In wet AMD:* PDT combined with IVTA injections have considerably improved the results both visually and angiographic.
- *Triamcinolone assisted vitreous surgery:* IVTA is injected into the vitreous cavity during the surgery to help in identifying the vitreoretinal tissue planes, and membrane peeling, thereby facilitating complete removal of vitreous membranes and easy induction of PVD.

Ideal Dose of Intravitreal Triamcinolone Acetonide

- The dose of IVTA used internationally varies from 1 to 25 mg.
- The most widely used dose is 4 mg in 0.1 mL.
- Two important studies to ascertain the optimum dose are DRCR study and SCORE study.

Complications

- *Defined risks include:* Endophthalmitis (incidence of 0.16%), retinal detachment (0.15%), and lens trauma/acute cataract (0.07%).
- *Rare complications include:* Hemorrhage, precipitated angle closure, elevated IOP, wound leak and hypotony, and anaphylactic reaction.
- *Noninfectious endophthalmitis due to IVTA:*
  - Incidence 0.87–5%.
  - Due to reaction to the diluent in which triamcinolone crystals are suspended.
  - Crystalline deposits in the AC could be due to migration of crystals into AC.
- *Ocular hypertension:* Mild-to-moderate rise in IOP was seen in 28–42% cases.
- *Steroid-induced cataract:* Seen in 10–30%.

29. Write a short note on posterior vitreous detachment.

- Posterior vitreous detachment (PVD) is defined as separation of the posterior vitreous cortex from the inner limiting membrane of the retina.
- This separation may be complete or partial. Vitreous traction at sites of significant vitreoretinal adhesion is responsible for most retinal breaks that lead to retinal detachment.
- PVD results from gel liquefaction and concurrent dehiscence of vitreoretinal adhesion. In the absence of vitreoretinal dehiscence, gel liquefaction causes anomalous PVD.
- It is estimated to occur in two-thirds of people older than 65 years.

Effects of Posterior Vitreous Detachment

- Posterior vitreous detachment which can place traction on the peripheral retina, resulting in rhegmatogenous sequelae: can pull on the macula, optic disc, and retinal blood vessels.
- Can create premacular membranes (via vitreoschisis) contributing to macular pucker and holes through tangential traction.
- Elevated intravitreal oxygen partial pressure, contributing to cataracts and possibly glaucoma.
- *Optical effects of PVD:* Degradation of contrast sensitivity function, which results in vision degrading vitreopathy if severe.

Risk Factors

- Posterior vitreous detachment is rare in people under the age of 40 years, and is increasingly common during advanced age.
- Myopia
- Trauma
- Recent eye surgery such as a cataract operation
- Patients who experience PVD in one eye will often experience PVD in the other eye within 1 year.

Various Theories of Posterior Vitreous Detachment

- The classic theory describes acute vitreoretinal separation at the posterior pole that then dissects peripherally.

- Another theory proposed that PVD is an insidious process beginning earlier in life at the perifoveal region, with later separation from the optic disc.
- Recent theory states that PVD was noted first more anteriorly in the paramacular area to peripheral fundus, not the posterior pole.

Classification of Posterior Vitreous Detachment

- *By slit-lamp biomicroscopy:*
  - *Complete posterior vitreous detachment (C-PVD):*
    - C-PVD with collapse
    - C-PVD without collapse
  - *Partial posterior vitreous detachment (P-PVD):*
    - P-PVD with shrinkage of the posterior hyaloid membrane (P-PVD with shrinkage)
    - P-PVD without shrinkage of the posterior hyaloid membrane (P-PVD without shrinkage)
- *By OCT:* A shallow PVD is classified as:
  - Absence of a shallow PVD
  - *A shallow PVD:*
    - *Shallow PVD without shrinkage of the posterior vitreous cortex:*
      - An age-related shallow PVD
      - A perifoveal PVD associated with a MH.
    - A shallow PVD with shrinkage of the posterior vitreous cortex,
    - A peripheral shallow PVD.

Stages of Posterior Vitreous Detachment

- Perifoveal separation with adhesion of vitreous to the fovea.
- Complete separation of the vitreous from the macula.
- Extensive vitreous separation with adhesion of the vitreous to the disc.
- C-PVD.

Clinical Implications of Posterior Vitreous Detachment

- *Symptoms of a PVD include:*
  - *Floaters (mobile blurry shadows that obscure the vision):* These may be due to blood from a torn or avulsed retinal vessel, condensations of vitreous collagen, or the epipapillary glial tissue (Weiss ring) that is torn from the ONH and area adjacent to the ONH.
  - *Flashes (streaks of light, usually at the side of the vision):* These are likely the result of vitreous traction on the retina.
- Methods for detecting PVD include slit-lamp biomicroscopy, ultrasonography, and OCT.
- PVD is important for predicting the prognosis and determining the indication for vitreoretinal surgery in many vitreoretinal diseases.
- In DR, a P-PVD or the absence of a PVD is a risk factor for retinal neovascularization, but a C-PVD is a strong negative risk factor for retinal neovascularization as vitreous attachment to the retina acts as a scaffold for neovascularization arising from the retina.
- OCT can visualize perifoveal PVDs with pinpoint vitreo-foveal traction in cases with an idiopathic macular hole.
- Approximately 8% and 22% of patients with acute PVD symptoms have a retinal tear at the time of the initial examination.

Management of Posterior Vitreous Detachment

- It is non sight-threatening and the symptoms subside in the vast majority of patients. Most patients no longer notice flashes or floaters 3 months later.
- There are no effective methods of preventing the vitreous syneresis and liquefaction—a careful peripheral fundus examination is recommended in patients with high-risk factors.
- Patients presenting with an acute PVD and no retinal breaks have a small chance (approximately 2%) of developing retinal breaks.
- Appropriate reassurance and precautions regarding the symptoms of retinal detachment should be given.

- The impact of floaters or floater-related visual symptoms may have an adverse effect on a person's vision-related quality of life. Pars plana vitrectomy is an option if symptomatic floaters are still bothersome after several months.
- Pars plana vitrectomy showed evidence of greater patient satisfaction compared with only moderate resolution of symptoms following the Nd:YAG laser procedure.

Follow-up

- *Symptomatic PVD with no retinal break:* Follow-up within 2 months depending on clinical findings then 6–12 months.
- Symptomatic PVD with no retinal break but with some retinal or vitreous hemorrhage:
  - Depending on the severity of retinal hemorrhage 1–2 weeks.
  - For VH-weekly until resolved.
  - Ultrasound to check for retinal breaks.

 30. Discuss evaluation and management of traumatic subretinal hemorrhage.

Subretinal hemorrhage/SMH is an accumulation of blood between the neurosensory retina and the RPE arising from the choroidal or retinal circulation.

Causes

- Choroidal neovascularization (CNV)
- Trauma
- Inflammation of the retina/choroid
- Vascular malformations
- Complication of intraocular surgeries
- Traumatic SMH can be as a result of blunt or penetrating injuries. SMH, subsequent to choroidal rupture in macular region, is a sight-threatening condition, and is associated with poor visual outcome, if it persists for several days.

Symptoms

The patient usually presents with sudden loss of vision. Visual loss is immediate and profound if the blood clot is thick and involves the fovea.

Damage to retina and RPE can be due to various mechanisms such as:
- Iron toxicity to photoreceptors from hemoglobin breakdown
- Photoreceptors damage due to sheering force by fibrin clots
- Impaired metabolic exchange between the photoreceptors and RPE due to clot, subretinal fibrosis, and fibrocellular scar formation.

Classification of Submacular Hemorrhage

According to the size:
- Small SMH measures less than four disc diameters
- Medium-size SMH has a diameter >4 disc diameters but does not extend beyond the temporal vascular arcade
- Massive SMH—overspreads the temporal vascular arcade

Management

- *Treatment options include:*
  - Vitrectomy with modifications such as a retinotomy
  - Mechanical removal of subretinal clot
  - Tissue-type plasminogen activator (tPA)
  - PFCL
- *Surgical approach includes:* Pars plana vitrectomy with evacuation of the clot was directly through one or more retinotomies either with or without adjuvant subretinal tPA injection.

- *Good surgical prognosis is expected in:*
  - Patients who had good VA before the hemorrhage
  - Duration of hemorrhage is <2 weeks
  - Size larger than 3 disc diameters in greatest linear dimension
- Postoperative complications—retinal detachment, recurrent hemorrhage, and subretinal fibrosis.
- Poor outcome is most probably due to damage to the overlying retinal photoreceptors and underlying RPE during surgical manipulation due to the tight adherence of the RPE and photoreceptors to the hemorrhagic clot.
- *Pneumatic displacement:* Has proved to be an effective treatment modality for traumatic submacular hemorrhage. It may be considered as first-line management. Subretinal rtPA and perfluoropropane gas are used to displace hemorrhage out of the subretinal space.
- *Perfluoropropane (C_3F_8):*
  - It is a colorless, odorless, and inert gas with high surface tension.
  - Interfacial tension at the gas-vitreous interface is responsible for the displacement of subretinal fluid.
  - Gravity may also play a role in subretinal fluid displacement with appropriate positioning of the patient.
  - Pure C_3F_8 bubble can expand to four times its original volume within 72–96 hours, persisting in the vitreous cavity for 6–8 weeks.
  - Complications of pneumatic displacement include vitreous hemorrhage, suprachoroidal gas displacement, endophthalmitis, iatrogenic retinal break, retinal detachment, glaucoma, and recurrent hemorrhage.
- *tPA:* 0.1–0.2 mL of intravitreal tPA (either 25 µg or 50 µg/mL) can be beneficial, especially for AMD-related SMH.

31. Discuss differential diagnosis, investigation, and management in a 22-year-old male with unilateral sudden diminution of vision.

The differential diagnosis of a patient with such presentation would include the following:

Painful:
- Giant cell arteritis
- Optic neuritis
- Angle-closure glaucoma (ACG)
- Corneal ulcer.

Painless:
- Nonarteritic ischemic optic neuropathy
- Most other retinal disorders such as retinal detachment, vitreous hemorrhage, and vitritis.

History and examination are the key in dealing with sudden diminution of vision in young male.

History

Description of visual symptoms differentiates whether there is ocular pathology or optic nerve pathology.
- Monocular metamorphopsia (wavy, warped images) and positive phenomena such as flashes or colored lights symbolizes retinal pathology.
- Colors look washed out or faded and signifies optic nerve dysfunction.
- *Tempo of visual loss:*
  - Ischemic optic neuritis—may quickly evolve and subsequently improve.
  - Ischemic optic neuropathy—sudden presentation has static course.
  - Compressive—insidious onset, suddenly noticed, and slowly progressive.
  - RD—may start from one quadrant and progress to complete lost over hours to days.
  - VH—usually sudden onset and complete loss.
- Presence or absence of associated orbital, neurologic, or systemic symptoms.

Examination

The following signs must be looked for:
- VA—reduced both in ocular and optic nerve pathology.
- Color vision and contrast sensitivity—disproportionately decreased in optic nerve pathology.
- Amsler grid—useful for macular pathology.

- *Visual fields:*
  - Central depression—maculopathy and optic neuropathy.
  - Nerve fiber bundle defect—more specific for optic neuropathy.
  - Homonymous field loss—retrochiasmal lesion.
  - Ciliary congestion—ACG.
- Cornea—edematous in ACG and ulcer.
- Pupil—rapid afferent pupillary defect (RAPD) signifies optic nerve pathology.
- IOP—spike will be seen in ACG.
- Angle—obliterated in ACG.
- *Fundus examination:*
  - Vitreous reaction—infective or inflammatory uveitis, vitreous hemorrhage
  - Normal—retrobulbar pathology
  - Disc edema—ischemia or inflammation of optic disc
  - Pallor disc—compressive pathology (incidentally noticed)
  - Hemorrhages, macular star, and retinal detachment.

Work-up

- *Orbital MRI sequence:* Coronal T2-weighted images and fat-saturated postgadolinium images typically provide excellent views of the prechiasmatic optic nerve. It differentiates between inflammatory, ischemic, and neoplastic optic neuropathies. Increased T2 signal distinguishes demyelination from nonarteritic anterior ischemic optic neuropathy (NAION).
- *OCT:* It differentiates between retinal pathology from optic nerve pathology.
- *FFA:* It is used in cases of occult maculopathy, e.g., ischemic lesion secondary to diabetes.
- *Visual-evoked potential:* It is not routinely used, P100 response with prolonged latency s/o optic nerve demyelination.
- *ERG:* If retinal dysfunction is suspected based on history, but no lesion is evident, based on this acute outer retinal dysfunction can be ruled out.
- *Serology and CSF tests:* These tests differentiate infectious inflammatory and neoplastic illnesses.
- *Genetic testing:* This test confirms the diagnosis of lever hereditary optic neuropathy (LHON).

Differentiating Features

Retinal Diseases

- Central retinal artery occlusion—retinal whitening, and CRS
- Branch retinal artery occlusion—segmental retinal whitening
- Retinal vein occlusion—retinal hemorrhages, and engorged veins
- Central serous retinopathy—subretinal fluid in macula, and confirmation by OCT
- Retinal detachment—billowing, and elevated retina
- Cystoid macular edema—subtle macular elevation, and confirmed by OCT
- Acute idiopathic blind spot enlargement syndrome and multiple evanescent white dot syndrome—blind spot enlargement, and subtle peripapillary retinal changes.

Optic Nerve Diseases

- *Hereditary:*
  - Leber hereditary optic neuropathy—painless sequential visual loss
  - Pseudopapilledema
  - Peripapillary telangiectasia
- *Infections:*
  - Neuroretinitis—macular star
- Inflammatory—uveitis, systemic inflammatory symptoms
- *Optic neuritis:*
  - Pain in eye movements
  - Normal appearance of disc or maybe mild swelling
  - Spontaneous recovery

- *Nonarteritic ischemic optic neuropathy:*
  - Painless
  - Altitudinal visual field defects
  - Optic disc edema, may be sectoral
  - Small C:D ratio in fellow eye
  - Increased age and vascular factors
  - Nocturnal hypotension
- *Arteritic ischemic optic neuropathy:*
  - Systemic symptoms (myalgia, jaw claudications, fever, scalp tenderness, and weight loss)
  - Optic disc edema, cotton-wool spots.

Angle-closure Glaucoma
- Painful acute vision loss
- Red eye, shallow chamber, fixed and dilated pupil, and increased IOP.

Trauma
Painful loss of vision.

Corneal Ulcer
Painful loss of vision, stain positive.

Management
Management depends upon the underlying cause.

 32. Discuss wide-angle viewing system (WAVS).

Wide-angle viewing system provides a panoramic view of fundus. It improves surgical efficiency and safety. Principles are similar to indirect ophthalmoscope.

All WAVS have two components:
1. First is an indirect ophthalmoscopic lens system that is placed on (contact) or above the cornea as a preplaced lens (noncontact).
2. Second will be a separate removable prismatic stereo-inverter mounted on the surgical microscope for inverting the fundus image.

Advantages
- Helps in easy evaluation of fundus and location of retinal pathologies without excessive rotation of eyeball during surgery compared to conventional floating prismatic lenses.
- In conjunction with chandelier lighting bimanual maneuvers can be easily performed.
- As it requires less globe rotation the flexibility of microincision vitrectomy surgical instruments is not problematic anymore.

Types
Noncontact WAVS are:
- BIOM (Binocular Indirect Ophthalmo Microscope)
- Merlin
- OFFISS (Optical Fiber-Free Intravitreal Surgery System)
- Resight
- Penman-Wessels-Landers semi wide-angle viewing system

Contact WAVS are:
- Clarivit
- HRX

Angle view is around 95° in fluid-filled conditions and 125° in air-filled conditions.

Contact WAVS have different magnification and based on that have fixed-field angle of views, but noncontact WAVS has the field angle of view in noncontact viewing system can be changed by changing distance between preplaced lens and the corneal surface.

Both contact and noncontact viewing system can gain magnified views by zooming surgical microscope.

Contact viewing system is directly placed on cornea hence often require experienced assistants to hold as well there is complexity in the inverted footswitch control for the x–y imaging movement but it gives better imaging quality because the aberrations and reflections from the corneal surface are compensated.

Factors affecting angle of view are:
- *Status of lens:* Aphakic eye has a wider angle of view than phakic and pseudophakic.
- Air-filled eye has 10–15° more field view than fluid-filled eye.
- Pupil size.

 33. Discuss Terson syndrome.

It is basically a subarachnoid hemorrhage or intracerebral hemorrhage or traumatic brain injury which is associated with intraocular hemorrhages which can be vitreous hemorrhage, subhyaloid, or intraretinal. It usually occurs in adults, and occasionally in children. It can present both as unilateral and bilateral.

Etiology

- Causes of sudden increase in intracranial pressure
- Cortical venous sinus thrombosis
- Carotid artery occlusion
- Intra-arterial angiography
- Epidural saline injection
- Moyamoya disease
- Lumbosacral myelomeningocele
- Iatrogenic (during endoscopic third ventriculostomy).

Pathogenesis

- Exact cause unknown
- Several possible mechanisms
- First is, may be direct transmission of subarachnoid blood through optic nerve sheath (less likely).
- Second, sudden spike in intracranial pressure—rapid effusion of CSF into optic nerve sheath—mechanical dilation of retrobulbar optic nerve—compression over central retinal vein—venous hypertension—rupture of thin retinal vessels (more likely).

Clinical Manifestations

- Mostly present within an hour of onset of subarachnoid hemorrhage, but can be delayed up to a few days.
- Dome-shaped hemorrhage in macula with double ring sign (inner ring caused by sub-ILM hemorrhage and outer ring caused by subhyaloid hemorrhage.
- Neurological outcomes are worse in patients who have associated Terson syndrome.

Diagnosis

- Usually delayed because of late reference to ophthalmologist because of neurological impairment.
- Fundus examination
- B-scan—in hazy media secondary to vitreous hemorrhage
- Orbital CT scan—can be helpful.

Treatment

- Mostly resolve on its own.
- Observation can be done up to 3 months before going for a vitrectomy. In bilateral presentation within 4–8 weeks intervention is required.

Prognosis

- Younger age has better prognosis.
- VA is better in patients who got operated within 3 months than patients who got operated after 3 months.

Complications

- ERM—most common sequel (15-78%), because of induced glial proliferation and disruption of ILM
- Retinal folds/premacular folds
- Retinal detachment
- Ghost cell glaucoma
- Proliferative vitreoretinopathies
- Macular hole (iatrogenic)
- Preretinal fibrosis
- Dissociated optic nerve fiber layer appearance.

34. Discuss recent advances in choroidal assessment OCT, in which situations has it been applied.

The choroid is the posterior portion of the uveal tract that provides oxygen and nourishment to the outer portion of the retina and photoreceptors and hence an important role to play in various retinal pathologies. Its main functions include blood supply to the RPE, outer retina, and prelaminar portion of the optic nerve. Also, it acts as a heat sink as the choroidal melanocytes absorb excess light. Therefore, assessment of choroid thickness has become an important part of assessment of patients presenting with various macular disorders and the pachychoroid disease. The various tools that are useful in measurement of choroidal thickness are ultrasonography, magnetic resonance imaging (MRI), and OCT. Enhanced depth imaging (EDI) on spectral domain OCT and newer swept source OCT can tell even the fine details of choroidal anatomy.

Enhanced Depth Imaging Optical Coherence Tomography

Enhanced depth imaging OCT is a novel technique that takes advantage of the increased depth of field from the inverted image obtained by placing a SD-OCT device close to eye. This helps in better visualization of choroid and choroid scleral junction.

- EDI allows evaluation of anatomy and thickness of the choroid.
- EDI displaces the zero delay line which is the point of maximal OCT signal sensitivity.
- With conventional OCT the zero delay line is positioned at the posterior vitreous level to provide a clear image of vitreoretinal structures. Here with EDI the zero delay line is displaced deeper in the tissue to provide choroidal images with great resolution.
- Image averaging, high-speed scanning, eye tracking, and low speckle noise result in an enhanced visualization of the choroidal morphology and enables quantitative measurements.
- With the help of EDI studies has shown with age-choroidal thickness decreases by approximately 15 µm with every decade of life.
- Even in the same age group choroidal thickness can vary.
- Choroidal thickness is maximum at central macula and becomes thinner in all directions especially nasally.
- Choroid is thinner in myopic eyes.
- Diurnal variation can be seen, slightly thicker in morning compared to evening.
- Choroid is thinnest at inferonasal to the optic nerve, this thinning corresponds to the optic fissure during development.
- Defining choroidal scleral junction (CSJ) is important, in some patients it is distinct, while in others it is broad hyporeflective band which corresponds to laminate fiscal which correlate to suprachoroidal layer histologically.

Swept-source Optical Coherence Tomography

It is a Fourier domain depth resolved method which is distinct from SD-OCT.

- It uses a frequency swept laser with a narrow band light sources that is rapidly turned over.
- Swept-source optical coherence tomography is a Fourier domain depth-resolved method distinct from SD-OCT. It uses a frequency swept laser with a narrow band light source that is, rapidly tuned over a broad optical bandwidth that enables the measurement of interference at different optical frequencies or wavelengths sequentially over time.

- No spectrometer or line camera is needed for the Fourier transformation. This increases the imaging speed up to 300,000 axial scans per second and allows a deeper penetration of the sampling beam. SS-OCT offers several potential advantages over SD-OCT, including increased sensitivity through the full imaging depth, decreased fringe washout, better axial resolution over a broad imaging range, and higher detection efficiencies.
- Since it uses a longer wavelength, it has the potential to image the choroid and even the scleral tissue better than conventional SD-OCT.
- Multiple studies have evaluated the image quality between these two deep-penetration OCT techniques, and other studies have assessed the agreement between these EDI-OCT and SS-OCT in measuring choroidal thickness, which is the most used parameter to study and differentiate primarily choroidal diseases.
- The subfoveal choroidal thickness measurements taken using SS-OCT and SD-OCT devices were very similar, with mean differences ranging from only 7 to 15 μ between the two OCT systems. With EDI, as the point of maximum sensitivity (zero delay line) moves to the choroid, detection of the inner retinal surface is reduced, and the posterior vitreous is not visible. To overcome this limitation and to obtain a single comprehensive image of both vitreoretinal interface and choroid a novel imaging method called combined depth imaging can be performed.
- Using a commercially available SD-OCT device, which is easy, fast, and sensitive to visualize posterior vitreo-retino-choroidal structures into a single, comprehensive image.

Applications

Central Serous Chorioretinopathy

- Increased choroidal thickness is a common finding in CSCR, especially in the areas of increased choroidal permeability on ICG angiography. This supports the role of the choroidal vasculature in CSCR. In particular, visualizing an extremely thick choroid in CSCR can be helpful in the differential diagnosis with AMD, where choroidal thickness is generally decreased compared to age-matched healthy subjects.
- Decrease in choroidal thickness following PDT but no change in choroidal thickness after LPC has been noted. Considering that CSCR arises from an abnormally thick choroid due to increased choroidal permeability, choroidal thinning after PDT supports its role in CSCR treatment. Fellow eyes of CSCR patients have also an increased choroidal thickness compared with normal eyes. Thus, choroidal thickness assessment using deep-penetration OCT would be useful for monitoring this disease over time.

Age-related Macular Degeneration

- Choroidal changes on SD-OCT in early AMD may not be very obvious; however, in the later stage of the disease, choroidal thinning has been reported compared to age-matched healthy individuals.
- In reticular pseudodrusen, loss of small choroidal veins on histopathology can be seen as choroidal thinning in the areas where pseudodrusen are located. Also, eyes with reticular pseudodrusen have a generally thinner choroid compared to eyes with early AMD. This differentiation is important as the eyes with reticular pseudodrusen are at a higher risk of developing wet AMD.
- It also helps in differentiating AMD from polypoidal choroidal vasculopathy (PCV).
- Retinal angiomatous proliferans (RAP), here choroidal imaging showed a thinner subfoveal choroidal thickness compared to typical wet AMD.
- Advanced form of dry AMD, subfoveal choroidal thickness may be a better predictor of disease progression.
- After multiple injections of anti-VEGF in wet AMD, a reduction in choroidal thickness has been reported.
- The subfoveal choroidal thickness may be a predictive factor for visual outcome and treatment response in typical wet AMD after intravitreal anti-VEGF injections.
- Foveomacular vitelliform dystrophy adult onset, one of the major differential diagnosis of wet AMD. In case of AMD, subretinal fluid is related to abnormal permeability of the CNV complex. In adult-onset foveomacular vitelliform dystrophy (AOFVD), subretinal fluid is because of lipofuscin material reabsorption without evidence of CNV complex.
- OCT angiography helps to visualize the stromal choroidal vessels as well as choriocapillaris. In addition to choriocapillaris, it can help in delineating CNV complex as well as quantitative estimation of flow.

Vogt–Koyanagi–Harada Syndrome

Choroid is the primary tissue involved. A significant increase in choroidal thickness happens during the acute stage of the disease, whereas during treatment progressive thinning occurs and correlates with decreasing inflammatory activity. OCT can help in diagnosis recurrence and could guide physicians in the early diagnosis of disease activity recurrence.

Sarcoidosis

It is primarily a choroidal inflammatory lesion. Hyporeflective well-demarcated choroidal lesion can be seen on EDI OCT which clinically correlates with noncaseating inflammatory infiltrates or granuloma.

Toxoplasma Retinochoroiditis

The assessment of choroidal involvement during and after toxoplasma retinochoroiditis can be simply performed by the use of OCT, which can provide useful information about the treatment response for active toxoplasmosis.

Retinitis Pigmentosa

If we can measure choroidal thickness with help of OCT, suprachoroidal implantation of electrode arrays will be possible then.

Diabetic Retinopathy

Subfoveal choroidal thickness is a predictor of response to anti-VEGF.

Pathologic Myopia

Thinning of choroid in pathological myopia can predispose for formation of CNV complex.

Choroidal Masses

It is very important to differentiate between benign and malignant tumors. EDI OCT plays a vital role. Melanocytic tumors demonstrate a highly reflective band within the choriocapillaris with posterior shadowing, whilst amelanotic nevi appears homogeneous with a medium reflective band associated with visible choroidal vessels within the tumor. In addition, choroidal nevi show smooth moderate dome-shaped with overlying retinal pigment epithelial alterations, subretinal cleft, and photoreceptor loss. Choroidal melanomas have a highly reflective band in the anterior choroid with lack of visibility of either the choroidal vessels or inner sclera, and they are smooth, moderately dome-shaped, and with overlying shaggy photoreceptors. Choroidal hemangiomas appear as a medium-to-low reflective band with a homogeneous signal and intrinsic spaces as well as smooth, acutely dome-shaped, and with subretinal fluid and/or cystoid retinal edema.

Uveal Effusion Syndrome

It is an idiopathic condition where there is exudative of transudative fluid escapes from the choriocapillaris into the surrounding potential space causing choroidal thickening and engorgement which leads to serous retinal detachment later. It is a rare disease which is related to impaired scleral permeability to proteins and compression of the vortex veins. EDI OCT helps in diagnosis as well and postsurgical assessment.

5.2 Photoreceptors

Mahesh Kumar MH, Navneet Sidhu, Monika Kapoor

1. Discuss anatomy and physiology of rods and cones, their distribution over retina. What are the implications in vision quality with rod and cone dysfunction?

Introduction

Rod and cone photoreceptors are specialized light-sensitive neurons in the retina which kick-start the process of vision. They are highly compartmentalized in structure and function, involving five principal regions:
1. Outer segment (OS)
2. Connecting cilium
3. Inner segment
4. Nuclear region
5. Synaptic region.

The OS captures light and performs the function of phototransduction, i.e., converting it into electrical signals. The connecting cilium, as the name implies, connects the OS with the inner segment, acting as a pipeline for the movement of substances via itself. The inner segment contains cell organelles, i.e., mitochondria, endoplasmic reticulum, Golgi complex, and lysosomes. The nucleus of the cell lies within the nuclear region. The photoreceptor terminates in the synaptic region, which contains synaptic vesicles housing the neurotransmitter glutamate, which is involved in the transmission of impulses from photoreceptors to bipolar cells and other secondary neurons.

Rods

There are about 120 million rods in the human retina, each being 40–60 μm long. Named on the basis of their cylindrical (rod-shaped) OSs, they contain visual purple (rhodopsin) which is specialized in peripheral vision and scotopic vision.
- Rod OSs are cylindrical and striated transversely, and contain rhodopsin pigment. There are around 600–1000 lipid-protein lamellar discs stacked on top of each other in the rod OS.
- The inner segment of rods is thicker as compared to the OS. It consists of two zones:
    1. Ellipsoid zone—outer zone consisting of mitochondria
    2. Myoid zone—inner zone consisting of glycogen and other organelles.

    Rods terminate in a rod spherule which is a bulb-like structure in contact with the cone foot.

Cones

There are about 6.5 million cones in the human retina. They contain iodopsin which is responsible for photopic vision and color vision. Cones have a wide range of lengths, ranging from 80 μm at the fovea to 40 μm at the periphery.
- Outer segment is conical in shape, with lamellar discs narrower than those in rods
- *Inner segment is divided into*:
    - Outer ellipsoid zone—which is densely packed with mitochondria and is metabolically very active
    - Inner myoid zone—contains other organelles

    Cone end has lateral processes called cone foot or cone pedicle which is located in the outer plexiform layer.

Physiology

Photoreceptor OSs house bilipid membranous discs that contain visual pigment consisting of a protein called opsin and a vitamin A-derived chromophore known as retinal. In the dark, the photoreceptor cell is partially depolarized by the "dark current", a steady current carried primarily by Na^+ ions, and releases neurotransmitter glutamate from its synaptic terminals onto second-order neurons.

On light stimulation: The dark current stops, resulting in the hyperpolarization of photoreceptor cell membrane, and cessation of neurotransmitter release to second-order neurons.

In the conventional visual cycle, photoexcitation causes release of all-*trans*-retinal from rhodopsin, which is then reduced to all-*trans*-retinol. Interphotoreceptor retinoid-binding protein (IRBP) shuttles all-*trans*-retinol to retinal pigment epithelium (RPE) cells where it is first converted to its retinyl esters by lecithin retinol acyltransferase (LRAT), after which it is isomerized to 11-*cis*-retinol, oxidized to 11-*cis*-retinal, and delivered back to photoreceptors by IRBP for the regeneration of rhodopsin.

In addition to the conventional visual cycle, cones also use a modified visual cycle in which 11-*cis*-retinal is resynthesized from all-*trans*-retinol through a series of reactions occurring in cones as well as Müller cells.

Spatial Distribution of Rods and Cones

Photoreceptors in the retina are assembled in a fairly exact mosaic, which, at the fovea, is a hexagonal packing of cones, that is broken outside the fovea by the rods, i.e., extrafoveal cones are surrounded by rings of rods. The optic nerve is photoreceptor free, hence forming the physiological blind spot.
- *Cone density:* Highest at the fovea. Cones are higher in number on the nasal than on the temporal retina.
- *Rod distribution:* Peaks in a ring around the fovea at about 4.5 mm or 18° from the foveal pit. Rods are absent at the fovea in an area of 0.35 mm.

The nasal retina has 20–25% more rods than temporal retina. Superior retina has 2% more rods than inferior retina.

Dysfunction of Rods and Cones

These are a heterogeneous group of disorders inherited as autosomal recessive, autosomal dominant, or X-linked (XL) recessive traits, and present at birth or in early infancy **(Table 1)**.

TABLE 1: Photoreceptor dysfunction.

Photoreceptor dysfunction	Inheritance	Impact on vision
Cone dysfunctions		
Complete achromatopsia/typical achromatopsia/rod monochromatism	AR	Usually hypermetropic refractive error with nystagmus and absent color vision
Incomplete achromatopsia, synonym atypical achromatopsia	AR	Usually hypermetropic refractive error with nystagmus and reduced color vision
Blue-cone monochromatism, synonym S-cone monochromatism; X-linked incomplete achromatopsia; X-linked atypical achromatopsia	XLR	Usually myopic refractive error with nystagmus and residual tritan discrimination
Oligocone trichromacy	AR	Equal prevalence of myopia and hypermetropia, with normal fundus and color vision, nystagmus is often absent
Bornholm eye disease, synonym X-linked cone dysfunction syndrome with dichromacy and myopia	XLR	Moderate-high myopia with astigmatism, protanopia or deuteranopia, with no nystagmus
Bradyopsia, also known as RGS9/R9AP-retinopathy	AR	Equal prevalence of myopia and hypermetropia, with normal fundus and color vision, nystagmus is often absent
Rod dysfunctions		
Congenital stationary night blindness (AD CSNB)	AD	No nystagmus, usually with no refractive error. Cone function is normal
Congenital stationary night blindness (AR CSNB)	AR	Nystagmus, usually with myopic refractive error. Cone function is reduced
Congenital stationary night blindness (XL CSNB)	X-linked	Nystagmus, usually with myopic refractive error. Cone function is reduced
Oguchi disease	AR	Visual acuity is often normal or mildly reduced, no nystagmus. Cone function is normal. Mizuo Nakamura phenomenon is characteristic
Fundus albipunctatus without cone dystrophy	AR	Visual acuity and cone function are normal. Multiple white dots are seen scattered throughout the retinal pigment epithelium
Fundus albipunctatus with cone dystrophy	AR	Visual acuity is normal, cone function is reduced. Multiple white dots are seen scattered throughout the retinal pigment epithelium

(AD: autosomal dominant; AR: autosomal recessive; XLR: X-linked recessive)

- **Rod dysfunction syndromes** such as congenital stationary night blindness, Oguchi disease, fundus albipunctatus usually have reduced visual acuity, nystagmus, and symptomatic night blindness.
- **Cone dysfunction syndromes** such as incomplete achromatopsia, complete achromatopsia, blue cone monochromatism, oligocone trichromacy, and X-linked cone dysfunction with dichromacy and myopia present with reduced visual acuity, photophobia, nystagmus, and color vision disturbance.

5.3 Vitreous Hemorrhage

Mahesh Kumar MH, Monika Kapoor

 1. Discuss vitreous hemorrhage.

The presence of extravasated blood within the closed space demarcated anteriorly by the zonular fibers of the lens and posterior capsule, posteriorly and laterally by the internal limiting membrane (ILM) of the retina, the nonpigmented epithelium of the ciliary body laterally is defined as vitreous hemorrhage (VH).

Types of Vitreous Hemorrhage

Based on the location of the blood, VH can be classified as follows:
- Preretinal hemorrhage:
  - *Subhyaloid hemorrhage:* Boat-shaped, generally immobile pool of blood between nondetached hyaloid and ILM. It is usually seen in proliferative diabetic retinopathy. If the hemorrhage lies between extensively detached hyaloid and ILM, it contains altered blood and can shift with the position.

- *Sub-ILM hemorrhage:* Though located between the nerve fiber layer of the retina and ILM, it is considered a type of VH because clinical differentiation from subhyaloid hemorrhage is difficult, owing to its boat-shaped appearance with a horizontal upper level, and immobility. It is seen in retinal macroaneurysm, Terson syndrome, valsalva retinopathy, penetrating ocular injury, anemia, shaken baby syndrome, branch retinal vein occlusion (BRVO), and diabetic retinopathy. In patients with sickle-cell retinopathy, it occurs when aggregated sickled red blood cells (RBCs) abruptly occlude and cause blowout of an arteriole, resulting in what is commonly called a "salmon patch".

- *Intravitreal or intragel hemorrhage:* The blood is dispersed in the gel and clots rapidly. Massive and recurrent hemorrhage resolves slowly and incompletely, and may form yellowish fluffy vitreous opacities and dense white and yellowish vitreous membranes (chicken fat VH). Blood in synthetic cavities remains mostly unclotted and accumulates in the dependent part of the globe. Blood in the gel vitreous itself promotes vitreous degeneration, liquefaction, and cavity formation. The color of the blood is determined by the extent of the degeneration of red blood cells, and may vary from red to yellow.

There are aqueous-filled spaces lying anterior to the border of formed vitreous, i.e.,:

- The canal of Hannover between orbiculo-anterocapsular and orbiculo-posterocapsular parts of zonular fibers
- Berger's canal (retrolental space of Erggelet) and canal of Petit between the anterior hyaloid membrane and posterior capsular surface and orbiculo-posterocapsular part of zonular fibers, separated from each other by Wieger's ligament. Blood within Berger's space collects in a crescent shape with the hyaloideocapsular ligament as its inferior border. Hemorrhage into the canal of Petit has a crescent-shaped superior border, which is also formed by the hyaloideocapsular ligament.
- Cloquet's canal and bursa premacularis are fluid-filled spaces within formed vitreous.

Hemorrhage into Berger's space, the canal of Petit, and Cloquet's canal have also been included in VH.

Clinical Features

The most common presenting feature is a sudden onset of vision loss which is usually painless. Other complaints could be floaters, photopsias, and the perception of shadows and cobwebs. Visual acuity in eyes with VH and retained macular function is primarily determined by the location and density of the hemorrhage and may range from sudden painless loss of vision to mildly impaired vision.

Conditions Simulating Vitreous Hemorrhage (Differential Diagnoses)

- Uveitis (vitritis)
- Asteroid hyalosis
- Amyloidosis of the vitreous
- Ocular or systemic lymphoma.

Causes of Vitreous Hemorrhage

Vitreous hemorrhage can be caused by pathological disruption of normal retinal vessels, bleeding from diseased retinal vessels or abnormal new vessels, and extension of hemorrhage through the retina from other sources. The various causes are summarized in **Table 1**.

TABLE 1: Etiology of vitreous hemorrhage.

Pathological disruption of normal retinal vessels	Bleeding from diseased retinal vessels or abnormal new vessels	Extension of hemorrhage through retina or other sources
• Anticoagulant therapy • Avulsed retinal vessel syndrome • Blunt or penetrating trauma • Bridging retinal vessel across retinal tear • Posterior vitreous detachment • Hyperviscosity syndromes • Terson syndrome • Valsalva retinopathy	• Diabetic retinopathy • Retinal neovascularization following retinal vein occlusions (BRVO, CRVO) • Subretinal neovascularization • Blood dyscrasias • Eales disease • Arteriovenous malformation of the retina • Coats' disease • Hypertensive retinopathy • Persistent hyaloid artery • Retinoblastoma • Retinal astrocytic hamartoma • Retinal angioma	• Age-related macular degeneration • Choroidal melanoma • Intrusion of scleral buckle • Multiple hemorrhagic retinal pigment epithelium (RPE) detachments (posterior uveal bleeding syndrome)

(BRVO: branch retinal vein occlusion; CRVO: central retinal vein occlusion)

- Vitreous hemorrhages clear from the eye at varying rates, depending on the volume of the blood and the status of the vitreous gel, i.e., a hemorrhage in a vitrectomized eye may clear rapidly.
- Spontaneous resolution may occur, the process involving clot formation, fibrinolysis, RBC hemolysis, absorption of blood byproducts by macrophage-assisted phagocytosis.
- Once the vitreous gel undergoes syneresis and begins to liquefy, the lysed blood can be efficiently reabsorbed. Vitreous liquefaction occurs more easily in the aphakic eye.
- Blood may remain in the vitreous cavity and form an intravitreal cyst or chocolate cyst.
- In addition, some of the blood may move through the anterior chamber and trabecular meshwork.

Diagnosis of Vitreous Hemorrhage

The underlying cause can be detected by retinal examination. In case of dense VH, history and examination of fellow eye can give suggestive clues.

Ultrasound: In cases where the posterior segment is not visible due to dense VH, a B-scan (brightness scan) with A-scan (amplitude scan) is done to find out the etiology and features of the hemorrhage.
- Fresh unclotted blood cannot be identified, as cellular accumulation occurs, reflectivity increases proportionately.
- In mild hemorrhage a chain of low amplitude spikes is seen on A-scan and dots and short lines are displayed on B-scan.
- If intravitreal blood gets organized, higher reflectivity on A-scan and membranous surfaces on B-scan can be noted.
- Kinetic B-scan ultrasonography (USG) typically shows an undulating after movement in posterior vitreous detachment (PVD).
- Subhyaloid (subvitreal) blood shows a smooth membrane on A-scan with a highly reflective spike, simulating a retinal detachment is found. This is known as posterior hyphema.

Optical coherence tomography (OCT): It is used to differentiate between subhyaloid or sub-ILM bleed in cases of premacular hemorrhage.

Fundus fluorescein angiography (FFA)/Indocyanine green angiography (ICGA): FFA helps in localizing areas with capillary nonperfusion and neovascularization to plan laser therapy. ICGA has the advantage of better clarity in VH due to the longer wavelength used.

Magnetic resonance imaging (MRI):
- Contrast-enhanced (Gd-DTPA) MRI is very helpful to differentiate subacute VH with retinal detachment from uveal melanoma in adults and retinoblastoma in children.
- Acute hemorrhagic retinal detachment appears isointense on T1-weighted (T1W) images and it is markedly hypointense on T2W images with respect to vitreous.
- In chronic stage of hemorrhage, there is accumulation of ferritin and hemosiderin causing changes in MRI features. The area of hyperintensity decreases to marked hypointensity in both T1W and T2W images.

Treatment of Vitreous Hemorrhage

- *Mild VH:* Often clears spontaneously within a matter of days to weeks, but if it persists, initial or supplemental panretinal laser photocoagulation (without vitrectomy) can be delivered. If laser is not possible, anti-vascular endothelial growth factor (VEGF) injection and early vitrectomy should be considered.
- Retinal laser photocoagulation can successfully give prophylaxis against VH in vascular retinopathies particularly in diabetic retinopathy, Eales' disease, BRVO, etc.
- Early vitrectomy is considered in cases of bilateral VH causing blindness, tight preretinal macular hemorrhage, chronically recurring hemorrhage, acute VH with retinal detachment, and VH with known tractional retinal detachment close to the macula.
- The goal of the surgery is to release all anterior-posterior vitreous traction and to perform retinal photocoagulation if indicated to prevent recurrent hemorrhage.
- *Nonclearing postvitrectomy hemorrhage:* If it persists beyond 3–4 weeks, revision surgery with vitreous cavity lavage and possible supplemental endolaser should be considered.
- *Dense premacular hemorrhage:* Early vitrectomy should be considered; anti-VEGF can also be considered as preoperative adjunct 1 week prior to surgery.

- *Laser hyaloidotomy:* Premacular subvitreal hemorrhage causing significant visual loss can be drained with argon green laser or YAG laser; the blood is drained into the dependent part of the vitreous cavity and there is immediate visual restoration.

Complications of Vitreous Hemorrhage

- Vitreous syneresis
- Hemosiderosis bulbi
- Vitreous bands and membranes causing cellophane retinopathy or fixed retinal folds
- *Glaucoma:*
  - Ghost cell glaucoma
  - Hemolytic glaucoma
  - Hemosiderotic glaucoma
- Necrosis of ganglion cell layer of retina and optic atrophy
- Cataract
- Siderotic changes in cornea and retina.

5.4 Pars Plana Vitrectomy

Mahesh Kumar MH, Monika Kapoor

 1. Discuss pars plana surgery and its indications.

- Pars plana vitrectomy (PPV) is a technique in vitreoretinal surgery that enables access to the posterior segment surgically.
- *Indications:*
  - Removal of vitreous opacities
  - Relieving vitreoretinal traction
  - Restoring normal anatomical relationship of the retina and retinal pigment epithelium (RPE)
  - Accessing subretinal space
  - *Specific conditions include:*
    - Macular hole
    - Epiretinal membrane
    - Vitreomacular traction
    - Vitreous hemorrhage
    - Tractional retinal detachment
    - Rhegmatogenous retinal detachment
    - Refractory macular edema
    - Vitreous biopsy
    - Endophthalmitis
    - Dislocated intraocular lens
    - Retained lens material
    - Intraocular foreign body
- *Basic components of vitrectomy setup are:*
  - Vitrectomy machine
  - Surgical microscope
  - Infusion cannula
  - Endoillumination light source
  - *Vitrectomy cutter:*
    - 20G has 0.9 mm diameter
    - 23G has 0.6 mm diameter
    - 27G has 0.4 mm diameter
    - 25G has 0.5 mm diameter

- *Surgical viewing systems:* Two main categories are:
  - Noncontact viewing system—includes Zeiss RESIGHT and Oculus BIOM wide-angle viewing systems.
  - Contact lens systems—include advanced visual instruments—offer one with 68° view to the equator and another with a 130° view up to ora serrata.
  - For macular surgery, special contact lens such as DORC flat vitrectomy lens enables higher resolution.
- *Surgical principles:* Three common surgeries that utilize PPV are:
  1. Retinal detachment repair
  2. Membrane peeling
  3. Crystalline lens removal
  - For pars plana lensectomy, soft lenses can be removed using vitrectomy cutter, but denser lenses may require fragmentome.
- *Complications:* Cataract, glaucoma, endophthalmitis, retinal tear, retinal detachment, hypotony, suprachoroidal effusion, cystoids macular edema, optic neuropathy, and phototoxicity.

5.5 Posteriorly Dislocated Nucleus

Mahesh Kumar MH, Monika Kapoor

1. Describe approach to a case of posteriorly dislocated nucleus.

Or

Discuss the management of posteriorly dislocated nucleus fragment into vitreous in a 65-year-old male 1 month postoperative after phacoemulsification.

Approach to a case of posteriorly dislocated nucleus includes the following:
- Incidence of posteriorly displaced lens fragments is probably 0.3%.
- Posterior loss of lens fragments is usually recognized after posterior capsular rupture.
- Common predisposing factors for posterior capsular rupture include:
  - Posterior polar cataract (PPC) and the cataract associated with posterior lenticonus or lentiglobus
  - Postvitrectomy cataract
  - Traumatic cataract
  - White cataract
  - Black cataract
- *Signs of early posterior capsular tear or zonular dehiscence include:*
  - Sudden deepening of the anterior chamber with momentary dilatation of the pupil
  - Sudden transitory appearance of a clear red reflex peripherally
  - Newly apparent inability to rotate a previously mobile nucleus
  - Excessive lateral mobility or displacement of the nucleus and loss of nucleus followability
  - Excessive tipping of one pole of the nucleus
  - Partial descent of the nucleus into the anterior vitreous space
- *Rescuing partially dropped nucleus:*
  - Posterior capsule or zonular rupture should be recognized early enough to avoid a dropped nucleus.
  - Continued phaco maneuvers and forces will expand the initial defect thereby creating a big hiatus to permit the nucleus to drop.
  - No attempt should be made to chase and spear the descending nucleus with the phaco tip.
  - Nucleus can be levitated into the pupillary plane or anterior chamber for subsequent management by extraction through a standard extracapsular cataract extraction (ECCE) incision.
  - The "PAL" technique (posterior assisted levitation), utilizes a cyclodialysis spatula through a pars plana stab incision to push the nucleus up into the anterior chamber from below.
  - Modified PAL includes inserting a viscoat cannula through a pars plana stab incision located 3.5 mm behind the limbus. Through a combination of injecting viscoat and maneuvering the cannula tip itself, the nucleus can be elevated through the capsulorhexis and pupil and into the anterior chamber.

Evaluation includes:
- Best corrected visual acuity (BCVA)
- *Slit-lamp biomicroscopy (pre- and postdilation):*
  - Degree of corneal edema
  - Uveitis
  - Cortex at pupil
  - Extent of posterior capsular rupture and integrity of capsular zonular apparatus
- Applanation tonometry
- Fundus examination/B-scan ultrasonography (USG)
- *Indications for removal of a dislocated crystalline lens:*
  - Impaired visual acuity
  - Phacolytic uveitis, glaucoma
  - Retinal detachment
  - Vitreous herniation into the anterior chamber resulting in a cystoid macular edema
  - Severe monocular diplopia (relative indication)
- *Indications for removal of lens fragments:*
  - Eyes with small retained lens fragments may be observed without treatment. Careful observation for 1–2 weeks, especially with smaller fragments and can be extended beyond this depending on clinical progress.
  - Surgery is indicated in eyes with moderate or severe inflammation or retention of 25% or more of lens material.
  - Elevated IOP calls for immediate surgery.
  - Associated retinal detachments, retinal tears, or endophthalmitis are all urgent indications for surgery.
- *Surgical options:*
  - The common technique currently used to remove a crystalline lens dislocated into the vitreous cavity includes performing a three-port pars plana vitrectomy (PPV). It includes PPV→ fragmentation of nucleus with a fragmentome along with usage of perfluorocarbon liquid (PFCL).
  - For very hard dislocated crystalline lens—preferable to remove it through the anterior (limbal route) using either a cryo or an irrigating vectis.
  - For dislocated crystalline lens with an associated rhegmatogenous retinal detachment, the scleral buckle is placed prior to the lens removal.
  - *Timing of vitrectomy:* Surgery to remove the retained lens fragments is performed within 2 weeks of the original cataract surgery to aid in:
    - Visual rehabilitation
    - To break the cycle of progressive lens-induced inflammation
    - To avoid long-term glaucoma
- *There are three basic approaches to removing lens fragments by PPV:*
  1. By ultrasonic fragmentation
  2. (A) Crushing the nuclear fragments between the endoilluminator and cutter; (B) retrieval through the limbal route.
  3. Using the vitrectomy cutter for soft nucleus or cortical matter.
- *Complications associated with vitrectomy includes:*
  - Retinal detachment (0–45%)
  - Cystoid macular edema (5–22%)
  - Elevated intraocular pressure (25–52%).

5.6 Photodynamic Therapy

Mahesh Kumar MH, Monika Kapoor

 1. Write a short note on verteporfin and photodynamic therapy.

Verteporfin

- Light-activated drug used in photodynamic therapy
- Lyophilized dark green cake
- The molecular formula is $C_{41}H_{42}N_4O_8$ with a molecular weight of approximately 718.8.

Mechanism of Action
- Two-stage process requiring injection and nonthermal red light, transported in the plasma by lipoproteins.
- Once activated by light in the presence of oxygen, it generates highly reactive, short-lived singlet oxygen, and reactive oxygen radicals.
- These oxygen radicals preferentially accumulate in neovasculature, including choroidal neovasculature and result in local damage to neovascular endothelium, resulting in vessel occlusion.
- Damaged endothelium in turn release procoagulant and vasoactive factors through the lipoxygenase (leukotriene) and cyclooxygenase (eicosanoids such as thromboxane) pathways, resulting in platelet aggregation, fibrin clot formation, and vasoconstriction.

Pharmacokinetics
Elimination half-life—5–6 hours mainly by hepatic metabolism.

Administration
- Reconstituted with 7 mL of sterile water for injection—2 mg/mL in 7.5 mL
- Reconstituted solution must be protected from light and used within 4 hours. Inspected for particulate matter and discoloration prior to administration—opaque dark green solution.
- Normal saline or other parenteral solutions are avoided as it may form precipitate in saline except 5% dextrose for injection, for dilution of the reconstituted Visudyne.
- The volume of reconstituted Visudyne required to achieve the desired dose of 6 mg/m^2 body surface area is withdrawn from the vial and diluted with 5% dextrose for injection to a total infusion volume of 30 mL.
- The full infusion volume is administered intravenously over 10 minutes at a rate of 3 mL/min, using an appropriate syringe pump and in-line filter (1.2 µm).
- Precautions should be taken to prevent extravasation at the injection site and if it occurs thoroughly protect it from direct light until swelling and discoloration have faded in order to prevent the occurrence of a local burn.

Lesion Size Determination
- The greatest linear dimension (GLD) of the lesion is estimated by fluorescein angiography and color fundus photography.
- All classic and occult choroidal neovascularization (CNV), blood and/or blocked fluorescence, and any serous detachments of the retinal pigment epithelium should be included for this measurement.

Spot Size Determination
- The treatment spot size should be 1,000 µm larger than the GLD of the lesion on the retina to allow a 500 µm border.
- Maximum spot size used in the clinical trials was 6,400 µm. The nasal edge of the treatment spot must be positioned at least 200 µm from the temporal edge of the optic disc.

Laser Delivery
- Initiate 689 nm wavelength laser light delivery to the patient 15 minutes after the start of the 10 minutes infusion with Visudyne as a single circular spot via a fiber optic and a slit lamp, using a suitable ophthalmic magnification lens.
- Recommended light dose is 50 J/cm^2 of neovascular lesion intensity of 600 mW/cm^2. Duration—over 83 seconds.

5.7 Macular Function Tests in Opaque Media

Mahesh Kumar MH, Monika Kapoor

 1. Evaluate macular function tests in opaque media.

Preoperative estimation of macular function in a patient with opaque media, e.g., in a dense vitreous hemorrhage or mature cataract, is imperative to predict the postoperative improvement in vision, to assess the risk–benefit ratio of a high-risk surgery, and to measure the relative contribution of retinal and optical disease to the loss of vision when the two coexist. A preliminary B-scan ultrasonography can give a fair idea about the anatomy of the posterior pole but macular function tests must be performed to assess the physiological status of the macula.

Macular Function Tests

In the presence of clear media, macular status can be assessed using tests such as color vision, contrast sensitivity, two-point discrimination, Amsler grid, and microperimetry, but macular function tests in the presence of opaque media must satisfy the following prerequisites:
- It must be able to project the image on the retina through the density or must be able to bypass the opacity.
- It should not obligate the visual system to assemble a high-quality image.

The tests that satisfy the above criteria and are useful in assessment of retinal and neural physiological status in the presence of media opacity are:
- Maddox rod
- Two-point discrimination
- Focal electroretinogram (ERG)
- Visually evoked potential (VEP)
- Laser interferometry
- Potential visual acuity meter test
- Entopic phenomena
- Preferential hyperacuity perimeter.

Maddox Rod Test

This is a simple, straightforward, and reliable test that can be used in semi-opaque media. The patient is asked to observe a light placed at a distance of 1/3 meter through a Maddox rod. The ability to visualize a straight unbroken line hints at normal macular function, and any break/hole, discoloration/distortion indicates a macular lesion.

Two-Point Discrimination

Crude assessment of macular function can be performed by asking the patient to look at two-point sources of light that are 2 inches apart, placed at a distance of 2 feet away from the patient in a darkened room, and his ability to appreciate the presence of two lights suggests normal functioning of the central area of the retina.

Focal Electroretinogram

Electroretinogram is the recording of the electrical potential waveform generated by the preganglionic retina in response to a flash or pattern, with the flash being an ideal stimulus as it can penetrate dense media opacities. It consists of three waves: a-wave (negative waveform arising from rods and cones), b-wave (positive wave representing the activity of bipolar cells), and c-wave (second positive wave representing the metabolic activity of the retinal pigment epithelium). A simple and convenient ERG is the Maxwell ophthalmoscope, a handheld foveal ERG, which uses a 3–4° white flickering light onto the fovea with a 10° annulus of constant white light to desensitize the surrounding retina, and can give a gross idea of the macular function.

Visually Evoked Potential

The other electrophysical test, that primarily reflects macular function by measuring the electric potential generated in the macula in response to a stimulus, and is more useful than ERG which mainly mirrors the response of rods to a stimulus, is VEP. But since it represents the integrity of the entire visual pathway from retina to occipital lobe, it cannot differentiate between macula, optic nerve head, and cortical pathology.

Laser Interferometry

Coherent white light or helium-neon laser is used to generate interference fringes which are onto the retina, where they are perceived as alternate dark and light bands, through a clear part of the lens. The resolving power is calculated from the minimum separation between an adjacent dark and light band at which they are seen separately. Overestimation of visual potential can take place in amblyopia, macular hole, cystoid macular edema, glaucomatous field loss cutting through fixation, and underestimation can occur in dense cataracts, poorly dilating pupils, and dense vitreous hemorrhage.

Potential Visual Acuity Meter Test

It is a slit lamp-mounted instrument that projects an aerial image of a reduced Snellen's chart via narrow beam of light of about 0.15 mm diameter through the pupil toward the macula. The ability of the patient to read the optotypes reflects the postoperative success rates, but since the beam cannot penetrate dense cataracts, potential acuity meter (PAM) usually gives a poorer prediction than the actual postoperative result. Its other limitations are the fact that it is a subjective test, and can only be done in an alert, oriented, and motivated patient.

Entoptic (Entopic) Phenomenon

Entoptic phenomena are the visual perceptions that have their origin within the structure of the eye. Three types are used for testing in an opaque media:
1. *Purkinje vascular entopic phenomenon:* If the eyes are closed and the globe is steadily and firmly massaged through the lower lid with a lighted torch, the entire vascular tree of the retina can be visualized on an orange background. Any blank area or scotomata can be particularly noted by oriented patients.
2. *Flying spot (blue-field entoptic phenomenon):* It relies on the observation of the leukocytes flowing in the parafoveal capillaries, when viewed against a background illuminated by a blue light (430 nm) produced by a 500W tungsten bulb or a Blue-Field Entoptoscope BFE 100.
3. *Haidinger's brushes:* The patient views a surface illuminated with blue light through a polarizer. Hourglass-shaped yellowish brushes, which rotate on rotating the polarizer, are seen radiating from the point of fixation.

These tests are also subjective and rely on the intelligence and cooperation of the patient.

Preferential Hyperacuity Perimeter

Hyperacuity refers to the visual performance level above that achieved by customary measurements of maximum visual acuity, and the ability to discern a subtle misalignment of the object. Hyperacuity thresholds are resistant to image degradation by optical blur and mild cataracts since the human visual system is able to calculate the centroid, or the so-called center of gravity of retinal light distribution of the target, and are raised only in case of impairment of the neural system behind the cataract. Vernier acuity, stereoacuity, displacement detection, and bisection of acuity are examples of hyperacuity. The test stimuli consist of two outer reference bars separated by a gap of 30 minutes arc, and thresholds are determined by a yes-no staircase procedure.

CHAPTER 6

Uvea

6.1 Uveitis

Gitanjli Sood Sirkek, Devesh Kumawat, Mahesh Kumar MH

Q 1. Discuss anatomy of the uveal tissue.

Taxonomy: "Uvea" is derived from a Greek word meaning "grape".
It can be divided into three parts: Iris, ciliary body, and choroid and the relevant anatomy is as described here.

Iris

Iris is the anterior most part of the uveal tract. It is a thin and circular part of the uvea, which forms a diaphragm-like structure in front of the crystalline lens with a central aperture called pupil. Iris is attached to the middle of anterior surface of ciliary body where the iris is thinnest (~0.5 mm). The iris divides the space in front of the lens into anterior chamber and posterior chamber. Anterior surface of the iris is divided into a pupillary zone and a ciliary zone by a circular ridge, located 1.5 mm away from pupillary margin, called collarette (also known as iris frill), which also is the thickest portion of iris (~1.5 mm).

- *Pupillary zone:* Pupillary zone extends from pupillary margin to collarette. Pupillary zone is relatively flat. Pupillary margin is marked by a dark border, known as pupillary ruff (anterior termination of the pigmented layer).
- *Ciliary zone:* Ciliary zone of iris extends from collarette to the iris root. There are some depressions or pit arranged in rows present in this area known as crypts. Crypts are found in two locations. Those present near collarette are relatively larger and known as Fuchs's crypt and few are seen in periphery of the iris.
- *Posterior surface of iris:* Posterior surface of the iris is much more uniform with numerous radial contraction folds. However, circular folds are also seen.

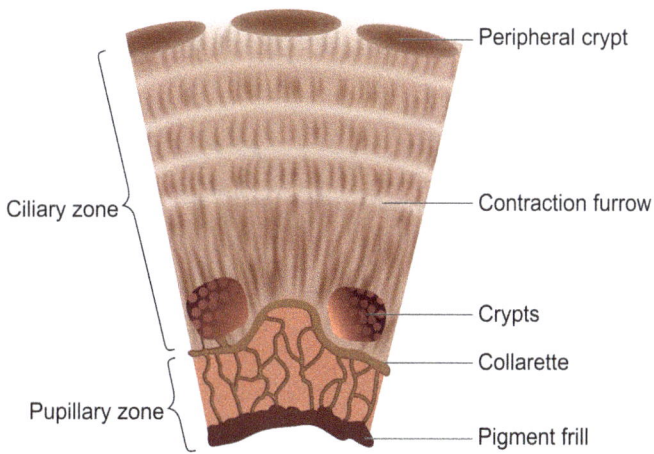

Microscopic Structure

- *Anterior limiting layer:* Anterior limiting layer lines the iris and is the anterior most condensations of iris stroma. The layer consists of mainly fibroblasts and melanocytes. These cells are arranged in a meshwork; fibroblasts are located

TABLE 1: Differences between muscles of the iris.

Sphincter pupillae	Dilator pupillae
Circular muscle, 0.75–1 mm wide, composed of smooth-muscle cells. It is thicker than the dilator pupillae. It encircles the pupil and is located in the pupillary zone of the stroma	It extends from the iris root to a point in the stroma below the midpoint of the sphincter. A dense band of connective tissue separates the sphincter and dilator muscles from each other
Is composed of spindle-shaped cells that are oriented parallel to the pupillary margin, so, contraction of the sphincter causes the pupil to constrict (a process known as miosis)	Because of the radial arrangement of the fibers of the muscle, contraction of the dilator pupillae muscle pulls the pupillary portion toward the root, thereby causing pupil to dilate (a process known as mydriasis)
The muscle is innervated by the parasympathetic system	The muscle is sympathetically innervated

on the surface and melanocyte beneath them. The color of the iris is largely determined by the pigment content (granules) within the anterior limiting layer and the melanocytes in the pigment epithelium. Anterior limiting layer is absent at the areas of crypts and very thin at the contraction furrows.

- *Iris stroma:* Iris stroma forms the main bulk of iris tissue and contains sphincter pupillae, dilator pupillae muscles, vessels, and nerves. It has pigmented melanocytes and clump cells, whereas the nonpigmented cells are fibroblasts, lymphocytes, macrophages, and mast cells. Fibroblasts are the most prominent cells in iris stroma. These cells are located in close association with blood vessels, muscles, and nerves. Melanocytes can be found around the adventitia of blood vessels. They have long processes with the help of which they form plexuses with fibroblasts and adjacent melanocytes.
  - *Muscles in iris stroma:* **Table 1** shows the muscles in iris stroma.
  - *Blood vessels in iris stroma:* Iris vessels include arterioles, venules, and capillaries. The iris arteries are branches of major circle of the iris, located in the ciliary body near the iris root. The iris vessels usually follow a radial course from the iris root to the pupil margin. Arrangement of collagen network prevents the iris vessels from kinking and compression during the extensive iris movement during constriction and dilatation of pupil. Iris veins have very thin walls consisting of endothelium surrounded by a thin layer of collagen. Capillaries are formed by a single layer of unfenestrated epithelium, which forms a part of the blood–aqueous barrier.
- *Anterior pigment epithelium:* The cells in anterior pigment epithelial layer of the iris have two distinct portions. Muscular basal portion anteriorly (lies next to stroma)—composed of elongated, contractile, smooth muscle fibers, and forms part of dilator muscle.

  The epithelial apical portion of anterior pigment epithelium is in close apposition with the apical surface of the posterior pigment epithelium. Similar kind of apex-to-apex arrangement is seen between the pigmented and nonpigmented epithelium (NPE) of ciliary body. The cause of this apex-to-apex arrangement is due to their common embryologic precursor, the optic cup.
- *Posterior pigment epithelium of iris:* Second layer of pigmented epithelium (PE) is situated posterior to the anterior epithelium. The cells are rectangular or pyramidal in shape with round cell nucleus and their cytoplasm contains large

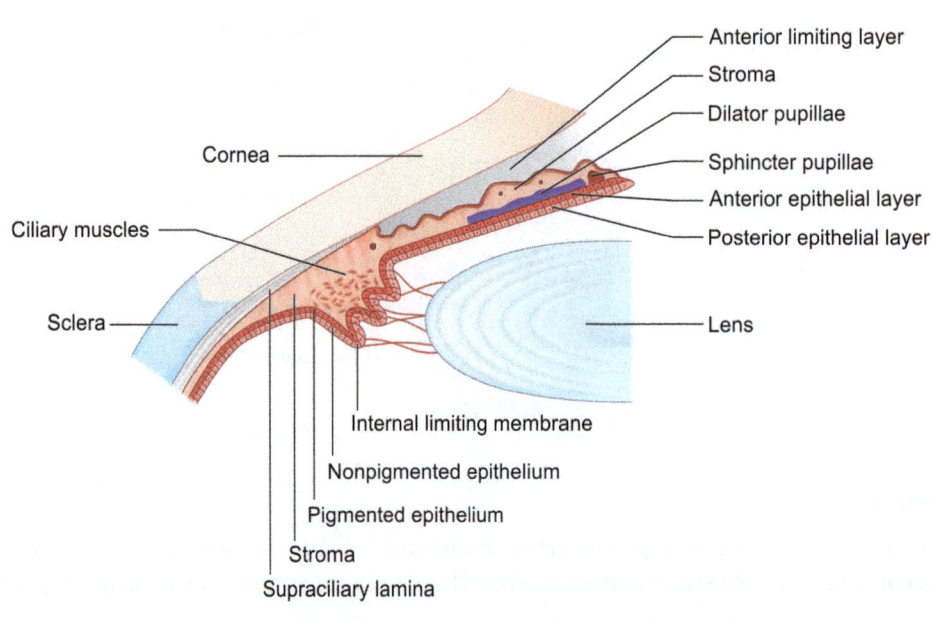

pigment granules. These are more heavily pigmented than anterior pigment epithelium. The cells are joined to each other by maculae adherens and occludens. These cells rest on a thin layer of basement membrane situated posteriorly.

Ciliary Body

Ciliary body is the middle part of the uveal tract. It is brown in color due to melanin pigment. Anteriorly, it is confluent with the periphery of the iris (iris root) and anterior part of the ciliary body bounds a part of the anterior chamber angle. Posteriorly, ciliary body has a crenated or scalloped periphery, known as ora serrata, where it is continuous with the choroid and retina. The ora serrata exhibits forward extensions, known as dentate process, which are well defined on the nasal side and less so temporally. Ciliary body has a width of approximately 5.9 mm on the nasal side and 6.7 mm on the temporal side.

Extension of the Ciliary Body

On the outside of the eyeball, the ciliary body extends from a point about 1.5 mm posterior to the corneal limbus to a point 6.5–7.5 mm posterior to this point on the temporal side and 6.5 mm posterior on the nasal side.

Parts of Ciliary Body

Ciliary body, in cross-section, is a triangular structure with outer surface attached to sclera with suprachoroidal space in-between. Anterior surface forms part of anterior and posterior chamber to which iris is attached. The inner side is divided into pars plicata and plana. The anterior part (2 mm) with finger-like processes is known as pars plicata (corona ciliaris) and posterior smooth (4 mm) is known as pars plana (orbicularis ciliaris).

- *Pars plicata:* It contains the ciliary processes (finger-like projections), which extend into the posterior chamber. The regions between ciliary processes are called valleys of Kuhnt. They are approximately 70–80 in numbers. A ciliary process measures approximately 2 mm in length, 0.5 mm in width, and 1 mm in height.
- *Pars plana:* It is the flat or smooth part of the ciliary body. It terminates at the ora serrata, which is the transitional zone between ciliary body and choroid. Histologically, the pars plana consists of a double layer of epithelial cells: the inner, NPE, which is continuous with neurosensory retina; and the outer, PE, which is continuous with the retinal pigment epithelium (RPE). The pars plana provides surgical access to the vitreous and retina.

Layers of Ciliary Body

From inside to outside (from vitread to sclerad), ciliary body consists of following layers as described here.

Ciliary Epithelium

Ciliary epithelium consists of two layers which cover the inner surface of the ciliary body:

1. *Nonpigmented epithelium of ciliary body:* It extends from the iris root to ora serrata. Cells are smaller and there are few melanin granules in the cells. At pars plicata, cells are cuboidal and they gradually become columnar with increasing age. At ora serrata, the NPE continues as sensory retina. The internal limiting membrane is secreted by the basal lamina of the NPE on its basal surface. It gives origin to parts of the suspensory lens ligament.
2. *Pigmented epithelium of ciliary body:* The cells of the PE are 8–10 micron wide and contain large pigment granules. These pigment granules are three to four times larger than those of the choroid. It continues posteriorly with the RPE.

   Ciliary epithelium has a greater number of mitochondria and thus it has a higher degree of metabolic activity, with a significant role in the active secretion of aqueous humor.

Ciliary Stroma

Ciliary stroma consists of bundles of loose connective tissue. Ciliary stroma contains blood vessels, nerves, and ciliary muscle. Ciliary stroma continues anteriorly with iris stroma and continues posteriorly with choroidal stroma after thinning out at pars plana. Ciliary stroma also consists of numerous capillaries which are fenestrated and large in size. The capillaries are more in numbers in ciliary processes, making them the most vascular organ of the eye.

Muscle in ciliary stroma: Ciliary muscle: Ciliary muscle is a nonstriated or smooth muscle primarily situated in the anterior two-thirds of the ciliary body stroma. The muscle has three parts:

1. *Outer longitudinal or meridional portion (Brücke's muscle):* This is the most external part (nearest to the sclera) of the ciliary muscle. This part of the muscle is V-shaped, the base is attached to the scleral spur and limbs are inserted into the stroma of choroid.

2. *Middle oblique portion (also called reticular or radial)*: This part of the muscle also originates from the scleral spur and the muscle fibers are attached to the collagenous substances near ciliary processes.
3. *Inner circular portion (Müller's muscle):* Here, the muscle bundles are circular in shape (that is why it is also called annular part of ciliary muscle) and act as a sphincter. It lies close to the periphery of lens and embedded in ciliary stroma near the major arterial circle of iris.

Contraction of the ciliary muscle, especially of the longitudinal and circular fibers, pulls the ciliary body forward during accommodation. This forward movement of ciliary body relieves the tension in the suspensory lens ligament (zonules), making the elastic lens more convex and thereby helps the eye in accommodation by increasing the refractive power of the lens.

Ciliary muscle is innervated by the autonomic nervous system, parasympathetic postganglionic fibers derived from the oculomotor nerve. The nerve fibers reach the muscle via short ciliary nerve. The parasympathetic stimulation activates the muscle for contraction.

Supraciliary Lamina

Supraciliary lamina is the outermost layer of ciliary body, which lies adjacent to the sclera. It is composed of loose connective tissue with collagen strands, fibroblasts, and melanocytes. Supraciliary lamina acts as a potential space. Thus, it also helps aqueous humor to exit by the unconventional pathway.

Ciliary Process

Ciliary processes are finger-like projections seen in pars plicata of ciliary body. Ciliary processes are approximately 70–80 in numbers in each eye and extend into the posterior chamber, and the regions between these ciliary processes are called valleys of Kuhnt. Zonules of lens (suspensory ligaments of lens) are inserted in these valleys. Each of these ciliary processes are 2 mm in length and 0.5 mm in diameter. The ciliary process lies 0.5 mm from the periphery (equator) of the crystalline lens. The ciliary processes are white whereas the valleys of Kuhnt are dark in color.

Microscopic Structure of Ciliary Process

- *Capillaries:* Each ciliary process contains a network of capillaries in its center. These capillaries consist of a thin endothelium which is characterized by numerous fenestrations or pores.
- *Stroma:* Connective tissue stroma is very thin and consists of ground substances, which include mucopolysaccharides, proteins, collagen connective tissue fibrils, mainly collagen type III, etc.
- *Ciliary epitheliums:* The outer PE has an atypical basement membrane which is a continuation of Bruch's membrane of choroid. The NPE consists of columnar cells. The basement membrane of the NPE faces aqueous humor and is also called internal limiting membrane.

Choroid

Choroid is a thin but highly vascular membrane lining the inner surface of sclera. It extends from ora serrata anteriorly to the optic nerve posteriorly. It has a rough outer surface which is attached to sclera at the optic nerve and at the exit of the vortex veins. The smooth inner surface of choroid is attached to the RPE. Choroid becomes continuous with pia and arachnoid at the optic nerve.

The choroid has the following layers (sclerad to vitread):
- *Suprachoroidal lamina (lamina fusca):* Suprachoroidal lamina consists of collagen fibers, fibroblasts, and melanocytes. Suprachoroidal lamina underlies a potential space between sclera and choroid known as suprachoroidal space. This potential space contains the long posterior ciliary arteries and nerves.
- *Choroidal stroma:* Unlike iris, where stroma occupies a major part of the tissue, choroidal stroma is sparse as major bulk of choroid is made up of choriocapillaris. The choroidal stroma is a pigmented loose connective tissue which contains following elements:
  - *Vessels:* The vessels of choroid are arranged in layers. Larger vessels are located on the outer side and the layer is called Haller's layer. The vessels of this layer branch and form medium-sized vessels, Sattler's layer. These vessels again branch forming smaller vessels and capillaries. Venues of choroid drain into veins which ultimately drain into four to eight vortex veins (one–two from each quadrant of the eye).
  - *Cells:* Melanocytes, fibrocytes, mast cells, and plasma cells are the predominant cells found in choroidal stroma. Melanocytes are distributed heavily in outer part of the layer and near optic disk. Among the nonpigmented cells, fibroblasts are the most common.
  - *Connective tissue:* Collagen fibrils are dispersed in all directions and surround the blood vessels.

- *Layer of choriocapillaris:* It is a single layer of capillaries which is larger than the normal capillaries of our body. It has been estimated that the lumen of these capillaries is three to four times larger than normal capillaries. The capillary walls are fenestrated and contains pericytes. Choriocapillaris layer contains a basement membrane. Experimentally, it has been found that choriocapillaris is arranged in a lobular structure where the feeding arterioles are in the center and draining veins are in the periphery.

Bruch's Membrane

Bruch's membrane is the innermost layer of choroid and it is also known as lamina vitrea. Bruch's membrane is thickest near optic disk (2-4 micron) and the thickness decreases toward periphery. Bruch's membrane is composed of five layers and from internal to external, these are:
1. Basement membrane of the RPE
2. Inner collagenous zone
3. Elastic tissue layer
4. Outer collagenous zone
5. Basement membrane of the choriocapillaris.

Blood Supply of Uveal Tract

The blood supply of the uveal tract is mainly from three arteries namely short posterior ciliary arteries, long posterior ciliary arteries, and anterior ciliary arteries. The posterior ciliary arteries are branches of the ophthalmic artery, and much variation can occur in their distribution.
1. *Short posterior ciliary arteries:* 15-20 short posterior ciliary arteries arise from the ophthalmic artery, form branches, enter the sclera in a ring around the optic nerve, and anastomose with other branches from the short posterior ciliary arteries to form the circle of Zinn (Zinn–Haller) which encircles the optic nerve at the level of the choroid. These arteries run in suprachoroidal space between sclera and choroid, branch and supply the choroid.
2. *Long posterior ciliary arteries:* Two long posterior ciliary arteries enter the sclera: one lateral and one medial to the ring of short ciliary arteries, run between the sclera and the choroid anteriorly, enter the ciliary body and branch superiorly and inferiorly, anastomose with each other and with the anterior ciliary arteries to form a circular blood vessel network, the major arterial circle of the iris.
3. *Anterior ciliary arteries:* Seven anterior ciliary arteries are derived from muscular branches of ophthalmic artery (two each from arteries of superior rectus, medial rectus, inferior rectus, and only one from lateral rectus muscle). These arteries reach episclera, form plexus and give branches, which in turn pierce sclera near the limbus, and anastomose with long posterior ciliary arteries to form major arterial circle of iris. Branches from major arterial circle enter the iris, run radially, and anastomose with each other to form minor arterial circle of iris at the collarette.

Blood Supply of Ciliary Process

Several branches from the major arterial circle of iris supply the ciliary processes. These are mainly precapillary arterioles and they divide into a network of capillary plexuses in each of the ciliary processes. These vessels drain into the choroidal and intrascleral veins. The precapillary arterioles supplying the ciliary processes have sphincters which are responsible for the autoregulation of blood supply to the tissue.

 2. Describe the embryology of iris. Describe the congenital abnormalities of the iris.

Embryology of Iris

Iris development starts in the 9th week of gestational period. Iris develops from two layers:
1. Mesenchyme forms the anterior stroma
2. Neuroectoderm of optic cup forms the iris pigment epithelium and muscles (sphincter and dilator pupillae).

Iris begins to develop by condensation of second wave of mesenchyme to form a pupillary membrane. The two layers of neuroectoderm (PE and NPE) from the edge of optic cup extend to the posterior surface of pupillary membrane. These three structures (PE, NPE, and pupillary membrane) ultimately fuse to become an iris.

At third month, the cells of anterior epithelium layer differentiate into myofibrils and form sphincter and dilator muscles. The cells of pupillary membrane differentiate into fibroblast-like cells and secret collagen fibrils and extracellular matrix

TABLE 2: Embryology of iris.	
9th week of gestation	Ciliary body begins to appear
12th week of gestation	Sphincter pupillae begins to appear
4th month of gestation	Ciliary processes are fully formed
5th month of gestation	Iris and choroid are formed
6th month of gestation	Dilator muscles begin to form. Sphincter muscle is fully formed
Postnatal period	Dilator muscles reach adult size by 5 years

which form the anterior stroma of iris. The pigmentation of posterior epithelial cell layer begins at the pupillary margin at midterm and by 7th month, the iris is fully pigmented.

Pupillary membrane begins to degenerate at about 8th month of gestation with formation of an opening in the central part of iris called pupil. The iris stroma and dilator muscle are still immature at birth and, therefore, the pupil appears miotic in newborns **(Table 2)**.

Congenital Anomalies of Iris

- *Hypoplasia/absence of an iris:* It is an inadequate inductive interaction between optic cup, surface ectoderm, and neural crest cell due to defect in PAX6 genes. It occurs as sporadic or autosomal dominant condition.
- *Persistent pupillary membrane:* It is most common congenital iris anomaly due to failure of degeneration of pupillary membrane.
- *Iris coloboma:* It is failure of embryonic fissure to close in 5th week of gestation. Pupil appears like inverted tear drop with peaking usually at the inferonasal quadrant. It can be associated with coloboma of choroid, ciliary body, and optic nerve. It may have syndromic associations such as trisomy 13, Klinefelter syndrome, Turner syndrome, and CHARGE (ocular coloboma, heart defects, choanal atresia, mental retardation, genitourinary, and ear anomalies).
- *Polycoria:* Accessory iris opening. It is associated with Axenfeld–Rieger syndrome (autosomal dominant disorder) due to mutation of PAX and FOXC1 genes.
- *Corectopia:* It is displacement of pupil from the usual central position. It may be associated with sectoral iris hypoplasia or coloboma or lens subluxation (ectopia lentis et pupillae).
- *Microcoria:* Congenital miosis. It occurs due to malformation of dilator pupillae muscle. It can be associated with microcornea, lens subluxation, iris atrophy, and glaucoma.
- *Congenital mydriasis:* It occurs due to malformation of iris sphincter muscle.

 3. Discuss classification, causes, clinical manifestation, and management of uveitis.

Uveitis is defined as inflammation of the uveal tract of the eye.

Classification of Uveitis

Clinicopathological or Woods Classification

Uveitis is classified as granulomatous or nongranulomatous on the basis of the predominant clinical characteristics **(Table 3)**.

Standardization of Uveitis Nomenclature (SUN) Classification

The most recent and widely accepted version of classifying uveitis is the SUN classification according to their primary site of inflammation **(Table 4)**.

Various descriptors for defining onset, duration, and course of uveitis have been proposed in SUN classification **(Tables 5 and 6)**.

Systemic History and Examination

Table 7 shows systemic history and examination.

TABLE 3: Differences between granulomatous and nongranulomatous uveitis.

	Granulomatous uveitis	Nongranulomatous uveitis
Onset and course	Insidious onset and chronic course	Sudden onset and acute course
Congestion	Absent or mild congestion	Severe episcleral congestion
Iris nodules	Keoppe's and Bussaca's nodules are common	Uncommon
Keratic precipitates (KPs)	Medium to large (Mutton fat KPs)	Fine, small KPs
Posterior segment involvement	Common	Uncommon

TABLE 4: Standardization of uveitis nomenclature (SUN) classification based on primary site of inflammation.

Type	Primary site of inflammation	Includes
Anterior uveitis	Anterior chamber	Iritis, iridocyclitis, anterior cyclitis
Intermediate uveitis	Vitreous	Pars planitis, posterior cyclitis, hyalitis
Posterior uveitis	Retina/choroid	Focal, multifocal, diffuse choroiditis chorioretinitis, retinochoroiditis, retinitis, neuroretinitis
Panuveitis	Anterior chamber, vitreous and retina or choroid	–

TABLE 5: Standardization of uveitis nomenclature (SUN) classification based on onset, duration, and course of disease.

Category	Descriptor	Description
Onset	• Sudden • Insidious	• Acute onset • Slow onset
Duration	• Limited • Persistent	• ≤3 months duration • >3 months duration
Course	• Acute • Recurrent • Chronic	• Episode characterized by a sudden onset and limited duration • Repeated episodes separated by periods of inactivity without treatment (inactivity >3 months in duration) • Persistent uveitis with relapse in <3 months after discontinuing treatment

TABLE 6: Standardization of uveitis nomenclature (SUN) classification based on activity of disease.

Term	Description
Inactive	Grade 0 cells (anterior uveitis)
Worsening activity	Two-step increase in the level of inflammation (e.g., anterior chamber cells, vitreous haze) or increase from grade 3 to 4
Improved activity	Two step decrease in the level of inflammation (e.g., anterior chamber cells, vitreous haze) or decrease to grade 0
Remission	Inactive disease for 3 months after discontinuing all treatments for eye disease

TABLE 7: Systemic history and examination in uveitis.

Signs	Uveitic entities
Arthralgias	Behçet's disease, sarcoidosis, systemic lupus erythematosus (SLE), juvenile idiopathic arthritis (JIA), Lyme disease, syphilis, psoriatic arthritis, Reiter syndrome, ulcerative colitis
Skin lesions	**Uveitis entities**
Nodules	Sarcoidosis, SLE, leprosy, Crohn's disease, ulcerative colitis
Rash	Syphilis, Lyme disease, Reiter syndrome, leprosy, sarcoidosis, Herpes zoster, Behçet's disease, psoriasis, SLE, Kawasaki disease
Erythema nodosum	Behçet's disease, sarcoidosis, acute posterior multifocal placoid pigment epitheliopathy (APMPPE), tuberculosis
Vitiligo, Poliosis	Vogt–Koyanagi–Harada syndrome (VKH)
Keratoderma blennorrhagicum	Reactive arthritis
Hair loss	VKH, SLE, syphilis
Oral ulcers	Behçet's disease, reactive arthritis, SLE, herpes simplex, Reiter syndrome, ulcerative colitis

Contd...

Contd...

CNS	Uveitis entities
Headache	VKH, tuberculosis, Herpes zoster, large cell lymphoma, cryptococcus meningitis, toxoplasmosis
Auditory/vestibular	VKH disease
Cranial neuropathy	Lyme disease, sarcoidosis, multiple sclerosis, syphilis, Herpes simplex virus
Cerebral vasculitis	Acute posterior multifocal placoid pigment epitheliopathy (APMPPE)
Ear, nose, and throat	**Uveitis entities**
Bilateral ear pinna inflammation	Relapsing polychondritis
Saddle nose deformity	Syphilis, Wegener's granulomatosis, SLE, relapsing polychondritis
Sinusitis	Sarcoidosis, Wegener's granulomatosis
Salivary/lacrimal gland swelling	Sarcoidosis, lymphoma
Lymphadenopathy	Lymphoma, human immunodeficiency virus (HIV)
Pulmonary	
Cough/breathlessness	Tuberculosis, sarcoidosis, *Pneumocystis carinii*, Wegener's granulomatosis
Nodules/hilar adenopathy/infiltrates	Ocular histoplasmosis, sarcoidosis (hilar adenopathy), malignancy, tuberculosis, *Pneumocystis carinii* pneumonia
Genitourinary	
Genital ulcers	Behçet's disease, Reiter syndrome, syphilis
Hematuria	Wegener's granulomatosis, polyarteritis nodosa (PAN), SLE
Circinate balanitis	Ankylosing spondylitis, Reiter syndrome
Nephritis	PAN, Wegener's granulomatosis, tubulointerstitial nephritis, and uveitis (TINU)

(CNS: central nervous system)

Examination of Case With Uveitis

- *Lids and adnexa:* Kaposi's sarcoma; enlargement of the lacrimal gland can be seen in sarcoidosis; characteristic skin lesions or scar mark can be seen in a case of herpes zoster ophthalmicus (HZO).
- *Conjunctiva:* Ciliary injection or "ciliary flush" is manifested by a ring of dilated episcleral vessels radiating from the limbus. Perilimbal vitiligo is often observed in patients with Vogt–Koyanagi–Harada's (VKH) syndrome and is known as Sugiura's sign. Subconjunctival hemorrhage can be seen in patients with leptospirosis. Look for nodules in sarcoidosis.
- *Anterior chamber:* Look for cells, flare, hypopyon, and hyphema.
  - *Causes of hypopyon uveitis:* Human leukocyte antigen B27 (HLA-B27)-associated anterior uveitis [ankylosing spondylitis (AS) and others], Behçet's disease, endophthalmitis, and drugs (rifabutin).
  - *Hyphema:* Viral uveitis, trauma, malignancies, Fuchs heterochromic uveitis, chronic uveitis with rubeosis, any severe uveitis **(Table 8)**
- *Cornea:*
  - *Keratic precipitates:* Mutton-fat or large keratic precipitates (KPs) can be seen in granulomatous uveitis. Fine KPs are seen in herpetic eye diseases and in other nongranulomatous conditions. Stellate or star-shaped KPs are seen in Fuchs heterochromic iridocyclitis (FHI). Old KPs are pigmented and have crenate margins.
     Band-shaped keratopathy (BSK) may occur in chronic uveitis. Look for corneal scars and ulceration.
  - *Pupil:* Presence of festooned pupil, occlusion pupillae (blocking of pupil by exudates), and seclusion pupillae (pupillary margin plastered to lens all around).
- *Iris:* Nodules seen in pupillary borders are known as Koeppe nodules and nodules on the iris surface are known as Busacca's nodules. Iris nodules are seen in granulomatous uveitis. Comparison of the color of iris between two eyes can detect heterochromia of iris which can be either hypochromic (abnormal eye is lighter than fellow eye) as seen in FHI or hyperchromic (abnormal eye is darker than fellow eye) as seen in melanosis of iris. Iris atrophy is a characteristic feature of herpetic uveitis. Herpesviruses generally produce sectoral iris atrophy due to an occlusive vasculitis.

TABLE 8: Standardization of uveitis nomenclature (SUN) working group grading scheme.

Grade	Cells in field of 1 mm by 1 mm slit beam (AC)	Vitreous haze	Flare
0	<1	Nil	None
0.5+	1–5	Trace	—
1+	6–15	Few opacities, mild blurring	Faint
2+	16–25	Significant blurring, but still visible	Moderate (iris and lens details clear)
3+	26–50	Optic nerve visible, no vessels visible	Marked (iris and lens details hazy)
4+	>50	Dense opacity obscures optic nerve head	Intense (fibrin or plastic aqueous)

TABLE 9: Differences between retinitis and choroiditis.

Retinitis	Choroiditis
Appears as a whitish patch	Appears as yellowish patches
Ill-defined margins	Relatively well-defined margins
Superficial	Deeper (deep to the retinal blood vessels)

- *Intraocular pressure (IOP):*
    - *Rise*—can occur from clogging of trabecular meshwork with inflammatory cells, inflammation of trabecular meshwork fibers ("trabeculitis"), peripheral anterior synechiae (PAS), pupillary block from posterior synechiae, and corticosteroid (CS)-induced IOP rise (steroid response).
    - *Hypotony:* In acute cases—ciliary body hyposecretion; in chronic cases—cyclitic membrane formation
- *Lens:* Posterior subcapsular cataract (PSC)
- *Vitreous:* Grading of vitritis/vitreous haze is given above.
- *Fundus:* Careful examination of the posterior segment can reveal inflammatory patches in the fundus. It is important to distinguish such lesions whether it involves retina or choroid or both. Sometimes, these lesions are associated with subretinal fluid or localized haze in vitreous **(Table 9)**.

Associated vasculitis should also be noted and whether predominantly involving arteries (arteritis), veins (phlebitis), or both.

Often a patient with posterior or panuveitis can present with an exudative retinal detachment one should be able to distinguish rhegmatogenous retinal detachment from such cases, which requires surgical management. Sequelae of retinal vasculitis can lead to the development of traction retinal detachment and should be dealt properly.

Meticulous examination of the fovea with slit lamp biomicroscopy often helps to identify cystoid macular edema (CME), choroidal neovascular membrane (CNVM), or sight-threatening inflammatory lesions such as serpiginous choroiditis. CME is common in patients with uveitis which if long-standing can lead to macular atrophy or macular hole.

Goals of Treatment

- Relief of symptoms
- Minimizing sequels
- Prevention of irreversible vision loss
- Prevention of recurrence
- Limit the side effects of drug therapies.

Topical Cycloplegics

Cycloplegic agents (e.g., tropicamide 1% QID, cyclopentolate 1% TID, homatropine 2% TID, atropine BID) are often prescribed for acute anterior uveitis (AAU), for exacerbations of chronic anterior uveitis (CAU) and for anterior component of panuveitis. They are usually given according to the severity of inflammation.

The clinical usefulness of cycloplegic agents in AAU is due to:
- Symptomatic relief of pain and photophobia, by relieving ciliary muscle spasm

- Prevention of formation of synechiae and/or synechiolysis. Frequent instillation at presentation may be given to either prevent or rapidly break any posterior synechiae that may be developing. In established posterior synechiae or in chronic cases, the cycloplegic may not relive the adhesion and, therefore, early instillation is important in AAU.
- This may also be useful for detailed assessment of the fundus by allowing more mydriasis.

Topical Corticosteroids

It is useful in the management of anterior uveitis and anterior component of panuveitis. Generally, steroid therapy should be given in high doses initially and then slowly tapered according to clinical evolution.

- *Mild inflammation:* It can be managed with a topical formulation q6h (e.g., prednisolone acetate 1% or dexamethasone 0.1%).
- *Moderate to severe uveitis:* Topical CS q1-2h dosing initially (e.g., prednisolone acetate 1%, dexamethasone 0.1%), and a steroid ophthalmic ointment can be given at night.
- In cases of severe uveitis, a loading dose can be considered (e.g., prednisolone acetate 1% q1min for 5 minutes, then q30min-1h). A commonly adopted regimen might consist of one drop q1h for 3 days, then one drop q2h for 3 days, then one drop q6h for 3 days, then one drop q8h for 7 days, then one drop q12h for 7 days, then one drop OD for 7 days, and then stop **(Table 10)**.

Indications and uses of periocular steroids and systemic steroids are discussed in subsequent questions. Noncorticosteroid immunomodulatory therapy (NCSIT) has also been discussed.

4. Explain investigative profile in uveitis.

Investigations should be tailored toward the most probable diagnosis based on history and examination as discussed above. **Table 11** summarizes various laboratory tests used in uveitis.

TABLE 10: Relative potencies of corticosteroids.

Corticosteroid	Systemic equivalent (mg)	Relative glucocorticoid potency
Betamethasone	0.6	33.0
Dexamethasone	0.75	26.0
Methylprednisolone	4	5.0
Triamcinolone	4	5.0
Prednisolone	5	4.0
Prednisone	5	4.0
Hydrocortisone	20	1.0
Cortisone	25	0.8

TABLE 11: Laboratory studies in uveitis.

Etiology	Laboratory studies	Others
Acute anterior uveitis:		
Behçet's syndrome	HLA-B51	
Glaucomatocyclitic crisis	Aqueous fluid PCR	
Viral	Aqueous fluid PCR	
Kawasaki disease		ECG, Echo
Post-streptococcal	Anti-streptolysin O titer	
Relapsing polychondritis	–	
Seronegative spondyloarthropathies	HLA-B27	Sacroiliac and lumbosacral X-ray
Tubulointerstitial nephritis and uveitis syndrome	Serum BUN, creatinine, and urine β2 microglobulin	Urinalysis

Contd...

Contd...

Etiology	Laboratory studies	Others
Chronic anterior uveitis:		
Fuchs heterochromic iridocyclitis	–	–
Viral	Aqueous fluid PCR	
Juvenile idiopathic arthritis	ANA	
Sarcoidosis	ACE, lysozyme	CXR/chest HRCT
Syphilis	RPR/FTA-ABS, CSF	
Tuberculosis	PPD, QuantiFERON	CXR/chest HRCT
Intermediate uveitis:		
Lyme disease	ELISA or Western blot	
Multiple sclerosis	CSF analysis	Brain MRI
Sarcoidosis	ACE, lysozyme	CXR/chest HRCT
Posterior uveitis:		
Birdshot chorioretinopathy	HLA-A29	FA, ICGA, FAF, ERG, and OCT
Cat-scratch disease	Bartonella serology	FA, ICGA, FAF, OCT
Multifocal choroiditis/panuveitis		FA, ICGA, FAF, OCT
Presumed ocular histoplasmosis syndrome		FA, ICGA, FAF, OCT
Sarcoidosis	ACE, lysozyme	CXR/chest HRCT
Serpiginous chorioretinopathy		FA, ICGA, FAF, OCT
Syphilis	RPR/FTA-ABS, CSF	
Toxocariasis	Serology	
Toxoplasmosis	Serology, aqueous PCR	
Tuberculosis	PPD, QuantiFERON	CXR/chest HRCT
Viral	Aqueous/vitreous PCR	
West Nile virus	IgM serology, CSF analysis	FA, ICGA, FAF, and OCT
Panuveitis:		
Endophthalmitis	Vitreous culture, blood culture	
Sarcoidosis	ACE, lysozyme	CXR/chest HRCT
Sympathetic ophthalmitis		FA, USG, OCT
Syphilis	RPR/FTA-ABS, CSF	
Toxocariasis	Serology	
Toxoplasmosis	Serology, aqueous PCR	
Tuberculosis	PPD, QuantiFERON	CXR/chest HRCT
Vogt–Koyanagi–Harada disease	CSF analysis	FA, USG, OCT

(ACE: angiotensin-converting enzyme; ANA: antinuclear antibody; BUN: blood urea nitrogen; CSF: cerebrospinal fluid; CXR: chest X-ray; ECG: electrocardiography; ELISA: enzyme-linked immunosorbent assay; ERG: electroretinogram; FA: fluorescein angiography; FAF: fundus autofluorescence; HRCT: high-resolution computed tomography; HLA: human leukocyte antigen; ICGA: indocyanine green angiography; OCT: optical coherence tomography; PCR: polymerase chain reaction; PPD: purified protein derivative; USG: ultrasonography)

5. Enumerate the role of various investigations in uveitis with respect to management modalities.

Imaging Studies in Uveitis

Fluorescein Angiography

Angiography may be performed to **Flowchart 1**:
- Confirm elements already revealed by clinical examination or other investigational methods such as optical coherence tomography (OCT).
- For better grading of the inflammation of the fundus and to make a good baseline inventory of inflammatory involvement to subsequently use it for follow-up purposes.
- In follow-up situations, angiography is usually performed to monitor disease activity and impact of therapy.
The flowcharts depict the various angiographic signs in uveitis:

Indocyanine Green Angiography

Inflammatory lesions of the choriocapillaris and choroidal stroma are best visualized on indocyanine green angiography (ICGA). Occult choroidal lesions that are missed on fundoscopy and fluorescein angiography can be picked up on ICGA.

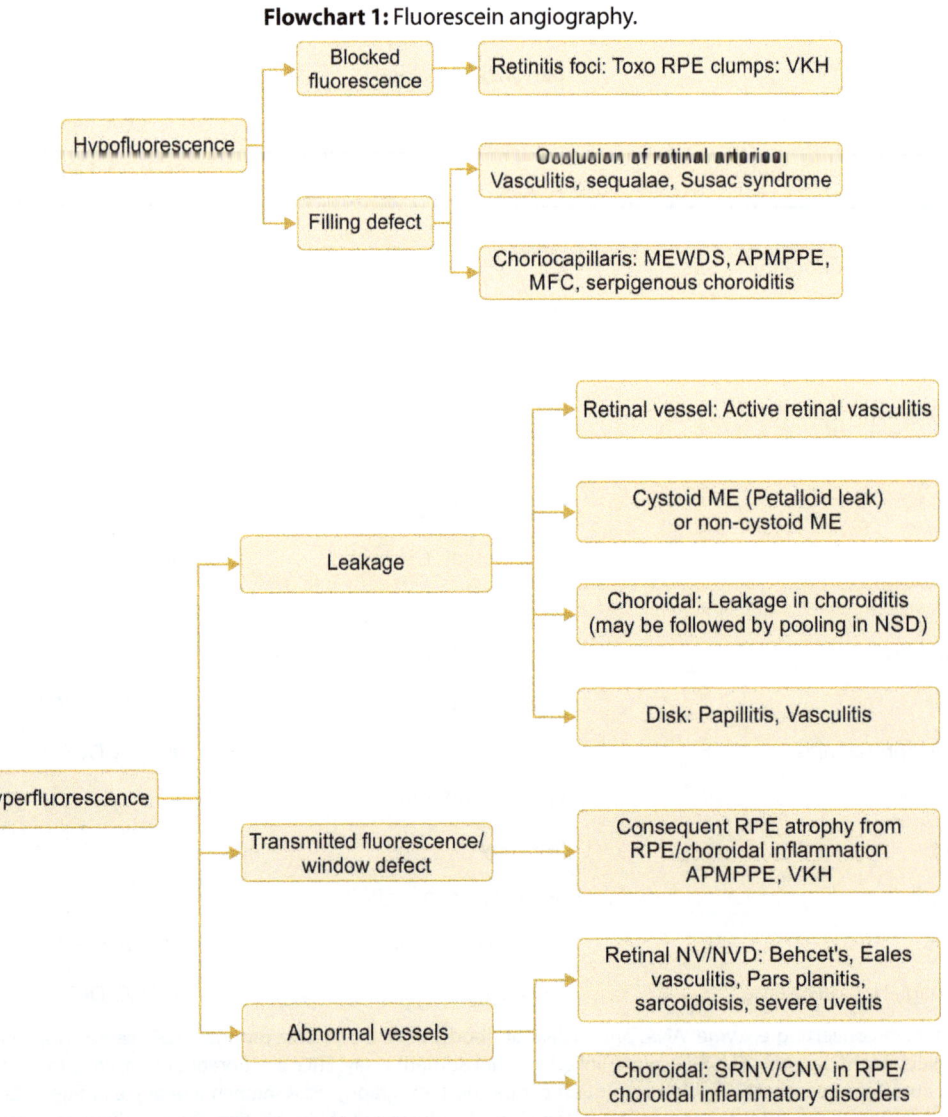

Flowchart 1: Fluorescein angiography.

(APMPPE: acute posterior multifocal placoid pigment epitheliopathy; CNV: choroidal neovascularization; MEWDS: multiple evanescent white dot syndrome; MFC: multifocal choroiditis; NVD: neovascularization on disk; RPE: retinal pigment epithelium; SRNV: subretinal neovascularization)

Hypofluorescence may be seen in eyes with choroidal nonperfusion and in early phase in cases of stromal inflammatory lesions. Hyperfluorescence may occur from inflamed disk or from stromal inflammatory lesions in late phase.

Ultra-wide-field Fluorescein Angiography

The peripheral retina is the site of pathology in many ocular diseases. With the advent of ultra-wide-field fluorescein angiography, it is now possible to view up to 200° of the retina in a single photograph measured from the ocular center. This is helpful in imaging peripheral ischemic retina in occlusive retinal vasculitis, which can be targeted with laser therapy.

Fundus Autofluorescence

Fundus autofluorescence (FAF) imaging depicts the status of metabolic activity of the RPE. This is useful in evaluation of activity of the choroiditis lesions. While active lesions show hyperautofluorescence due to stressed our RPE, healed lesions show hypoautofluorescence due to RPE attenuation or loss.

Optical Coherence Tomography

Optical coherence tomography has become an indispensable ancillary test in the diagnosis and management of inflammatory diseases involving the retina and choroid.

Macular edema is a common cause of visual loss in patients with uveitis. OCT can be used to document and monitor CME. OCT is particularly helpful in cases with toxoplasma retinitis.

Spectral domain OCT with enhanced depth imaging (EDI) images choroid with clarity. With the introduction of EDI, visualization of the choriocapillaris and choroid has become possible. Choroidal granuloma can be picked up on OCT and this can also be used to monitor treatment.

Optical coherence tomography can be used for evaluation of vitreous inflammation intensity. OCT can be used to measure vitreous (VIT) signal intensity and compared with intensity of RPE, generating a ratio of "VIT/RPE-relative intensity". This ratio is significantly higher in uveitic eyes than in uveitic eyes without vitreous haze or in healthy controls. The VIT/RPE-relative intensity shows a significant, positive correlation with clinical vitreous haze scores.

Anterior segment optical coherence tomography (AS–OCT) can be used to measure anterior chamber inflammation to identify responses to treatment in patients with uveitis.

Optical Coherence Tomography Angiography

Optical coherence tomography angiography (OCT-A) as a noninvasive, depth-resolution imaging tool of retinal and choroidal vessels adds detailed qualitative and quantitative information of the status of retinal and choroidal vessels and bridges the gap between the conventional diagnostic tools used in uveitis. It is important, though, to be aware of its limitations, such as its susceptibility to motion artifacts, limited comparability among different devices, and restricted contribution of information regarding the grade of disease activity.

 6. What are the types, ocular clinical features, differential diagnosis, and management of a case of juvenile idiopathic arthritis?

Juvenile Idiopathic Arthritis

Definition

A chronic arthritis with at least 6 weeks duration in a child <16 years of age. It is the most common cause of uveitis of childhood in Europe and North America. The criteria published by the International League of Associations of Rheumatology (ILAR) cover all childhood arthritides under the name juvenile idiopathic arthritis (JIA). Apart from unifying the name, it has established that the disease duration for the diagnosis should be 6 weeks and includes juvenile ankylosing spondylitis (JAS), juvenile psoriatic arthritis (JPsA), and arthropathy associated with inflammatory bowel disease (IBD) under this broad definition.

The new classification of JIA has divided it into seven subtypes, defined after the first 6 months of disease. Oligoarthritis is the most common subtype (50–70%), followed by polyarthritis (30%), with the great majority being rheumatoid factor (RF) negative. Systemic onset and enthesitis-related arthritis each occurs in about 5% of patients.

Uveitis in JIA

As much as 80% of anterior uveitis in the pediatric population is associated with JIA. A recent meta-analysis revealed that the cumulative incidence of JIA-associated uveitis is 8.3%.

TABLE 12: Clinical features of juvenile idiopathic arthritis.			
Oligoarthritis	**Rheumatoid factor-negative polyarthritis**	**Psoriatic arthritis**	**Enthesitis-related arthritis**
Four or fewer (large) joints; Most common: Knee	Chronic course; More than four joints (small and large) in first 6 months of disease	Oligo- or polyarticular disease; Diagnosis based on psoriasis and arthritis	Chronic inflammation of entheses and particularly foot, knee, and pelvis
Predominantly in young girls	More common in girls; older age at onset		Predominantly adolescent and adult boys
First 6 months of disease: 40–50% of all cases of JIA and includes the vast majority (80–90%) of patients with JIA-associated uveitis	40% of JIA cases overall but only about 10% of cases of JIA-associated anterior uveitis	• No increase in frequency of HLA-B27 • Rarely have sacroiliitis or LS spine arthritis	• HLA-B27 positivity • Develop sacroiliitis and LS spine disease

(HLA: human leukocyte antigen; JIA: juvenile idiopathic arthritis; LS: lumbosacral)

Clinical Features

Table 12 shows clinical features of juvenile idiopathic arthritis.

Oligoarticular-onset JIA is further subdivided into:
- *Type 1 disease:* It is observed in girls under the age of 5 years who are typically positive for antinuclear antibody (ANA); CAU occurs in up to 25% of these patients.
- *Type 2 disease:* It is found in older boys, many of whom develop evidence of seronegative spondyloarthropathy (75% are HLA-B27 positive). The uveitis in these patients is more likely to be acute and recurrent rather than chronic, unlike in type 1 disease.

Risk factors for development of uveitis include:
- *Oligoarticular arthritis type:* Triple the risk when compared to polyarticular disease
- Early age at onset of arthritis
- Positive ANAs, negative RF, and female sex.

Factors associated with long-term complications: Severe disease at presentation, short interval between onset of arthritis and the diagnosis of uveitis, male sex, presence of complications at initial presentation, and early age at onset of uveitis.

Ocular features: In 80% of patients, the uveitis is insidious, asymptomatic, and may result in blindness if left untreated. During exacerbations, patients may manifest discomfort and redness. This picture is most frequently bilateral, with either simultaneous presentation or with second eye involvement generally occurring after a few months and rarely after 1 year.

Examination shows bilateral, nongranulomatous chronic iridocyclitis with small KPs in the inferior half of the cornea and mild-to-severe anterior chamber flare and cells and anterior vitreous cells. Granulomatous presentation has been rarely reported (should rule out sarcoidosis and other causes). An AAU may be seen in enthesitis-related arthritis and tends to occur in older HLA-B27-positive boys, with pain, redness, and photophobia.

Most cases of uveitis are diagnosed within 4 years of the onset of arthritis but may occur sooner, especially in those with extended oligoarthritis, who tend to fall ill quite early on.

Many patients with uveitis continue to show disease activity in adult life and this is usually associated with activity of the joint disease. An elevated erythrocyte sedimentation rate (ESR) appeared to be a predictor for the occurrence of uveitis in patients with JIA.

Differential Diagnosis

The differential diagnosis includes TINU, Fuchs heterochromic uveitis, Behçet's disease, seronegative spondyloarthropathies, herpetic uveitis, and Lyme disease.

Complications and Prognosis

Chronic nature of the disease, with periods of exacerbation, causes complications. Most complications occur in the anterior segment but may also occur in the posterior segment.

Cataract: PSC (complicated cataract) results from chronic inflammation and chronic use of CS therapy. Anterior subcapsular opacities will also appear in places where posterior synechiae develop. The reported prevalence is variable but approaches 50%.

Secondary glaucoma: In the majority of affected eyes, the IOP increases shortly after control of inflammation is achieved, suggesting recovery of ciliary body function and chronic damage to trabecular meshwork from chronic inflammation, PAS, and CSs. The prevalence ranges from 14% to 42%.

Band-shaped keratopathy: It occurs due to long-standing inflammation and tends to affect the interpalpebral area, with a cumulative incidence of 15.7%.

Hypotony: It is not common and usually reflects severe and poorly controlled uveitis.

Posterior segment complications: Vitreous haze, CME, disk edema, and disk neovascularization (NV). In severe cases, retinal detachment, hypotony, and phthisis bulbi may occur, indicating poor prognosis.

Management

Early identification with prompt and aggressive therapy is the only step to prevent complications and visual loss **(Table 13)**. Management should be done with the help of pediatric rheumatologist. Even with aggressive and early therapy, long-term visual loss can result.

High-potency *CS eyedrops*, initially at a high frequency, associated with short-acting mydriatic drops, such as *tropicamide or cyclopentolate* (to prevent posterior synechiae), should be used. Long-acting mydriatics such as atropine should be avoided as can lead to synechiae in dilated position and amblyopia if the child is young. Cases not responding to topical steroids need *periocular steroids*. It is important to remember that systemic absorption of ocular steroid therapy can cause systemic adverse reactions including Cushing's syndrome. Some recalcitrant cases can be managed with *intravitreal steroids,* but cataract and raised IOP are common side effects.

Some patients will require systemic therapy. Early introduction of *immunosuppressive agents* will result in better disease control apart from being CS-sparing. Methotrexate, azathioprine, and cyclosporine have been used for JIA-associated uveitis. Biological agents offer a new modality of treatment. Tumor necrosis factor-α (TNF-α) blockers (infliximab and adalimumab) are the preferred biological drug for the treatment of uveitis associated with JIA.

Management of Complications

Cataract: Management is a special challenge, especially in younger children. The visual outcomes are worse and the postoperative course is complicated when compared to pediatric cataract surgery for complicated cataract due to other reasons. Control of the inflammatory process is essential for a favorable outcome, but young patients need quick intervention to prevent the development of amblyopia.

The uveitis should be inactive/quiescent, for at least 3 months preceding cataract surgery. Immunosuppressive therapy, in the perioperative and postoperative period, improves the visual outcomes.

Cataract surgery can be difficult due to poor visualization from BSK, poor pupillary dilation, posterior synechiae, and inflammatory membranes over the anterior capsule. The postoperative complications may include fibrinous reaction, glaucoma, CME, epimacular membrane, posterior capsular opacification, cyclitic membrane formation, hypotony, and phthisis. Immunomodulator treatment may need escalation in the perioperative and postoperative period to prevent and manage these complications.

Intraocular lens (IOL) implantation in the primary surgery is controversial. The feared complications include pigment and fibrin deposition over IOL and posterior lens capsule, synechiae with the IOL, secondary cataract, and cyclitic membrane formation. An intact posterior capsule and anterior vitreous are reported by some authors to be associated with a higher incidence of cyclitic membrane formation and progression to hypotony and phthisis. Thus, some surgeons favor posterior capsulorhexis and anterior vitrectomy following cataract extraction and leave the eye aphakic. However, recent studies report no difference in complication rate between aphakia and IOL implantation, if inflammation is well controlled for 3 months prior to surgery. Acrylic IOLs provide better results than poly(methyl methacrylate) (PMMA) and silicone IOLs.

Good outcomes, with visual acuity of 20/40 or better, can be achieved in 75% of the eyes with adequate control of uveitis before and following cataract surgery.

Secondary glaucoma: It is often refractory to medical therapy, with a poor response to topical β-blockers, sympathomimetics, and carbonic anhydrase inhibitors. Conventional filtering surgery may be used but will require antimetabolites. Implants also provide good results.

Cystoid macular edema: CME can be treated with a topical combination of CS and nonsteroidal anti-inflammatory drug (NSAID), with the option of periocular CSs in case of failure. Systemic therapy including immunosuppression can be used in resistant cases, especially if sight is threatened. Vitrectomy may be helpful in handful of recalcitrant cases.

Symptomatic band keratopathy: It may be treated by chelating agents or excimer laser.

Prognosis

Poor visual acuity is found in as many as 20% of the children, and as many as 10% of eyes are blind. Poor visual outcome is more common in those who have developed uveitis prior to or at the same time as arthritis. Eyes with ocular hypertension or secondary glaucoma have close to threefold higher incidence of legal blindness, and this risk can be reduced by early introduction of immunosuppressive therapy.

The Systemic Immunosuppressive Therapy for Eye Diseases (SITE) study assessed the incidence of—and risk factors for—visual acuity loss and ocular complications in patients with JIA-associated uveitis. It found that 60% of the patients had at least one ocular complication. Increasing uveitis activity was associated with increased risk of vision loss, and the risk was reduced by the use of immunosuppressive drugs.

Follow-up: See Table 13

TABLE 13: Ocular screening criteria for children with JIA.

Type	ANA	Age at onset (years)	Duration of disease (years)	Risk category	Eye examination frequency (months)
Oligoarthritis/polyarthritis	+	<6	<4	High	3
	+	<6	>4	Moderate	6
	+	<6	>7	Low	12
	+	>6	<4	Moderate	6
	+	>6	>4	Low	12
	–	<6	<4	Moderate	6
	–	<6	>4	Low	12
	–	>6	Not applicable	Low	12
Systemic disease (fever, rash)	Not applicable	Not applicable	Not applicable	Low	12

(ANA: antinuclear antibody; JIA: juvenile idiopathic arthritis)

7. Discuss Still's disease.

Juvenile idiopathic arthritis with systemic onset is known as Still's disease. This type, usually observed in children under age of 5 years, accounts for approximately 10–15% of all cases of JIA. It occurs with similar frequency in boys and girls. It is characterized by fever, rash, lymphadenopathy, hepatosplenomegaly, pericarditis, and peritonitis. Joint involvement may be minimal or absent initially. The arthritis in systemic JIA can affect any number of joints, is classically polyarticular and destructive, and can affect the hip, cervical spine, and temporomandibular joint. Ocular involvement is rare; fewer than 6% of patients have uveitis. Rest of the features of JIA are discussed above.

8. Discuss differential diagnosis and management of a 10-year-old boy presenting with bilateral diminution of vision and swelling of the right knee.

In a 10-year-old boy presenting with bilateral diminution of vision and swelling of right knee, the differential diagnosis can be uveitis associated with:
- JIA
- Juvenile-onset spondyloarthropathies (JOSpAs)
- Sarcoidosis
- Blau syndrome.
  Juvenile idiopathic arthritis is discussed above.

Juvenile-onset Spondyloarthropathies

Juvenile-onset spondyloarthropathies represent a group of HLA-B27-associated pediatric rheumatic diseases characterized by inflammatory peripheral arthritis, enthesitis, sacroiliitis, absence of RF and ANA, and tendency for acute ocular inflammation and variable mucocutaneous lesions. This group includes JAS, reactive arthritis, IBD-related arthritis, and psoriatic arthritis.

Juvenile Ankylosing Spondylitis

It is a chronic arthropathy that predominantly affects boys after the age of 10 years. Patients have a history of back pain, radiographic involvement of the sacroiliac joint and sometimes the lumbosacral spine, and peripheral arthritis together with enthesitis. More than 91% of patients are HLA-B27 positive. Recurrent attacks of symptomatic AAU can develop, in contrast to the chronic asymptomatic iridocyclitis of JIA. Uveitis is seen in 10–15% of patients and the attacks typically involve only one eye at a time, although the inflammation can switch back and forth between eyes. The typical presentation is of severe AAU, often with fibrin and hypopyon.

Juvenile reactive arthritis and IBD-related arthritis are uncommon in children.

Reactive arthritis in children has the same pathogenic and clinical characteristics as in adults, with a classic triad of nonspecific urethritis, polyarthritis, and conjunctival inflammation accompanied by iritis. The uveitis attacks are typically unilateral, resembling those seen with AS.

Inflammatory bowel disease-associated arthritis is typically mild, pauciarticular, and affects large joints. Less frequently, spondylitis and sacroiliitis are seen, often associated with the presence of HLA-B27. Children with IBD can develop any type of ocular inflammation, including acute or CAU, scleritis, CME, or retinal vasculitis. Chronic uveitis is more commonly seen in children with peripheral joint disease.

Juvenile psoriatic arthritis is defined as arthritis occurring with psoriasis, dactylitis, or nail pitting or a family history of psoriasis. If psoriatic arthritis is seen before 3 years of age, it clinically resembles the ANA-positive oligoarthritis subtype of JIA. Anterior uveitis occurs in approximately 10–20%. When the onset of arthritis is in early childhood, the uveitis is typically chronic. When the arthritis develops in later childhood, recurrent, AAU is typical.

Sarcoidosis and Blau Syndrome

These tend to present with granulomatous ocular inflammation and can have posterior segment involvement, which is atypical in JIA-related uveitis.

9. Discuss (a) differential diagnosis of heterochromia iridis, and (b) features, complications, and management of a case of Fuchs uveitis syndrome.

Definition of Heterochromia

Heterochromia is a clinical situation when there is a difference in the color and pattern of iris. Heterochromia iridis or sectoral/segmental heterochromia refers to difference in the color of a sector of iris from the rest of it, whereas, heterochromia iridium or complete heterochromia is difference in color of both eyes. The abnormal iris can be of darker (hyperchromia) or lighter (hypochromia) hue **(Table 14)**.

It can also be classified as to whether the abnormal iris is hypo- or hyperpigmented **(Table 15)**.

TABLE 14: Causes of heterochromia.

Congenital	Acquired
Horner's syndrome	Hyphema
Benign heterochromia	Iritis or uveitis
Sturge–Weber syndrome	Surgical trauma
Waardenburg syndrome	Fuchs' heterochromic cyclitis
Piebaldism	Acquired Horner's syndrome
Hirschsprung disease	Latanoprost and other PG analogs
Bloch–Sulzberger syndrome	Pigment dispersion syndrome
Von Recklinghausen disease	Ocular melanosis
Bourneville disease	Posner–Schlossman syndrome
Parry–Romberg syndrome	Iris ectropion syndrome
Chediak–Higashi syndrome	• Benign and malignant tumors of the iris • Ocular siderosis

(PG: prostaglandin)

TABLE 15: Causes based on chromicity of iris.

Hypochromic	Hyperchromic	Hypo-/hyperchromic
Idiopathic congenital	*Unilateral:* Use of a topical prostaglandin analog	Fuchs uveitis syndrome
Horner syndrome, particularly if congenital	Oculodermal melanocytosis (naevus of Ota)	Other causes of chronic anterior uveitis
Waardenburg syndrome	Ocular siderosis	
Posner–Schlossman syndrome	• Diffuse iris naevus or melanoma • Sturge–Weber syndrome • Post-traumatic • Melanotic • Neovascular	

Features, Complications, and Management of Fuchs Uveitis Syndrome

Fuchs uveitis syndrome (FUS) (also known as Fuchs heterochromic iridocyclitis) is a low-grade, chronic, nongranulomatous uveitis of unknown origin. It is mostly a unilateral disease but can be bilateral in 10% of cases with no racial and genetic predisposition. Characteristically, the eye is not red. There are diffuse small stellate KPs scattered on the entire corneal endothelium, iris atrophy with or without heterochromia, abnormal angle vessels, and a lack of posterior synechiae. Cataract and glaucoma are considered to be the major complications.

Amsler Sign

Bleeding from the fragile blood vessels in the iridocorneal angle and iris that may occur following paracentesis during cataract surgery or spontaneously.

Previously the disease was called "Fuchs heterochromic iridocyclitis". But the presence of heterochromia is variable. People with darker color of iris develop hypochromia due to progressive iris atrophy whereas those with light-colored iris develop hyperchromia as iris atrophy leads to better visibility of underlying pigment epithelium.

Etiology

There is no HLA association but various studies have found an association with infectious etiologies such as toxoplasma, rubella, and cytomegalovirus (CMV).

Clinical Features

- Usually presents in young patients.
- Patients can present with history of floaters or gradual decrease in vision. Pain and redness are not a typical feature. Some patients are aware of heterochromia. Infrequently blurred vision and floaters are due to recurrent hyphema. Symptoms of glaucoma may include mild pain, blurred vision, and colored haloes around lights.

Examination

- Presence of small, white, stellate KPs distributed across the endothelium
- Low-grade anterior chamber inflammation
- Diffuse iris stromal atrophy with or without heterochromia
- Absence of posterior synechiae prior to cataract surgery
- Presence of cells and opacities in the anterior vitreous.

Complications of a Case with FUS

- *Cataract:* Usually posterior subcapsular type that progresses variably.
- *Glaucoma:* The prevalence is as high as 60%. This is the most common cause of visual impairment and permanent vision loss. The etiology can be chronic open angle type, or secondary glaucoma due to PAS, NV, steroid induced, phacolytic glaucoma, or due to trabeculitis.

- *Vitreous opacities:* These also can be of any grade and are common in most of the cases. Anterior vitreous is more commonly involved. Macular edema is not a feature of FHI.
- *Chorioretinal atrophic scars:* Peripheral scars resembling toxoplasma or histoplasmosis are noted in 7.2–65% of cases.

Management

- Most of the patients are asymptomatic with mild anterior chamber reaction that does not need treatment with topical steroids. Long-term side effects of therapy are more and it does not alter the course of disease.
- In presence of an episode of severe inflammation with associated pain and rise in IOP, topical steroids should be used and tapered slowly.
- *Cataract surgery:* Routine microincisional cataract surgery with IOL in the bag has good visual outcome. Preoperative and postoperative topical steroids are given to control inflammation.
- Intraocular bleed can occur (Amsler sign) but is not severe to hamper surgery. These patients have more risk of developing glaucoma after surgery and posterior capsule opacification.
- *Vitreous opacities:* Deposits in vitreous are sometimes dense enough to require pars plana vitrectomy (PPV).
- *Glaucoma:* Initially manage with topical medication. In patients who are unresponsive to topical medication, glaucoma filtering surgery is required with adjuncts such as mitomycin C and 5-fluorouracil, due to high risk of failure in presence of inflammation.

10. What are the causes of heterochromia iridocyclitis?

Fuchs uveitis syndrome is the most common etiology of heterochromia iridocyclitis.

Other causes of heterochromic iritis are:
- Posner–Schlossmann syndrome or glaucomatocyclitic crisis—resembles FHI and is complicated by secondary glaucoma.
- Lymphoid hyperplasia of uveal tract, malignancy such as melanoma and leukemia can cause heterochromia and masquerade as uveitis.
- Juvenile xanthogranuloma can affect any of the ocular structures. Iris is mostly involved with fleshy iris nodule, spontaneous hyphema, unilateral glaucoma, heterochromia iridis, and red eye with signs of uveitis.
- Intermediate uveitis (IU)—frequently presents with symptoms of floaters and blurred vision, often unilaterally in an age group similar to that for FHI. Furthermore, nongranulomatous anterior chamber inflammation and inflammatory aggregates in the anterior vitreous and peripheral retina are the hallmark of the disease. However, neither the pars plana exudates nor the macular edema is noted in FHI.

11. What are the various presentations of uveitis in spondyloarthropathies?

Definition

Several autoimmune diseases known as seronegative spondyloarthropathies are strongly associated with both acute nongranulomatous anterior uveitis and HLA-B27. Patients are RF negative. The seronegative spondyloarthropathies include:
- Ankylosing spondylitis
- Reactive arthritis syndrome
- Inflammatory bowel disease
- Psoriatic arthritis.

These entities are sometimes clinically indistinguishable, and all may be associated with spondylitis and sacroiliitis. Women are more likely than men to experience atypical spondyloarthropathies. HLA-B27 is a major histocompatibility complex (MHC) class I antigen.

Ankylosing Spondylitis

Up to 90% of patients with AS test positive for HLA-B27, although most HLA-B27-positive individuals do not develop the disease. Symptoms ranges in severity from asymptomatic to crippling include lower back pain and morning stiffness. The chance that an HLA-B27-positive patient will develop spondyloarthritis or eye disease is 1 in 4. Often, persons with anterior uveitis lack symptoms of back disease.

Sacroiliac imaging studies should be obtained when indicated by a suggestive history of morning lower back stiffness that improves with exertion. Patients should be informed of the risk of deformity and referred to a rheumatologist. Pulmonary apical fibrosis and cardiovascular disease (aortic valvular insufficiency) may also develop.

Reactive Arthritis

Reactive arthritis syndrome, formerly known as Reiter syndrome, consists of the classic diagnostic triad of nonspecific urethritis, polyarthritis, and conjunctival inflammation, often accompanied by nongranulomatous anterior uveitis. The HLA-B27 marker is found in up to 95% of patients. The condition constitutes <2% of all spondyloarthropathies and occurs most frequently in young adult men. Only 10% of the patients are female.

Reactive arthritis syndrome may be triggered by episodes of diarrhea or dysentery without urethritis. Ureaplasma urealyticum as well as *Chlamydia, Shigella, Salmonella,* and *Yersinia* species have all been implicated as triggering infections, although pathogens cannot be isolated from affected joints. Arthritis begins within a month of infection in 80% of patients. The knees, ankles, feet, and wrists are affected asymmetrically and in an oligoarticular (4 or fewer joints) distribution. Sacroiliitis is present in as many as 70% of patients.

In addition to the classic triad, two other conditions are considered major diagnostic criteria:
1. *Keratoderma blennorrhagicum:* A scaly, erythematous, irritating disorder of the palms and soles of the feet
2. *Circinate balanitis:* A persistent, scaly, erythematous, circumferential rash of the distal penis.

Extra-articular findings such as nail bed pitting, oral ulcers, conjunctivitis, uveitis, and constitutional symptoms help establish a diagnosis of reactive arthritis syndrome, according to criteria established by the Assessment of Spondylo Arthritis International Society (ASAS). Eye involvement occurs in approximately 20% patients. Conjunctivitis is the most common eye finding, and it is usually mucopurulent and papillary. Punctate and subepithelial keratitis may also occur, occasionally leaving permanent corneal scars. Acute nongranulomatous anterior uveitis occurs in up to 10% of patients and may become bilateral and chronic.

Inflammatory Bowel Disease

Ulcerative colitis and Crohn's disease (granulomatous ileocolitis) are both associated with AAU. Up to 12% of patients with ulcerative colitis and 2.4% of patients with Crohn's disease develop AAU. Occasionally, bowel disease is asymptomatic and follows the onset of uveitis. 20% of patients with IBD have sacroiliitis; of these, 60% are HLA-B27 positive. Patients with both AAU and IBD are more likely to be HLA-B27 positive and have sacroiliitis. Patients with IBD who are HLA-B27 negative may develop sclerouveitis or features of IU.

Psoriatic Arthritis

Diagnosis of psoriatic arthritis is made according to findings of typical cutaneous changes, terminal phalangeal joint inflammation, and ungual involvement. Up to 25% of patients develop anterior uveitis, which tends to be insidious and bilateral; it is also more likely to be chronic than is the uveitis associated with other spondyloarthropathies. Uveitis may be more severe in HLA-B27-positive patients. The mean age of onset is older than in idiopathic or HLA-B27-associated uveitis and may be bilateral and of longer duration. Posterior segment involvement can also be present.

Treatment of Seronegative Spondyloarthropathies

It consists of cycloplegic and mydriatic agents and CSs, which are usually given topically. In severe cases, periocular or systemic CSs may be required, and chronic cases may need immunomodulatory therapy. AS needs treatment with NSAIDs for enthesopathy. Sulfasalazine may be used in patients whose joint disease is not controlled with NSAIDs and it reduces the recurrences of uveitis. Recalcitrant cases need anti-TNF drugs.

 12. Describe etiopathogenesis, clinical features, and management of intermediate uveitis.

Intermediate Uveitis

Definition

According to International Uveitis Study Group (IUSG) and the "SUN" Working Group, "intermediate uveitis" is described as an intraocular inflammatory disease with the vitreous as the primary site of inflammation. Inflammation may be concentrated in the anterior vitreous and in the vitreous base overlying the peripheral retina-pars plana region and ciliary body, characterized by vitreal inflammatory aggregates, i.e., "snowballs", inflammatory exudate on the inferior pars plana, i.e., "snowbanking" and not infrequently, retinal phlebitis.

Pars Planitis

It refers to that subset of IU where snowbank or snowball formation is found without an associated infection or underlying systemic disease and so, is "idiopathic".

Clinical Features

Symptoms: Typically, a bilateral disease (80%) with a chronic, slowly progressive course and episodes of relapses in some patients. Most frequently, patient presents with blurred vision or floaters. Unlike anterior uveitis, there is not much pain, photophobia, or redness in eyes. More severe cases with macular edema and severe vitritis can have marked diminution in vision. Sudden drop in vision can be due to vitreous hemorrhage or retinal detachment.

Signs: Anterior segment may be normal or there may be mild reaction, few KPs and posterior synechiae rarely. Thus, one should look for vitreous cells in all cases of anterior uveitis so as not to miss the cases with IU. Some cases may manifest a linear line of KPs similar to that seen in endothelial rejection. There may also be concomitant corneal edema.

Vitritis may range from 1+ to 4+ (grading) depending on severity. Vitreous aggregates called "snowballs" are mostly seen in inferior vitreous periphery. Vasculitis may be seen in 10–32% of patients and includes vascular venous sheathing (periphlebitis) that may lead to occlusion and sometimes peripheral retinal NV. Snowbank refers to the presence of exudates over pars plana or the peripheral retina, which is also noted more commonly inferiorly but spreads circumferentially. Inactive disease with organized exudates and no overlying inflammation is called pars plana fibrosis. Inferior peripheral retina may develop retinoschisis, and/or tractional or exudative detachment.

Diagnosis

Diagnosis is basically clinical with careful indentation of eyes to look for snowballs and pars plana exudates.

History

Ask for duration of symptoms, treatment, and number of recurrences. Ask for disease-specific history such as fever, fatigue, or night sweats [sarcoidosis and tuberculosis (TB)], loss of sensitivity or paresthesia of the hands, arms, or legs [multiple sclerosis (MS)], dermatitis (Lyme disease, TB, or syphilis), arthritis of the knee (Lyme disease), or contact with cats (Bartonella infection). Patients with MS may have had previous episodes of neurological involvement, such as optic neuritis. The importance of diagnosing these on time is to start the systemic therapy early so as to decrease disease morbidity.

The following investigations are done to rule out common causes of IU:

Chest X-ray/CT chest	Tuberculosis/sarcoidosis
Serum ACE	Sarcoidosis
Gallium scan	Combination of a positive gallium scan and an elevated ACE increases the specificity for sarcoidosis diagnosis to 100%
Serum lysozyme	Sarcoidosis, tuberculosis, and leprosy
Serology	Cat scratch disease, Lyme's disease
RPR, VDRL	Syphilis
Mantoux test	Tuberculosis
MRI brain	MS, CNS lymphoma
Vitreous biopsy	Lymphoma

(ACE: angiotensin-converting enzyme; CNS: central nervous system; CT: computed tomography; MS: multiple sclerosis; RPR: rapid plasma reagin; VDRL: venereal diseases research laboratory)

In case an elderly patient presents with features of IU, one must rule out intraocular lymphoma. Definitive diagnosis is by vitreous biopsy followed by molecular analysis and interleukin-10 (IL-10)/IL-6 ratio.

Management

The traditional Kaplan regimen (four-step treatment) is as follows:
- Corticosteroid therapy
- Cryotherapy or indirect laser photocoagulation
- Pars plana vitrectomy
- Systemic immunosuppressive agents.

However, as ophthalmologists have currently been gaining more experience with the use of immunosuppressive agents and new biological treatments, the preferred strategy places steroids as the mainstay of initial treatment followed by IMT and then surgical intervention.

Step 1: Periocular steroids may be used as first choice in unilateral cases of IU. The duration of action is around 4 weeks and 3–4 injections of sub-Tenon triamcinolone can be administered before shifting to oral therapy. They usually result in resolution of features of IU and CME. In refractory cases of CME, one can inject steroids intravitreally as well.

Step 2: Oral steroids are given in bilateral disease or unilateral disease unresponsive to local therapy.

Step 3: Systemic immunomodulatory therapy is added in case patient is nonresponding to systemic steroids or is dependent on systemic steroids or steroids are causing side effects or are contraindicated.

Step 4: In case of NV and sequelae, peripheral ablation with cryotherapy or indirect laser photocoagulation to the peripheral retina can be done.

Step 5: If all the treatment modalities fail to control inflammation, PPV with induction of posterior hyaloidal separation and peripheral laser photocoagulation may be performed, along with immunomodulatory therapy.

Medical

Corticosteroids: These are the mainstay of treatment—
- *Systemic:* For binocular involvement or uniocular not improving with periocular injections: oral prednisolone 1–2 mg/kg/day
- *Periocular:* Posterior sub-Tenon or transseptal—triamcinolone acetonide (2–4 mg/0.1 mL), methylprednisolone acetate (40–80 mg)
- *Intravitreal:* Triamcinolone (2–4 mg/0.1 mL)
- *Intravitreal implants:* Fluocinolone (Retisert), Dexamethasone (Ozurdex), when the patient needs more than two to three periocular injections and for recurrent CME
- Intravenous methylprednisolone is very rarely required
  In case of spillover anterior uveitis, one may use topical steroid drops and cycloplegics.

Immunomodulator agents
- *Antimetabolites:*
  - *Azathioprine:* Nucleoside analog interferes with DNA replication and RNA transcription (up to 2 mg/kg/day)
  - *Methotrexate:* Folic acid analog inhibits dihydrofolate (starting 10–15 mg/week gradually increasing to 15–25 mg/week)
  - Mycophenolate mofetil: Inosine monophosphate inhibitor (1–1.5 g/BD)
- *T-cell inhibitors:*
  - Cyclosporine—IL-2 inhibitor (1–5 mg/kg/day)

Following biological agents can be used in IU in consultation with rheumatologist:
- Etanercept, TNF-α receptor blocker
- Infliximab, TNF-α inhibitor.

Surgical

- Cryopexy of peripheral retina—in recalcitrant disease or peripheral retinal NV with vitreous hemorrhage.
- Pars plana vitrectomy—for chronic cases, and those with vitreomacular traction (VMT) or epiretinal membrane (ERM).
- Separate surgery may be needed in case of cataract, glaucoma, hypotony, and BSK.

Immunomodulators	Peri-/intraocular steroids	Vitrectomy
• Long-term steroid therapy dependence (≥10 mg/day for 3 months) • Recurrent disease • Unacceptable steroid side effects/contraindication of steroids • Inadequate response to corticosteroids alone • Failure of therapy to steroids alone/severe inflammation	• Posterior uveitis • Retinal vein occlusion • Uniocular uveitis • Contraindications for systemic steroids • Recurrent CME	• Uveitic CME in presence of hyaloid traction on macula, dense epiretinal membranes • Dense vitreous opacities • Persistent vitreous hemorrhage • Resistance to medical therapy • Diagnostic in case of suspected lymphoma

(CME: cystoid macular edema)

13. What is pars planitis?

Pars planitis or idiopathic IU is characterized by formation of snowbanking or snowballs without any associated underlying infection or systemic disease. So, the diagnosis is made after ruling out various infective and noninfective causes of IU.

Clinical features, complications, and management of disease are discussed above.

14. What is vision loss in intermediate uveitis?

Chronic disease and recurrent episodes of IU can cause many sight-threatening complications.
- *Macular edema and maculopathy* are the most common causes of vision loss. Around 60% of cases with long-term IU develop macular edema.
- *Cataract:* Complicated cataract formation is as common as 50%. It is more in patients treated with long-term steroids than with immunosuppressives.
- *Ocular hypertension or glaucoma*—seen in 8–10% of cases and is mostly related to CSs use.
- *Retinal vasculitis:* Predominantly a phlebitis, is common manifestation of disease. Sometimes, vessel occlusion leads to NV (5–15%) and cyclitic membrane formation. Vitreous hemorrhage is more common in children than adults.
- *Retinal detachment in IU*—can be exudative, tractional, or combined retinal detachment. Some cases with IU also have retinoschisis (13%), mostly involving inferior retina.
- *Epiretinal membrane formation*
- *Optic disk edema*—is more common in younger patients with IU. Rarely, optic atrophy or optic disk NV and optic neuritis associated with MS can be found.

Management of complications is discussed subsequently on question in medical and surgical management of uveitis.

15. What are the indications and modes of application of periocular steroids for uveitis? What are their advantages and complications and what steps can be taken to prevent them?

Periocular Steroids

Indications for the injection are:
- Severe unilateral anterior uveitis
- Anterior uveitis with hypopyon
- Anterior uveitis complicated by CME
- Unilateral intermediated uveitis
- Unilateral posterior uveitis (preferably not involving the disk and macula, i.e., not sight threatening; sight-threatening cases required high-dose systemic steroids)
- Contraindications for systemic steroid treatment
- Poor patient compliance to topical medications posing a likely factor for unresponsiveness to topical treatment.

Following drugs are used:
- Subconjunctival betamethasone sodium phosphate solution (4 mg in 1 mL) alone or in combination with betamethasone acetate suspension (6 mg in 1 mL).
- Sub-Tenon triamcinolone (0.5–1.0 mL sub-Tenon injection of triamcinolone acetonide 40 mg/mL).

Sub-Tenon injection is administered by any of the following two techniques:

Inferior transseptal injection	*Posterior sub-Tenon approach*
1. Topical anesthesia (e.g., tetracaine)	1. Topical anesthesia
2. Disinfection of the skin of the lower eyelid and maxillary area (e.g., povidone–iodine)	2. Place a small cotton pledget impregnated with an anesthetic agent (e.g., tetracaine, lidocaine 2% gel) in the superior fornix at the site of injection for 2 minutes
3. Shake the vial containing the steroid	3. Shake the vial containing the steroid
4. Draw 1 mL steroid (triamcinolone acetonide or methylprednisolone acetate 40 mg/mL) into a 2-mL syringe	4. Draw 1 mL steroid (triamcinolone acetonide or methylprednisolone acetate 40 mg/mL) into a 2-mL syringe
5. Replace the drawing-up needle with a 26-gauge needle	5. Replace the drawing-up needle with a 26-gauge needle
6. Instruct the patient to look straight ahead	6. Instruct the patient to look in the nasal inferior direction (i.e., the direction opposite to the superotemporal injection site)
7. Insert the 26-gauge needle through the skin at the junction of the other third and the inner two-thirds of the lower orbital rim, entering close to the bony margin while clearing the margin itself (Note: some inject via the conjunctiva)	7. Penetrate the bulbar conjunctiva with the needle tip, bevel toward the eye globe
8. Advance the needle slowly and tangentially to the globe	8. Slowly insert the needle posteriorly, following the contour of the globe, making side-to-side motions to prevent globe penetration
9. Slightly withdraw the plunger to ascertain no blood enters the syringe, and inject the full 1 mL of steroid in a slow fashion	9. Slightly withdraw the plunger to ascertain no blood enters the syringe, and inject the full 1 mL of steroid in a slow fashion
10. Withdraw the needle carefully	10. Withdraw the needle carefully

Complications that may arise of the periocular steroid injection are subconjunctival hemorrhage, globe perforation, optic nerve injury, subcutaneous fat atrophy, ptosis, and skin depigmentation.

Long-term effects of steroids such as cataract, glaucoma, scleral melting, and retinal vein occlusion may also occur.

Using an intravenous catheter made of polytetrafluoroethylene (PFTE), steroids can be safely injected in sub-Tenon space. This avoids the risks of needle injury.

 16. What are the indications, advantages, and disadvantages of intraocular steroids?

Intraocular steroids are injected in cases with noninfectious uveitis (NIU) to control inflammation or in cases of NIU with macular edema in two settings:
1. *Corticosteroids in acute inflammatory outbreak:* Intravitreal injections of CSs are reserved for severe recurrences involving the macula and/or the optic nerve which are the most sight-threatening uveitis. Triamcinolone acetonide (4 mg in 0.1 mL) and dexamethasone phosphate (0.4 mg in 0.1 mL) have been the most commonly used intravitreal CSs for the treatment of uveitis and uveitic macular edema, although they have limited duration of action. Their possible complications are IOP increase (glaucoma), cataract formation, and infectious or sterile endophthalmitis.
2. *Long-term maintenance corticosteroids:* For sustained long release of steroids into the eye, some implants can be surgically implanted in the eye.

Fluocinolone Acetonide Intravitreal Implants

Retisert® (Bausch and Lomb, Rochester, NY): It was the first FDA-approved implantable device for the treatment of severe noninfectious posterior uveitis. It contains 590 µg of FA, which is slowly released over the course of 30 months. Patients treated with the Retisert implant show significant decreased recurrences of inflammation at 1, 2, and 3 years following implantation. However, it has consistently shown marked induction of cataract formation in all cases, and significant IOP increase in two-thirds of the cases. Other less common side effects include hypotony, retinal detachment, and endophthalmitis. The implant is not biodegradable and must be surgically removed if clinically indicated in the setting of significant adverse events.

Iluvien: It is a cylindrical polyimide tube that contains 190 g of fluocinolone acetonide (FA). Iluvien has been evaluated in patients with diabetic macular edema showing a similar local safety profile to Retisert: cataract progression (80%) and significant IOP increase (40%).

Dexamethasone Intravitreal Implants

Ozurdex: It is a biodegradable dexamethasone drug delivery system, made of a solid biodegradable polymer composed of a polylactic acid-co-glycolic acid (PLGA) matrix. This matrix is saturated with 0.7 mg of dexamethasone. As the polymer dissolves, dexamethasone is slowly released into the vitreous and the retina. In patients with posterior uveitis, Ozurdex achieves a significant decrease of the intraocular inflammation peaked at week 8 following the intravitreal implantation, which is maintained for up to week 26. Throughout this period, 23% of eyes require IOP-lowering medications, and cataract formation is reported in around 15% of eyes. Ozurdex is FDA approved for the treatment of noninfectious intermediate and posterior uveitis.

Commercial name	Generic name	Biodegradation	Dose	Expected efficacy	Side effects
Ozurdex	Dexamethasone	Yes	0.7 mg	3–6 months	Significant IOP increase (23%) Cataract (15%)
Iluvien	Fluocinolone acetonide	No	0.19 mg	24–36 months	Significant IOP increase (40%) Cataract (80%)
Retisert	Fluocinolone acetonide	No	0.59 mg	24–36 months	Significant IOP increase (66%) Cataract (100%)

(IOP: intraocular pressure)

Multicenter Uveitis Steroid Treatment (MUST) Trial

It was a randomized clinical trial, which compared the safety and effectiveness of the FA implant vs. systemic therapy with CSs, plus immunosuppression among 255 patients (497 eyes) with noninfectious intermediate, posterior, or panuveitis. At 2 and 4.5 years, the visual acuity improvement was similar with either treatment. But at 7 years' time point, the visual acuity improvement was greater with systemic treatment. Both treatment options were well tolerated. FA implant group had more ocular complications such as rise in IOP and significant cataract.

 17. Discuss retinal vasculitis and describe Wegener's granulomatosis (WG).

Definition

Retinal vasculitis is inflammation of the retinal vessel wall that can lead to perivascular sheathing/cuffing, cotton wool spots (CWS), retinal hemorrhages, vascular leakage, and/or occlusion that may lead to retinal ischemia, subsequent NV, and sequelae. There can be involvement of retinal veins (phlebitis) or arteries (arteriolitis) or both simultaneously.

It can be a part of ocular or systemic disease or an isolated entity. It is more common under the age of 40 years. It is usually a bilateral disease with both eyes either involved simultaneously or subsequently.

Classification

Classification can be done according to whether predominantly the disease affects veins or arteries or both.

Arteries	Vein	Both
Acute retinal necrosis	Eales disease	Behçet's disease
IRVAN	Sarcoidosis	Frosted branch angiitis
SLE	Intermediate uveitis	Toxoplasmosis
PAN	Multiple sclerosis (MS)	Relapsing polychondritis
Syphilis	Tuberculosis	Wegener's granulomatosis
PORN	Birdshot chorioretinopathy	Crohn's disease
Churg–Strauss syndrome	HIV-paraviral syndrome	

(HIV: human immunodeficiency virus; IRVAN: idiopathic retinal vasculitis, aneurysms, and neuroretinitis; PAN: polyarteritis nodosa; PORN: progressive outer retinal necrosis; SLE: systemic lupus erythematosus)

Stages of retinal vasculitis:

I: Stage of inflammation	• Active inflammation has features of segmental perivascular infiltrates (cuffing), sometimes causing vascular occlusion • Retinal hemorrhages, retinal edema, macular edema • Vitritis • Associated features (±): Active choroiditis (Birdshot choroiditis), retinitis (CMV retinitis), intermediate uveitis
II: Stage of ischemia	• Sclerosed vessels and presence of capillary nonperfusion areas on fluorescein angiography • Collateral vessels • Healed paravascular pigmented choroiditis patches.
III: Stage of neovascularization	• NVE, NVD
IV: Stage of complications	• Vitreous hemorrhage • Tractional retinal detachment • Epiretinal membrane • Neovascular glaucoma

(CMV: cytomegalovirus; NVD: neovascularization of the disk; NVE: neovascularization elsewhere)

Occlusive Retinal Vasculitis

This type has poor prognosis with higher incidence of macular edema, ERM formation, and NV. Causes include TB, Eales disease, systemic lupus erythematosus (SLE), MS, Behçet's disease, relapsing polychondritis, and Susac syndrome.

Diagnosis

Patient profile: Idiopathic form of disease affects young adults whereas those associated with underlying etiology can have variable presentation for age and gender.

Clinical Features

Involvement of retinal veins or arteries or both should be noted. Retinal arteritis is mostly associated with systemic disease or acute retinal necrosis (ARN). The vessel involvement may be focal, diffuse, or segmental. Perivascular white fluffy cuff may be seen due to inflammation of vessel wall and exudation surrounding it. Sarcoidosis is characterized by perivascular exuberant exudation termed as "candle wax dripping".

- *Intraretinal infiltrates:* Seen in cases with ARN and CMV which lead to retinal necrosis and breaks. Also seen in Adamantiades–Behçet's disease (ABD), where the retinal infiltrates are transient.
- *Cotton wool spots:* Retinal precapillary arteriolar occlusion leads to microinfarcts in nerve fiber layer, more in disorders such as SLE, polyarteritis nodosa (PAN), and Churg–Strauss syndrome.
- *Retinal necrosis:* Seen in infectious disorders such as toxoplasmosis, varicella zoster, herpes simplex, CMV, and human T-lymphotropic virus (HTLV).
- *Frosted branch angiitis:* Associated with disorder such as CMV, lymphoma, leukemia, SLE, Crohn's disease, and toxoplasmosis. There is severe infiltration of the perivascular space by lymphocytes.
- *Neovascularization:* Due to retinal ischemia
- *Symptoms:* Blurring of vision, floaters, flashes, scotoma, and metamorphopsia.

Diagnosis

Diagnosis is usually clinical, supported by ancillary tests such as fundus fluorescein angiography (FFA).

Features on FFA: Vascular leakage (diffuse, segmental, or focal) involving veins or arteries or both in active disease; vascular occlusion and capillary drop out and capillary nonperfusion (CNP) areas; leakage from retinal NV; pooling of dye at macula due to edema; disk leakage due to NV or staining in late phase of active disease.

Investigations of a case of vasculitis need to be tailored as per the systemic and ocular findings suggestive of a particular disease. These may include one or more of the following:

Ocular imaging evaluation	- FFA (indications mentioned above) - OCT (CME) - USG (VH or TRD)
Systemic imaging	- X-ray chest (tuberculosis, sarcoidosis) - CT chest (tuberculosis, sarcoidosis)
Hematology and biochemistry	- CBC - ESR - CRP - LFT/KFT - Blood sugar - Blood smear (leukemia/lymphoma) - Bone marrow biopsy (leukemia)
Serology	- VDRL (syphilis) - PPD (tuberculosis) - Toxoplasma serology - Lyme disease - Cat scratch - Weil–Felix test (Rickettsial infection) - HIV serology - Viral serology (herpes and CMV)
Serum autoantibodies	- Anti-ds DNA (SLE) - Antinuclear antibody (SLE) - RA factor (RA) - ANCA (WG and CSS) - APLA (SLE)
Miscellaneous	- Vitreous biopsy (Eales, lymphoma) - HLA testing - Complement analysis - CSF analysis

(ANCA: antineutrophil cytoplasmic antibody; APLA: antiphospholipid antibody; CBC: complete blood count; CME: cystoid macular edema; CMV: cytomegalovirus; CRP: C-reactive protein; CSS: Churg Strauss syndrome; CT: computed tomography; ESR: erythrocyte sedimentation rate; FFA: fundus fluorescein angiography; HLA: human leukocyte antigen; LFT/KFT: liver function test/kidney function test; PPD: purified protein derivative; OCT: optical coherence tomography; SLE: systemic lupus erythematosus; TRD: tractional retinal detachment; USG: ultrasonography; VDRL: venereal diseases research laboratory; VH: vitreous hemorrhage; WG: Wegener's granulomatosis)

Management

Infectious retinal vasculitis needs treatment with appropriate antimicrobial agents. In noninfectious cases, the stage of inflammation requires treatment with steroids/immuno modulator therapy (IMT). Unilateral cases are managed with posterior subtenon injection/periocular steroids (PST) and bilateral cases are treated with systemic steroids. The vasculitis usually starts to respond within 2 weeks of treatment. Treatment response is characterized by resolution of cuffing, vitritis, retinal edema, and organization of the perivascular exudation and later on sclerosis of the affected vessel. Systemic steroid therapy may be tapered gradually once the active vasculitis settles. Nonresponsive cases or steroid responders may require immunosuppressive therapy. Systemic connective tissue disorders and autoimmune disorders generally need IMT or biologic agents to control the inflammation. Commonly used immunosuppressive agents are azathioprine, cyclosporine, mycophenolate mofetil, and cyclophosphamide.

The stage of ischemia requires close monitoring for the development of neovascularization elsewhere (NVE)/neovascularization of the disk (NVD)/neovascularization index (NVI). Prophylactic laser photocoagulation of CNP areas on FFA may be performed in one-eyed patients, patients with poor compliance, and those with extensive peripheral ischemia such as in Behçet's disease, SLE, WG, and IRVAN (idiopathic retinal vasculitis, aneurysms, and neuroretinitis).

The stage of NV requires prompt laser photocoagulation of the ischemic retina. FFA can be used to guide targeted retinal photocoagulation. Ultrawide field angiography may help in locating peripheral CNP areas in eyes with persistent NV.

The complications such as nonresolving vitreous hemorrhage and tractional retinal detachment involving or threatening the macula require vitrectomy.

Wegener's Granulomatosis (Granulomatosis with Polyangiitis)

It is an autoimmune disorder of small- and medium-sized vessels (arterioles, venules, capillaries, and small arteries) affecting orbit, nose, sinuses, kidney, lungs, and throat and less commonly skin, joints, and nerves. It is associated with the presence of diffuse staining antineutrophil cytoplasmic antibody (c-ANCA) against serine proteinase-3 antigen.

Ocular features: These seen in around 60% of patients and result in vision loss in around 8% of cases and increase to 37%, if treated inadequately. Any structure in eye or orbit may be involved.

Orbit: Orbit can be involved in continuation with nasal and sinus involvement. Orbital involvement can present as proptosis, diplopia, watering, redness, and pain. Optic nerve involvement with ischemic optic neuropathy and progressive proptosis are a cause of visual decline. Painful ophthalmoplegia is also a feature of disease.

Eyelid involvement: Diffuse eyelid involvement is called "yellow lid sign".

Conjunctiva: Noninfectious chronic conjunctivitis (ulcerative and necrotic) may be seen.

Sclera: Nodular scleritis or episcleritis is one of the most common initial presentations in around half of the cases. Patient will have dull boring pain and history of redness in eyes.

Cornea: Peripheral ulcerative keratitis is a common feature of the disease.

Uveitis: Uveitis is an uncommon manifestation. Some cases may have retinal hemorrhages and CWS and rarely manifest with retinal vascular occlusions.

18. Describe chorioretinitis.

Chorioretinitis is a type of posterior uveitis characterized by inflammation of the choroid and the retina. Based on the etiology, chorioretinitis can be classified as infectious or noninfectious. Noninfectious causes may have systemic associations.

Infective causes	Noninfectious etiology with systemic association	Noninfectious etiology without any systemic association
Tuberculosis	Sarcoidosis	Multifocal choroiditis and panuveitis
Toxoplasmosis	Behçet's disease	Punctate inner choroidopathy
Toxocara		Multiple evanescent white dots syndrome
Syphilis		Birdshot choroidopathy
Bartonella		Serpiginous choroidopathy
Candida		
Histoplasmosis		
Viruses—herpes, CMV		

(CMV: cytomegalovirus)

19. Discuss posterior uveitis.

Here we shall briefly discuss the various etiological presentations of the disease. The individual diseases are discussed in relevant questions.

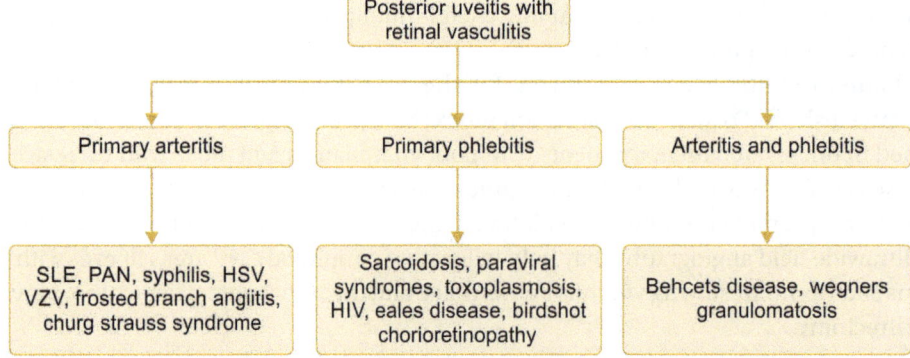

(HIV: human immunodeficiency virus; HSV: herpes simplex virus; PAN: polyarteritis nodosa; SLE: systemic lupus erythematosus; VZV: varicella zoster virus)

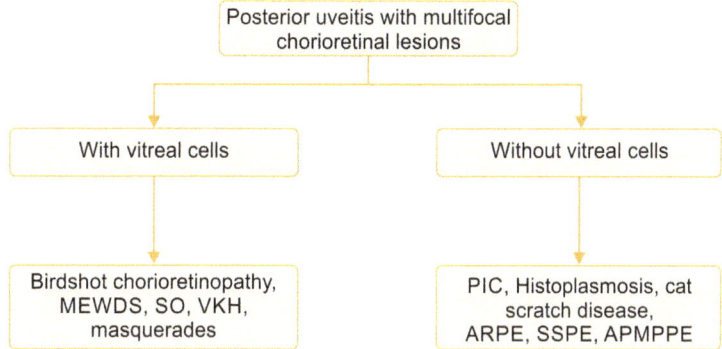

(APMPPE: acute posterior multifocal placoid pigment epitheliopathy; ARPE: acute retinal pigment epitheliitis; MCP: multifocal choroiditis and panuveitis; MEWDS: multiple evanescent white dot syndrome; PIC: punctate inner choroidopathy; SO: sympathetic ophthalmitis; SSPE: subacute sclerosing panencephalitis; VKH: Vogt–Koyanagi–Harada syndrome)

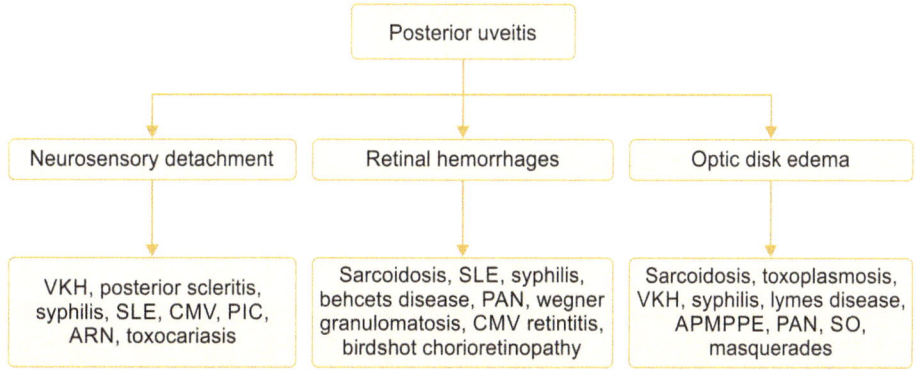

(APMPPE: acute posterior multifocal placoid pigment epitheliopathy; ARN: acute retinal necrosis; CMV: cytomegalovirus; PAN: polyarteritis nodosa; PIC: punctate inner choroidopathy; SLE: systemic lupus erythematosus; SO: sympathetic ophthalmitis; VKH: Vogt–Koyanagi–Harada syndrome)

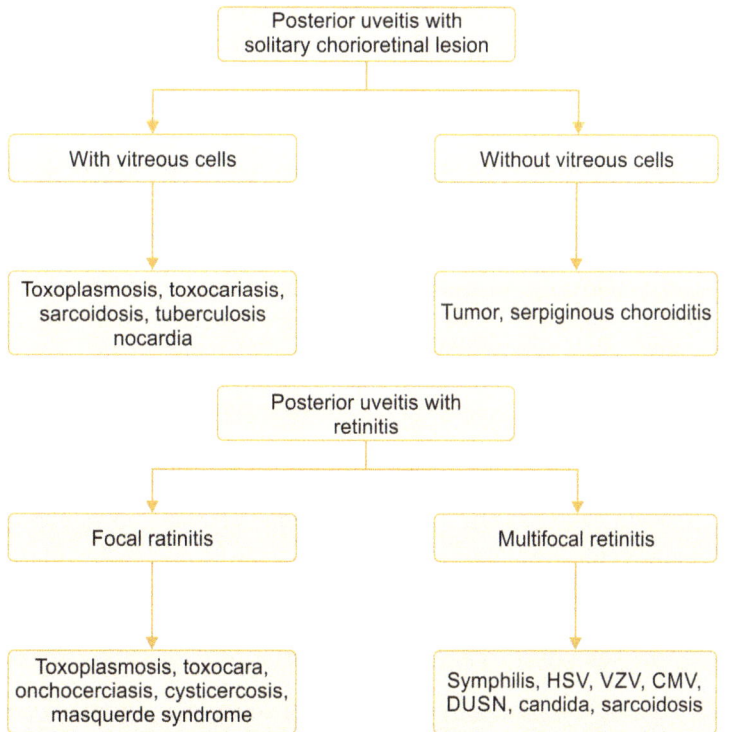

(CMV: cytomegalovirus; DUSN: diffuse unilateral subacute neuroretinitis; HSV: herpes simplex virus; VZV: varicella zoster virus)

20. Discuss the differentials and management of posterior parasitic uveitis.

The following parasitic diseases can affect the eye:
- Toxoplasmosis
- Toxocariasis
- Cysticercosis
- Diffuse unilateral subacute neuroretinitis (DUSN)
- Malaria
- Gnathostomiasis
- Amebiasis
- Giardiasis.

Clinical manifestations often include characteristic ocular lesions, dermatological involvement, and other extraocular sites affection.

Toxoplasma, toxocara, and cysticercosis are discussed subsequently in relevant questions.

Diffuse Unilateral Subacute Neuroretinitis

It is also called unilateral wipe-out syndrome. It is caused by a number of motile, nematode roundworms including *Toxocara canis, Gnathostoma, Brugia malayi, Ancylostoma caninum,* and the trematode Altaria. Males are more frequently affected than females. These nematodes first of all invade the skin and then through bloodstream they reach the retinochoroidal complex. The features in retina and choroid are due to toxic, inflammatory, and autoimmune reaction to the parasitic antigen.

Clinical Features

Symptom: Paracentral scotomas, floaters, and visual field defect without any significant ocular pain.

Clinical features: Optic disk edema, mild-to-moderate vitritis, and retinal gray yellowish tract like lesions. During late stage, there can be optic atrophy, narrowing of retinal arteries, increased reflection of internal limiting membrane (Oréfice's sign), and subretinal tunnels (Garcia's sign), RPE degeneration, and chorioretinal atrophy.

Diagnosis

Diagnosis is mostly clinical based on characteristic features.

Fluorescein angiography (FA): Disk leakage, atrophic tracts reveal increase choroidal fluorescence.

Indocyanine green angiography: Sometimes useful to locate the lesions as hypofluorescent spots and corresponding choroidal infiltration and inflammation.

Electroretinogram (ERG) and electro-oculogram (EOG): In ERG, a/b ratio can be normal in early stages of the disease. But "b" wave can be defective when significant retinal involvement is present.

Optical coherence tomography is an important tool to demonstrate degeneration of retinal nerve fiber layer (RFNL) and thinning of the macula.

Hematological evaluation: Eosinophilia

Treatment

Management of DUSN depends on whether the worm is visible. Visible live nematodes are treated with retinal photocoagulation. Systemic treatment involves 400 mg albendazole daily for 1 month with oral CS 1 mg/kg/day in tapering dose for 1 month. The course of the disease depends on the disease stage.

Malaria

Ocular complications are more common in *Plasmodium falciparum* infection. Almost all the structures of the eye may be involved in malaria.

Clinical Features

Conjunctival hyperemia, subconjunctival hemorrhage, conjunctival pigmentation, dendritic ulcer, interstitial keratitis, uveitis, vitreous hemorrhage, retinal hemorrhage, retinal detachment, optic neuritis, paralysis of extraocular muscles, and orbital cellulitis have been reported.

Retinal hemorrhage is considered to be due to rheological complications—the parasitized erythrocytes tend to clump along the vessel wall leading to occlusion. Other ocular lesions are transient ocular nerve palsies, orbital edema, choroiditis, retinal embolism, papilledema, paralysis of the pupillary light reflex, and accommodation.

Therefore, a patient with unexplained large retinal hemorrhages should always be investigated thoroughly for malaria, especially in an endemic country such as India.

Gnathostomiasis

It is due to parasite known as Gnathostome, ingested by eating semicooked fish, usually found in dirty shallow drains.

Clinical Features

Features occur due to migration of the larvae as well as host response to the toxins. The most common presenting feature is anterior uveitis. Other features include lid swelling, iritis, iris atrophy, iris holes, and rarely glaucoma. Intravitreal gnathostomiasis is a very rare entity. Macular scarring or retinal tear with choroidal hemorrhage near the optic disk points to the posterior retina as a possible route of entry to the eye. Movement of worm in the eye causes retinal hemorrhage and subsequent chorioretinitis. Surgical removal of the live worm may be done while it is visible in the anterior chamber.

21. What are differential diagnosis and management of bilateral panuveitis?

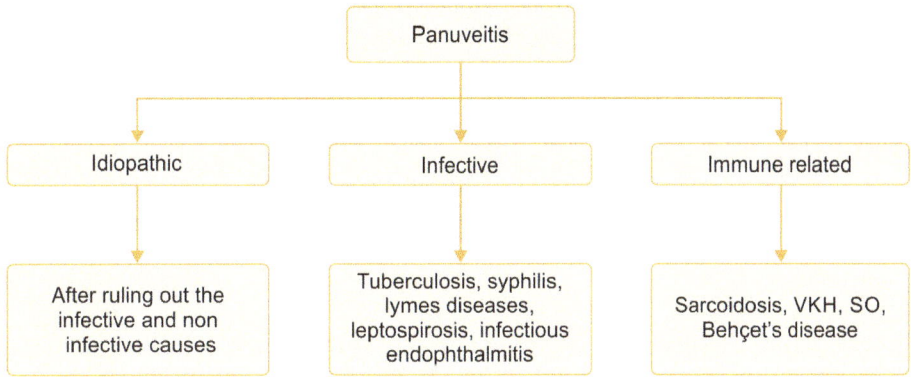

(VKH: Vogt–Koyanagi–Harada; SO: sympathetic ophthalmitis)

The individual disease entities and management of panuveitis are discussed under individual headings. Here we discuss Behçet's disease.

Behçet's Disease

A multisystem vasculitis of unknown cause primarily involving the eyes, the mucosal surfaces, and the skin. Males are affected in their 3rd to 5th decade of life. The uveitis of Behçet's disease is believed to be most severe in young men between 15 and 25 years of age. Disease has long been associated with the HLA-B51 allele.

Ocular Features

These are seen in 70% of cases with Behçet's disease. In most cases, uveitis follows the onset of recurrent oral ulcers after 3–4 years, although ocular disease is the initial manifestation in about 20% of cases. It starts with a unilateral disease and progresses to bilateral disease in two-thirds of cases.

Symptoms

Decreased vision due to anterior chamber inflammation with or without hypopyon. Pain, redness, and/or photophobia may be present.

Examination

Mobile hypopyon is seen in Behçet's disease. Very small hypopyon is noted on gonioscopic examination. Synechiae can develop after repeated bouts of anterior segment inflammation. The IOP is often normal or low. Mild vitreous cells or mild-to-moderate vitreous opacification commonly occurs. Fundus examination may show transient yellow–white retinal infiltrates, retinal hemorrhages, vascular engorgement, and/or disk hyperemia. Fundus may be entirely normal during an episode of anterior segment inflammation.

Complications

Anterior segment complications include iris NV, glaucoma, and cataract. In the posterior segment, retinal vascular sheathing or occlusion, retinal or disk NV, vitreous hemorrhage, progressive vitreous opacification, and optic atrophy.

Diagnostic Criteria

International study group criteria for diagnosing Behçet's disease.

Criteria	Description
Recurrent oral ulcerations	Minor or major aphthous ulcerations or herpetiform ulcerations observed at least 3 times in 12-month period
Plus 2 of the following in the absence of other clinical explanation	
Recurrent genital ulceration	Aphthous ulcerations or scarring
Eye lesions	Anterior or posterior uveitis or vitreous cells seen on SLE; retinal vasculitis
Skin lesions	Erythema nodosum; Pseudofolliculitis; papulopustular lesions; acneiform nodules
Positive results from pathergy test	Oblique insertion of a 20–22-G needle 5 mm into skin, read after 24–48 hours. Development of a papule 2 mm or larger denotes positive test

(SLE: systemic lupus erythematosus)

Differential Diagnosis

Rule out other causes of hypopyon uveitis such as HLA-B27, AAU, and infectious endophthalmitis. Differentials for posterior segment involvement are TB, sarcoidosis, toxoplasmosis, and syphilis.

Treatment

Anterior segment disease requires topical CSs. Posterior segment involvement needs periocular and systemic steroid therapy. Oral steroids are often needed for few years.

Thus, IMT can be started early in disease considering the aggressive and long-term course of disease. Cases refractory to steroid require antimetabolites and alkylating agents. Triple therapy, consisting of CSs, cyclosporine, and azathioprine, has been reported to successfully induce remission in refractory cases. Biologicals are also used with success in managing refractory cases.

 22. Discuss sympathetic ophthalmitis (SO)—etiopathogenesis, clinical features, and management.

Bilateral granulomatous non-necrotizing panuveitis that may develop after either surgical or accidental trauma to eye (called the exciting eye), followed by a latent period and the appearance of uveitis in the injured as well as the uninjured fellow eye (the sympathizing eye).

Previously, the incidence after trauma was 0.5% and following intraocular surgery was 10/100,000 cases. With better understanding of the disease and use of immunomodulators, the incidence now is around 0.03/100,000. Ocular surgery (mostly vitreoretinal surgery) has emerged as the main risk for the development of SO. In the early 1980s, the prevalence of SO in patients undergoing PPV was 0.01%, increasing to 0.06% when surgery was performed for trauma. Recent studies report an increased incidence of SO following vitrectomy, which can be attributed to increased rate for which these surgeries are performed in cases with trauma and other diseases.

Traditionally, it has been widely accepted that SO develops in around 80% of patients within 3 months of injury and in 90% within 1 year. This observation has also changed recently, with only one-third of patients developing SO within 3 months and less than one-half within 1 year of injury.

Etiopathogenesis

Altered T-lymphocyte responses to previously sequestered ocular self-antigens and antigens derived from the RPE or choroid. The penetrating wound facilitates exposure of uveoretinal antigens to conjunctival lymphatic channels and thereby initiates this immunopathologic response. There may be a genetic predisposition as patients with SO are more likely to express HLA-DR4, -DRw53, and -DQw3 haplotypes.

Symptoms—vary from minimal problems in near vision, mild photophobia, and slight redness to severe pain and blurring of vision.

Clinical Features

Typically present with asymmetric bilateral granulomatous panuveitis, in which the exciting eye exhibits more severe inflammation than the sympathizing eye, at least initially.

Anterior segment: Mutton-fat KPs, thickening of the iris from lymphocytic infiltration, posterior synechiae formation, and elevated IOP due to trabeculitis or hypotony as a result of ciliary body shutdown.

Posterior segment: Moderate to severe vitritis with characteristic yellowish white, midperipheral choroidal lesions (so-called Dalen–Fuchs nodules) that may become confluent.

Peripapillary choroidal lesions, exudative retinal detachment may also develop. Structural complications of SO include cataract, chronic CME, peripapillary and macular choroidal neovascularization (CNV), and optic atrophy. The presence of active intraocular inflammation and exudative retinal detachment correlate with poorer vision in the sympathizing eye.

Extraocular findings similar to those observed with VKH syndrome may be seen. Although uncommon, cerebral spinal fluid pleocytosis, sensory neural hearing disturbance, alopecia, poliosis, and vitiligo may be noted.

Diagnosis

The diagnosis of SO is clinical, and the disorder should be suspected in the presence of bilateral uveitis following any ocular trauma or surgery.

Fluorescein angiography: In acute stage, multiple hyperfluorescent sites of leakage may be seen at the level of the RPE during the venous phase, which persists into the late stage. Pooling of dye may occur beneath areas of exudative retinal detachment. Chorioretinal lesions (clinically Dalen–Fuchs nodules) show either hypofluorescence (blockage of choroidal fluorescence by nodule and granulomatous inflammation) or hyperfluorescence (breakdown of overlying RPE) in early phase and staining in late phase.

Indocyanine green angiography—reveals numerous hypofluorescent foci in intermediate phase, some of these foci may become isofluorescent in the late stage of the study.

Optical coherence tomography: Shallow serous retinal detachment, intraretinal edema, septae between the neurosensory retina and RPE, exudation in subretinal space, bumpy RPE layer, and thick choroid.

B-scan ultrasonography—reveals choroidal thickening.

Histologic features—are similar for both the exciting and sympathizing eyes. Findings include diffuse, granulomatous, and non-necrotizing infiltration of the choroid that classically spares the choriocapillaris in the early stage. Dalen–Fuchs nodules are present in about one-third of patients (also seen in VKH and sarcoidosis).

Differential Diagnosis

Other causes of panuveitis as TB, sarcoidosis, syphilis, and fungal infections, as well as traumatic or postoperative endophthalmitis. Lens-associated uveitis has been reported with SO in up to 25% of cases and may present with a similar clinical picture. The clinical presentations of SO and VKH syndrome may be strikingly similar; however, a prior ocular injury is by definition absent in VKH syndrome.

Treatment

The course is chronic, with frequent exacerbations; left untreated, SO leads to loss of vision and phthisis bulbi. Every attempt should be made to salvage eyes with a reasonable prognosis for useful vision through meticulous and prompt closure of penetrating injuries. Enucleation within 2 weeks of injury to prevent the development of SO should be considered in patients with grossly disorganized globes with no discernible visual function.

Enucleation may still be preferred to evisceration as some residual tissue may remain after evisceration in traumatic eyes that may cause SO later. Regardless of visual potential, once SO is established, enucleation of the exciting eye is not beneficial. In fact, the exciting eye may eventually become the better-seeing eye.

The initial treatment is systemic CSs, with the frequent addition of CS-sparing drugs such as azathioprine, methotrexate, mycophenolate mofetil, cyclosporine, chlorambucil, and cyclophosphamide, as extended therapy for 6 months to 1 year is anticipated in most patients. Topical CSs, together with cycloplegic and mydriatic agents, are essential in the treatment of the AAU associated with SO. Periocular CSs are used to manage inflammatory recurrences and CME. Intravitreal CSs may be used for patients intolerant of systemic CS therapy. With prompt and aggressive systemic therapy, the visual prognosis of SO is good; 60% of patients achieve a final visual acuity of 20/40, although up to 25% may decline to 20/200 or worse in the sympathizing eye.

 23. Discuss Vogt–Koyanagi–Harada disease.

Vogt–Koyanagi–Harada Disease

It is also known as uveomeningitic syndrome, it is an autoimmune disorder involving eye, ears, nervous, and the integumentary system.

Ocular involvement is characterized by chronic, bilateral, diffuse, granulomatous panuveitis with exudative retinal detachment. It was Vogt (1906) who reported whitening of the eyelashes, eyebrows, and hair (poliosis) that was associated with ocular inflammation. Harada (1926) described a type of posterior uveitis associated with exudative retinal detachment and cerebrospinal fluid (CSF) pleocytosis. Koyanagi (1929) reported association of bilateral iridocyclitis with vitiligo, alopecia, and poliosis accompanied by tinnitus and deafness. Later, the three were known to be a spectrum of same disease and thus the term VKH.

There are four stages of VKH syndrome: Prodromal, acute uveitic, convalescent, and chronic recurrent.

Etiopathogenesis

A cell-mediated autoimmune process is driven by T lymphocytes directed against self-antigens associated with melanocytes of all organ systems in a genetically susceptible individual. A strong association with HLA-DR4 and HLA-DR1 is present.

Histologic findings vary depending on the stage.

Acute uveitic stage: Diffuse, non-necrotizing, granulomatous inflammation identical to SO (lymphocytes, macrophages admixed with epithelioid and multinucleate giant cells, with preservation of the choriocapillaris). Proteinaceous exudation is observed in the subretinal space. Peripapillary choroid is the predominant site of the granulomatous inflammation. The ciliary body and iris may also be affected.

Convalescent stage: There is infiltration of uveal tissue by lymphocytes and plasma cells and there is a nongranulomatous inflammation. There are no epithelioid histiocytes. The number of choroidal melanocytes and melanin pigment decreases. This corresponds with the characteristic clinical feature known as sunset-glow fundus. Peripheral retina can have nummular chorioretinal scars.

Chronic recurrent stage: There is granulomatous choroiditis with destruction of the choriocapillaris.

Clinical Features

These vary depending on the stage of the disease.

Prodromal stage: Flu-like symptoms occur several days preceding the onset of ocular symptoms. The symptoms include headache, nausea, fever, tinnitus, meningismus, dysacusis, orbital pain, photophobia, and hypersensitivity of the skin and hair to touch.

Focal neurologic signs may include cranial neuropathies, aphasia, hemiparesis, and transverse myelitis. CSF lymphocytic pleocytosis with normal levels of glucose is seen in >80% of patients and persists for up to 8 weeks. Auditory manifestations include dysacusis, which occurs in up to 75% patients and involves higher frequencies or tinnitus, typically improving within 2-3 months; however, persistent deficits may remain.

Acute uveitic stage: Sequential blurring of vision occurs in both eyes, starting 1-2 days after the onset of central nervous system (CNS) signs. This stage is marked by bilateral granulomatous anterior uveitis, a variable degree of vitritis, thickening of the posterior choroid with elevation of the peripapillary retinal choroidal layer, hyperemia and edema of the optic nerve, and multiple serous retinal detachments. These focal areas of shallow serous detachment may become confluent to form bullous detachment. Profound vision loss may occur. IOP may be high due to forward displacement of lens iris diaphragm or may be low due to ciliary body shutdown.

Convalescent stage: Several weeks later, with resolution of the exudative retinal detachments and gradual depigmentation of the choroid, there occurs a classic orange-red discoloration of fundus, or sunset-glow fundus with small, round, discrete depigmented lesions in the inferior peripheral fundus. Juxtapapillary depigmentation may also be seen. Perilimbal vitiligo (Sugiura sign) may be present in up to 85% of Japanese patients but is rarely observed among white patients. Integumentary changes are vitiligo, alopecia, and poliosis. These may occur weeks to months after ocular inflammation, or simultaneously. Between 10% and 63% of patients develop vitiligo, depending on ethnic background; among Hispanic patients, the incidence of cutaneous and other extraocular manifestations is relatively low.

Chronic recurrent stage: Repeated bouts of granulomatous anterior uveitis (KPs, posterior synechiae, iris nodules, iris depigmentation, and stromal atrophy) may occur. Posterior recurrence is uncommon. This stage requires systemic therapy. Complications develop in this phase and include PSC, glaucoma, CNV, and subretinal fibrosis.

Imaging

Optical coherence tomography: It is helpful in diagnosis and monitoring of serous macular detachments, CME, and CNVMs. Characteristic fibrin bands extending from the retina to the RPE may be seen in the acute phase. Spectral domain OCT (SD-OCT) using EDI demonstrates choroidal thickening in the acute phase that decreases with treatment. The combined use of SD-OCT and FAF imaging, which shows granular hyperautofluorescence in areas of inflammation, offers a noninvasive assessment of RPE and outer retinal inflammation that may not be apparent on clinical examination in patients with chronic VKH syndrome.

Fundus fluorescein angiography: In early venous phase, patchy hypofluorescence may be seen due to delayed choroidal perfusion. In mid phase, there occurs multiple punctate areas of hyperfluorescence (sometimes in the form of a starry sky) in the area of choroiditis (leakage from RPE). Pooling occurs later within the serous retinal detachments in the form of lobules, separated by hypofluorescent rim from subretinal septae. In chronic disease, there occurs RPE window defect and spotted hypo- or hyperfluorescence.

The ICGA features include patchy hypofluorescence in very early phase from delayed choroidal perfusion, large stromal vessel hyperfluorescence in early phase, hypofluorescent dots from granulomas in intermediate phase and diffuse choroidal hyperfluorescence in late phase.

The optic disk appears "hot" on FFA as well as ICGA in active disease suggesting papillitis.

Diagnosis

Diagnostic criteria for VKH syndrome are as follows:
- No history of penetrating ocular trauma or surgery preceding the initial onset of uveitis
- No clinical or laboratory evidence suggestive of other ocular disease entities
- Bilateral ocular involvement (A or B must be met, depending on the stage of disease)
  - *Early manifestations of disease:*
    - There must be evidence of a diffuse choroiditis (with or without anterior uveitis, vitreous inflammatory reaction, or optic disk hyperemia), which may manifest as one of the following:
      a. Focal areas of subretinal fluid, or
      b. Bullous serous retinal detachments

- With equivocal fundus findings, both of the following must be present as well:
  - Focal areas of delay in choroidal perfusion, multifocal areas of pinpoint leakage, large placoid areas of hyperfluorescence, pooling within subretinal fluid and optic nerve staining (listed in order of sequential appearance) by fluorescein angiography
  - Diffuse choroidal thickening without evidence of posterior scleritis by ultrasonography
- *Late manifestations of disease:*
  - History suggestive of prior presence of findings from 3a, and either both 2 and 3, or multiple signs from 3
  - *Ocular depigmentation (either of the following manifestations is sufficient):*
    - Sunset glow fundus
    - Sugiura sign
  - *Other ocular signs:*
    - Nummular chorioretinal depigmented scars
    - Retinal pigment epithelium clumping and/or migration
    - Recurrent or CAU
- *Neurological/auditory findings (may have resolved by the time of examination):*
  - Meningismus (malaise, fever, headache, nausea, abdominal pain, stiffness of the neck and back, or a combination of these factors; headache alone is not sufficient to meet definition of meningismus, however)
  - Tinnitus
  - Cerebrospinal fluid pleocytosis
- Integumentary finding (not preceding onset of CNS or ocular disease):
  - Alopecia
  - Poliosis
  - Vitiligo

Probable VKH (isolated ocular disease); criteria I–III must be present
Incomplete VKH; criteria I–III and either IV or V must be present
Complete VKH; criteria I–V must be present.

Differential Diagnosis

SO, uveal effusion syndrome, posterior scleritis, primary intraocular lymphoma, uveal lymphoid infiltration, acute posterior multifocal placoid pigment epitheliopathy (APMPPE), and sarcoidosis.

Treatment

Acute stage: CSs are started early and high dose is given, typically 1–1.5 mg/kg/day of oral prednisone or 1 g/day of intravenous methylprednisolone for 3 days followed by oral steroids. Steroids are slowly tapered over 6–12 months. In cases that develop side effects from oral steroid therapy, intravitreal steroids or IMT can be used. Tapering CSs too soon can result in early recurrence.

Recurrent disease: It requires IMT (including cyclosporine, azathioprine, mycophenolate mofetil, chlorambucil, cyclophosphamide, and infliximab) earlier to achieve more prompt inflammatory control and to facilitate more rapid tapering of CSs.

Prognosis and Complications

The overall visual prognosis for patients treated timely and aggressively is fair, with up to 70% of patients retaining visual acuity of 20/40 or better. Complications include cataract, glaucoma, optic atrophy, CNV, and subretinal fibrosis.

 24. Discuss various ophthalmic manifestations of Hansen's disease.

Ocular Lesions

Ocular involvement depends on the form of leprosy, the duration of disease, and the previous systemic and local treatment. Ocular complications in leprosy have decreased due to timely diagnosis and highly effective multi drug therapy (MDT).

Ocular lesions may occur by four mechanisms:
1. Spread from adjacent skin or nasal mucosa
2. Corneal damage from neuritis with infranuclear facial nerve palsy or 5th nerve involvement

3. Direct intraocular infection with *Mycobacterium leprae*
4. Allergic reaction to *M. leprae* antigen.

Lepromatous leprosy (LL) tends to be associated with more severe intraocular involvement, whereas patients with tuberculoid (TT) leprosy typically present with early involvement of the motor and sensory nerves with resulting corneal problems.

Lids, Cornea, and Conjunctiva

Eyebrow hair loss and loss of lashes (madarosis): These are most common manifestations of leprosy. Lagophthalmos is caused by seventh nerve paralysis, often accompanied by ectropion, occurs in about 20% of patients. Lagophthalmos may result in corneal disease (exposure keratitis, ulcer, or opacity) which is accentuated by corneal hypesthesia (trigeminal nerve involvement).

Denervation of the lacrimal gland and infiltration of the meibomian glands of lids result in tear film abnormalities that further contribute to corneal morbidity.

Cornea: Pathognomonic of disease is focally enlarged corneal nerves that may resemble beads on a string. Direct bacterial invasion of superior cornea may cause asymptomatic, avascular, punctate keratitis. Rarely, interstitial keratitis may develop. Lepromatous pannus with microlepromata can develop. Pterygium formation associated with lepromatous granuloma of the conjunctiva has been reported to occur in leprosy patients.

Sclera: Cases may develop either nodular or diffuse episcleritis and scleritis. It usually occurs during the leprosy reactions and often associated with keratitis or iridocyclitis. Chronic cases may have necrosis of sclera and subsequent melting and staphyloma formation.

Iris and ciliary body: Uveal tract involvement is primarily seen in LL leprosy due to direct invasion, neuroparalysis, or uveal hypersensitivity. Early subtle signs are diminished pupillary reactions with denervation hypersensitivity to adrenergic agents, and reduced accommodation with early presbyopia.

Iris involvement can be divided into four main groups: (1) acute iridocyclitis, (2) chronic iridocyclitis, (3) miliary iris lepromas, and (4) nodular iris lepromas.

1. *Acute iridocyclitis:* It is nongranulomatous, often bilateral, and accompanies type II [erythema nodosum leprosum (ENL)] reaction. The signs may include conjunctival hyperemia, KPs, aqueous cells and flare, hypopyon, posterior synechiae, secondary glaucoma, and spontaneous hyphema.
2. *Chronic iridocyclitis:* It is a blinding form of low-grade granulomatous or nongranulomatous iridocyclitis common in LL leprosy. It is usually asymptomatic with aqueous cells and flare with fine or mutton-fat KPs scattered all over the corneal endothelium. It eventually leads to severe iris atrophy and polycoria.
3. *Miliary iris lepromas:* Small, glistening, and white lesions *(iris pearls)* are pathognomonic for leprosy. These represent aggregates of living and dead bacilli lying within mononuclear cells (foam or lepra cells). These are located at the pupil margin around the collarette, resembling a necklace or beads of a rosary. They may become pedunculated and eventually drop off into the anterior chamber.
4. *Nodular iris lepromas:* These are yellow, globular, polymorphic masses which are less frequent.

Posterior segment lesions: Choroid is usually spared due to organism's predilection for cooler parts of the body. Rarely, leprosy "pearls" have been described in the anterior choroid or as retinal pearls situated near the posterior pole of the eye.

Ocular changes during leprosy reactions: Type I reactions occur during treatment, especially in borderline-tuberculoid (BT) patients. Lagophthalmos is a feature of Type I reaction. *Type II reactions (ENL)* may develop in multibacillary patients with long-standing untreated disease, but up to 50% of patients develop ENL within the first year of antileprosy treatment. Borderline-lepromatous (BL) and LL leprosy patients are, in particular, at risk of acute iridocyclitis and (epi-)scleritis during treatment and early follow-up. However, once an eye has had acute iridocyclitis, it seems more prone to recurrent uveitis, without generalized signs of type II reaction.

Treatment

Treatment of leprosy involves rifampicin, dapsone, and clofazimine for a period of 6–12 months. Uveitis requires intensive treatment with topical CSs, while oral CSs may be required in more severe cases in conjunction with antileprosy agents. Phenylephrine is preferred for the management of miosis.

25. Discuss clinical features, diagnostic investigations, and management of ocular tuberculosis.

Tuberculosis

Choroid is most commonly affected in intraocular TB. Uveitis is most common ocular manifestation of TB. Any of the ocular structures may be involved and present as retinal vasculitis, choroiditis, neuroretinitis, optic neuritis, conjunctivitis, scleritis, keratitis, phlyctenulosis, and several forms of orbital disease such as dacryoadenitis, orbital mass, eyelid, and nasolacrimal duct involvement. Ocular TB is extrapulmonary form of disease and is paucibacillary in nature. Thus, it is difficult to isolate organism in smear or culture from ocular fluids using the conventional techniques.

Clinical Spectrum
- Multifocal choroidal tubercles
- Solitary choroidal tuberculoma
- Subretinal abscess
- Serpiginous-like choroiditis (SLC)
- Neuroretinitis
- Retinal vasculitis
- Endophthalmitis/Panophthalmitis.

Choroidal Tubercles
Most characteristic of intraocular TB due to dissemination of bacilli from systemic source. Unilateral or bilateral and multiple (≤5) discrete grayish yellow subretinal lesions with indistinct borders at the posterior pole up to midperiphery. Once healed, they produce scars with pale, atrophic, sharply demarcated borders, and variable pigmentation.

Investigation:
Fundus fluorescein angiography: Hypofluorescent in early and transit phase with hyperfluorescent in late phase.

Indocyanine green: It is used to monitor course of disease. There are two types of lesions. Type I lesions remain hypo in early and intermediate phase and hyper in late phase. Type II lesions remain hypo in late phase as well and indicate healing.

Optical coherence tomography: It is used to differentiate tubercle from granuloma. Presence of subretinal fluid and "contact sign" between RPE-choriocapillaris layer and overlying neurosensory retina goes in favor of granuloma. Tubercular granuloma is more well defined, has lower reflectivity, is more homogenous, and allows more transmission through them.

Choroidal Tuberculoma/Subretinal Abscess
Solitary choroidal granuloma is larger in size than tubercules and presents as subretinal yellowish lesion with overlying fluid. It occurs due to disseminated systemic TB.

Abscess: It occurs due to rapid multiplication of bacilli followed by liquefactive necrosis; a more larger and yellowish lesion with overlying hemorrhages.

Imaging of abscess:
- *Fluorescein angiography:* Hypofluorescent in early phase with hyperfluorescent in late phase.
- *Indocyanine green:* Hypofluorescent in early and late phase
- *Ultrasound:* Noted as dome-like lesion with high surface spike and low internal reflectivity.

Serpiginous-like Choroiditis
Usual presentation is bilateral at slightly younger age as compared to serpiginous choroiditis and associated with vitritis, in people from TB-endemic regions. It may be a manifestation of hypersensitivity reaction to bacilli sequestered in RPE. Clinical presentation is:
- Multifocal discrete yellowish lesion of varying size from 0.25–1DD with raised edges. As the lesions grow, they become confluent and show a wave-like progression over 1–4 weeks. On FA, the lesions are hypo in early phase and hyper later. On ICGA, the lesions remain hypo throughout.

- A diffuse pattern with amoeboid shape and active serpiginous-like edge at presentation. The edge is yellowish, fluffy, and raised and the center shows variable pigmentation. On FA, the active edge is hypo in early phase and hyper later, whereas center of lesion has variable fluorescence.
- Mixed type of above patterns.

The OCT pattern can vary in different stages of SLC. In early stages, there is increased hyperreflectivity in the external layers with no backscattering from choroid. As lesions heal, there is loss or photoreceptors and RPE with increased scatter from choroid.

Retinal Vasculitis

Venules are more common involved than arterioles. These are associated with moderate vitritis, perivascular cuffing with infiltrates, retinal hemorrhages, peripheral CNP causing NV of the optic disk or elsewhere in the retina. It may also be associated with neuroretinitis. The presence of choroiditis lesions (active or healed) under the retinal vessels indicates a strong possibility of tubercular etiology.

Diagnosis

The diagnosis of intraocular TB is often presumptive as intraocular fluid/tissue sampling to demonstrate bacilli is not routinely performed. However, the demonstration of organism from ocular sample along with clinical findings confirms the diagnosis. In most cases, one uses clinical clues supported by indirect evidence to diagnose and treat intraocular TB. The characteristic findings in tubercular uveitis are broad-based anterior synechiae, choroidal tubercles/tuberculoma/abscess, and serpiginous-like choroiditis.

Definitive evidence: If demonstration of bacilli by acid-fast stain or culture from ocular fluid or tissue sample is reported. Difficulty in sampling and low yield from sample makes these less preferred methods. Polymerase chain reaction (PCR) of the fluid/tissue may demonstrate DNA segments but is not available readily.

Indirect evidence: Tuberculin sensitivity test: 0.1 mL of 5 tuberculin units of purified protein derivative (PPD) is injected intradermally in the forearm. The amount of induration (and not erythema) is measured after 48–72 hours. A person who has been exposed to the bacteria is expected to mount an immune response in the skin containing the bacterial protein. An induration of >10 mm indicates positive test. This is type IV immune response characterizing delayed type hypersensitivity. Though has low sensitivity and specificity, a positive tuberculin skin test (TST) along with presence of any of the characteristic signs suggests the diagnosis of intraocular TB.

Interferon-γ-release assays (IGRAs/QuantiFERON-TB Gold/ELISpotPLUS/T-SPOT.TB): These tests measure and compare the IFN-γ response of T cells to *Mycobacterium tuberculosis* antigen.

However, a positive TST or IGRA result only indicates lasting immune response to tubercle bacilli but not necessarily true "latent TB infection" with viable bacilli.

Chest X-ray/CT: These are not helpful as intraocular TB often occurs in absence of pulmonary involvement. A negative X-ray or CT of chest does not refute the diagnosis of intraocular TB.

Treatment

Anti-TB therapy (ATT) can be started in cases with high index of clinical suspicion and positive Mantoux test. The treatment for ocular TB comprises the same four-drug regimen: isoniazid 5 mg/kg/day, rifampicin 10 mg/kg/day, ethambutol 15 mg/kg/day, and pyrazinamide 20–25 mg/kg/day) in the intensive phase of 3–4 months followed by rifampicin and isoniazid. The duration of treatment varies 12–18 months. Systemic steroids are given along with the ATT in tapering dose. It should be started in consultation with internist.

 26. Elaborate ocular manifestation of human immunodeficiency virus (HIV) and its management. What is the impact of highly active antiretroviral therapy (HAART) on ocular features?

Human immunodeficiency virus can have varied manifestation involving any part of eye (ocular adnexa and globe). HIV retinopathy is the most frequent ocular manifestation of HIV-AIDS. The most common opportunistic infection is CMV retinitis (CMVR). The following are the manifestations of the disease:

Eyelids

- *Herpes zoster ophthalmicus:* One should suspect HIV in any individual under the age of 50 years who presents with HZO. Vesicular rash along the division of the ophthalmic branch of trigeminal nerve can be associated with conjunctivitis and keratitis.
    - *Treatment:* Parenteral acyclovir 10 mg/kg 8 hourly for 10 days followed by oral maintenance therapy.
- *Kaposi's sarcoma:* It presents as flat or very slightly raised purple papules on the eyelid. These lesions are sometimes part of multifocal presentation including viscera and may also present within the conjunctiva or orbit.
    - Treatment of eyelid lesion: Excision, intralesional chemotherapy/radiation. If there is associated systemic involvement, systemic chemotherapy may be all that is indicated.
- *Molluscum contagiosum:* A DNA poxvirus that causes raised lesions with umbilicated centers presents along the eyelid may be associated with follicular conjunctivitis. Patients with AIDS may have numerous larger lesions.
    - *Treatment:* Excision, curettage, or cryotherapy.

Conjunctiva

Nonspecific conjunctivitis	Dry eyes	Microvasculopathy	Kaposi's sarcoma
10% cases with AIDS	Around 10% of cases	Immune complex deposition in vessel wall and endothelial damage by virus	<1% of cases
Usually, culture negative	Systemic medication side effect or malabsorption of nutrients	Dilated capillary segments, microaneurysms, and sludging of blood flow similar to sickle-cell disease	Reddish plaque, usually located in cul-de-sac
Rx: Topical antibiotics, good lid hygiene	Rx: Tear substitute		*Differential:* Hemorrhage

(AIDS: acquired immunodeficiency syndrome)

Cornea

- Bacterial or fungal corneal ulcers
- Herpes simplex keratitis has been documented in AIDS patients, but whether there is an increased risk of such infection is uncertain. Lesions tend to have a predilection for the peripheral cornea and may respond to conventional topical therapy. However, a lengthy course of disease with multiple recurrences has been noted in AIDS patients.

Anterior Uveitis

People with AIDS can frequently develop iritis. Need to rule out spillover uveitis from posterior segment conditions such as ARN, toxoplasma retinochoroiditis, and syphilitic retinochoroiditis. Flare is present in eyes with CMVR although it does not seem to predict the development of the retinitis. There have been several reports of anterior uveitis associated with the rifabutin treatment of atypical mycobacterial infection in AIDS patients. This iritis may be severe and associated with hypopyon. Intensive topical CS therapy is needed. If unsuccessful, lowering the dose of rifabutin is effective.

Retina and Vitreous

- *Cotton wool spots/HIV retinopathy:* The most common ocular manifestation of AIDS is CWS, which occur in about 50% of patients. CWS are manifestation of the microvasculopathy arising out of endothelial damage caused by circulating immune complexes. Resulting from occlusion of precapillary arterioles, generally these do not compromise visual acuity and do not require treatment. These may indicate a greater risk for the onset of CMVR. Moreover, the appearance of CWS is sometimes confused with those seen in CMVR, that is, a progressive disease. Thus, one needs to carefully follow up cases with CWS.
- *Intraretinal hemorrhages:* Various types including Roth spots are commonly seen in AIDS patients due to noninfectious microvascular retinopathy. These hemorrhages may be present posteriorly or peripherally, within different layers of the retina, and are generally innocuous.
- *Retinal infections:* Retinal infections in patients with AIDS include CMV, syphilis, toxoplasmosis, candida, varicella zoster, TB, and herpes simplex.
    - *Cytomegalovirus retinitis:* It is most common intraocular infection in AIDS, affecting about 25% of patients. CMV is a neurotropic virus and is less likely to infect retinal vascular endothelium. HIV causes endothelial damage, allowing

CMV access to retinal tissue. This explains the high incidence of CMVR in AIDS. It presents as hemorrhagic necrosis of retina often extending along the vascular arcade, and may be associated with a mild anterior and vitreal inflammation, granular infiltration along with the vascular arcade, or perivascular sheathing. Multicentric origin and bilateral disease are frequently seen. As the lesions mature, they become more granular and ultimately become transparent. Faint pigment stippling is seen at the level of the RPE. Inactive lesions have focal deposits of lipid, calcium, and glial tissue; the retinal vessels become markedly attenuated, and secondary optic atrophy develops. A zone of active necrotizing retinitis remains at the margin of the inactive lesion. CMV can also cause papillitis. CMVR tends to affect patients with CD4 counts of <50/mL, and survival after the initial diagnosis ranges from 8 to 12 months.

- *Treatment options:* Intravenous ganciclovir, which can lead to myelosuppression, or intravenous foscarnet, which is associated with renal insufficiency. Ganciclovir can be given by direct injection into the vitreous cavity but multiple injections are necessary. A sustained intravitreal ganciclovir-releasing device, which is surgically implanted, can be used even in patients who are resistant to intravenous ganciclovir. In resistant cases, cidofovir therapy may be used but the dose-dependent complications are iritis and hypotonia.

  Relapses and recurrences necessitate life-long treatment of this condition, which can be further complicated by retinal detachment. Prophylactic laser coagulation of the retina to prevent subsequent retinal detachment is controversial.

- *Syphilis:* It has varied presentations including uveitis, choroiditis, retinitis, papillitis, and papilledema. The retinitis manifests as a deep yellow lesion, sometimes associated with intraocular inflammation or retinal vasculitis. Serological tests for syphilis should be done in patients with any of these presentations; if positive, neurosyphilis should be ruled out. Since syphilis follows a more aggressive course in AIDS patients, vigorous therapy should be initiated with intravenous penicillin.

- *Toxoplasma retinochoroiditis:* It comprises 1–3% of ocular infections in AIDS patients; the manifestation being deep yellow–white intraretinal lesions. In contrast to immunocompetent patients, there are no associated retinochoroidal scars, nor is dense vitritis invariably present. Lesions may be bilateral and/or multifocal. Treatment is with oral pyrimethamine, sulfadiazine, and folinic acid.

- *Candidial endophthalmitis:* No increased association with AIDS patients. However, AIDS patients with predisposing factors for fungal infection such as intravenous drug use or the presence of a long-term indwelling catheter, may be at greater risk of ocular candidiasis. It presents as focal white choroidal infiltrate that may break through the retina into the vitreous causing an overlying vitritis. If this disease is strongly suspected, intravenous amphotericin should be given. Vitrectomy with culture and cytological testing of the vitreous specimen and subsequent intravitreal injection of amphotericin may also be required.

- Acute retinal necrosis is an infectious condition that may affect immunocompetent as well as immunosuppressed individuals. ARN manifests as whitish retinitis patches in periphery that have a circumferential spread in addition to occlusive arteriolitis and severe vitritis. As the infection spreads to the posterior pole, a path of retinal scarring is left behind. At the junction of scarred and infected retina, there is high incidence of retinal detachment. Etiological factors include herpes zoster and simplex, so acyclovir should be given intravenously.

With progression, there is clearing of lesions initially around blood vessels, giving a "cracked mud" appearance. With large infected areas getting necrotic, retinal breaks develop which lead to a retinal detachment with poor visual prognosis. The diagnosis of this condition is clinical. Treatment includes early institution of intravenous acyclovir followed by oral acyclovir for 6–8 weeks. Alternate treatment option is use of oral valacyclovir. Systemic steroids are usually started 24–48 hours after starting antivirals in ARN, but in patients with AIDS, an internist consult should be done to start these or as an alternative periocular steroid may be used.

Choroid

Choroidal infiltrates can be due to infective (TB, syphilis, *Pneumocystis carinii*, *Candida*, *Cryptococcus*) or noninfective causes such as lymphoma and present as deep yellow or white lesions.

Impact of HAART on Ocular Features

With introduction of HAART, the following has happened to the ocular features:
- Incidence of infective uveitis [CMV, varicella zoster virus (VZV), TB, and toxoplasmosis] has decreased.
- Immune recovery uveitis (IRU) after starting HAART has become a major visually threatening condition. As the patient's immune response builds up, there is an increase in absolute CD4 cell count following renewed production of naïve CD4 T cells. HIV-infected individuals experience clinical deterioration after initiating antiretroviral therapy that is believed to be a result of the restored immune system to mount an exuberant inflammatory response. Immune reconstitution

syndrome can cause posterior segment inflammation (worsening) in CMVR and can lead to visual morbidity in patients with AIDS.
- High rates of ocular syphilis have been documented as well among patients receiving HAART.

 27. Describe diagnostic features of HIV retinopathy and relationship to CD4 counts.

The features of HIV retinopathy are given above.

Etiology of HIV Retinopathy

HIV-associated retinal vascular endothelial infection. Hematological abnormalities such as leukocyte activation and rigidity and red blood cell (RBC) aggregation lead to disease or there can be immune complexes deposited in retinal capillaries.

Clinical Features

Clinical features are usually asymptomatic, may be associated with scotoma/visual field defects.

Ocular examination: CWS, retinal hemorrhages, and microaneurysm can be seen.

Differential diagnosis: Diabetic retinopathy, radiation retinopathy, hypertensive retinopathy, and CMVR (large CWS can look retinitis patches).

Management

Nonspecific:
- Patient needs to restore the immune function with HAART therapy.
- Patient should have a dilated fundus examination every 3 months, if CD4 count <50 and early if symptomatic.
- *Differentiating from CMV:* The lesions in HIV retinopathy do not enlarge and resolve in 4–6 weeks. CWS are <750 microns. Not associated with contiguous areas of hemorrhage and not associated with vitritis.

Other etiologies of HIV retinopathy are discussed above, there relationship to CD4 count is as below.

Stage of HIV	CD4 count cells/mm^3	Immunity/eye disease
Seroconversion	1,000	Normal immune function, normal eye
Early	500–1,000	Sporadic autoimmune disease, allergic eye disease and uveitis
Intermediate	200–500	Sporadic autoimmune disease, milder opportunistic infection: blepharitis, follicular conjunctivitis, bacterial conjunctivitis, molluscum contagiosum, Kaposi sarcoma, herpes, TB uveitis, optic neuropathy, lymphoma, and HIV retinopathy
Late	0–200	CMV retinitis, severe opportunistic infections, and aggressive neoplasms

(CMV: cytomegalovirus; HIV: human immunodeficiency virus; TB: tuberculosis)

 28. Discuss ocular toxoplasmosis/toxoplasma retinitis.

Toxoplasmosis is most common infectious posterior uveitis in adults and children caused by parasite *Toxoplasma gondii*, a single-cell obligate intracellular parasite. Cats are the definitive hosts of *T. gondii*, and humans and a variety of other animals serve as intermediate hosts.

Life cycle: Toxoplasma gondii has a complex life cycle and exists in three major forms. Transmission to humans and other animals may occur with all three forms.
1. Oocyst, or soil form (10-12 μm), which contains sporozoites: Result of sexual reproduction in the intestinal mucosa of cat and shed in feces contaminating the environment. After maturation in the soil, these oocysts may then be ingested by intermediate hosts or reingested by cats.
2. *Tachyzoite, or infectious form (4-8 μm):* The proliferative form in the circulatory system and may invade nearly all host tissue.
3. *Tissue cyst, or latent form (10-200 μm), which contains as many as 3,000 bradyzoites:* In an immunocompetent host, replication of tachyzoites eventually ceases, with some microorganisms persisting as dormant bradyzoites within intercellular tissue cysts.

Modes of transmission:
- Ingestion of undercooked infected meat containing tissue cysts
- Ingestion of contaminated water, fruit, or vegetables with oocysts
- Inadvertent contact with cat feces, cat litter, or soil containing oocysts
- Transplacental transmission with primary infection during pregnancy
- Blood transfusion or organ transplantation.

Pregnant women should be extremely cautious of acquiring infection especially in endemic regions such as Brazil. Around 40% of primary maternal infections result in congenital infection; transplacental transmission is highest during the third trimester. The risk of severe disease in the fetus is inversely proportional to gestational age. In first trimester, this may result in spontaneous abortion, stillbirth, or severe congenital disease, whereas that acquired later in gestation may produce an asymptomatic, normal-appearing infant with latent infection.

Congenital toxoplasmosis: Features include retinochoroiditis, hydrocephalus or microcephaly, intracranial calcifications, and cognitive impairment (Sabin's tetrad occurring in <10% of infected children). Retinochoroidal lesions, which can be found in up to 80% of cases, are the most common abnormality in patients with congenital toxoplasmosis; they are bilateral in approximately 85% and carry a predilection for the posterior pole and macula. Most experts recommend antiparasitic therapy for newborns with congenital toxoplasmosis during the first year of life to reduce disease burden, regardless of the presence of ocular and/or systemic signs.

Acquired Toxoplasmosis

Initially, onset of toxoplasma after infancy was thought to be reactivation of congenital disease but now the disease is thought to be acquired one even in children.

Clinical Features

Symptoms: Dependent on the location of the lesion—blurred vision, loss of vision, and floaters.

Examination: Mild to moderate granulomatous anterior uveitis; 20% of patients have acutely elevated IOP at presentation. Classically, lesion is a focal, white retinochoroiditis, with overlying moderate vitreous inflammation ("headlight in the fog"), often adjacent to a pigmented retinochoroidal scar. Mostly, these occur in the posterior pole but may occur adjacent to or directly involving the optic nerve. Retinal vasculitis may be present adjacent to lesion as perivasculitis with diffuse venous sheathing and segmental arterial plaques (Kyrieleis arteriolitis). Vascular occlusions may also be present.

Complications: Cataract, persistent vitreous opacities, CME, retinal detachment, ERMs, optic atrophy, and CNV.

Retinochoroiditis in immunocompromised and older patients: It may present with atypical findings, including large, multiple, and/or bilateral lesions, with or without associated retinochoroidal scars. This more severe clinical picture can also occur in patients receiving steroids without concomitant antiparasitic therapy.

Other atypical presentations include neuroretinitis, punctate outer retinal toxoplasmosis (PORT), unilateral pigmentary retinopathy simulating retinitis pigmentosa, and other forms of intraocular inflammation in the absence of retinochoroiditis. PORT is characterized by small, multifocal lesions at the level of the outer retina, with exudation to subretinal space and scant overlying vitreal inflammation.

Diagnosis

Diagnosis is mostly clinical on the basis of the appearance of the characteristic lesion on indirect ophthalmoscopy. Serologic evaluation using indirect fluorescent antibody and enzyme-linked immunosorbent assay (ELISA) tests to detect specific anti-*T. gondii* antibodies is commonly used to confirm exposure to the parasite. Intraocular production of specific anti-*Toxoplasma* antibodies may be computed by using the Goldmann-Witmer (GW) coefficient. A ratio of greater than 3 is considered diagnostic of local antibody production. Highly sensitive and specific PCR-based techniques have been used to detect *T. gondii* DNA in the aqueous humor and vitreous fluid of patients with ocular toxoplasmosis.

Optical coherence tomography: Features include increased hyperreflective signals in the overlying vitreous, thickening of the posterior hyaloid, inner retinal hyperreflectivity with "smudge effect", inner/middle highly reflective layers (HRLs) around active focus, posterior optical shadowing, subretinal fluid, and focal thickening of underlying choroid.

Treatment

In immunocompetent patients, the lesions are known to self-heal and treatment does not alter the course of disease. The relative indications of treatment are:

- Lesions threatening the optic nerve or fovea
- Lesions associated with moderate to severe vitreous inflammation
- Lesions greater than 1 disk diameter in size
- Persistence of disease for >1 month
- Presence of multiple active lesions.

Treatment is indicated in immunocompromised patients (those with HIV/AIDS, with neoplastic disease, or undergoing IMT), patients with congenital toxoplasmosis, and pregnant women with recently acquired disease.

Drug and dosage	Precautions and observations
Sulfadiazine: • 1 g QID in adults • 50–100 mg/kg/day in children	• Caution and dose correction for hepatic and renal failure • Contraindicated in G6PDH deficiency • Hydration and alkalinization of urine may prevent crystalluria • Avoid at the end of gestation (risk of kernicterus) • Hypersensitivity and allergies demand suspension • Stevens–Johnson syndrome possible but rare • Bone marrow suppression in <0.1%
Pyrimethamine: • Loading dose of 100 mg, followed • by 25–50 mg/day • 1 mg/kg/day in children	• Caution in hepatic or renal failure • Contraindicated in first trimester (teratogenic) • Common gastrointestinal disturbances • Risk of bone marrow depression demands concomitant use of folinic acid (5–7.5 mg/day or 15 mg 3×/week) and periodic CBC monitoring
Clindamycin: • 300 mg QID • 10–25 mg/kg/day in children	• Caution in hepatic or renal failure • Common gastrointestinal disturbances • Risk of pseudomembranous colitis (suspend if bloody diarrhea)
Azithromycin: • 250–500 mg/day • 5 mg/kg/day in children	• Food decreases oral absorption • Gastrointestinal disturbances in <10% • May be used in pregnancy
Sulfamethoxazole/trimethoprim: • 800 mg/160 mg BID • 40–50 mg/8–10 mg/kg/day in children	• Better tolerated than classic therapy but probably less effective • Caution and dose correction in case of hepatic/renal failure • Contraindicated in G6PDH deficiency • Avoid during gestation (risk of teratogenicity and kernicterus) • Risk of sulfa hypersensitivity • Bone marrow suppression uncommon
Spiramycin: • 1.5 million IU (500 mg) QID	• High levels in placenta • Safest antiparasitic drug in pregnancy • Limited intraocular penetration • Gastrointestinal disturbances and hypersensitivity
Atovaquone: • 750 mg QID • 30 mg/kg/day in children	• Caution with liver failure • Food increases drug absorption • Maculopapular rash in up to 20% • No safety studies concerning gestation/lactation

(CBC: complete blood count; G6PDH: glucose-6-phosphate dehydrogenase)

Oral CS (0.5–1 mg/kg/day of prednisone or equivalent) is used in a tapering regimen, with favorable effect on inflammation of the vitreous, retina, and optic nerve. It should be initiated at least 24 hours after starting antiparasitic drugs and tapered off before stopping them. Caution should be taken to avoid CSs without concomitant antiparasitic coverage because of risk of progressive/devastating intraocular inflammation. The use of periocular or intravitreal depot CSs is relatively contraindicated for the same reasons. Treatment duration is often 5–6 weeks but may be longer for larger active lesions and persistent intraocular inflammation. Resolution of the active lesion is typically centripetal, with progressive flattening of the margins and decreased exudation. Lesion pigmentation may be delayed, and is a variable and unreliable feature.

 29. Describe ocular toxocara.

Toxocariasis is an uncommon disease of children and young adults that may cause significant loss of vision.

Life Cycle

It results from tissue invasion by the second-stage larvae of *Toxocara canis* or *Toxocara cati,* roundworm parasites that complete their life cycles in the small intestines of dogs and cats, respectively. Transmission occurs through ingestion of soil or contaminated food, or the fecal–oral route. The eating disorder pica and contact with puppies or kittens are common among children with toxocariasis. The organisms grow in the small intestine, enter the portal circulation, disseminate throughout the body by hematogenous and lymphatic routes, and ultimately reside in target tissues, including the eye. Maturation of the adult worm does not occur in humans; consequently, ova are not shed in the alimentary tract, rendering stool analysis for larvae unproductive. Ocular toxocariasis (OT) and the systemic disease visceral larvae migrans (VLM) rarely present contemporaneously. VLM typically affects children younger than age of 3 years, possibly because of an increased rate of pica among this group; whereas, OT is found most often in older children or young adults. Finally, there is a direct relationship between the degree of peripheral eosinophilia and the parasitic burden in the systemic disease but not in OT.

Clinical Features

Patients with OT present with unilateral decreased vision that may be accompanied by pain, photophobia, floaters, strabismus, or leukocoria. Bilateral disease is exceedingly rare. The eye is typically white and the anterior segment is quiet. However, nongranulomatous anterior uveitis and posterior synechiae may be present in severe disease. Posterior segment findings include three recognizable ocular syndromes:
1. *Chronic endophthalmitis (2–9 years):* Leukocoria results from moderate to severe vitreous inflammation (25% of cases)
2. *Localized macular granuloma (6–14 years):* 25% of cases; solitary white elevated lesion with minimal reaction, 1–2 DD in size, in the macula or peripapillary region.
3. *Peripheral granuloma (6–40 years):* 50% of cases; peripheral hemispheric mass with dense connective tissue strands in vitreous cavity that may connect to optic nerve hypoplasia (ONH).

Uncommon variants include unilateral pars planitis with diffuse peripheral inflammatory exudates and granulomas involving the optic nerve. Vision loss depends on the amount of inflammation, CME, tractional detachment, and foveal involvement. Eyes with endophthalmitis have worst prognosis.

The diagnosis is essentially clinical, supported by laboratory data, and findings on imaging studies. The serum ELISA titer of 1:8 is 91% sensitive and 90% specific for prior exposure to the organism. Up to one-third of patients with OT may have negative ELISA results. In these cases, examination of intraocular fluids with ELISA may reveal specific *T. canis* antibodies and results leading to a positive GW coefficient, providing evidence of primary ocular involvement. *Toxocara* larvae have been recovered from the vitreous during PPV. PCR testing of vitreous is not successful.

B-scan ultrasonography and CT are useful in the presence of media opacity; they may reveal vitreous membranes and tractional retinal detachment and confirm the absence of calcium, a characteristic finding in retinoblastoma (other finding to differentiate both are younger age at presentation, paucity of inflammation, and lesion growth in retinoblastoma)

Differential Diagnosis

Infectious endophthalmitis, toxoplasmosis, and pars planitis, as well as congenital retinovascular abnormalities such as retinopathy of prematurity, persistent fetal vasculature, Coats disease, and familial exudative vitreoretinopathy.

Treatment

Medical therapy with periocular and systemic CSs is aimed at reducing the inflammatory response in an effort to prevent structural complications. Anthelminthic therapy has not been established, although albendazole or thiabendazole can be used in concert with CSs. Laser photocoagulation of the larvae may be considered if identified on clinical examination. Vitreoretinal surgical techniques have been used successfully to manage tractional and rhegmatogenous complications.

 30. Explain clinical feature, evaluation, and management of ocular cysticercosis.

Ocular cysticercosis is the most common tapeworm infection caused by *Cysticercus cellulosae,* which is a larval form of the pork tapeworm *Taenia solium.* Sometimes, it may be caused by beef tapeworm. Consumption of undercooked pork and use of contaminated vegetables or water can cause this infection. Cysticercosis primarily affects the CNS, subcutaneous tissue, external eye structures, muscles, and intraocular structures such as vitreous and retina.

Clinical Features

Symptoms: Loss of vision, periorbital pain, scotoma, and photopsia. May be asymptomatic in the early stages when parasite is small and alive. May present as neurocysticercosis features (neurological symptoms and seizures) or subcutaneous or muscular cysticercosis.

Examination

The cyst may be localized to the subconjunctival space or orbit or may invade the globe and present in the anterior or posterior segment. Intravitreal cysticercosis presents as a translucent white cyst with a dense spot (invaginated scolex). The shape and undulating movements are typical. Subretinal cysticercosis may present as acute central retinitis with retinal edema and subretinal exudates. The subretinal organism eventually develops into a cyst. The macular area is the common site of subretinal cysticercus because of vascularity of the area. The movements of the cysticercus are easily seen through the thin macular tissues. The cyst often migrates into the vitreous, leaving behind a chorioretinal scar. One mode of presentation is that of fibrinous anterior uveitis with secondary glaucoma; the uveitis resolves with removal of the cyst. The posterior segment manifestation of ocular cysticercosis can be variable, ranging from mild to intense vitritis with evidence of cystic larvae. Retinal break, rhegmatogenous retinal detachment, exudative retinal detachment, chorioretinal scar, or atrophy with epimacular membrane can be seen. Optic atrophy, optic disk edema, and sometimes atypical optic neuritis may be the remote presentation. Death of parasite cause very intense inflammatory response and results in painful blind eye.

Diagnosis

B-scan ultrasound with identification of an intralesional scolex is diagnostic in cases of intraocular cysticercosis. It demonstrates the complete cyst with an eccentric high-reflective opacity (scolex). Other diagnostic modalities include imaging such as CT imaging or magnetic resonance imaging (MRI) of brain and orbit. Coin-shaped lesion(s) with perilesional edema can be picked up in an MRI scan of the brain.

Serologically, cysticercosis can be diagnosed by precipitin reaction, complement fixation, or indirect hemagglutination assay. Anti-cysticercus antibodies can be detected by ELISA in approximately 80% cases of neurocysticercosis, 57% of ocular cysticercosis, and 50% with myocysticercosis.

Differential Diagnosis

Differential diagnosis includes conditions associated with leukocoria (retinoblastoma, Coats disease, retinopathy of prematurity, persistent fetal vasculature, toxocariasis, and retinal detachment) and DUSN.

Treatment

Surgical removal of the intraocular cyst is recommended.

Transscleral approach may be used for subretinal cysts positioned anterior to the equator.

Pars plana vitrectomy—for intravitreal and subretinal cysts located posterior to the equator. In presence of both intraocular and CNS lesion, surgery must be done prior to starting medical therapy. Use of anthelminthic medication in intraocular cysticercosis without surgical removal can kill the intraocular live parasite and thereby can induce severe intraocular reaction causing eventual blindness. Steroids may be considered to prevent this inflammatory reaction and should be started a few days prior to starting anthelminthic treatment. Albendazole and praziquantel are principal antiparasitic drugs that are used in treating neurocysticercosis and primary external ocular disease.

 31. What are clinical features, investigations, treatment, and prognosis in a case of CMV retinitis.

Cytomegalovirus is a member of *Herpesviridae* family. Primary infection is often asymptomatic in general population. However, CMV causes severe infections in immunocompromised patients. The infection affects both genders equally and is very common in both children and adult. CMV can reactivate in the setting of immunosuppressed states (particularly T-cell dysfunction) leading to involvement of a variety of organ systems. CMV causes necrotizing retinitis in immunocompromised host. CMVR is tightly linked to the AIDS epidemic, with the majority of patients having $CD4^+$ lymphocyte counts of <50. CMV can also cause anterior uveitis. Occasionally, it is associated with FUS and Posner–Schlossman syndrome (glaucomatocyclitic crisis).

Clinical Features

Symptoms: Photopsia, loss of vision, and floaters or asymptomatic (detected incidentally).

Examination

Cytomegalovirus retinitis typically starts as a solitary white retinitis lesion with a granular border.

Vasculitis is usually prominent resulting in ischemia and hemorrhages with mild vitritis. If optic nerve is involved, one must rule out CNS involvement. Stellate KP may be observed. CMVR subsequently may involve the fellow eye.

The two less common forms of CMVR are:
1. Indolent form, involving the periphery; more granular and with less hemorrhage
2. Fulminant form, may involve macula, more intense retinal infiltration with lot of retinal hemorrhage.

Cytomegalovirus-associated anterior uveitis has a chronic recurrent course characterized by episodes of elevated IOP with active inflammation characterized by mild anterior chamber cell and flare. Corneal edema and nummular corneal endotheliitis may be seen. Iris atrophy is frequently present.

Diagnosis

Clinically especially in patients at high risk for the disease, such as those with AIDS. PCR is the confirmatory test in cases of dilemma.

Differential Diagnosis

- *Posterior uveitis:* ARN, toxoplasma retinitis, Behçet's disease, syphilitic retinitis, TB, and rarely, ocular lymphoma or leukemia, endogenous bacterial or fungal endophthalmitis, and sarcoidosis.
- *Anterior uveitis:* HSV and VZV anterior uveitis, HLA-B27–associated disease, and Fuchs' heterochromic iridocyclitis.

Treatment

Highly active antiretroviral therapy is crucial in the treatment of CMVR. Immune recovery (CD4 cells above 100/mm^3) allows discontinuation of anti-CMV treatment that otherwise may be required indefinitely.

Cytomegalovirus retinitis is treated with systemic or intravitreal administration of antiviral agents. Systemic therapy can control the disease at extraocular sites and prevent involvement of the fellow eye but has systemic adverse effects.

Intravenous ganciclovir is effective in treating CMVR, starting with 5 mg/kg twice daily for 2 weeks in induction phase and maintaining later on 5 mg/kg/day. Bone marrow suppression with neutropenia is a serious side effect. Valganciclovir offers improved bioavailability and can be used both for induction and maintenance therapy. It is typically started at 900 mg BID. Foscarnet and cidofovir are other therapeutic options. Renal toxicity is a common and serious side effect of both agents.

Intravitreal ganciclovir injections (2 mg, weekly or twice a week) are a therapeutic alternative. When injected intravitreal, foscarnet is administered as 2.4 mg once or twice a week. Intravitreous cidofovir is administered as a 20-μg dose given every 5 weeks. Both local and systemic uses of cidofovir are associated with ocular toxicity, including iritis and hypotony.

Glaucoma medications and topical CSs are employed to control IOP and inflammation.

32. Discuss acute retinal necrosis.

Etiopathogenesis

Acute retinal necrosis can be caused by—HSV type 1 and 2, VZV, and CMV viruses. It is equally common in males and females. It is necrotizing viral retinitis involving all layers of retina. The retinal vessels show fibrinoid necrosis of the vessel wall and vascular occlusion.

Clinical Features

It is a disease of immunocompetent adolescents or adults, though cases in immunocompromised patients (HIV/organ transplant/systemic steroids/IMT) have been reported.

Symptoms: Redness, photophobia, blurring of vision, and pain which may be worse on moving the eye. Severe vision loss at presentation indicates posterior pole retinitis or optic nerve involvement.

Examination

Acute retinal necrosis presents within 2 weeks of symptoms with as a classic triad of peripheral retinitis, vitritis, and occlusive retinal arteriolitis. In addition, posterior retinitis may also be present. Retinitis patches are deep at the level of RPE and begin in the periphery and have a circumferential spread. The necrosis spreads circumferentially and posteriorly very rapidly. The macula is often spared. There is vascular sheathing and attenuation of arterioles. Sheathing of venules is less conspicuous. Often, vascular nonperfusion may be found especially in the periphery which may result in retinal NV. Multiple small intraretinal hemorrhages can also be seen. There is associated intense vitritis with spillover reaction in anterior segment. Scleritis can also be a feature of ARN. Retrobulbar optic neuritis can cause visual loss which is out of proportion to the macular involvement.

Regression starts initially around vessels giving a cracked mud or "Swiss cheese" pattern. There occurs retinal necrosis and breaks can form in the necrotic retina. Demarcation line can form between area affected by ARN and healthy retina. Optic atrophy may develop in patients who have disk edema or retrobulbar optic neuritis.

In AIDS, 59–70% patients may have bilateral disease.

Diagnosis

Clinical picture is characteristic of disease and confirmed by PCR of ocular fluid sampling. Intraocular fluid analysis is indicated in patients with atypical presentation. Negative tests still do not rule out ARN. In cases where PCR is negative and there is a high suspicion of ARN, a retinochoroidal biopsy may provide additional information.

Fluorescein angiography: Dye leakage from retinal vessels and sometimes from the optic disk. In the affected retina, vascular occlusions are seen especially affecting the venules and the capillaries.

Differential Diagnosis

Differential diagnosis includes cytomegalovirus retinitis, progressive outer retinal necrosis (PORN), toxoplasma, and Behçet's disease.

Clinical features	ARN	PORN	CMV retinitis
Immune status	Healthy	Immunosuppressed	Immunosuppressed
Laterality	B/L, 30–80%	B/L, 70%	B/L, 30–50%
Visual loss	Initial mild, later gross	Early loss of central vision	Variable, depends on site
Anterior segment	Moderate AU	Mild nongranulomatous uveitis	Mild nongranulomatous uveitis
IOP	Normal/raised	Normal	Normal
Vitritis	Significant	Minimum	Minimum
Retinal involvement	Full thickness	Deep retinal involvement without granular border	Full thickness involvement with granular border
Pattern of involvement	Multifocal, predominantly peripheral	Multifocal, early macular involvement	Unifocal, fovea relatively spared
Classic appearance	Swiss cheese (late)	Cracked mud	Cottage cheese with ketch-up or pizza pie
Vasculitis	Common	Uncommon	Seen but uncommon
Retinal hemorrhage	Common	Uncommon	Common in active lesion
Retinal detachment	Common	Common	Less common
Optic nerve involvement	Common	Uncommon	Seen but uncommon
Progression	Rapid	Rapid	Slow

(ARN: acute retinal necrosis; CMV: cytomegalovirus; IOP: intraocular pressure; PORN: progressive outer retinal necrosis)

Treatment

The major goals of treatment of ARN include stoppage of retinal necrosis so as to avoid retinal detachment and optic atrophy; to minimize collateral damage caused by severe inflammation and occlusive vasculitis; to protect the fellow eye.

- *Antiviral agents:* Antivirals may be started even before a laboratory diagnosis of viral infection is sought. HSV and VZV are the most common causative viruses and hence intravenous acyclovir is recommended in a dose of 1,500 mg/m^2/day for 10 days followed by oral acyclovir 800 mg 5 times a day for 6–14 weeks for adults. Oral famciclovir 500 mg 3 times a day is an alternative. Valaciclovir can also be given in a dose of 1,000 mg orally every 8 hours during induction followed by 1,000 mg orally once daily for maintenance.

  Other drugs used are ganciclovir, valganciclovir, and foscarnet. Intravitreal ganciclovir with or without foscarnet can be used in patients who are not responding to intravenous or oral therapy. Duration of maintenance therapy in ARN is usually 3 months but may be longer in cases of immunosuppression or multiple recurrences.
- *Antithrombotic therapy:* Since ARN is an occlusive vasculitis, aspirin has been recommended in the dose of 125–650 mg once or twice a day. However, no clinical trials have proved its efficacy till now.
- *Corticosteroids:* Vitritis associated with ARN may reduce the visual acuity of the patient and make examination difficult. Steroids (periocular or systemic) should be started after 24 hours of starting acyclovir therapy. Steroids suppress intraocular inflammation and aid in improvement of vision and evaluation of fundus.
- *Prophylactic laser photocoagulation:* Prophylactic application of laser photocoagulation to the area of retinitis or surrounding the necrotic retina is controversial.
- *Vitrectomy:* Early vitrectomy combined with endolaser photocoagulation has been proposed to eliminate the role of vitreous traction on the necrotic retina.
- *Retinal detachment surgery:* Internal repair through vitrectomy and the use of silicone oil may be more successful in reattaching the detached retina than standard scleral buckling procedures because of extensive vitreous traction and multiple posterior retinal tears.

33. What are clinical presentation, investigation, and management of pediatric uveitis?

The most common cause of pediatric uveitis is JIA, accounting for 80–90% of the cases (discussed above).

The other causes are:
- Juvenile-onset spondyloarthropathies
- *Tubulointerstitial nephritis and uveitis (TINU):* Ocular signs and symptoms can precede, develop concurrently with, or follow the onset of interstitial nephritis. Patient can have pain, redness, photophobia, or decrease in vision at presentation. TINU presents mostly as anterior bilateral nongranulomatous uveitis, but granulomatous form has also been reported. Posterior or panuveitis occurs in about 20% of the cases.
- *Early onset sarcoidosis/Blau syndrome:* Blau syndrome presents in early childhood as a triad of granulomatous dermatitis, polyarthritis, and uveitis.
- *Infective causes:* Infectious uveitis in children accounts for 6–33% of all cases of pediatric uveitis. These include ocular toxoplasmosis, OT, and viral causes (HSV, VZV, CMV, and EBV).
- *Masquerade syndromes:* Juvenile xanthogranuloma, retinoblastoma, and leukemia
- *Traumatic uveitis:* If severe inflammation is noted after minor injury, one must suspect HLA-B27 positivity. Penetrating injuries usually lead to severe inflammation which can be infective or noninfective. One must search for entrance wound in case of persistent unexplained inflammation after injury and any hidden foreign body in angle or ciliary body. Ultrasound biomicroscopy (UBM), X-ray, and CT are important investigations in this regard.

34. What are white dot syndromes and differential diagnosis?

Definition

White dot syndromes are heterogeneous group of inflammatory chorioretinopathies, with overlapping clinical features such as discrete, multiple, well-circumscribed, yellow-white lesions at the level of the retina, outer retina, RPE, choriocapillaris, and/or choroid during some phase of their course. Usually with a self-limiting course, the prognosis is variable depending on the disease. The cause is often unknown with negative serological evaluation.

Usually bilateral involvement, though asymmetric involvement [except multiple evanescent white dot syndrome (MEWDS)] is the rule. It is usually in young age <50 years (except birdshot uveitis or serpiginous choroiditis). A female predominance is observed in patients with MEWDS, birdshot uveitis, multifocal choroiditis (MFC) and panuveitis, punctate inner choroiditis (PIC), subretinal fibrosis and uveitis syndrome, and acute zonal occult outer retinopathy.

Differential Diagnosis

Differential diagnosis is systemic and ocular infections such as syphilis, DUSN, and ocular histoplasmosis syndrome (OHS), as well noninfectious entities such as sarcoidosis, sympathetic ophthalmia, VKH syndrome, and intraocular lymphoma.

Symptoms

Symptoms are photopsia, blurred vision, nyctalopia, floaters, and visual field loss contiguous with the blind spot. History of prodromal viral syndrome may be present.

The etiology of the white dot syndromes is unknown. Some investigators have postulated an infectious cause; others have suggested an autoimmune/inflammatory pathogenesis arising in individuals with common nondisease-specific genetics, triggered by some exogenous agent.

Birdshot Chorioretinopathy/Retinochoroidopathy/Vitiliginous Chorioretinitis

It is a disorder usually found in healthy females in their third to sixth decade of life and around 90% of cases are positive for human lymphocyte antigen A*29 (HLA-A*29) allele. This is the highest HLA association with any disease by far. The primary lesions occur at the level of choroid.

Ocular Features

Symptoms: Blurred vision, floaters, central and peripheral photopsia, and, later, nyctalopia and color blindness.

Examination

Lesions are scattered around the optic disk and radiate to the equator in a "shotgun" pattern; they sometimes appear to follow choroidal vessels. The creamy lesions are small and <1 disk diameter in size. They can be oval or round in shape and are located deep to the retina. They tend to cluster near the nerve, especially nasal and inferiorly to it. Vitreous inflammation is present. Associated disk edema, narrowed retinal vessels, and CME may be noted.

Diagnosis

Diagnosis is mainly clinical and based on history. Imaging is done to monitor the disease and treatment response.

Fluorescein angiography (FA): It reveals disk staining, vascular leakage, and, often, late macular leakage suggestive of CME. The birdshot lesions have variable appearance with this mode of imaging and generally are seen better clinically. The lesions are hypofluorescent in early phase and in the late phases, the lesions are mildly hyperfluorescent.

Indocyanine green angiography—in acute disease—demonstrates hypofluorescent lesions in the intermediate phase of the angiography, and the lesions are bordered by medium-to-large vessels even before apparent clinical lesions.

Spectral domain OCT: In later phase, circular patches of chorioretinal atrophy, ellipsoid zone disruption, outer retinal atrophy, and chronic retinal thinning. EDI-OCT shows reduction in choroidal thickness and volume with increased disease duration. It is also useful in monitoring CME, a common cause of vision loss in birdshot chorioretinopathy (BCR).

Optical coherence tomography angiography: Reduction of retinal capillary density at the deep retinal capillary plexus level, may explain the development of retinal NV, retinal thinning, and reduction of visual function.

Fundus autofluorescence: It reveals more extensive hypoautofluorescent lesions than are seen clinically.

Electroretinography: It is important in the diagnosis of BCR. It may show moderate to severely depressed rod and cone function. Severe cases often demonstrate an extinguished response on ERG.

Electro-oculography: It is usually normal but can be variably subnormal in some cases.

Visual field: Enlargement of blind spot, central or centrocecal scotoma and constriction of visual field. Visual field analysis can be used for disease monitoring.

Differential diagnosis: Intermediate uveitis, sarcoidosis, intraocular lymphoma, MFC, VKH syndrome, OHS, syphilis, sympathetic uveitis, and metastasis

Complications

Macular edema and photoreceptor loss lead to permanent vision loss. Optic disk edema causing late optic atrophy can also cause visual deterioration. Rarely, CNV can form. Retinal vascular attenuation and chorioretinal atrophy may eventually occur. It is a chronic disease with lingering course that does not remit. The long-term visual prognosis is guarded.

Treatment

Corticosteroids: Short-term mainstay of therapy as oral, sub-Tenon's, intraocular, or sustained-release administrations of FA.
Corticosteroid-sparing immunomodulatory agents for long-term management of refractory cases.
Systemic cyclosporine, azathioprine, mycophenolate mofetil, or low-dose methotrexate may be administered. Biologicals such as adalimumab have a good response.

Choroidal neovascularization: Anti-vascular endothelial growth factor (VEGF) therapy

Monitor disease activity: Visual acuity, Goldmann visual fields (at least yearly), ERG (yearly), and OCT to evaluate for integrity of photoreceptors, ERMs, and CME.

Acute Posterior Multifocal Placoid Pigment Epitheliopathy

Acute posterior multifocal placoid pigment epitheliopathy is a bilateral inflammatory disease that affects the choriocapillaris, RPE, and outer retina of otherwise healthy young adults, often in the second and third decades of life, that may be preceded by a viral prodrome. Men and women are affected equally.

Clinical Features

Symptoms: These are unilateral or bilateral sudden, painless diminution of vision. Symptoms of meningismus, headaches, and transient hearing loss are also reported. Cerebral vasculitis can occur. If the placoid lesions are central, they lead to reduction in visual acuity.

Ocular Examination

There are no features of anterior uveitis. There is minimal to no vitreous cellular reaction. Multiple, yellow, creamy-colored, flat-to-placoid (plate-like) lesions of variable size are seen and involve the posterior pole. Fresh lesions may present over the course of a few weeks, so lesions of differing ages can be seen. Associated exudative detachments may be there. As the lesions resolve, they clear centrally and they become hypopigmented. Later pigment clumping occurs. An association with retinal vasculitis, retinal vein occlusions, CNV, optic disk edema has been noted.

Investigations

Fluorescein angiography: Early hypofluorescence with later staining

Indocyanine green: Hypofluorescent lesions in the acute phase are more numerous than seen clinically.

Fundus autofluorescence: It delineates the extent of lesions better than clinical examination.

Optical coherence tomography: Disruption of external limiting membrane (ELM), IS/OS junctions, and the ellipsoid zone in active lesions. As lesions heal, there is hyperreflectivity in photoreceptor layer and RPE disruption.

Optical coherence tomography angiography: Patchy area of choriocapillaris ischemia at lesion site, which improves with regression

Cerebrospinal fluid: Protein and cells in CSF; cerebral involvement should dictate neurological consultation because death may result from cerebral vasculitis.

Differential Diagnosis

- Serpiginous choroiditis—suspected if disease is recurrent and chronic
- Relentless placoid chorioretinitis (RPC)—if severe, persistent, and recurrent cases.
- Harada disease, metastatic tumors, viral retinitis, syphilis, and toxoplasma retinochoroiditis—the lesions are not flat and are associated with significant vitritis.

Management

Usually, no treatment is necessary; the disease is self-limiting. Steroids do not alter the course of disease.

Serpiginous Choroiditis

Definition

It is also called—*helicoid peripapillary chorioretinal degeneration, geographical helicoid peripapillary choroidopathy,* and *geographical choroidopathy.*

Serpiginous choroiditis is a recurrent bilateral inflammatory disease involving the RPE, the choriocapillaris, and the choroid. The condition affects healthy patients from the second to seventh decades of life. Men and women are affected equally. It is usually bilateral, recurrent, and progressive. This disease affects the outer retina and RPE, perhaps associated with impaired circulation in choriocapillaris and inner choroid.

The disease is characterized acutely by irregular, gray–white or cream–yellow subretinal infiltrates at the level of the choriocapillaris and the RPE. These lesions show a propensity for developing near the optic disk, extending centrifugally in a pseudopodial or serpentine fashion.

A pattern of inflammatory quiescence followed by recurrence is common with the recurrences appearing at the edges of the atrophic chorioretinal scars from prior attacks, occurring weeks, months, or even years after a prior attack. With time, atrophy of the RPE, choriocapillaris, and overlying retina occur, leaving scarred tissue in the wake of the lesions.

Clinical Features

Mostly whites, male to female ratio is 1:1, 30–60 years old

Symptoms: Blurred vision, metamorphopsia, and central or paracentral scotomas. Although a bilateral disease, the patient usually presents with unilateral symptoms when a lesion affects the fovea. Unlike in APMPPE, usually one eye is actively involved at a time.

Ocular Examination

Anterior segment is quiet or mild reaction may be present, vitreous may have cells/pigments in 50% of cases. Sharply demarcated gray-green or cream-colored deep-within-the-retina lesions with irregular borders, involving the RPE and choriocapillaris; lesions develop first in the peripapillary area and tend to spread centrifugally. Lesions extend in a pseudopodial pattern, leaving extensive chorioretinal atrophy.

With time, these lesions become atrophic, with disappearance of the RPE, choriocapillaris, and choroid. In patients who have macular SC, the initial lesions are seen in the macula. Subretinal hemorrhage and serous retinal detachment as a result of CNV can occur in eyes with SC.

Ampiginous Choroiditis

Patients with isolated round plaque-like lesions similar to APMPPE which coalesce producing typical serpiginous lesions with RPE and choroidal atrophy, suggesting this that this condition termed "ampiginous choroiditis" is a variant of serpiginous choroiditis.

Diagnosis

Fluorescein angiography:
- *Active phase:* Early hypofluorescence and late hyperfluorescence (leakage) at borders of lesions.
- *Inactive phase:* Mottled hyperfluorescence and late staining of the scar. Retinal vascular staining may occur adjacent to active lesions.

Indocyanine green angiography: ICGA also shows hypofluorescent active and healed lesions.

Optical coherence tomography: SD-OCT has shown hyperreflective outer retina, with disruption of ellipsoid zone in acute lesions and eventual retinal thinning and RPE atrophy with resolution.

Optical coherence tomography angiography: OCTA demonstrates multiple small geographical areas of inner choroidal/choriocapillaris nonperfusion within active lesions that improve with treatment. Older atrophic lesions are marked by decreased or absent inner choroidal vessels.

Fundus autofluorescence: New lesions as hyperautofluorescent, appearing at the edge of old lesions, which are hypoautofluorescent. Furthermore, FAF seems to be useful in distinguishing TB-related disease from SC. TB lesions that mimic SC appear more stippled compared with the more homogeneous lesions of SC.

Visual field: Absolute scotomas (active phase), relative scotomas (resolution) corresponding precisely to visible funduscopic lesions

Differential Diagnosis

White dot syndromes	Infectious diseases	Miscellaneous
Acute posterior multifocal placoid pigment epitheliopathy	Outer-layer retinal toxoplasmosis	Sarcoidosis
Multifocal choroiditis and panuveitis	Tuberculous choroiditis	Harada's disease
Presumed ocular histoplasmosis syndrome		Sympathetic ophthalmia
Acute retinal pigment epitheliitis		

Treatment

Because of the relapsing and progressive nature of this disease, therapy is aimed at treating acute episodes as well as at preventing recurrences that can lead to foveal involvement. Corticosteroids are a mainstay of treatment and have been given via multiple routes of administration (oral, sub-Tenon's, intravenous, intravitreal injections, and via intravitreal implant).

Aggressive management with CSs is useful in treating acute attacks but not in preventing recurrence. Treatment with other immunosuppressive therapy may be necessary for long-term management of SC. Cyclosporine, azathioprine, and other cytotoxic agents have been used to treat SC. CNV is common in this disease, which responds to anti-VEGF injection.

Relentless Placoid Chorioretinitis

Definition

Rare, often bilateral disease of unknown etiology presenting between the second and sixth decades of life with no gender predisposition. It comes under the differentials of APMPPE and SC.

Symptoms

These are decreased vision, pericentral scotomas, photopsia, floaters, and, rarely, pain.

Ocular Manifestations

Varying numbers of anterior chamber and vitreous cells may be seen.

Active retinal lesions are creamy white and located at the level of the outer retina. They may be smaller than those of APMPPE (1–2 disk area). The lesions can be active bilaterally and may affect the mid- and far periphery prior to involvement of the posterior pole, unlike APMPPE or SC. Lesions heal over weeks, resulting in chorioretinal atrophy. Some lesions progressively enlarge and new lesions appear. The presence of multiple lesions (>50) at same time in the fundus is hallmark of RPC. When macula becomes involved, it leads to vision loss, metamorphopsia, or scotoma. When these lesions heal, visual acuity is often preserved even with macular involvement.

Diagnosis

It is based on clinical appearance and prolonged course of disease that resolves with IMT.

Fluorescein angiography: It shows early hypofluorescence and late staining.

Indocyanine green angiography—shows hypofluorescence in the areas corresponding to the clinical lesions.

Spectral domain OCT: Active lesions have photoreceptor layer disruption in ellipsoid zone with associated fluid. Healed lesions have RPE atrophy with ellipsoid zone rarefaction.

Optical coherence tomography angiography: Multifocal areas of inner choroidal ischemia, which improve with treatment but recur in adjacent and noncontiguous areas.

Fundus autofluorescence: Three concentric zones with a central round area of dense hypoautofluorescence, surrounded by a narrow ring of hyperautofluorescence, which is surrounded by a faint wider ring of hypoautofluorescence. With time, lesions become more hyperautofluorescent with central hypoautofluorescence (RPE hyperplasia).

Differential diagnosis: APMPPE, serpiginous choroiditis, persistent placoid maculopathy, MFC, viral retinitis, choroidal vasculitis (e.g., SLE and PAN), neoplastic infiltration of the choroid, syphilis, sarcoid, and TB.

Treatment

Oral CSs cause healing of lesions with improvement in visual acuity. IMT slows the progression of disease activity. Relapses are common. New lesions can appear till 2 years of disease onset. Long-term visual prognosis is fair to good.

Multifocal Choroiditis and Punctate Inner Choroidopathy

Definition

Multifocal choroiditis and punctate inner choroidopathy (PIC) are essentially same entity. PIC term is used when lesions are at posterior pole and MFC when they extend to periphery as well. Some lesions may have significant fibrosis associated with them and are called *subretinal fibrosis with uveitis (SFU).*

Multifocal choroiditis can be secondary to other processes, including infectious [TB, syphilis, fungal/presumed ocular histoplasmosis syndrome (POHS), and viral infections], and noninfectious etiologies (sarcoidosis).

Multifocal choroiditis: Predominantly in myopic women between second and sixth decades; bilateral presentation. MFC and PIC are characterized by inflammation at the level of the RPE and outer retina, so "choroiditis" may be a misnomer.

Ocular Manifestations

Symptom: Decreased visual acuity in one eye or both eyes, photopsia, and enlarged blind spot

Ocular Examination

Variable amount of anterior segment inflammation and vitritis. When there is a significant amount of vitritis, the terms *MFC and panuveitis* have been used. Peripapillary RPE mottling may be seen. An area of fibrosis in the shape of a "napkin ring" may surround the disk. Acute lesions are multiple in number, are yellowish to gray in color, and located at the level of the RPE and outer retina; they range in size from 50 to 1,000 microns. They can occur in linear clusters or as streak lesions at posterior pole, around disk or nasally. Peripapillary and macular CNV occurs in up to 70% of the eyes.

Diagnosis

Diagnosis is based on clinical examination findings.

Fluorescein angiography: Acute stage—hypofluorescent; later phase—these lesions stain. Healed lesions may show a window defect. Peripapillary or sub-foveal CNV may be seen. CME may be noted.

Indocyanine green angiography: Hypofluorescent lesions, far more numerous than those seen on FA or clinical examination.

Spectral domain OCT: Elevation of the RPE corresponding to active lesion with loss of the ellipsoid layer, outer photoreceptor damage, choroidal thickening, and subretinal material that may erupt through the RPE with an intact Bruch's membrane.

Optical coherence tomography angiography: It helps to distinguish inflammatory lesions from CNV.

Fundus autofluorescence: Diffuse zone of peripapillary and/or multiple posterior-pole hyperautofluorescent acute lesions, even in areas that appear clinically uninvolved, and that can resolve with treatment

Visual field: Enlarged blind spot

Differential diagnosis: Evanescent lesions may resemble MEWDS. Other differentials include POHS, sarcoidosis, VKH syndrome, SO, SC, infectious etiologies (syphilis, TB, septic choroiditis, metastatic endophthalmitis, histoplasmosis, cryptococcosis, candidiasis, toxoplasmosis, and DUSN), and intraocular lymphoma.

Treatment

Treatment aims at controlling inflammation and its complications (CME and CNV). MFC can present with significant anterior and posterior inflammation. CSs (topical, periocular, intraocular, and systemic) are used. CS-sparing immunomodulatory agents become necessary when CSs are not tolerated or recurrence is frequent. CNV is primarily managed with anti-VEGF injections.

 35. Describe the clinical features, evaluation, and management of serpiginous choroidopathy.

Serpiginous choroiditis is discussed above in white dot syndrome.

 36. Describe clinical features, diagnosis, and management of ocular sarcoidosis.

Sarcoidosis

It is a multisystem granulomatous disorder of unknown etiology with systemic and ocular manifestations.

Systemic involvement occurs most frequently of the lungs (90%); others include lymph nodes, skin, bones and joint, CNS, liver, and heart. Eye involvement is seen in half of the cases of sarcoidosis. The basic lesion of sarcoidosis is a noncaseating granuloma without histologic evidence of infection or foreign body.

Sarcoidosis can affect any ocular tissue, including the orbit and adnexa. Cutaneous involvement is frequent, and orbital and eyelid granulomas are common. Palpebral and bulbar conjunctival nodules may also be observed and provide a readily accessible site for tissue biopsy. Lacrimal gland infiltration may cause keratoconjunctivitis sicca.

Ocular involvement in systemic sarcoidosis may be a feature of acute disease or chronic (>2 years) disease. Uveitis in acute disease is associated with two syndromes:

1. *Lofgren syndrome:* Erythema nodosum, febrile arthropathy, bilateral hilar adenopathy, and acute iritis that is responsive to systemic CSs.
2. *Heerfordt syndrome (uveoparotid fever):* It is characterized by uveitis, parotitis, fever, and facial nerve palsy.

Anterior Uveitis

It is the most common ocular manifestation, occurring in around two-thirds of cases with ocular sarcoidosis. Patient presents with mild to moderate blurring of vision and pain in the eyes.

Examination: Anterior segment may show mutton-fat KPs, Koeppe and Busacca nodules on the iris, nodules involving the anterior chamber angle (Berlin nodule), peripheral anterior tent-shaped synechiae, and white clumps of cells ("snowballs") in the inferior–anterior vitreous. Extensive posterior synechiae may lead to iris bombé and angle-closure glaucoma. Infrequent nummular corneal infiltrates and inferior corneal endothelial opacification may be present; band keratopathy may occur in cases of chronic uveitis.

Posterior Segment Involvement

It occurs in 20% of patients with ocular sarcoidosis. Vitreous commonly has clumps of snowballs with or without diffuse cellular infiltration. Cells may form linear strands known as "string of pearls". Nodular granulomas measuring ¼–1 disk diameter may be present on—optic nerve, retina and choroid, either posteriorly or peripherally. Perivascular sheathing is also common, appearing most often as either a linear or segmental periphlebitis. Relatively well-defined, discrete chorioretinal exudates with granuloma may occur along with venules and have been termed *candle-wax drippings,* or *taches de bougie.* Occlusive retinal vascular disease, especially branch retinal vein occlusion and, less commonly, central retinal vein occlusion may also occur. The resultant retinal NV can cause vitreous hemorrhage. CME is frequently present, and optic disk edema without granulomatous invasion of the optic nerve may be observed in patients with papilledema and neurosarcoidosis.

Seven intraocular signs that are suggestive of ocular sarcoidosis are:

1. Mutton-fat KPs (large or small) and/or iris nodules at the pupillary margin (Koeppe) or in the stroma (Bussacca)
2. TM nodules and/or tent-shaped PAS
3. Snowballs/string of pearls vitreous opacities
4. Multiple chorioretinal peripheral lesions (active and atrophic)
5. Nodular and/or segmental periphlebitis (± candle wax drippings) and/or macroaneurysm in an inflamed eye
6. Optic disk nodule(s)/granuloma(s) and/or solitary choroidal nodule
7. Bilaterality (assessed by clinical examination or laboratory tests showing subclinical inflammation)

Diagnosis

Diagnostic criteria for ocular sarcoidosis were proposed in an international workshop of ophthalmologists but have yet to be validated. These criteria consist of diagnostic grades ranging from "definitive" (based on tissue biopsy), to "presumed" (based on typical ocular findings with bilateral hilar adenopathy), to "probable" or "possible" disease (with supporting ancillary evidence).

Biopsy: Definite diagnosis is made by histologically examination from tissue obtained from the lungs, mediastinal lymph nodes, skin, peripheral lymph nodes, liver, conjunctiva, minor salivary glands, or lacrimal glands.

Chest X-ray: Abnormalities are present at some point in up to 90% of sarcoid patients, but do not persist throughout the disease course and thus may be absent at the time of workup.

High-resolution CT: It is more sensitive imaging modality and valuable in patients with a normal X-ray but a high clinical index of suspicion remains.

Serum angiotensin-converting enzyme (ACE): ACE and lysozyme levels may be abnormally elevated; neither result is diagnostic nor specific. They reflect total-body granuloma content and are useful in tracking active disease. (Note that the ACE levels may be falsely low in patients taking ACE-inhibitor medications.)

Serum and urinary calcium levels and liver function.

Gallium scanning: It detects occult disease activity, but has limited sensitivity.

Bronchoalveolar lavage: Mononuclear alveolitis with increased CD4+ lymphocytes is supportive of diagnosis.

Five laboratory tests that are carried out on suspected ocular sarcoidosis patients are:
- Negative tuberculin test in a BCG-vaccinated patient or having had a positive PPD previously
- Elevated serum ACE and/or elevated serum lysozyme[a]
- Abnormal liver enzyme tests[b]
- Chest X-ray; look for bilateral hilar lymphadenopathy (BHL)
- Chest CT scan in patients with negative chest X-ray.

Treatment

Corticosteroids: Topical, periocular, and systemic CSs are the mainstays of therapy for ocular sarcoidosis. Cycloplegia is useful for relieving the pain and for prevention of posterior synechiae. Vision-threatening posterior segment lesions generally require and are responsive to systemic CSs (prednisone, 40–80 mg/day). Intravitreal CSs, including the Flucinolone Acetonide (FA) implant, are potential treatment options for patients intolerant of systemic therapy, but they leave the systemic disease untreated.

Systemic IMT with methotrexate, azathioprine, mycophenolate mofetil, or cyclosporine can provide good control of the disease while minimizing the risks of long-term CS therapy. Recently, the TNF-α inhibitors infliximab and adalimumab have been shown to be effective in the treatment of sarcoidosis-associated uveitis. Paradoxically, the TNF-α inhibitor etanercept has been reported to cause a sarcoid-like syndrome in some patients.

37. Discuss surgical management of complications of uveitis.

Following are the indications of surgery in a case with uveitis:
- *For visual rehabilitation:* For BSK, complicated cataract, or dense vitreous haze/membranes left after resolution of inflammation
- Diagnostic procedures in cases where it is not proved by the conventional investigations; vitreous biopsy or aqueous tap can be sent for analysis. In case of choroidal lesions that are unresponsive to management, choroidal biopsy can be taken.
- *Others:* Glaucoma filtering surgery in cases unresponsive to topical medications; vitrectomy for recurrent or nonresolving vitreous hemorrhage and tractional retinal detachment. Some cases with persistent hypotony can be managed by removal of ciliary body membranes and infusion of silicone oil.

---

[a]: Test required in patients treated with ACE inhibitors.
[b]: Positive when serum levels of alkaline phosphatase are more than three times the upper limit of normal; or when two of the following liver enzymes, alkaline phosphatase, (AST: aspartate aminotransferase; ALT: alanine transaminase) are more than twice the upper limit of normal.

Cataract Management

The eye should be quiet off treatment for 3 months prior to surgery (exception is FUS). Anterior chamber should be quiet (0–5 cells), vitreous haze should be absent or decreased as difficult to have clear vitreous once inflammation sets in. There are several factors in addition to cataract that will hamper the surgery (posterior synechiae, nondilating pupil, BSK) or visual outcome postoperatively like macular edema, ERM, optic atrophy, and vitreous opacities.

Indications of cataract surgery in a case with uveitis are:
- Visually significant cataract in presence of well-controlled inflammation without treatment for 3 months.
- Phacoantigenic uveitis
- Cataract that obscures view of posterior segment in case of active disease in posterior segment that needs medical or surgical management. Thus, cataract surgery is done in presence of steroids.

Surgical Technique

Phacoemulsification or extracapsular cataract extraction remains the choice of surgery depending on surgeon's comfort and patient factors such as presence of nondilating pupil, posterior synechiae, membranes, and hazy view due to BSK. IOL can be implanted in quite eyes. Special consideration against IOL implantation in eyes with JIA as IOL acts as scaffold for formation of membranes, cyclitic membranes, and resultant hypotony. However, with aggressive control of inflammation prior to and following surgery, this complication may be avoided.

Complications

Surgery should be done by an experienced surgeon as the following complications are anticipated intraoperatively—nondilating pupil with difficult capsulorhexis, shallow anterior chamber, posterior capsular rent, and zonular dehiscence. Postoperatively, there can be inflammation flare-up, hyphema, exacerbation of CME, and secondary glaucoma. In long term, there is increased risk of posterior capsule opacification, optic capture, pupillary and cyclitic membrane formation, and hypotony.

Role of systemic steroids in pre- and postoperative period: They can be given depending on disease severity and history of recurrences.

Band-shaped Keratopathy

It develops in patients with chronic uveitis, with deposition of calcium at the level of corneal epithelial basement membrane and Bowman's membrane. The deposits usually start in corneal periphery and slowly encroach on the pupillary axis. BSK is most commonly seen in children with JIA and may require early treatment as this can lead to visual deprivation amblyopia.

Current modalities in approaching this problem are:
- Phototherapeutic keratectomy (PTK)
- Chemical chelation with ethylenediaminetetraacetic acid (EDTA)—scraping the epithelium and applying 0.05 mol, 1.5% EDTA for 3–5 minutes followed by copious irrigation with normal saline and removal of loosened epithelium and calcium debris manually with a number 15 surgical blade. This is followed by application of a bandage contact lens.
- Superficial keratectomy with or without adjuvant amniotic membrane transplant (AMT).

Glaucoma Surgery

The incidence of glaucoma is around 20% as a complication of uveitis. Medical therapy is often insufficient and glaucoma surgery needs to be considered as vision salvageable procedure and not an end-stage procedure. There are several mechanisms of secondary glaucoma:
- Severe anterior segment inflammation resulting in decreased trabecular filtration
- Pupillary block glaucoma (posterior synechiae)
- Angle-closure glaucoma—from formation of peripheral anterior synechia
- Steroid response.

There is increased risk of bleb failure after surgery due to enhanced fibrosis and scarring. Thus, antimetabolites should be used with glaucoma filtering surgery. Glaucoma drainage implant may be used as primary procedure in those below 30 years. The success rates range from 94% to 74% at the end of 1 year with implants.

Refractory glaucoma: Transscleral cyclo-photocoagulation or cryotherapy, transscleral diode cyclophotocoagulation.

Vitreoretinal Surgery in Uveitis

Pars plana vitrectomy has been increasingly performed both for diagnostic and therapeutic purposes in management of patients with uveitis. The indications can be:
- Diagnostic
- Therapeutic
- Both.

Whereas cataract surgery in uveitis is ordinarily performed only after complete quiescence of the uveitis for 3 months, vitrectomy may often be required in active disease. For nonurgent elective procedures, quiescence of anterior segment inflammation is advisable. Inflammatory choroidal effusion or exudative retinal detachments are commonly considered contraindications. Active pars plana exudation may increase the risk of retinal injury from the pars plana sclerotomy sites.

Diagnostic vitrectomy	Therapeutic vitrectomy
Indications	Indications
1. Atypical clinical presentations 2. Nonresponsive to empirical treatment with corticosteroids/immunosuppressants 3. Rapidly progressive disease with inconclusive noninvasive work-up 4. Strong suspicion of malignancy	1. Media opacities obscuring the visual axis 2. Tractional or combined retinal detachment 3. Nonresolving CME 4. ERM as consequence of inflammation 5. Cyclitic membrane removal for the treatment of nonresponding hypotony
Techniques	Techniques
1. Vitreous tap/aspiration 2. Vitreous biopsy 3. Chorioretinal biopsy	3-port pars plana vitrectomy (23G/25G) along with membrane peeling/endotamponade
(CME: cystoid macular edema; ERM: epiretinal membrane)	

It is important to promptly recognize cyclitic membranes preoperatively using UBM. Early removal of these membranes followed by appropriate intraocular tamponade can prevent recalcitrant hypotony in some of the patients.

Postoperative Complications of Vitrectomy in Uveitis

- *Hypotony:* It is related to shutdown of the aqueous humor production from acute, severe inflammation. Wound leakage and retinal detachment are other possibilities that need to be excluded. Management is with topical/periocular as well as systemic CSs.
- *Retinal detachment:* Doing surgery in inflamed posterior segment is fraught with the increased risk of retinal breaks that can occur at ora near sclerotomy sites and at edge of choroidal inflammation. Secondary contracture of left over vitreous may lead to new retinal breaks.
- *Recurrent vitreous hemorrhage:* It occurs due to persistent NV or port side proliferation.
- *Uveitis recurrence:* Recurrence of uveitis following PPV can occur. Transient increase in inflammation immediately after surgery is common and can be treated with oral CSs. Because the vitreous gel is absent, vitreous cells are sparser and are less likely to affect the visual acuity.

 38. Describe occlusive retinal vasculitis.

Occlusive Retinal Vasculitis

Vasculitis with poor prognosis due to higher incidence of retinal ischemia, NV, and macular edema. The following are the common causes:
- Intraocular TB
- Eales disease
- Syphilis
- Varicella zoster uveitis
- Behçet's disease
- Systemic lupus erythematosus

- Relapsing polychondritis
- Susac syndrome
- Multiple sclerosis.

The clinical features, diagnosis, investigation profile, and management are discussed with retinal vasculitis.

 39. Discuss role of biological agents in management of patient with bilateral chronic uveitis

Noncorticosteroid Immunomodulatory Therapy

Treatment with systemic NCSIT and biologic agents has become increasingly widespread in cases of uveitis not controlled with CS therapy alone.

The Fundamentals of Care for Uveitis (FOCUS) global Initiative group organized a consensus through evidence synthesis on the optimal systemic treatment of patients with NIU. This uveitis expert panel produced the following statements and concepts:

- Noncorticosteroid immunomodulatory therapy may be introduced for the management of NIU to control persistent or severe inflammation, or to prevent ocular structural complications.
- Indications for introducing NCSIT also include contraindications or intolerance to other medications, or a need for CS-sparing effect to maintain disease remission.
- Biologic agents are generally considered for patients whose disease is inadequately controlled by CS and NCSIT drug therapy.

The use of NCSIT is indicated in the following situations:
- Visual acuity < 20/100
- Increase of vitreous haze of grade 2 or higher
- Relapse of CME
- Disease that impacts quality of life

The SUN group has defined failure of NCSIT therapy as:
- Either a 2-step increase in the level of inflammation, or
- Lack of 2-step decrease in the level of inflammation and inability to decrease to inactive disease despite therapy

One must check for compliance before considering treatment failure/lack of benefit of NCSIT.

The choice of therapy for patients with NIU refractory to NCSIT must be individualized taking into account the patient's history, cause of uveitis, and comorbidities. The following strategies can be considered when a NCSIT is not adequately effective or tolerated:
- Dose escalation of the drug to the maximum tolerated therapeutic dose
- Switch to another NCSIT
- Add-on therapy with introduction of a novel NCSIT
- *Withdrawal of NCSIT:* The decision to stop a NCSIT must be made on an individual basis, and involves a risk–benefit assessment that considers the risk of disease recurrence or aggravation against the benefits derived from not being subjected to systemic immunosuppression (e.g., systemic side effects).
- Biologics.

The following table summarizes the NCSIT:

Class	Generic name	Mechanism of action	Dose	Side effects
Antimetabolite	• Azathioprine	• Purine metabolism	• 1 mg/kg/day Maximum: 2.5–4 mg/kg/day	• Bone marrow suppression; GI upset; hepatotoxic
	• Methotrexate	• Inhibitor of DHFR	• 7.5–12.5 mg/week; Maximum: 25 mg/week	• Hepatotoxic, Interstitial pneumonia; cytopenia
	• Mycophenolate mofetil	• IMP dehydrogenase inhibitor	• 500 mg BD; Maximum: 1.5 g BD	• Diarrhea, nausea, neutropenia, and infection
	• Leflunomide	• Dihydro-orotate dehydrogenase inhibition (pyrimidine synthesis)	• 100 mg QID × 3 days then 20 mg/day	

Contd...

Contd…

Class	Generic name	Mechanism of action	Dose	Side effects
Alkylating agent	• Cyclophosphamide	• DNA to DNA cross-linking. Inhibits cell replication and protein synthesis	• 2.5 mg/kg/day; Maximum 3 mg/kg/day	• Bone marrow suppression; Hemorrhagic cystitis, malignancy, infection, and infertility
	• Chlorambucil	• DNA to DNA cross-linking. Inhibits cell replication and protein synthesis	• 0.1 mg/kg/day; Maximum: 0.2 mg/kg/day	• Infertility, BM suppression, teratogenic, infections
T-cell inhibitor	• Cyclosporine	• T-cell inhibitor	• 2.5–5 mg/kg/day; Maximum: 10 mg/kg/day	• Renal dysfunction, tremor, hirsutism, hypertension, gum hyperplasia
	• Tacrolimus	• T-cell inhibitor	• 0.15–0.30 mg/kg/day	• Nephrotoxicity, Hypertension, neurotoxicity, Hyperkalemia, hepatitis, diabetes
	• Rapamycin	• Blocks response to IL-2 and thereby blocks T- and B-cell activation	• LD: 6 mg; MD: 2 mg/day	• Infections, lymphoma, hyperlipidosis
Calcineurin inhibitor	• Voclosporin	• Reversible inhibitor T-cell proliferation	• 0.25–4.5 mg/kg/day	• Diarrhea, headache, and hypertension
	• Colchicine	• Inhibits neutrophil chemotaxis by microtubule polymerization	• 1.5 mg/day	• Thrombocytopenia, anemia, hypokalemia, GI upset, anorexia, rash, hyperlipidemia

(BM: bone marrow; DHFR: dihydrofolate reductase; GI: gastrointestinal)

Biologicals

Generic name	Target	Route	Dosage	Side effects
TNF inhibitors				
Infliximab	TNF-α	IV	3–5 mg/kg LD @ 0, 2, 6 weeks then MD 3–10 mg/kg every 4–8 weeks (Maximum 20 mg/kg in children)	• Infections • Hypersensitivity reactions; demyelinating disease, lupus-like syndrome, malignancy, thromboembolic events, congestive heart failure
Adalimumab	TNF-α	SC	40 mg every 1–2 weeks; (LD 80–160 mg)	
Etanercept	TNF-α/β	SC	Adults: 50 mg weekly; Children: 0.8 mg/kg/week (Maximum 50 mg/week)	
Golimumab	TNF-α	SC	50 mg monthly	
Certolizumab	TNF-α	SC	400 mg at week 0, 2, 4 then 200 mg every 2 weeks or 400 mg every 4 weeks	
Anti-interleukin therapy				
Daclizumab	IL-2	IV/SC	1–2 mg/kg every 2–4 weeks	Hypersensitivity reactions; headache, GI upset
Anakinra	IL-1 receptor	SC	100 mg daily	Infections; neutropenia, injection site reaction
Tocilizumab	IL-6 receptor	IV	4 mg/kg infusion over 1 hour every 4 weeks	Infections; neutropenia, thrombocytopenia
Rituximab	CD20; B cells	IV	500/1,000 mg at week 0 and 2	Infusion reactions, severe mucocutaneous reactions, hypertension, bronchospasm, progressive multifocal leukoencephalopathy
Interferons				
Interferons-α-2a		SC	3–6 million IU/day tapering over 6 months	Flu-like reaction, inject site reaction; bone marrow suppression
Fusion protein of CTLA-4				
Abatacept	CTLA-4	IV	500/1,000 mg at week 0, 2, 4 then every 4 weeks	Infections, allergic reactions, malignancy, respiratory problems

(CTLA: cytotoxic T lymphocyte antigen; IL: interleukin; IV: intravenous; SC: subcutaneous; TNF: tumor necrosis factor)

40. (a) Discuss indications, routes of administration, dosage schedule, and complication of steroids in uveitis. (b) Describe role of alternative drugs used in uveitis.

Topical Corticosteroids

These are useful in the management of anterior uveitis and anterior component of panuveitis. Generally, steroid therapy should be given in high doses initially and then slowly tapered according to clinical evolution.

- *Mild inflammation*—can be managed with a topical formulation q6h (e.g., prednisolone acetate 1% or dexamethasone 0.1%)
- *Moderate to severe uveitis*—topical CS q1-2h dosing initially (e.g., prednisolone acetate 1%, dexamethasone 0.1%), and a steroid ophthalmic ointment can be given at night
- In cases of severe uveitis, a loading dose can be considered (e.g., prednisolone acetate 1% q1min for 5 minutes, then q30min-1h). A commonly adopted regimen might consist of—one drop q1h for 3 days, then one drop q2h for 3 days, then one drop q6h for 3 days, then one drop q8h for 7 days, then one drop q12h for 7 days, then one drop OD for 7 days, and then stop.

Corticosteroid	Systemic equivalent (mg)	Relative potency
Betamethasone	0.6	33.0
Dexamethasone	0.75	26.0
Methylprednisolone	4	5.0
Triamcinolone	4	5.0
Prednisolone	4	5.0
Prednisone	5	4.0
Hydrocortisone	20	1.0
Cortisone	25	0.8

Periocular Steroids

Indications for periocular steroids are:
- Severe unilateral anterior uveitis
- Anterior uveitis with hypopyon
- Anterior uveitis complicated by CME
- Unilateral IU
- Unilateral posterior uveitis (preferably not involving the disk and macula, i.e., not sight threatening; sight-threatening cases required high-dose systemic steroids)
- Contraindications for systemic steroid treatment
- Poor patient compliance to topical medications posing a likely factor for unresponsiveness to topical treatment.

Following drugs are used:
- Subconjunctival betamethasone sodium phosphate solution (4 mg in 1 mL) alone or in combination with betamethasone acetate suspension (6 mg in 1 mL)
- Sub-Tenon triamcinolone (0.5–1.0 mL sub-Tenon injection of triamcinolone acetonide 40 mg/mL).

Systemic Therapy

Systemic steroids are the mainstay of therapy for noninfectious posterior or panuveitis. Initially, these are given as high dosage than tapered according to clinical effects. Initial dosing can be 1.0–1.5 mg/kg body weight/day of prednisolone, and maintenance doses may be 10–20 mg/day or as low a dose as possible; for chronic diseases, the target dose is <7.5 mg/day.

A typically adopted steroid-tapering schedule is as follows:

		Taper interval	
Prednisone dose (mg/day)	Decrement (mg/day)	Rapid	Standard
60–30	10	2 days	Weekly
30–15	5	2 days	Weekly
15–7.5	2.5	2 days	Weekly
<7.5	2.5–1	2–7 days	Weekly–monthly

Ocular Side-effects

- Cataract, usually a PSC
- *Elevation of IOP and glaucoma:* up to 30% of CS-treated patients
- Central serous chorioretinopathy (CSCR).

Systemic Side-effects

Common (oral route)	• Cushingoid changes • Moon facies • Weight gain • Fat redistribution • Increased acne • Suppression of hypothalamic pituitary axis • Delay in pubertal growth • Infections • Hypertension • Diabetes mellitus • Fluid retention • Hyperlipidemia • Atherosclerosis • Osteoporosis • Anxiety, mood changes • Easy bruising • Poor wound healing • Gastric ulcerations
With intravenous route	• Arrhythmias • CVS collapse • Myocardial infarction • Severe infection

(CVS: cardiovascular)

The MUST trial: It compared sustained-release intravitreous FA implant with systemic therapy (steroids supplemented with immunomodulatory therapy and biologic agents). The systemic and local therapies were comparable in visual outcomes, controlling inflammation, and reducing macular edema in patients with IU, posterior uveitis, or panuveitis. Cases with implant though had better inflammation control. Oral CSs and immunosuppression can be administered relatively safely for at least 7 years.

Interestingly, a Cochrane systematic review was unable to conclude that the implants are superior to traditional systemic therapy for the treatment of NIU, and findings regarding safety outcomes suggest increased risks of postimplant surgery for cataract and high IOP compared with standard-of-care systemic therapy including CS.

 41. A 30-year-old male presented with genital lesions and complained of sudden diminution of vision is one eye followed 6 weeks later by similar diminution in the other eye. What are the possible diagnoses? Give broad guidelines in the management of each situation.

The differential diagnoses are:
- Behçet's disease
- Reiter's syndrome
- Syphilis.

Behçet's disease and Reiter's disease have already been discussed. Here, syphilis is discussed.

Syphilis

A multisystem, chronic bacterial infection caused by the spirochete *Treponema pallidum* that is associated with numerous ocular manifestations in both the acquired and congenital forms of the disease. Transmission occurs most often through sexual contact; however, transplacental infection of the fetus may occur after the 10th week of pregnancy. Although syphilis is thought to be responsible for <2% of all uveitis cases, it is one of the great masquerades and should always be considered in the differential diagnosis of any intraocular inflammatory disease. Delay in the diagnosis may lead not only to permanent vision loss but also to significant neurologic and cardiac morbidity.

Acquired Syphilis

Primary syphilis occurs after an incubation period of 3 weeks. The characteristic lesion is chancre, a painless solitary lesion at the site of inoculation, resolving spontaneously within 12 weeks regardless of treatment. CNS is seeded with treponemes during this period.

Secondary syphilis occurs 6-8 weeks later. There is lymphadenopathy and generalized maculopapular rash more prominent on palms and soles. Uveitis occurs in approximately 10% of cases. Followed by latent period ranging from 1 year (early latency) to decades (late latency).

Tertiary syphilis occurs in one-third of the untreated patients. It may be further subcategorized as benign tertiary syphilis (the characteristic lesion being gumma, most frequently found on the skin and mucous membranes but also in the choroid and iris), cardiovascular syphilis, and neurosyphilis.

Although uveitis may occur in up to 5% of patients whose disease has progressed to tertiary syphilis, it can occur at any stage of infection, including primary disease. Because the eye is an extension of the CNS, ocular syphilis is best regarded as a variant of neurosyphilis, a notion that has important diagnostic and therapeutic implications.

Clinical Features

Syphilis affects all ocular structures—conjunctiva, cornea, sclera, lens, uveal tract, retina, retinal vasculature, optic nerve, pupillomotor pathways, and cranial nerves.

Symptoms are pain, redness, photophobia, blurred vision, or floaters.

Examination: Intraocular inflammation may be granulomatous or nongranulomatous, unilateral or bilateral, and it may affect the anterior or posterior segments.

Anterior segment findings can include iris roseola, vascularized papules (iris papulosa), larger red nodules (iris nodosa), and gummata. Interstitial keratitis, posterior synechiae, lens dislocation, and iris atrophy can also occur.

Posterior segment: It can mimic any of the disorders with vitritis, chorioretinitis, focal retinitis, necrotizing retinitis, retinal vasculitis, exudative retinal detachment, isolated papillitis, and neuroretinitis. A focal or multifocal chorioretinitis, associated with vitritis, is the most common manifestation. These lesions are typically small, grayish yellow, and located in the postequatorial fundus, but they may become confluent. Retinal vasculitis and disk edema, with exudates appearing around the disk and the retinal arterioles, together with serous retinal detachment, may accompany the chorioretinitis. Solitary or multifocal, macular or papillary, placoid, yellowish gray lesions may occur at the level of the RPE.

Syphilis is an important entity to consider in the differential diagnosis of patients with neuroretinitis and papillitis. Patients with syphilis who are immunocompromised or who have HIV/AIDS, optic neuritis, and neuroretinitis are more common in the initial presentation. Neuro-ophthalmic manifestations of syphilis are Argyll Robertson pupil, ocular motor nerve palsies, optic atrophy, and retrobulbar optic neuritis.

Diagnosis

- *Nonspecific tests:* Rapid plasma reagin (RPR), venereal disease research laboratory (VDRL)
- *Specific tests:* Fluorescent treponemal antibody absorption test (FTA-ABS), micro-hemagglutination assay for T. pallidum (MHATP)
- *T. pallidum* immobilization test (TPI)
- Darkfield microscopy
- Polymerase chain reaction.

Treatment

- Intravenous penicillin G 18-24 million units daily for 10-14 days
- *For penicillin-allergic patients:*
  - Tetracycline hydrochloride 500 mg PO QID for 30 days
  - Doxycycline 100 mg PO BID for 14 days
  - Consider penicillin desensitization in certain individuals.

Glaucoma

7.1 Developmental Anomalies of the Angle

Dewang Angmo, Ritweez Sahu, Karthikeyan Mahalingam, Kanchangouri Satpute

 1. Briefly discuss disorders exhibiting developmental anomalies of the angle.

The following disorders exhibit some degree of goniodysgenesis.

Primary Congenital Glaucoma

Primary congenital glaucoma (PCG) is characterized by isolated maldevelopment of trabecular meshwork with or without other anomalies of the eye that can raise intraocular pressure (IOP). Approximately 80% of the affected children develop signs of glaucoma in the first year of life.

Genetics
- Most cases occur sporadically, with autosomal recessive hereditary patterns seen in 10% of cases.
- PCG caused by pathogenic variants in CYP1B1 (GLC3A) or LTBP2 is inherited in an autosomal recessive manner while
- When caused by a pathogenic variant in TEK it is inherited in an apparently autosomal dominant manner.

Pathophysiology
There have been various proposals aiming to explain the pathogenesis of PCG including:
- Failure of posterior recession of iris and ciliary body during fetal development and
- The presence of a membrane covering the trabecular meshwork.

Clinical Presentation
- Parents usually present with the complaint of the infant having epiphora, blepharospasm, and photophobia.
- Clinically, an enlarged cornea with haze, horizontal breaks in Descemet's membrane (Haab's striae), optic nerve cupping, and corneal edema may be present. Vision is typically reduced due to corneal edema, myopia, astigmatism, or setting in off amblyopia. Intraocular pressure is typically raised.

Management
- Control of IOP and treatment of secondary complications is the aim of treatment, with angle surgery being the mainstay mode of treatment.
- Goniotomy is the preferred modality in clear cornea, with trabeculotomy being preferred in hazy corneas.
- Concurrent trabeculectomy with mitomycin C improves the success rate of trabeculotomy.
- Drainage implant procedures may be planned in refractive cases.
- Laser cycloablation and cyclocryotherapy are the reserve options.
- Medical therapy is usually temporary to decrease preoperative corneal haze and to provide immediate postoperative support.

Posterior Embryotoxon

Anterior displacement and thickening of Schwalbe's line usually occur as an isolated anomaly with limited clinical significance and is relatively common in the population **(Fig. 1)**. It is usually detected on gonioscopy although it may be prominent enough to be detected on the slit lamp.

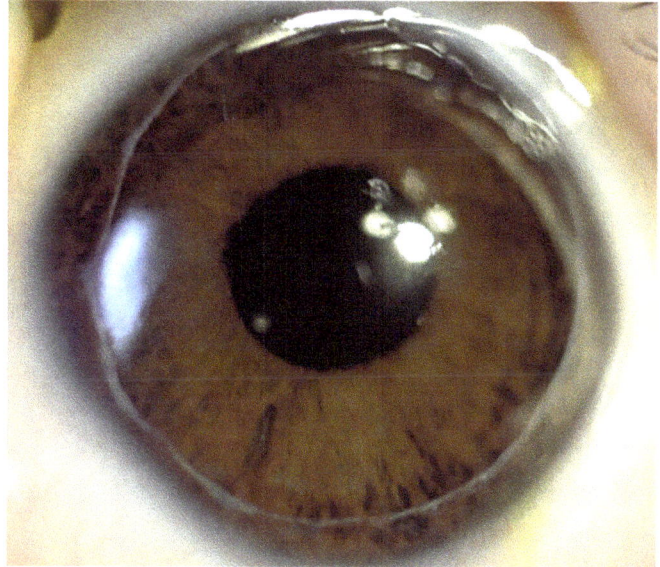

Fig. 1: Posterior embryotoxon.

Axenfeld–Rieger Syndrome

Axenfeld–Rieger (A-R) syndrome comprises a spectrum of bilateral anterior segment anomalies including:
- *Axenfeld anomaly:* Prominent, anteriorly displaced Schwalbe's line with iridocorneal adhesions.
- *Rieger anomaly:* Iris stromal atrophy with corectopia, pseudocornea, and ectropion uvea.
- Associated dental anomalies including microdontia, oligodontia, and hypodontia. Facial anomalies include midfacial hypoplasia, hypertelorism, and telecanthus.

More than half of the patients with A-R syndrome have associated glaucoma, manifesting mainly in childhood or early adulthood.

Pathophysiology

- It is believed to be caused because of developmental arrest of structures formed from neural crest cells leading to abnormal retention of endothelium and associated basement membrane, represented by a membrane over iris and the angle.
- The neural crest origin explains the associated facial anomalies. A-R syndrome is associated with FOXC1 and PITX2 genes and is inherited in an autosomal dominant fashion.

Management

Detection and control of glaucoma remain the primary goal in management. Medical therapy is instituted before surgical modalities are considered. Drugs reducing aqueous production, i.e., beta blockers, carbonic anhydrase inhibitors, and alpha-2 agonists are most likely to be beneficial. Among surgical options, goniotomy and trabeculotomy have been tried in infantile cases with limited success. Trabeculectomy is the preferred procedure in most cases.

Aniridia

Aniridia is a bilateral developmental disorder characterized by the congenital absence of a normal iris **(Fig. 2)**.

Genetics

- Aniridia is inherited in an autosomal dominant fashion with almost complete penetrance but variable expression in about two-thirds of cases.

- The remaining one-third of cases are sporadic-associated with deletion or mutation of PAX6 gene which is telomeric to WT1 gene associated with Wilms tumor.

Clinicopathologic Features
- A rudimentary iris stump is present, which is visible on gonioscopic examination although in some cases it may be visible on the slit lamp. This stump comes to lie over the trabecular meshwork and undergoes contracture leading to progressive angle closure.
- It is almost always associated with foveal hypoplasia and early over nystagmus.

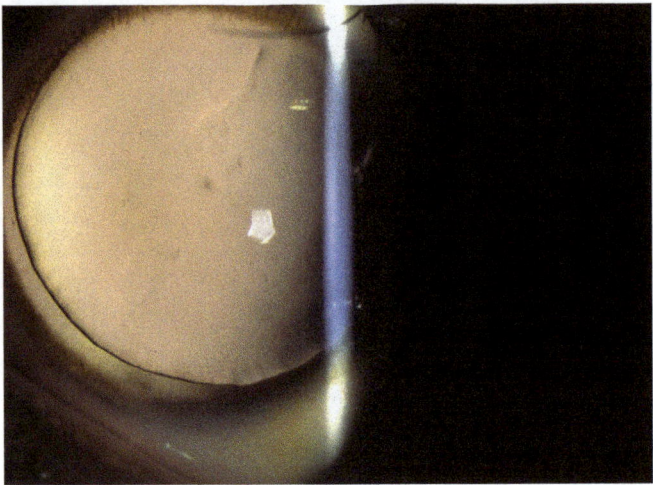

Fig. 2: Aniridia.

Management
- Children with aniridia must undergo regular eye examinations to check for ocular hypertension throughout childhood.
- Trabeculectomy is the preferred procedure for those refractory to medical management.
- Drainage tube surgeries and cyclodiode laser remain the last resort.
- Correction of amblyopia and refractive errors are simple and essential measures.
- Regular renal ultrasound in childhood is imperative to detect Wilms tumor.

Peters Anomaly

Peters anomaly is a sporadic, bilateral anterior dysgenesis of the anterior segment. Peters anomaly can be caused by mutation in the *PAX6* gene, the *PITX2* gene, the *CYP1B1* gene, or the *FOXC1* gene.

Pathophysiology
- The hallmark of Peters anomaly is a central defect in Descemet's membrane and corneal endothelium with thinning and opacification of the corresponding area of corneal stroma.

These are the three major clinical forms of Peters anomaly **(Figs. 3A to C)**.

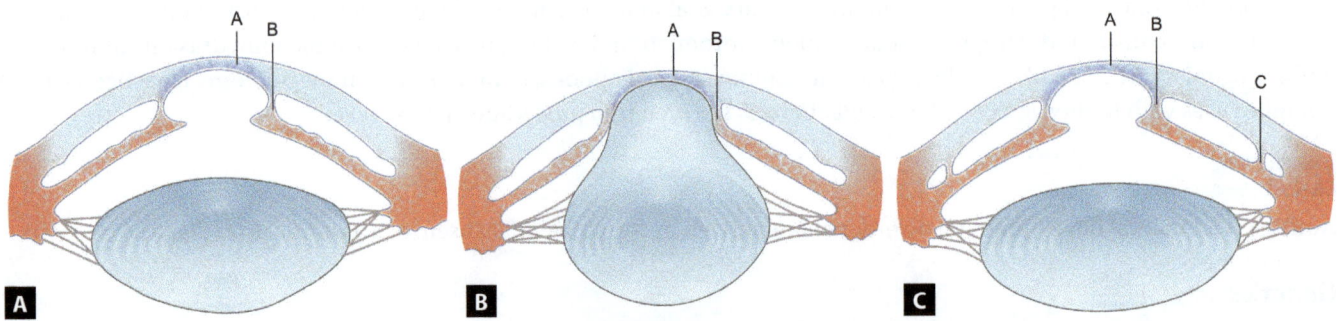

Figs. 3A to C: (A) Peters anomaly without keratolenticular contract; (B) Peters anomalies with keratolenticular contract; (C) Peters anomalies with peripheral defects of Axenfeld–Rieger syndrome.

1. In the presence of other systemic anomalies, it is placed under the group Peters plus syndrome.
2. Approximately one-half of the patients with Peters anomaly will develop glaucoma, frequently presenting in early childhood.
3. Angles are characteristically open, but on ultrastructural studies, aging changes of the trabecular meshwork are seen.

Management

- Treatment aims at clearing the central visual axis through keratoplasty, iridoplasty, and cataract extraction, with medical management of rise in intraocular pressure.
- However, while medical management and filtering surgeries are effective in mild cases, filtering surgeries and cyclodestructive procedures are required in majority of cases.

Suggested Reading

1. Allingham RR, Bruce Shields M (Eds). Shields' Textbook of Glaucoma. Philadelphia: Lippincott Williams & Wilkins; 2005.
2. Bowling B. Kanski's Clinical Ophthalmology, 8th edition. WB Saunders; 2015.
3. Krishnadas R, Ramakrishnan R. Congenital glaucoma—a brief review. J Curr Glaucoma Pract. 2008;2(2):17-25.
4. Stampert RL, Lieberman MF, Drake MV (Eds). Becker-Shaffer's Diagnosis and Therapy of the Glaucomas. Elsevier; 2009.

7.2 Anterior Cleavage Syndromes

Dewang Angmo, Akshaya Balaji, Karthikeyan Mahalingam, Kanchangouri Satpute

1. Discuss the stepladder classification of anterior cleavage syndromes and its management.

Abnormalities of anterior chamber cleavage syndromes, now termed as anterior segment dysgenesis, are due to developmental mesodermal dysgenesis of iris and cornea. They are grouped as central (involving cornea), peripheral (involving angle), and combination of both central and peripheral.[1]

Anatomical findings of anterior cleavage syndromes are tabulated in a stepladder from simple to complex manifestations **(Fig. 1)**:

Posterior Embryotoxon

Prominent, anteriorly displaced Schwalbe's line that appears as gray-white arcuate ridge adjacent to the limbus on the inner surface of the cornea. It occurs as an isolated finding in 8–15% of the population. It can also be a part of Axenfeld–Rieger anomaly.[2]

Axenfeld Anomaly (Fig. 2)

- Caused by defective neural crest cell-related processes during fetal development.
- Characteristic features—posterior embryotoxon and attached strands of peripheral iris viewed on gonioscopy.
- Developmental glaucoma is seen in 50% of the cases.[3]
- Gonioscopy shows broad leaves of iris strands adherent to cornea anterior to Schwalbe's line.

Rieger Anomaly

- Caused by defective neural crest cell related processes during fetal development.
- *Features:*
  - Posterior embryotoxon
  - Iris stromal hypoplasia
  - Ectropion uvea
  - Corectopia and full thickness iris defects
- Manifests with features similar to iridocorneal endothelial syndrome (ICE).
- It is termed as *Rieger syndrome* when associated with extraocular malformations—dental anomalies such as microdontia and hypodontia; facial anomalies such as maxillary hypoplasia, telecanthus, hypertelorism, and broad nasal bridge; renal anomalies and other features—redundant paraumbilical skin, hypospadias, etc.
- Developmental glaucoma is seen in 50% of the cases.[3]

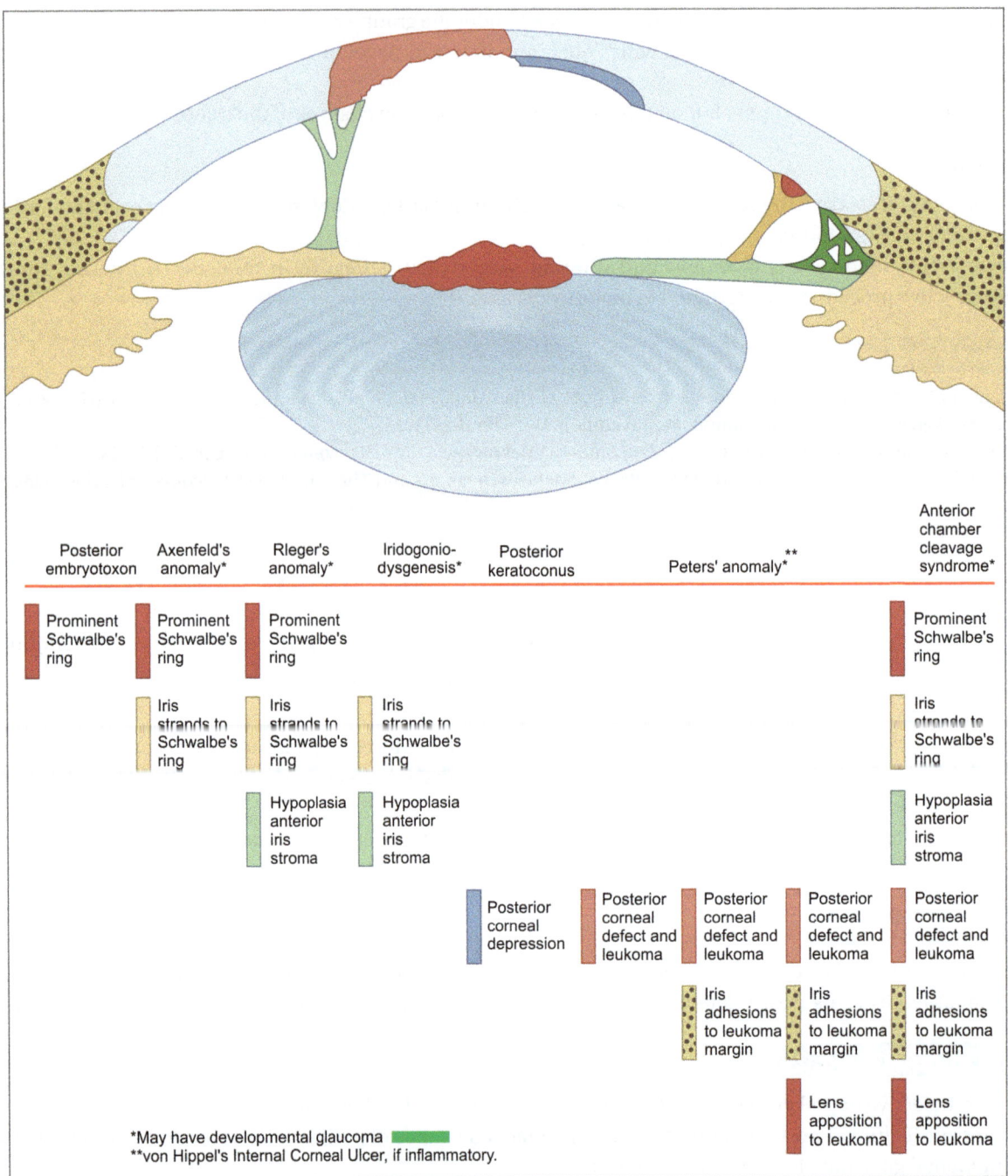

Fig. 1: Stepladder classification.

Peters Anomaly (Fig. 3)

Bilateral rare condition occurs due to defective neural crest cell migration during fetal development. Mostly sporadic can be autosomal recessively inherited. There are two types: type 1 affects cornea only whereas type 2 shows both corneal and lenticular abnormalities.
- *Clinical features:*
    - Central corneal opacity
    - Posterior corneal defect involving Descemet membrane, posterior stroma, and endothelium with or without corneal or lenticulo-corneal adhesions.
    - Glaucoma in 50% cases is associated with angle anomaly.
- Peters-plus syndrome is associated with systemic associations including craniofacial and central nervous system (CNS) anomalies.[4]

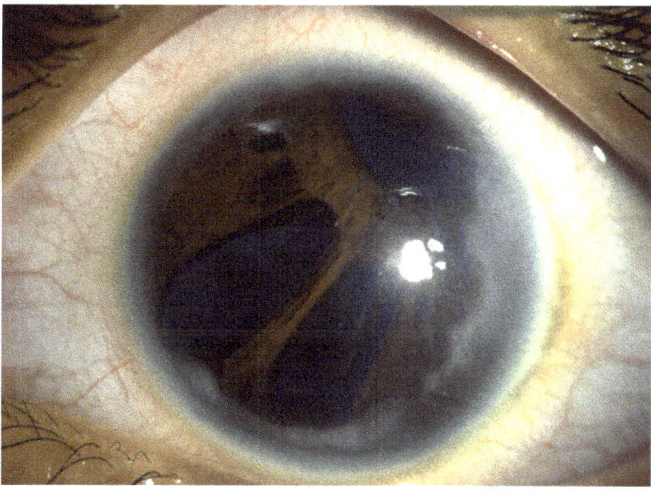

Fig. 2: Axenfeld–Rieger anomaly.

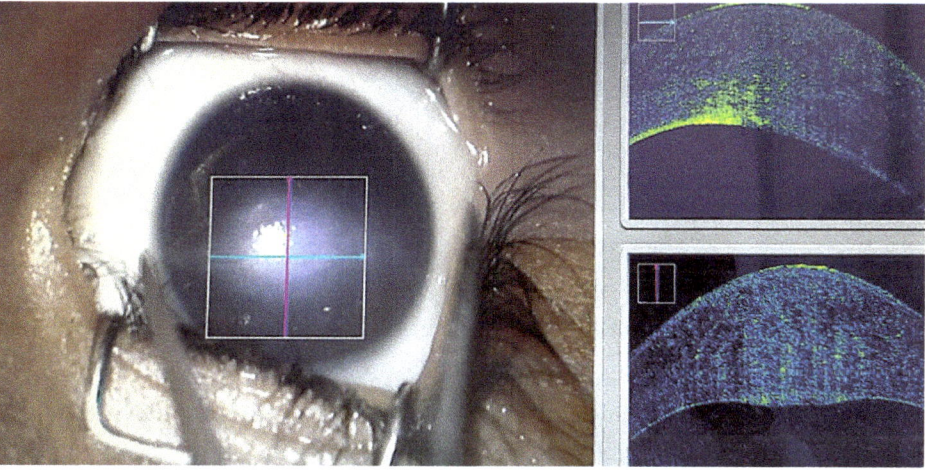

Fig. 3: Peters anomaly.

Aniridia (Fig. 4)[5]

- A rare bilateral condition often having associated systemic manifestations.
- Due to abnormal neuroectodermal development secondary to *PAX 6* gene adjacent to *WT1* mutation.
- Autosomal dominant aniridia has no systemic associations—about two-thirds cases.
- Sporadic cases are a part of WAGR syndrome (Wilms tumor, aniridia, mental retardation, and genitourinary anomalies): 30% of cases have risk of developing Wilms tumor.
- Presentation is at birth with photophobia, decreased visual acuity, and nystagmus.
- Gonioscopy shows rudimentary or hypoplastic iris tissue.
- Glaucoma is seen in 75% cases presenting late in childhood due to synechial angle closure.
- Associated cataract, amblyopia, and subluxation of the lens can be seen.

Management

Peripheral Abnormalities

- Usually mild where glaucoma is the only vision-threatening complication.
- Routine examination with intraocular pressure (IOP) measurement is to be recorded.
- Medical management of glaucoma is not usually adequate.
- May require surgical options for managing IOP.
- Lifelong follow-up is mandatory.
- Family screening is advised routinely.

Central Abnormalities

- Infants are brought with leukocoria—examination under anesthesia is to be done with IOP measurement using Mackay-Marg tonometer.
- Ultra-biomicroscopy is done to rule out lenticular adhesions and look for angle anomalies.
- Cases with central corneal opacity generally have poor visual outcomes where penetrating keratoplasty has a role to prevent amblyopia and improve vision.
- If patient presents later, refractive error correction in the form of spectacles, and contact lens are given.
- Refractory glaucoma is seen in most cases which do not respond to medical management requiring surgical options early in life such as trabeculectomy with trabeculotomy with mitomycin-C application. Shunt procedures also have a role.

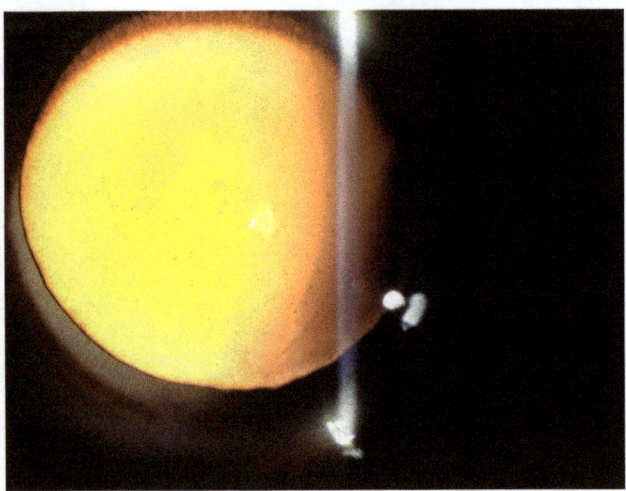

Fig. 4: Aniridia.[5]

Aniridia

- Glaucoma management with various surgical options such as trabeculectomy with trabeculotomy, glaucoma drainage devices, and diode laser cyclophotocoagulation are done.[6]
- Painted contact lenses for cosmesis.
- Lubricants for associated keratopathy.
- Prosthetic iris implantation in pseudophakics.
- Refractive error, amblyopia, and squint to be managed aggressively.

References

1. Waring GO, Rodrigues MM, Laibson PR. Anterior chamber cleavage syndrome. A stepladder classification. Surv Ophthalmol. 1975;20(1):3-27.
2. Burian HM, Braley AE, Allen L. Visibility of the ring of Schwalbe and the trabecular zone; an interpretation of the posterior corneal embryotoxon and the so-called congenital hyaline membranes on the posterior corneal surface. AMA Arch Ophthalmol. 1955;53(6):767-82.
3. Tanwar M, Dada T, Dada R. Axenfeld-Rieger syndrome associated with congenital glaucoma and cytochrome P4501B1 gene mutations. Case Rep Med. 2010;2010:212656.
4. Lesnik Oberstein SA, Ruivenkamp CA, Hennekam RC. Peters plus syndrome. In: Adam MP, Ardinger HH, Pagon RA, Wallace SE, Bean LJ, Stephens K, et al. (Eds). GeneReviews®. Seattle (WA): University of Washington; 1993.
5. Bremond-Gignac D. Congenital aniridia in children. Rev Prat. 2019;69(1):67-70.
6. Soyugelen Demirok G, Ekşioğlu Ü, Yakın M, Kaderli A, Kaderli ST, Örnek F. Short- and long-term results of glaucoma valve implantation for aniridia-related glaucoma: a case series and literature review. Turk J Ophthalmol. 2019;49(4):183-7.

7.3 Epidemiology of Glaucoma

Neha Midha, Dewang Angmo

Q 1. Write a note on epidemiology of glaucoma in India.

Glaucoma is the leading cause of irreversible blindness in India with at least 12 million people affected and nearly 1.2 million people blind from the disease. An additional 28 million are diagnosed with ocular hypertension, primary angle-closure or primary angle-closure suspect. Every 1 out of 8 people above the age of 40 years in India is either suffering from glaucoma or is at risk of the disease. India accounts for a minimum of 12.9% of primary open-angle glaucoma (POAG) blindness and 12.7% of primary angle-closure glaucoma (PACG) blindness in the world.[1,2]

The prevalence and risk factors of glaucoma have been studied by many population-based studies such as the Central India Eye and Medical Study (CIEMS), Chennai Glaucoma Study (CGS) for rural and urban populations, Vellore Eye Study (VES), Andhra Pradesh Eye Disease Study (APEDS), West Bengal Glaucoma Study (WBGS), Hooghly River Glaucoma Study (HRGS), and Aravind Comprehensive Eye Survey (ACES).

The prevalence of POAG ranges from 0.4% in VES to 3.5% in CGS (urban) and PACG from 0.2% in WBGS to 4.32% in VES. Except VES, all other population studies have shown higher prevalence of POAG as compared to PACG this disparity is possibly due to differences in case definitions and inclusion criteria of each study.

More than 90% of patients (rural > urban) are unaware about the disease at the time of recruitment in the study, highlighting inadequacy of glaucoma awareness and screening programs in India.

Risk factors:
- Age has been found to be an important risk factor and patients over the age of 70 years were five times more likely to have POAG than those younger than 50 years (CGS).
- *Gender:* Most studies have found higher prevalence of POAG in men (ACES and HRGS) while CGS found no gender predilection. PACG was found to be more common in females.
- *Refractive error:* POAG is more common in myopes while PACG is more common in hyperopes.
- Higher vertical cup-disc ratio (CDR) >0.6:1 is found to be an important predictor (CGS and HRGS).
- *Genetic:* POAG is a multifactorial disease caused by the interactions among genetic, systemic, and environmental factors, a substantial fraction of POAG (5%) has genetic basis. The four most commonly involved genes include Myocilin, *CYP1B1*, Optineurin, and *WDR36*.
- First-degree relatives (FDRs) of glaucoma patients have a 10-fold increase in the risk of glaucoma.

Secondary glaucoma: The prevalence of secondary glaucoma ranges from 0.15% to 0.3% (HRGS and ACES). Most common causes include pseudoexfoliation, pigment dispersion syndrome, uveitic, neovascular, and phacomorphic.

Childhood glaucoma: Primary congenital glaucoma (PCG) is the most common childhood glaucoma. The prevalence of PCG is one in 3,300 live births and it accounts for 4.2% of all childhood blindness in Indian population. It is most commonly bilateral and male:female ratio almost equal to 1.[3]

Common secondary childhood glaucoma are: glaucoma associated with ocular anomalies, traumatic glaucoma, and steroid-induced glaucoma.

References

1. George R, Ve RS, Vijaya L. Glaucoma in India: estimated burden of disease. J Glaucoma. 2010;19(6):391-39.
2. George R, Vijaya L. Prevalence of glaucoma in India: a review. J Curr Glaucoma Pract. 2007;1(2):7-11.
3. Senthil S, Badakere S, Ganesh J, Krishnamurthy R, Dikshit S, Choudhari N, et al. Profile of childhood glaucoma at a tertiary center in South India. Indian J Ophthalmol. 2019;67(3):358-65.

7.4. Optic Nerve Head Damage and Visual Field Changes

Priyanka Mishra, Dewang Angmo

 1. Discuss the different types of visual field defect seen in open-angle glaucoma.

Structural changes in glaucoma usually precede functional loss. Visual field defects (VFD) are picked up in standard automated perimetry only after the loss of 25–35% of retinal ganglion cells (RGCs), and ≤10% axons remain by the stage of severe field loss. The defects usually follow the topographical arrangement of axons in the optic nerve.

Table depicting visual field defects in glaucoma.

Localized NFL defect	Peripheral field loss	Generalized or central depression
• Paracentral	• Nasal step	• Concentric contraction
• Seidel	• Vertical step	• Enlargement of blind spot
• Arcuate	• Temporal sector defect	• Angioscotomata
• Double arcuate		
(NFL: nerve fiber layer)		

Visual field defects can be divided into three groups:
1. *Localized nerve fiber layer defect:*
   a. Initial damage to ≥1 axon bundles
   b. Most definitive early evidence of visual field defect from glaucoma.
   c. Follows retinal topography.

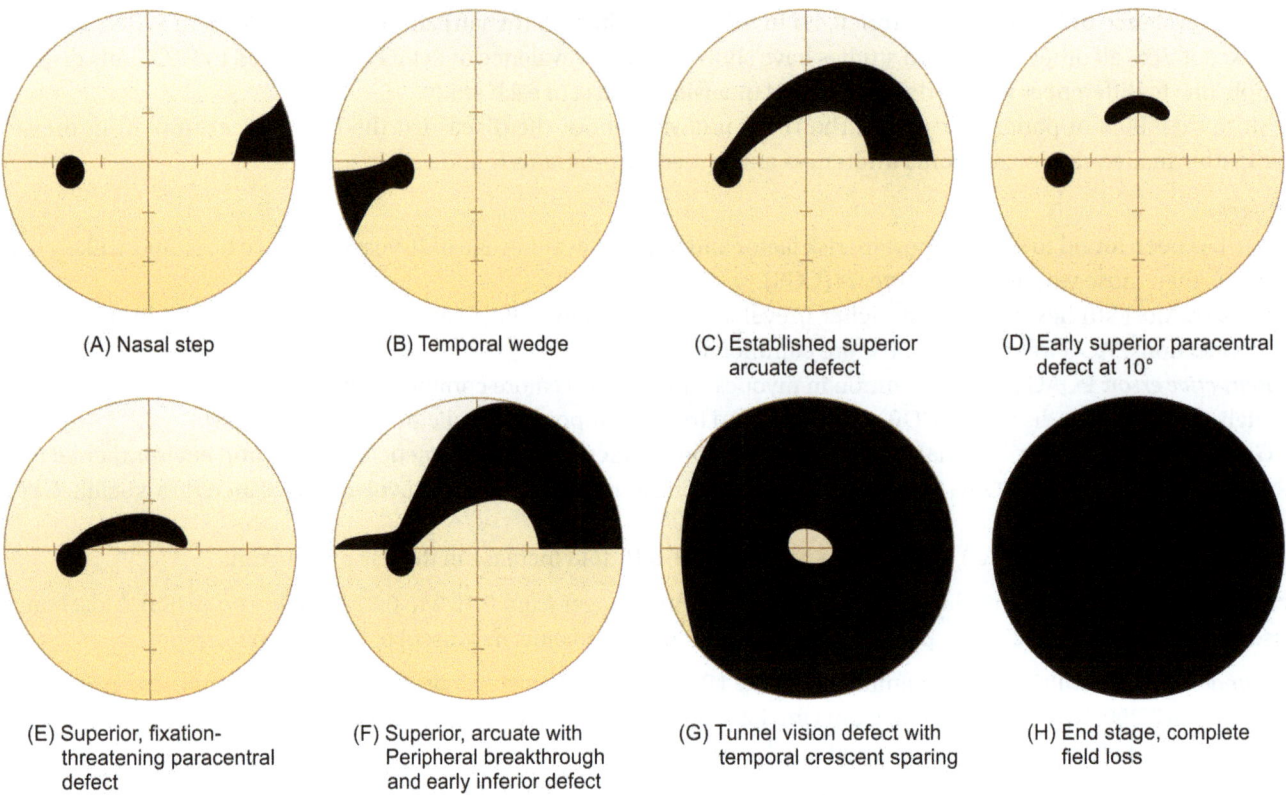

Fig. 1: Types of visual field defect.

Types of localized defects **(Fig. 1)**:
a. *Paracentral scotoma:* Shallow paracentral depression which becomes larger and denser to give absolute surrounded by relative scotoma.
b. *Seidel scotoma:* Early arcuate defect; it may connect to the blind spot and taper to a point in slightly curved course.
c. *Arcuate/Bjerrum scotoma:*
   i. It starts from the blind spot and arches above or/and below the fixation to the horizontal median raphe, corresponding to the arcuate retinal nerve fiber layer (RNFL).
   ii. Nasal extreme can involve up to 1° from fixation, extending to 10-20° nasally.
   iii. Superior field involvement is more common.
d. Double arcuate/ring scotoma.
2. *Peripheral visual field loss:*
   a. Usually associated with more central field defect
   b. Isolated defect in 3–11% cases
   c. Can be missed in standard achromatic perimetry (SAP).

Types of peripheral defect:
a. *Nasal step:*
   i. Most common peripheral defect
   ii. Common in acute or early chronic angle closure glaucoma (CACG)
   iii. Forms due to disparity of defect in between hemispheres
   iv. Can be central, peripheral or isolated scotoma in periphery
   v. *Central:* Due to unequal double arcuate field loss closer to fixation
   vi. *Peripheral nasal step of Ronne:* Formed due to unequal contraction of fields on the peripheral side of defect; there is loss of corresponding peripheral arcuate defect.
b. *Vertical steps or hemianopic offset:*
   i. Rare
   ii. More seen nasally

iii. It should be considered with suspicion only if located temporally as nasal defect can be seen in normal population also
iv. It is related to the segregation of axons from either side of vertical midline in the optic nerve head (ONH).
c. *Temporal sector or wedge defect:*
    i. Usually appears late, but can be presenting defect
    ii. Due to the lesion involving the nerve fibers nasal to the disc coursing straight.
3. *Generalized and central depression of visual field:*
    a. It is related to diffuse RNFL loss

    Types:
    a. *Concentric/isopter contraction:*
        i. Early visual field defect
        ii. More marked in nasal field, which has been called as "crowding of the peripheral nasal isopters"
    b. *Enlargement of blind spot:*
        i. Due to depression of peripapillary retinal sensitivity
        ii. Early glaucomatous field change
        iii. *Differential diagnosis:* AIBSE (acute idiopathic blind spot enlargement), papilledema, healthy persons with threshold targets
    c. *Angioscotomata:*
        i. May represent early glaucomatous field defect but not diagnostic
        ii. Seen as long branching scotoma above and below blind spot
        iii. Presumed to be due to the shadows of large retinal vessels, which may have representation in the visual cortex
    d. *Advanced glaucomatous field defect:*
        i. Double arcuate scotoma, coalescing nasally, and may extend peripherally to involve the peripheral limits in all areas, except temporally.
        ii. The temporal island of vision is more resistant and may persist long after central vision is lost.

 2. Describe the various concepts that explain the pathogenesis of optic nerve damage in glaucoma.

Theories for glaucomatous optic neuropathy (GON):
- *Mechanical theory of Muller:* Elevated intraocular pressure (IOP) causes direct compression and death of RGCs.
- Vascular theory of Jaeger
- Schnabel cavernous atrophy of optic neuropathy (ON).

The present evidences suggest the role of obstruction of axoplasmic flow in the pathogenesis. However, it is unclear whether mechanical, vascular or any other factor is responsible for the axoplasmic obstruction.

Other speculations involve the possible role of excitotoxicity, apoptosis, neurotrophin deprivation, and autoimmunity.

Mechanical theory **(Flowchart 1)**:
- The posterior and lateral displacement of lamina cribrosa (LC), and the misalignment of the fenestrae of the multilayered LC.
- There is greater displacement in the periphery, corresponding to the early axonal loss in the inferior and superior axonal bundles.
- The larger fibers are more prone, probably due to the higher proportion in the superior and inferior segments.
- Innate constriction at LC may be a factor in glaucoma wherein IOP is not elevated. The extracellular matrix of LC plays important role in progression.

Vascular theory **(Flowchart 2)**:
- Probably, less role than mechanical
- Explains the association of disc hemorrhage in cases of normal-tension glaucoma (NTG) and its association with vasospastic episodes
- Systemic hypotension and autonomic dysregulation related to glaucoma progression
- *Autoregulation in retinal blood vessels:* Normally retinal vessels alter their tone to maintain a constant blood flow independent of IOP. This has been seen to be impaired in cases of glaucoma.

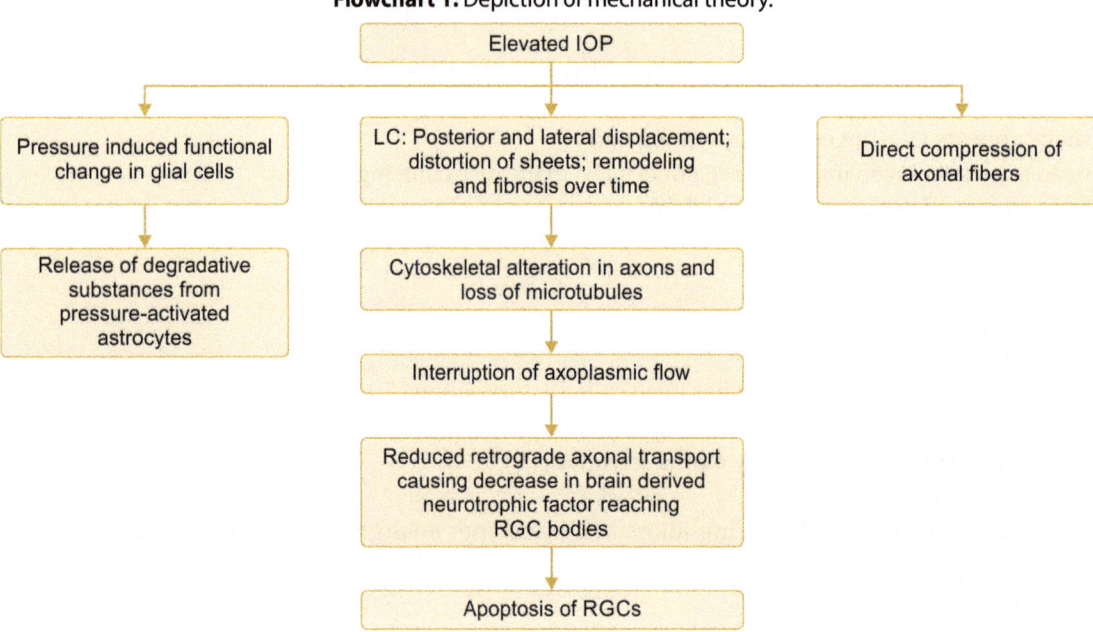

Flowchart 1: Depiction of mechanical theory.

(IOP: intraocular pressure; LC: lamina cribrosa; RGC: retinal ganglion cell)

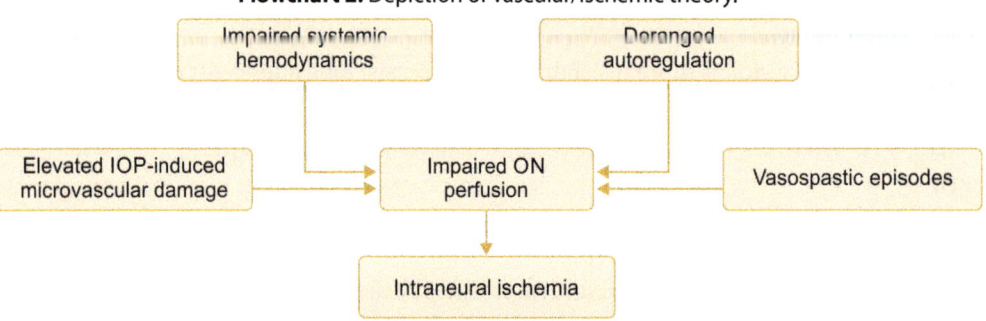

Flowchart 2: Depiction of vascular/ischemic theory.

(IOP: intraocular pressure; ON: optic neuropathy)

Cerebrospinal fluid (CSF) pressure and GON:
- Cerebrospinal fluid (CSF) extends anteriorly to the ON sheath and the subarachnoid space to the posterior aspect of LC.
- *Translaminar pressure:* The difference between IOP and CSF pressure has been demonstrated to play important role in the pathogenesis of GON.
- CSF pressure has been found to be significantly decreased in patients with chronic open-angle glaucoma (COAG) and NTG; and higher in ocular hypertension (OHT).

Excitotoxicity and role of glutamate: Altered delivery of neurotrophin + impaired nutrition → stressed metabolism → impaired Muller cells function → increased extracellular glutamate → RGC toxicity

 3. Discuss preperimetric glaucoma, its diagnosis, and factors in progression of field defects.

Preperimetric glaucoma is defined as the presence of characteristic glaucomatous optic disc and RNFL damage, in the absence of detectable visual field defect on conventional SAP.
- It may be said to represent the mild/early stage of glaucoma.
- It has been reported that up to 40% of RGCs can be lost before white-on-white perimetry will show an abnormality.
- In most of the cases, structural changes can be picked up prior to the functional changes.

Diagnosis: Following tests are useful in the diagnosis of preperimetric glaucoma.

Structural tests	**Functional tests**	
1. Clinical examination	*Perimetry techniques*	*Electrophysiological*
2. ONH photography:	1. SWAP	1. ERG (PERG, mfERG)
a. Two-dimensional	2. FDT	2. VEP
b. Stereoscopic	3. FDF	3. Afferent pupillary reaction
3. USG B scan	4. High pass resolution perimetry	
4. *Computed analysis of ONH and RNFL:*	5. Motion detection perimetry	
a. CSLO		
b. SLP		
c. OCT		

(CSLO: confocal scanning laser ophthalmoscopy; ERG: electroretinography; FDF: Flicker defined form; FDT: frequency doubling technology; mfERG: multifocal electroretinography; OCT: optical coherence tomography; ONH: optic nerve head; PERG: pattern electroretinography; RNFL: retinal nerve fiber layer; SLP: scanning laser polarimetry; SWAP: short-wavelength automated perimetry; USG B scan: ultrasonography B scan; VEP: visual-evoked potentials)

Structural Tests

1. *Clinical examination of ONH and RNFL:*
   a. Subjective with mild interobserver agreement and can be inconclusive in early cases; but progressive changes denote glaucomatous damage
   b. Using direct ophthalmoscopy, slit lamp biomicroscopy
   c. *Size of ONH: This includes the use of:*
      i. Direct ophthalmoscope using either a graticule incorporated in the instrument or the smallest round white light spot of Welch Allen model, which projects a 1.5 mm diameter spot on retina in most eyes
      ii. Binocular indirect ophthalmoscope (BIO) with a spacing device on condensing lens
      iii. Slit lamp biomicroscopy with a condensing or contact lens, using an appropriate correction factor
   d. Red-free filter for RNFL defects
   e. Findings can be depicted with drawing.

Disc patterns in early GON	
Focal atrophy	Usually IT and ST region, vertical or oblique enlargement of cup; violation of ISNT rule; focal notch, bayoneting
Concentric atrophy	Usually directed IT or ST; temporal unfolding; crescentic shadow adjacent to disc margin; difficult to distinguish from physiologic cup; look for symmetry in fellow eye
Deepening of cup	Laminar dot sign
Pallor-cup discrepancy	May occur with focal or diffuse enlargement of cup; Saucerization (diffuse, shallow cupping extending to disc margins with the retention of central cup); focal Saucerization (usually IT, with "tinted hollow") shadow sign, laminar dot sign

(GON: glaucomatous optic neuropathy)

Vascular signs in early GON	
Optic disc hemorrhage	• Most commonly inferiorly; especially in NTG; Frequency declines in the advanced stage • Associated with progression
Overpass cupping	Vessels bridge the cup
Baring of circumciliary vessels	May be occasionally seen normally; its presence in glaucoma suspect is associated with development of VFD
Vertical eccentricity of central retinal vessel trunk	
Proximal constriction of retinal arteries near disc	In 42% patients with normal- and high-tension glaucomas; corresponding to sectors of greatest cupping

(GON: glaucomatous optic neuropathy; NTG: normal-tension glaucoma; VFD: visual field defect)

Vascular signs in early GON	
Optic disc hemorrhage	• Most commonly inferiorly; especially in NTG; Frequency declines in the advanced stage • Associated with progression
Overpass cupping	Vessels bridge the cup
Baring of circumciliary vessels	May be occasionally seen normally; its presence in glaucoma suspect is associated with development of VFD
Vertical eccentricity of central retinal vessel trunk	
Proximal constriction of retinal arteries near disc	In 42% patients with normal- and high-tension glaucomas; corresponding to sectors of greatest cupping

(GON: glaucomatous optic neuropathy; NTG: normal-tension glaucoma; VFD: visual field defect)

Peripapillary changes associated with early GON	
RNFL defects	Focal loss appears as wedge-shaped defect in peripapillary area, paralleling the retinal striations, or as diffuse loss of striations; often following disc hemorrhages
Peripapillary pigmentary changes	• Larger beta area-to-disc area ratio was found to be associated with an increased risk of glaucomatous damage • Both alpha and beta zones occur more frequently and are larger in eyes with glaucoma and increase progressively with an increase in damage

(GON: glaucomatous optic neuropathy; RNFL: retinal nerve fiber layer)

2. *Photographic techniques:* It is helpful for recording the findings of ONH, RNFL defect (especially with red-free filter), and peripapillary area
   This is helpful for longitudinal follow-up. It allows looking for progressive changes.
3. *Ultrasonography:* Not useful for early GON; can detect cup-to-disc ratio (CDR) of ≥0.7:1.
4. *Computed analysis of ONH and RNFL:*
   a. Some patients demonstrate structural alterations in the ONH, parapapillary RNFL, and macular RNFL before functional changes are detectable.
   b. Can help in early diagnosis and detection of glaucoma
   c. Results must be interpreted in context of clinical examination and other tests to avoid concluding a statistically abnormal result as true disease.
   d. Progression analysis may be helpful.
   e. The different methods are as follows:
      i. *Confocal scanning laser tomography (ONH evaluated):*
         1. High-resolution images are obtained by using confocal laser beams to measure several reflected light intensities at different focal planes in different depths, for each location.
         2. HRT (Heidelberg retina tomography) produces quantitative measurements of the morphometric parameters of ONH that can be used to classify it as normal or glaucomatous, or to compare topographic images to quantify progression [Topographic Change Analysis (TCA) or change probability map].
         3. The parameters that are most useful are cup shape measure, rim area, variation of height contour line, and RNFL thickness. Other less useful parameters include disc and cup area and volume, mean and maximum cup depth.
      ii. *Confocal scanning laser polarimetry (RNFL evaluated):*
         1. It is a CSLO with an integrated polarimeter that measures the amount of retardation (phase shift) of polarized light (λ = 780 nm) as it passes through birefringent tissue (e.g., RNFL).
         2. The variable/enhanced corneal compensator (GDxVCC, GDxECC) corrects for the polarization induced by the cornea and lens.
      iii. *Optical coherence tomography (ONH, RNFL, Macula evaluated)*

Functional Tests

- *FDT (frequency doubling technology):* It has demonstrated high sensitivity and specificity in glaucoma suspects for detecting VFDs that are predictive functional loss detected on SAP later. These newer methods target the redundancy of the visual system.

- *Short-wavelength automated perimetry:* It tests a small subgroup of small ganglion cells, called bistratified blue-yellow ganglion cells, which are sensitive to blue stimuli. It has been demonstrated to predict the development of glaucoma in patients with ocular hypertension, and the patients in which the VFD is likely to progress.
- *Frequency doubling field:* It is based on the frequency doubling illusion and targets a subset of large diameter ganglion cells, called My ganglion cells, projecting to the magnocellular pathway. These cells detect motion and contrast and are thought to get affected early.
- *High-pass resolution perimetry or ring perimetry:* It is essentially a peripheral visual acuity test using vanishing optotypes. It tests the parvocellular system. It was demonstrated to identify glaucomatous VFD in early and moderate stages.
- *Random dot motion automated perimetry:* It targets the reduced motion sense in glaucoma by presenting a directional shift in position of dots in a defined circular area against a background of fixed dots. The VFDs correspond to focal changes in ONH topography.

Electrophysiological Tests

- *Electroretinogram:*
  - Reduced pattern electroretinography (PERG) amplitudes may be seen in the early stages of glaucoma, and in some eyes with ocular hypertension which are at risk of developing glaucoma.
  - Multifocal electroretinography (mfERG) may be able to detect abnormalities before SAP.
- *Visual-evoked potentials (VEP):*
  - More variable than PERG
  - It has been suggested that the signal in multifocal visual evoked potential (mfVEP) and the sensitivity of Humphrey visual fields (HVF) are linearly related to RGC loss.

Afferent pupillary defect: It has been shown to be proportional to the amount of visual field defect. It may precede the VFD detected on SAP.

4. Short note on criteria of glaucomatous visual field changes.

The Hoddap–Parrish–Anderson classification system considers mean deviation (MD) value and the number of depressed points in the Humphrey Statpac-2 pattern deviation (PD) probability map of the 24-2, SITA (Swedish Interactive Threshold Algorithm) STANDARD test **(Table 1)**.

Criteria for early disease:
- MD < –6 dB
- <25% of the points (18) depressed below the 5% level; and <10 points depressed below the 1% level on the PD plot
- All points in central 5° must have sensitivity of at least 15 dB.

Criteria for early disease:
- MD < –12 dB
- <50% of the points (37) depressed below the 5% level; and <20 points depressed below the 1% level on the PD plot
- No point in central 5° can have sensitivity of 0 dB.
- Only one hemifield may have a point of sensitivity of <15 dB within 5° of fixation.

Criteria for early disease:
- MD > –12 dB
- >50% of the points (37) depressed below the 5% level; and >20 points depressed below the 1% level on the PD plot
- At least one point in central 5° has a sensitivity of 0 dB.
- Points within central 5° with sensitivity <15 dB in both hemifield.

TABLE 1: Hoddap–Parrish–Anderson classification system.

Stage	MD (in dB)	Points below 5%*	Points below 1%*	Points in central 5°	GH
Early	<–6	<25%	<15%	No point <15 dB	–
Moderate	–6 to –12	<50%	<25%	No point ≤0 dB	One GH has point <15 dB within central 5°
Severe	>–12	>50%	>25%	Any point ≤0 dB	Both GHs have points <15 dB within central 5°

(GH: glaucoma hemifield; MD: mean deviation)
*On pattern deviation plot.

5. Short note on epidemic dropsy glaucoma.

It refers to a hypersecretory glaucoma, occurring in association of epidemic dropsy. Epidemic dropsy refers to an acute toxic multisystem disease resulting from unintentional ingestion of alkaloids, sanguinarine, and dihydrosanguinarine in *Argemone mexicana*. This is an adulterant of cooking oil, usually mustard oil.

Epidemiology:
- Incidence among epidemic dropsy patients: 1–12%
- Predominantly affects young individuals (21–40 years)
- Male > female
- Clustering of cases to a community or a family
- History/risk of ingestion of particularly adulterated food item
- Usually occurs after 4–6 weeks of systemic involvement.

Pathophysiology:
- Hypersecretory
- Aqueous assay reveals elevated prostaglandin E_2 (PGE_2) levels, histamine activity, and increased osmolarity due to increased extravasation of low-molecular-weight proteins with normal globulin fraction.
- Dilatation and increased permeability of capillaries in the whole uveal tract
- Open angles, normal outflow facility, normal trabecular meshwork by histopathologic and histochemical tests
- Antiadrenaline action of sanguinarine is also proposed to be responsible.

Symptoms: Burning sensation, ocular irritation, diminution of vision associated with colored halos

Ocular findings:
- Bilateral, may be asymmetric
- Corneal edema
- Presenting IOP is usually high approximately 50 mm Hg in a white eye
- *Associated findings:* Retinal vascular dilation and tortuosity (40–90%), superficial retinal hemorrhages (10–60% approximately), subconjunctival hemorrhage, macular edema, subhyaloid hemorrhage, anemic retinopathy, disc edema, and central retinal vein occlusion (CRVO)
- Retinal vascular changes correlate more with the systemic disease rather than the increase in IOP

Visual field changes:
- It is supposed to be due to retinal toxicity and leaking microangiopathy.
- More frequent in early part of disease, with gradual improvement with the recovery of retinal cells.
- Independent of increase in IOP; occurred in epidemic dropsy patients without ocular symptoms or increased IOP.
- Central and nasal defects predominate
- Advanced and permanent field changes can occur in eyes with prolonged high IOP.

Associated systemic findings: Explosive onset of leg edema, with tenderness, erythema, and rash over edematous parts, gastrointestinal (GI) symptoms, pallor, low-grade fever, hepatomegaly, congestive heart failure that may be fatal.

Tests: Such as nitric oxide, ferric chloride tests silica gel chromatography, spectrophotometric assay in oil, serum, and urine samples

Treatment:
- Glaucoma is self-limited; filtering surgery can be done when maximal tolerable medical therapy fails.
- Topical and systemic aqueous suppressant are preferred; drugs targeting outflow, are usually ineffective.
- Topical clonidine, a centrally acting drug, or sympathomimetic agent can be useful.
- Systemic or topical nonsteroidal anti-inflammatory drugs (NSAIDs), especially indomethacin, aspirin, and topical steroids, can be used due to their antiprostaglandin action.

Suggested Reading

1. Allingham RR, Damji KF, Shields MB. Shields Textbook of Glaucoma. Philadelphia: Wolters Kluwer Health/Lippincott Williams & Wilkins; 2011.
2. Gessesse GW, Damji KF. Advanced glaucoma: management pearls. Middle East Afr J Ophthalmol. 2013;20(2):131-41.
3. Hakim SA. Argemone oil, sanguinarine, and epidemic-dropsy glaucoma. Br J Ophthalmol. 1954;38(4):193-216.

4. Jonas JB, Budde WM. Diagnosis and pathogenesis of glaucomatous optic neuropathy: morphological aspects. Prog Retin Eye Res. 2000;19(1):1-40.
5. Rosenberg LF, Gedde SJ, Mansberger SL, Stein JD, Moroi SE, Herndon Jr LW, et al. Primary Open-Angle Glaucoma Preferred Practice Pattern® guidelines. Ophthalmology. 2016;123(1):P41-111.
6. Sachdev MS, Sood NN, Verma LK, Gupta SK, Jaffery NF. Pathogenesis of epidemic dropsy glaucoma. Arch Ophthalmol. 1988;106(9): 1221-3.
7. Singh K, Singh MJ, Das JC. Visual field defects in epidemic dropsy. Clin Toxicol (Phila). 2006;44(2):159-63.
8. Susanna Jr R, Vessani RM. Staging glaucoma patient: why and how? Open Ophthalmol J. 2009;3:59-64.
9. Weinreb RN, Aung T, Medeiros FA. The pathophysiology and treatment of glaucoma: a review. JAMA. 2014;311(18):1901-11.

7.4.1 Short-wavelength Automated Perimetry

Dewang Angmo, Karthikeyan Mahalingam

Q 1. Short note on short-wavelength automated perimetry.

The standard automated white-on-white perimetry (SAP) is the gold standard for the functional assessment of ganglion cells. But it does not show an abnormality unless 25–50% of ganglion cells have been lost.[1] Thus, it is less sensitive to detect early glaucoma. Certain ganglion cells damaged by glaucoma have less redundancy (fewer partner cells that cover up their function when they are lost).[2] So, tests such as short-wavelength automated perimetry (SWAP) and frequency-doubling technology (FDT) which target the ganglion cells which have little redundancy can detect early glaucoma.

Short-wavelength Automated Perimetry

It tests the blue-cone mechanisms and the konio ganglion cells that carry this information. Color vision is affected in glaucoma and tests that include the blue-yellow end of the spectrum will be more specific for glaucomatous damage.[3]

Testing

- The background is bright yellow (500 nm) and a blue-violet (440 nm), Goldmann size V stimulus is projected onto it.
- This stimulus size is significantly larger than that usually used in white-on-white threshold perimetry (Goldmann size III).
- The determination of threshold in the standard SWAP test is the same as used in the full-threshold SAP **(Fig. 1)**.

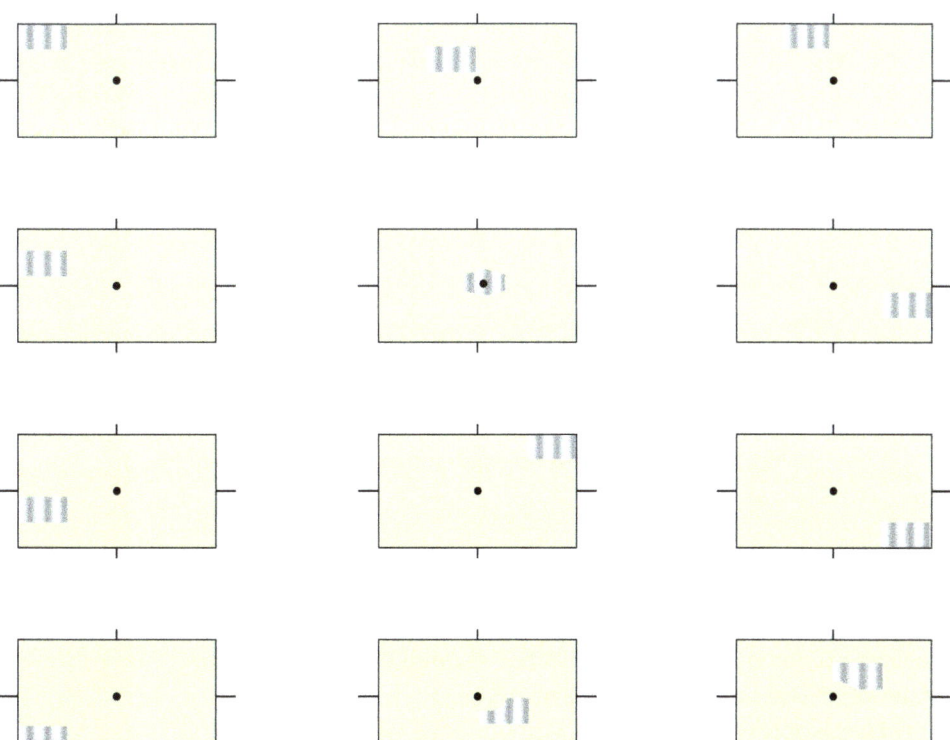

Fig. 1: Alternating dark and light stripes are presented in 17 different parts of the visual field in the original device, and 64 in the matrix. The contrast between the dark and light stripes is varied to define the threshold.

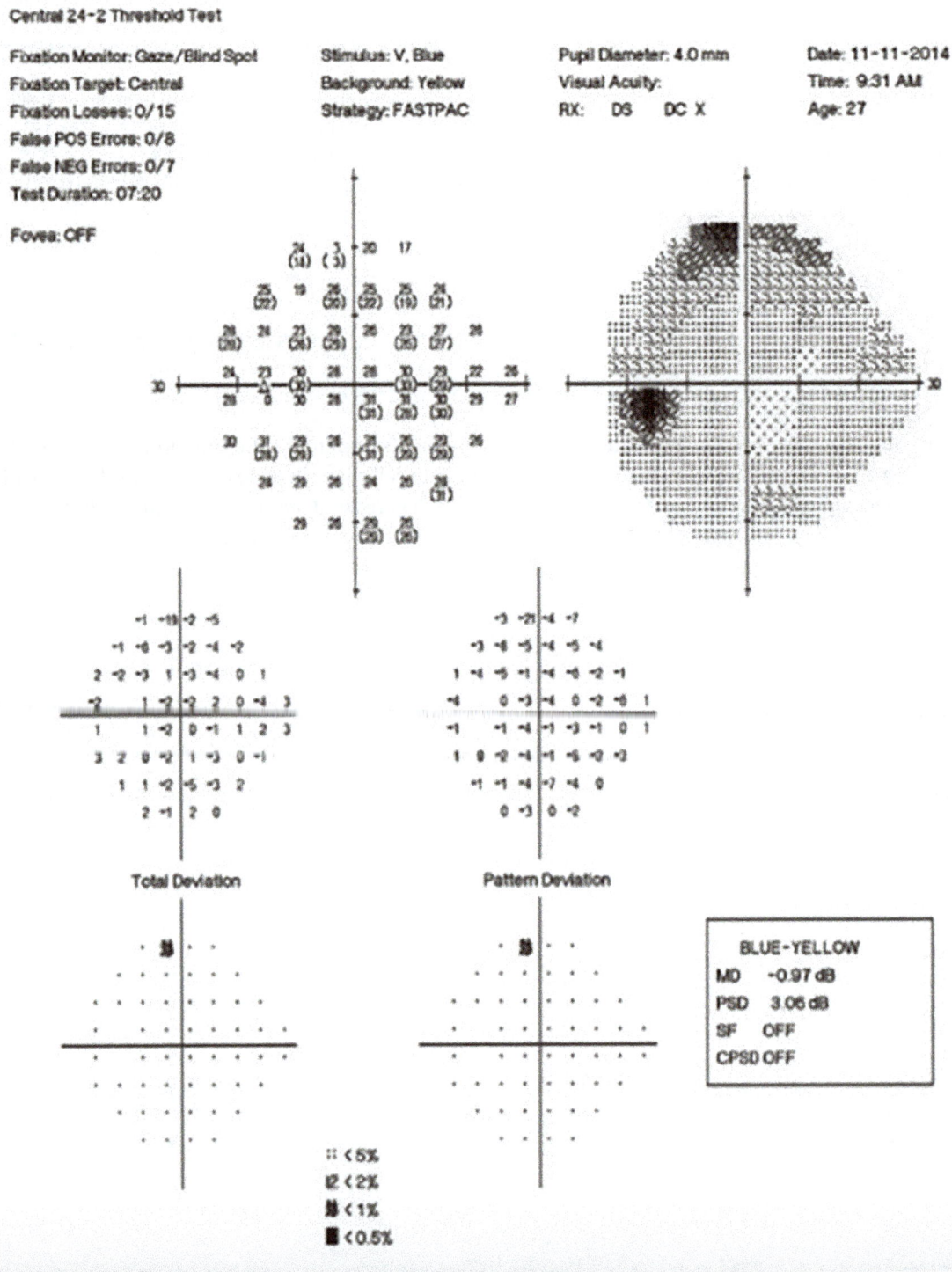

Fig. 2: Output of short-wavelength automated perimetry (SWAP).

- The probability of abnormality is indicated with the help of STATPAC as it contains normative database for SWAP. Abnormalities detected in SWAP are predictive of ultimate defects in SAP. Several studies have demonstrated the superiority of SWAP over SAP in both early detections of glaucoma and its progression.[4,5] A SWAP **(Fig. 2)** is considered abnormal if the following criteria are met on at least two examinations:[6]
- Pattern standard deviation is abnormal at worse than 1% level
- Glaucoma hemifield test is outside normal limits
- There is one hemifield cluster with sensitivity below the 1% level, there are two hemifield clusters below the 5% level, there are four abnormal (<0.05%) points, or there are five abnormal (<0.05%) points on the pattern deviation plot.

TABLE 1: Advantages and disadvantages of short-wavelength automated perimetry (SWAP).

Advantages	Disadvantages
Early detection of glaucoma defects	Tedious
Tracking progression	Takes 20–30 minutes per eye
Can be done in most of the available perimeters	Affected by media opacities
Familiar format on results	Affected by refractive error

Short-wavelength automated perimetry is likely to detect functional glaucomatous damage and progression before SAP. However, problems with media opacities, length of test, fatigue, tediousness, high long-term fluctuation, and repeatability compared to SAP limit its usefulness, especially in the elderly **(Table 1)**. The advent of SITA (Swedish Interactive Threshold Algorithm) SWAP may reduce the tediousness, duration, and noise level of SWAP, but this remains to be independently verified.

References

1. Quigley HA, Dunkelberger GR, Green WR. Retinal ganglion cell atrophy correlated with automated perimetry in human eyes with glaucoma. Am J Ophthalmol. 1989;107(5):453-64.
2. Guo L, Moss SE, Alexander RA, Ali RR, Fitzke FW, Cordeiro MF. Retinal ganglion cell apoptosis in glaucoma is related to intraocular pressure and IOP-induced effects on extracellular matrix. Invest Ophthalmol Vis Sci. 2005;46(1):175-82.
3. Stamper RL, Lieberman MF, Drake MV, Becker B, Shaffer RN, Stamper RL, et al. (Eds). Becker and Shaffer's Diagnosis and Therapy of the Glaucomas, 8th edition. Mosby/Elsevier; 2009.
4. Johnson CA, Adams AJ, Casson EJ, Brandt JD. Progression of early glaucomatous visual field loss as detected by blue-on-yellow and standard white-on-white automated perimetry. Arch Ophthalmol. 1993;111(5):651-6.
5. Girkin CA, Emdadi A, Sample PA, Blumenthal EZ, Lee AC, Zangwill LM, et al. Short-wavelength automated perimetry and standard perimetry in the detection of progressive optic disc cupping. Arch Ophthalmol. 2000;118(9):1231-6.
6. Johnson CA, Sample PA, Cioffi GA, Liebmann JR, Weinreb RN. Structure and function evaluation (SAFE): I. Criteria for glaucomatous visual field loss using standard automated perimetry (SAP) and short wavelength automated perimetry (SWAP). Am J Ophthalmol. 2002;134(2):177-85.

7.5 Optical Coherence Tomography in Glaucoma

Bhagabat Nayak, Dewang Angmo

 1. Discuss the uses and pitfalls of optical coherence tomography (OCT) in glaucoma.

We will discuss first the uses of the OCT in glaucoma and then the pitfalls of OCT in glaucoma.

Uses of Glaucoma

- It is more useful in early diseases where the visual field cannot give any clue about the damage, by detecting retinal nerve fiber layer thickness (RNFLT) and ganglion cell loss (GCC).[1]
- It is also very useful for diagnosis during the stages when ocular hypertension turns to glaucoma or glaucoma suspect turns into glaucoma.
- It is also useful in early glaucoma progression.
- Apart from the optic nerve assessment, OCT also comes to help in identifying the narrow-angle, plateau iris configuration, and also bleb morphology through anterior segment optical coherence tomography (ASOCT).
- Recent advancement of OCT in spectral domain optical coherence tomography (SD-OCT) and swept source optical coherence tomography (SS-OCT) has power of better acquisition of image and resolution of 5–8 μm.[2] These high-resolution tomography help in imaging and morphometry of ganglion cell (GCL) and retinal nerve fiber (RNF) layer thickness and Bruch's membrane-based minimum neuroretinal rim width (BMO-MRW) measurement which allow the detection of early pathologic changes.
- Recent advancements in OCT angiography can assess the microcirculation around the optic nerve, which is an indirect way of assessing the damage also.

Pitfalls of Optical Coherence Tomography in Glaucoma

- It does not give accurate data if the glaucoma is advanced because of the "floor effect" that is when the RNFLT reaches about 40–50 μm, it bottoms out and does not decrease any further even though the damage continues to worsen. At that time, for glaucoma progression, the visual field and other functional tests should be relied on.
- The accuracy of the OCT scan depends on factors such as signal quality, scan alignment, scan centration, and opacities.
- OCT shows poor signal quality in case of significant cataract, vitreous hemorrhage, corneal opacity, corneal edema, and dry eye.
- If the scan is not properly aligned, it will give false information. Not only does the eye have to be aligned on the visual axis, but the depth of the scan must be correct. In axial myopia, the scan alignment problem occurs.
- If the scan circle is not centered around the optic nerve, the part of the circle that is too close to the nerve will measure thicker than it is, and the part that is farther away from the center will measure thinner. So that a focal defect in the thin area may be appreciated. If there is difficulty in maintaining fixation, this can happen so the technician or doctor should be aware of it. It becomes a problem in optic disc dysplasia, tilted disc, and also in the myopic disc.[3]
- Opacities can disturb the scan, especially the floaters due to vitreous opacity. It also cannot diagnose in cases of nerve fiber layer disorder such as thick myelinated nerve fiber around optic nerve head.[4]
- There may be a segmentation error. The software tries to segment out the nerve fiber layer, but if the quality of the scan is not good the segmentation is thrown off and gives the inaccurate value of RNFLT.
- In event-based progression analysis, there may be intertest machine reliability although it is easy to compare.
- If trend-based analysis is better than event-based analysis, it must test a greater number of tests and good baseline test to see the rate of change in time. It may not be feasible always to stick to one software or a machine.[5]
- An analysis of the OCT print outlook for the focal defect not the overall changes such as a new defect or widening of a defect. As the deepening of the existing RNFL defect may also occur without widening.
- The age-matched control data is in the software. As the machine has not stored less than 16-year-old normal population data, it is difficult to assess the children. Also, the age matched loss of retinal nerve fiber layer optical coherence tomography (RNFLOCT) should be considered when you are comparing two OCT data of the same individual after a long gap.

Best Utilization of Optical Coherence Tomography

Optical coherence tomography can help us diagnose and monitor glaucoma patients, especially those with early or moderate disease.

But we can best utilize the machine if we focus on the following lines:
- Maintain good quality scans by proper alignment, proper centration, rule out segmentation error, and opacity.[6]
- Look at the entire readout, not just one or two numbers.
- Look for focal change, not just overall change.
- The aging effect should be accounted for.
- For progression analysis, trend-based analysis should be used whenever possible. Even if we use event-based analysis, be aware of its potential problems so you get the best possible information from the data comparison.

References

1. Optic nerve, retina and choroid. In: Allingham RR (Ed). Shields Textbook of Glaucoma, 6th edition. Philadelphia, USA: Lippincott Williams & Wilkins; 2011. pp. 77-8.
2. Yang Z, Tatham AJ, Zangwill LM, Weinreb RN, Zhang C, Medeiros FA. Diagnostic ability of retinal nerve fiber layer imaging by swept-source optical coherence tomography in glaucoma. Am J Ophthalmol. 2015;159(1):193-201.
3. Tan NYQ, Sng CCA, Jonas JB, Wong TY, Jansonius NM, Ang M. Glaucoma in myopia: diagnostic dilemmas. Br J Ophthalmol. 2019;103(10):1347-55.
4. Mackenzie PJ, Mikelberg FS. Evaluating optic nerve damage: pearls and pitfalls. Open Ophthalmol J. 2009;3:54-8.
5. Kotowski J, Wollstein G, Folio LS, Ishikawa H, Schuman JS. Clinical use of OCT in assessing glaucoma progression. Ophthalmic Surg Lasers Imaging. 2011;42:S6-14.
6. Dharwadkar S, Nayak BK. Optical coherence tomography-I. Clin Ophthalmol Res. 2017;5:51-67.

7.6 Juvenile Open-angle Glaucoma

Harathy Selvan, Dewang Angmo, Karthikeyan Mahalingam

  1. Discuss juvenile open-angle glaucoma.

Introduction

Juvenile open-angle glaucoma (JOAG) is a subset of primary glaucoma.[1] It is usually diagnosed when a patient of age 10–40 years presents with an intraocular pressure (IOP) of >21 mm Hg on two separate occasions associated with open angles on gonioscopy and glaucomatous optic disc cupping with corresponding repeatable visual field defects. It is more common in the Asian countries as compared to the western population, constituting 3.3% of glaucoma referrals to a tertiary care center in India.[2] Being midway in the spectrum between the congenital glaucoma and primary open-angle glaucoma, they carry their own genetic and clinical peculiarities as detailed below.

Etiology

They can be broadly subdivided into inherited and sporadic cases. Most cases are inherited; predominantly by autosomal dominant pattern while a few follow autosomal recessive pattern. The common genes involved in the causation of JOAG are:[1,3]

- Myocilin *(MYOC)*
- Cytochrome P450 1B1 *(CYP1B1)*
- Optineurin *(OPTN)*
- Neurotrophin 4 *(NTF4)*
- WD repeat domain 36 *(WDR36)*
- Ankyrin repeat and SOCS box containing 10 *(ASB10)*.

Pro370Leu is the most common myocilin mutation detected in JOAG patients. Many other genes contributing to minor proportions of JOAG also exist. Most of these genes are also identified as a causative of primary open-angle glaucoma (POAG), reinforcing the fact that JOAG is a part of the POAG spectrum. Family histories of JOAG or POAG, both are identified as risk factors for JOAG.

Clinical Features

Symptoms

It is largely asymptomatic during the initial stages. Hence, nonfamilial patients usually present late at the advanced stages as compared to the familial cases who are picked up early due to family screening and increased awareness among the affected families. They usually present with diffuse ocular pain/headache due to increased IOP or blurred vision due to associated myopia. Rarely they may present with redness, foreign body sensation, tearing, or incidental trauma.[4]

Signs

- *Cornea:* Usually clear with normal thickness
- *Anterior chamber:* Deep
- *Angle:* Open. Other associated features:
  - High iris insertion
  - Prominent iris processes
  - Featureless angles
- *Iris:* Normal pattern
- *Pupils:* Normal ruff. Relative afferent pupillary defect (RAPD) may be present if glaucomatous optic atrophy ensues.
- *IOP:* High baseline IOPs poorly responsive to medical management.
- *Optic nerve head (ONH):* Larger in size as compared to POAG patients. Concentric enlargement of the cup occurs with circumferential thinning of the neuroretinal rim (NRR).
- *Peripapillary retina:* Arcuate retinal nerve fiber layer defects may be seen. Peripapillary atrophy may be seen.
- *Refractive status:* Associated with myopia.

Differential Diagnosis

Lately Diagnosed Primary Congenital Glaucoma
They may display classic features of congenital glaucoma such as increased size of the eyeball, enlarged corneal diameter, Descemet tears, corneal opacity secondary to chronic corneal edema, blue sclera, and prominent angle dysgenesis.

Glaucoma Associated with Other Ocular Developmental Anomalies
- Axenfeld–Rieger syndrome
- Peters' anomaly
- Aniridia
- Nanophthalmos
- Congenital ectropion uvea.

Glaucoma Associated with Systemic Disorders
- Sturge–Weber syndrome
- Neurofibromatosis type 1
- Lowe syndrome
- Marfan syndrome
- Homocystinuria.

Secondary Glaucoma
- Steroid-induced glaucoma
- Traumatic glaucoma
- Inflammatory glaucoma
- Postsurgical glaucoma
- Pigmentary glaucoma.

Work-up

History
The specific histories related to a JOAG patient have been elaborated below.
- *Age of onset:* 10–40 years of age. Mean age of diagnosis ~25 years of age.
- *Common complaints:* Ocular pain/headache/blurred vision
- History of spectacle use and frequency of age of glasses.
- *Family history of glaucoma:* JOAG/POAG in siblings/parents/other relatives. History of consanguinity within the family. A pedigree chart should be drawn in patients with positive family history to assess the mode of inheritance.
- Previous diagnosis of glaucoma elsewhere, and if so, the treatment taken. The number and type of medications, their frequency, compliance, and adequacy of treatment should also be evaluated.
- History of any laser or surgical procedures and subsequent IOP control.
- Socioeconomic status of the patient should be assessed. It is important to judge if the patient would be able to continue medical management life-long, or else surgical treatment can be sorted too.

Examination
To be examined for signs explained under the heading "Signs".
No phenotypic differences are known to occur between familial and sporadic JOAG patients.[5]

Investigation
- *Applanation tonometry:* IOP > 21 mm Hg on two separate occasions. Usually associated with high baseline IOP refractory to medical therapy.
- *Pachymetry:* Usually normal central corneal thickness
- *Diurnal variation:* To assess the IOP every 3 hours over a period of 24 hours to identify the variations and peaks attained throughout the day.

- *Perimetry:* Humphrey field analyzer Swedish Interactive Threshold Algorithm (SITA) standard may show visual field defects consistent with glaucoma. A glaucomatous field defect is one where ≥3 nonedge points occur in the Bjerrum's area, with all showing p< 5% and one point p <1% on pattern deviation plot, on at least two consecutive visual field tests 6 months apart.
- *Anterior segment optical coherence tomography (OCT) to assess the angle:* Up to 40% of eyes may show abnormal tissue or a hyperreflective membrane, suggestive of angle dysgenesis. The Schlemm's canal is recognizable in roughly 60% of patients as compared to 90% in normal individuals.[6]
- *Disc stereo-photography:* To capture the baseline status of the ONH, i.e., cup-disc ratio, NRR, and the RNFL status. It helps in assessing structural progression.
- *Posterior segment OCT to assess the retinal nerve fiber layer thickness:* This can be sorted to in doubtful situations where a thin RNFL would be suggestive of glaucoma.
- *Heidelberg retinal tomography (HRT):* This test is used to measure the area and volumes of the disc, optic cup, and the NRR. Stereoparametric trend graph plotted from the above on subsequent visits can be used to assess progression.

Assessment of Progression

The sole strategy for treatment in glaucoma is to avoid its progression. Progression can be assessed in two ways, the structural and functional progression. The former is assessed by studying the structure of the ONH with respect to its baseline (comparing the size of cup and NRR in different quadrants) in serial optic disc photographs. They can also be assessed through OCT or HRT studies, with trends assessed over time. Functional progression is assessed from the visual fields when the preexisting defects spread over the adjacent points on pattern deviation plot. Over 5 years, 9.5% of treated JOAG progress.[7] The risk factors for faster progression include:[4]
- Positive family history
- Uncontrolled IOP
- Long-term IOP fluctuations
- Advanced disease at diagnosis.

Management

Nonsurgical Management

- Medical management has been explained in the Chapter of POAG. The features that need special mention are:
  - Aqueous suppressants fare better than outflow enhancers.
  - Avoiding Brimonidine eye drops in young children.
  - Higher resistance to medical management.
- *Laser trabeculoplasty:* Recent studies have shown that up to 43% of JOAG benefit from selective laser trabeculoplasty. Patient with normal appearing angles had greater chances of success as compared to those with angle dysgenesis.[8]

Surgical Management

The various options include:
- Goniotomy (rarely)
- Trabeculotomy
- Trabeculectomy [±Mitomycin-C (MMC)]
- Trabeculotomy + trabeculectomy
- Minimally invasive glaucoma surgery.
  At 5 years, the success of trabeculectomy without MMC in JOAG is 79%.[9]

Key Points

- Juvenile open-angle glaucoma is a form of POAG diagnosed between the ages of 10 and 40 years.
- It maybe familial (autosomal dominant > recessive) or sporadic.
- The present with very high IOP and concentric enlargement of the cup.
- Progression is faster and is less responsive to medical or laser therapy as compared to surgical management.

References

1. Turalba AV, Chen TC. Clinical and genetic characteristics of primary juvenile-onset open-angle glaucoma (JOAG). Semin Ophthalmol. 2008;23(1):19-25.

2. Das J, Bhomaj S, Chaudhuri Z, Sharma P, Negi A, Dasgupta A. Profile of glaucoma in a major eye hospital in North India. Indian J Ophthalmol. 2001;49(1):25.
3. Gupta V, Somarajan BI, Gupta S, Chaurasia AK, Kumar S, Dutta P, et al. The inheritance of juvenile onset primary open angle glaucoma. Clin Genet. 2017;92(2):134-42.
4. Kwun Y, Lee EJ, Han JC, Kee C. Clinical characteristics of juvenile-onset open angle glaucoma. Korean J Ophthalmol. 2016;30(2):127-33.
5. Gupta V, Markan A, Somarajan BI, Sihota R, Gupta A, Gupta S, et al. Phenotypic differences between familial versus non-familial Juvenile onset open angle glaucoma patients. Ophthalmic Genet. 2018;39(1):63-7.
6. Gupta V, Chaurasia AK, Gupta S, Gorimanipalli B, Sharma A, Gupta A. In vivo analysis of angle dysgenesis in primary congenital, juvenile, and adult-onset open angle glaucoma. Invest Ophthalmol Vis Sci. 2017;58(13):6000-5.
7. Gupta V, Ov M, Rao A, Sharma A, Sihota R. Long-term structural and functional outcomes of therapy in juvenile-onset primary open-angle glaucoma: a five-year follow-up. Ophthalmologica. 2012;228(1):19-25.
8. Gupta V, Ghosh S, Sujeeth M, Chaudhary S, Gupta S, Chaurasia AK, et al. Selective laser trabeculoplasty for primary open-angle glaucoma patients younger than 40 years. Can J Ophthalmol. 2018;53(1):P81-5.
9. Pathania D, Senthil S, Rao HL, Mandal AK, Garudadari CS. Outcomes of trabeculectomy in juvenile open angle glaucoma. Indian J Ophthalmol. 2014;62(2):224-8.

7.7 Medical Management of Glaucoma

Vaishali Rakheja, Dewang Angmo

1. Classify the pharmacological agents used in the management of glaucoma.

The different classes of antiglaucoma medications are summarized below:

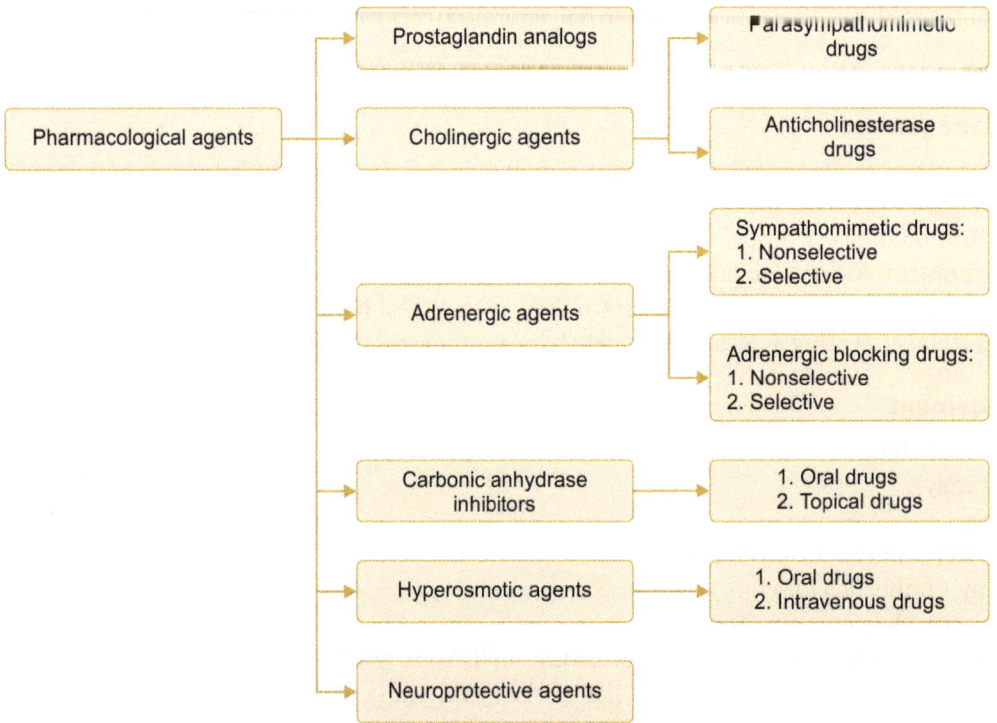

- *Cholinergic agents:*
  - *Parasympathomimetic drugs:* Pilocarpine (1%, 2%, 4%) and carbachol (0.75%, 3%)
  - *Anticholinesterase drugs:* Echothiopahate iodide and physostigmine
- *Prostaglandin analogs:* Latanoprost (0.005%), bimatoprost (0.03%, 0.01%), travoprost (0.004%), and tafluprost (0.0015%)
- *Adrenergic agents:*
  - Sympathomimetic drugs which may be nonselective drugs such as epinephrine (0.5%, 1%, 2%), dipivefrine (0.1%), or selective alfa agonists such as clonidine (0.06%, 0.125%), apraclonidine (0.5%, 1%), and brimonidine (0.1%, 0.15%, 0.2%)

- Adrenergic blocking drugs which may be nonselective drugs such as timolol (0.25%, 0.5%), levobunolol (0.25%, 0.5%), and carteolol (1%, 2%) or selective beta-1 antagonists such as betaxolol (0.25%, 0.5%)
- *Carbonic anhydrase inhibitors (CAIs):*
  - *Oral drugs:* Acetazolamide and methazolamide
  - *Topical drugs:* Dorzolamide (2%) and brinzolamide (1%)
- *Hyperosmotic agents:*
  - *Oral drugs:* Glycerol
  - *Intravenous drugs:* Mannitol and urea
- *Neuroprotective agents*
- *Newer drugs:* Rho kinase (ROCK inhibitors) (Ripatec 0.4%), latanoprostene bunod (Vyzulta 0.024%), ROCKLACTAN (Netarsudil 0.02% + Latanoprost 0.005%)

2. What is the mechanism of action of various classes of topical agents?

Prostaglandin Analogs

The prostaglandin analogs exert their intraocular pressure (IOP)-lowering effect by enhancing the outflow of the aqueous via the uveoscleral pathway. The maximal IOP-lowering effect exerted is 25–32% and this class of drugs is used as the first-line medication. Two mechanisms have been proposed for the same:
1. Remodeling of the extracellular matrix of the ciliary muscles by upregulating the matrix metalloproteinases
2. Relaxation of the ciliary muscles.

Cholinergic Agents

Parasympathomimetic agents such as *pilocarpine* have a beneficial effect in both open- and closed-angle glaucoma. In the case of *open-angle glaucoma*, it acts by stimulating the muscarinic receptors located on the ciliary muscles. The contraction of the longitudinal ciliary muscles causes traction on the scleral spur and causes an alteration in the angle configuration improving the aqueous outflow. In cases of *angle-closure glaucoma*, the miotic effect of pilocarpine due to the contraction of the sphincter pupillae muscle helps to open the angle recess and may aid in relieving the pupillary block. They are used as the second-line medications and exert an IOP-lowering effect of 18–25%.

Beta-adrenergic Receptor Antagonists

They decrease the IOP by an antagonistic effect on the beta-adrenergic receptors present in the ciliary processes. They inhibit the catecholamine stimulated synthesis of the cyclic adenosine monophosphates (cAMP), thus reducing the aqueous humor production and decreasing the IOP. Beta-adrenergic receptor antagonists can also be used as first-line medications and exert an IOP-lowering effect of about 20–28% from the baseline.

Alfa-adrenergic Receptor Agonists

The IOP-lowering effect of medications such as apraclonidine, clonidine, and brimonidine is by decreasing adenylate cyclase-mediated aqueous production mediated through their action on alfa-2A receptors on the ciliary epithelium. Brimonidine also has an additive neuroprotective effect and IOP-lowering effect by improving the aqueous outflow via the uveoscleral pathway. They decrease the IOP by 20–25%.

Carbonic Anhydrase Inhibitors

They act by decreasing the aqueous humor formation by inhibiting the catalytic step mediated by carbonic anhydrase II isoenzyme which is critical in the ion transport for aqueous secretion.

3. What is the mechanism of action of systemic agents?

Oral Carbonic Anhydrase Inhibitors

Oral CAIs work in the same way as the topical CAI and exert their IOP-lowering effect by reducing the aqueous formation. They interfere with the ion transport and aqueous secretion by inhibiting the carbonic anhydrase isoenzyme II. Acetazolamide is the most commonly used oral CAI. The adult dose is 250 mg 6 hourly or 500 mg sustained-release capsules twice daily. In children, a dose of 5–10 mg/kg body weight is administered 6 hourly.

Hyperosmotic Agents

The hyperosmotic agents work by reducing the vitreous volume by altering the osmotic gradient between the blood and ocular tissues. This leads to a shift of fluid to the extracellular compartment which decreases the IOP. Depending upon the route of administration they are classified as:
- *Oral:* Glycerol (50%): 1–1.5 mg/kg per dose 6–8 hourly, Isosorbide
- *Intravenous:* Mannitol (20%): 1–2 mg/kg per dose 8–12 hourly.

 4. What are the principles of medical management of glaucoma?

Following are the principles that guide the medical management of glaucoma:
- *Establish diagnosis:* Ascertain the type of glaucoma as the management differs for various types. For an open-angle glaucoma medical treatment is instituted whereas for glaucoma due to angle-closure mechanism may need adjunctive interventions in the form of laser iridotomy.
- Baseline IOP and visual field analysis should be documented as it helps to estimate the severity of the disease at presentation. This will help in formulating a suitable management plan for the patient.
- *Risk factors:* Family history of glaucoma, pseudoexfoliation, and pigment dispersion syndrome, any associated ocular morbidity, diabetes mellitus, disc hemorrhage, and thin cornea.
- *Comorbidities:* Systemic hypertension and hypotension, chronic obstructive pulmonary disease (COPD)/asthma, and cardiac issues should be ruled out as they have a bearing on the medical treatment.
- *Target IOP:* As it is known that IOP is the only key modifiable factor it can be targeted to monitor the progression of the disease and the success of the treatment. According to the landmark AGIS (Advanced Glaucoma Intervention Study), a consistent low IOP with minimal fluctuations was associated with a reduced progression. This forms the basis of establishing a target IOP range for each new patient. It is based on the amount of neuroretinal rim loss and associated risk factors at presentation. For an eye with minimal damage that is early neuroretinal rim loss without visual field defect, the target IOP should lie in middle to high teens, and in eyes, with moderate disc damage and early field loss, the target IOP should be set in low to middle teens. Whereas for a patient with advanced neuro-retinal rim loss and central visual field defects the target IOP should be below 10–12 mm Hg.
- *Starting medical therapy:* In order to achieve and maintain the target IOP, medication with the least possible side effects and maximal IOP-lowering effect should be chosen keeping in mind the systemic history of the patient. Monotherapy at minimal concentration and frequency should be initiated and response should be observed at a follow-up of 3–4 weeks. In case of intolerance due to side-effects another congener of the same class should be administered before switching to a different category of drugs. When the target IOP is not being maintained on a single drug another drug can be added to the existing regime.
- *When to go in for surgery?*
  The indications for quitting the medical therapy and moving to surgical intervention are:
  - Inability to maintain target IOP on maximal tolerable medications
  - Progression of the glaucomatous damage despite ongoing maximal medical therapy
  - Poor patient compliance or inability to adhere to medical therapy due to profound side-effects or cost factors.

 5. What are the adverse effects and contraindications of various classes of antiglaucoma medications?

Prostaglandin Analogs

Ocular Side-effects
- Periocular fat atrophy
- Increased pigmentation of periocular skin which is reversible
- Eyelashes become elongated, thickened, hyperpigmented, and occasionally hypertrichosis may occur.
- Conjunctival hyperemia is a very common side effect.

- Irreversible hyperpigmentation of iris which is most noticeable in green-brown irides
- May lead to a reactivation of herpetic keratitis.
- Rarely may lead to a flaring up of anterior uveitis in inflamed eyes.
- Perioperative use in patients undergoing cataract surgery is associated with an increased incidence of cystoid macular edema.

Systemic Side-effects

- *Flu-like symptoms:* Myalgia, malaise, skin rash, symptoms of upper respiratory tract infection
- Precipitation of migraine
- Rarely may cause allergic contact dermatitis specifically seen with latanoprost.

Beta-adrenergic Blockers

Ocular Side-effects

- Burning and conjunctival hyperemia are rare.
- Superficial punctate keratopathy and corneal anesthesia
- *A rare but vision-threatening reaction:* Ocular cicatricial pemphigoid
- Metipranolol is associated with troublesome granulomatous anterior uveitis.

Systemic Side-effects

- *Respiratory system:* May lead to aggravation of bronchospasm in patients with asthma and COPD.
- *Cardiovascular system:* Due to effects such as bradycardia, heart block, hypotension, and worsening of heart failure, the mortality is higher in predisposed individuals.
- *Central nervous system:* May lead to depression, confusion, sleep disorders, rarely hallucinations.
- *Integumentary system:* Few cases of reversible alopecia and maculopapular rash have been reported.
- Also known to cause dyslipidemia.

Alfa-adrenergic Agonists

Ocular Side-effects

- Follicular and allergic conjunctivitis
- Conjunctival hyperemia
- Rarely may lead to granulomatous anterior uveitis
- Apraclonidine is known to cause lid retraction and mydriasis.

Systemic Side-effects

- Xerostomia
- Headache and fatigue
- Sedation
- Bradycardia, vasovagal attack, and postural hypotension

Carbonic Anhydrase Inhibitors

This is the only class of drugs that is available in both oral and topical formulations.

Ocular Side-effects

- The most common side-effect seen with topical formulations is stinging and irritation immediately on instillation.
- Periorbital dermatitis is also observed with topical agents.
- Systemic agents lead to ciliary body effusion and induce transient myopia by moving the iris-lens diaphragm anteriorly.

Systemic Side-effects

- *Electrolyte imbalance:* Such as metabolic acidosis and hypokalemia
- *Gastrointestinal tract disturbances:* Such as nausea, vomiting, abdominal discomfort, and metallic taste

- *CNS disturbances:* Such as paraesthesias, vertigo, and insomnia.
- *Bone marrow suppression:* Aplastic anemia
- Steven Johnson Syndrome in rare cases
- *Contraindications:* CAIs should be avoided in patients with chronic kidney disease, chronic liver disease, known allergy to sulfonamides, and those who have undergone renal transplant.

Miotic Agents

Ocular Side-effects

- Browache and headache
- Transient myopic shift due to anterior shifting of the lens
- Dim vision and visual field defects appear denser and larger
- Corneal epithelial staining and haze
- Increased risk of retinal tears and detachments
- Postoperative inflammation
- Iris cysts and cataract
- Rarely may lead to ocular cicatricial pemphigoid.

Systemic Side-effects

- Lacrimation and salivation
- Nausea, vomiting, and bronchospasm due to increased secretions
- Third-degree atrioventricular (AV) heart block.

Hyperosmotic Agents

Ocular Side-effects

- A rapid rebound of IOP on cessation of effect.

Systemic Side-effects

- Sudden postural hypotension is most commonly seen with intravenous mannitol.
- Nausea, vomiting, and diarrhea
- Electrolyte imbalance and dehydration
- Pulmonary edema and congestive cardiac failure
- Hyperglycemia can occur after the administration of glycerol.

 6. Write a short note on prostaglandin analogs used to treat glaucoma.

Prostaglandins are the metabolic end products of the C-20 arachidonic acid pathway. The ocular hypotensive effect is exerted by action on the prostaglandin F-2-alfa receptors.

Mechanism of action: IOP-lowering effect is produced by enhancing the outflow of the aqueous via the uveoscleral pathway. Two mechanisms have been proposed for the same:
1. Remodeling of the extracellular matrix of the ciliary muscles by upregulating the matrix metalloproteinases.
2. Relaxation of the ciliary muscles

Their IOP-lowering effect is the maximum for a single agent: *27–35%* and they are administered as *once-daily dosage before bedtime.*

Various prostaglandin analogs that are available for use are:
- Latanoprost (0.005%) is the most commonly used prostaglandin analog and is often used as the first-line agent.
- Bimatoprost (0.01% and 0.03%) less hyperemia with lower concentration with an almost similar ocular hypotensive effect.
- Travoprost (0.004%) is associated with a very high incidence of conjunctival hyperemia as compared to the other two drugs of this class.

- Tafluprost (0.0015%) is the first prostaglandin analog available in preservative free form and hence is more tolerated by the patients.

  The adverse effects associated with the use of prostaglandin analogs are enlisted below:
- *Ocular side effects:*
  - Periocular fat atrophy
  - Increased pigmentation of periocular skin which is reversible
  - Eyelashes become elongated, thickened, hyperpigmented, and occasionally hypertrichosis may occur.
  - Conjunctival hyperemia is a very common side effect.
  - Irreversible hyperpigmentation of iris which is most noticeable in green-brown irides
  - May lead to a reactivation of herpetic keratitis
  - Rarely may lead to a flaring up of anterior uveitis in inflamed eyes
  - Perioperative use in patients undergoing cataract surgery is associated with an increased incidence of cystoid macular edema.
- *Systemic side-effects:*
  - *Flu-like symptoms:* Myalgia, malaise, skin rash, and symptoms of upper respiratory tract infection
  - Precipitation of migraine
  - Rarely may cause allergic contact dermatitis specifically seen with latanoprost.

 7. Write a short note on dorzolamide.

Dorzolamide is a topical CAI that reduces IOP by decreasing the aqueous humor formation by inhibiting the catalytic step mediated by carbonic anhydrase II isoenzyme which is critical in the ion transport for aqueous secretion.
- It is available in a solution form with a concentration of *2%* and can be administered as a *twice or thrice daily regime*. Better adherence has been reported with the twice-daily dosing and the thrice-daily dosing offers a greater IOP-lowering effect.
- At 2 hours from administration a *15–20% reduction in IOP* is observed and it decreases to 12–17% reduction at hours from dosing.
- It is known to be well tolerated by the pediatric population and can be used in neonatal and developmental glaucomas.
- The most common side-effect associated with this formulation is an intense stinging and bitter taste in the mouth, that occurs shortly after the administration of the drug. Few cases of allergic blepharoconjunctivitis have also been reported.

7.8 Laser Peripheral Iridotomy

Barkha Gupta, Dewang Angmo

 1. Write a short note on laser peripheral iridotomy.

Laser Peripheral Iridotomy

Laser peripheral iridotomy (LPI) is a medical laser procedure that attempts to open up a narrow angle wherein a hole is created in peripheral iris allowing aqueous humor to traverse directly from posterior to anterior chamber (AC) permitting equalization of pressure in both the chambers.

It is indicated for all forms of *angle-closure glaucoma*, primary and secondary, involving pupillary block and as a prophylactic measure for patients with occludable angles. LPI is the preferred procedure for treating *angle-closure glaucoma* caused by relative or absolute pupillary block.

The first iridotomy was done by Meyer Schwickerath in 1956 using a broad-spectrum incoherent light source and xenon arc lamp.

Mechanism of Action

Laser peripheral iridotomy eliminates pupillary block by allowing the aqueous to pass directly from the posterior chamber into the AC, bypassing the pupil. This allows the iris to fall back exposing areas that had iridotrabecular functional apposition, not organic synechiae. An iridotomy also prevents further attacks of angle closure seen on dark room prone provocative test or mydriatic tests. Laser iridotomy itself is not expected to reduce intraocular pressure (IOP), as that depends on preexisting damage to outflow channels.

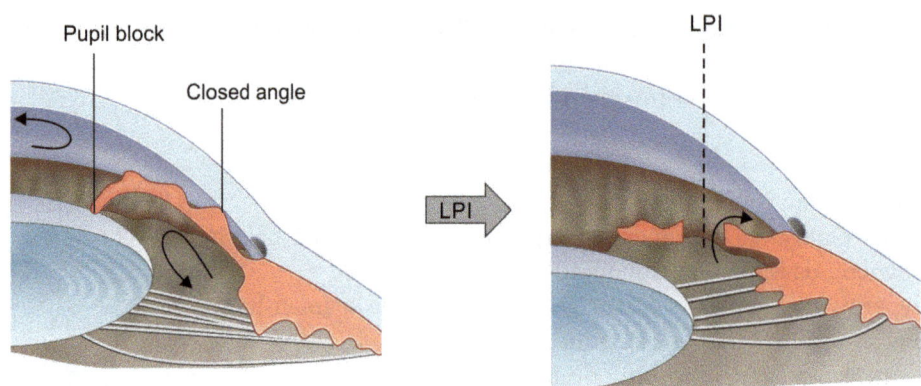

(LPI: laser peripheral iridotomy)

Indications
- Primary angle closure glaucoma (PACG)
- Primary angle closure (PAC)
- Fellow eyes of patients having PACG
- *PACS with risk factors:*
  - Family history of PACG
  - Frequent dilation required, as in diabetic retinopathy
  - Noncompliant patient, not willing to follow-up
  - Difficult to access laser
  - Positive provocative tests
- All secondary angle closure—e.g., uveitis, aphakic, or pseudophakic pupillary block.
- Combined mechanism glaucoma
- In the diagnosis of aqueous misdirection syndrome
- Phakic intraocular lenses (IOLs), anterior chamber intraocular lens (ACIOL)
- Pigmentary glaucoma, if a reverse pupillary block is demonstrated.

Contraindications
- Widely dilated pupil
- Media opacity (marked corneal edema/opaque cornea)
- Flat AC
- Active uveitis/inflammation
- Rubeosis iridis
- Angle closure due to other mechanisms [neovascular glaucoma (NVG), iridocorneal endothelial syndrome (ICE)]
- Uncooperative patient.

Technique

Instruments
- Contact lens—a contact lens with antireflective coating is used.
  - Most commonly used is *Abraham iridotomy* lens which is a modified Goldmann type of fundus lens with a +66D planoconvex button bonded into a decentered 8 mm hole.
  - *Wise iridotomy lens (+103D)* can also be used, providing higher magnification which causes difficulty in focusing and decreased depth of focus.
  - The advantages of contact lens are:
    - It acts as a speculum, and keeps the lids apart.
    - Controls eye movements and blinking, provides stability for the procedure.
    - Minimizes corneal epithelial burns and retinal burns by acting as a heat sink. It causes relative divergence of light at the cornea and retina, which reduces the power density to one fourth.
    - Allows concentrated laser energy at desired location. Focuses and increases the power density on the iris surface by a factor of four.

- Provides the magnification of the target site with less loss of depth of field that occurs with increase magnification of slit lamp.
- *Lasers*—LPI can be performed with an argon laser (514 nm continuous/pulsed), with a Q-switched neodymium-doped:yttrium-aluminum-garnet (Nd:YAG 1064 nm) laser, or in certain circumstances, with both. Nd:YAG is the laser of choice by most of the ophthalmologists and is most appropriate for dark-colored irides that are thicker than light irides. It is a photodisruptive laser, where an intense focal laser beam is delivered onto a tissue over a period of nano- or picoseconds causing optical breakdown and a resultant shock wave that disrupts independent of pigmentation.

- *Selection of treatment site:* LPI is performed in a peripheral iris crypt or a thin area in superior quadrant usually from 11 to 1 o'clock, covered beneath the upper eyelid to prevent a second pupil effect. The best site is superonasal quadrant to prevent direct injury to macula. 12 o'clock position is to be avoided because gas bubbles prelude adequate visualization if argon laser is used and site can be left for future iridectomy during filtering surgery.

  In silicon oil-filled eyes, iridotomy is made inferiorly to avoid blockage by the oil.

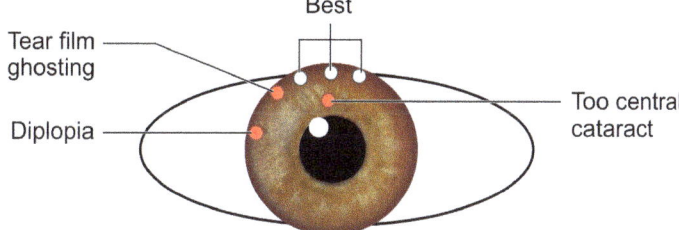

- *Prelaser patient preparation:* A written, informed consent should be obtained. A history of anticoagulant/ecosprin use should be checked for and consider stopping them after a physician consult. A couple of drops of pilocarpine 2% are instilled 15–30 minutes before the procedure to maximally thin and stretch peripheral iris. 1% apraclonidine or 0.2% brimonidine is instilled 6 hours before to prevent postoperative IOP spikes. Topical anesthesia is given with proparacaine hydrochloride (0.5%).
- *Method:* Most Nd:YAG lasers come with He–Ne/diode laser aiming beams. The two aiming spots are brought to focus and then they are defocused slightly posteriorly in the iris stroma. Laser is fired at a focusing angle (cone angle) of 18° after appropriate selection of the site. An initial energy level of 4–6 mJ may be used in a 1–3 pulses per burst. A gush of pigment (smoke signals) and aqueous with deepening of the AC is noted on penetration. The size of the opening is then enlarged with lower energy levels, a size of about 300–500 µm is considered adequate.

  Sequential argon laser pretreatment can be done in cases of thick iris, so that a drumhead is created using argon laser and then a central Nd:YAG spot can easily perforate the stretched-out iris.
- *Post laser therapy:* To control the inflammation and possible IOP spike post laser, administer topical steroids qid and add one glaucoma medication eye drop for 5–7 days post laser on preexisting glaucoma therapy. The eye should be monitored for IOP spikes 1–2 hours post laser, especially in eyes with advanced glaucomatous optic neuropathy or prior raised IOP. Such eyes prone to a significant rise in IOP should be done under cover of systemic acetazolamide. Mild iris candle wax-like bleeding can be controlled by gentle pressure with the iridotomy lens. The patency of the LPI should be checked by retroillumination on a slit lamp and gonioscopy performed on follow-up. After 2–3 weeks, at least three tonometry readings should be taken, preferably at different times of the day, and a "target" IOP planned accordingly.

Complications

Transient IOP spike and low-grade anterior uveitis are seen commonly after LPI, amenable to medical therapy. Other complications include corneal burn, iris bleed, cataract which is usually nonprogressive, glare, dysphotopsia, and ghost images. Closure of iridotomy can occur, usually within 6–8 weeks and is more common with argon laser. Other rare complications include pupillary distortion and retinal burns.

 2. Write a short note on laser peripheral iridoplasty.

Laser Peripheral Iridoplasty

Iridoplasty, also known as gonioplasty, uses low-energy laser burns to the peripheral iris in order to widen the AC angle and/or break peripheral anterior synechiae (PAS). It was first described by Krasnov as gonioplasty in 1977 and has been refined over time by Kimbrough and others. The effort changed from a penetrating to a slower-burn contraction technique (i.e., iridoplasty).

Iridoplasty is useful as a stand-alone procedure for the treatment of *nonpupillary block angle closure*. It may also be used adjunctively for pupillary block angle closure and for open-angle glaucoma in the presence of narrow angles.

Mechanism of Action

The contraction burns of iridoplasty pull the peripheral iris stroma away from the angle structures to deepen the angle recess. The application of continuous-wave laser energy causes contracture of the pigmented epithelium of the anterior iris with thinning and flattening of the peripheral iris. These changes facilitate mechanical widening of the angle, visualization of the angle structures, and possibly a release of PAS.

Indications

- Iridoplasty effectively treats conditions involving *appositional angle closure such as plateau iris, nanophthalmos, and iris cysts*.
- Acute angle-closure glaucoma can be effectively treated initially with laser iridoplasty as an adjunctive therapy, followed by definitive treatment with laser iridotomy, especially in cases of corneal edema, extremely shallow/flat AC or extensive inflammation which precludes immediate iridotomy.
- Acute angle closure crisis not responsive to medical therapy or in cases where medical therapy is contraindicated such as in patients with renal disease, on dialysis, etc.
- As an initial treatment to break an attack of acute phacomorphic angle closure.

Technique

A written informed consent is taken. Preoperatively, pilocarpine 4% eye drops is instilled to constrict the pupil, and brimonidine/apraclonidine drops to minimize a postoperative pressure spike. Under topical anesthesia, argon laser light is delivered through an Abraham iridotomy lens/single mirror lens using a 500-μm spot size for 0.5–0.7 s duration. Treatment is initiated at 240 mW of power and increased until the surgeon sees the tissue contract. If bubbles form or pigment is released, then power is reduced. The aiming beam should be directed as far peripherally as possible, even overlapping slightly onto the adjacent sclera. Approximately, 24 spots over 360°, six to eight spots in each quadrant are placed depending on the spot size, with a gap of two spot diameters between each application.

Postoperatively, a drop each of brimonidine and a topical steroid is prescribed at least for 3–5 days. The postoperative IOP is monitored closely and treated as needed.

Complications

Argon laser iridoplasty is a safe and effective procedure with few common complications which include low-grade inflammation responsive to topical steroids, transient IOP spikes. Additional rare complications reported are diffuse corneal endothelial burns, pigment scars, intraoperative hemorrhage (very rare with use of low-power settings), iris necrosis, or Urrets-Zavalia syndrome.

Suggested Reading

1. Belcher III CD, Greff LJ. Laser therapy of angle-closure glaucoma. In: Albert DM, Jakobiec FA (Eds). Principles and Practice of Ophthalmology. Philadelphia: WB Saunders; 2000.
2. Fleck BW. How large must an iridotomy be? Br J Ophthalmol. 1990;74(10):583-8.
3. Higginbotham EJ. Laser peripheral iridotomy for pupillary-block glaucoma. Ophthalmology. 1994;101:1749-58.
4. Kumar H, Mansoori T, Warjri GB, Somarajan BI, Bandil S, Gupta V. Lasers in glaucoma. Indian J Ophthalmol. 2018;66(11):1539.
5. Lam DSC, Tham CCY, Congdon N. Peripheral iridotomy for angle-closure glaucoma. In: Shaarawy TM, Sherwood MB, Hitchings RA, Crowston JG (Eds). Glaucoma, volume 2. China: Saunders; 2009. pp. 61-9.
6. Nolan W. Argon laser peripheral iridoplasty. Asian J Ophthalmol. 2008;10:211.
7. Ritch R, Tham C, Lam D. Argon laser peripheral iridoplasty (ALPI): Na update. Surv Ophthalmol. 2007;52(3):279-88.
8. See JL, Aquino MC, Aduan J, Chew PT. Management of angle closure glaucoma. Indian J Ophthalmol. 2011;59(Suppl. 1):S82-7.
9. Zhang X, Peng D. Combined argon and Nd:YAG laser peripheral iridectomy: a new approach in clinical practice. Eye Sci. 1996;12(3):158-62.

7.9 Newer Antiglaucoma Medications

Aafreen Bari, Dewang Angmo

Q 1. Discuss newer antiglaucoma medications.

The current research aims at the development of new drug formulations which have improved efficacy and duration of action, decreasing the need for multiple medications, thereby decreasing side effect profile and improving adherence and overall quality of life. The last decade has seen the advent of many novel drugs exerting the favorable ocular hypotensive effect useful in the management of glaucoma. These are as follows:

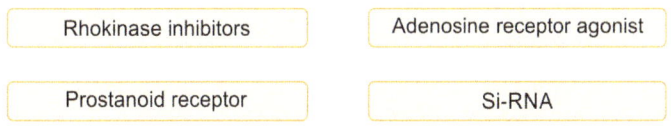

(Si-RNA: small-interfering ribonucleic acid)

- *Rhokinase inhibitors:* Rhokinase is a serine/threonine kinase whose activity increases actomyosin contraction in smooth muscle cells, including the smooth muscle-like cells of the trabecular meshwork (TM). On activation by binding to GTP (guanosine triphosphate), rho activates its effector molecules ROCK (rhokinase) which polymerize actin fibers inducing vasoconstriction and decrease cell migration. ROCK inhibitors depolymerize filamentous actin leading to enhanced TM outflow presumably by wider empty spaces in the juxtacanalicular region and increased vacuoles in endothelial cells.[1-3]
    - *Mechanism of action:*
        - *ROCK 1 and 2 inhibition:* Alterations in the extracellular matrix (ECM)-surrounding cells and alterations within the cells of TM and Schlemm canal's inner wall that modulate cellular contractility and tension, thus increasing TM outflow and decreasing episcleral venous pressure.
        - *Norepinephrine transporter (NET) inhibition:* Decreased aqueous humor production
    - *Commercial availability:* Rhopressa™ (Netarsudil ophthalmic solution 0.02%), Roclatan (fixed-dose combination of netarsudil and latanoprost), Glanatec™ (Ripasudil 0.4%; K-115), Vyzulta (Latanoprostene Bunod 0.024%)
    - *Indications:* Open-angle glaucoma and ocular hypertension
    - *Adverse drug reactions:* Conjunctival hyperemia (most common ocular ADR): 53% cases
        - *Others:* Corneal verticillate (seen in 20% cases), instillation site pain, and conjunctival hemorrhage. Instillation site erythema, corneal staining, blurred vision, increased lacrimation, erythema of eyelid, and reduced visual acuity were reported in 5–10% of patients.

Name of drug	Mechanism of action	Dosage	Mean IOP reduction
Rhopressa™	• Improves trabecular outflow • Decreasing episcleral venous pressure • Decreases aqueous production	OD (bedtime)	5.5 mm Hg
Rhoclatan™	Increases trabecular and uveoscleral outflow	OD (bedtime)	2.7 mm Hg greater reduction than Rhopressa
Glanatec	Improved trabecular outflow	BD	2.7–3.7 mm Hg
Vyzulta™	Enhances uveoscleral and trabecular outflow	OD	7.5–9 mm Hg (22%)

(IOP: intraocular pressure)

- *Adenosine receptor agonist:*
    - *Mechanism of action:* Adenosine receptor agonists stimulate secretion of matrix metalloproteinases (MMPs) in the endothelial cells lining the TM. This causes cell volume shrinkage and ECM remodeling, which ultimately facilitates conventional aqueous outflow.[4]
    - *Commercial availability:* Trabodenoson (INO 8875) and CF-101 (Can-Fite Biopharma)
    - *Indications:* Normal-tension glaucoma and open-angle glaucoma
    - *Adverse drug reactions:* Conjunctival hyperemia, constipation, headache, and palpitations

Name of drug	Mechanism of action	Dosage	Mean IOP reduction
Trabodenoson (INO 8875)	• Adenosine A1 receptor agonist • Enhances trabecular outflow	500 µg OD oral	4 mm Hg
CF-101 (Can-Fite)	Adenosine A3 receptor agonist Improves trabecular outflow	1 mg BD oral	1.1 mm Hg (12 weeks)

(IOP: intraocular pressure)

- *Prostanoid receptor agonist:* Prostaglandin analogs, latanoprost and travoprost, act on prostanoid prostaglandin F receptor (FP receptor), a receptor for Prostaglandin F2 alpha (PGF2α). Bimatoprost is a synthetic PGF2α ethanolamide mimetic, termed prostamide F2α. These drugs enhance aqueous outflow through the uveoscleral pathway and cause intraocular pressure (IOP) lowering. Recently, EP2 and EP3 receptors have emerged as new targets of interest for IOP-lowering therapy.[4]
    - *Mechanism of action:*
        - Relaxation of endothelial cells in the Schlemm's canal, facilitating uveoscleral outflow
        - Increase conventional outflow by acting on the TM, decreasing cell contractility and collagen deposition
    - *Commercial availability:* DE-117, Taprenepag isopropyl, and ONO-9054 (0.003%)
    - *Indications:* Open-angle glaucoma, normal-tension glaucoma, and ocular hypertension
    - *Adverse drug reactions:* Conjunctival hyperemia, iritis, dry eye, and photophobia

Name of drug	Mechanism of action	Dosage	Mean IOP reduction
Taprenepag isopropyl	• EP 2 agonist • Increases uveoscleral outflow	BD	30–50%
ONO-9054	EP 3 agonist Improves uveoscleral outflow	OD	28–31%

(IOP: intraocular pressure)

- Small-interfering ribonucleic acid (Si-RNA)
    - *Mechanism of action:* It acts through specific gene silencing and causes beta-2 adrenergic receptor blockade, thereby decreasing aqueous production by the ciliary body.
    - *Commercially availability:* Bamosiran (SYL040012)
    - *Indications:* Ocular hypertension and open-angle glaucoma
    - *Adverse drug reactions:* Darkening of iris color, lash growth, periocular pigmentation, and conjunctival hyperemia

Name of drug	Mechanism of action	Dosage	Mean IOP reduction
Bamosiran (SYL040012)	Si-RNA → beta 2 adrenergic receptor blockade → decreasing aqueous production	BD	30–50%

(IOP: intraocular pressure; Si-RNA: small-interfering ribonucleic acid)

Suggested Reading

1. Chen J, Runyan SA, Robinson MR. Novel ocular antihypertensive compounds in clinical trials. Clin Ophthalmol. 2011;5:667-77.
2. Dhillon J. Rhokinase inhibitors novel potential treatment modality for glaucoma. Delhi J Ophthalmol. 2016;26:272-4.
3. [online] Available from https://www.accessdata.fda.gov/drugsatfda_docs/label/2017/208254lbl.pdf. [Last accessed June, 2022].
4. Kadambi SV, George R. Newer drugs in glaucoma management. TNOA J Ophthalmic Sci Res. 2017;55:134-9.

7.10 Advances in Management of Glaucoma

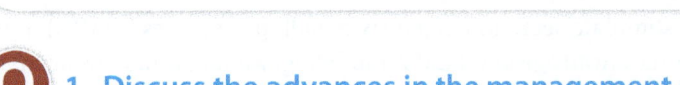

Dewang Angmo, Karthikeyan Mahalingam

  1. Discuss the advances in the management of glaucoma and their limitations.

As glaucoma is the irreversible disease, the treatment plan has been developed for the most modifiable risk factor that is intraocular pressure (IOP). As both peak of IOP and fluctuation of IOP are known to impact the disease development and progression, even in cases with statistically normal pressures.[1,2]

The most crucial barrier in the health-seeking behavior of patients and causes for failure of treatment is adherence and persistence to medical therapy. It is mainly due to complex multiple drug regimen, side effects on long-term use and poor tolerability profile, difficulty administering drops due to essential tremors and lack of ability, lack of health education, inability to comprehend nature of the disease, financial constraints, and travel issues.[3]

So, there is always research ongoing for new drug formulations which will have a long duration of action, less dosing formulation, safe and efficient so that there will be better adherence to the treatment.

Apart from the drugs to control IOP, the newer surgery and the newer diagnostic tool for glaucoma combinedly help in better management of glaucoma.

Following are some newer drug formulations; some of these are used by the patients:
- *Topical drugs:*
  - *Rho-associated coiled-coil-forming protein kinase (ROCK) inhibitors:* Rho-associated coiled-coil-forming protein kinase (ROCK) is serine/threonine inhibitor which acts as selective inhibitors of the actin cytoskeleton contractile tone of smooth muscle in the trabecular meshwork (TM). This results in increased aqueous outflow directly through the conventional pathway, thereby lowering IOP.[4]
    - *Ripasudil:* Already, patients started using it. It acts mainly by increasing the trabecular pathway of aqueous drainage.
    - *Netarsudil:* It has a dual-action as ROCK inhibitor and norepinephrine transporter inhibitor. It facilitates both trabecular and uveoscleral pathways and decreases the episcleral venous pressure.
  - *Adenosine receptor agonist:* Adenosine receptor agonists stimulate secretion of matrix metalloproteinases (MMPs) in the endothelial cells lining the TM. This causes cell volume shrinkage and extracellular matrix remodeling, which ultimately facilitates the conventional aqueous outflow.
  - *Prostanoid receptor agonist:* Apart from the prostaglandin F (FP) receptor where prostaglandin analogs such as travoprost and latanoprost work there are new receptors coming now as EP2 and EP3 receptors. These agonists cause relaxation of endothelial cells in the Schlemm's canal (SC), facilitating uveoscleral outflow. They also increase conventional outflow by acting on the TM, decreasing cell contractility and collagen deposition.[5] DE-117, Taprenepag isopropyl, and ONO-9054 (Ono Pharmaceuticals, Japan) are three upcoming drugs undergoing trial.
  - *Small interfering RNA:* Bamosiran is a new drug which acts as aqueous suppressor through specific gene silencing and causes beta-2 adrenergic receptor blockade, thereby decreasing aqueous production by the ciliary body.
  - *Neuroprotection:* Current research is ongoing for the drugs, which will prevent retinal ganglion cell (RGC) loss despite having normal IOP.
    Memantine is N-methyl-D-aspartate (NMDA) receptor antagonist which will reduce glutamate-induced-excitatory cytotoxicity of RGC, although a randomized clinical control failed to establish this effect.[6,7]
    Brimonidine 0.2% also acts as neuroprotector.
  - Preservative-free, newer preservatives, and self-preserved IOP-lowering medications: As glaucoma medications already have ocular surface side effects to add that the preservative used such as benzalkonium chloride cause more side effects and irritation to eye and damage to the cornea. So newer less toxic preservative is coming now.
    Purite (stabilized oxychloro complex), polyquad, and sofZia are new preservatives and are some newer less toxic preservative.
- *Newer drug delivery system:* Nanoparticle-based topical drug formulation contact lens-based drug delivery, drugs through ocular insert or punctal plug, and intracameral sustained-release prostaglandin analog are the new hopes. It will decrease the frequency of medication and will increase the adherence among patients.
- *Gene therapy in glaucoma:* Both viral and nonviral vectors are used to deliver genes to target tissue of interest such as TM, ciliary epithelium, ciliary body, and RGC. Gene therapy may delete, replace/inactivate an aberrant gene, or introduce a new gene which helps in targeted therapeutic protein expression.
  Adeno-associated viral vectors (AAV) have been used to deliver antiapoptotic genes to the retina in rodent glaucoma models. Intravitreal injections of AAV expressing brain-derived neurotrophic factor have resulted in RGC survival for a month in rodent models with induced ocular hypertension.[8]
  These promising newer models of drugs and delivery systems are not without side effects which will be better evaluated after prolong use by patients for some time but hope for future glaucoma treatment.
- *Newer surgical approach:* Two conventional procedures are continuing for years; one is trabeculectomy with or without augmentation with either mitomycin C (MMC), fluorouracil or ologen (crossed collagen matrix) implant. Another is shunt surgery where a silicon tube is entered the anterior chamber for aqueous humor to be drained. But as these two commonly done procedures also have some complications. So constant research is ongoing to find better alternative invasive or noninvasive surgery.

Trabeculectomy with MMC has better bleb survival rate than conventional trabeculectomy alone but is associated with complication with thinning of bleb, hypotony and endophthalmitis, etc.

Trabeculectomy with Ologen implant has the same success as with trabeculectomy with MMC but the complications due to MMC are less here apart from the cost of the Ologen implant.

Microinvasive Glaucoma Surgery (*MIGS*) encompasses the group of glaucoma surgeries that causes less damage and scarring to conjunctiva with various effect on IOP reduction. These surgeries have minimal impact on the quality of life of patients and at least show modest efficacy initially. They cause minimal trauma to target tissue anatomically and physiologically.

The mechanism of MIGS for lowering IOP are:
- Increase outflow by creating a new drainage channel into the subconjunctival space by forming an external bleb such as Ex-PRESS glaucoma implant, and Fugo blade transciliary filtration.
- Increase the conventional trabecular outflow pathway into the SC as with trabecular micro-bypass stent (Glaukos iStent), trabectome, Excimer laser trabeculotomy (ELT), canaloplasty, and Fugo Blade goniotomy.
- Increase the uveoscleral outflow into the suprachoroidal space (CyPass Shunt, SOLX Gold shunt).

Some common examples of these are described below:
- *EX-PRESS Glaucoma Filtration Device:* It is a small, stainless steel implant <3 mm in size which diverts aqueous from the anterior chamber into the subconjunctival space such as a conventional trabeculectomy.

  Studies have found similar IOP-lowering efficacy of Ex-PRESS shunt as compared to conventional trabeculectomy.[9] This implant is indicated for patients who are poor candidates for iridotomy due to the risk of bleeding or inflammation. Those patients who have very narrow angles, neovascular glaucoma, uveitis, or severe dry eye are not good candidates for this implant. The higher cost of this implant is a matter of consideration when deciding for primary Ex-PRESS implant insertion.
- *Glaukos iStent:* This is a 1 × 0.3 mm heparin-coated titanium implant for insertion through the TM into SC. It is US FDA approved for use in open angle glaucoma with cataract extraction. The study has shown that iStent, along with cataract extraction, has shown a 20% reduction of IOP.[10]
- *Trabectome:* It is a 19.5-gauze electrocautery device with a disposable handpiece connected to a console, with irrigation and aspiration controlled by a foot pedal. Under gonioscopic guidance, 90–120° of TM and inner walls of SC is cauterized and stripped to create a direct communication between the anterior chamber of the eye and SC. Studies have reported similar efficacy to trabeculectomy either alone or combined with phacoemulsification.[10] Intraoperative blood reflux is seen in 100% of cases.
- *Canaloplasty:* It is a nonpenetrating and bleb independent procedure; aqueous outflow is enhanced by circumferential 360-degree distension of the SC by a microcatheter with visco material such as Healon GV. This is US FDA approved. The study showed it lowers IOP to lower to mid-teens alone or combined with cataract surgery in open-angle glaucoma.10 It is a technique to learn more difficult, expensive, and time-consuming procedures. Complications include microhyphema, elevated IOP, and Descemet's detachment. Other side effects such as conjunctival scarring and bleb formation in some patients.

  Although from above procedure some are US FDA approved, the cost, the learning curve of the technique, their complication, the modest decrease of IOP in comparison to conventional trabeculectomy, most are done along with cataract surgery, these procedures are suited for early and moderate uncomplicated glaucoma. They are not best suited for advanced and complicated glaucoma where the target IOP is in low teens. Current operative techniques for ab-interno MIGS require direct gonioscopy, intraoperative manipulation of microscope, and patient head tilting. Better intraoperative surgical techniques may reduce the existing complications with these newer procedures.
- *Newer diagnostic tools:* Apart from the IOP, optic disc evaluation, and visual field now some newer tools can diagnose the preperimetric glaucoma and help in assessing the progression.

  Optical coherence tomography (OCT): Recent advancement of OCT in spectral-domain optical coherence tomography (SD-OCT) and swept-source optical coherence tomography (SS-OCT) has the power of better acquisition of image and resolution of 5–8 μm.[11] These high-resolution tomographies help in the imaging and morphometry of ganglion cell layer (GCL) and retinal nerve fiber (RNF) layer thickness and Bruch's membrane-based minimum neuroretinal rim width (BMO-MRW) measurement which allow the detection of early pathologic changes.

  Recent advancement in OCT angiography can assess the microcirculation around the optic nerve, which is an indirect way of determining the damage also.

  At the same time, it has some pitfalls also. The accuracy of the OCT scan depends on factors such as signal quality, scan alignment, scan centration, and opacities.

Heidelberg retinal tomography (HRT) and *glaucoma* diagnostics (GDx) are also other less used procedure which can analyze the optic nerve head and early loss of RNFL respectively. Still, they need accuracy while doing it and cost is another hindrance to these newer tools.

References

1. Collaborative Normal-Tension Glaucoma Study Group. Comparison of glaucomatous progression between untreated patients with normal-tension glaucoma and patients with therapeutically reduced intraocular pressures. Am J Ophthalmol. 1998;126: 487-97.
2. Leske MC, Heijl A, Hyman L, Bengtsson B, Dong L, Yang Z, et al. Predictors of long-term progression in the early manifest glaucoma trial. Ophthalmology. 2007;114:1965-72.
3. Schwartz GF, Quigley HA. Adherence and persistence with glaucoma therapy. Surv Ophthalmol. 2008;53(Suppl. 1):S57-68.
4. Wang SK, Chang RT. An emerging treatment option for glaucoma: rho kinase inhibitors. Clin Ophthalmol. 2014;8:883-90.
5. Wang JW, Woodward DF, Stamer WD. Differential effects of prostaglandin E2-sensitive receptors on contractility of human ocular cells that regulate conventional outflow. Invest Ophthalmol Vis Sci. 2013;54:4782-90.
6. Osborne NN. Recent clinical findings with memantine should not mean that the idea of neuroprotection in glaucoma is abandoned. Acta Ophthalmol. 2009;87:450-4.
7. Sena DF, Lindsley K. Neuroprotection for treatment of glaucoma in adults. Cochrane Database Syst Rev. 2013:CD006539.
8. Martin KR, Quigley HA, Zack DJ, Levkovitch-Verbin H, Kielczewski J, Valenta D, et al. Gene therapy with brain-derived neurotrophic factor as a protection: retinal ganglion cells in a rat glaucoma model. Invest Ophthalmol Vis Sci. 2003;44:4357-65.
9. Maris Jr PJ, Ishida K, Netland PA. Comparison of trabeculectomy with Ex-PRESS miniature glaucoma device implanted under scleral flap. J Glaucoma. 2007;16:14-9.
10. Samuelson TW, Katz LJ, Wells JM, Duh Y-J, Giamporcaro JE, for the US iStent Study Group. Randomized evaluation of the trabecular microbypass stent with phacoemulsification in patients with glaucoma and cataract. Ophthalmology. 2011;118:459-67.
11. Yang Z, Tatham AJ, Zangwill LM, Weinreb RN, Zhang C, Medeiros FA. Diagnostic ability of retinal nerve fiber layer imaging by swept-source optical coherence tomography in glaucoma. Am J Ophthalmol. 2015;159(1):193-201.

7.11 Nonpenetrating Glaucoma Surgery

Neha Midha, Dewang Angmo

1. Write a note on nonpenetrating glaucoma surgery, its types, advantages, and limitations.

Nonpenetrating glaucoma surgery (NPGS) refers to surgical procedures which do not involve full-thickness penetration of sclera into anterior chamber as in trabeculectomy.[1] They facilitate passage of aqueous humor via Schlemm's canal and bypass the juxtacanalicular meshwork, which is the site of the highest resistance. Other possible mechanisms include transscleral flow, uveoscleral outflow, and opening of nonfunctional areas of Schlemm's canal.[2]

Types of NPGS

- *Deep sclerectomy:* This is the most commonly performed NPGS. It involves creating a superficial scleral flap similar to trabeculectomy after which a deep scleral flap (90% depth of sclera) is dissected, leaving only a thin layer of scleral tissue over the underlying uvea. Schlemm's canal is now identified and unroofed. The dissection of the deep flap is advanced farther onto the cornea and then excised. This step creates an exquisitely thin trabeculo-Descemet's membrane (TDM) that allows the egress of aqueous from the anterior chamber in a more controlled manner as compared to trabeculectomy. To make the TDM more permeable, trabecular forceps are used to peel off Schlemm's canal endothelium and the juxtacanalicular trabecular meshwork. In high-risk cases, this technique is augmented with mitomycin-C and collagen implant such as Ologen.
- *Viscocanalostomy:* This technique is essentially similar to deep sclerectomy except after unroofing the Schlemm's canal, a viscoelastic is injected (Healon GV) to dilate its lumen and facilitate aqueous outflow.

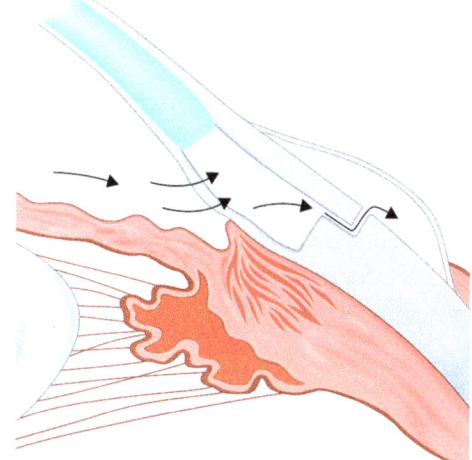

Source: With permission from Caretti L, Buratto L. Non-penetrating glaucoma surgery (NPGS): viscocanalostomy, deep sclerectomy and canaloplasty. In: Caretti L, Buratto L (Eds). Glaucoma Surgery. Springer, Cham; 2018.

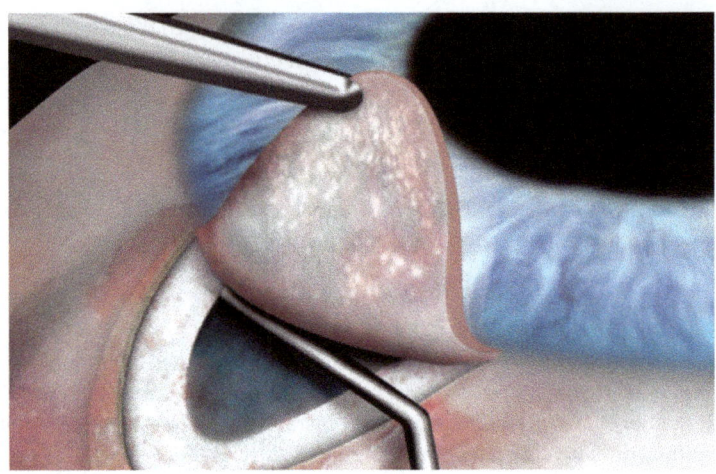

- *Canaloplasty:* The initial steps are similar to viscocanalostomy. After dilation of Schlemm's canal with a viscoelastic agent, 360° cannulation of the canal with 10-0 prolene suture is done using a flexible illuminated microcatheter as a guide wire. The 10-0 prolene suture is then tightened to apply a long-term, moderate tension to the tissues of the inner wall of Schlemm's canal.

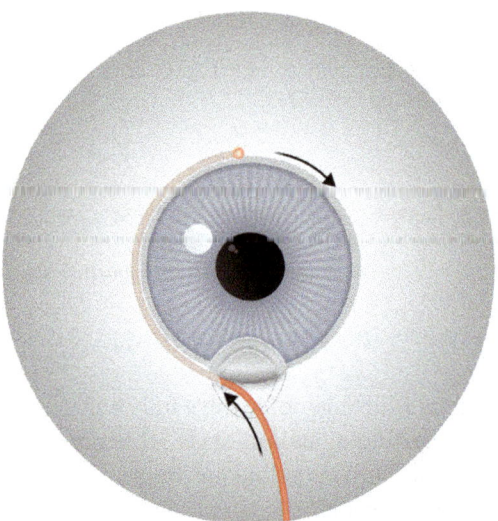
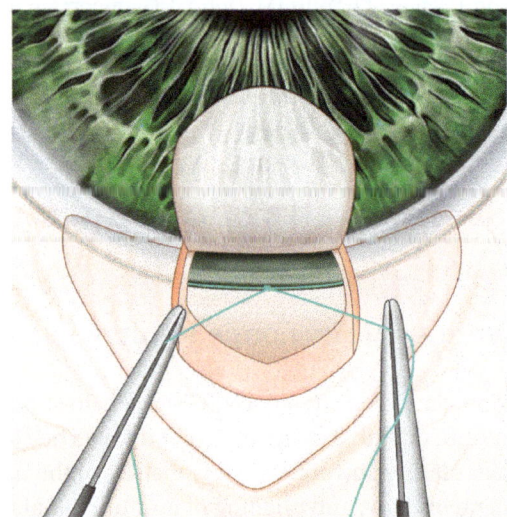

Indications

- Early to moderate open-angle glaucoma where target IOP is in high to mid-teens.
- Conditions where penetrating surgeries have high risk of choroidal effusions such as Sturge–Weber syndrome and high myopia.
- One-eyed patients.
- Pseudoexfoliative glaucoma, uveitic glaucoma (without extensive synechial angle closure) to prevent excess inflammation associated with penetrating surgeries.
- Aphakic glaucoma, to prevent risk of vitreous prolapse.

Contraindications

- Angle-closure glaucoma as iris root is very close to the trabecular meshwork effective filtration might not occur.
- Neovascular glaucoma as new vessels grow in the angle and trabeculum loses its function.
- Angle recession glaucoma as some degree of trabecular meshwork fibrosis has occurred.
- Postselective laser trabeculoplasty as trabeculum might not be intact and may rupture during the surgery.
- Advanced glaucomas where target IOP is in low teens.
- Patient noncooperative for goniopuncture, if needed at a later stage.

Advantages of NPGS

- Early postoperative complications such as shallow anterior chamber and hypotony are rare.
- Bleb-related complications are extremely uncommon. More diffuse and shallow blebs are seen.
- Less inflammation (as anterior chamber not penetrated and no iridectomy), early recovery, and decreased chances of cataract progression.
- Closed globe surgery, less chances of endophthalmitis.

Limitations

- Less efficacy in comparison to trabeculectomy, suitable for patients with target IOP in mid to high teens.
- Learning curve is steep: Inability to localize Schlemm's canal, perforation of TDM, and iris prolapse are common intraoperative complications.
- Postoperative failure rate is high compared to trabeculectomy. Laser goniopuncture of TDM can be done to improve outflow.
- Use limited to open-angle glaucoma.
- Postoperative conjunctival scarring limits future surgical options.

References

1. Eldaly MA, Bunce C, Elsheikha OZ, Wormald R. Non-penetrating filtration surgery versus trabeculectomy for open-angle glaucoma. Cochrane Database Syst Rev. 2014;(2):CD007059.
2. Shaarawy T, Flammer J. Pro: non-penetrating glaucoma surgery—a fair chance. Graefes Arch Clin Exp Ophthalmol. 2003;241(9):699-702.

7.12 Selective Laser Trabeculoplasty

Barkha Gupta, Dewang Angmo

1. Write a short note on selective laser trabeculoplasty.

Selective laser trabeculoplasty (SLT), a laser therapy for open-angle glaucoma, was designed to selectively target pigmented trabecular meshwork (TM) cells while sparing adjacent cells and tissues from thermal damage and maintaining TM architecture.[1] It was first introduced by Latina and Park in 1995.

Mechanism of Action

Selective laser trabeculoplasty is based on the concept of selective photothermolysis, which ensures confinement of thermally mediated radiation damage to a selected pigmented cell population within a tissue with no collateral damage. Selective targeting of pigmented TM cells can be obtained with pulse duration of 3 ns or less and low energy, approximately 1% of the total energy used by argon laser trabeculoplasty (ALT). These low parameters used in SLT are too short for melanin (chromophore) to convert the electromagnetic energy to thermal energy, and hence no heat is generated.[2]

The mechanism by which SLT reduces intraocular pressure (IOP) is unknown; however, the three main theories proposed by Van Buskirk et al., which apply to both SLT and ALT, include a mechanical, biochemical, and cellular effect on TM. According to mechanical theory, SLT results in a stretching and separation of the TM beam and increased mobility following SLT. The biological theory states that SLT causes the release of chemical mediators and stimulates endothelial cell replication. Cellular changes reported following SLT include increased reactive oxygen metabolites that amplify an inflammatory cascade and have direct cytotoxic effects on TM cells. Also, an increase in the monocyte population has been noted in TM which in turn then releases cytokines, such as tumor necrosis factor alfa (TNFα), that could modulate TM cells or alter the Schlemm's canal permeability. Therefore, it is likely that a combination of all these mechanisms could lead to decrease in IOP after SLT.

Procedure

The commercially available SLT device uses a Q-switched, frequency-doubled, 532-nm Nd:YAG laser, 400 μm diameter spot size and delivers energy in 3 ns. Latina SLT single-mirror goniolens is used with methylcellulose as a coupling medium.

The laser is focused on the TM using the helium–neon (He-Ne) aiming beams. An initial energy level of 0.7–0.8 mJ is typically used (with typical settings of 0.4–1.2 mJ) for lightly pigmented TM. The energy level used is titrated to the degree of trabecular pigmentation, that is, with the greater pigmentation, less energy is required. In more heavily pigmented TM, around 0.6 mJ initial energy may be used. If cavitation bubbles ("champagne bubbles") appear, the laser energy is reduced by 0.1 mJ increments until no bubble formation is observed and the treatment is continued at the same energy level. If no cavitation bubbles are observed at the TM after laser application, the pulse energy is increased by increments of 0.1 mJ until bubble formation is seen and then decreased as described above. An energy level just below that of bubble formation is then maintained. Confluent spots are applied for the best results. Whole 360° is lasered (100 spots; 25 spots per quadrant), except in an eye with a heavily pigmented TM, when 180° is done first, and the remaining 180° later, if needed.

Complications

Redness, discomfort, and anterior chamber (AC) reaction in the first week after SLT are very common. Other complications seen after SLT include transient IOP spike, iritis, hyphema, and macular edema. In addition, some uncommon complications of transient corneal thinning, changes in endothelial cell count, foveal burn, and corneal haze have been reported.

References

1. Jha B, Bhartiya S, Sharma R, Arora T, Dada T. Selective laser trabeculoplasty: an overview. J Curr Glaucoma Pract. 2012;6(2):79-90.
2. Kumar H, Mansoori T, Warjri GB, Somarajan BI, Bandil S, Gupta V. Lasers in glaucoma. Indian J Ophthalmol. 2018;66:1539-53.

7.13 Bleb

Dewang Angmo, Niranjana Balasubramaniam, Karthikeyan Mahalingam

1. How will you assess a filtration surgery bleb?

Introduction

Trabeculectomy first described by Cairns, continues to be the preferred method of surgical management of glaucoma.[1] The outcome of this guarded filtration surgery depends on the balance between the formation of a functional shunt to egress the aqueous and the wound healing factors.[2] Bleb morphology is a crucial parameter in deciding the long-term surgical success. The important morphological characteristics include:
- Presence of microcysts
- Conjunctival vascularity
- Extent of the bleb
- Height of the bleb
- Encapsulation of the bleb.

Favorable and Unfavorable Bleb Features

Picht and Grehn in a retrospective study found the favorable and unfavorable morphological features influencing the surgical success.[3]

Favorable	Unfavorable
Microcysts of conjunctiva	Increased vascularization
Paucity of vessels	Corkscrew vessels
Diffuse bleb	Encapsulation of the bleb
Moderate elevation of the bleb	High-doomed appearance

Ideal Bleb

A good functional bleb should be diffuse in appearance, slightly elevated above the scleral flap, with the presence of microcysts in the conjunctival epithelium and should have low conjunctival vascularity similar to that of the surrounding conjunctiva **(Fig. 1)**.[4]

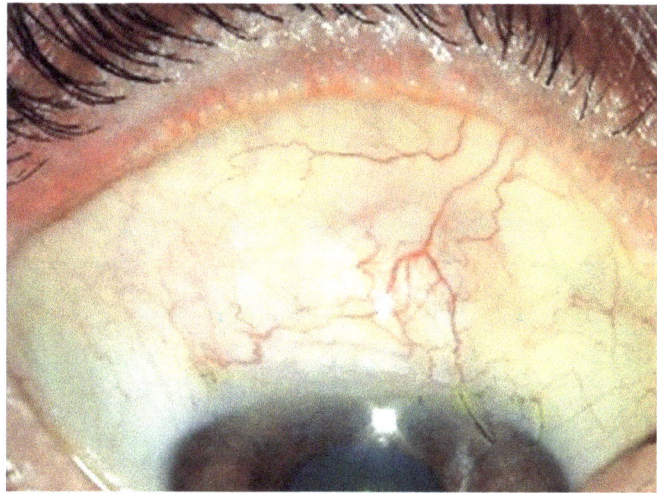

Fig. 1: An ideal bleb.

Assessment of the Bleb

- Clinical assessment—slit-lamp biomicroscopy
- Imaging modalities.

Slit-lamp Biomicroscopy Bleb Grading Systems

The Indiana Bleb Appearance Grading Scale (IBAGS)[5]

This consists of slit-lamp photographic standards and the parameters assessed include bleb height, extent, vascularity, and Siedel's test (HEVS). It was found that slit-lamp and both stereo and mono photographs had high levels of agreement **(Fig. 2)**.[6]

Height standards

	H_0	Flat bleb with no visible elevation
	H_1	Low bleb elevation
	H_2	Moderate bleb elevation
	H_3	High bleb elevation

Extent standards

	E_0	No visible bleb to less than 1 clock hour
	E_1	≥1 clock hour to <2 clock hours
	E_2	≥2 clock hours to <4 clock hours
	E_3	≥4 clock hours

Vascularity standards

	V_0	Avascular (no visible microcysts)
	V_1	Avascular/cystic
	V_2	Mild vascularity
	V_3	Moderate vascularity
	V_4	Extensive vascularity

Siedel's test

	S_0	No bleb leak
	S_1	Pinpoint transconjunctival leakage within 5 seconds
	S_2	Streaming of aqueous within 5 seconds

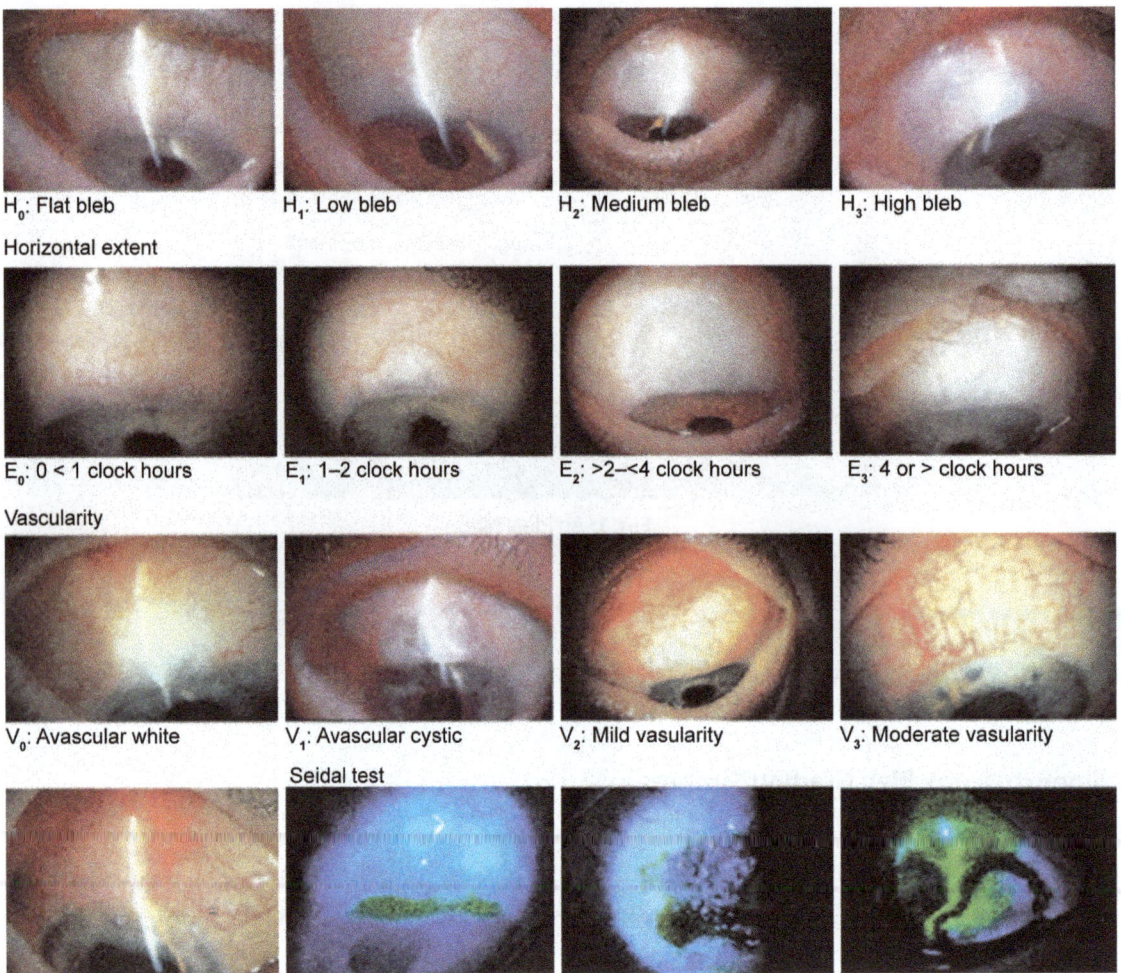

Fig. 2: Photographic standards of the Indiana Bleb Appearance Grading Scale (IBAGS).

The Moorfields Bleb Grading System (MBGS)

Six criteria are assessed pertaining to three main aspects of bleb **(Fig. 3)**.
1. *Area:* Assessment of both the main bleb area (1A, marked by arrows) and the central demarcation area of the bleb (1B, marked by arrows) are to be done. Scoring is done in comparison with the reference photographs.[7]

Score	Extent
1	0%
2	25%
3	50%
4	75%
5	100%

2. *Height:* This represents the highest point of the bleb, given a score of 1-4 in comparison with the reference photographs. Score 1 being the least height and score 4 being the greatest height.
3. *Vascularity:* Vascularity is assessed under three criteria:
   - 3a—Vascularity at the central demarcation area of the bleb
   - 3b—Vascularity at the peripheral part of the bleb
   - 3c—Vascularity at the peripheral nonbleb conjunctiva

Score of 1-5 is made comparing with the reference photographs, with 1 being avascular and 5 being severe vessel inflammation.

Also, the Siedel's test and the presence of subconjunctival blood are included in MBGS.

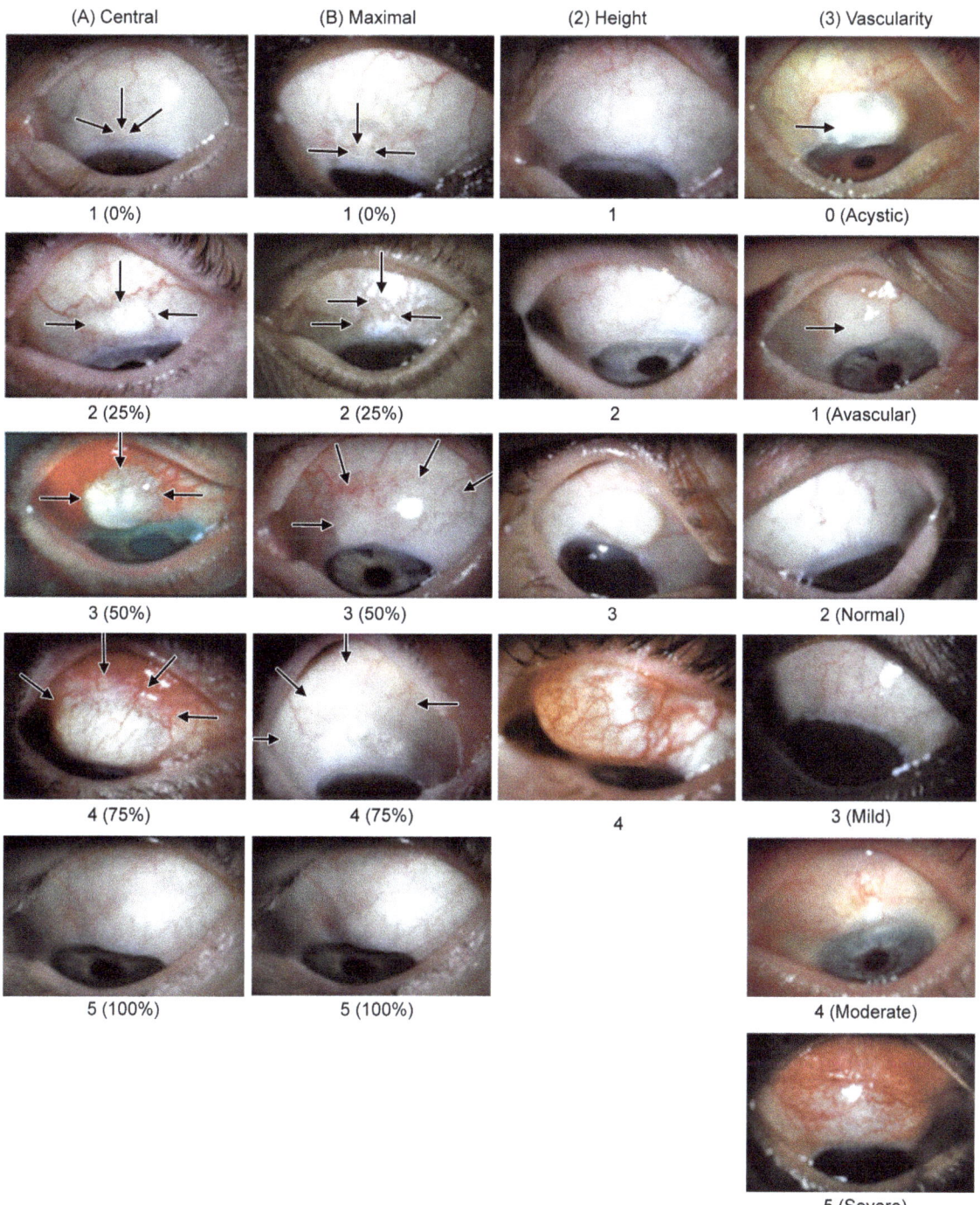

Fig. 3: Moorfields bleb grading system (MBGS).

Some of the other slit-lamp-based clinical bleb grading systems include:
- MaBGS—Mainz bleb appearance grading system[7]
- WBCS—Wuerzburg bleb classification score[8]
- Migdal and Hitchings bleb classification.[9]

Bleb Classification Based on Newer Imaging Modalities

Anterior Segment Optical Coherence Tomography

Anterior segment optical coherence tomography (AS-OCT) provides a more detailed and an ultrastructural imaging of the bleb. The biometric parameters that can be studied include bleb wall thickness, radial length and height, as well as the reflectivity of the bleb wall **(Figs. 4 and 5)**.[10]

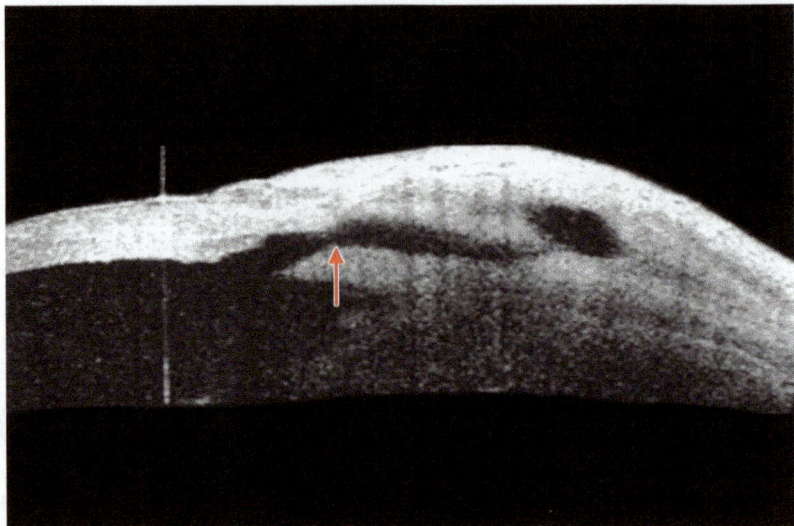

Fig. 4: Patent fistula beneath the sclera (arrow).

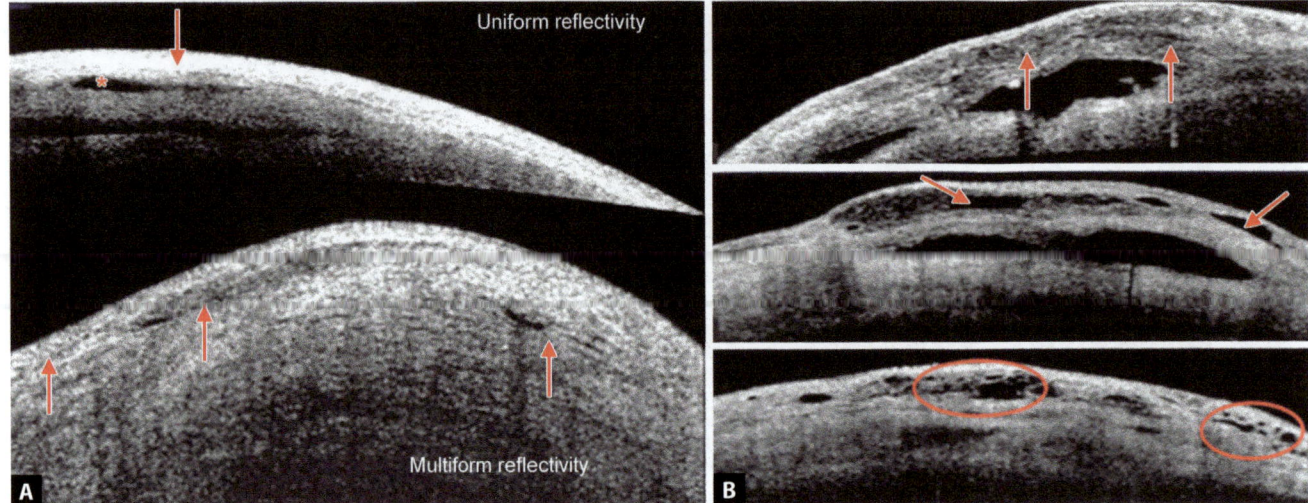

Figs. 5A and B: Anterior segment optical coherence tomography (AS-OCT) images—red arrows indicating reflectivity and red circles indicate cystic changes.

In Vivo Confocal Microscopy

In vivo confocal microscopy (IVCM) enables real-time internal tissue assessment of the bleb. The structural network of conjunctival stroma, epithelial stromal cystic changes, and the vascularity can be studied in detail using IVCM.[4]

Polarization-sensitive Optical Coherence Tomography

Polarization-sensitive optical coherence tomography (PS-OCT) is an extension of OCT that can be used to measure the polarization property of the bleb. This reveals the fibrosis and scarring of the bleb, as collagen is known to have strong birefringence. This enables assessment of the functionality of the filtering blebs.[11]

References

1. Cairns JE. Trabeculectomy: preliminary report of a new method. Am J Ophthalmol. 1968;66(4):673-9.
2. Singh M, Chew PT, Dada T, Singh K, Spaeth GL. Bleb morphology assessment and imaging. J Curr Glaucoma Pract. 2008;50-5.
3. Picht G, Grehn F. Classification of filtering blebs in trabeculectomy: biomicroscopy and functionality. Curr Opin Ophthalmol. 1998;9(2):2-8.
4. Güven Yılmaz S, Değirmenci C, Palamar M, Yağcı A. Evaluation of filtering bleb function after trabeculectomy with mitomycin C using biomicroscopy, anterior segment optical coherence tomography and in vivo confocal microscopy. Turk J Ophthalmol. 2015;45(4):132-7.

5. Cantor LB, Mantravadi A, WuDunn D, Swamynathan K, Cortes A. Morphologic classification of filtering blebs after glaucoma filtration surgery: the Indiana Bleb Appearance Grading Scale. J Glaucoma. 2003;12(3):266-71.
6. Wells AP, Crowston JG, Marks J, Kirwan JF, Smith G, Clarke JCK, et al. A pilot study of a system for grading of drainage blebs after glaucoma surgery. J Glaucoma. 2004;13(6):454-60.
7. Hoffmann EM, Herzog D, Wasielica-Poslednik J, Butsch C, Schuster AK. Bleb grading by photographs versus bleb grading by slit-lamp examination. Acta Ophthalmol. 2019;98(5):e607-10.
8. Furrer S, Menke MN, Funk J, Töteberg-Harms M. Evaluation of filtering blebs using the 'Wuerzburg bleb classification score' compared to clinical findings. BMC Ophthalmol. 2012;12(1):24.
9. Migdal C, Hitchings R. The developing bleb: effect of topical antiprostaglandins on the outcome of glaucoma fistulising surgery. Br J Ophthalmol. 1983;67(10):655-60.
10. Paulaviciute-Baikstiene D, Vaiciuliene R, Januleviciene I. Filtering blebs structure and function evaluation using optical coherence tomography. J Model Ophthalmol. 2016;1(2):10-9.
11. Kasaragod D, Fukuda S, Ueno Y, Hoshi S, Oshika T, Yasuno Y. Objective evaluation of functionality of filtering bleb based on polarization-sensitive optical coherence tomography. Invest Ophthalmol Vis Sci. 2016;57(4):2305-10.

7.14 Complications of Glaucoma Surgery

Bhagabat Nayak, Dewang Angmo

1. Diagnosis, management, and prevention of complications of trabeculectomy arising within 6 weeks after surgery.

Early Postoperative Complication

After the surgery, the most common complications from next day to earlier weeks are intraocular pressure (IOP)-related complications. The IOP may be low or high. In either case, the anterior chamber (AC) may be shallow to flat or deep. The mechanism behind this should be identified and treated accordingly.[1]

Hypotony and Shallow Anterior Chamber

Low IOP <6 mm Hg or nonrecordable IOP with shallow AC should be checked in slit-lamp biomicroscope to see the grade of shallow AC. Usually, shallow AC mostly occurred on second or third day and gradually recovered after 1 week.[2]

- If there is only peripheral iris touch with cornea without central corneal touch with the lens and without central corneal edema then no intervention should be done **(Fig. 1)**.[3]
- If there is central corneal lenticular touch with corneal edema **(Fig. 2)** then intervention should be done to increase the AC depth with air, viscoadaptives such as Healon 5, or only viscocohesive such as Healon or Healon GV if Healon 5 is not available.
- Other causes of the shallow AC such as leak from wound margin, conjunctival defect, or buttonholing should be checked by Seidel's test.
- If there is leak found then it can be (1) pad bandaged for 8–12 hours or overnight with a rolled pad over lid and then a gauze pad over it to secure tight tamponade. (2) If still there is leak, a large-diameter therapeutic soft contact lens can be placed. (3) The conjunctiva can be sutured with 10'0 round body Vicryl suture which is placed intraconjunctively. (4) If there is large conjunctival gap that can be covered by new conjunctival graft from the tissue posterior to the defect or conjunctival autograft. (5) Autologous blood serum or fibrinogen can be injected into the bleb.[4,5]
- If there is no leak or defect and the bleb height is good, then the hypotony is due to *overfiltration*. It is either due to the loose or insufficient nylon suture placed over the partial-thickness scleral flap or the use of antimetabolites leading to overfiltration through the scleral flap or through the conjunctival layer. The postoperative dose of steroid eye drops can be reduced temporarily to promote some fibrosis to increase IOP.
- The *choroidal detachment (CD)* should be ruled out as it occurs due to hypotony and may be due to inflammation, but again it causes persistent hypotony. If there is minimal CD, it may resolve spontaneously. A short course of systemic steroid with increased topical dose along with mydriatics will take care of the inflammatory component and CD may resolve within 4–5 days. If it is large CD or CD with bloody effusion that pushing lens–iris diaphragm anteriorly and cornea is decompensating, then it should be drained through inferior quadrant sclerotomy at the site of maximum height of CD.

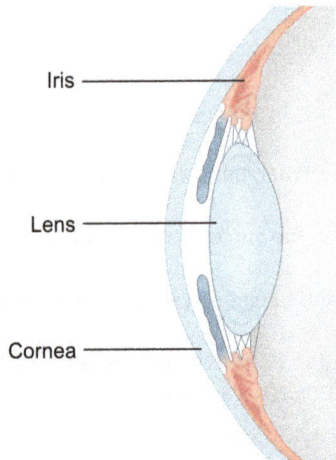

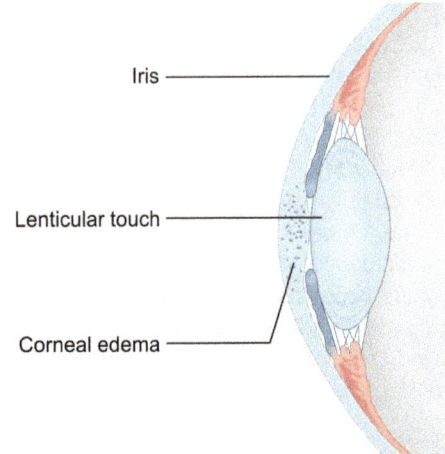

Fig. 1: Peripheral iridocorneal touch but central shallow anterior chamber (AC) without corneolenticular touch.

Fig. 2: Flat anterior chamber (AC) with both peripheral and central iridocorneal and central corneolenticular touch with central corneal edema.

Prevention of flat AC: Careful closure of scleral flap with meticulous conjunctival closure and putting of releasable suture in phakic patients with angle-closure glaucoma is enough to prevent hypotony and flat AC. Sometimes the use of some viscoelastics may be needed to deepen AC while doing surgery or closing the wound to prevent sudden postoperative shallow AC.

Hypotony and Deep Anterior Chamber

If there is low IOP for some days without bleb leak, inflammation, flat AC, and posterior segment complication, no special intervention is required. The dose of topical steroid can be reduced temporarily for allowing some fibrosis to the wound. If there are posterior pole complications such as hypotonic maculopathy such as macular striae with choroidal folds, tortuous vessels, and blurring of disc it is difficult to treat. So preventive measures such as minimum use of antimetabolites and tight wound closure should be done in high-risk patients like young age and those with myopia.[6] Once this complication occurs, standard measures such as pressure patching, oversized bandage contact lens over bleb, combination of autologous blood injection and the bleb, and bleb compression suture should be tried. Application of trichloroacetic acid or cryotherapy to bleb can also be tried, although not so effective if antimetabolites have been used.

If all those above measures fail, surgical revision is considered. Surgical approaches such as resuturing of scleral flap, patch grafting with a donor sclera or pericardium, or transconjunctival sutures through scleral flap can be considered. Visual loss can be reversed with the overfiltration treated within 6 months of the complication.[7]

Elevated Intraocular Pressure with Flat Anterior Chamber

There may be three causes to it.
1. Aqueous misdirection syndrome
2. Incomplete iridectomy with pupillary block
3. Delayed suprachoroidal hemorrhages.

Management

Aqueous misdirection syndrome/malignant glaucoma

Medical Management
- Mydriatic cycloplegics such as the topical atropine three to four times[8]
- Hyperosmotic agents such as intravenous mannitol[9]
- Aqueous suppressants such as beta-blocker and alpha-2 agonist.

Surgical Management

Argon laser photocoagulation of ciliary process through an iridectomy or transscleral diode laser cyclophotocoagulation may relieve by breaking ciliolenticular block.[10]

- Nd:YAG laser of anterior disrupting the anterior hyaloid face in aphakic and pseudophakic malignant glaucoma[11]
- Slit-lamp needle revision where laser not possible by needling of anterior hyaloid face
- Posterior sclerotomy and air injection in AC[12] (**Fig. 3**)
- Pars plana anterior vitrectomy to break anterior hyaloid face[13]
- Lastly, lens extraction with anterior hyaloidotomy should be considered when all other measure fails.[1]

These should be followed by use of atropine to prevent recurrence.

Delayed suprachoroidal hemorrhages: Patients present with severe pain, nausea, and diminution of vision during first few postoperative days. Ultrasonography (USG) can detect this and its extent whether it is 360°, kissing choroid, associated retinal detachment, vitreoretinal adhesion, etc. Drainage of blood is required in these severe cases but has to wait at least 7–10 days till the clot lysis occurs.[1-3]

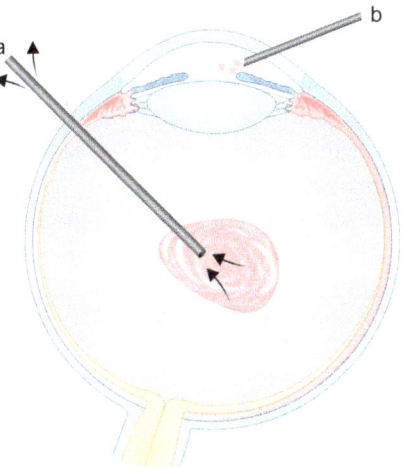

Fig. 3: Posterior sclerotomy and air injection in the management of malignant glaucoma. Fluid is drained or aspirated from the vitreous by means of a pars plana incision (a) and the anterior chamber is deepened with air (b).

Elevated Intraocular Pressure and Deep Anterior Chamber

It indicates that inadequate filtration may be due to tight scleral flap and obstruction of the ostium by iris tissue, blood, lens, or vitreous.

- Gonioscopy should be done to see the ostium. If there is internal blockage it can be relieved by Nd:YAG laser disruption or retraction of the tissue from the ostium by argon laser therapy.
- If not relieved by laser revision surgery may be needed. Sometimes, there may be scarred tissue at the side of flap may obstruct the fistula, but there is still filtering bleb, then internal bleb revision should be done with a spatula entering into the fistula through the ostium from 90 to 180° from the wound site. It will elevate the flap margin and relieve the obstruction. Postoperatively, 5-fluorouracil (5-FU) injection may be required to prevent scarring.
- Intracameral or subconjunctival tissue plasminogen activator (TPA) may be used if there is blood or clot in AC or near scleral flap, respectively.
- If there is no adhesion or fistula obstruction then the *bleb failure* is anticipated.

Failing Bleb and Management

The filtering bleb is typically low to flat and heavily vascularized with corkscrew vessel with no microcysts. Immediate measures should be taken before it permanently fails.

Treatment

- Frequency of topical steroid drop should be increased in addition with subconjunctival steroid injection.
- Subconjuctival 5-FU injection can be given away from the filtering bleb.
- Scleral flap sutures should be lysed or removed in case of releasable suture.
- Application of mitomycin C (MMC) in higher concentration of 0.04% soaked with Merocel sponge can be applied for 3 minutes over the failing bleb on alternate days for three times.
- Intermittent digital massage of globe with index finger for 15 seconds once or twice a day if successful in elevating the bleb may continue for some days to relieve any obstruction or fibrosis and allowing aqueous humor pass through the fistula can solve the problem sometimes.
- If suture lysis or release is ineffective, or if a blood or fibrin clot appears to block the fistula, intracameral TPA may be beneficial.[1,5] Subconjunctival TPA can be given to free a scleral flap from fibrin clot.
- If all these measures fail, antiglaucoma medication can be resumed to control IOP and retrabeculectomy with MMC or 5FU may be tried in a different quadrant or implantation of glaucoma drainage device (GDD) may be required.

Encapsulated Filtering Bleb

Encapsulated filtering bleb, also called Tenon capsule cyst, is characterized by highly elevated, smooth, dome-shaped bleb with large vessels but intervening avascular spaces and no microcysts. More importantly, movement of conjunctiva revealed a second set of stationary vessels beneath the conjunctiva, which is in the layer of fibrous tissue that lines the bleb.

Management includes increased frequency of steroids, bleb massage digitally, and bleb needling through 25–30 G needle with 5 mg of 5FU injection near bleb or MMC injection near bleb. Lastly, dissect the conjunctiva from the fibrous tissue, completely excise it, and resuture the conjunctiva.

Other early postoperative complications include the following:
- *Uveitis and hyphema:* Uveitis can be managed conservatively with more frequency of steroids. Hyphema although less common can be managed conservatively with elevation of head and limited activity.
- *Dellen adjacent to the bleb:* Can be managed by frequent artificial tear and bandaged contact lens. Corneal ulcer can complicate the dellen. Persistent dellen from overhanging blebs should be excised.
- *Loss of central vision:* Central loss of vision or "snuff out" phenomena happens when the remaining central island of vision wipe out after sudden reduction of IOP. Although rare, it occurs in the cases of old age, macular split fixation in the visual field preoperatively, and hypotony.[1] So measures should be taken not to reduce IOP to extremely low postoperatively in these cases.
- *Decompression retinopathy:* Retinal hemorrhage or hemorrhage at macula can occur due to sudden hypotony and decompression of globe. That can be managed conservatively.

2. Management of postoperative shallow AC following filtering surgery.

Kindly refer to Answer 1.

3. Management of encapsulated bleb following filtering surgery.

Encapsulated filtering bleb, also called Tenon capsule cyst, is characterized by highly elevated, smooth dome-shaped bleb with large vessels but intervening avascular spaces and no microcysts. It is typical to see a patent ostium on gonioscopy. More importantly, the movement of conjunctiva revealed a second set of stationary vessels beneath the conjunctiva, which is in the layer of fibrous tissue that lines the bleb. It is important to distinguish it from the typical failing bleb which is low to flat and heavily vascularized with no microcysts where the risk of failure is high if immediate, aggressive steps are not taken.

Both are associated with high IOP and deep AC in the early postoperative period, but the prognosis and management differ.

Management

The physician should be aware that most encapsulated bleb begin functioning well within a few months.[14]
- The mainstay of the treatment is to resume antiglaucoma medications until the improvement occurs.
- Increase the frequency of steroids to reduce inflammation and fibrosis. But one study says that the prolonged steroid therapy may increase the incidence of the encapsulated bleb.[15]
- *Digital bleb massage:* Intermittent digital massage of the globe with index finger for 15 seconds once or twice a day may relieve any obstruction or fibrosis and allowing aqueous humor pass through the fistula can solve the problem sometimes **(Figs. 4A and B)**. But some study says that digital pressure may further reduce aqueous flow through the encapsulated bleb by compressing the subconjunctival layer of tissue.[16]
- Early needling in which a 25–30 G needle is passed beneath the conjunctiva about 5–10 mm from the bleb **(Fig. 5)**. It usually balloon up the conjunctiva and further advances into the bleb to puncture the encapsulation and incise the fibrous episcleral tissue.[17] It may be added with 5 mg of 5FU injection near bleb or MMC injection near bleb.
- Bleb needling with transconjunctival scleral flap suture may also serve the purpose without the complication of sudden hypotony and followed by subchoroidal hemorrhage.[18]
- Lastly, dissect the conjunctiva from the fibrous tissue, completely excise it, and resuture the conjunctiva.[19]
  As invasive procedures are having some complications, it should be done if the conservative management fails.[1]

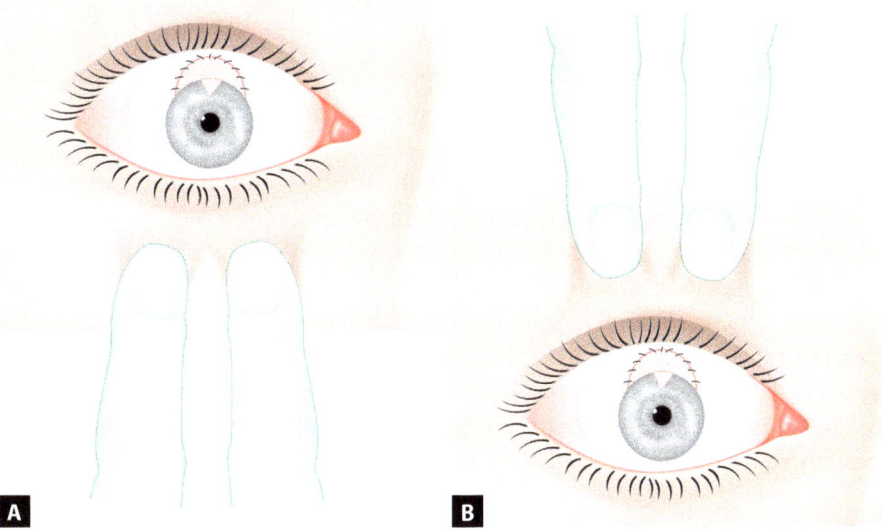

Figs. 4A and B: (A) Digital massage by two index fingers alternatively depressing the globe through the lid from the inferior side. (B) Digital massage by two index fingers alternatively depressing the globe through the lid from superior side of globe distant from the bleb.

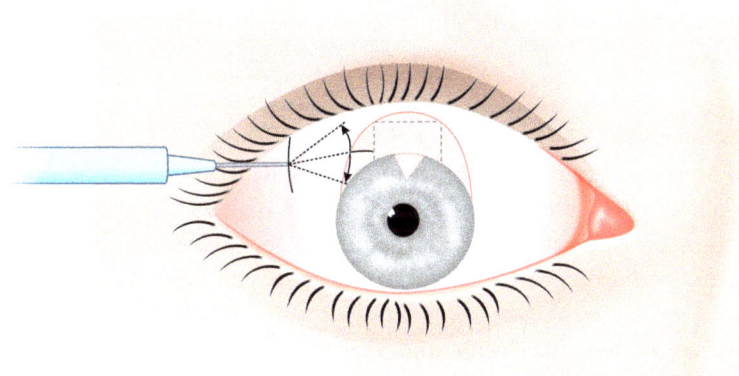

Fig. 5: A 26 or 30 G needle is inserted under conjunctiva 5–10 mm from the bleb margin through the sidewise movements to break the adhesions till it reaches the scleral flap and punctures the encapsulated fibrosis and ensures a free flow of aqueous through the fistula.

 4. Surgical management of failed trabeculectomy.

Once the bleb is failed, then it is difficult to revive the same bleb. Also, there is more chance of failure in making a second trabeculectomy. So some intervention should be tried to save the same bleb before going for the resurgery. Failed trabeculectomy is either due to vascularized flat bleb or encapsulated nonfunctional bleb. Always resume the antiglaucoma medications to achieve the target pressure. If the target IOP is achieved with a stable field and optic disc, then the resurgery should be delayed or avoided.

There are a few surgical options:
- Intervention to revive the same bleb if detected very early
- Retrabeculectomy with antimetabolites or Ologen implant augmentation at the different quadrant if there is normal conjunctiva
- GDD if repeat trabeculectomy not possible
- Cyclodestructive surgery

Intervention to Revive the Same Bleb if Detected Very Early

If there is encapsulated bleb:
The physician should be aware that most encapsulated bleb begin functioning well within a few months.[14] As invasive procedures are having some complications it should be done if the conservative management fails.[1]

- Increase the frequency of steroids to reduce inflammation and fibrosis. But one study says that the prolonged steroid therapy may increase the incidence of the encapsulated bleb.[15]
- *Digital bleb massage:* Intermittent digital massage of the globe with index finger for 15 seconds once or twice a day may relieve any obstruction or fibrosis and allowing aqueous humor pass through the fistula can solve the problem sometimes.
- Early needling in which a 25–30 G needle is passed beneath the conjunctiva about 5–10 mm from the bleb **(Fig. 5)**. It usually balloons up the conjunctiva and further advances into the bleb to puncture the encapsulation and incise the fibrous episcleral tissue.[17] It may be added with 5 mg of 5FU injection near bleb or MMC injection near bleb.
- Bleb needling with transconjunctival scleral flap suture may also serve the purpose without the complication of sudden hypotony and followed by subchoroidal hemorrhage.[18]
- Opening of the obstruction by translimbal ab interno penetration of sclerostomy spatula with pretreatment of mitomycin injection near bleb which is moderately elevated, before 7 days sometimes helps in reviving of the bleb.[20]
- Lastly, dissect the conjunctiva from the fibrous tissue, completely excise it, and resuture the conjunctiva.[19]

Retrabeculectomy with Antimetabolites or Ologen Implant at the Different Quadrant if there is Normal Conjunctiva

When the measures to revive the failed bleb fails, then another trabeculectomy at a different site to the original bleb is advised provided there is normal conjunctiva. In these cases, always there are more chances of failure than the primary bleb. So either antimetabolites such as MMC 0.02–0.04% should be applied during trabeculectomy or Ologen implant can be put to prevent fibrosis in these cases.

Glaucoma Drainage Device if Repeat Trabeculectomy not Possible

When there is difficulty to do second trabeculectomy due to nonavailability of good conjunctiva, scarred conjunctiva due to previous surgery such as vitreoretinal surgery, or there is high-risk cases such as young age, postpenetrating keratoplasty glaucoma, neovascular glaucoma, postvitreoretinal surgery glaucoma, uveitic glaucoma, glaucoma in aphakia and pseudoaphakia, refractory pediatric glaucoma, and iridocorneal endothelial syndrome, then plan for GDD should be done.

It may be nonvalved such as Molteno, Baerveldt, and Sochet or valved such as Ahmed **(Fig. 6)** and Krupin glaucoma valve.

Cyclodestructive Surgery

When all the medical management and surgeries fail, and glaucomas are refractory such as aphakic or pseudophakic glaucoma, neovascular glaucoma, inflammatory glaucoma, chronic angle-closure glaucoma, tumor-associated glaucoma, and postkeratoplasty glaucoma with poor visual prognosis, cyclodestructive procedure is required. It usually reduces the IOP by destructing the ciliary process. There are many techniques described, but the most effective and popular are transscleral cyclophotocoagulation and cyclocryotherapy.[21] Endoscopic cyclophotocoagulation is also an upcoming and promising method. The described methods are the following:

- Beta-irradiation therapy
- Cycloelectrolysis
- Therapeutic USG
- Transscleral microwave cyclodestruction
- Excision of the ciliary body
- Transscleral cyclophotocoagulation: By Nd:YAG laser, diode laser, or krypton laser. It destroys pars plicata with ciliary epithelium thereby decreases the aqueous production and also enhances aqueous outflow.
- *Cyclocryotherapy:* It destroys the ability of the ciliary process to produce aqueous humor by a biphasic mechanism of intracellular ice crystal formation and ischemic necrosis **(Figs. 7A to C)**.

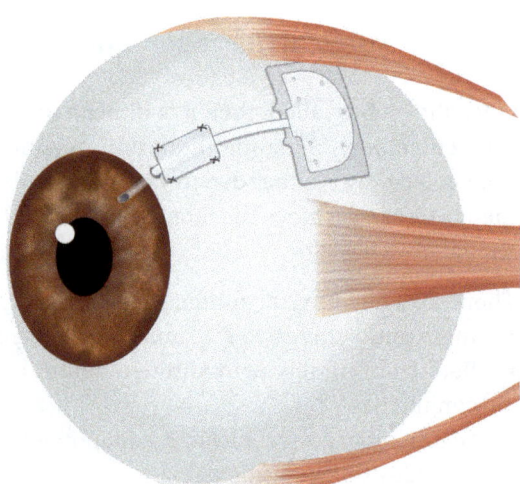

Fig. 6: Ahmed glaucoma drainage device.

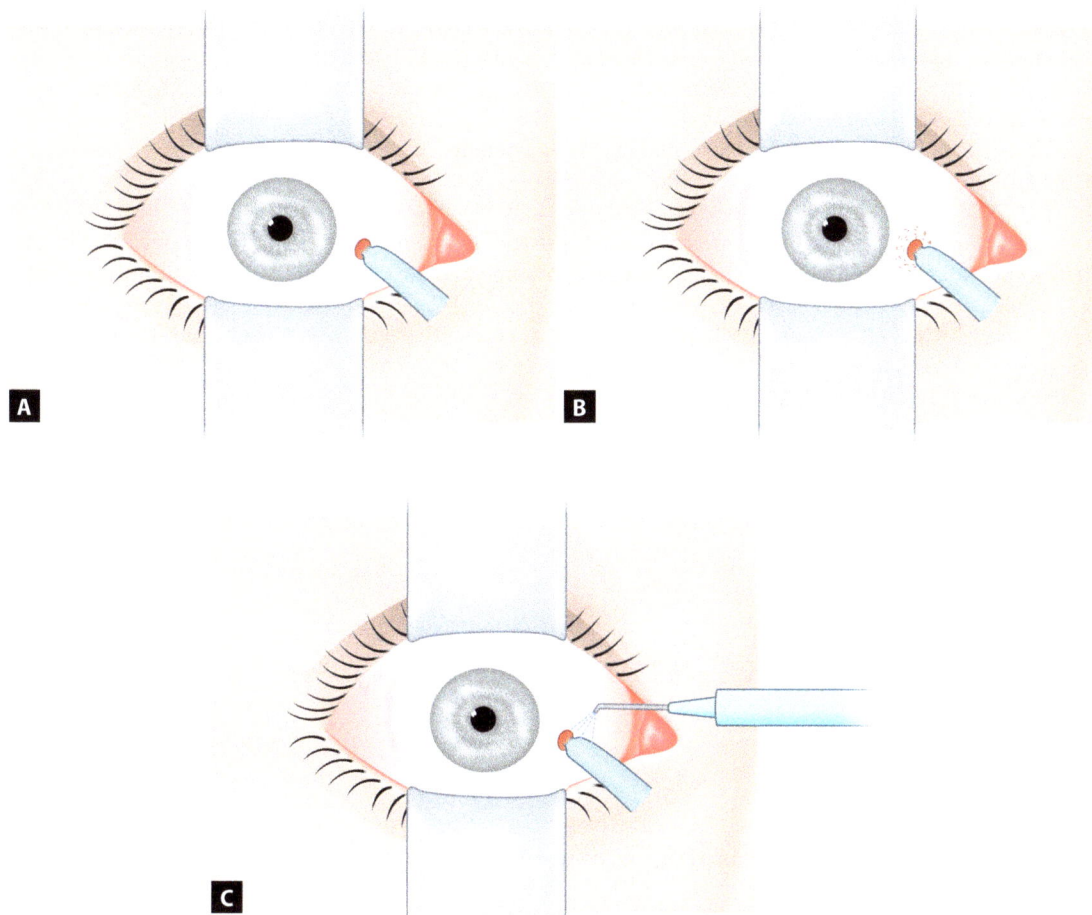

Figs. 7A to C: Cyclocryotherapy technique. (A) The probe tip is placed roughly 2.5 mm from the limbus. The temperature at the probe tip is reduced to approximately −80°C and maintained for 60 seconds. (B) Typical ice ball 30 seconds after initiating freezing. (C) The probe is irrigated with saline solution before removing the probe from the conjunctiva.

 5. **A patient with chronic angle-closure glaucoma undergoes a trabeculectomy and has a shallow AC on the first postoperative day. Describe the process by which you would discern the cause of postoperative AC shallowing and how you would manage this situation.**

Kindly see the above Answers.

References

1. Filtering surgery. In: Rand Allingham R (Ed). Shields Textbook of Glaucoma, 6th edition. Philadelphia, USA: Lippincott Williams & Wilkins; 2011. pp. 502-5.
2. Kao SF, Lichter PR, Musch DC. Anterior chamber depth following filtration surgery. Ophthalmic Surg. 1989;20(5):332-6.
3. Stewart WC, Shields MB. Management of anterior chamber depth after trabeculectomy. Am J Ophthalmol. 1988;106(1):41-4.
4. Zalta AH, Weider RH. Closure of leaking filtering bleb with cyanoacrylate tissue adhesives. Br J Ophthalmol. 1991;75(3):170-3.
5. Graham SL, Murray B, Goldberg I. Closure of fornix-based posttrabeculectomy conjunctival wound leaks with autologous fibrin glue. Am J Ophthalmol. 1992;114(2):221-2.
6. Chandler PA, Grant WM. Mydriatic-cycloplegic treatment in malignant glaucoma. Arch Ophthalmol. 1962;68:353-9.
7. Weiss DI, Shaffer RN, Harrington DO. Treatment of malignant glaucoma with intravenous mannitol infusion: medical reformation of the anterior chamber by means of an osmotic agent—a preliminary report. Arch Ophthalmol. 1963;69:154-8.
8. Stumpf TH, Austin M, Bloom PA, McNaught A, Morgan JE. Transscleral cyclodiode laser photocoagulation in the treatment of aqueous misdirection syndrome. Ophthalmology. 2008;115(11):2058-61.
9. Epstein DL, Steinert RF, Puliafito CA. Neodymium-YAG laser therapy to the anterior hyaloid in aphakic malignant (ciliovitreal block) glaucoma. Am J Ophthalmol. 1984;98:137-43.

10. Chandler PA, Simmons RJ, Grant WM. Malignant glaucoma: medical and surgical treatment. Am J Ophthalmol. 1968;66:495-502.
11. Koerner FH. Anterior pars plana vitrectomy in ciliary and iris block glaucoma. Graefes Arch Clin Exp Ophthalmol. 1980;214:119-27.
12. Bastian A, Kohler U. Therapy and functional results in malignant glaucoma. Klin Monatsbl Augenheilkd. 1972;161:316-21.
13. Freeman WR, Schneiderman TE, Weinreb RN, Baerveldt G. Hemorrhagic choroidal detachment with anterior vitreoretinal adhesions. Ophthalmic Surg. 1991;22(11):670-5.
14. Mandal AK. Results of medical management and mitomycin C-augmented excisional bleb revision for encapsulated filtering blebs. Ophthalmic Surg Lasers. 1999;30(4):276-84.
15. Loftfield K, Ball SF. Filtering bleb encapsulation increased by steroid injection. Ophthalmic Surg. 1990;21(4):282-7.
16. Scott DR, Quigley HA. Medical management of a high bleb phase after trabeculectomies. Ophthalmology. 1988;95(9):1169-73.
17. Ewing RH, Stamper RL. Needle revision with and without 5-fluorouracil for the treatment of failed filtering blebs. Am J Ophthalmol. 1990;110(3):254-9.
18. Laspas P, Culmann PD, Grus FH, Prokosch-Willing V, Poplawksi A, Pfeiffer N, et al. A new method for revision of encapsulated blebs after trabeculectomy: combination of standard bleb needling with transconjunctival scleral flap sutures prevents early postoperative hypotony. PLoS One. 2016;11(6):e0157320.
19. Van Buskirk EM. Cysts of Tenon's capsule following filtration surgery. Am J Ophthalmol. 1982;94(4):522-7.
20. Grover DS, Fellman RL. Outcomes for ab interno bleb revision with a novel translimbal sclerostomy spatula. J Glaucoma. 2017;26(7):633-7.
21. Cyclodestructive surgery. In: Rand Allingham R (Ed). Shields Textbook of Glaucoma, 6th edition. Philadelphia, USA: Lippincott Williams & Wilkins; 2011. pp. 565-74.

7.15 Releasable Sutures in Trabeculectomy

Dewang Angmo, Vatsala Nidi, Karthikeyan Mahalingam

 1. Discuss releasable sutures in trabeculectomy.

Trabeculectomy can have complications based on both overfiltration and underfiltration.[1,2] This can be dealt with by regulating flow through the ostium.

Complications of hypotony and shallow anterior chamber are as follows:
- Peripheral anterior and posterior synechiae
- Corneal decompensation
- Cataract formation
- Choroidal detachment
- Macular edema
- Suprachoroidal hemorrhage.

Various methods have been used to titrate flow through the ostium such as:
- Laser suture lysis[3]
- Removal of externalized scleral flap sutures
- Adjustable sutures
- Releasable sutures.
Releasable sutures have gained the most popularity because of less inherent complications.

Mechanism by which releasable sutures prevent overfiltration: The suture position and tension in trabeculectomy determine the apposition of the flap to the sclera adjacent to the sclerostomy leading to resistance to the flow of aqueous.
- If the flap is loose, the flow through sclerostomy is high, which can lead to hypotony.
- If the scleral flap is too tight, the flow through sclerostomy is low leading to high intraocular pressure (IOP).
  This can lead to ganglion cell loss worsening of glaucomatous optic neuropathy or a sudden loss of remaining field if the glaucoma is advanced known as "snuff out".
  Manipulation of the suture tension could, therefore, alter the flow beneath the flap and also the IOP which can be done by the use of releasable suture techniques.
  Releasable sutures were introduced by Schaffer et al. but popularized by Cohen and Osher.[4] Various techniques of putting releasable sutures are as follows:
- *Wilson's technique:*[4] Wilson described a mattress-type scleral suture, with the knot externalized on the cornea. The suture is first passed through clear cornea to intact sclera passing under the limbus, beginning just anterior to the limbus

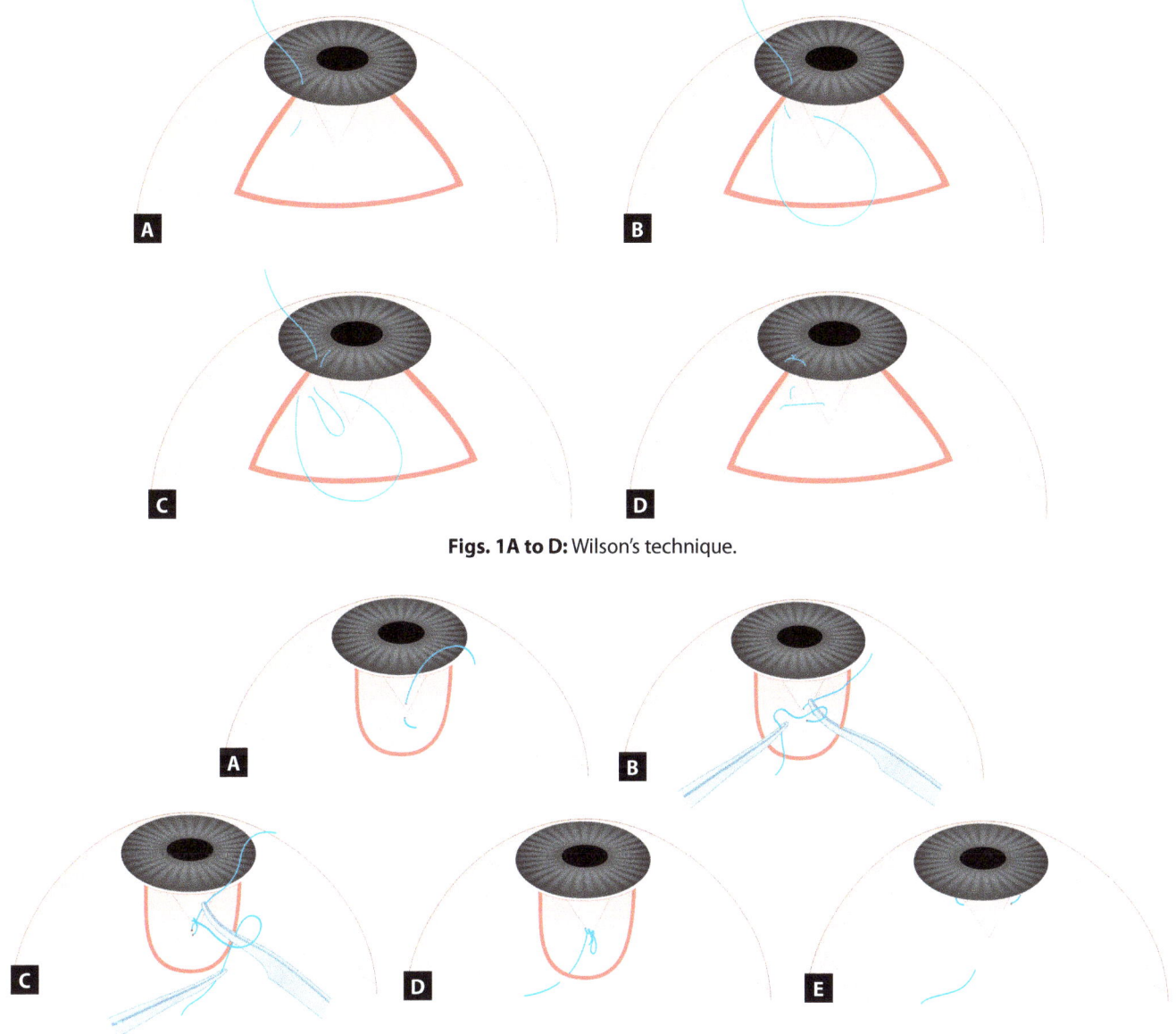

Figs. 1A to D: Wilson's technique.

Figs. 2A to E: Shin's technique.

(**Fig. 1A**). The suture is passed through the periphery of the scleral flap to the adjacent intact sclera (**Fig. 1B**). The third and final pass of the suture is through intact sclera back under the limbus to clear cornea (**Fig. 1C**). The suture is tied to the cornea and adjusted to the desired tension (**Fig. 1D**).

- *Shin's technique:*[5] Shin fashioned a scleral flap suture utilizing a releasable knot, which was passed through the conjunctival bleb approximately 7–8 mm away from the limbus (**Figs. 2A to E**). This technique risks subsequent wound leakage.
- *Cohen and Osher's technique:*[6] These scleral flap sutures can be removed predictably even in the presence of hemorrhagic, thickened, or edematous conjunctiva. The suture is first passed in a reverse fashion through the intact sclera to the apex of a triangular scleral flap (**Fig. 3A**). Next, the suture is passed through the center of the base of the triangular scleral flap to the clear cornea (**Fig. 3B**). A four throw is performed, holding the long tail of the suture with the straight tie in the left hand and throwing four times over the curved tie held in the surgeon's right hand (**Fig. 3C**). Adjust the suture to the desired tension and the excess tail of the suture is cut, leaving approximately 3 mm of suture resting freely on the cornea (**Fig. 3D**).
- *Kolker's technique:*[7] This technique is a modification of Cohen's technique. The suture is passed through the scleral flap to clear cornea, passing under the limbus (**Fig. 4A**). A four throw is performed with the suture, holding the long tail of the suture with the straight tie in the left hand and throwing four times over the curved tie held in the right hand (**Fig. 4B**). A slipknot is created, the suture is adjusted to the desired tension and the excess tail of suture is cut. The suture is then passed back through the clear cornea to clear cornea laterally (**Fig. 4C**). The needle end of the suture is cut flush with the cornea (**Fig. 4D**).

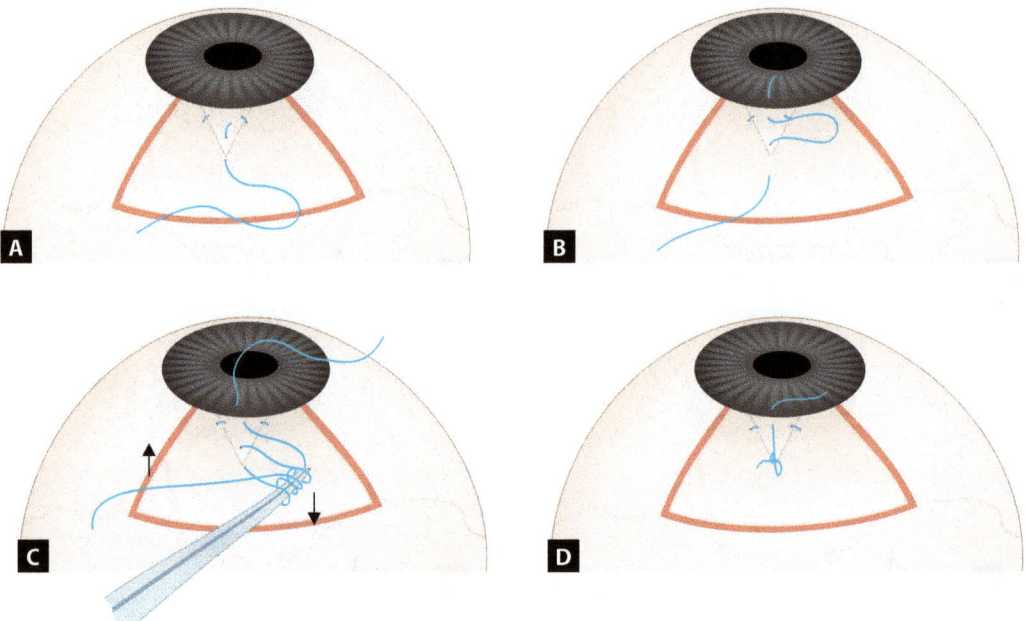

Figs. 3A to D: Cohen and Osher's technique.

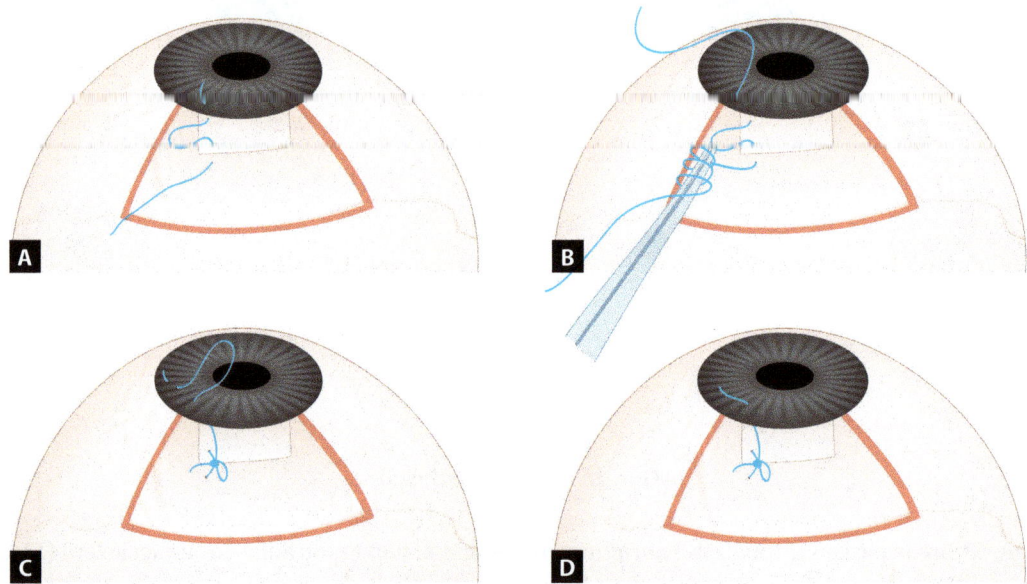

Figs. 4A to D: Kolker's technique.

- *Johnstone's technique:*[8] In this technique, both arms of the suture are used. They are passed through the clear cornea to the intact sclera and the knot is buried beneath the right posterior corner of the quadrangular flap **(Figs. 5A to D)**.

  After putting one releasable suture, the amount of leakage should be checked using sponges after irrigation into the anterior chamber. Depending on the amount of aqueous flow, a second releasable suture may be added for a high-flow state.

Timing of the release of the releasable suture: It depends on the:
- IOP
- Bleb morphology
- Amount of filtration desired for the patient.

The IOP-lowering effect is maximum if the sutures are released within the first three postoperative weeks, especially the first week. With a fornix-based flap, suture release should be deferred until the conjunctival flap is tightly healed, usually around fifth postoperative day.

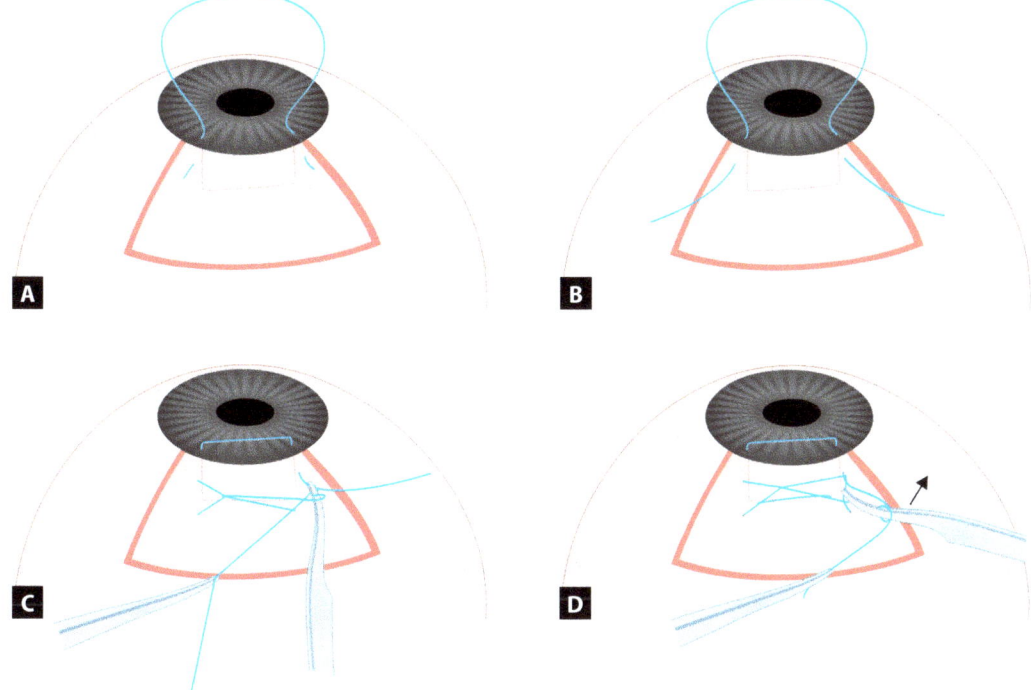

Figs. 5A to D: Johnstone's technique.

Technique of Suture Removal

With upper lid elevated, with a fine forceps, grasp the suture where it changes direction at the elbow between the first (intracorneal) and second (sublimbal) bites of the releasable suture. The intracorneal segment of the loop is teased out using a 23-G needle and pulled with constant, gentle traction to release the loop knot.

Assessment after Suture Release

- After suture release, IOP should be measured.
- If IOP has reduced, it is rechecked after 30 minutes to see if the reduction persists.
- If the IOP remains unchanged, slight digital pressure can be applied to initiate or promote filtration. The patient should be followed up the next day to see the effect of suture release on IOP and bleb morphology.

Advantages

- Releasable sutures reduce the incidence of shallow and flat anterior chamber and iridocorneal touch after trabeculectomy without compromising long-term control of IOP.[9]
- Suture removal is done with minimal equipment and is therefore inexpensive.
- It is easier and less time consuming than performing laser suture lysis, especially in case of a subconjunctival hemorrhage.
- Lens-induced pain, trauma, or risk of a perforated conjunctival flap during laser suture lysis are avoided, and access to a laser is not required.

Disadvantages

- Increased surgery time
- Because of fibrosis, the slipknot can become embedded in the episcleral tissue, making its release difficult.
- "Windshield-wiper keratopathy" occurs if an unburied releasable suture causes corneal abrasions. It resembles the pattern on a car windscreen after the use of wiper blades and happens due to the rubbing of the suture on the cornea with the movement of the lids.
- Release of sutures can lead to subconjunctival hematoma.
- There is always the risk of bleb infection if a track remains where the suture is trimmed.
- Astigmatism

- Excessive shearing stress can result in flap tears since releasable sutures are full-thickness bites near the base of the scleral flap.
- Excess filtration can result after removal of suture.

Therefore, to conclude, releasable sutures ensure the safety of more secure wound closure after filtering surgery without affecting the success of the operation in lowering the IOP for long-term control of glaucoma.

References

1. Dreyer EB. Post-trabeculectomy hypotony. Ophthalmology. 1997;104(9):1367.
2. Alemu B. Trabeculectomy: complications and success in IOP control. Ethiop Med J. 1997;35(1):1-11.
3. Savage JA, Condon GP, Lytle RA, Simmons RJ. Laser suture lysis after trabeculectomy. Ophthalmology. 1988;95(12):1631-8.
4. Wilson RP. Technical advances in filtration surgery. In: McAllister JA, Wilson RP (Eds). Glaucoma. Boston: Butterworths; 1986. pp. 243-50.
5. Shin DH. Removable-suture closure of the lamellar scleral flap in trabeculectomy. Ann Ophthalmol. 1987;19(2):51-3, 55.
6. Cohen JS, Osher RH. Releasable scleral flap suture. Ophthalmol Clin North Am. 1988;1:187-97.
7. Kolker AE, Kass MA, Ratt JL. Trabeculectomy with releasable sutures. Arch Ophthalmol. 1994;112:62-6.
8. Johnstone MA, Wellington DP, Ziel CJ. A releasable scleral-flap tamponade suture for guarded filtration surgery. Arch Ophthalmol. 1993;111(3):398-403.
9. Aykan U, Bilge AH, Akin T, Certel I, Bayer A. Laser suture lysis or releasable sutures after trabeculectomy. J Glaucoma. 2007;16(2):240-5.

7.16 Classification of Secondary Glaucoma

Gazella Bruce Warjri, Dewang Angmo

 1. Outline the classification of secondary glaucoma.

Secondary glaucoma can be classified as described here.

Secondary Childhood Glaucoma

- *Associated with systemic abnormalities:*
  - *Chromosomal disorders:*
    - Trisomy 21 (Down syndrome)
    - Trisomy 18 (Edwards syndrome)
    - Trisomy 13-15 (trisomy D syndrome)
    - Turner syndrome (XO)
  - *Connective tissue disorders:*
    - Marfan syndrome
    - Weill-Marchesani syndrome
    - Stickler syndrome
  - *Metabolic disorders:*
    - Homocystinuria
    - Oculocerebrorenal syndrome (Lowe syndrome)
    - Mucopolysaccharidoses (Hurler syndrome)
  - *Phakomatosis:*
    - Neurofibromatosis
    - Sturge-Weber syndrome
    - von Hippel-Lindau syndrome
  - *Others:*
    - Cystinosis
    - Zellweger syndrome
    - Lowe syndrome
    - Rubinstein-Taybi syndrome
    - Wagner syndrome
    - Walker-Warburg syndrome

- *Glaucoma associated with acquired conditions:*
  - Traumatic glaucoma
  - Steroid induced glaucoma
  - *Secondary to intraocular neoplasm:*
    - Retinoblastoma
    - Juvenile xanthogranuloma
    - Leukemia
    - Melanoma
    - Iris rhabdomyosarcoma
    - Melanocytoma
  - *Lens induced glaucoma:*
    - *Subluxation-dislocation:*
      - Marfan syndrome
      - Weill–Marchesani
      - Homocystinuria
    - Pupillary block—spherophakia
  - Postsurgery for congenital cataract
  - Uveitic glaucoma
  - *Secondary to rubeosis:*
    - Retinoblastoma
    - Coats disease
    - Familial exudative vitreoretinopathy
    - Medulloepithelioma
    - Chronic retinal detachment
  - Retinopathy of maturity
  - Secondary to intraocular infection
  - Secondary to maternal rubella
  - Persistent fetal vasculature

Secondary Adult Glaucoma

- *Secondary open-angle glaucoma:*
  - Pseudoexfoliation glaucoma
  - Pigmentary glaucoma
  - Lens induced glaucoma:
    - Phacolytic glaucoma
    - Lens particle glaucoma
    - Phacoanaphylactic glaucoma
  - Steroid induced glaucoma
  - *Glaucoma associated with intraocular hemorrhage:*
    - Hyphema
    - Microhyphema
    - Hemolytic glaucoma
    - Ghost cell glaucoma
    - Hemosiderotic glaucoma
  - *Traumatic glaucoma:*
    - Contusion injuries
    - Angle recession glaucoma
    - Chemical burns
  - *Glaucoma caused by increased episcleral venous pressure:*
    - *Episcleral and orbital causes:*
      - Hemangioma in Sturge–Weber syndrome
      - Nevus of Ota

- Orbital varices
- Endocrine orbitopathy
- Orbital tumors (retrobulbar)
- Pseudotumor
- Orbital phlebitis
- Orbital arteriovenous fistula
- Chemical burn or radiation damage of the episcleral veins
- Radius-Maumenee syndrome
- *Neurologic conditions:*
  - Cavernous sinus thrombosis
  - Dural shunts
- *Other systemic causes:*
  - Superior vena cava obstruction
  - Jugular vein obstruction
  - Pulmonary venous obstruction
  - Congestive heart failure
- Idiopathic forms
- *Glaucoma due to ocular surgery and laser:*
  - *Aphakic glaucoma/Pseudophakic glaucoma:*
    - Retained viscoelastic material
    - Inflammatory debris and hemorrhage
    - Vitreous in the anterior chamber
    - Lens particles in the anterior chamber
    - Pigment dispersion
    - Pupillary block
  - Postlaser iridotomy
  - Postlaser capsulotomy
  - Postlaser trabeculoplasty
  - Postvitrectomy with silicon oil implantation
  - Uveitis-glaucoma-hyphema (UGH) syndrome
- *Secondary angle-closure glaucoma:*
  - *With pupillary block:*
    - *Enlarged, swollen lens:*
      - Traumatic cataract
      - Phacomorphic glaucoma
      - Phacotopic glaucoma
    - *Anterior lens dislocation:*
      - Traumatic
      - Pseudoexfoliation syndrome
      - Simple ectopia lentis
      - Ectopia lentis et papilla
      - Weill-Marchesani syndrome
      - Marfan's syndrome
      - Homocystinuria
    - Posterior synechia with seclusion or occlusion of the pupil
    - *Aphakia:*
      - Protruding vitreous face
      - Protruding intravitreal silicone oil
    - Microspherophakia
    - *Intraocular lens (IOL) induced:*
      - Anterior chamber IOL
      - Phakic IOL
      - Anteriorly dislocated posterior chamber IOL

- *Secondary angle closure with anterior pulling mechanism without pupillary block:*
  - Neovascular glaucoma
  - Iridocorneal endothelial (ICE) syndrome
  - Posterior polymorphous dystrophy
  - Epithelial and fibrous ingrowth after anterior segment surgery
  - Epithelial and fibrous ingrowth after penetrating trauma
  - Postargon laser trabeculoplasty (ALT) peripheral anterior synechiae (PAS) and endothelial membrane covering the trabecular meshwork
- *Secondary angle closure with posterior pushing mechanism without pupillary block:*
  - Malignant glaucoma (also known as aqueous misdirection, cilio-lenticular block, ciliary block)
  - Iris and ciliary body cysts or tumors
  - Suprachoroidal hemorrhage
  - Uveal effusion
  - Silicon oil or other tamponading fluids or gas implanted in the vitreous cavity
  - Retinopathy of prematurity (stage V)
- *Glaucoma's with mixed mechanisms:*
  - *Glaucoma associated with corneal procedures:*
    - Postpenetrating keratoplasty
    - Postkeratoprosthesis
  - *Glaucoma associated with retinal and vitreous procedures:*
    - Postpars plana vitrectomy
    - Postscleral buckling
  - *Glaucoma associated with intraocular tumors:*
    - Anterior uveal malignant melanoma
    - Ring melanoma of the angle
    - Ciliary body melanoma
    - Posterior uveal malignant melanoma
    - Melanocytoma
    - Melanosis iridis/melanosis oculi
    - Oculodermal melanocytosis
    - Metastasis to anterior segment, posterior segment, or the whole globe
    - Leukemia
    - Primary intraocular lymphoma
    - Histiocytosis X
    - Multiple myeloma
    - Myelodysplastic syndrome
    - Retinoblastoma
    - Juvenile Xanthogranuloma
    - Medulloepithelioma
    - Rhabdomyosarcoma
  - *Uveitic glaucoma:*
    - Posner–Schlossman syndrome
    - Herpes simplex virus (HSV) keratouveitis
    - Varicella zoster virus (VZV) keratouveitis
    - Fuchs heterochromic iridocyclitis
    - Sarcoidosis
    - Human leukocyte antigen B27 (HLA-B27) positive acute anterior uveitis
    - Juvenile rheumatoid arthritis
    - Ankylosing Spondylitis
    - Behçet disease
    - Reiter syndrome
    - Grant syndrome
    - Pars planitis

- Sympathetic ophthalmia
- Syphilis
- *Glaucoma due to infectious diseases:*
  - Congenital rubella
  - Congenital syphilis
  - Hansen disease
  - Acquired immune deficiency syndrome (AIDS)
  - Listeria monocytogenes.

7.17 Drug-induced Glaucoma

Gazella Bruce Warjri, Dewang Angmo

 1. Write a short note on drug-induced glaucoma.

Most of the drug-induced glaucoma is due to an attack of angle closure, which occurs more in predisposed individuals with narrow iridocorneal angle.[1] These medications either stimulate sympathetic or inhibit parasympathetic activation causing pupillary dilation, which can precipitate angle closure (pupillary block). Choroidal volume expansion is also a contributing factor in inducing angle closure by slight forward movement of the lens, especially in predisposed eyes with short axial length and narrow iridocorneal angle.[2] The other mechanism for angle closure is thickening and forward movement of lens, ciliary body rotation, and choroidal effusion. This seems to be an idiosyncratic reaction to certain systemic medications.

Adrenergic Agents

- Topical phenylephrine, its prodrug dipivefrin, and apraclonidine are sympathomimetics, with α-1 agonist activity. They can cause mydriasis and precipitate angle-closure glaucoma in predisposed patients.[3,4] There have been reports of acute angle-closure glaucoma after systemic administration of epinephrine (adrenaline) to treat anaphylactic shock or after nasal ephedrine in the acute management of epistaxis.[5]
- Nebulized β2-adrenergic agonists such as salbutamol, albuterol, or terbutaline can increase intraocular pressure and induce transient angle closure. The stimulus of ciliary body β2-adrenergic receptors can lead to an increase in aqueous humor secretion. These drugs may sometimes get absorbed through the cornea and conjunctiva, because of improper fitting masks during nebulization, and then lead to partial dilatation of the pupil which then induces pupillary block, which occurs mainly in patients with preexisting shallow anterior chamber angles.[6] These can be avoided by using properly fitted masks and handheld nebulizers, with protective eyewear. Ipratropium has a parasympathetic inhibitory effect which can lead to pupil dilatation.[7]
- Amphetamine, dextroamphetamine, and methamphetamine are noncatecholamine adrenergic agonists which are used in some cases of obesity or narcolepsy. In toxic doses, they can cause mydriasis and induce angle-closure glaucoma.[8]

Cholinergic Agents

- Cholinergic agents, pilocarpine, intraocular acetylcholine, and carbachol can cause anterior movement of the iris–lens diaphragm and induce angle closure.[1] Moreover, aqueous misdirection or malignant glaucoma can also be induced by these agents.[9] Eyes with zonular weakness or pseudoexfoliation syndrome seem to be prone to develop miotic-induced angle closure.[10]
- Acetylcholine and carbachol were used to constrict the pupil during intraocular surgery, as in cataract surgery. They can also induce pupillary block in predisposed individuals.[11]

Anticholinergic Agents

- Short-acting anticholinergic such as tropicamide used for pupillary dilation and long-acting ones such as atropine, homatropine, and cyclopentolate used for cycloplegia and pupillary dilation can induce acute angle-closure glaucoma.[12]

- Atropine is often used in general anesthesia as well and can induce angle-closure glaucoma, especially if used with other drugs such as scopolamine, muscle relaxants, ephedrine, and epinephrine. These coupled with psychological stress of surgery and darkness-induced mydriasis may increase the risk.[13]

Sulfa-based Drugs

- Acetazolamide, an oral carbonic anhydrase inhibitor (CAI), is capable of causing a nonpupillary block angle-closure glaucoma, due to ciliary body edema, choroidal detachment, and anterior displacement of the lens–iris diaphragm.[14]
- Hydrochlorothiazide, a diuretic and cotrimoxazole, an antibiotic are also sulfa-based drugs. These also cause rare reactions leading to angle-closure glaucoma.[15,16]
- Another sulfa-based drug is topiramate. It is a sulfamate substituted monosaccharide antiepileptic used in the management of migraine, neuropathic pain, and depression and has also caused glaucoma with the same mechanism.[17]

Antidepressants

- Selective serotonin reuptake inhibitors (SSRIs) such as fluoxetine, paroxetine, fluvoxamine, citalopram, and escitalopram have been associated with acute angle-closure glaucoma.[18] The mechanisms hypothesized are that the glaucoma is induced by the anticholinergic effects or the increased levels of serotonin that cause partial pupillary dilation, as it has been noted that episodes of acute angle-closure glaucoma have been reported to occur within a short period of starting the drugs and also after several days.
- Tricyclic antidepressants such as imipramine, also have this anticholinergic adverse effect and therefore causes the acute angle-closure glaucoma in predisposed individuals.[19]

Histamine H1 and H2 Receptor Antagonists

- Pheniramine, brompheniramine, dexbrompheniramine, chlorpheniramine, dexchlorpheniramine, dimethindene, and triprolidine are histamine H1 receptor antagonists used to treat allergic conditions.
- While cimetidine and ranitidine are H2 receptor antagonists used for gastric and duodenal ulcers and gastroesophageal reflux. Both these groups show a weak anticholinergic effect which can cause mydriasis and induce acute angle-closure glaucoma in predisposed patients.[20]

Anticoagulants

- A rare complication of anticoagulants is massive vitreous, choroidal, or subretinal hemorrhage, especially in cases of overtreatment with anticoagulants, exudative age-related macular degeneration, or nanophthalmos.[21-23]
- Heparin, low-molecular-weight heparin (enoxaparin), and warfarin have all been reported to cause acute angle-closure glaucoma. In most cases, surgery may be needed to drain the choroidal hemorrhage or effusion.

Other Drugs

- The prostaglandin analog, latanoprost, had induced ciliochoroidal effusion in a patient with Sturge–Weber syndrome and in two other separate cases as well.[24,25] It has been speculated that the increased uveoscleral outflow caused swelling of the ciliary body leading to pushing of the iris lens diaphragm anteriorly.[25]
- There has been a case reported of candesartan cilexetil (angiotensin receptor blocker) induced angioedema in the choroid. This caused choroidal effusion followed by shallow anterior chamber and eventually malignant glaucoma.[26]

References

1. Lachkar Y, Bouassida W. Drug-induced acute angle closure glaucoma. Curr Opin Ophthalmol. 2007;18(2):129-33.
2. Quigley HA. Angle-closure glaucoma-simpler answers to complex mechanisms: LXVI Edward Jackson Memorial Lecture. Am J Ophthalmol. 2009;148(5):657-69.
3. Zenzen CT, Eliott D, Balok EM, Watnick RL, German P. Acute angle-closure glaucoma associated with intranasal phenylephrine to treat epistaxis. Arch Ophthalmol. 2004;122(4):655-6.
4. Wolfs RC, Grobbee DE, Hofman A, de Jong PT. Risk of acute angle-closure glaucoma after diagnostic mydriasis in nonselected subjects: the Rotterdam study. Invest Ophthalmol Vis Sci. 1997;38(12):2683-7.
5. Zenzen CT, Eliott D, Balok EM. Acute angle-closure glaucoma associated with intranasal phenylephrine to treat epistaxis. Arch Ophthalmol. 2004;122:655-6.

6. Rho QS. Acute angle-closure glaucoma after albutolol nebulizer treatment. Am J Ophthalmol. 2000;130:123-4.
7. Shah P, Dhurjon L, Metcalfe T, Gibson JM. Acute angle closure glaucoma associated with nebulised ipratropium bromide and salbutamol. BMJ. 1992;304:40-1.
8. Fraunfelder FT, Fraunfelder FW. Drug-induced ocular side effects for optic nerve degeneration. The Recognition of Facts. Boston (MA): Butterworth-Heinemann; 2001.
9. Rieser JC, Schwartz B. Miotic-induced malignant glaucoma. Arch Ophthalmol. 1972;87(6):706-12.
10. Ritch R, Lowe R. Angle-closure glaucoma: clinical types. In: Ritch R, Shields M, Krupin T (Eds). The Glaucomas. St. Louis: Mosby; 1996; pp. 829-30.
11. American Academy of Ophthalmology. Basic and clinical meshwork cells. Invest Ophthalmol Vis Sci. 1997;38(6):1229-40.
12. Brooks AM, West RH, Gillies WE. The risk of precipitating acute angle closure glaucoma with the clinical use of mydriatic agents. Med J Aust. 1986;145:34-6.
13. Lentschener C, Ghimouz A, Bonnichon P, Parc C, Ozier Y. Acute postoperative glaucoma after nonocular surgery remains a diagnostic challenge. Anesth Analg. 2002;94:1034-5.
14. Fan JT, Johnson DH, Burk RR. Transient myopia, angle-closure glaucoma, and choroidal detachment after oral acetazolamide. Am J Ophthalmol. 1993;115(6):813-4.
15. Geanon JD, Perkins TW. Bilateral acute angle-closure glaucoma associated with drug sensitivity to hydrochlorothiazide. Arch Ophthalmol. 1995;113(10):1231-2.
16. Grinbaum A, Ashkenazi I, Gutman I, Blumenthal M. Suggested mechanism for acute transient myopia after sulfonamide treatment. Ann Ophthalmol. 1993;25(6):224-6.
17. Banta JT, Hoffman K, Budenz DL, Ceballos E, Greenfield DS. Presumed topiramate bilateral acute angle-closure glaucoma. Am J Ophthalmol. 2001;132(1):112-4.
18. Eke T, Carr S. Acute glaucoma, chronic glaucoma and serotoninergic drugs. Br J Ophthalmol. 1998;82(8):976-8.
19. Ritch R, Krupin T, Henry C, Kurata F. Oral imipramine and acute angle closure glaucoma. Arch Ophthalmol. 1994;112(1):67-8.
20. Tripathi RC, Triathi BJ, Haggerty C. Drug-induced glaucomas: mechanism and management. Drug Saf. 2003;26:749-67.
21. Schlote T, Freudenthaler N, Gelisken F. Anticoagulative therapy in patients with exudative age-related macular degeneration: acute angle closure glaucoma after massive intraocular hemorrhage. Ophthalmologe. 2005;102:1090-6.
22. Neudorfer M, Leibovitch I, Goldstein M, Loewenstein A. Massive choroidal hemorrhage associated with low molecular weight heparin therapy. Blood Coagul Fibrinolysis. 2002;13:257-9.
23. Caronia RM, Sturm RT, Fastenberg DM, Berke SJ, Weintraub J. Bilateral secondary angle-closure glaucoma as a complication of anticoagulation in a nanophthalmic patient. Am J Ophthalmol. 1998;126:307-9.
24. Sakai H, Sakima N, Nakamura Y, Hayakawa K, Sawaguchi S. Ciliochoroidal effusion induced by topical latanoprost in a patient with Sturge-Weber syndrome. Jpn J Ophthalmol. 2002;46(5):553-5.
25. Yalvac IS, Tamcelik N, Duman S. Acute angle-closure glaucoma associated with latanoprost. Jpn J Ophthalmol. 2003;47(5):530-1.
26. Hille K, Hille A, Ruprecht KW. Malignant glaucoma due to drug-related angioedema. Am J Ophthalmol. 2003;135(2):224-6.

7.18 Lens-induced Glaucoma

Gazella Bruce Warjri, Dewang Angmo

1. Write a short note on lens-induced glaucoma.

Lens-induced glaucoma can be of following types as described here.

Open-angle Glaucoma

Phacolytic Glaucoma

Pathogenesis

When it was first described it was thought that the glaucoma was due to obstruction of the trabecular meshwork by a combination of swollen macrophages, distended by engulfed lens material and lens debris.[1] It was later proved that in this acute open-angle glaucoma there is a role of high-molecular-weight (HMW) proteins in causing obstruction.[2] It was also interesting to note that phacolytic glaucoma does not occur in children or young adults, as HMW proteins are not present in the lenses of patients in this age group.[3]

Clinical Features and Diagnosis

Patients present with a painful red eye, photophobia with a history of acute reduction of vision (due to the corneal edema and associated glaucoma), preceded by a period of gradual diminution of vision for months or years. On examination, circumcorneal congestion, microcystic edema in the cornea, endothelial precipitates, cells and flare in the anterior chamber, and high intraocular pressure (IOP) are seen. An open anterior chamber angle is seen on gonioscopy. Aspirated anterior chamber fluid can be examined microscopically. Biochemical studies can also be done to identify HMW proteins.

Treatment

Phacolytic glaucoma is an ocular emergency. The high recalcitrant IOP can be brought down initially by systemic carbonic anhydrase inhibitors (CAI) and osmotic agents. Topical β-blockers, CAIs, and α-2-agonists along with topical cycloplegics, topical steroids (to reduce the inflammation) are prescribed. The definitive treatment is extraction of the cataract.

Lens Particle Glaucoma

Pathogenesis

Unlike phacolytic glaucoma, the glaucoma here is caused by liberated lens particles due to a disrupted lens capsule.[4] It can occur after trauma to the lens, postcataract surgery, or postneodymium-doped yttrium aluminum garnet (Nd:YAG) posterior capsulotomy.

Clinical Features and Diagnosis

A history of trauma, previous cataract surgery, or Nd:YAG posterior capsulotomy will be present. Clinical findings are similar to phacolytic glaucoma. The inflammation may be greater here and lead to formation of anterior and posterior synechiae with pupillary membranes.

Treatment

Topical steroids with topical mydriatics are given to prevent synechiae formation, along with topical glaucoma medications. If the lens material does not resorb, then surgical removal of the material has to be done. Permanent damage to the trabecular meshwork may occur if timely intervention is not done. Cystoid macular edema and even traction retinal detachments may also occur.[5]

Phacoantigenic Glaucoma

Pathogenesis

It is also known as phacoanaphylactic glaucoma and is the most difficult to diagnose clinically. The term is a misnomer as the underlying mechanism is thought to be an Arthus-type immune complex reaction, mediated by immunoglobulin G (IgG) and the complement system, against lens proteins, and not an allergic reaction.[6] It usually occurs after an ocular surgery or trauma to the lens capsule.

Clinical Features and Diagnosis

The time interval between the trauma and the onset of inflammation is 24 hours to 2 weeks. On examination, there is eyelid edema, circumcorneal congestion, corneal edema, mutton fat keratic precipitates (KPs), severe anterior chamber reaction, posterior synechia with occasional anterior vitritis.[7]

A conclusive diagnosis is by checking for the presence of polymorphonuclear leukocytes in the aqueous along with lens proteins, the amount of which is inadequate to account for the severity of the glaucoma.

Treatment

Topical steroids are given to reduce the inflammation and glaucoma medications to reduce the IOP. Surgical intervention is usually required to remove the lens material.

Angle-closure Glaucoma

Phacomorphic Glaucoma

Pathogenesis

Initially pupillary block occurs due to the intumescent cataractous lens, especially in the mid-dilated state when the posterior component of the dilator papillae muscle reaches maximum effort.[8] With this force, the iris is pushed against the lens leading to a pupillary block. Aqueous humor accumulates in the posterior chamber, pushing the iris further forwards until the iris root comes in contact with the trabecular meshwork, leading to angle-closure glaucoma. A shallow anterior chamber as in hyperopia predisposes to this condition.

Clinical Features and Diagnosis

The clinical features are quite similar to acute angle-closure glaucoma. Patients present with severe ocular pain with headache, which may be associated with nausea and vomiting, perception of haloes around lights (due to corneal edema). There is also a history of diminution of vision for months or years followed by a recent acute decrease in vision. On examination, features are circumcorneal congestion, corneal edema, shallow anterior chamber, mid-dilated pupil, intumescent mature cataractous lens, and minimal anterior chamber cells and flare. Gonioscopy reveals a closed angle.

Treatment

The high IOP has to be reduced on an emergency basis by systemic CAIs, osmotic agents, topical β-blockers, topical α-2-agonists, and topical CAIs. This is immediately followed by cataract extraction, the definitive treatment. The fellow eye is also usually predisposed, so a prophylactic laser iridotomy should be done if the eye is not pseudophakic.

Ectopia Lentis

Pathogenesis

It may be present as an isolated inherited form such as simple ectopia lentis or ectopia lentis et papillae, or there may be systemic associations such as Marfan syndrome, homocystinuria, or Weill-Marchesani syndrome. Subluxation or dislocation of the lens occurs either spontaneously or after trauma.

Clinical Features and Diagnosis

Minimal subluxation may be asymptomatic. Symptoms include ocular pain, redness, decrease in visual acuity, and sometimes headache, nausea, and vomiting, when the dislocation results in pupillary block and angle-closure glaucoma.

Clinical findings would include iridodonesis, phacodonesis, asymmetric or symmetric shallowing of the anterior chamber. Examination of the fellow eye might show differences in the depth of the anterior chamber with the affected eye.

Treatment

Pupillary block with consequent angle-closure glaucoma, and total anterior dislocation of the lens would require removal of the lens. Procedures that can be performed include lensectomy/vitrectomy with aphakic contact lens or spectacles, iris fixated intraocular lens, or scleral fixated posterior intraocular lens.

Note: Topical miotic agents and topical prostaglandin analogs are to be avoided in all lens-induced glaucomas.

References

1. Flocks M, Littwin CS, Zimmerman LE. Phacolytic glaucoma. A clinicopathologic study of one hundred thirty-eight cases of glaucoma associated with hypermature cataract. Arch Ophthalmol. 1955;5437-45.
2. Epstein DL, Jedziniak JA, Grant WM. Obstruction of aqueous outflow by lens particles and by heavy-molecular-weight soluble lens proteins. Invest Ophthalmol Vis Sci. 1978;17:272-7.
3. Yanoff M, Scheie HG. Cytology of human lens aspirate. Its relationship to phacolytic glaucoma and phacoanaphylactic endophthalmitis. Arch Ophthalmol. 1968;80:166-70.
4. Chandler PA, Grant WM. Glaucoma, 2nd edition. Philadelphia: Lea & Febiger; 1979. pp. 216-23.
5. Conner IP, et al. Lens-induced glaucoma. In: Epstein DL, Schuman JS, Kahook MY (Eds). *Chandler and Grant's Glaucoma,* 5th edition. Thorofare, N.J.: Slack; 2013. pp. 441-7.
6. Thach AB, Marak Jr GE, McLean IW, Green WR. Phacoanaphylactic endophthalmitis: a clinicopathologic review. Int Ophthalmol. 1991;15:271-9.
7. Papaconstantinou D, Georgalas I, Kourtis N, Krassas A, Diagourtas A, Koutsandrea C, et al. Lens-induced glaucoma in the elderly. Clin Interv Aging. 2009;4:331-6.
8. Mapstone R. Acute shallowing of the anterior chamber. Br J Ophthalmol. 1981;65:446-51.

7.19 Normal-tension Glaucoma

Neha Midha, Dewang Angmo

 1. **What is normal-tension glaucoma? Discuss its etiopathogenesis, clinical characteristics, differential diagnosis, and management of a case of normal-tension glaucoma.**

Normal-tension glaucoma (NTG) is a diagnosis of exclusion and is characterized by glaucomatous optic neuropathy with intraocular pressure (IOP) measurements consistently below 21 mm Hg.

Etiopathogenesis

Etiopathogenesis of NTG is unclear, however, the postulated hypothesis is:[1]
- Reduced ocular blood flow (OBF) causing ischemia and death of retinal ganglion cells (RGCs). This hypoperfusion has been attributed to systemic hypotension/nocturnal hypotension, disturbed autoregulation, vascular dysregulation/Flammer syndrome.
- Vascular dysregulation is partly mediated by endothelial dysfunction which causes raised levels of endothelin-1 (vasoconstrictor) and decreased levels of nitric oxide (vasodilator).
- Systemic conditions such as Raynaud's disease, migraine, and obstructive sleep apnea are also associated with impaired OBF.
- This unstable oxygen tissue supply due to impaired OBF contributes to glaucomatous damage. This phenomenon is known as ischemia–reperfusion injury (IRI). The main effect of IRI is the induction of chronic oxidative stress, particularly in local mitochondria of RGCs and their axons.
- An elevated retrograde translaminar pressure gradient due to reduction in intracranial pressure can also induce optic nerve damage, either due to barotrauma or through damage to the capillaries, resulting in a posteriorly displaced lamina cribrosa.
- NTG also has a genetic predisposition and runs in families.

Clinical Characteristics

Normal-tension glaucoma has optic nerve cupping, open angles, and visual field loss similar to primary open-angle glaucoma (POAG) with few distinguishing features:[2]
- IOP < 21 mm Hg at all visits and on diurnal variation curve without any treatment.
- Presence of disc hemorrhages—their presence signify poor control and high likelihood of progression.
- Field defects are deeper, steeper, and closer to fixation.

Differential Diagnosis

- *Burnt out open-angle glaucoma:* Steroid induced, posttraumatic
- *Pseudo glaucoma (mimicking glaucomatous optic neuropathy):*
  - Anterior ischemic optic neuropathy
  - Branch retina vein occlusion
  - Disc drusen
  - Physiological cupping
  - Drug induced optic neuropathy—isoniazid and ethambutol
  - Systemic diseases such as syphilis and tuberculosis
  - Orbital or intracranial tumor
  - Shock-induced optic neuropathy
- *High pressure glaucoma misdiagnosed as NTG due to:*
  - Thin central corneal thickness (CCT)
  - History of refractive surgery
  - Missing the IOP peak in diurnal curve.

Management

Detailed history: Questions to look for signs and symptoms of vascular dysregulation (cold hands and migraine), past history of corticosteroid eye drops, history of a hemodynamic crisis, major surgery with a difficult recovery, or a blood transfusion, and family history of glaucoma.

A comprehensive examination to look for: Signs of ocular allergy (to rule out prolonged steroid use), signs of trauma, presence of collateral vessels suggesting old vascular occlusions, disc pallor, color vision, and contrast sensitivity.

Investigations: Applanation tonometry, pachymetry, visual field examination, and retinal nerve fiber layer optical coherence tomography (RNFL OCT) (if needed).

Once the diagnosis has been established:[3]
- Lower IOP by 30% as recommended by collaborative NTG study.
- Topical medications or selective laser trabeculoplasty can be chosen as primary mode of treatment.
- Principles of medical management are similar as for primary open-angle glaucoma—prostaglandin (PG) analogs, α-agonist, and carbonic anhydrase inhibitors can be used. Use of β-blockers as first line is avoided as there is some controversy over whether they decrease perfusion.
- Low pressure glaucoma treatment study showed lower rates of progression with brimonidine 0.2% as compared to timolol 0.5%.
- Surgical treatment (filtering surgery) should be offered only when progression is documented on maximal tolerable medical therapy or noncompliance to medical therapy.

References

1. Trivli A, Koliarakis I, Terzidou C, Goulielmos GN, Siganos CS, Spandidos DA, et al. Normaltension glaucoma: pathogenesis and genetics (review). Exp Ther Med. 2018;17:563-74.
2. Anderson DR. Normal-tension glaucoma (low-tension glaucoma). Indian J Ophthalmol. 2011;59(Suppl. 1);S97-101.
3. Stein JD, Challa P. (2007). Diagnosis and Treatment of Normal-Tension Glaucoma. [online] Available from https://www.aao.org/eyenet/article/diagnosis-treatment-of-normal-tension-glaucoma. [Last accessed June, 2022].

7.20 Refractory Glaucoma

Dewang Angmo, Nikitha Ayyadurai, Karthikeyan Mahalingam

 1. Write a short note on refractory glaucoma.

Certain types of glaucoma and certain patients respond to treatment poorly leading to inability to achieve target intraocular pressure (IOP) and progression of field defect.

Causes

- Neovascular glaucoma
- Postpenetrating keratoplasty glaucoma
- Pseudophakic/aphakic glaucoma
- Silicon oil induced glaucoma (postvitreoretinal surgery)
- Traumatic glaucoma
- Chronic uveitis
- Primary congenital glaucoma
- Anterior segment dysgenesis—Peters, iridocorneal endothelial (ICE), Axenfeld–Rieger syndrome, and aniridia
- Congenital hereditary endothelial dystrophy (CHED) associated glaucoma.

Pathogenesis

The most common cause of failure in glaucoma filtering surgery is scarring of the filtering bleb with increased amount of collagen and proliferation of fibroblasts. Newer antifibrotic agents and drug delivery systems are under development in an effort to improve efficacy and safety. Aqueous humor contains transforming growth factor-β (TGF-β), a potent modulator of tissue repair, in human aqueous and plays a role in the healing process after glaucoma filtering surgery. Aqueous humor has chemoattractant activity for ocular fibroblasts, and this activity is significantly greater in eyes with previously failed glaucoma surgery. Therefore, components of normal aqueous humor and its alterations in some glaucoma patients are likely to influence both success and failure of the filtering bleb.[1]

Predisposing Factors

Young age, chronic topical glaucoma medication usage before trabeculectomy has been identified as a risk factor for failure of trabeculectomy because of subclinical inflammation. Conjunctival impression cytology correlated significant degrees of metaplasia with the number of glaucoma medications used. The number of conjunctival fibroblasts and inflammatory cells increases after previous ocular surgery involving the conjunctiva.

Primary Congenital Glaucoma

As the fibroblastic activity and wound healing response are very robust at young age, children are more prone to bleb failure. As such the functioning of the underdeveloped trabecular meshwork (TM) also contribute to the poor outcome post-trabeculectomy. Mitomycin C (MMC) when used should be used at a higher concentration say 0.4 mg/mL for a comparatively longer time than adults.

Anterior Segment Dysgenesis

Entities such as Peters' anomaly, ICE, CHED, aniridia, ectropion, and uvea are associated with refractory glaucoma despite surgical management due to reasons similar to congenital glaucoma.

Adult Refractory Glaucomas

Pseudophakic/aphakic glaucoma, traumatic glaucoma, postpenetrating keratoplasty glaucoma, and epithelial downgrowth are associated with high IOP and poor outcomes post-trabeculectomy might require multiple procedures before achieving target IOP.

Postpars Plana Vitrectomy Surgery Glaucoma

Incidence of glaucoma after vitreoretinal (VR) surgery and silicone oil injection—56% at 8 months. Incidence of glaucoma after pars plana vitrectomy (PPV)—15–20%.[2]

Mechanism of glaucoma after VR surgery:
- Inflammation
- Overfill of silicone oil
- Pupillary block in aphakia and synechial angle closure.
- Migration of emulsified oil into the anterior chamber (AC) and blockage of trabecular meshwork.
- In post-PPV—damage to TM due to diffusion of oxygen from vitreous to aqueous.

In Buckling—compression of the vortex veins, swelling of the ciliary body, and anterior displacement of lens iris diaphragm.

Poorer outcomes reported compared to other secondary glaucoma.

Causes—severe inflammation due to silicone oil, subconjunctival fibrosis and scarring (especially with peritomy), fibrosis of the scleral ostium. Singh et al. reported an absolute success rate of 15.8% and a total success rate of 36.9% at 1 year. Bleb was flat and nonfunctional in 52.6%, required needling in 63.1%.[3]

Management

Modes of Management (Flowchart 1)
- Antifibroblast agents augmented trabeculectomy
- Retrabeculectomy
- Glaucoma drainage devices (GDDs)
- Cyclophotocoagulation (trans-scleral and endoscopic)
- Cyclocryotherapy.

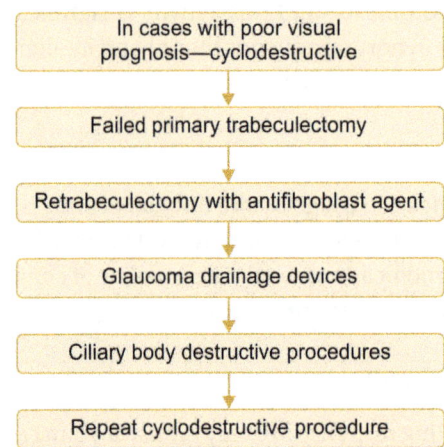

Flowchart 1: Protocol for refractory glaucoma.

Antifibrotic Agents

Corticosteroids:
- Prevents bleb failure by modulating the wound healing process.
- The first of the antifibrotic to be used clinically were the corticosteroids. It inhibits cell attachment and proliferation.
- Subconjunctival triamcinolone before filtering surgery may improve the success rate.[4]

Fluorouracil:
- It is a pyrimidine antimetabolite, which blocks deoxyribonucleic acid (DNA) synthesis through the inhibition of thymidylate synthesis and inhibits fibroblast proliferation.
- Complications included conjunctival wound leaks and corneal epithelial defects in the early postoperative course, plus an increased risk for late-onset bleb leakage.
- Used intraoperatively as surgical sponge soaked in 25–50 mg/mL of the drug and applied to the surgical site for 5 minutes.[5]

Mitomycin C:
- MMC is an antineoplastic antibiotic isolated from Streptomyces caespitosus.
- MMC is more efficacious and less likely to cause the postoperative complications that are typically associated with 5-FU, such as corneal epithelial toxicity and wound leaks and others such as hypotony maculopathy, AC reaction, and corneal endothelial toxicity if the MMC gains entry into the eye.
- MMC 0.4 or 0.2 mg/mL applied for 2 minutes may be as effective as higher doses but are associated with fewer complications.[6]

Glaucoma Drainage Devices

In refractory glaucoma, GDDs appear to be a better choice because they create an alternate pathway by shunting aqueous from the AC to an equatorial plate through a long tube resulting in a posterior bleb.[7,8]

Cyclodestructive Procedures

- Cyclophotocoagulation or cryotherapy is resorted as the last way of management in most of the refractory glaucomas.
- It is sorted earlier if visual prognosis is guarded. As the chances of reduction in vision post-treatment, severe inflammation, risk of phthisis although low is a deciding factor in choosing this option of management.

References

1. Addicks EM, Quigley HA, Green WR, Robin AL. Histologic characteristics of filtering blebs in glaucomatous eyes. Arch Ophthalmol. 1983;101(5):795-8.
2. Kornmann HL, Gedde SJ. Glaucoma management after vitreoretinal surgeries. Curr Opin Ophthalmol. 2016;27(2):125-31.
3. Singh D, Chandra A, Sihota R, Kumar S, Gupta V. Long-term success of mitomycin-augmented trabeculectomy for glaucoma after vitreoretinal surgery with silicone oil insertion: a prospective case series. Retina. 2014;34(1):123-8.
4. Sugar HS. Clinical effect of corticosteroids on conjunctival filtering blebs; a case report. Am J Ophthalmol. 1965;59:854-60.
5. Al Habash A, Aljasim L, Owaidhah O, Edward D. A review of the efficacy of mitomycin C in glaucoma filtration surgery. Clin Ophthalmol. 2015;9:1945-51.

6. The Fluorouracil Filtering Surgery Study Group. Five-year follow-up of the fluorouracil filtering surgery study. Am J Ophthalmol. 1996;121:349-66.
7. Roy S, Ravinet E, Mermoud A. Baerveldt implant in refractory glaucoma: long-term results and factors influencing outcome. Int Ophthalmol. 2001;2:93-100.
8. Desai MA, Gedde SJ, Feuer WJ, Shi W, Chen PP, Parrish 2nd RK. Practice preferences for glaucoma surgery: a survey of the American Glaucoma Society in 2008. Ophthalmic Surg Lasers Imaging. 2011;42:202-8.

7.21 Primary Congenital Glaucoma and its Associated Syndromes

Dewang Angmo, Karthikeyan Mahalingam

 1. Discuss the genetics, pathophysiology, differential diagnosis, and management of primary congenital glaucoma and its associated syndromes.

Primary congenital glaucoma (PCG) is characterized by isolated maldevelopment of trabecular meshwork with or without other anomalies of the eye that can raise intraocular pressure (IOP). Incidence varies from 1 in 1,250 in Slovakian Gypsy to 1 in 20,000 in western population.[1] Approximately, 80% of affected children develop signs of glaucoma in first year of life. Anatomically, it is classified by Hoskins et al. as:[2]

- Isolated trabeculodysgenesis
- Iridodysgenesis (iris anomaly + trabeculodysgenesis)
- Corneodysgenesis (corneal anomaly + iridodysgenesis).

Genetics

Most cases occur sporadically. Autosomal recessive hereditary pattern is seen in 10% of cases. There is variable penetrance of 40–80% in offsprings.[3] Other researchers believe that there is a polygenetic pattern of inheritance. PCG caused by pathogenic variants in *CYP1B1* or *LTBP2* is inherited in an autosomal recessive manner. PCG caused by a pathogenic variant in *TEK* is inherited in an apparent autosomal dominant manner.[4]

Pathophysiology

- Anderson believed that the trabecular meshwork becomes exposed to the anterior chamber by means of posterior sliding of the iris, ciliary muscle, and ciliary processes.
- Iris and ciliary body in PCG appear like an eye that is in the seventh or eighth month of gestation rather than one at full-term development. As the iris and ciliary body have failed to recede posteriorly, the iris insertion and anterior ciliary body overlap the posterior portion of the trabecular meshwork.
- Furthermore, histologic studies by Maumenee found an anterior insertion of the ciliary body muscle.
- Histologic abnormalities found in the trabecular meshwork: Thickening of the trabecular beams, thickened cords of the uveal meshwork, and compression of the meshwork with a resultant decrease of trabecular spaces.
- Barkan and Worst proposed that the surface of the trabecular meshwork is covered by a thin membrane (Barkan's membrane).[5]
- Schlemm's canal is open in early cases of PCG. It may be obliterated in advanced cases, but this is believed to be a secondary alteration caused by the effect of pressure elevation on the ocular tissues.

Clinical Features

Patients usually present with epiphora, blepharospasm, photophobia, enlarged cornea or eyeball, and cloudy cornea.[6] Stretching of limbus, Haab's striae (breaks in Descemet's membrane), optic nerve head cupping, and myopia are seen.

Differential Diagnosis

- Other secondary glaucomas
- *Conditions causing enlarged cornea or clouding:*
  - Megalocornea
  - Posterior polymorphous dystrophy

- Congenital hereditary endothelial dystrophy
- Trauma or keratitis
- *Conditions causing epiphora or photophobia:*
  - Nasolacrimal duct obstruction
  - Chemical conjunctivitis (due to silver nitrate)
  - Corneal abrasions
  - Corneal dystrophies such as Meesman's corneal dystrophy, Reis–Buckler dystrophy
- *Other optic nerve abnormalities:*
  - Congenital malformations include congenital pits, colobomata, and optic nerve hypoplasia.
  - Tilted disc in axial myopia
  - Large physiological cups.

Management

Medical Management

As surgery is the treatment of choice for PCG, medications are used to control IOP in the waiting period.[7] β-blockers, such as timolol 0.25% or betaxolol suspension 0.25%, may be administered. Topical carbonic anhydrase inhibitors (dorzolamide) can be used. For short-term use, acetazolamide (5–10 mg/kg body weight every 6–8 hours) orally in suspension form may be considered. Other drugs can be used but are not efficacious as they are in adult glaucomas. Brimonidine is contraindicated because it causes central nervous system depression.

Surgical Management

- Goniotomy is performed when the cornea is clear and in milder forms of PCG.
- Trabeculotomy can also be performed as an initial surgical procedure.
- Glaucoma filtering surgery is considered when goniotomy, trabeculotomy, or both fail to control the glaucoma.
- Trabeculectomy along with trabeculotomy with mitomycin C is usually done to improve the success rate of surgery.
- Glaucoma drainage devices can also be used to treat PCG. They provide a promising alternative in intractable childhood glaucomas.
- Cyclodestructive procedures are used when all other treatment modalities fail or in case of painful blind eye.

Follow-up

- Parents of the child should be counseled regarding life long follow-up.
- Examination under anesthesia (EUA) must be done to look at IOP, status of bleb, and to remove releasable sutures if any.
- First EUA must be done at 4–6 weeks. Subsequent EUA can be done after 3–6 months as required till the patient is old enough for routine examination.

Associated Syndromes

- Sturge–Webers syndrome
- Neurofibromatosis
- Pierre Robin and Stickler syndromes
- Skeletal dysplastic syndromes
- Aniridia-WAGR syndrome
- Rubinstein–Taybi syndrome
- Trisomies (13,14,15)
- Lowe syndrome
- Rubella
- Peters anomaly
- Axenfeld–Rieger syndrome.

References

1. Genčík A. Epidemiology and genetics of primary congenital glaucoma in Slovakia. Description of a form of primary congenital glaucoma in gypsies with autosomal-recessive inheritance and complete penetrance. Dev Ophthalmol. 1989;16:76-115.

2. Hoskins HD, Shaffer RN, Hetherington J. Anatomical classification of the developmental glaucomas. Arch Ophthalmol. 1984;102(9):1331-6.
3. Stamper RL, Lieberman MF, Drake MV. Becker and Shaffer's Diagnosis and Therapy of the Glaucomas, 8th edition. Mosby; 2009.
4. Abu-Amero KK, Edward DP. Primary congenital glaucoma. In: Adam MP, Ardinger HH, Pagon RA, Wallace SE, Bean LJ, Stephens K, et al. (Eds). GeneReviews®. Seattle (WA): University of Washington, Seattle; 1993.
5. Worst JGF. Pathogenesis and treatment of congenital glaucoma. Ophthalmologica. 1965;149(2):118-20.
6. Allingham RR. Shields Text Book of Glaucoma, 6th edition. Lippincott Williams and Wilkins; 2011.
7. Mandal AK, Chakrabarti D. Update on congenital glaucoma. Indian J Ophthalmol. 2011;59(Suppl. 1):S148-57.

7.22 Surgical Management of Congenital Glaucoma

Dewang Angmo, Karthikeyan Mahalingam

Q 1. Discuss surgical management of congenital glaucoma.

Preoperatively glaucoma medications should be started to lower the intraocular pressure (IOP) and to clear the cornea. Many factors such as a smaller palpebral fissure, relatively less rigid and thinned sclera, stretched limbus, and clouding of the cornea make the surgery in congenital glaucoma challenging. There are various surgical procedures available to treat congenital glaucoma. They are summarized in **Flowchart 1**.

Goniotomy

Goniotomy is performed when the cornea is clear and in milder forms of congenital glaucoma.[1] Incision is made superficial into the anterior trabecular meshwork **(Fig. 1)**. The aim is to open a route for aqueous humor to exit the anterior chamber into the Schlemm's canal by removing obstructing tissue, but the precise mechanism by which pressure reduction occurs remains obscure. Studies suggest that goniotomy has a success rate of 72–90% after one or two attempts.[2]

Trabeculotomy

It is indicated when angle structures cannot be visualized through a cloudy cornea or after the failure of two goniotomies.[3] Either trabeculotome or 6-0 Prolene suture (for 360° trabeculotomy) is passed in to Schlemm's canal and subsequent centripetal rupture through the trabecular meshwork into the anterior chamber is made to create a passage for aqueous flow **(Fig. 2)**.

Some studies suggest that trabeculotomy is superior to goniotomy as an initial surgical procedure, other studies suggest vice-versa.[4] Both goniotomy and trabeculotomy have success rate of more than 80% and can be used as an initial surgical procedure.

Trabeculectomy

- It is done in an eye with reasonable visual potential and unscarred conjunctiva after angle surgery has failed, with guaranteed faithful follow-up.[5]
- It is usually combined with trabeculotomy to increase its success rate. Antimetabolites are used in addition to increase the success rate. Studies report that combined trabeculectomy and trabeculotomy has a success rate of more than 90%.[6]
- In trabeculectomy, after peritomy, a scleral flap is made, sclerostomy and iridectomy is done. Scleral flap and conjunctiva is closed and thus an alternate path for aqueous outflow is created.

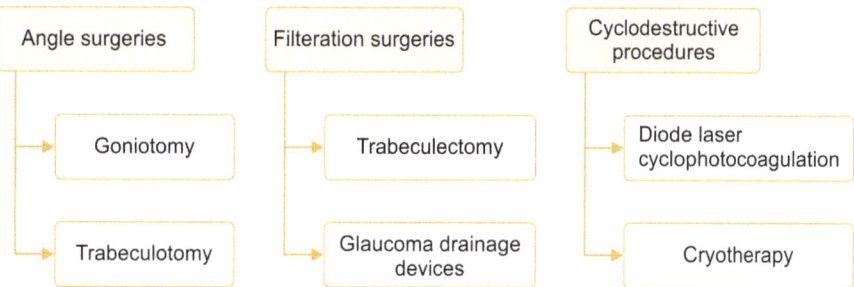

Flowchart 1: Various surgical procedures for congenital glaucoma.

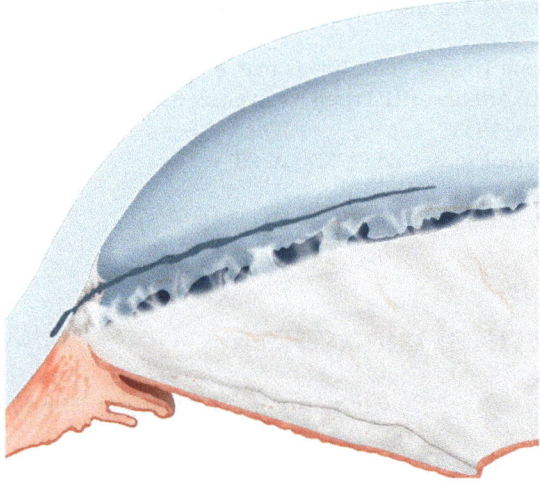

Fig. 1: Goniotomy.

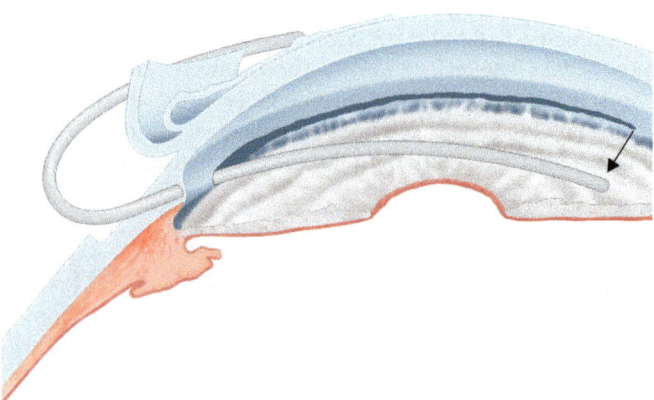

Fig. 2: Trabeculotomy using trabeculotome.

Follow-up

Parents of the child should be counseled regarding lifelong follow-up. Examination under anesthesia (EUA) must be done to look at IOP, status of bleb, to remove releasable sutures if any. First EUA must be done at 4–6 weeks. Subsequent EUA can be done after 3–6 months as required till the patient is old enough for routine examination.

Glaucoma Drainage Devices

- It is indicated in eyes with multiple failed trabeculectomy with antimetabolites or in aphakic glaucoma.
- They provide a promising alternative to intractable childhood glaucomas.[7]
- Initially, Molteno implant was being used for two decades, but now Baerveldt and Ahmed drainage implants are also being used.

Cyclodestructive Procedures

- It is used when all other treatment modalities fail or in case of painful blind eye.
- It is an alternative approach to reducing IOP, by partially eliminating the function of the ciliary processes and decreasing the rate of aqueous production.
- Laser cyclophotocoagulation has replaced cryotherapy because of its advantage over the latter technique.
- Newer approaches with micropulse transscleral and endoscopic diode laser appear to be associated with reasonable efficacy and fewer vision-threatening complications and may be considered in eyes with better vision.[8]

References

1. Yu Chan JY, Choy BN, Ng AL, Shum JW. Review on the management of primary congenital glaucoma. J Curr Glaucoma Pract. 2015;9(3):92-9.
2. Gramer E, Tausch M, Kraemer C. Time of diagnosis, reoperations and long-term results of goniotomy in the treatment of primary congenital glaucoma: a clinical study. Int Ophthalmol. 1996-1997;20(1-3):117-23.
3. Stamper RL, Lieberman MF, Drake MV. Becker and Shaffer's Diagnosis and Therapy of the Glaucomas, 8th edition. Mosby; 2009.
4. Girkin CA, Rhodes L, McGwin G, Marchase N, Cogen MS. Goniotomy versus circumferential trabeculotomy with an illuminated microcatheter in congenital glaucoma. J AAPOS. 2012;16(5):424-7.
5. Allingham RR. Shields Text Book of Glaucoma, 6th edition. Lippincott Williams and Wilkins; 2011.
6. Elder MJ. Combined trabeculotomy-trabeculectomy compared with primary trabeculectomy for congenital glaucoma. Br J Ophthalmol. 1994;78(10):745-8.
7. Chen A, Yu F, Law SK, Giaconi JA, Coleman AL, Caprioli J. Valved glaucoma drainage devices in pediatric glaucoma: retrospective long-term outcomes. JAMA Ophthalmol. 2015;133(9):1030-5.
8. Lee JH, Shi Y, Amoozgar B, Aderman C, De Alba Campomanes A, Lin S, et al. Outcome of micropulse laser transscleral cyclophotocoagulation on pediatric versus adult glaucoma patients. J Glaucoma. 2017;26(10):936-9.

7.23 Ocular Blood Flow and Glaucoma

Neha Midha, Dewang Angmo

Q 1. Describe in detail the role of ocular blood flow in glaucoma pathogenesis.

Two important theories in glaucoma pathogenesis are:
1. *Mechanical theory:* Increased intraocular pressure (IOP) causes stretching of the laminar beams and damages retinal ganglion cell (RGC) axons.
2. *Vascular theory:* Insufficient blood supply due to either increased IOP or other risk factors reducing ocular blood flow (OBF).

A certain percentage of glaucoma patients continue to progress even after the IOP is well controlled. Impaired OBF has been postulated as an important cause in these cases. Studies have shown that glaucoma patients have lower OBF compared to healthy subjects and the effect is more pronounced in eyes with normal-tension glaucoma.

Good irrigation of the ocular tissues is ensured by an adequate ocular perfusion pressure (OPP) which can be estimated as the difference between the arterial pressure and IOP **(Flowchart 1)**.[1] In the Barbados Eye Study and Early Manifest Glaucoma Study, increased incidence and progression of glaucoma were seen in patients with low systolic blood pressure (BP).

Flowchart 1: Role of ocular perfusion pressure in glaucoma.

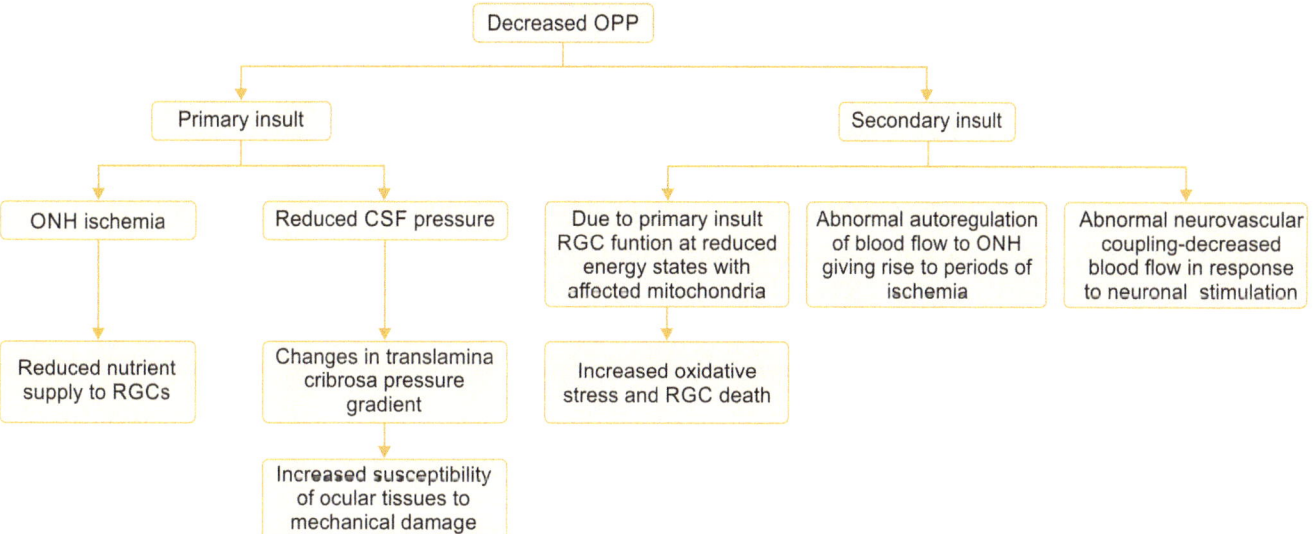

(CSF: cerebrospinal fluid; ONH: optic nerve head; OPP: ocular perfusion pressure; RGC: retinal ganglion cell)

Since measurement of OBF is currently difficult in routine clinical practice, a detailed systemic history must be taken from all glaucoma patients to identify signs of vascular dysregulation such as cold hands and migraine. Measurement of 24-hour ambulatory blood pressure together with a 24-hour IOP profile is ideal for identification of periods of nocturnal hypotension and low OPP.[2]

Methods to study OBF include See **Table 2**:

TABLE 1: Methods of measuring ocular perfusion pressure (OPP).	
Instrument	**Principle**
OCT angiography	Color Doppler imaging
Retinal oximetry	Laser Doppler velocimetry
Retinal vessel analyzer	Laser Doppler flowmetry
SLO angiography/FFA/ICGA	Laser speckle technique
Doppler OCT	Blue field entoptic technique
(FFA: fundus fluorescein angiography; ICGA: indocyanine green angiography; OCT: optical coherence tomography; SLO: scanning laser ophthalmoscopy)	

There are no concrete methods to improve OBF; however, few important measures are:[3]
- Decreasing antihypertensive medication in patients with nocturnal hypotension
- Treatment of systemic vascular dysregulation disorder
- Drugs which are nitric oxide (NO) donors such as latanoprostene bunod
- Other drugs postulated to improve ocular hemodynamics include dorzolamide, betaxolol, latanoprost, bimatoprost, and timolol.

References

1. Cherecheanu AP, Garhofer G, Schmidl D, Werkmeister R, Schmetterer L. Ocular perfusion pressure and ocular blood flow in glaucoma. Curr Opin Pharmacol. 2013;13(1):36-42.
2. Maram J, Srinivas S, Sadda SR. Evaluating ocular blood flow [published correction appears in Indian J Ophthalmol. 2018;66(1):181]. Indian J Ophthalmol. 2017;65(5):337-46.
3. Stewart WC, Feldman R, Mychaskiw MA. Ocular blood flow in glaucoma: the need for further clinical evidence and patient outcomes research. Br J Ophthalmol. 2007;91(10):1263-4.

7.24 Neuroprotective Agents

Aafreen Bari, Dewang Angmo

  1. Write a short note on the neuroprotective agents.

Glaucoma is a neurodegenerative disease characterized by progressive loss of retinal ganglion cells (RGCs) leading to irreversible optic neuropathy.

Glaucoma is characterized by central neurodegenerative changes in the visual pathway which contributes to the progression of glaucoma. Therefore, therapies combining intraocular pressure (IOP)-lowering approaches with neuroprotective agents would confer protection of local and central visual neurons, thus preserving vision.[1-3]

The following diagram shows a simplified pathway of RGC death and assumed mechanisms of neuroprotective agents:

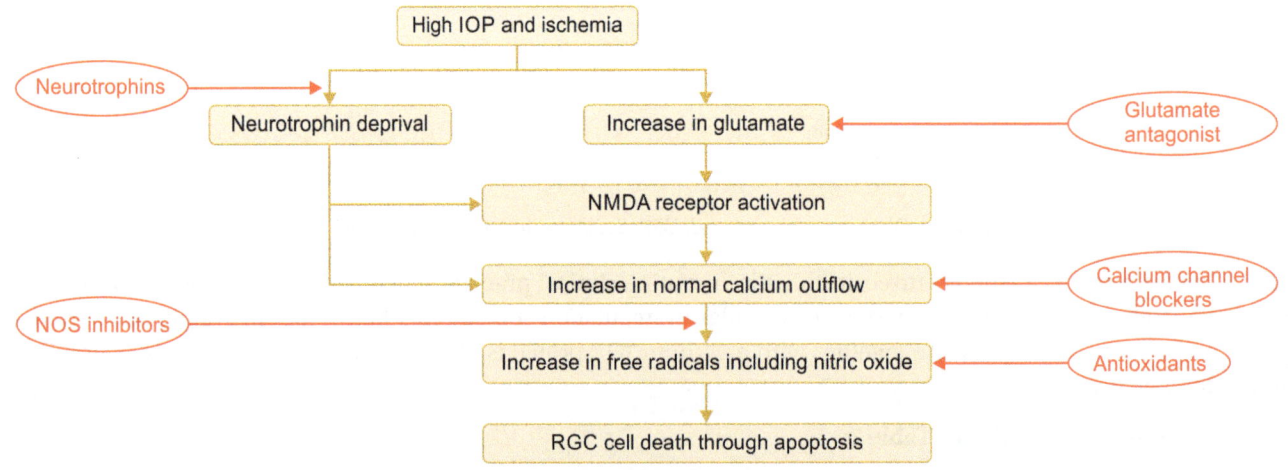

Flowchart 1: Neuroprotective agents and their possible site of action.

(IOP: intraocular pressure; NMDA: N-methyl-D-aspartate; NOS: nitric oxide synthase; RGC: retinal ganglion cell)

Neurotrophic Factors

- The hypothalamic neuropeptide, ciliary neurotrophic factor (CNTF), is a neuronal survival factor that confers neuroprotection in glaucoma and trials are on to study efficacy and safety of intravitreal implantation of this neurotrophic factor.
- Recombinant human nerve growth factor (rhNGF) is another effective neuroprotective agent with a favorable safety and efficacy profile and the ophthalmic formulations of rhNGF are Food and Drug Administration (FDA)-approved for treating neurotrophic keratitis. Clinical trials investigating the role of rhNGF in glaucoma are being done.

- The brain-derived neurotrophic factor was reported to be decreased in early glaucoma, and therefore can be tapped as a biomarker for detecting early. disease.

Brimonidine

- Brimonidine is an α-2 adrenergic agonist commonly used as an antiglaucoma, IOP-lowering agent.
- Brimonidine also protects RGCs from somatic, axonal, and dendritic degeneration in optic injuries involving ischemia, N-methyl-d-aspartate (NMDA)-induced neurotoxicity, ocular hypertension, optic crush, and optic neuritis.
- Various mechanisms for brimonidine's neuroprotective effects have been purported including neurotrophic factor activation, vasomodulation, glutamate inhibition, and cell-survival signal upregulation as well as apoptosis downregulation.
- The Low-Pressure Glaucoma Treatment Study (LoGTS) compared the effects of brimonidine and timolol on visual field progression in low-pressure glaucoma and showed that the incidence of visual field progression was significantly lower for patients receiving brimonidine monotherapy relative to the timolol group (9.1% and 39.2%, respectively), despite similar IOP-lowering effects.

Calcium Channel Blockers

- Calcium channel blockers (CCBs) have been implicated in glaucoma neuroprotection by preventing calcium-mediated apoptosis and improving ocular blood flow.
- Brovincamine and nilvadipine are two such CCBs that permeate the blood–brain barrier and, thus, selectively influence the optic nerve circulation without appreciably affecting systemic circulation.
- Randomized clinical trials have demonstrated the therapeutic effects of brovincamine and nilvadipine, whereby normal tension glaucoma (NTG) patients treated with CCBs showed improved ocular blood flow and delayed progression of visual field defects.

Antioxidants

- Decreased antioxidant levels along with increased oxidative free radical damage have been implicated in glaucoma pathogenesis. Studies have also demonstrated trabecular meshwork (TM) degeneration followed by IOP elevation and subsequent glaucomatous damage in human tissues.
- A significant correlation between oxidative damage in TM gene expression and increased IOP as well as visual field loss has been reported.
- Among the various antioxidants, coenzyme Q10 (CoQ10), a cofactor of the mitochondrial respiratory chain, may be useful in scavenging free radicals and minimizing oxidative stress.
- Glaucoma patients receiving the combined regimen featured improved inner retinal function and visual cortical responses, as determined by pattern electroretinography (PERG) and visual evoked potential (VEP), respectively.

Nicotinamide (Vitamin B3 or NAM)

- Nicotinamide (NAM) is an important precursor for nicotinamide adenine dinucleotide (NAD), and has a favorable neuroprotective profile in glaucoma given its integral roles in calcium homeostasis, endothelin-mediated vascular regulation, and maintenance of mitochondrial function.
- NAM neuroprotection in glaucoma has largely been demonstrated in animal models and independently of IOP.

Ginkgo Biloba

- Ginkgo biloba extract (GBE) has various antioxidant effects and has been suggested as a neuroprotective agent in neurodegenerative diseases including cognitive impairment and Alzheimer's disease (AD). Mitochondrial dysfunction and oxidative stress have both been purported in dementia and glaucoma pathogenesis.
- In a 4-year longitudinal study conducted by Lee et al., NTG patients treated with GBE also showed marked improvement in visual field performance and without significant IOP changes.[4]
- In addition to its antioxidant effects, GBE also has vascular regulatory effects and has been shown to improve ocular blood flow.

Memantine

Memantine is a noncompetitive NMDA antagonist with antiglutamate excitotoxicity effects. Though typically indicated in moderate to severe AD, memantine has also been shown to protect against RGC loss in animal models of glaucoma.

Citicoline

- Topical administration of citicoline eye drops has also been shown to improve retinal function and neural conduction along the visual pathway, as measured by PERG and VEP.
- Citicoline is approved in the European Union (EU) and Italian Ministry of Health, as a novel food ingredient in food supplements and in dietary foods for special medical purposes in glaucoma patients.

References

1. Doozandeh A, Yazdani S. Neuroprotection in glaucoma. J Ophthalmic Vis Res. 2016;11(2):209-20.
2. Nucci C, Martucci A, Giannini C, Morrone LA, Bagetta G, Mancino R. Neuroprotective agents in the management of glaucoma. Eye. 2018;32:938-45.
3. Vasudevan SK, Gupta V, Crowston JG. Neuroprotection in glaucoma. Indian J Ophthalmol. 2011;59(Suppl. S1):102-13.
4. Lee J, Sohn SW, Kee C. Effect of Ginkgo biloba extract on visual field progression in normal tension glaucoma. J Glaucoma. 2013; 22(9):780-4.

7.25 Advanced Glaucoma and Painful Blind Eye

Bhagabat Nayak, Dewang Angmo

 1. What is advanced glaucoma? How would you follow-up a case of advanced glaucoma? Discuss the various treatment options.

Patients with advanced glaucoma can be defined as near total cupping of the optic nerve with or without severe visual field loss within 10° of fixation, i.e., scotoma encroaching or splitting fixation.

Difficulties in Management

- Worse visual prognosis and accelerated progression
- Imminent danger of losing remaining field
- Socioeconomic, mental health difficulties, increased chances of falls, and driving accidents.

Clinical Evaluation and Follow-up

- Look for risk factors for progression

Ocular risk factors		Nonocular
Strong evidence	*Moderate evidence*	African race
Initial advanced loss	Disc hemorrhage	Increasing (POAG) or young (JOAG) age
High IOP	Thin cornea	Strong family history of blindness
Marked visit-to-visit IOP fluctuation	Damage to fellow eye	Decreased ocular perfusion pressure (DBP-IOP ≤55 mm Hg)
Exfoliation		Socioeconomic background
Myopia		

(DBP: diastolic blood pressure; IOP: intraocular pressure; JOAG: juvenile open-angle glaucoma; POAG: primary open-angle glaucoma)

- *Look for secondary causes if not already, or is suspected:*
    - Such as neovascularization and uveitis
    - Dilated examination to look for subtle exfoliation, peripheral fundus (neovascularization, inflammation, etc.)
    - Gonioscopy

- Systemic factors contributing to progressions such as nocturnal hypotension, or hypotension in general, obstructive sleep apnea, and faulty yoga/exercise techniques.
- *Monitoring structure and function:*
  - Diurnal control or variation of intraocular pressure (IOP)
  - Optic nerve head (ONH) changes
  - Imaging devices
  - Visual field changes
- *ONH changes:*
  - Difficult to assess subtle changes on nerve.
  - Visual field (VF) changes may have less correlation with ONH changes.
  - Examine and document any remaining neuroretinal rim (NRR), especially temporally for the papillomacular bundle (responsible for central visual acuity) as well as presence of disc hemorrhage.
- *Imaging devices:*
  - Not very helpful as minimal NRR and retinal nerve fiber layer (RNFL) tissue left (floor effect, noise in measurement).
  - Macular nerve fiber layer (NFL) thickness may be helpful.
- *Visual field changes:*
  - Important, maybe the only evidence of progression
  - Consider central Humphrey 10-2 program with size III or size V (if having difficulty with size III), either alone or together with 24-2 or 30-2
  - Cardinal points around fixation and quadrant totals should be examined carefully

Long-term follow-up:
- Every 3–4 months, or earlier if unstable
- Target IOP should be in low teens or high singles.

Management

Medical Therapy

- Assess for compliance, affordability, tolerance, and caregiver support.
- Education regarding correct application of medication, importance of regular follow-up and medication usage, what to expect from therapy, and the expected course of action.
- The least amount of medication(s), preferably combination, with most likelihood of lowering IOP, while keeping the cost to minimum, and tolerable/minimal side effects.
- Prostaglandin analogs, combination of carbonic anhydrase inhibitors (CAIs) and β-blockers are associated with lower level of IOP fluctuations compared with β-blockers alone.
- Brimonidine and betaxolol can be considered for their beneficial effects on neuroprotection and ONH perfusion, respectively.

Laser Treatment (LTP with Argon, Diode, or Selective Laser Treatment)

- Unlikely to achieve adequate IOP
- Can be used to reduce the number of medications, as an adjunct, or while awaiting incisional surgery, or when surgery is not possible
- *Concerns:*
  - Immediate postoperative rise in IOP (IOP spikes may threaten fixation)
  - Sustained inflammation
  - Weaning of effect
  - Unpredictable result, e.g., in patients with exfoliation glaucoma.

Cyclodestructive Procedures

- Reserved for refractory cases with poor prognosis
- Endoscopic cyclophotocoagulation (CPC) and micropulse laser may be preferable over trans-scleral diode CPC

Surgical Management

- Usually resorted to when medical therapy which is maximally tolerated is unable to achieve target IOP.
- Role of newer microinvasive glaucoma surgery (MIGS) surgeries is limited in advanced glaucomas.
- Trabeculectomy has been reported to have less diurnal IOP fluctuations, less marked peak IOP, and lower mean diurnal IOP values compared to maximum medical therapy.
- Special concern regarding trabeculectomy in advanced glaucoma is "wipe-out or snuff out" with incidence of 0–7%.
- Combined surgery (cataract and trabeculectomy) in cases of visually significant cataract.
- Peribulbar or retrobulbar blocks should be avoided, instead topical or subtenon/sub-conjunctival, or intracameral anesthesia with preservative-free lignocaine can be administered.

Visual Rehabilitation and Psychosocial Support

- *Near work:* Handheld or stand magnifiers, electronic magnifiers, computer screen readers, reading machines, and handheld scanner/reader.
- Field expanders such as optical minifiers, reverse telescopes, prisms, and electronic field enhancement.
- Glare control using environmental modifications, polarizing glasses, and tinted lenses.
- *Nonoptical devices:* Typoscopes, signature guides, tactile dots, labels, etc., to help in daily activities.
- Trainings such as orientation and mobility training, preferred retinal locus (PRL) and eccentric fixation training.

 2. How will you manage a patient of painful blind eye with medically uncontrolled intraocular pressure (IOP) of 50 mm Hg.

In a case of painful blind eye with high IOP, the pain may be caused by:
- Increased IOP
- Inflammation due to underlying cause
- Bullous keratopathy with epithelial defect/ulcer.

In this case, as given in question, the IOP is 50 mm Hg, which means the pain would be most likely due to increased IOP. But patients should be examined for the other causes also.

Measures to Control Intraocular Pressure

- *Antiglaucoma medications:* Usually first line, if tolerable. In our case already it has been tried.
- *Panretinal photocoagulation (PRP):*
  - If media clarity and pupil dilation permits, it can be done in cases of neovascular glaucoma (NVG); it might lead to regression of neovascularization
  - But still control of IOP is unlikely, without filtration surgery, as increased IOP is usually caused in the angle-closure stage of NVG.
- *Cyclodestruction:*
  - No need of media clarity; relieves pain by decreasing aqueous production and destruction of corneal nerves.
  - Using laser such as trans-scleral neodymium-yttrium aluminum garnet (Nd:YAG) cyclophotocoagulation (contact or noncontact), diode laser cyclophotocoagulation (TS-DLCP); or cyclocryotherapy.
  - Cyclocryotherapy is less predictable and causes more inflammation than laser cyclodestructive procedures.
  - The TS-DLCP causes less postoperative inflammation and better IOP control than the Nd:YAG, and has become the surgical procedure of choice for NVG, when filtering surgery is not indicated.
  - Complications include postoperative pain and inflammation, hyperemia, hyphema, hypotony, phthisis bulbi, and sympathetic ophthalmitis (caution if the other eye has vision).
- *Transconjunctival anterior retinal cryotherapy (ARC):*
  - For neovascular glaucoma
- *Retrobulbar injection:*
  - It causes the destruction of long and short ciliary nerves and ciliary ganglion.
  - Provides pain relief for prolonged variable period (1–12 months)
  - Agents used include absolute alcohol, chlorpromazine, and phenol.
  - *Complications:* hematoma, restrictive strabismus, ptosis, external ophthalmoplegia, cellulitis, neurotrophic keratopathy, eyelid edema, and conjunctival chemosis.

- Intravitreal triamcinolone acetonide injection
- *Evisceration or enucleation with ocular prosthesis:*
  - Former preferred over the latter.
  - Usually resorted to when patient agrees, and otherwise there is unacceptable cosmesis of the blind eye.
- Intraocular procedures such as filtering surgery, glaucoma drainage-device surgery, pars plana vitrectomy with lamina cribrosa puncture, endoscopic cyclophotocoagulation, and stereotactic surgery are not advised in our case in view of blind eye and risk of endophthalmitis.

In Case of Associated Inflammation

- Administer topical steroids such as prednisolone acetate/phosphate or difluprednate, topical NSAIDs, strong cycloplegics such as atropine 1%.
- Look out for corneal epithelial damage/ulcer when patient is receiving topical steroids or NSAIDs.

In Case of Bullous Keratopathy

- Withdraw topical CAI, if any
- Control IOP, inflammation
- Anterior stromal puncture
- Contact lens
- Hypertonic saline
- Gunderson flap.

Suggested Reading

1. Allingham RR, Damji KF, Shields MB (Eds). Shields Textbook of Glaucoma. Philadelphia: Wolters Kluwer Health/Lippincott Williams & Wilkins; 2011.
2. Gessesse GW, Damji KF. Advanced glaucoma: management pearls. Middle East Afr J Ophthalmol. 2013;20(2):131-41.
3. Prum Jr BE, Rosenberg LF, Gedde SJ, Mansberger SL, Stein JD, Moroi SE, et al. Primary Open-Angle Glaucoma Preferred Practice Pattern® guidelines. Ophthalmology. 2016;123(1):P41-111.
4. Schacknow PN, Samples JR. The Glaucoma Book: A Practical, Evidence-Based Approach to Patient Care. New York, NY: Springer; 2010.

CHAPTER 8: Cornea and Conjunctiva

8.1 Anatomy and Physiology of Cornea

Sohini Mondal, Ritu Nagpal

Q 1. Discuss the embryology and anatomy of corneal endothelium.

Embryology

Endothelium and Descemet membrane (DM) are formed from mesenchymal cells derived from neural crest (at margins of the rim of optic cup).

Wave Theory

Three waves of tissue arise at the edge of the optic cup from the neural crest cells between the surface ectoderm and lens to form various anterior segment structures. The wave theory has been depicted in **Flowchart 1**.

- *40 days of gestation:* Endothelium consists of two layers of flattened cells.
- *3rd month of gestation:* Fuses to form a single layer of flattened cells occupying central cornea resting on future DM (interrupted basal lamina).
- *4th month of gestation:* Apices of endothelial cells are connected by zonula occludentes.
- *6th month of gestation:* Distinct demarcation of DM.

Gross Anatomy

Corneal endothelium forms the posterior (inner) most layer of cornea. It is a single layer of polygonal (mostly hexagonal) cells covering the posterior surface of DM in a well-arranged mosaic pattern. These cells are uniformly 5 μm in thickness and 20 μm in width. Cell density of endothelium at birth is around 7,500 cells/mm^2 which falls by 26% in first year of life and another 26% by next 11 years. Therefore, the cell density reduces to around 3,000–3,500 cells/mm^2 by 35 years of age.

Microscopic Anatomy

Descemet membrane forms the basement membrane of endothelium and is primarily composed of collagen type IV and VIII; laminin and fibronectin. Type VIII collagen produced by corneal endothelium forms a hexagonal lattice which is structurally different from type IV collagen. Although endothelial cells are attached to DM by hemidesmosomes and laterally to each

Flowchart 1: Wave theory.

First wave: Differentiates into endothelium and DM by 8th week

↓

Second wave: Forms the corneal stroma

↓

Third wave: Forms pupillary membrane and iris stroma

(DM: Descemet membrane)

TABLE 1: Endothelial cell indices and their implication.	
Polymegathism	Variability in cell size. The defect left by the dying cells is filled by enlargement of residual adjacent cells resulting in variable size
Coefficient of variation	• Marker for degree of polymegathism • *Normal value:* 0.27–0.30 • More the value, more is the number of variable cells
Pleomorphism	• Variability in cell shape. Looses its hexagonality
Hexagonality	• Marker for degree of pleomorphism • *Normal value:* 50–60% • Lower the value, more is the number of non-hexagonal cells

other by junctional complexes: zonula occludens, macula occludens, and macula adherens, they provide a leaky barrier to aqueous humor, small molecules, and electrolytes. These cells contain a large nucleus and numerous organelles such as mitochondria, endoplasmic reticulum, free ribosomes, and Golgi apparatus making them second most metabolically highly active structure in the eye next to photoreceptors. These cells are incapable of regenerating and proliferating as they are arrested in G1 phase of cell cycle under normal conditions.[1,2] Critical count of endothelial cells is 300–500 cells/mm^2, below which corneal decompensation occurs.

The various endothelial cell indices have been depicted in **Table 1**.

Physiology

Corneal endothelium has a barrier and a pump function that are vital for maintenance of corneal clarity. The barrier function is mediated by proteins such as zonula occludens-1 and pump function mediated by an active Na$^+$K$^+$-ATPase pump.

 2. Discuss the anatomy of limbus and its surgical importance.

Depicted in **Flowchart 2 and Figure 1**.

Application of Surgical Limbus In Cataract Surgery

Small Incision Cataract Surgery (SICS)

The sclerocorneal tunnel incision comprises three parts:
1. *External scleral incision:* 1/3rd–1/2 scleral thickness, 1.5–2 mm from limbus, 5.5–7.5 mm in length incision is constructed with the help of 11 or 15 no. blade depending on the grade of cataract. Various configurations may be:
   • *Frown/antismile incision (Singer):*
     ◆ Preferred for SICS
     ◆ Curved away from limbus → More stability and less astigmatism

Flowchart 2: Anatomy of the limbus.

- Bulbar conjunctiva is firmly adherent to the underlying structures
- Epithelium is 7–10 layers thick containing melanin
- Undulated basement membrane containing basal stem cells (pallisade of Vogt)
- Insertion of conjunctiva and Tenon's capsule into the cornea
- Termination of Bowman's membrane

Limbus
- Anatomical
  - Conjunctivo-corneal junction
  - Corneoscleral junction
- Surgical
  - Blue limbal zone → Anterior limbal border
  - White limbal zone → Mid limbal line
  - 2 mm wide circumcorneal transition zone → Posterior limbal border

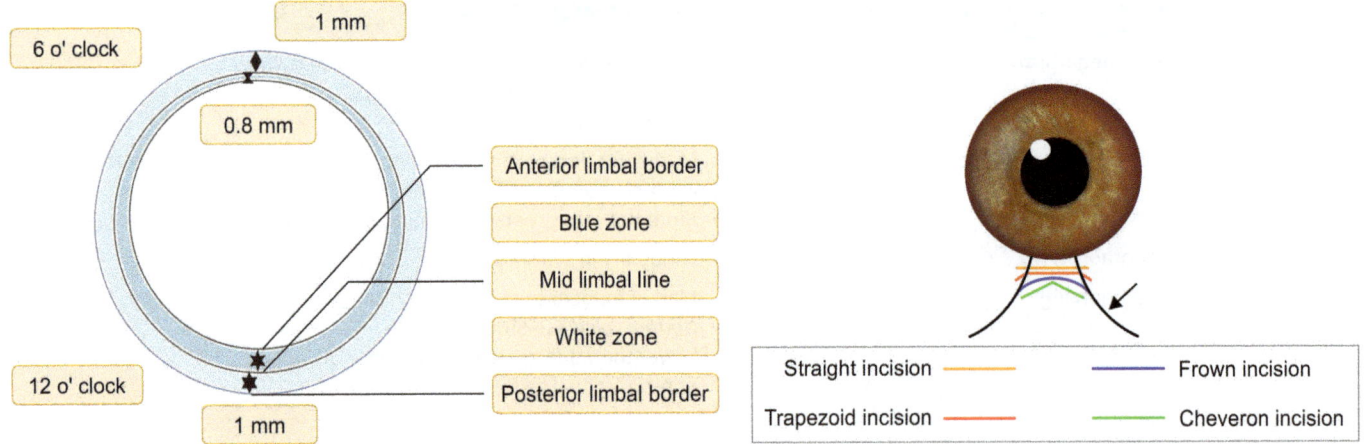

Fig. 1: Surgical anatomy of the limbus.

Fig. 2: Various type of external scleral incisions used in SICS.

- *Chevron/reverse V incision (Gills):*
    - More stability and less astigmatism
- *Trapezoid incision:*
    - Suitable for hard cataract/large nucleus
    - Central straight part with radiating cuts at both ends
- *Straight incision:*
    - Not preferred → extends beyond the astigmatic neutral funnel producing significant astigmatism postoperatively.
    - To counteract this, the incision is placed quite posterior to the limbus to fit in the funnel resulting in difficult instrumentation.

Various types of external scleral incisions have been depicted in **Figure 2**.

2. *Sclerocorneal tunnel:*
   - Made with 2.8 mm crescent blade
   - Extend till 1–1.5 mm of clear cornea
   - Depth of dissection is such that the blade is just visible beneath the sclera
   - Uniform thickness flap
   - Avoid button holing of flap (superficial dissection) and premature entry into anterior chamber (deep dissection)
   - Scleral pockets are optional only for large nucleus and dissected with the side edges of the blade
3. *Internal corneal incision:*
   - With sharp 2.8- or 3.0- or 3.2 mm angled keratome
   - Parallel to the iris plane
   - Linear self-sealing incision.

Phacoemulsification

The wound construction may be classified into three types which is illustrated in **Flowchart 3**.

The advantages and disadvantages of various types of incisions are depicted in **Tables 2 to 4**.

The types of clear corneal incisions have been shown in **Figures 3 to 6** and **Flowchart 4**.

Application of surgical limbus in scleral buckling surgery: Various types of peritomy and their advantages and disadvantages have been illustrated in **Flowchart 5**.

Application of surgical limbus in pars plana vitrectomy surgery/intravitreal injections: Placement of trocar or needle at various distances from the limbus according to lens status has been depicted in **Table 5**.

Flowchart 3: Types of wound construction in phacoemulsification.

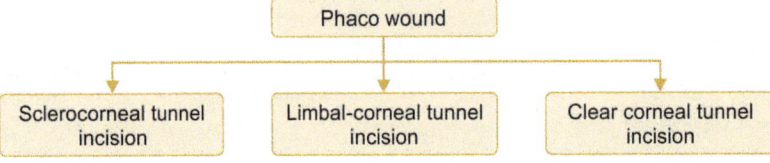

TABLE 2: Sclerocorneal tunnel incision—Constructed in similar way as that of SICS wound.

Advantages
- Less astigmatism
- Less chances of tunnel infection
- Faster healing and wound stabilization

Disadvantages
- Requires local anesthesia
- Time consuming
- Bleeding occurs
- Difficult instrumentation
- Chances of iris prolapse

(SICS: small incision cataract surgery)

TABLE 3: Limbal corneal tunnel incision.

Advantages
- Less astigmatism
- Faster wound healing
- Self-sealing

Disadvantages
- Ballooning of conjunctiva
- Bleeding into anterior chamber

TABLE 4: Clear corneal tunnel incision (Preferred for modern day phacoemulsification with foldable IOL).

Advantages
- Only topical anesthesia is required
- No risk of bleeding
- Easier instrumentation
- No corneal distortion

Disadvantages
- May not be self-sealing
- May cause astigmatism
- Risk of Descemet membrane detachment

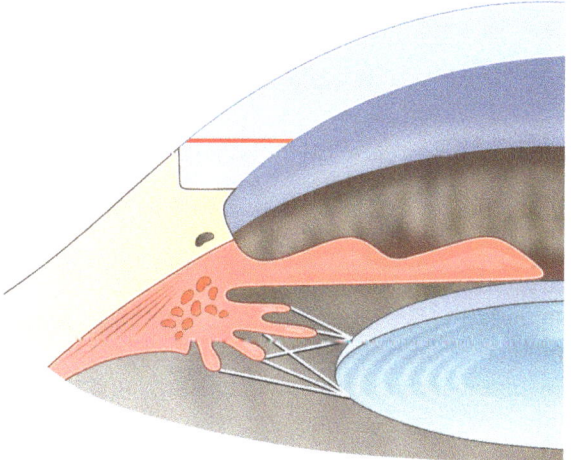

Fig. 3: Uniplanar incision.

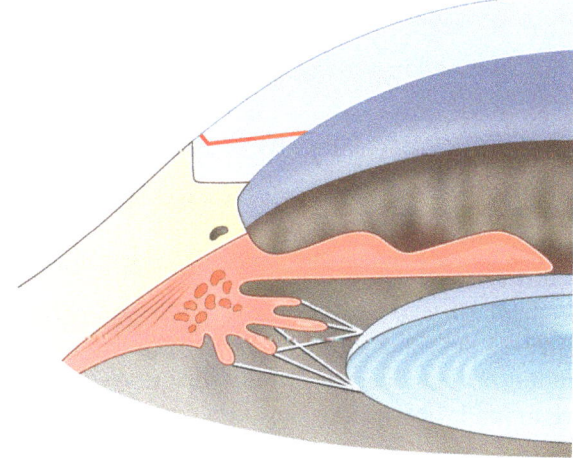

Fig. 4: Biplanar incision.

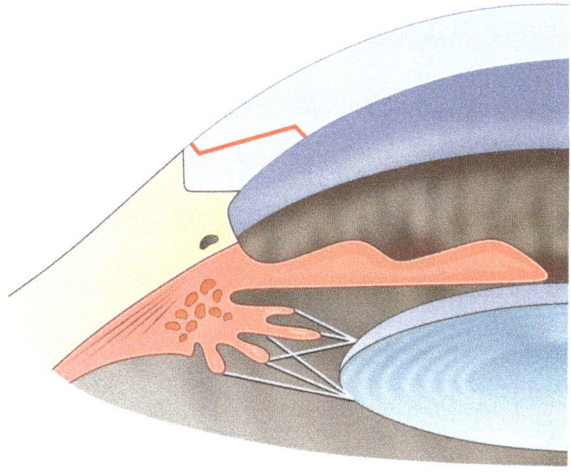

Fig. 5: Triplanar incision.

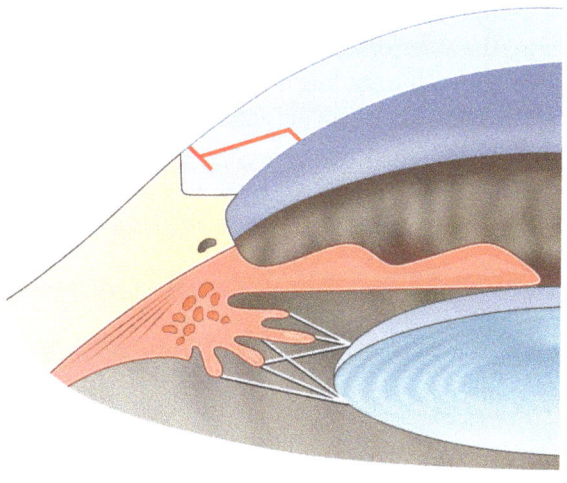

Fig. 6: Hinged incision.

Flowchart 4: Types of clear corneal incision.

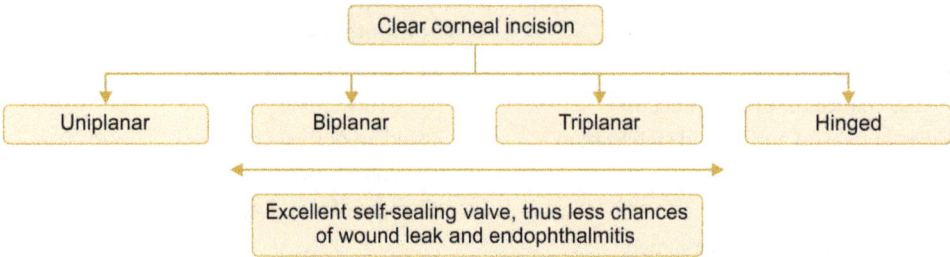

Flowchart 5: Advantages and disadvantages of types of conjunctival peritomy.

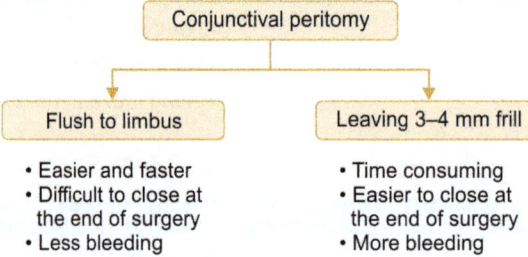

- Easier and faster
- Difficult to close at the end of surgery
- Less bleeding

- Time consuming
- Easier to close at the end of surgery
- More bleeding

TABLE 5: Trocar placement.	
Lens status	**Placement of trocar or needle (Distance from limbus)**
Phakic	4 mm
Pseudophakic	3.5 mm
Aphakic	3 mm

Q 3. Write a short note on pre-Descemet membrane or Dua's layer.

Gross Anatomy

This layer has been discovered in 2013 by Dr Harminder Singh Dua, an Indian origin ophthalmologist currently working in Nottingham, UK. It is a tough, impervious to air, well-defined, acellular layer (devoid of keratocytes—CD 34 negative) only about 10–15 µm thick sandwiched between the corneal stroma and DM. It occupies central 7.5–9 mm of central cornea depending on an individual's corneal diameters and is continuous with trabecular meshwork. The bursting pressure of this layer is around 700–900 mm Hg.

Microscopic anatomy has been illustrated in **Flowchart 6**.
- Provides a cleavage plane useful in lamellar keratoplasty—accessed by air or mechanically
- Forms the posterior wall of type I big bubble (BB)
- Forms the anterior wall of type II BB
- Helps our understanding of mixed BB
- Explains how air enters the anterior chamber during BB deep anterior lamellar keratoplasty (DALK)

Flowchart 6: Microscopic anatomy of pre-Descemet membrane.

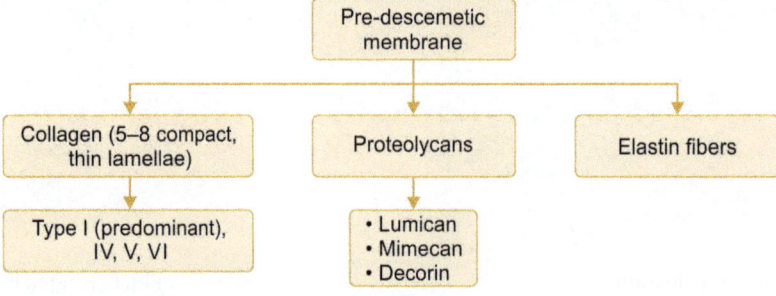

- Confers strength to the eye after DALK
- Improves understanding of DALK and makes it safer
- Improves understanding of posterior corneal pathology, e.g., descemetocele and acute hydrops
- *Forms the basis of innovations in surgery:* DALK triple, pre-Descemet's endothelial keratoplasty, and management of acute hydrops.
- Presence of elastin fibers explains pre-Descemet layer (PDL) reverts to its original dimension on deflation of the bubble during BB DALK.

 4. Discuss corneal transparency.

Apart from structural function, the main physiologic function of the cornea is to act as a major refractive medium besides our natural crystalline lens. It contributes almost three-fourths of total refractive power of the eye. Therefore, maintaining corneal transparency is a prerequisite to obtain a clear and sharp retinal image.

Factors maintaining corneal transparency: The various anatomical and physiological factors have been depicted in **Flowchart 7**.

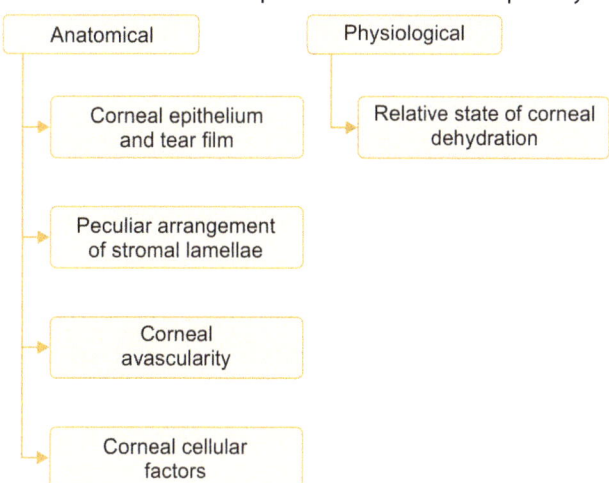

Flowchart 7: Factors responsible for corneal transparency.

Corneal Epithelium and Tear Film

- Epithelium is transparent due to homogenicity of its refractive index.
- Tight intercellular junctions such as macula occludentes and desmosomes provide resistance to the flow of water, electrolytes, and glucose (unlike endothelium).
- Tear film keeps the corneal surface smooth and provides high-quality optical surface.

Clinical implication: Conditions associated with epithelial abnormality (defect, bullae, erosion) and tear film abnormality (evaporative or aqueous or mixed form of dry eye disease) may result in loss of transparency.

Peculiar Arrangement of Stromal Lamellae

The various theories contributing to corneal transparency are depicted in **Figure 7**. **Figure 8A** depicts the cross-sectional view showing regular arrangement of the corneal fibrils on the basis of corneal transparency (Maurice theory) and **Figure 8B** depicts the cross-sectional view showing irregular arrangement of corneal fibrils on the basis of loss of corneal transparency (Maurice theory).

Corneal Avascularity

Cornea is avascular except for the perilimbal 1 mm of cornea which is invaded by small loops of anterior ciliary vessels. This vascular system is responsible for:
- Defense mechanism against noxious agents
- Provides nutrition
- Allows transport of systemic drugs.

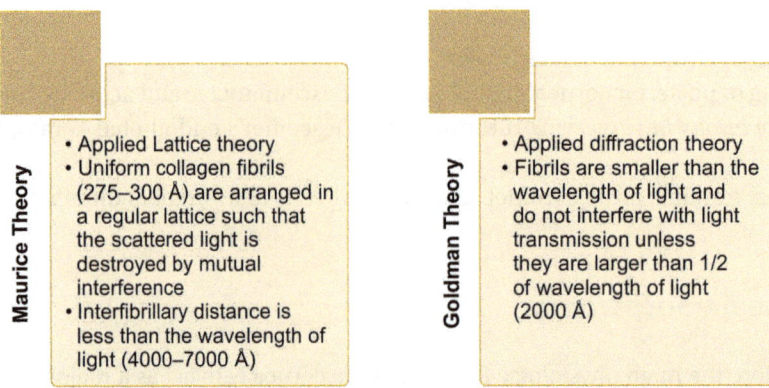

Fig. 7: Theories responsible for corneal transparency.
(IOP: intraocular pressure)

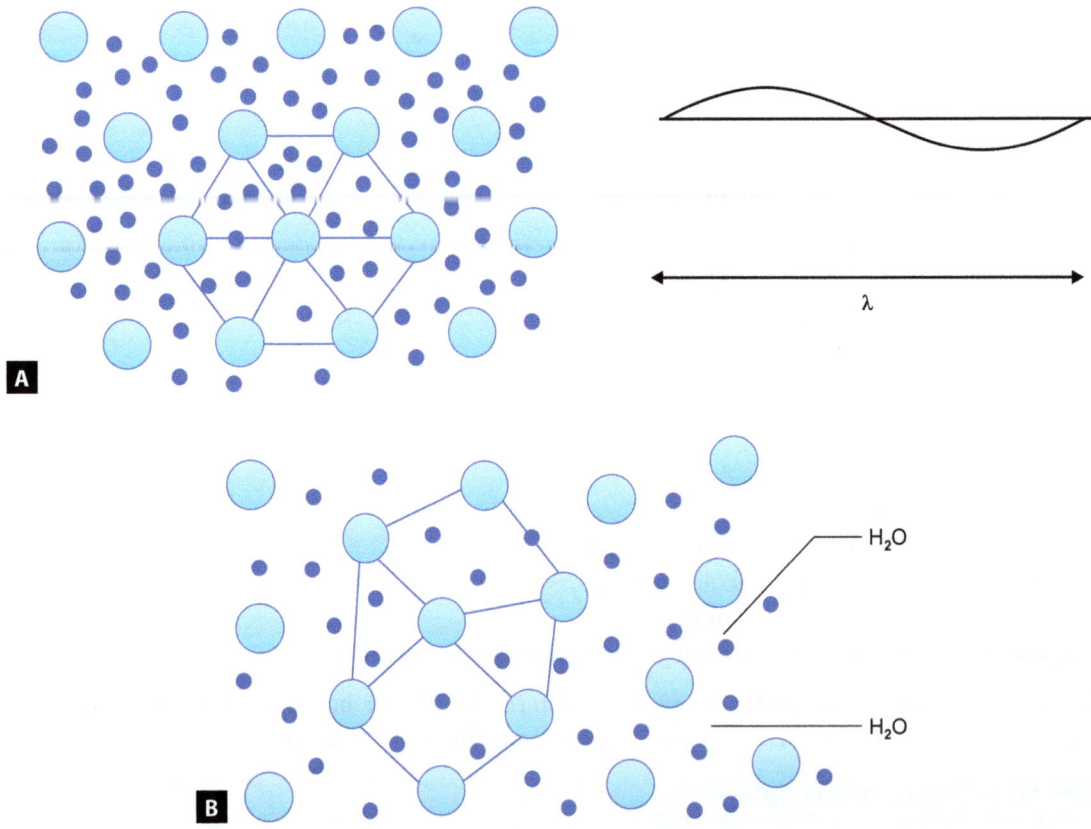

Figs. 8A and B: Regular and irregular arrangement of collagen fibrils depicted using Maurice theory.

Theories of Corneal Vascularization

Various theories have come forward to explain vascularization of cornea in pathologic conditions.
- *Chemical theory:*
  - *Presence of vasostimulatory factor (VSF) (Campbell and Michelson):* Low–molecular-weight amine. **Flowchart 8** illustrates the mechanism of action of VSF.
  - *Absence of vasoinhibitory factor (VIF) (Meyer and Chafre):* Sulfate ester of hyaluronic acid.
- *Mechanical theory (Cogan):* Blood vessels are unable to invade the structurally compact normal cornea. Therefore, loosening of stromal collagen lamellae caused by corneal edema is a prerequisite for neovascularization.

Flowchart 8: Mechanism of action of vasostimulatory factor.

Release of VSF at the site of lesion → VSF diffuses through the stroma and reaches limbus → VSF stimulates the limbal plexus for growth of new vessels

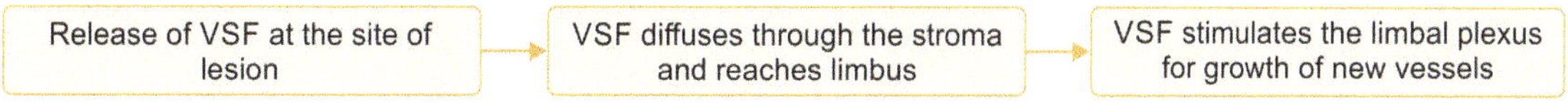

(VSF: vasostimulatory factor)

- Factors which draw water into the cornea

  Stroma swelling pressure, IOP

- Factor which prevent flow of water into the cornea

  Mechanical barrier function of epithelium

- Factor which draw water out of the cornea

  Active pump of endothelium

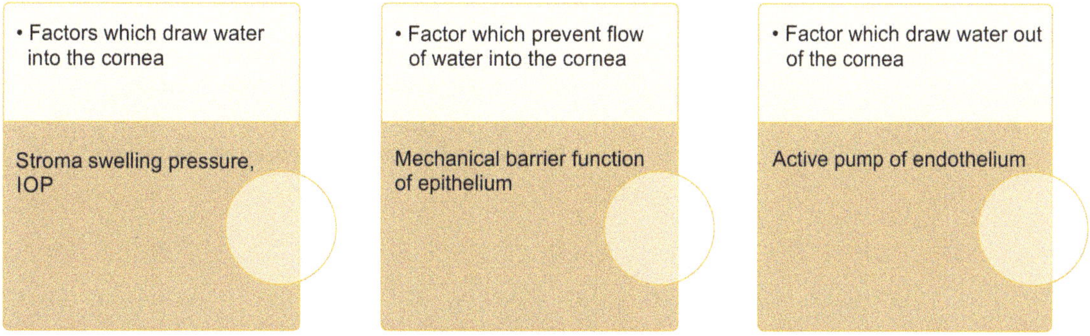

Fig. 9: Factors responsible for maintaining relative state of corneal dehydration.
(IOP: intraocular pressure)

(*Point against:* Absence of corneal vascularization in aphakic/pseudophakic bullous keratopathy and Fuchs endothelial dystrophy)
- *Combined theory (Maurice):* Both chemical and mechanical factors are mandatory for neovascularization.
- *Role of leukocytes:* Corneal vascularization occurs in response to release of inflammatory mediators predominantly leukocytes.

Corneal Cellular Factors

Fibroblasts (keratocytes) are the source of stromal collagen and proteoglycans. They contain:
- Enzymes*
- *Water-soluble proteins:* Transketolase and aldehyde dehydrogenase

(*Clinical implication:* Specific enzyme defects result in corneal opacification such as mucopolysaccharidosis)

Relative State of Dehydration

The water content of normal cornea is around 80% (highest water content in any connective tissue). The various factors responsible for maintaining the relative state of dehydration of cornea are depicted in **Figure 9**.

Disturbance of any one of the factors will result in corneal edema, increase in corneal thickness, and loss of transparency.
- *Stromal swelling pressure (SSP):* It is defined as the positive pressure exerted by the glycosaminoglycans (GAGs) of corneal stroma (mean: 60 mm Hg).
  - *Imbibition pressure (IP):* Negative pressure is created by the anionic charges of the GAGs which cause sucking of the fluid out of the stroma.
  - *Intraocular pressure (IOP):* Positive fluid pressure inside the eye (mean: 17 mm Hg).
    IP = IOP − SSP
       = 17 − 60 = −43 mm Hg
    (*Clinical implication:* When IOP > SSP as in glaucoma, or SSP < IOP as in endothelial dystrophy, IP becomes positive pressure resulting in drawing of fluid into the stroma and corneal edema)
- *Mechanical barrier function of epithelium and endothelium:* Corneal epithelium acts as a perfect semipermeable membrane to both small solutes (NaCl, urea) and water, whereas the barrier function of endothelium being calcium dependent restricts only water and not solutes.
  (*Clinical implication:* When endothelium is damaged, corneal transparency is lost much more than when epithelium is damaged)
- *Active pump of endothelium:* The various active pumps (energy dependent) are illustrated in **Table 6**.
  Endothelial active pump mechanisms controlling the corneal hydration is depicted in **Figure 10**.

TABLE 6: Various energy dependant active pumps of corneal endothelium.	
Na^+K^+-ATPase pump	• Located in the basolateral cell membrane • Pumps Na^+ out from the stroma • Inhibited by Oubain
Bicarbonate dependent ATPase pump	• Present in mitochondria • Inhibited by thiocyanate
Carbonic anhydrase enzyme	• Produces HCO_3^- and H^+ ions • Mediates flow of fluid from stroma to aqueous • Inhibited by acetazolamide and dorzolamide
Na^+/H^+ pump	• Located in lateral cell membrane • Pumps out Na^+ into aqueous and H^+ into stroma

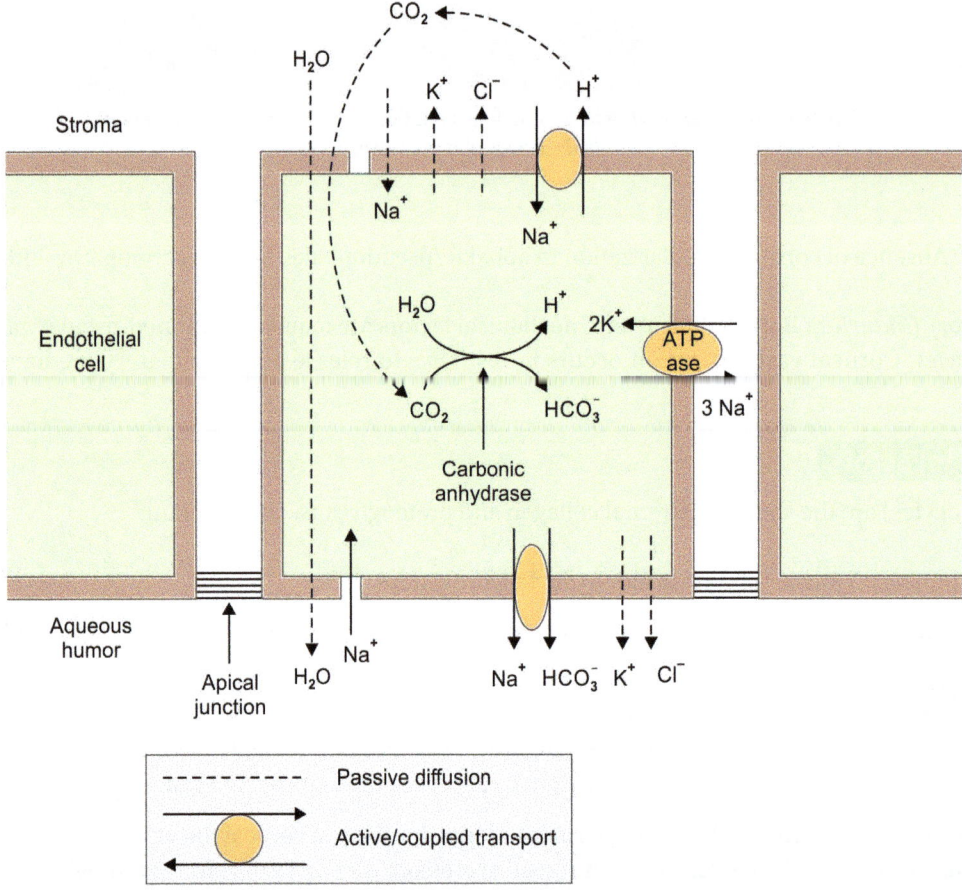

Fig. 10: Mechanism of action of corneal endothelial pumps.

- *Passive ion movements:*
  - K^+, Cl^-, HCO_3^- diffuses into aqueous humor
  - Na^+, Cl^-, HCO_3^- diffuses in the contralateral direction
- *Hypoxia, pH, and changes in temperature:* These can alter the metabolic activity and thereby can cause alteration in corneal thickness and loss of transparency.
- *Evaporation of water from corneal surface:* Illustrated in **Figure 11**.

5. Discuss corneal wound healing.

The anatomical regions of the cornea can be divided into four zones for the purpose of discussing pathologic responses:
1. Epithelium
2. Subepithelium (epithelial basement membrane and Bowman's layer)

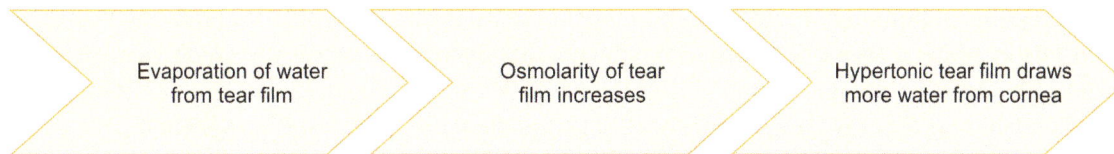

Fig. 11: Maintaining relative state of dehydration by tear film evaporation.

3. Stroma
4. Endothelium and DM.

A spectrum of pathological processes can interrupt the structural integrity of the above-mentioned zones and interfere with the function. These responses can be divided into six categories:
1. Defects and their repair
2. Fibrosis and vascularization
3. Edema and cysts
4. Inflammation and immune responses
5. Deposits
6. Proliferation.

Pathological Responses on Corneal Epithelium

- *Defects and their repair:* In physiological conditions, epithelium is continuously replaced every 4–7 days by a process that involves: (1) Basal cell differentiation toward the surface; (2) centripetal movement of limbal and peripheral cells; (3) desquamation of epithelial cells from the surface. The common causes may be corneal abrasion, focal foreign bodies, and neurotrophic keratopathy. Factors required in maintaining normal epithelial integrity are: normal basement membrane, vitamin A, normal tear film, and intact sensory innervation.
- *Fibrosis and vascularization:* This process does not take place in this layer owing to the absence of connective tissue.
- *Edema and cysts:* This can cause reduction in visual acuity due to creation of irregular surface which diffracts and scatters light. Edema in this layer is mainly attributed to endothelial dysfunction and epithelial hypoxia and trauma (contact lens induced). When fluid accumulates between the basement membrane and overlying cells thus causing a breach in the desmosomal connections, bullae appear. Cysts can result from accumulation of rapidly multiplying or degenerating epithelial cells.
- *Inflammation and immune responses:* In corneal allograft rejection, the donor epithelium is attacked by cytotoxic T-lymphocytes which clinically appear as a serpentine line that starts from the graft host junction toward the center of cornea. This may be a self-limiting, asymptomatic process as epithelial healing runs parallels cell death.
- *Deposits:*
  - *Elements:* Iron deposits in the lysosomes of the basal epithelial cells in a linear pattern. Various types of iron lines in the corneal epithelium are depicted in **Table 7**.
    Other conditions are: Salzmann nodular degeneration, elevated corneal scar, keratoplasty, and radial keratotomy.
  - *Drugs:* Amiodarone (antiarrhythmic) is the most common drug causing characteristic whorl-like pattern. The severity is usually dose-dependent and disappears on withdrawal of the drug. They rarely interfere with patient's vision with exceptions of mucopolysaccharidosis type VI-A, Maroteaux–Lamy, Fabry disease, multiple myeloma, and cystinosis.
  - *Corneal dystrophies and degenerations:* They rarely form deposits in the epithelial layer with the exception of Meesmann epithelial dystrophy.

TABLE 7: Iron deposition lines in various conditions.

Condition	Location	Terminology
Normal eyelid closure	Upper two-thirds and lower one-third junction	Hudson–Stahli line
Keratoconus	Base of the cone	Fleischer ring
Pterygium	In front of the cap	Stocker's line
Filtering bleb	Anterior edge of the bleb	Ferry's line

- *Proliferation:* Epithelial thinning occurs over elevations (over Salzmann's nodules) whereas thickening occurs when epithelium fills in defects. These compensatory adjustments occur to preserve a smooth corneal surface so as to maintain an optimal optical function. Metaplasia into abnormal keratin-producing epithelium occurs in Stevens–Johnson syndrome. Epithelium is the only layer bearing neoplastic potential thus may result in squamous cell carcinoma at the limbus where stem cells reside. Therefore, intraepithelial neoplasia usually presents as gray intraepithelial sheet onto the clear cornea or as raised limbal mass. Ectopic migration of epithelium can also occur through a corneal fistula to form a cyst or downgrowth sheet in the anterior chamber after an episode of perforating injury or surgical trauma. Epithelial proliferation and ingrowth can be visible underneath a laser-assisted in situ keratomileusis (LASIK) flap usually when a flap lift has been done for repeat LASIK procedure.

Pathological Responses of Subepithelial Zone

- *Defects and their repair:* The epithelial basement membrane is secreted by the basal epithelial cells and thus can be regenerated in excess form when damaged whereas, the Bowman's membrane lacks regenerative potential. So, any defect in Bowman's layer is repaired with fibroblasts and hence scar formation.
- *Fibrosis and vascularization:* This can occur between the epithelial basement membrane and Bowman's layer as avascular pannus (advanced Fuchs' endothelial dystrophy, postphotorefractive keratectomy, and Salzmann nodular degeneration) or vascular pannus (extended wear soft contact lens, trachomatous eyelid scarring, and alkali burns).
- *Edema and cysts:* These arise from endothelial dysfunction and stromal edema can result in epithelial basement membrane folds.
- *Inflammation and immune response:* This is characterized by epithelial defect and superficial infiltrate which causes damage to the Bowman's layer and anterior stroma which is usually seen in infection and trauma. Subepithelial infiltrates can also be caused by antigens and toxins as in adenoviral keratoconjunctivitis. These infiltrates might also be seen following penetrating keratoplasty as an allograft rejection.
- *Deposits:* Various deposits with their associated disorders are illustrated in **Table 8**.
- *Proliferation:* This is seen in primary epithelial disorders (epithelial basement membrane dystrophy), as a nonspecific response (Salzmann nodular degeneration), as systemic disease (diabetes mellitus).

TABLE 8: Types of deposits in various pathological conditions.

Material	Causative agent/disorder
Adenochrome pigment	Epinephrine
Hemosiderin rust ring	Iron containing foreign bodies
Amyloid	Gelatinous drop-like dystrophy
Fine curled filaments	Thiel–Behnke corneal dystrophy
Calcium	Band-shaped keratopathy

Pathological Responses of Corneal Stroma

- *Defects and their repair:* Stromal defects can occur from accidental, surgical trauma or microbial invasion where repair involves microorganism elimination and control of inflammation. Progressive thinning without epithelial ulceration occurs in ectatic disorders such as keratoconus and pellucid marginal degeneration. This results in alteration in corneal curvature, visual instability, and loss. Insults such as alkali burns, autoimmune diseases, and infection will set off a series of destructive and enzymatic events finally ending up in descemetocele and corneal perforation.
- *Fibrosis and vascularization:* Wound healing in this layer is relatively slower owing to the avascular tissue and its rate decreases with age. The scar tissue is weaker than the normal stroma as seen by the traumatic dehiscence of keratoplasty wounds after surgery. There are three phases in wound healing—(1) *Destructive phase:* Removal of abnormal tissues by polymorphonuclear leukocytes (PMNL), macrophages, collagenase, and proteoglycans; if not contained, melting of stroma can result in corneal perforation; (2) *Synthetic phase:* New collagen and proteoglycan synthesis by stromal fibroblasts aiding in wound closure; if inhibited by drugs (steroids) or disease (rheumatoid arthritis) wound strength will decrease; if progresses uncontrolled, visually significant scarring will occur; (3) *Remodeling phase:* Transformation of the initial scar into a clearer structure through collagen structural changes. **Flowchart 9** shows the series of events following anterior stromal injury.

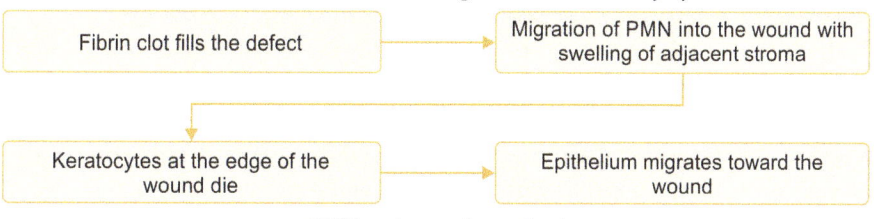

Flowchart 9: Events following anterior stromal injury.

(PMN: polymorphonuclear)

The healing epithelium expresses cytokines [interleukin-1 (IL-1), transforming growth factor-β (TGF-β)] which stimulate stromal keratocytes to transform into fibroblasts and myofibroblasts and to secrete extracellular matrix.

Stromal fibrosis: Irregular alignment of collagen fibrils cause scattering of light and appear as stromal opacity. The severity, duration, and extent of healing depends on the degree of corneal scarring. Bacterial and fungal keratitis usually leave a focal, well-delineated scar while alkali burns leave diffuse, opaque scars.

Stromal vascularization: It is a nonspecific response of wound healing. The location and number of vessels gives a hint of the location and severity of the inflammation. They can disrupt the normal stromal architecture, allow lipid leakage, and can increase the chances of allograft rejection in corneal transplant cases. Stromal vessels can grow at three levels: (1) Subepithelial and superficial stroma (superficial corneal disease); (2) Middle stroma (chronic inflammation); (3) Deep stroma (keratouveitis). They arise from superficial conjunctival vessels, deep scleral vessels, or iris vessels when iris is in contact with cornea and spread along corneal lamellar planes unless scarring is present. In inflammatory conditions, the pattern of vessels follows the trail of leukocytic infiltrate. Triangular tufts grow toward focal inflammation while in penetrating keratoplasty, ring of vessels surrounds the graft host junction. Stromal vessels dilate during active stage of inflammation and shrink to endothelium lined tubes without blood flow (i.e., ghost vessels) when inflammation subsides. These can refill with blood if recurrence occurs or ischemia develops.

- *Edema and cysts:* These occur as a result of endothelial or epithelial pump failure leading to increase in corneal thickness. Fluid accumulates in the glycosaminoglycans of the stroma thus changing the regular collagen fibril arrangement, clinically visible as ground-glass haze with or without cysts. As the edema progresses, corneal striae develop as the DM is displaced posteriorly. The various reasons may be: surgical trauma, Fuchs endothelial dystrophy, severe iridocyclitis, acute hydrops, and acute angle-closure glaucoma. Stromal edema remains confined to the area of endothelial or epithelial damage.
- *Inflammation and immune responses:* Infective keratitis, immunologic diseases, and trauma can lead to accumulation of leukocytes in the stroma which if severe can create foci of yellow-white suppuration. The stroma thickens with edema and pus, becomes gelatinous and starts to melt. This destructive activity is usually balanced by fibrosis with or without vascularization. Gram-negative bacteria such as *Pseudomonas* species can cause severe stromal suppuration and destruction due to secretion of proteolytic enzymes from bacteria and PMNs. On the contrary, immune-based stromal inflammation can result from deposition of antigen antibody complex and complement-mediated hypersensitivity such as in herpes simplex immune stromal keratitis.
- *Deposits:*
  - Gold (ocular chrysiasis)—accumulates in cytoplasm of keratocytes
  - Blood staining of cornea following hyphema and persistent IOP rise
  - Arcus senilis/juvenilis—lipid deposition in old age/hyperlipoproteinemia
  - Lipid keratopathy—lipid deposition secondary to interstitial viral keratitis
  - Retained stromal foreign bodies such as wood if not removed are auto-extruded as a part of inflammatory response
  - Mucopolysaccharidosis—excess of dermatan and keratan sulfate create ground glass appearance
  - Globulin crystals in multiple myeloma
  - Lecithin-cholesterol acyltransferase (LCAT) deficiency—central corneal lipid deposits
  - Lattice corneal dystrophy—amyloid
  - Macular corneal dystrophy—glycosaminoglycans
  - Schnyder central crystalline dystrophy—lipid
- *Proliferation:* This usually occurs in the peripheral cornea which may be of two types:
  1. *Congenital*—dermoid choristoma (histologically normal tissue in an abnormal location)
  2. *Acquired*—proliferate at a surgical or accidental wound without vascularization; can occur anteriorly or posteriorly when a defect in Bowman's membrane persists or through a keratoplasty wound, respectively

Pathological Responses of Corneal Endothelium and Descemet Membrane

- *Defects and their repair:* Defects in the endothelium can occur alone or in combination with defects in DM. In either case, aqueous humor seeps into the stroma resulting in stromal and/or epithelial edema.
    - *Defects in endothelium:* This may occur—(A) *Acute:* After trauma or surgery (DMEK/DSAEK); (B) *Chronic:* In Fuchs endothelial dystrophy. The damaged endothelium repairs itself by migration and hypertrophy mainly. This layer does not undergo cell division under normal circumstances but can be stimulated by injury. Only the cells adjacent to the injured cells participate directly in wound healing, although cells in the peripheral endothelium may be a source of regenerative cells. Stromal edema resolves when the barrier and pump functions are re-established. Changes in cell size and shape occur during healing thus decreasing the hexagonality. Enlarged cells represent those which had spread out to cover the defect, whereas the smaller cells represent those desquamating or those resultant from cell division. If the count drops below the critical endothelial cell count (i.e., 500 cells/mm^2), the capacity to maintain corneal detergence is exceeded and decompensation results.
    - *Defects in DM:* This layer being elastic tends to break and recoil under tension as seen in acute hydrops. In birth trauma, due to forceps injury, DM breaks vertically as a result of globe compression. During healing phase, the split ends of DM do not reapproximate but the endothelium continuity is reestablished owing to the young age of the patient.
- *Fibrosis and vascularization posterior to DM:* Endothelium and DM lack connective tissue and thus do not develop fibrosis or vascularization. However, as a response to injury or disorder, it secretes a layer of abnormal fibrillar tissue (posterior collagenous layer) which may lead to visual compromise. Clinically, this PCL appears as a gray sheet at the level of DM. With light microscopy, the normal DM gets stained with periodic acid-Schiff (PAS) with the PCL behind it with multiple lamellae of variable thickness and staining. Immunohistochemistry revealed five different types of collagen and proteoglycans in PCL. PCL is also used to date the onset of endothelial or DM disease with transmission electron microscopy. For example, in corneas affected by iridocorneal endothelial (ICE) syndrome, the layers of normal banded and nonbanded DM are presently lined posteriorly by abnormal PCL indicating adult onset of the disorder. Likewise, abnormalities in the anterior portion of the nonbanded layer of DM indicates congenital etiology. Vascularization is absent in the DM and PCL.
- *Edema and cysts:* DM is a compact water-permeable layer with traces of glycosaminoglycans because of which it does not become edematous. However, intra- and extracellular fluid accumulation in the endothelial cells creates a dew drop, beaten metal appearance known as pseudo-guttata. Posterior polymorphous corneal dystrophy (PPMD) is characterized by focal, small lesions like a group of vesicles which are small pits in the posterior stroma lined by a thin DM.
- *Inflammation and immune responses:* In inflammatory disorders such as microbial keratitis and iridocyclitis, vasodilatory and chemotactic factors bring the endothelium in contact with leukocytes, forming keratic precipitates (KPs). KPs may form variety of patterns: (1) diffuse spattering (ankylosing spondylitis); (2) focal aggregation (HSV disciform endotheliitis); and (3) central, inferior, elliptical (sarcoid uveitis). In allograft rejection, antigens on the endothelial cell surface stimulate an immune reaction (Khodadoust rejection line). PMNs bind to the endothelial cells through cell surface receptors → penetrate between the cells → migrate between the DM and endothelium. **Figure 12** illustrates the series of events occurring following mild and severe inflammation at level of DM and endothelium. DM is highly resistant to proteolytic and collagenolytic enzymes released during keratitis or iridocyclitis, which enables protection to the passage of leukocytes and most microorganisms. Fungi are an exception as they release enzymes which enable them to penetrate intact DM.
- *Deposits:* The various deposits with their associated conditions are depicted in **Table 9**.
- *Proliferation:* Neoplastic or dysplastic disorders of endothelium does not exist. However, endothelial cells are capable of differentiating into fibroblast and epithelial-like cells (ICE syndrome, PPMD). Endothelium can proliferate over

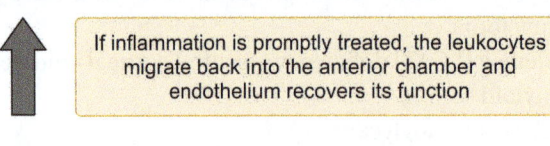

Fig. 12: Events following inflammation at DM-endothelium complex level.

TABLE 9: Types of deposits in various conditions at DM-endothelial level.

Condition	Material	Level
Silver containing drugs (Argyrol)	Silver	DM
Wilson's disease	Copper (Kayser-Fleischer ring)	DM
Arcus senilis	Lipid	DM
Pigment dispersion syndrome	Melanin (Krukenberg spindle)	Endothelium
Hyphema	Red blood cells	Endothelium
Anterior uveitis	KPs (lymphocytes and PMNs)	Endothelium
Lymphoproliferative disorders	Tumor cells	Endothelium
Pseudoexfoliation syndrome	Fibrillary whitish flakes	Endothelium
Post-cataract surgery	Lens cortex	Endothelium
Macular corneal dystrophy	Glycosaminoglycans	DM and endothelium

(PMN: polymorphonuclear; DM: Descemet membrane; KP: keratic precipitate)

trabecular meshwork, iris and vitreous in specific situations and is clinically visible as a glass or hyaline membrane. This is known as endothelialization or descemetization of the anterior chamber thus resulting in secondary glaucoma and corectopia.

References

1. Engelmann K, Böhnke M, Friedl P. Isolation and long-term cultivation of human corneal endothelial cells. Invest Ophthalmol Vis Sci. 1988;29(11):1656-62.
2. Joyce NC, Meklir B, Joyce SJ, Zieske JD. Cell cycle protein expression and proliferative status in human corneal cells. Invest Ophthalmol Vis Sci. 1996;37(4):645-55.

8.2 Acute Conjunctivitis

Siddhi Goel, Ritu Nagpal

 1. Describe the etiology, clinical features, approach, and management of acute conjunctivitis.

Introduction

The conjunctiva is a thin, transparent mucus membrane lining the anterior part of the sclera and inside of the eyelids. It consists of three parts—bulbar, forniceal, and palpebral. The bulbar portion begins at the edge of the cornea and covers the visible part of the sclera; the forniceal part lines the fornices and is loose and redundant and the palpebral part lines the inside of the eyelids. Conjunctivitis is an inflammation that affects the conjunctiva primarily. It is characterized by dilatation of the conjunctival vessels, resulting in hyperemia and edema of the conjunctiva, typically with associated discharge.[1] It is estimated that acute conjunctivitis affects 6 million people annually in the United States.[2] The prevalence of conjunctivitis varies according to the underlying cause, and is influenced by the patient's age, as well as the season of the year. Viral conjunctivitis is the most common cause of infectious conjunctivitis followed by bacterial conjunctivitis.[3] Allergic conjunctivitis is the most frequent cause, affecting 15–40% of the population,[4] and is observed more frequently in spring and summer.

Etiology

Acute conjunctivitis can be broadly classified into infective and noninfective causes. **Table 1** highlights the various causes of conjunctivitis.

Approximately 80% of acute cases of conjunctivitis are viral in etiology, the most common pathogen being *Adenovirus*. Herpetic conjunctivitis, though not often seen in the Indian scenario, is prevalent in the western world. Bacterial conjunctivitis is far more common in children than in adults. In adults, the most frequently encountered etiological agents are *Staphylococcus* species, mainly *Staphylococcus aureus*, *Streptococcus pneumoniae*, and *Haemophilus influenzae*, while in children the disease

TABLE 1: Causes of conjunctivitis.	
Infective	*Noninfective*
Viral • Adenoviral conjunctivitis • Herpes simplex virus (HSV) conjunctivitis • Varicella (herpes) zoster virus (VZV) • Molluscum contagiosum	Allergic • Seasonal allergic conjunctivitis • Vernal conjunctivitis • Atopic conjunctivitis • Giant papillary conjunctivitis (GPC), which also has a mechanical component
Bacterial • Bacterial conjunctivitis (including non-gonococcal and gonococcal) • Chlamydial conjunctivitis	Immune-mediated • Ocular mucous membrane pemphigoid (OMMP) • Graft-versus-host disease (GVHD) • Stevens–Johnson syndrome

is more often caused by *H. influenza, S. pneumoniae,* and *Moraxella catarrhalis*. Neonatal conjunctivitis could be chemical (occurring within 24 hours of birth), gonococcal (first week of life), or chlamydial (second week of life) in etiology.

Lately, the novel coronavirus, i.e., COVID-19, has also been reported to cause conjunctivitis as the only manifestation, or the presenting feature, preceding fever, cough, respiratory distress, and death.

Clinical Features

Symptoms

A case of acute conjunctivitis can present with the following symptoms:
- *Discharge:* It may be watery, mucoid, mucopurulent, or severe purulent based on the underlying etiology.
- Red eye—conjunctival hyperemia and chemosis
- *Itching:* It is the hallmark of allergic disease.
- Photophobia
- Blurred vision, colored haloes
- Irritation, grittiness.

Signs

The various signs of conjunctivitis which should be looked for are:
- Conjunctiva—pattern of injection, subconjunctival hemorrhage, chemosis, cicatricial change, and type of discharge
- Eyelids—any signs of inflammation or cicatrization
- Presence and size of papillae, follicles
- Membranes—whether true membranes or pseudomembranes
- Regional lymphadenopathy, particularly preauricular is commonly associated with viral infection.

Differential Diagnosis

The various causes of acute red eye in addition to acute conjunctivitis are uveitis, acute angle-closure glaucoma, acute endophthalmitis, subconjunctival hemorrhage, scleritis, episcleritis, and cellulitis. **Table 2** differentiates conjunctivitis from other causes of red eye.

It is also necessary to distinguish an infective conjunctivitis from an allergic conjunctivitis, since the management changes significantly. **Table 3** enumerates the features differentiating the former from the latter.

Work-up

Focused ocular examination and history are crucial for making appropriate decisions about the treatment and management of any eye condition, including conjunctivitis.

History

The patient should be inquired about the following:
- Onset and duration of symptoms
- Unilateral or bilateral presentation
- Character of discharge

TABLE 2: Distinguishing features of important causes of red eye.

Characteristics	Acute conjunctivitis	Acute iridocyclitis	Acute congestive glaucoma
Pain	Usually absent to mild discomfort	Moderate intensity	Severe intensity
Discharge	Watery, mucoid, or mucopurulent based on cause	Watery	Watery
Visual acuity	Usually normal	Mildly impaired	Markedly impaired
Pattern of congestion	Superficial, conjunctival	Deep ciliary	Deep ciliary
Pupil	Normal	Small and irregular due to synechiae	Large, vertically oval
Media	Clear	May be hazy due to KPs, AC reaction, and exudates	Hazy due to corneal edema
Anterior chamber depth	Normal	Variable	Extremely shallow
Intraocular pressure	Normal	Usually normal, maybe elevated	Very high
Constitutional symptoms	Absent	Usually absent	Prostration and vomiting

(AC: anterior chamber; KPs: keratic precipitates)

TABLE 3: Differences bzetween infective and allergic conjunctivitis.

	Infective conjunctivitis	Allergic conjunctivitis
Itching	Absent/minimal	Marked
Discharge	Mucopurulent in bacterial, watery in viral conjunctivitis	Mild watery discharge
Laterality	Mostly unilateral to begin with, may spread to fellow eye	Always bilateral
Concurrent otitis media	May be present	Absent
History of eczema/asthma/family history of atopy	Not relevant	Usually present
Course	Self resolving, complete resolution within 1–2 weeks	Waxing and waning course, with flare-ups in allergic season

- Recent exposure to an infected individual
- Allergy or family history of atopy
- Any history of trauma: mechanical, chemical, and ultraviolet radiation
- Any exacerbating factors
- Use of topical and systemic medications.

Examination

The initial eye examination should include measurement of visual acuity, torch light examination, and slit-lamp biomicroscopy.
- Eyelids—any swelling, malposition, associated skin conditions like seborrhea, eczema
- Eyelashes—matting of lashes, any loss of lashes
- Conjunctiva—any follicles/papillae, hemorrhages, mucus discharge, membranes or pseudomembranes, chemosis, any foreign body
- Cornea—any epithelial defect, punctate keratopathy, associated dry eye, filaments, and keratic precipitates
- Anterior chamber—for any signs of inflammation.

Investigations

Many cases of conjunctivitis can be diagnosed on the basis of history and examination only. Additional diagnostic tests may be helpful in cases of suspected infectious neonatal conjunctivitis, recurrent conjunctivitis, conjunctivitis recalcitrant to therapy, conjunctivitis presenting with severe purulent discharge, and cases suspicious of gonococcal or chlamydial infection.[5] The various tests include:
- Culture—for severe bacterial conjunctivitis not responsive to conventional management

- Viral diagnostic tests—a rapid, in-office immunodiagnostic test using antigen detection is available for adenovirus conjunctivitis.[5] Polymerase chain reaction (PCR) can also be used for viral detection.
- Tests for chlamydia—various immunologically-based diagnostic tests are available, including a direct immunofluorescent antibody test and enzyme-linked immunosorbent assay (ELISA).
- Confocal microscopy—noninvasive modality may have a role in atopic conjunctivitis
- Smears/cytology—Gram's/Giemsa stains can be used to identify the underlying organism.

Management

Prevention

Early detection of conjunctivitis is crucial as it helps in prompt and appropriate treatment, speeds up the disease resolution, minimizing both the sequelae of untreated conjunctivitis and time away from work or school. Infective conjunctivitis is highly contagious with a high risk of transmission. The pathogen spreads through direct contact via contaminated fingers, medical instruments, swimming pool water, or personal items (fomites). Thus, hand washing, strict instrument disinfection, and isolation of the infected patients from the rest of the family should be advised. During an active epidemic, consideration should be given to triaging patients upon arrival at the hospital and directing those who appear infected to a dedicated "red-eye room."

Treatment

Conjunctivitis is the most common cause of red or pink eye in patients seeking primary care treatment. Most cases of conjunctivitis are self-limiting[6] and indiscriminate use of topical antibiotics or corticosteroids should be avoided. Corticosteroids can potentially prolong adenoviral infections and worsen herpes simplex virus (HSV) infections. Treatment methods are described below for the most common types of acute conjunctivitis in clinical practice.[7]

Viral Conjunctivitis

Adenoviral Conjunctivitis

Though adenoviral conjunctivitis resolves even without treatment within 1–2 weeks, patients with adenoviral conjunctivitis should be explained about the highly contagious nature of this disease and about appropriate measures to reduce the risk of spreading the infection to their other eye or to other people. Because of its ability to infect multiple members of a family or a classroom, this infection is often termed as epidemic keratoconjunctivitis. It is also necessary to identify patients infected during an outbreak of such an epidemic, who may only have a mild disease but can act as chronic carriers/reservoirs of the virus, shedding it in the community.

Symptomatic treatment: Artificial tears, topical antihistamines, and vasoconstrictors, or cold compresses may be useful in alleviating some of the symptoms.

Antiviral therapy: Available antiviral medications are not useful.

Antibiotic therapy: Topical antibiotics do not protect against secondary infections, and their use may complicate the clinical presentation by causing drug allergy and toxicity, leading to delay in diagnosis of other possible ocular diseases.[8]

Topical corticosteroids: The role of steroids in adenoviral conjunctivitis is controversial. Though known to provide early relief in severely symptomatic patients, there persists a theoretical risk of increased duration of viral shedding that could be hazardous. Steroids at minimum effective doses are indicated over a long duration in case of remnant subepithelial infiltrates.

Topical steroid-sparing agents: Long-term steroids given to a patient with subepithelial infiltrates could act as a double-edged sword, giving rise to its known complications such as cataract and glaucoma. In patients in whom steroids are contraindicated, topical steroid-sparing agents such as cyclosporine or tacrolimus are known to be beneficial in alleviating the visual complaints.

Recent advances in treatment of adenoviral conjunctivitis: Currently, a novel topical ophthalmic suspension of povidone-iodine (PVP-I) 0.6% and dexamethasone 0.1%, which can not only treat both viral and inflammatory components but also the immune-related sequelae such as subepithelial infiltrates, is undergoing phase 3 randomized control trial.

Herpes Conjunctivitis

Topical and/or oral antiviral treatment is recommended for HSV conjunctivitis to prevent corneal infection. The various available antivirals include topical ganciclovir 0.15% gel used 3–5 times per day, trifluridine 1% solution 5–8 times per day, or topical acyclovir 3% ointment 5 times per day. Oral acyclovir (200–400 mg 5 times per day), oral valacyclovir (500 mg 2 or 3 times a day) and famciclovir (250 mg twice a day) can also be used.[5] Care should be taken regarding the epithelial toxicity of these medications. Topical corticosteroids potentiate HSV infection and should be avoided.

Herpes zoster virus, responsible for shingles, can involve ocular tissue, especially if the first and second branches of the trigeminal nerve are involved. Oral antivirals are recommended at a dose of 800 mg five times daily for 7 days for acyclovir, 1,000 mg every 8 hours for 7 days for valacyclovir, or 500 mg three times daily for 7 days for famciclovir. Immunocompromised patients need to be treated more aggressively.

Bacterial Conjunctivitis

Mild bacterial conjunctivitis is usually self-limited, and it typically resolves spontaneously without specific treatment in immune-competent adults.[6] Topical antibiotics help in achieving earlier clinical and microbiological remission compared with placebo; however, this benefit lessens over time.[6] Empirical broad-spectrum topical antibiotic is usually effective and the most convenient or least expensive option can be selected. We usually start our patients with eye drop moxifloxacin 0.5% 6 times a day or eye drop gatifloxacin 0.5% and monitor the response. Supportive therapy in the form of artificial tears can be added. Contact lens wear should be discontinued until at least 48 hours after complete resolution of symptoms.

Conjunctival cultures and slides for Gram staining should be obtained if gonococcal infection is a possibility and in cases with poor response to empirical therapy. In these cases, the choice of antibiotic is guided by the results of laboratory tests. *Methicillin-resistant Staphylococcus aureus* (MRSA) has been isolated with increasing frequency from patients with bacterial conjunctivitis.[9] Cases of MRSA should be managed with fortified vancomycin. Conjunctivitis caused by *Neisseria gonorrhoeae* is a frequent source of hyperacute conjunctivitis in neonates and sexually active adults and young adolescents. Systemic antibiotic therapy is necessary to treat conjunctivitis due to *N. gonorrhoeae* and *Chlamydia trachomatis*. The drug of choice for gonococcal conjunctivitis is ceftriaxone 250 mg IM, single dose, or azithromycin 1 g single oral dose or doxycycline 100 mg orally, twice a day for 7 days. For chlamydial conjunctivitis, azithromycin or doxycycline in the same above-mentioned dose can be used.[10,11]

References

1. Leibowitz HM. The red eye. N Engl J Med. 2000;343(5):345-51.
2. Udeh BL, Schneider JE, Ohsfeldt RL. Cost effectiveness of a point-of-care test for adenoviral conjunctivitis. Am J Med Sci. 2008;336(3):254-64.
3. Fitch CP, Rapoza PA, Owens S, Murillo-Lopez F, Johnson RA, Quinn TC, et al. Epidemiology and diagnosis of acute conjunctivitis at an inner-city hospital. Ophthalmology. 1989;96(8):1215-20.
4. Bielory BP, O'Brien TP, Bielory L. Management of seasonal allergic conjunctivitis: guide to therapy. Acta Ophthalmol (Copenh). 2012;90(5):399-407.
5. American Academy of Ophthalmology. Cornea/External Disease Panel. Preferred Practice Pattern Guidelines: Conjunctivitis-Limited Revision. San Francisco, CA: American Academy of Ophthalmology; 2011.
6. Sheikh A, Hurwitz B, van Schayck CP, McLean S, Nurmatov U. Antibiotics versus placebo for acute bacterial conjunctivitis. Cochrane Database Syst Rev. 2012;(9):CD001211.
7. Skevaki CL, Galani IE, Pararas MV, Giannopoulou KP, Tsakris A. Treatment of viral conjunctivitis with antiviral drugs. Drugs. 2011;71(3):331-47.
8. O'Brien TP, Jeng BH, McDonald M, Raizman MB. Acute conjunctivitis: truth and misconceptions. Curr Med Res Opin. 2009;25(8):1953-61.
9. Freidlin J, Acharya N, Lietman TM, Cevallos V, Whitcher JP, Margolis TP. Spectrum of eye disease caused by methicillin-resistant *Staphylococcus aureus*. Am J Ophthalmol. 2007;144(2):313-5.
10. Borazan M, Karalezli A, Akova YA, Akman A, Kiyici H, Erbek SS. Efficacy of olopatadine HCl 0.1%, ketotifen fumarate 0.025%, epinastine HCl 0.05%, emedastine 0.05% and fluorometholone acetate 0.1% ophthalmic solutions for seasonal allergic conjunctivitis: a placebo-controlled environmental trial. Acta Ophthalmol (Copenh). 2009;87(5):549-54.
11. Holland EJ, Brilakis HS, Schwartz GS. Herpes simplex keratitis. In: Krachmer JH, Mannis MJ, Holland EJ (Eds). Cornea, 2nd edition. St Louis: Mosby; 2004. pp. 1043-74.

8.3 Ophthalmia Neonatorum

Ritika Mukhija, Prafulla Kumar Maharana, Ritu Nagpal

 1. Describe the etiology, clinical features, approach, and management of ophthalmia neonatorum.

Introduction

Ophthalmia neonatorum, also known as neonatal conjunctivitis, refers to conjunctival inflammation along with discharge during the first month of life. This condition can be caused by bacterial, viral, and chemical agents. Widespread effective prophylaxis has contracted its occurrence to very low levels in industrialized countries, but ophthalmia neonatorum remains a significant cause of ocular infection, blindness, and even death in medically underserved areas around the world.

Worldwide, the incidence of ophthalmia neonatorum is greater in areas with poor health care and a high prevalence of sexually transmitted diseases. The prevalence ranges from 0.1% in highly developed countries with effective prenatal and perinatal care to 10% in areas such as East Africa.

In India, the incidence of neonatal conjunctivitis varies from 1 to 24% depending upon the geographical region. Prior to Crede's prophylaxis, ophthalmia neonatorum was the main cause of neonatal blindness (60–75%); it can be sight-threatening if specific treatment is not provided immediately.[1-5]

Etiopathogenesis

Neonatal conjunctivitis manifests as a diffuse, often hyperacute conjunctivitis with a papillary reaction, as a follicular response is not seen prior to 6–8 weeks of life. It may result from both chemical and microbial agents, with severity of the inflammatory response depending mainly on the inciting agent.

Risk Factors

There are various perinatal risk factors associated with the development of ophthalmia neonatorum. Prolonged exposure to the vaginal flora in cases of vaginal delivery and premature rupture of membranes (PROM) may predispose the neonate to infection, even in cases of delivery by cesarean section. Prolonged intrauterine exposure due to retrograde transmission of microbes in case of PROM also leads to errors in relating the time of onset of conjunctivitis to the etiologic agent. Further, prolonged delivery time coupled with any instrumentation during delivery may lead to ocular trauma in terms of epithelial breakdown and exposure, and facilitate the invasion by infectious organisms.

Sexually transmitted infections in the mother also play an important role and these account for *Chlamydia trachomatis* being the most common cause of infectious neonatal conjunctivitis in industrialized countries. Approximately 60% of infants exposed to *C. trachomatis* and 40% of neonates exposed to *Neisseria gonorrhoeae* during delivery contract the infection. Neonatal infection from herpes simplex virus occurs in 40–60% of neonates exposed to active genital herpes virus, with the highest risk being when the mother has primary genital herpes involving the cervix at delivery.

Additionally, there are inherent factors in the neonatal immune system, such as lack of local secretory immunoglobulin A (IgA) (unless provided by adequate breastfeeding), abnormally low tear secretion in most preterm and about 20% of full-term infants, absence of lymphoid tissue in conjunctiva, and decreased concentration of tear lysozymes in premature infants that further put them at risk of developing ophthalmia neonatorum. After birth, infection can be contracted from the caregiver (cold sores, nasopharyngeal bacteria, etc.) or even nosocomial infections from prolonged duration of neonatal intensive care.

Causes

- *Chemical conjunctivitis:* Also known as aseptic conjunctivitis, it is usually characterized by a mild and transient conjunctival injection and watering, which typically resolves in 24–48 hours. This is caused by instillation of silver nitrate into the conjunctival fornix, which was recommended by Crede in 1881 as a prophylactic measure for gonococcal neonatal conjunctivitis. Though this prophylaxis played a major role in reducing ocular morbidity from neonatal conjunctivitis, it has been largely replaced by topical antibiotics now in view of the adverse effects.
- *Microbial conjunctivitis:* It is also known as septic conjunctivitis; it can be bacterial, viral, or fungal.

- *Bacterial:* The most commonly implicated organisms are *N. gonorrhoeae* and *C. trachomatis* which are implicated in sexually transmitted infections. Apart from these, *Haemophilus* species, *Streptococcus pneumoniae*, and *Staphylococcus aureus* are also implicated. Rare causes include *Streptococcus viridans*, *Pseudomonas aeruginosa*, *Escherichia coli*, and *Klebsiella* pneumonia.
- *Viral:* Herpes simplex virus (both HSV I and II) and adenovirus may cause neonatal conjunctivitis. HSV II, which is the genital strain, is responsible for around 80% of neonatal herpes infections.
- *Fungal:* An infrequent cause of neonatal conjunctivitis is *Candida*, which may present in the eye as a pseudomembranous conjunctivitis or as a white conjunctival plaque. The time of onset after exposure is 5 days or more.

The age of the baby provides an important clue toward the etiology of disease; although it should be noted that bacterial infections can occur anytime. Chemicals such as silver nitrate or other prophylactic topical medicines such as erythromycin and gentamicin usually cause symptoms in the first 24 hours of life. Bacterial causes are most likely (*N. gonorrhoeae* is the most common cause, *S. aureus*) in 24–48 hours of life. After 5 days of life, *C. trachomatis* is more common followed by herpes keratoconjunctivitis.

Clinical Features

Conjunctival hyperemia and discharge, along with lid erythema and edema are the common features of conjunctivitis. It is important to note that papillary conjunctival response is most common as follicular hypertrophic response is not seen in the infant prior to 6–8 weeks of age because of the immaturity of the lymphoid system. The commonly implicated organisms are discussed in detail here:

- *Gonococcal conjunctivitis:* Symptoms due to *N. gonorrhoeae* classically appear 2–5 days after birth. While an earlier onset may be due to cases of PROM, a later onset suggests postnatal exposure to the organism. An initial serosanguineous discharge progresses rapidly, usually over 24 hours to a thick and purulent discharge, associated with markedly edematous eyelids and prominent chemosis. The involvement is usually bilateral. Gonococci with their ability to penetrate intact epithelial cells and replicate rapidly, may lead to corneal ulceration and perforation if the diagnosis and subsequent treatment is delayed. Gonococcal infection can also give rise to systemic complications such as stomatitis, arthritis, rhinitis, septicemia, and meningitis.
- *Chlamydial conjunctivitis:* With incubation period of 5–14 days, the onset is later than gonococcal conjunctivitis. The genital serovar types D-K of *C. trachomatis* are responsible for causing neonatal conjunctivitis. More than a third neonates infected with the organism develop watery conjunctivitis which later becomes more copious and purulent. Most of the cases are mild and self-limited, but occasionally severe involvement with eyelid swelling, chemosis, pseudomembrane, peripheral pannus, and corneal involvement has been noted. Untreated 10–20% of the cases develop infantile pneumonia, which is a major cause of morbidity and mortality. Other extraocular involvement of chlamydia includes nasopharyngeal, rectal, and vaginal colonization.
- *Herpes simplex keratoconjunctivitis:* It usually presents with generalized herpes infection, with about 80% of neonates with typical herpetic lesions of the skin, eye, or mouth. Conjunctivitis typically occurs within 6–14 days after birth and may be unilateral or bilateral. It is associated with eyelid edema and a serous discharge.[1] Microdendrites or geographic ulcers are the more prominent signs of corneal involvement. Neonatal keratoconjunctivitis may be the sole manifestation of herpes infection, but is frequently associated with systemic infection, with mortality rate for disseminated disease as high as 50%.
- *Fungal:* Candida is an infrequent cause of neonatal conjunctivitis, with time of onset after exposure being 5 days or more. It may present in the eye as a pseudomembranous conjunctivitis or as a white conjunctival plaque.

Differential Diagnosis

Differential diagnoses of neonatal conjunctivitis include:
- *Congenital nasolacrimal duct obstruction and dacryocystitis:* Congenital lacrimal pathway obstruction also causes unilateral conjunctivitis in neonates and infants. Watering or collection of mucopurulent discharge over lower fornix in the affected eye is seen.
- *Congenital glaucoma:* The classic triad of manifestations includes epiphora, photophobia, and blepharospasm.
- *Preseptal/orbital cellulitis:* Periorbital erythema and edema and pain are usually more severe in these cases. Limitation of extraocular movement, chemosis, afferent pupil, or resistance to retropulsion indicates orbital extension of the infection.
- *Infectious keratitis:* It may be present with or without associated conjunctivitis.

Work-up

History

As mentioned before, the onset of symptoms and age of the baby provide important diagnostic clues. History related to various perinatal risk factors should also be meticulously taken.

Examination

- *Lids and adnexa:* To look for any evidence of dacryocystitis, blepharitis, preseptal cellulitis, etc.
- *Conjunctiva:* Severity of inflammation, type of discharge.
- *Cornea:* Corneal haze may be seen in gonococcal keratitis. Infectious keratitis should also be ruled out.

Investigations

- Conjunctival scraping for Gram stain should be done in all cases of neonatal conjunctivitis. Following findings are expected:
  - Chemical conjunctivitis—neutrophils, occasional lymphocytes
  - Bacterial conjunctivitis—bacteria, neutrophils
  - Gonococcal conjunctivitis—neutrophils, gram-negative intracellular diplococci.
  - Chlamydial conjunctivitis—neutrophils, lymphocytes, plasma cells
  - Herpetic conjunctivitis—lymphocytes, plasma cells, multinucleate giant cells
- Giemsa stain cases of chlamydial conjunctivitis show basophilic intracytoplasmic inclusions in epithelial cells.
- A Papanicolaou-stained smear, which shows eosinophilic intranuclear inclusions in epithelial cells, is necessary for suspected HSV infection.
- Bacterial cultures on blood and chocolate agar are indicated in every case of neonatal conjunctivitis and are the standard investigations of choice.
- In cases of suspected chlamydial and HSV involvement, culture of epithelial cells is required; corneal epithelial cells in case of associated HSV keratitis may also be taken.
- Conjunctival scraping for polymerase chain reaction (PCR) assay is accepted as a useful test to detect chlamydia and HSV.
- In cases of HSV, dermal or mucosal vesicular lesions, if present, should be scraped for cytologic evaluation with Papanicolaou stain, viral culture, or immunologic testing.
- Apart from these, newer diagnostic techniques such as transcription-mediated amplification (TMA), enzyme-linked immunosorbent assay (ELISA), and direct fluorescent antibody (DFA) studies are useful for detecting chlamydia and HSV.
- Cervical cultures from the mother may also be obtained if indicated.

Management

Approach Considerations

- Preliminary treatment should be started on the basis of clinical picture and the findings on Gram, Giemsa, and Papanicolaou stains; pending culture reports should not cause a delay in starting the treatment.
- The mother should be examined for sexually transmitted disease as appropriate, and treated, if required, along with her sexual partner(s). It is important to remember that sexually transmitted organisms often coexist, and hence diagnostic and therapeutic modalities should be used accordingly.
- Infants with a sexually transmitted disease, such as gonorrhea or chlamydia, should also undergo evaluation for other sexually transmitted diseases, such as syphilis and HIV.
- Neonates with conjunctivitis are at risk for developing secondary infections such as pneumonia, meningitis, and septicemia, which may be life-threatening. Therefore, a consultation should always be made with a pediatrician or pediatric infectious specialist and patient be admitted for full work-up and treatment.
- In cases of chemical conjunctivitis, withholding the offending agent suffices, and no additional treatment is required. Symptoms usually subside in 24–48 hours. Tear substitutes may be used to ease any discomfort.
- Emphasis should be laid on maintaining ocular hygiene, with as frequent as hourly saline irrigation in cases of gonococcal conjunctivitis with copious discharge. Eye patching is not recommended.

Specific Treatment

- *Gonococcal conjunctivitis:* Due to emergence of widespread penicillin resistance, ceftriaxone has replaced intravenous aqueous penicillin G as the recommended treatment. A single intramuscular dose of ceftriaxone 125 mg is highly effective against neonatal gonococcal conjunctivitis and also simultaneously treats extraocular infection. Cefotaxime is also effective against resistant *N. gonorrhoeae* organisms, the recommended dose for neonatal ophthalmia being 25 mg/kg IV or IM every 8–12 hours for 7 days.
- *Chlamydial conjunctivitis:* The treatment of choice for neonatal chlamydial conjunctivitis is oral erythromycin ethylsuccinate suspension, 50 mg/kg/day in three or four divided doses for 14 days. Topical erythromycin ointment, although clinically effective in conjunctivitis, plays only an adjunctive role as it does not eradicate nasopharyngeal colonization, which may be present in 50% or more infants with neonatal chlamydial conjunctivitis. Azithromycin suspension 20 mg/kg either as a single dose or once daily for 3 days is an alternative regimen. It is also important to treat the caregivers with *C. trachomatis* infection with oral doxycycline for 7 days or with a single dose of azithromycin.
- *HSV conjunctivitis:* All infections caused by herpes simplex in the neonatal period should be treated with systemic acyclovir or vidarabine. In addition, topical antivirals should be used in infants with HSV keratoconjunctivitis. Trifluorothymidine 1% solution topically every 2 hours for 7 days and no longer than 21 days, adenine arabinoside 3% ointment or acyclovir 5% ointment given five times daily are the various options. Neonates with HSV keratitis may also be treated with topical cycloplegic agents for the relief of ciliary spasm. Topical corticosteroids should be avoided in neonatal or primary HSV keratoconjunctivitis.
- *Other bacterial conjunctivitis:* Tetracycline 1% or erythromycin 0.5% ointment every 4 hours for 7 days is effective against Gram-positive cocci. *Methicillin-resistant staphylococcus aureus* (MRSA) neonatal conjunctivitis may be treated with bacitracin 500 IU/g ointment, chloramphenicol 1% ointment, or vancomycin 5–31 mg/mL depending upon bacterial sensitivity. Tobramycin 0.3% or ciprofloxacin 0.3% ointment every 4 hours for 7 days is effective against gram-negative bacilli.
- *Fungal conjunctivitis:* Natamycin 5% drops hourly for 10–14 days, or flucytosine 1% drops hourly for 10–14 days are recommended.

Prophylaxis

Ocular prophylaxis is largely aimed at preventing infected genital secretions of the mother from contaminating the neonates eyes at birth. Antenatal screening in third trimester of pregnancy to rule out herpetic, chlamydial, or gonococcal infection is critical. Delivery by elective cesarean section may be considered in cases of active herpes lesions at delivery.

Pharmacological prophylaxis has largely shifted from 2% silver nitrate drops to 2.5% povidone iodine, 1% tetracycline ointment, or 0.5% erythromycin ointment. Povidone iodine has been shown to be equal efficacy as compared to the other agents, with an added advantage of broad spectrum of action against all bacteria, fungi, chlamydia, and viruses.

Complications and Prognosis

Ocular complications of neonatal conjunctivitis range from thickened palpebral conjunctiva, pseudomembrane formation, peripheral pannus formation, corneal edema, and opacity to corneal perforation and staphyloma formation. Untreated cases may even progress to endophthalmitis and blindness.

Systemic complications of chlamydia conjunctivitis include pneumonitis (10–20% cases), otitis, and pharyngeal, and rectal colonization, while that of gonococcal conjunctivitis include arthritis, meningitis, anorectal infection, septicemia, and death.

Prognosis is generally considered to be good in cases that are diagnosed early and prompt medical therapy is initiated. Most cases of infectious conjunctivitis respond well to appropriate treatment; however, morbidity and mortality increases due to systemic involvement may require hospitalization and intensive care.

Key Points

- Development of ophthalmia neonatorum can be prevented by reducing the prevalence of sexually transmitted diseases and ensuring good antenatal and perinatal care.
- Risk of complications can be minimized with prompt diagnosis and appropriate antibiotic therapy.
- Both the pediatrician and ophthalmologist should be meticulously involved in the treatment.

Reference

1. Holland EJ, Brilakis HS, Schwartz GS. Herpes simplex keratitis. In: Krachmer JH, Mannis MJ, Holland EJ (Eds). Cornea, 2nd edition. St Louis: Mosby; 2004. pp. 1043-74.

2. Lindquist Thomas D. Chapter 46 – Ophthalmia Neonatorum. In: Cornea; Volume 1 - Fundamentals and Medical Aspects of Cornea and External Disease. 3rd ed. USA: Elsevier; 2011. p. 1222–34.
3. Ophthalmia neonatoum. BCSC series: Pediatric Ophthalmology and Strabismus. American Academy of Ophthalmology; 2017.
4. Loto O, Gharaibeh A, Mezer E, Stankovic B, Isenberg S, Wygnanski-Jaffe T. Ophthalmia neonatorum treatment and prophylaxis: IPOSC global study. Graefes Arch Clin Exp Ophthalmol. 2016;254(3):577-82.
5. Mohile M, Deorari AK, Satpathy G, Sharma A, Singh M. Microbiological study of neonatal conjunctivitis with special reference to Chlamydia trachomatis. Indian J Ophthalmol. 2002;50(4):295-9.

8.4 Corneal Infection and Inflammatory Disorders

Deepali Singhal, Pranita Sahay, Ananya Parampalli Ravindra, Siddhi Goel, Ritika Mukhija, Saumya Yadav, Alisha Kishore, Aafreen Bari, Ritu Nagpal

 1. Describe the etiology, clinical features, approach, and management of bacterial keratitis.

Introduction

An ulcer is any discontinuity of an epithelial surface. A corneal ulcer is defined as an epithelial defect with superficial tissue loss. It is also associated with variable degree of inflammation. An infective etiology usually presents with infiltrates in the stroma. Microbiological evidence remains the mainstay for confirmation of an infective etiology. Bacteria is the most common cause of infectious keratitis.

Etiology

The onset of keratitis depends on the presence of risk factors, virulence of the organism, and also the immune status of the patient. The various risk factors include:
- Trauma with vegetable matter, foreign body, and ocular medications
- Recent surgery
- Contact lens use—*Pseudomonas* being the most common organism
- Ocular surface disorder—dry eye, burns, Stevens–Johnson syndrome
- Tear film dysfunction
- History of topical steroids and antifungal drugs
- *Immunocompromised state:* Diabetes and human immunodeficiency virus (HIV)

The bacterial organism can be either gram-positive or gram-negative. Gram-positive bacteria have a thicker peptidoglycan layer compared to gram-negative. The most common organism identified is gram-positive bacteria which includes *Staphylococcus*. In India, the most common bacteria include *Staphylococcus epidermidis* and *Streptococcus*.

Clinical Features

Symptoms: A patient with bacterial keratitis will present with the general symptoms of:
- Decreased visual acuity
- Pain
- Photophobia
- Redness
- Discharge

Signs:
- Precorneal tear film has numerous cells and debris, especially in a case of active infection.
- Associated conjunctivitis is seen in case of *Gonococcal, Pneumococcal,* and *Hemophilus* infection
- Chemosis
- Conjunctival pseudomembrane
- Conjunctival papillae
- Epithelial defect

The intact cornea can be infected and invaded by certain organisms and include:
- *Neisseria*
- *Corynebacterium*

- *Haemophilus*
- *Shigella*
- *Listeria*

Specific characteristics of organisms are given here.
- *Staphylococcus:* Well defined, gray-white infiltrates and sometimes stromal abscess
- *Streptococcus:* Can be either purulent or crystalline. Purulent ulcer generally presents with sudden onset, fulminant course. Severe anterior chamber reaction with hypopyon formation. Crystalline keratopathy has an indolent course.
- *Pneumococcus:* History of trauma is present. They are generally associated with dacryocystitis. Start from the site of trauma and spread toward the center. They are associated with severe anterior chamber reaction and hypopyon formation. Fibrin deposition is seen on the endothelial side. A deep stromal abscess can be formed.
- *Pseudomonas:* Rapidly progressive, necrotic infiltrate. Profuse mucopurulent discharge with hypopyon. Generally presents with history of contact lens use
- *Moraxella:* In patients with ocular surface disorders and in immunocompromised patients. Indolent course and is generally located in the inferior part of the cornea.

Differential Diagnosis

See **Table 1**.

TABLE 1: Differential diagnosis of bacterial keratitis.

Diagnosis	Features
Fungal keratitis	• History of trauma with vegetable matter, contact lens use • Infiltrates have feathery borders and presence of satellite lesions
Acanthamoeba keratitis	• Extremely painful and is associated with perineural invasion • History of contact lens use, especially wearing of contact lens while swimming • In the early stages, it resembles herpetic keratitis and later becomes ring-shaped
Herpetic keratitis	• Associated skin lesions • Corneal epithelial dendrites • History of recurrent unilateral infection or known case of ocular herpes • Always rule out superadded bacterial infection
Staphylococcal hypersensitivity	• Peripheral corneal infiltrates with an overlying epithelial defect with clear space between the infiltrate and the limbus • Minimal anterior chamber reaction and localized conjunctival injection
Sterile corneal thinning and ulcers	• Minimal discharge, peripheral stromal infiltration with vascularization • Cultures are negative
Atypical mycobacteria	• Following trauma and ocular surgery (especially refractive surgeries) • Acid-fast bacillus smear • Löwenstein–Jensen media for at least 8 weeks
Residual corneal foreign body or rust ring	• History of foreign body injury • Corneal stromal inflammation, edema, and sterile infiltrate • Always rule out any superadded infection

Work-up

History:
- Onset, progression, and duration of all the symptoms
- Rule out all the predisposing risk factors:
  - *Contact lens use:*
    - Daily/extended wear
    - Conventional/frequent replacement/single use
    - Lens solutions used
    - Recent change in routine
    - Exposure of water with the lenses (swimming)
  - Trauma with vegetable matter, foreign body, and ocular medications
  - *Ocular surface disorder:* Dry eye, burns, and Stevens-Johnson syndrome

- Tear film dysfunction
- History of topical steroids and antifungal drugs
- *Immunocompromised state:* Diabetes and HIV
- *Occupation:* Farmers and gardeners (fungal)

Examination:
- *Visual acuity:* Decreased, especially if located in the center of the cornea or associated with hypopyon.
- *Eyelid:* Examine for any eyelid condition such as trichiasis, entropion, and ectropion to identify predisposing condition leading to keratitis.
- *Lacrimal sac:* Examine for dacryocystitis and canaliculitis (*Actinomyces* keratitis)
- *Conjunctiva:* Examine for—
  - Any papillae, follicles in case of vernal keratoconjunctivitis and atopic conjunctivitis
  - Discharge
  - Keratinization, cicatrization, poor ocular surface, dry eye disease, and limbal stem cell deficiency
  - Membrane, pseudomembrane, and foreign body
- *Cornea:*
  - *Slit lamp:*
    - *Location:* Gives an idea about the etiology and prognosis
      - Central—*Staphylococcus aureus, Pseudomonas, Fusarium*
      - Paracentral—*Staphylococcus aureus, Pseudomonas, Fusarium*
      - Peripheral—Coagulase negative *Staphylococcus aureus, Mycobacterium tuberculosis, herpes simplex*
      - Superior—Ulcer associated with shield ulcer [vernal keratoconjunctivitis (VKC)] or foreign body
      - Inferior—exposure keratopathy
    - *Size:* Measure the size along the two largest meridians. It can be measured with the micrometer in the slit lamp. The size of infiltrate and epithelial defect should be measured separately. The epithelial defect should be always measured after staining with fluorescein and looking under the cobalt blue filter.
    - *Shape:*
      - Dendritic shape—viral keratitis
      - Ring-shaped ulcer—*Acanthamoeba, Staphylococcus*
      - Oval—neurotrophic ulcer
    - *Margins of ulcer:* Margin can be—
      - Well defined—seen in healing infectious ulcer or sterile ulcer
      - Punched out—neurotrophic ulcer
      - Indistinct—seen in cases of progressive ulcer
      - Feathery—fungal corneal ulcer
      - Overhanging—Mooren's ulcer
    - *Base:* Infective is filled with necrotic slough. A dry looking ulcer is suggestive of fungal ulcer.
    - *Depth:* It is measured with help of a slit lamp. If more than 50% of the depth is involved, then systemic antibiotics should be started.
    - *Surrounding cornea:* Presence of any corneal scars or satellite lesions
    - *Vascularization:* Superficial or deep. It is a sign of healing.
- *Corneal sensations:* It is measured with the help of a cotton wisp or esthesiometer (Cochet–Bonnet). Proper documentation of the corneal ulcer should be done using clinical photographs or detailed schematic drawings. This is necessary for monitoring of the corneal ulcer on treatment.
- *Sclera:* Involvement of the sclera should be always examined as in such cases systemic antibiotics have to be added. Scleral involvement is generally seen in cases of acanthamoeba keratitis and immunological disorders.
- *Anterior chamber:* Examine the anterior chamber for the presence of any inflammatory reaction. Look for cells and flare if visible. Also, it is important to look for the presence of hypopyon. If present, the height should always be measured with the help of a micrometer on the slit lamp. This helps in monitoring and progression of the disease. Also, check for the mobility of hypopyon by asking the patient to lie supine for 10 minutes. Mobile hypopyon is found in a bacterial ulcer whereas fixed is found in fungal ulcer.
- *Iris:* Examine for the presence of synechiae, any new vessel formation, and in case of perforation for uveal tissue prolapsed.
- *Pupil:* In case of severe inflammation, the pupil can be atonic.

- *Intraocular pressure (IOP):* It should be always measured as in case of perforation, hypotony can occur. Also, many cases are associated with secondary glaucoma due to posterior synechiae.
- *Posterior segment:* Always look for any abnormality in the posterior segment with the help of indirect ophthalmoscopy. If not visible, then an ultrasonography should be done.
- *Fellow eye:* It should be always examined, especially when immunological disorder is suspected.

Investigations

Microbiological diagnosis:
- It remains the mainstay of diagnosis of microbial keratitis.
- Sample should be taken before starting the antimicrobial therapy.
- Samples needed for diagnosis include:
  - Corneal scraping
  - Contact lens, case, solution—in the case of contact lens use
  - Anterior chamber paracentesis—hypopyon and deep stromal ulceration
- *Corneal scraping:*
  - It is dinstruments used include a 26-gauge needle, hypodermic needle, and Bard–Parker blade No. 15.
  - The eyelids are separated using an eyelid speculum. Under topical anesthesia (0.5% proparacaine hydrochloride) and after removing mucus debris, sample is taken from the ulcer base and margins with the help of slit lamp.
  - Multiple samples are taken for smear and culture. It should be done carefully in case of descemetocele and deep keratitis.
  - Two slides for gram stain and 10-20% potassium hydroxide (KOH). Acid-fast stain is used when suspecting mycobacteria.
  - *Culture and sensitivity media:*
    - Peptone water and glucose broth are used for bacterial culture which is subcultured in blood agar.
    - Sabaroud's dextrose agar (SDA) is used for fungal culture.
    - Other culture media are used when suspecting some specific organism and include—chocolate agar for *Neisseria, Haemophilus, Moraxella*; cooked meat broth for anaerobic bacteria; Lowenstein-Jensen media for mycobacteria; and Thayer-Martin blood agar for *Neisseria.*
  - *Corneal specimens should be held for:*
    - 7 days for aerobic culture
    - 7–14 days for anaerobic culture
    - 4–6 weeks for mycobacterial and anaerobic culture before being reported as no growth
- Positive culture rates vary from 40 to 73%. Culture reports should always be correlated with clinical scenario.
- When the culture results are negative, antibiotic treatment can be stopped for 24 hours. Rescraping is done following that and culture is repeated.

Corneal biopsy: It is indicated in the following cases:
- Clinically infectious keratitis is suspected but the cultures are negative which have been repeated two times.
- No response to treatment
- Deep fungal keratitis and intrastromal abscess.

Partial thickness trephination is done using a trephine of appropriate size. Care should be taken that an adequate sample is taken. In case of midstromal keratitis, a sample beneath the lamellar flap can be taken.

Anterior chamber paracentesis: This procedure is not routinely done. It is indicated only when a clinically fungal infection is suspected but it comes negative on culture and smear.

Confocal microscopy: It is a noninvasive method for the diagnosis of bacterial keratitis. It has been used for the diagnosis of cysts of Acanthamoeba and fungal hyphae. Besides, it can detect the presence of inflammatory cells and keratocyte aggregation. It is a useful screening tool for bacterial and fungal keratitis but confirmation requires culture. Its usefulness lies in early institution of specific therapy when culture reports are still awaited, correlation with clinical diagnosis, and progress and response to ongoing therapy through inflammatory cell monitoring.

Newer modern techniques: These include immunohistochemistry, fluorescent microscopy, enzyme immunoassays, polymerase chain reaction, and molecular biology. With the help of these newer techniques, the diagnosis can be made in 1–6 hours.

Ultrasonography: It is important for the evaluation of the posterior segment when it is not visible with the help of indirect ophthalmoscopy.

Systemic work-up: Fasting/random blood sugar level should be done in all patients to rule out diabetes.

Management (Flowchart 1)

Medical Management

Antimicrobial therapy:
- For ulcers which are small in size (<3 mm) and in the periphery, monotherapy can be started. Fluoroquinolone is used for small ulcers instead of fortified drops as they have to be prepared, are more toxic, have a shelf life of about 1 week, and are more expensive. Fluoroquinolones are equally effective as fortified drops in small ulcers.
- In the case of large ulcers, an empirical antibiotic therapy is started to cover both gram-positive and gram-negative in the form of:
  - Fortified tobramycin 1.3% for gram-negative and fortified cefazoline 5 or 10% for gram-positive organism, or
  - Fluroquinolone moxifloxacin 0.5% or gatifloxacin 0.3% for gram-positive and tobramycin 1.3% for gram-negative organism
- Initially, a loading dose of one drop every 5 minutes is administered for the first 30 minutes. This is followed by one drop every 30 minutes for 24 hours. Then, the medication is tapered according to the response.
- The clinical response should be the mainstay for the monitoring of the therapy. But in the case of nonhealing ulcers, in vitro sensitivity is important. Before considering a change in therapy, certain factors such as poor compliance and debris covering the site of infection can result in poor penetration of the drug, and should be ruled out.
- Favorable signs which suggest a good response to therapy include:
  - Improvement in symptoms
  - Reduced activity at the margins of the ulcer

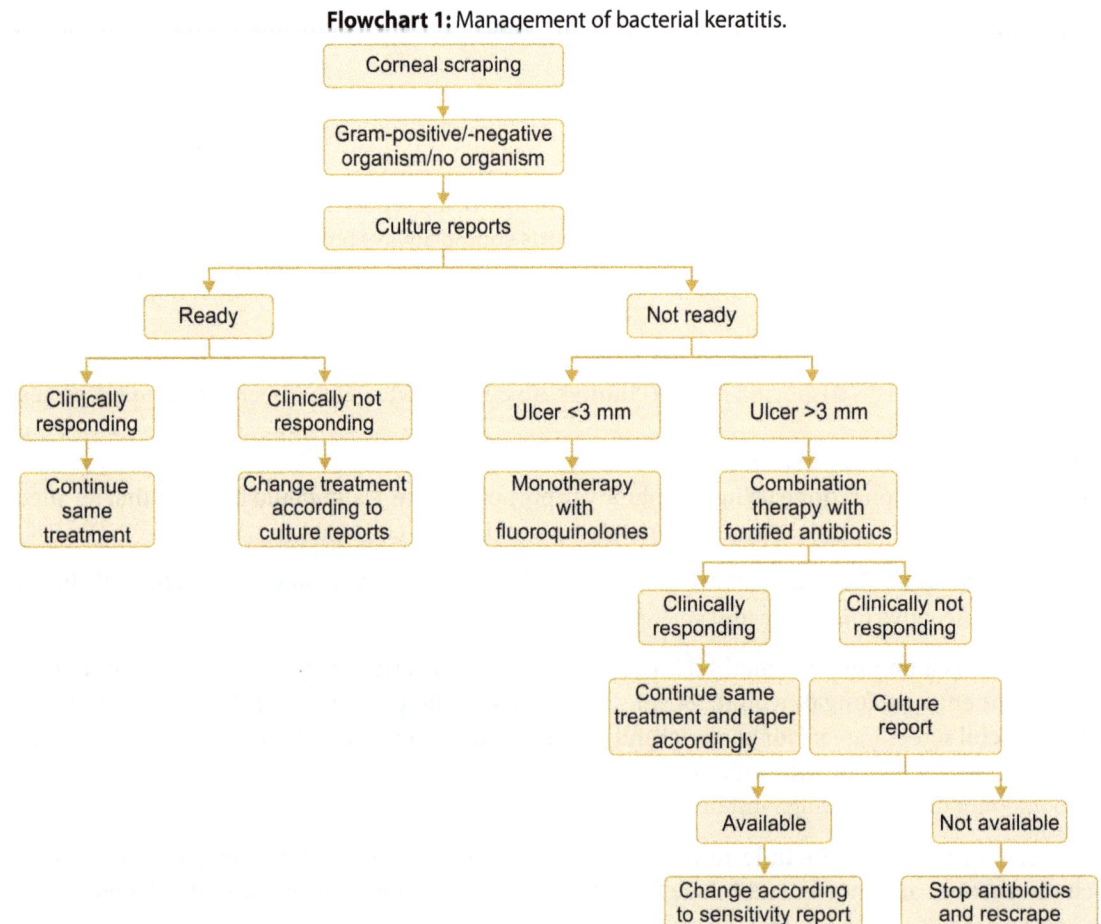

Flowchart 1: Management of bacterial keratitis.

- Healing of the epithelial defect
- Decrease in infiltration
- Reduction in hypopyon and anterior chamber reaction
- Vascularization.

Cycloplegic agents: Homatropine bromide 2% is started four times in a day to prevent the formation of posterior synechiae and to relieve pain due to ciliary body spasm.

Antiglaucoma drugs: To be started whenever keratitis is associated with raised IOP. Beta-blockers or a combination of beta-blocker with alpha-adrenergic agonist is generally used initially to control the IOP.

Tear drop supplements: To maintain the ocular surface, it is given in all cases of bacterial keratitis.

Topical corticosteroids: It is to be given only after starting the antimicrobial therapy for 24 hours in case of severe inflammatory reaction. According to the Steroids in Cornea Ulcer Trial (SCUT), adjunctive steroid may be associated with improved long-term clinical outcome in bacterial keratitis not caused by *Nocardia*. However, the final decision of whether to use steroid will depend upon the treating ophthalmologist and the case.

Systemic antibiotics: These are to be included in case of perforated ulcer, post-traumatic injury, scleral or posterior segment involvement, and highly virulent organisms. Oral ciprofloxacin 500 mg bd is given.

Surgical Management

The indications for surgical intervention include:
- Impending corneal perforation
- Perforated ulcer
- To decrease bacterial load in case of nonhealing ulcer.

The various surgical interventions include the following:

Tissue adhesives: It is helpful in case of small perforation (size up to 3 mm). Cyanoacrylate glue is used along with bandage contact lens. Cyanoacrylate provides support and, in addition, it has also got the bacteriostatic property for gram-positive organism. All the necrotic debris should be removed from the ulcer base before applying the tissue adhesive. It is placed until it loosens on its own or until any further intervention is done.

Patch graft: The following are the types of graft that can be done:
- *Tectonic patch graft:* For corneal perforation of size up to 3–5 mm, a small patch of corneal graft is used.
- *Multilayered amniotic membrane graft:* This is also done in case of small corneal perforation and severe thinning.
- *Tenon's patch graft:* This is done in case of peripheral corneal ulcer which heals by the fibroblastic proliferation.

Therapeutic penetrating keratoplasty: A full-thickness corneal graft is done in case of failure of medical therapy, impending or perforated ulcer, nonhealing corneal ulcer, large ulcer threatening to involve limbus and sclera, and sometimes to reduce the infective load in large and deep ulcer. In an acutely infected eye, the results of grafting are generally poor. A 0.5 mm margin of clear cornea should be removed to prevent the recurrence of infection in the graft. Results are better with donor graft size less than 8 mm. With larger grafts, there is a high risk of graft rejection and post-keratoplasty glaucoma.

Collagen cross-linking: This has been tried in case of refractory keratitis. It has direct bactericidal activity. Also, the cornea becomes more resistant to further damage by the organisms.

Conjunctival flap: It is done to stabilize the epithelial surface in case of persistent epithelial defect. In the late stage of corneal ulcer when the prognosis is very poor, the whole cornea can be covered with the conjunctiva which is known as Gundersen's flap.

References

1. Krachmer JH, Mannis MJ, Holland EJ. Cornea, 2nd edition, Volume 1. Philadelphia: Elsevier, Mosby; 2005. p. 955.
2. Vajpayee RB, Namrata S. Corneal ulcers: diagnosis and management, 1st edition. New Delhi: Jaypee Brothers Medical Publishers; 2008.
3. Gupta N, Tandon R. Investigative modalities in infectious keratitis. Indian J Ophthalmol. 2008;56(3):209-13.
4. Maharana PK, Namrata S, Kumar A. Ophthalmology clinics for postgraduates, 1st edition. New Delhi: Jaypee Brothers Medical Publishers; 2017.

2. A 30-year-old female got up at night with severe pain and watering in left eye. She gave a history of a nail injury to her eye 1 year back. How would you approach and manage such a case? or Describe the different types of recurrent corneal erosions. Give an outline of their treatment.

In a 30-year-old female with sudden onset of ocular pain and watering at night with past history of injury to the eye, the most likely diagnosis would be recurrent corneal erosions (RCEs).

A systematic approach to such a case is as described here.

History

A thorough history should include:
- *Symptoms:*
  - *Pain:* Most common, most bothersome clinical feature, that makes the patient seek medical help. Typically, sudden onset pain after the first awakening [due to rapid eye movement (REM) during early morning and shearing lid movement after nocturnal dryness], which can persist for several minutes to days.
  - *Associated symptoms:* Redness, watering, photophobia, and blurred vision
- *Past history:*
  - History of similar episodes in the past, with inciting and relieving factors
  - History of ocular trauma (corneal abrasions)
  - History of ocular surgeries/procedures, usage of bandage contact lenses
  - Systemic illnesses such as diabetes mellitus, juvenile X-linked Alport syndrome [which are secondary causes of recurrent corneal erosion syndrome (RCES)].
- Family history of similar complaints/diagnosed cases of epithelial dystrophies/RCES in the family.

Examination

The whole eye should be examined, with specific attention to corneal findings. The fellow eye should also be examined in great detail, to look for evidence of corneal dystrophies.
- *Conjunctiva:* Variable congestion present
- *Cornea:* Loose irregular (ragged) epithelium, most often in inferior, paracentral cornea. Touching the tip of a cellulose sponge to a topically anesthetized cornea causing it to be pushed into folds easily (cellulose sponge test) suggests loose adherence, denuded epithelium can be stained with vital dyes. Features of vital dyes are enumerated in **Table 1**.
- Depending upon size, erosions may be microform [(smaller, i.e., <1 mm, less severe, last only for hours, occur almost every few days and are commonly seen in association with anterior corneal dystrophies, most commonly in epithelial basement membrane dystrophy (EBMD)] or macroform [larger epithelial breaks with surrounding loosely adherent epithelium, persist longer (1–21 days), have few recurrences and most commonly seen following trauma]. Corneal epithelial microcysts, stromal infiltrates, and opacities may be present.
- Scars suggestive of previous ocular trauma or surgery may be seen.
- Since a plethora of etiologies can primarily or secondarily cause RCES, a thorough biomicroscopic examination should be performed to pinpoint the diagnosis. The root causes leading to RCES are enlisted in **Table 2**.

Differential Diagnosis of Recurrent Corneal Erosion Syndrome

- Herpes simplex viral keratitis
- Conjunctival foreign body

TABLE 1: Vital dyes and their characteristics.

Fluorescein stain	*Rose Bengal stain*	*Lissamine Green stain*
• Stains cornea to greater degree than conjunctiva • Exposure zone punctate or blotchy fluorescein staining observed in dry eye	• Performed using saline moistened 1% solution • Stains devitalized epithelial cells • More sensitive for staining the conjunctiva • Causes severe irritation, warranting the use of topical anesthetic before instillation	• Similar to Rose Bengal in staining characteristics • Least irritating dye • Better for visualization of the conjunctiva and the lid margins

TABLE 2: Etiology of recurrent corneal erosion syndrome.

Primary (Intrinsic defect present in the epithelial basement membrane)	• Epithelial basement membrane dystrophy (19–29%)—Cogan's microcystic (map-dot-finger) • Dystrophy involving Bowman's layer—Reis–Bucklers, Thiel–Behnke, lattice, and granular • Stromal dystrophy—macular dystrophy • Endothelial dystrophy—Fuch's dystrophy
Secondary (Acquired defect in epithelial basement membrane)	• Trauma is the most common cause which is seen in 45–64% cases. It may be caused by sharp, sudden abrading injury (finger nail, paper edge, tree branch), chemical, or thermal injury • Degeneration—band keratopathy and Salzmann's nodular degeneration • Infection—bacterial or viral keratitis • Eyelid abnormalities—entropion, ectropion, floppy eyelid, lagophthalmos, meibomian gland dysfunction, and blepharitis • Previous ocular surgery—LASIK, PRK (rare), cataract, and keratoplasty • Systemic causes—diabetes mellitus, epidermolysis bullosa, and juvenile X-linked Alport's syndrome • Miscellaneous—dry eyes, bullous keratopathy, idiopathic, and Munchausen syndrome

(LASER: laser assisted in situ keratomileusis; PRK: photorefractive keratectomy)

- Exposure keratopathy
- Neurotrophic keratitis
- Infectious keratitis
- Dry eye disease
- Self-inflicted corneal injury.

Investigations

Though the diagnosis is mainly clinical, investigations are performed to identify the primary cause, when diagnosis is doubtful, and prior to planning surgical management.
- *Corneal topography:* May show irregular astigmatism, corneal topographic lagoons (small, well-delineated areas of markedly reduced corneal dioptric power, i.e., >2D)
- *Anterior segment optical coherence tomography (ASOCT):* Useful in confirming the diagnosis, assessment of the structural changes occurring in eyes with EBMD, and differentiating acute from chronic RCES.
  - *Acute RCES:* ASOCT shows anterior stromal hyper-reflectivity, epithelial edema, and irregular breaks in the epithelium.
  - *Chronic RCES:* Absence of epithelial basement membrane, intraepithelial basement membrane or re-duplication of basement membrane, intraepithelial inclusions, and anterior stromal hyper-reflectivity may be seen.
- *Confocal microscopy:* Useful for supporting the diagnosis in doubtful cases. Shows deposits in basal corneal epithelial cells, microfolds in sub-basal nerve plexus, stromal scarring, streaks among the basal epithelial cells, damaged sub-basal nerves, altered morphology of the anterior stroma, and round brightly reflecting cells (suspected to be inflammatory cells) or cell nuclei within stroma.

Pathophysiology

Recurrent corneal erosions may be multifactorial, as shown in given flowchart:

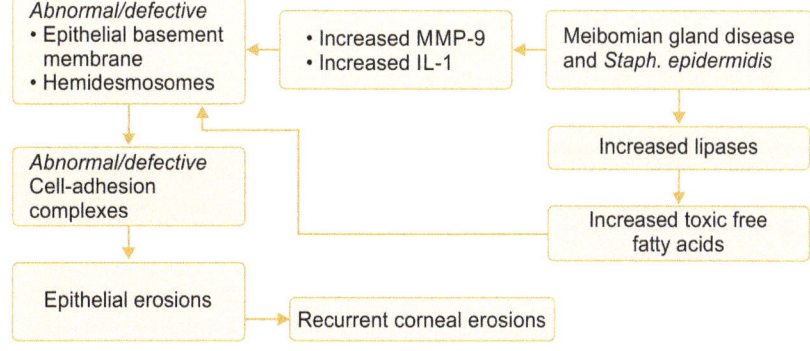

(IL-1: interleukin-1; MMP-9: matrix metalloproteinase-9)

Management of a Case of Recurrent Corneal Erosions

The primary goal is to hasten re-epithelialization and re-establishment of a competent basement membrane complex, while simultaneously providing adequate pain relief.

Nonsurgical Management

A patient presenting with RCES should be first managed medically. Medical management helps in the resolution of the epithelial defect, but may not prevent recurrences. On failure of the same, a multitude of noninvasive methods can be used. Different modalities of nonsurgical management are enumerated in **Table 3**.

Surgical Management

Surgical management should be reserved for failure of aggressive medical therapy. Different modalities of the same are described in **Table 4**.

Novel Approaches for RCES

These are modalities proposed by investigators which have shown success in small cohorts but lack adequate studies to show their benefit:
- Substance P-derived peptide (250 μg/mL) + Insulin-like growth factor (1 μg/mL) eye drops to promote re-epithelialization. Application of topical cocaine to cornea to facilitate epithelial debridement.
- Intramuscular botulinum toxin injection to reduce eye movements at night and prevent the development of erosions.

Complications

The following complications can occur in long run:
- Periodic recurrences
- Corneal scarring
- Superadded infections.

Clinical pearls:
- RCEs may present several days to years following trauma.
- Always examine the other eye for signs of corneal dystrophy.
- Erosions in RCES may be microform (commonly seen in association with anterior corneal dystrophies, most commonly in EBMD) or macroform (most commonly seen following trauma).
- Continue treatment for at least 6 weeks (formation and maturation of hemidesmosomes).

TABLE 3: Modalities of nonsurgical management of recurrent corneal erosion syndrome.

Episode	Medical management	Failure of medical management
Acute	• *Artificial tears (preservative-free) first line:* It promotes epithelial healing • *Night-time ointment:* It prevents nocturnal drying of ocular surface • *Broad-spectrum antibiotics (FQs, macrolides):* Given prophylactically, to prevent superadded infections • *Cycloplegics +/–, oral NSAIDs:* To relieve pain and ciliary spasm	Acute: • *Therapeutic soft BCL*—can be used for up to 6 weeks It relieves pain and provides a scaffold for healing
Chronic	In addition to the above-mentioned treatment, a chronic case also necessitates the use of: • *Hypertonic saline:* It promotes adhesion by transient osmotic gradient	Chronic: • *Punctal plugs (silicone/collagen):* They help in tear pooling • *Blood serum: (autogenic/allogenic/umbilical cord):* They provide growth factors and cytokines • *Topical steroids:* They decrease local inflammation • *MMP inhibitors* (oral tetracyclines; doxycycline 50 mg BD for 1–2 months; topical acetylcysteine 20%) ↓ MMP-9 → ↑collagen

(BCL: bandage contact lens; MMP: matrix metalloproteinase; NSAIDs: nonsteroidal anti-inflammatory drugs)

TABLE 4: Surgical line of management of a case of recurrent corneal erosion syndrome.

Surgical technique	Mechanism of action	Advantages	Disadvantages
1. Amniotic membrane graft (AMG)	Provides a protective barrier and growth factors to encourage epithelial regrowth and adhesion	• Good alternative to traditional BCL • Useful in acute episodes	• Difficult to procure • Expensive
2. *Epithelial debridement (ED):* Central 7–10 mm using cotton swab/cellulose sponge/blunt spatula/15 no. BP blade under topical anesthesia, followed by BCL placement	Hastens corneal epithelial turnover and normalizes surface epithelium	Simple, low cost, clinic procedure	• Limited efficacy in preventing recurrence • Not effective in dystrophies
3. *Diamond burr polishing:* 10–15 seconds of treatment with a diamond burr to smoothen Bowman's layer after ED	Removes abnormal basement membrane and provides a smooth surface for re-epithelialization, causes reactive fibrosis to allow scarring, and stronger epithelial adhesion and hence reduce recurrences	• Lowest rate of recurrence • Simple, low cost clinic procedure • Replicable	• Long recovery time • Corneal haze
4. *Alcohol delamination:* 50–75 μL 20% alcohol for 40 second: → peeling of epithelium into using a spatula, followed by thorough saline irrigation	Provides a smooth surface for re-epithelialization	• Bowman's layer is not disrupted • Epithelial sheet can be sent for histopathological examination	• Toxicity • OT procedure • Few reports
5. *Phototherapeutic keratectomy (PTK):* Excimer laser ablation of Bowman's layer and 5–7 μm of stroma	Smoothens the outer layer of cornea to a precise depth to encourage re-epithelialization	• Low recurrence rate • Accurate • Can be combined with PRK • Suitable for dystrophies	• Cost • OT procedure • Induced astigmatism/hyperopia • Corneal haze
6. *Anterior stromal puncture (ASP):* A bent 23–25-gauge needle is used to create multiple partial depth punctures (approximately 10–20% stromal depth or 0.1 mm) in the cornea, 0.5–1 mm apart Modifications of ASP: ASP by Nd:YAG laser (0.2–0.4 mJ/shot) ASOCT guided ASP	Induction of extracellular matrix proteins within the puncture sites and in the reactive subepithelial pannus adjacent to the puncture site, which promotes attachment of epithelial cells to the underlying stroma	• Simple, low cost • Clinic procedure • Minimal discomfort	• Scarring • Blurred vision • Glare • Risk of perforation • Failure to prevent recurrences

(ASOCT: anterior segment optical coherence tomography; BCL: bandage contact lens; Nd:YAG: neodymium-doped yttrium aluminum garnet; PRK: photorefractive keratectomy)

 3. Discuss presentation, pathogenesis, and management of Mooren's ulcer.

Introduction

Mooren's ulcer, otherwise called ulcer rodens or chronic serpiginous ulcer of cornea, is an idiopathic painful, relentless, chronic ulcerative keratitis that begins peripherally and progresses circumferentially and centrally. It is a relatively rare disorder, most commonly reported from Central and South Africa, China, and Asia.

Presentation

History

- A patient with Mooren's ulcer typically presents with the following symptoms:
  - *Pain:* Hallmark of Mooren's ulcer, incapacitating, out of proportion to the inflammation.
  - Associated redness, tearing, and photophobia are usually present.
  - *Reduced visual acuity:* Due to iritis/central corneal involvement/irregular astigmatism due to peripheral thinning and scarring.

- *Past history:* History of ocular trauma, infections, procedures or surgeries, hepatitis-C (which are associated risk factors of Mooren's ulcer).
- Systemic illnesses such as tuberculosis, syphilis, varicella zoster, sarcoidosis, collagen vascular diseases, rheumatoid arthritis, granulomatosis with polyangiitis, polyarteritis nodosa, systemic lupus erythematosus (since these are systemic diseases leading to peripheral corneal thinning and ulceration).
- *Personal history:* Including history of sexually transmitted diseases and IV drug abuse.

Examination

Following findings may be seen:
- *Eyelids:* Lid edema with associated mechanical ptosis, blepharophimosis
- *Conjunctiva:* Inflamed, hyperemia may be seen, ciliary congestion, especially at the area adjacent to the ulcer
- *Cornea:* In early stages, crescent-shaped gray-white infiltrates are seen in the peripheral cornea, concentric to the limbus. With disease progression, epithelial breakdown and stromal melting may be seen, and in long-standing cases, a chronic crescent-shaped peripheral ulcer, with undermined, overhanging edges is usually present. In advanced cases, most of the cornea is lost, leaving behind a central island of cloudy cornea surrounded by an area of grossly thinned, scarred, and vascularized tissue. Some patients may also present with a perforation.
- *Sclera:* Adjacent scleral hyperemia is seen, may be ulcerated in advanced cases.
- *Anterior chamber (AC):* Hypopyon may be seen if secondarily infected.
- *Iris:* Iritis may be present, variable degree of iris tissue prolapse may be noted in corneal melt and perforation.
- *Lens:* Cataract can occur secondary to persistent inflammation, long-term use of corticosteroids, and after surgical interventions.
- *Fundus:* Clinical assessment may not be possible in most cases, due to which ultrasonography may be performed, but when visible, a good fundus evaluation is imperative to rule out other causes.

Classification of Mooren's Ulcer

- According to Wood and Kaufman, there are two types:
    1. *Limited (typical or benign):* Unilateral entity with mild-moderate symptoms, affecting elderly responding to medical and surgical treatment.
    2. *Progressive (atypical or malignant):* Bilateral in 75% cases affecting young individuals with severe pain and poor response to therapy. Usually, bilateral progressive form occurs in older individuals.
- Watson and colleagues classified the disease based on clinical presentation and anterior segment fluorescein angiographic findings as shown in **Table 5**.

TABLE 5: Watson's classification of Mooren's ulcer.

Characteristics	Unilateral MU	Bilateral aggressive MU	Bilateral indolent MU
Age	Old	Young	Middle-aged or old
Gender	Usually female	Male	Male and female
Race	Usually white	Usually African/Indian/Chinese	Usually Indian
Triggering factor	Minor trauma/infection	Trauma/infection	• Chronic systemic infection • Minor ocular trauma or infection
Laterality	Unilateral	Bilateral	Bilateral
Pain	Excruciating	Painful	Less
Progression	Rapid	Slow	Slow
Anterior segment angiography	Vaso-obliteration of superficial vascular networks with leakage from large vessels. Intense deep leakage. Vascularization of ulcer, from superficial and deep vessels	Conjunctival and episcleral networks normal. Intense deep leakage. Ulcer vascularized from deep vessels	• Superficial networks normal • Vasodilation of deep network • Ulcer vascularized from deep vessels
Treatment	Unsatisfactory	Immunosuppression	Local immunosuppressive therapy + supportive general treatment
Keratoplasty	Recurrence common	Recurrence common	Recurrence rare
Perforation	Very rare	Can occur	Rare

TABLE 6: Causes of peripheral thinning and ulceration.

Ocular	Bacterial	• *Staphylococcus* • *Gonococcus* • *Moraxella* • *Hemophilus* • *Streptococcus*
	Viral	• Herpes simplex • Herpes zoster
	• Amebic • Fungal	*Acanthamoeba*
	Traumatic	Chemical, thermal, radiation burn
	Local, autoimmune	Allograft reaction
	Neurologic	Neurotrophic keratitis
Systemic	Autoimmune vasculitic diseases	• Rheumatoid arthritis • Wegener's granulomatosis • Relapsing polychondritis • Systemic lupus erythematosus • Polyarteritis nodosa • Sjögren's syndrome
	Dermatological disorders	• Acne rosacea • Cicatricial pemphigoid • Stevens–Johnson syndrome
	Inflammatory bowel disease	
	Malignancy	
	Bacterial	Tuberculosis, syphilis, gonorrhea, borreliosis, bacillary dysentery
	Viral	Varicella zoster, acquired immune deficiency syndrome, hepatitis

Differential Diagnosis of Mooren's Ulcer

Mooren's ulcer is a diagnosis of exclusion. All causes of peripheral ulcerative keratitis must be ruled out before diagnosing a Mooren's ulcer. Ocular and systemic causes of the same are enumerated in **Table 6**.

Investigations

A battery of investigations are performed mainly to rule out systemic causes of peripheral ulcerative keratitis and are as follows:
- *Laboratory studies:* Complete blood counts, erythrocyte sedimentation rate, rheumatoid factor, antinuclear antibody, antineutrophil cytoplasmic antibodies, liver enzymes, fluorescent treponemal antibody absorption test, hepatitis C antigen, urine, and stool examination.
- *Radiological examination:* X-ray examination of chest and sacroiliac joint

Pathogenesis

It still remains uncertain, with autoimmunity being the most likely cause due to the following evidence:
- Abnormal function of T-suppressor cells
- Increased level of IgA
- Increased concentration of plasma cells and lymphocytes in the conjunctiva adjacent to the ulcerated areas
- Increased $CD4^+:CD8^+$ and $B7-2^+:APC$ ratios and increased vascular cell adhesion molecule 1, very late antigen 4, and intercellular adhesion molecule 1 in the vascular endothelium of conjunctival vessels
- Tissue-fixed immunoglobulins and complement in the conjunctival epithelium and peripheral cornea.

Management

Aim of the treatment is to promote reepithelialization, prevent progression by controlling inflammation, and alleviate pain. Though a number of treatment modalities have been described, the best way to go about it would be to titrate the treatment according to the requirement of the affected eye, for which a stepwise approach has been given as follows:

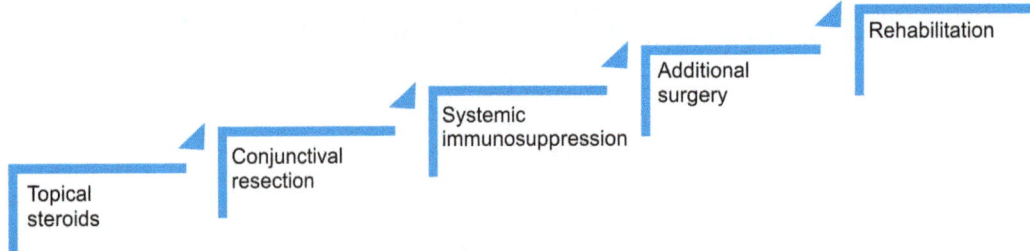

- *Local immunosuppression:*
  - *Topical steroids:*
    - These are used aggressively initially, along with low frequency topical prophylactic antibiotics and cycloplegic medications. Steroid therapy is tapered gradually over months with signs of corneal reepithelialization and halting of stromal melt. However, the patient should be closely monitored for signs of cataract and increase in intraocular pressure (IOP).
    - Topical cyclosporine (up to 2%) or tacrolimus 0.1% ointment can be used as steroid-sparing agents as well as in refractory cases, but their onset of action is slow. Subconjunctival interferon α-2b in cases of hepatitis-C can be effective. Topical tetracycline, medroxyprogesterone, and acetylcysteine have anticollagenolytic properties.
- *Conjunctival resection:*
  - If there is progression in spite of topical steroids, conjunctival resection can be done along with removal of necrotic tissue. This removes involved conjunctiva and blocks collagenase, inflammatory cells, and cytokines from reaching the cornea by acting as a biological barrier.
  - In this procedure, conjunctiva adjacent to the corneal ulcer is resected 4 mm from the limbus and 2 clock hours on either side.
- *Systemic immunosuppressives:* In nonresponsive, bilateral, or cases with advanced disease on presentation can be treated with oral prednisolone (1–1.5 mg/kg body) or cyclophosphamide (2 mg/kg/day), methotrexate (7.5–15 mg once weekly), azathioprine (2 mg/kg/day), and cyclosporine (5–10 mg/kg/day). Intravenous methylprednisolone and cyclophosphamide can be given in relentless progression.
- *Additional surgical procedure:*
  - *Keratoepithelioplasty:* A donor corneal lenticule is sutured onto the scleral bed so as to form a physical barrier against conjunctival regrowth and further melting.
  - *Lamellar keratectomy:* Residual central island in advanced disease is dissected to remove the corneal antigenic stimulus, a lamellar keratoplasty may be performed later for visual rehabilitation.
  - *Lamellar keratoplasty:* Size of the graft depends on the area of involvement, can be crescentic (<½ limbus), dough-nut (>2/3rd limbus), or full lamellar graft (central cornea).
  - *Tissue adhesives and bandage contact lenses:* In cases of small (<4 mm) perforation or impending perforation
  - *Tectonic graft:* Patch graft or penetrating keratoplasty can be done in large perforation, however being an autoimmune reaction, Mooren's type melt can be seen in donor tissue as well, requiring long-term immunosuppression.
- *Rehabilitation:* Cataract surgery or optical penetrating keratoplasty can be planned in the quiescent stage.

Clinical pearls:
- Mooren's ulcer is a diagnosis of exclusion, and all ocular and systemic causes of peripheral ulcerative keratitis (PUK) must be ruled out before diagnosing a Mooren's ulcer.
- Pain out of proportion to the inflammation is the hallmark of Mooren's ulcer.
- Absence of scleritis distinguishes Mooren's ulcer from systemic diseases associated with PUK.
- Steroids must be continued for months prior to tapering down to a halt.

 4. Describe the clinical features, evaluation, and management of microsporidial keratitis.

Introduction

Microsporidia are obligate, spore-forming intracellular, eukaryotes belonging to the phylum *Microspora* and kingdom Protista. Recently, based on morphological and molecular studies they have been classified as fungi.
- They are ubiquitous in nature and affect almost all organs, causing infections such as encephalitis, sinusitis, pneumonitis, myositis, and ocular infections.

TABLE 7: Microsporidial species and their clinical manifestations.

Microsporidial species	Clinical manifestations
Anncaliia algerae	Keratoconjunctivitis, skin, and deep muscle infection
Encephalitozoon (cuniculi and *hellem)*	Keratoconjunctivitis, UTI, URI
Nosema spp., *Anncaliia connori*	Ocular infection
Trachipleistophora hominis	Stromal keratitis, muscular infection
Vittaforma corneae (syn. *Nosema corneum*)	Ocular infection, UTI

(URI: upper respiratory infection; UTI: urinary tract infection)

- Ocular infections manifest as stromal keratitis and epithelial keratoconjunctivitis seen in immunocompetent and immunocompromised individuals, respectively and rarely endophthalmitis.
- However, unilateral epithelial involvement has been increasingly reported in the past decade among healthy individuals.

Table 7 lists out microsporidial species and their clinical manifestations.

Risk Factors

Trauma, exposure to soil/contaminated water/rainwater, contact lens, and topical steroids are important risk factors.

Clinical Features and Evaluation

- *Symptoms:* Redness, watering, irritation, photophobia, lid swelling, foreign-body sensation, and variable decrease in vision are major symptoms. Most of the patients present within 1 week of symptoms.
- *History:* A detailed history specifically to rule out the risk factors must be recorded. These include trauma, exposure to soil/contaminated water/rainwater, contact lens use, and topical steroids.
- *Signs:*
  - *Eyelids:* Lid edema with variable degree of mechanical ptosis may be noted.
  - *Conjunctiva:* Chemosed, with fusiform swelling of inferior fornix and reduced luster. Mild-moderate, nonpurulent, papillary/follicular conjunctivitis is seen.
  - *Cornea:* Superficial punctate keratopathy, i.e., coarse, multifocal, punctate, raised round to oval lesions of size <1 mm, mostly unilateral with "stuck-on" appearance and can be debrided. They can be diffuse, paracentral, or peripheral in location. Resolving superficial keratitis is accompanied with variable anterior stromal infiltrate, i.e., nummular keratitis and may have residual subepithelial scars, complete visual recovery is seen varying from 70 to 100%.
  - *AC:* White round-oval KPs and AC cells, suggestive of uveitis.
  - *Less common features:* Endotheliitis, limbitis, and endophthalmitis.
- *Differential diagnosis:* Adenoviral, Thygeson's superficial punctate keratitis, and herpes simplex virus (HSV) epithelial keratitis are common differentials. Features differentiating them from microsporidial keratitis are enumerated in **Table 8**.
- *Investigations:* Corneal scraping or corneal biopsy is sent. Microsporidial spores are identified as bright fluorescent rice grain-like, nonbudding structures against a relatively dark background, giving a typically "starry night sky" appearance on staining with 0.1% calcofluor white + 10% KOH; and as gram-positive stippled ovoid spores in Gram stain.
  - Being an obligate intracellular organism, microsporidium requires cell culture for growth and is not amenable to routine culture media. Madin–Darby canine kidney (MDCK), VeRo, HeLa, and statens seruminstitut rabbit cornea (SIRC) cell lines support growth of microsporidia.
  - Identification of species—transmission electron microscopy, polymerase chain reaction, immunofluorescent assay
  - In vivo techniques—ASOCT, confocal microscopy.

Management

Medical

- Epithelial disease can be managed with topical lubricants only. Few authors recommend debridement, however, studies have shown no benefit over lubricants. Topical fumagillin can be used in cases of epithelial disease. Stromal disease is treated with topical fumagillin and oral albendazole. Patients should be closely monitored for hepatotoxicity.
- Propamidine isethionate, polyhexamethylene biguanide (PHMB), chlorhexidine, ciprofloxacin, moxifloxacin, voriconazole, and oral itraconazole have also been tried with varied success rates.

TABLE 8: Differentiating features of microsporidia and adenoviral keratoconjunctivitis, and Thygeson's superficial punctate keratitis.

Features	Microsporidia	Adenoviral	Thygeson SPK
Laterality	Usually unilateral	Bilateral in 70% cases	Bilateral, may be asymmetric
Corneal lesion	Multifocal, elevated, coarse, round-oval epithelial/subepithelial lesions, "stuck-on" appearance	Multifocal, fine punctate subepithelial infiltrates	Coarse, oval-shaped, slightly raised epithelial/subepithelial lesions
Conjunctiva	Mild-to-moderate conjunctival congestion	Moderate-to-severe conjunctival congestion, petechial hemorrhages, pseudomembrane	Mild congestion
Fluorescein stain	Stains positively and negatively	Stains positively in acute stage. Negative in nummular scarring stage	Stains minimally
Evolution of corneal lesion	Monomorphic	Polymorphic	Evanescent pattern
Duration of symptoms	Days to few weeks	1–2 weeks, nummular scars persist for longer duration	Chronic, exacerbation and remission, months to years
Sequelae	Rarely scars only if subepithelial	Usually subepithelial haze and scarring noticed	Scars when Bowman's membrane and anterior stroma are involved
Associated systemic conditions	None	Pharyngoconjunctival fever	*Viral associations:* Varicella zoster, HSV, HLA-DR3

(HLA-DR: human leukocyte antigen-DR isotope; HSV: herpes simplex virus; SPK: superficial punctate keratitis)

- Topical steroids are indicated in cases with limbitis, corneal edema, uveitis or subepithelial infiltrates, and stroma keratitis.

Surgical

- Surgical treatment is indicated in cases unresponsive to medical management.
- Keratoplasty is useful in case of deep stromal microsporidiosis, although recurrence can occur in graft periphery.
- Cryotherapy to residual tissue may reduce the risk of recurrence.

> *Clinical pearls:*
> - Microsporidia generally manifest as stromal keratitis in immunocompetent and epithelial keratoconjunctivitis in immunocompromised individuals.
> - Affected cornea has typical coarse, multifocal, punctate, raised round to oval lesions of size <1 mm, mostly unilateral with "stuck-on" appearance.
> - Being an obligate intracellular organism, microsporidium requires cell culture for growth and is not amenable to routine culture media.
>   - Epithelial disease is treated with topical fumagillin or lubricants only, while stromal disease is treated with topical fumagillin and oral albendazole.
>   - Topical steroids are indicated in cases with limbitis, corneal edema, uveitis or subepithelial infiltrates, and stroma keratitis.

5. Discuss the role of steroids in keratitis.

Corticosteroids are the strongest anti-inflammatory drugs available for use. The use of steroids in keratitis is controversial. It is known to behave like a double-edged sword when given in a corneal ulcer. **Table 9** throws light on the pros and cons of steroids in corneal ulcers.

Multiple studies have been conducted to develop guidelines on the usage of steroids in corneal ulcers of various etiologies, and the results are summarized here.

Steroids in Bacterial Ulcers

The use of topical corticosteroids as adjunctive therapy in the treatment of bacterial corneal ulcers has been a matter of debate during the past few decades, to resolve which a National Eye Institute supported study was done between 2006 and 2010, which was named the Steroids for Corneal Ulcers Trial (SCUT).

TABLE 9: Advantages and disadvantages of steroids in corneal ulcers.

Desirable effects of steroids	Disadvantages of steroids
Decreasing the immune-mediated tissue damage	Delaying corneal epithelial and stromal healing
Resolving corneal inflammation	Increasing collagenolytic enzyme production and contribute to corneal thinning
Facilitating epithelial and stromal healing	Promoting recrudescence and slow recovery
Decreasing the scar formation, corneal opacification, and neovascularization	Accelerating stromal loss and increase the risk of perforation
Overall improving the visual acuity outcomes	Elevating the intraocular pressure

Steroids for Corneal Ulcers Trial

Objective

To look for possible benefits in clinical outcomes in the treatment of bacterial corneal ulcers with the use of topical corticosteroids as adjunctive therapy.

Trial Design

Randomized, placebo-controlled, double-masked, multicenter clinical trial comparing prednisolone sodium phosphate, 1.0%, to placebo (sodium chloride 0.9%) as adjunctive therapy for the treatment of bacterial corneal ulcers. Eligible patients (sample size—500, divided into two arms in a ratio of 1:1) had a culture-positive bacterial corneal ulcer and had received topical moxifloxacin for at least 48 hours before randomization.

Results

- Pilot study (primary endpoint at 3 months):
  - No significant difference was seen in 3-month best spectacle corrected visual acuity (BSCVA) between the two groups.
  - No obvious benefit was found in using corticosteroids in the overall study population.
  - No apparent serious safety concerns were observed (in particular, no apparent increased risk of corneal perforation).
- *12-month follow-up:* 399 out of the 500 participants were followed up at 1 year and the results were as follows:
  - For *Nocardia* ulcers, corticosteroid use was associated with larger scar sizes and lower BSCVA.
  - For *Pseudomonas* ulcers, steroid use was associated with better visual outcome.
  - For large ulcers not caused by *Nocardia* species, a reduction in scar size was seen, along with improved clinical outcome.

A recent Cochrane database review titled *"Topical Corticosteroids as Adjunctive Therapy for Bacterial Keratitis: A Review"* incorporated four RCTs, including SCUT, and came up with the following conclusions:

- No difference in reduction in ulcer size, change in visual acuity, adverse events, or quality of life between topical corticosteroid therapy and placebo or control treatment.
- Only one study reported that healing or cure time in the steroid group was slower than the placebo group.
- No difference between the two groups in adverse events, except that one study reported that more eyes in the control group developed IOP elevation.

Steroids in Fungal Keratitis

Steroid usage is contraindicated in fungal keratitis, since corticosteroids have been identified as a major risk factor for development of keratitis, so much so that they have been utilized to create experimental models of fungal keratitis in animals since fungi have been known to replicate more freely in the presence of steroids. Steroids may be responsible for delayed diagnosis because of their anti-inflammatory properties and are associated with a decreased response to antifungal agents. They have been found to worsen the course of existing fungal infection and also worsen the clinical outcome.

Steroids in Viral Keratitis

Corticosteroids are contraindicated in herpes epithelial keratitis where active viral replication is in progress at the surface, but oral and topical steroids have been shown to be beneficial in certain conditions, which are enumerated in **Table 10**. In case a patient is having both epithelial and stromal forms of keratitis, antiviral therapy should be started first and steroids should be introduced as soon as the epithelial defect heals.

TABLE 10: Indications of corticosteroids in viral keratitis.

Topical steroids	Oral steroids
Marginal keratitis	Severe immune stromal keratitis
Moderate immune stromal keratitis	Severe disciform keratitis
Moderate disciform endotheliitis	Severe diffuse endotheliitis
Moderate diffuse endotheliitis	All cases of linear endotheliitis
Inflamed neurotrophic keratopathy	Severe iridocyclitis/trabeculitis
Moderate iridocyclitis/trabeculitis	

Steroids in Acanthamoeba Keratitis

Steroids are a relative contraindication in cases of acanthamoeba keratitis (AK) and are indicated only in cases with deep vascularization, unbearable pain, and inflammatory complications (scleritis, persistent keratitis, AC inflammation).

The use of topical steroid without amoebicidal therapy produces proliferation of acanthamoeba trophozoites and increases the risk of corneal destruction.

Steroids after Keratoplasty

Immunosuppressive therapy is the main postoperative treatment for keratoplasty to prevent immunologic rejection, but should be started after the margin culture is proven sterile. In case of a keratoplasty performed for a fungal keratitis, it is imperative to wait for 10-14 days postsurgery prior to initiating steroids. It is important to continue antifungal therapy for at least 4-6 weeks in the postoperative period. They can then be safely administered in the absence of clinical signs of recurrence. Nonetheless, in cases where the complete removal of microorganisms is uncertain, topical steroids should only be utilized after the patient has been treated with appropriate antifungal medication. In the absence of complications, topical steroids should be tapered during the first 6 months following penetrating keratoplasty. IOP should be measured on every postoperative assessment.

Clinical pearls:
- Corticosteroids reduce inflammation, hence decreasing immune-mediated tissue damage, decreasing the scar formation, corneal opacification, and neovascularization, hence potentially improving visual outcome, but are associated with recrudescence and slow recovery, increased risk of corneal melt, and elevation of IOP.
- Corticosteroids are contraindicated in herpes epithelial keratitis and fungal keratitis.
- Can be used in bacterial keratitis except *Nocardia*; however, the patient must be on antibiotics, for at least 48 hours, to which the organism is sensitive.
- In acanthamoeba keratitis, steroids are indicated only in cases with deep vascularization, unbearable pain, scleritis, persistent keratitis, and AC inflammation.

 6. Discuss exposure keratitis.

Exposure keratopathy is the disease process that occurs primarily from prolonged exposure of the ocular surface to the outside environment which can lead to inadequate tear film, resulting in epithelial breakdown, followed by its complications such as ulceration, microbial keratitis, and permanent loss of vision from scarring.

Etiopathogenesis

Intact blink reflex with a normal blink rate, and complete eyelid closure during blinking and sleep are prerequisites for an even distribution of the tear film over the ocular surface. Disruption of any of these may lead to epithelial breakdown, making the cornea vulnerable to harmful external agents. The various etiologies leading to exposure keratitis can be classified as follows:
- *Anatomical causes:* Any malposition of the eyelids preventing complete closure of the eyelids, i.e.,
  - *Lagophthalmos* (inability to close the eyelids completely).
    - Paralytic lagophthalmos, which occurs as a result of facial nerve palsy and is the most common cause of lagophthalmos. Bell's palsy, which is an idiopathic, unilateral facial nerve paralysis, constitutes the vast majority

of cases. Other causes may be traumatic (secondary to fractures to the skull base, temporal bone, or mandible), iatrogenic (parotid gland surgery, acoustic neuroma resection, neurosurgery, etc.), infective [herpes zoster virus or Ramsay Hunt syndrome, human immunodeficiency virus (HIV), tuberculosis, leprosy, measles, polio, Lyme disease, cat-scratch disease] or neoplastic (acoustic neuroma, adenoid cystic neuroma of external auditory canal, metastasis from orbit, breast, lung or kidney).
- Cicatricial lagophthalmos, results from excessive scarring of the eyelid, and may occur after trauma or surgery, thermochemical injuries, lacerations, and chronic skin diseases such as xeroderma pigmentosa.
- Nocturnal lagophthalmos or incomplete eyelid closure during sleep, in the absence of Bell's phenomenon during sleep, can cause exposure keratopathy.
- *Proptosis* or anterior protrusion of eyeball may limit complete eye closure, and its causes include thyroid eye disease, craniosynostosis syndromes, orbital tumors, Cushing's syndrome, neurofibromatosis 1, aortic regurgitation, carotid-cavernous sinus fistula, arachnoid cysts, and trauma.
- *Lid margin abnormalities* such as ectropion and coloboma can also cause exposure keratitis.
- *Neurological causes:* These can be neurotrophic (decreased corneal sensation) or neuroparalytic (paralysis of facial nerve, leading to impaired lid closure). Causes include keratoconus, bullous keratopathy, atopic keratoconjuctivitis; systemic polyneuropathies as in cases of diabetes, vitamin B_{12} deficiency, amyloidosis, alcoholism; drug use like that of intranasal cocaine; autoimmune causes such as Graves' disease and Sjögren's syndrome; hereditary neuropathies such as Riley–Day syndrome, congenital aniridia, ocular-auriculo-vertebral dysplasia, and multiple endocrine neoplasia 2A and 2B; infectious causes such as herpes simplex or varicella zoster virus, *Mycobacterium leprae*, *Acanthamoeba*; Iatrogenic cases as seen after corneal refractive procedures.

Presentation

History

Chief complaints: Irritation of eyes, foreign body sensation, burning, watering, redness, photophobia, and intermittent blurry vision (due to an unstable tear film).

In cases of neurotrophic keratopathy, patients may not have many symptoms and may even present late with infective keratitis or corneal ulceration, or decreased vision due to corneal opacity. Patients with nocturnal lagophthalmos may complain that symptoms are worse in the morning.

Past history: History of recent trauma, surgery, or any infection, a previous episode of facial nerve palsy should be taken, to find out the root cause of lagophthalmos.

Systemic history: A detailed systemic history, with special emphasis on diabetes (associated with facial palsy) and thyroid disorder (which may cause proptosis) should also be taken.

Examination

- *Systemic Examination:* Apart from the routine systemic work-up, a complete neurological examination including assessment of all cranial nerves should be performed.
- *Ocular Examination:*
  - *Eyelids:* Patients can present with lagophthalmos, proptosis, eyelid malposition or deformity, or an impaired blink reflex. Lid position as well as interpalpebral distance should be assessed in a relaxed open and closed state. Appositional closure of the eyelids with each blink should be recorded. Obscure lagophthalmos, wherein the upper and lower eyelashes meet, either preventing complete closure of the lids, or obscuring the view of the true eyelid position, maybe better examined using a slit lamp. Bell's phenomenon should be recorded.
  - *Conjunctiva:* Conjunctiva should be examined for any areas of scarring or cicatrization. There may also be congestion/chemosis of the conjunctiva.
  - *Cornea:* Corneal involvement may range from punctate epitheliopathy in the inferior one-third of cornea in early stages to epithelial defects, edema, ulceration, and even perforation in later stages. Extent of corneal involvement, in terms of epithelial staining, presence of infiltrates, opacity, etc. should be documented.

Investigations

- Staining with fluorescein sodium dye may reveal any punctuate epithelial erosions, frank epithelial defects, or ulceration.
- Corneal sensations are assessed by using a wisp of cotton or measured using an esthesiometer.

Management

It includes both supportive therapy as well as treating the primary cause.
- *Conservative management:*
  - *Ocular lubricants:* They act by promoting reepithelialization, ameliorating persistent epitheliopathy, and by preventing recurrent erosions. Preservative-free artificial tear drops should be used, as the preservatives can be epitheliotoxic and can stimulate inflammation and further disrupt the tear film. Lubricating ointments should be used at night followed by taping the eyelid, in cases with lagophthalmos.
  - *Antibiotics:* Prophylactic broad-spectrum antibiotics are usually given in order to prevent secondary infections that may occur owing to a breach in the corneal epithelium. Chloramphenicol 0.5% or fluoroquinolones such as moxifloxacin 0.5% may be used.
  - *Anti-inflammatory agents:* Topical drugs, such as nonsteroidal anti-inflammatory drugs (NSAIDs) and steroids, may help in symptomatic relief, but should be used with extreme caution as they increase the risk of stromal melt, and may lead to secondary infections. Oral tetracyclines such as doxycycline are sometimes added for their anti-inflammatory and anticollagenolytic effects.
  - *Punctal occlusion:* Use of punctal plugs helps in better retention of the tear film and tear substitutes. Long-acting collagen or silicone punctal plugs may be used for temporary punctual occlusion, both prophylactically and therapeutically.
  - *Eyelid closure:* This can be achieved by simple taping or patching of the eyes. Other described techniques are use of a saline soaked or paraffin gauzes, polyacrylamide hydrogel dressing marketed as "Geliperm", use of a sterile polythene cover, or a moisture chamber.
  - *Bandage contact lens:* Although they are useful in promoting epithelial healing and providing comfort to the patient, they are associated with an increased risk of infection. Long-term use is not advocated, and concurrent antibiotic cover should always be given.
- *Surgical Management:*
  - Surgeries aimed at treating the primary cause: Canthoplasty, lid tightening procedures, ectropion correction, etc., for exposure secondary to lid malposition; orbital decompression for proptosis.
  - *Supportive strategies:*
    - Temporary tarsorrhaphy/frost suture for lagophthalmos expected to last >6 weeks.
    - Permanent tarsorrhaphy or gold weight implantation when lagophthalmos is presumed to be irreversible.
    - Amniotic membrane transplantation in cases of persistent epithelial defects. Currently, especially designed devices are available with a clipped piece of amniotic membrane tissue, e.g., PROKERA®
    - In cases of corneal ulcers with perforation, cyanoacrylate glue with a bandage contact lens or a tectonic graft may be used.

Clinical pearls:
In cases of neurotrophic keratopathy, patients may not have many symptoms and may even present late with infective keratitis or corneal ulceration, or decreased vision due to corneal opacity. In such cases, a complete neurological examination, including assessment of all cranial nerves, should be performed.

 7. Discuss neurotrophic keratopathy.

Introduction

Neurotrophic keratitis is a degenerative disease of cornea associated with impairment of corneal sensation, leading to increased susceptibility to trauma, reduced reflex tearing, and delayed epithelial healing, which occur as a result of defect in trigeminal corneal innervation, which may occur due to lesions at any level of this nerve pathway starting from its nucleus in pons, the Gasserian ganglion, the trigeminal ophthalmic branch, the nasociliary nerve, to the long ciliary nerve, and can result in corneal ulceration and stromal melt if not treated appropriately.

Etiopathogenesis

The cornea is the most richly innervated tissue of the human body. This sensory innervation plays an important role in maintaining the corneal epithelium. Various causes, both ocular and systemic, can lead to impaired corneal sensations **(Table 11)**.

TABLE 11: Causes of corneal hypesthesia.

Infection
- Herpes simplex
- Herpes zoster
- Leprosy

Fifth nerve palsy
- Surgery (as for trigeminal neuralgia)
- Neoplasia (such as acoustic neuroma)
- Aneurysms
- Facial trauma
- Congenital familial dysautonomia (Riley–Day syndrome)
- Goldenhar–Gorlin syndrome
- Möbius syndrome
- Familial corneal hypesthesia
- Congenital insensitivity to pain with anhidrosis

Topical medications
- Anesthetics
- Timolol
- Betaxolol
- Sulfacetamide 30%
- Diclofenac sodium

Corneal dystrophies
- Lattice
- Granular (rare)

Systemic disease
- Diabetes mellitus
- Vitamin A deficiency

Iatrogenic
- Contact lens wear
- Trauma to ciliary nerves by laser and surgery (primarily for retinal conditions)
- Corneal incisions
- Corneal refractive surgery

Toxic
- Chemical burns
- Carbon disulfide exposure
- Hydrogen sulfide exposure

Miscellaneous
- Increasing age
- Dark eye color
- Adie's syndrome

Neurotrophic keratitis involves various degrees of degenerative corneal and conjunctival changes secondary to loss corneal innervation with or without decreased tear production, as shown in flowchart given below:

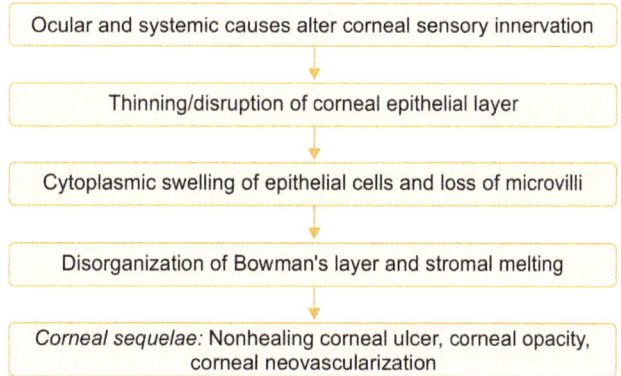

TABLE 12: Clinical stages of neurotrophic keratitis based on Mackie classification.

Stage	Clinical signs
Stage 1	• Rose Bengal staining of inferior palpebral conjunctiva (earliest sign of neurotrophic keratitis) • Decreased TBUT • Increased viscosity of tear mucous • Punctate epithelial staining with fluorescein • Scattered small facets of dried epithelium (Gaule spots), better seen on retroillumination in early cases
Stage 2	• Acute loss of epithelium surrounded by a rim of loose epithelium, usually over the area covered by the upper lid • Stromal edema • Aqueous flare and cells, rarely a sterile hypopyon may be present • Edges of the defect become smooth and rolled with time, forming punched-out horizontal, oval, or circular defect that is characteristic of neurotrophic keratitis
Stage 3	• Stromal lysis • Secondary bacterial infection • Corneal perforation

(TBUT: tear breakup time)

Clinical Features

- *Symptoms:* Patients are usually asymptomatic or may present with blurring of vision with or without dull aching pain.
- *Signs:* Mackie classified the ocular signs of neurotrophic keratitis into three stages, as given in **Table 12**.

Investigations

Though sterile, these ulcers but may be associated with bacterial superinfections. In such cases, corneal scraping is to be taken from the leading edge and base of the ulcer and sent for staining (Gram's, Giemsa, and Grocott's methenamine silver stain), culture and sensitivity testing or can be directly inoculated onto blood agar, chocolate agar, Sabouraud agar plate, and viral culture medium. Direct immunofluorescence staining can be done for herpes virus.

A magnetic resonance imaging of the brain and orbits can be done in cases of suspicion of any neurological cause.

Treatment

The selection of treatment modality depends on the stage of disease.

Stage 1: Treatment in this early stage involves withdrawal of epitheliotoxic drugs, use of ocular lubricants (preferably preservative free), and bandage contact lenses (used for short term in view of risk of infective keratitis). Oral tetracyclines may be used as adjuvant therapy as they can prevent stromal melt due to anticollagenase action and can reduce the amount of mucus produced. In cases of severe anesthesia, lateral tarsorrhaphy, palpebral spring, or botulinum A injection into the levator can be done to prevent epithelial defects.

Stage 2: Treatment of stage-2 neurotrophic keratitis involves use of growth factors and cell attachment factors [nerve growth factor (NGF), epidermal growth factor (EGF), laminin, fibronectin, insulin-like growth factor (IGF)-1, substance-P, and albumin)] in addition to copious lubrication as in stage 1. Patching or tarsorrhaphy (temporary or permanent) may be done to prevent recurrence.

Stage 3: During this stage, it is important to maintain the integrity of corneal surface. Collagenase inhibitors are used topically (acetylcysteine 20% and EDTA 0.2 mol/L) and orally (tetracycline 250 mg QID and doxycycline 100 mg BD) to prevent stromal melting.

Tissue adhesives (glue-BCL) may be used for corneal perforation up to 3 mm and for impending cases as tectonic support. Conjunctival flap (Gunderson flap) is indicated for extensively filling the ulcer cavity. A multilayered amniotic membrane grafting also serves the same purpose but in addition, provides anti-inflammatory factors to decrease inflammation and help in early healing. Small lamellar or full-thickness keratoplasty is done in large perforations (>3 mm).

Role of Cenegermin

A recombinant form of human nerve growth factor (rhNGF) has been recently approved by Food and Drug Administration (FDA) for the treatment of moderate-severe neurotrophic keratitis. It is available as 0.002% ophthalmic solution which is dosaged as one drop six times a day for 8 weeks.

Clinical pearls:
- Impairment of corneal sensations can occur any damage to trigeminal corneal innervation, which may occur due to lesions at any level of this nerve pathway starting from its nucleus in pons, the Gasserian ganglion, the trigeminal ophthalmic branch, the nasociliary nerve, to the long ciliary nerve.
- Corneal sensations should always be assessed in any case of nonhealing corneal ulcer.
- Scattered small facets of dried epithelium better seen on retroillumination in early cases of neurotrophic keratopathy are called Gaule spots.
- Early tarsorrhaphy or AMT should be considered if medical therapy fails to avoid melting.

(AMT: amniotic membrane transplant)

8. Elaborate the risk factors, clinical presentation diagnosis, and management of acanthamoeba keratitis.

Introduction

Acanthamoeba keratitis is the most common parasitic corneal infection. It is primarily associated with contact lens use in Western world, and exposure to contaminated water and soil in tropical countries and developing countries. Acanthamoeba are free-living protozoans ubiquitously found in water, soil, and air. It exists in two forms—infective, freely mobile trophozoite or dormant double-walled cyst which is resistant to extremes of temperature, desiccation, chlorine, and a wide range of antimicrobial agents.

Acanthamoeba castellani, Acanthamoeba polyphaga, Acanthamoeba culbertsoni are important pathogenic species. Other less important pathogenic species are *Acanthamoeba palestinensis, Acanthamoeba astronyxis, Acanthamoeba divionensis,* and *Acanthamoeba rhysodes*.

Pathogenesis

The pathogenesis can be described in three stages: epithelial adhesion and desquamation, stromal invasion, and neuritis.

1. *Epithelial adhesion and desquamation:* Acanthamoeba can adhere to a normal epithelium. Transmembrane proteins expressed by the parasite such as mannose-binding protein and laminin binding protein facilitate acanthamoeba binding to the glycoproteins and glycolipids present on the corneal epithelial cell after which acanthamoeba produces several contact-dependent metalloproteinases, superoxide dismutase, neuraminidase, ecto-ATPase, elastase, and phospholipase, which help the organism in causing direct epithelial cell cytolysis; phagocytosis; induction of apoptosis and stromal invasion.
2. *Stromal invasion:* The parasite breaches the epithelium and Bowman's membrane and further degradation of stroma occurs with upregulation of proteases (MIP-133) and collagenases, followed by the death of host tissue and deeper penetration of amoeba.
3. *Neuritis:* Trophozoites follow a chemotactic response to corneal nerves and can cause a cytolytic and apoptotic response, causing the characteristic radial neuritis. This is the final stage of inflammation in most cases. Trophozoites cannot disrupt corneal endothelial cells and enter the AC.

Risk Factors

Contact lens (soft > hard contact lenses) is the most common risk factor associated with AK in the Western world. Trauma accounts for the majority of cases in India. Other known risk factors are contaminated soil and water, swimming in contaminated ponds, immunocompromised state, using contaminated eye drops and contact lens solution, ocular surgery, orthokeratology, and poor socioeconomic status.

Clinical Features

History

In addition to the history of exposure to above risk factors, one of the characteristic features of AK is its waxing and waning course. The disease progression is relatively slow and the waxing and waning course due to conversion of cysts to trophozoite in active phase and back to dormant cyst during remission. The disease runs a protracted course often requiring therapy for >3–6 months.

Most cases are bilateral, rarely a contact lens user can present with bilateral keratitis.

Symptoms
- *Pain:* The amount of pain in AK is known to be out of proportion to the severity of clinical picture in initial stages, due to radial keratoneuritis, which is the hallmark of this disease.
- Foreign body sensation
- Redness
- Watering and mucoid discharge
- Photophobia
- Diminution of vision

Signs

Eyelids and Adnexa
Eyelids are edematous as in case of any corneal ulcer, and the patient can have features of dacryoadenitis.

Conjunctiva
Conjunctival congestion is present.

Cornea
Corneal signs expected in AK are:
- Radial keratoneuritis is an early sign and results from infiltration along corneal nerves. Infiltrates are present at mid stromal level starting paracentrally and extending toward the limbus in a radial pattern. There is no ulcer overlying these infiltrates. This is the cause of severe pain despite a seemingly mild corneal involvement in early stages. It is one of the pathognomonic sign of AK.
- Ring infiltrate, seen in about one half of the patients, is an important sign of advanced disease and is nearly pathognomonic. It is associated with a variable overlying epithelial defect.
- *Corneal epithelial abnormalities and punctate erosions:* AK in early stages present with epithelial swelling, or punctate erosions. This often confuses with HSV keratitis and in majority of AK one may find initial treatment in line of HSV keratitis.
- Epithelial haze
- Pseudodendrites
- Microcysts
- Stromal thinning
- Satellite lesions
- Stromal ulceration
- *Perforation:* In advanced cases, there could be stromal lysis and melting.

Limbus
Severe limbitis characterized by focal or diffuse ciliary congestion near limbus can also be there. Limbitis is one of the characteristic features of AK.

Anterior Chamber
Anterior chamber cells and a hypopyon may be present.

Iris
Iritis may be present.

Lens
The visual acuity may be worsened by subsequent development of a complicated cataract.
Clinical examination of the fundus is rarely possible due to hampered visibility.

Differential Diagnosis

A high index of suspicion is required for early diagnosis of AK, and a brief summary of the classical features of the differentials is given in **Table 13**. It is often confused with fungal or viral keratitis and the presence of secondary bacterial infections can further complicate the clinical diagnosis.

TABLE 13: Differential diagnosis of acanthamoeba keratitis.

Clinical characteristics	Differential diagnosis
Pseudo-dendriform epitheliopathy, epithelium defects without terminal knots, perineural infiltrates, ring infiltrates, endothelium is not involved	Herpes simplex keratitis
Usually restricted to cornea, absence of anterior chamber activity, stromal infiltrates are usually multifocal (not monofocal), ring infiltrates	Bacterial keratitis
Usually restricted to cornea, clear epithelium defects, perineural stromal infiltrates, ring infiltrates	Fungal keratitis

Investigations

Microbiology

- The cysts are seen on wet smears stained with iodine stain, Giemsa-Wright, gram, hematoxylin and eosin, calcofluor stain, acridine orange, Lugol solution, lactophenol cotton blue, and wheaty-trichome stains as double-walled structures with circular to oval outer wall and a hexagonal/irregular inner wall. The trophozoites are difficult to distinguish from inflammatory cells.
- Gold standard for diagnosis is culture of a superficial corneal scraping/biopsy/contact lens solution or case/contact lens itself, but the rate of obtaining a positive culture is only 50%. The preferred medium for culture is non-nutrient agar with *Escherichia coli* overlay at 35°C. In most of the cases, a positive culture is obtained within 4–5 days and is seen as a characteristic "snail track" appearance due to amoeba grazing on the *E. coli*. A waiting period of at least 2 weeks is recommended before declaring a culture negative.

Molecular Methods

Polymerase chain reaction can be applied on samples for detecting organisms. It has sensitivity similar to conventional microbiology. Recently described methods are isoenzyme analysis and mitochondrial and cellular DNA analysis, and direct amplification of acanthamoeba DNA without extraction.

Confocal Microscopy

It provides instantaneous in-vivo histological image to suggest the diagnosis. It is particularly useful for detecting organisms in the deep corneal infiltrate (such as acanthamoeba and fungal hyphae) which are inaccessible to scraping and can monitor response to treatment. Cysts are seen as double walled hyper-reflective structures, trophozoites are seen as ovoid to S-shaped structures, radial keratoneuritis can be seen as irregularly swollen nerves with probable infiltration.

Complications

It includes scleritis, iris atrophy, mid-dilated pupil and cataract, and rarely perforation and endophthalmitis.

Treatment

Depth of infiltration is the most important indicator of poor prognosis. Other poor prognostic factors are duration of disease and presence of immune ring at initial presentation. Cysts are highly resistant to treatment and may persist for years.

Medical

The various drugs used in AK are summarized in **Table 14**.
Most of the drugs act on free trophozoites and are less effective on cysts.

- *Biguanides:* They contain highly charged positive molecules and cause effect by increasing cytoplasmic membrane permeability.
    For example, PHMB 0.02–0.06%, effective against both cysts and trophozoites but possess significant epitheliotoxicity; chlorhexidine 0.02–0.2%, which is less epitheliotoxic than PHMB.
- *Diamidines:* Aromatic compounds which induce structural changes in the cell membrane due to the cationic surface-active properties, e.g., propamidine isethionate 0.1%, hexamidine 0.1%.
- *Azoles:* Inhibit the synthesis of ergosterol present in cell membrane of Acanthamoeba, e.g., voriconazole—oral (100 mg/day) or topical (1%).
- *Aminoglycoside:* Neomycin 1.0%.

Cornea and Conjunctiva

TABLE 14: Drugs used in acanthamoeba keratitis.

Class of drug	Mechanism of action	Drug	Cysticidal activity	Antitrophozoite activity	Special comments
Biguanide	Increasing cytoplasmic membrane permeability	Polyhexamethylene biguanide (PHMB) 0.02%	++	++	Epitheliotoxic
		Chlorhexidine 0.02%	++	++	Less epitheliotoxic than PHMB
Diamidines	Inhibit DNA synthesis	Propamidine isethionate 0.1%	–	++	
		Dibromopropamidine 0.15%	–	++	
		Hexamidine 0.1%	+	++	
Aminoglycoside	Inhibits protein synthesis by binding to 30s ribosome	Neomycin 1%	–	+	
Azoles	Inhibits ergosterol synthesis present in cell membrane	Voriconazole 1% Systemic voriconazole 200 mg BD	+	+	
All phospho-cholines	Inhibition of phosphatidyl choline biosynthesis and inhibition of Akt involved in regulation of cell cycle	Miltefosine 65 µg/mL in BD dose	+	+	

- *Miltefosine:* It has attained orphan drug status by FDA for AK. It is alkylphosphocholine which interacts with lipid in the cell wall and inhibits cytochrome C oxidase. Its topical dose is 65 µg/mL and oral dose is available as 50 mg capsule (BD/TDS depending on weight of patient) for 28 days.

Treatment Protocol

So far there is no single therapeutic agent that has shown good activity against both trophozoite and cystic forms. Trophozoites are easier to treat as they are metabolically active. Therapy is usually effective if initiated within 1 month of onset. Two-drug therapy with biguanides and diamidines is recommended by most authors compared to single-drug therapy with biguanides. Combination of PHMB (0.02%) and propamidine (0.1%) is most commonly used. They should be given hourly for first 72–96 hours, followed by 2 hourly for 2–4 weeks and then tapered to QID for 6 months to 1 year.

Long-term therapy is required because of the cysts that are present deep in the corneal stroma. Abrupt reduction in frequency of topical drugs can result in reactivation of cysts following which therapy needs to be scaled up and then tapered slowly. This approach called "pulse therapy" can help in reducing resistant cysts in stroma. However, if there is improvement in symptoms following abrupt reduction in frequency, it indicates drug toxicity and the treatment should then be continued at QID dosing.

Cycloplegics and NSAIDs are useful in managing pain and inflammation. Epithelial abrasion can help in penetration of above drugs. Any bacterial and fungal coinfection should be treated accordingly.

Role of Steroids

Steroids enhance the conversion of cysts to trophozoites which can help in eradication of pathogen, but they also reduce the killing power of macrophages which is important for killing the amoeba. Thus, it is generally recommended to use steroids only in cases with:
- Limbitis or associated scleritis
- Inflammatory complications (severe anterior uveitis, persistent corneal inflammation, stromal melt, severe pain)
- Postkeratoplasty
- Indolent ulcer
- Deep vascularization
- Out of proportion pain.

Steroid therapy is to be started after 2 weeks of antiamoebic therapy and the antiamoebic treatment should be continued for at least 4 weeks after stopping steroids. Oral steroids can be given in cases not responding to topical steroids.

Surgical

In severe cases, therapeutic penetrating keratoplasty (TPK) is performed to reduce the infectious load and hasten recovery. Due to high rate of recurrence, optimal control of infection is recommended before keratoplasty. A gap of 3–6 months is recommended between complete resolution of infection on medical therapy and optical keratoplasty.

For superficial involvement lamellar keratoplasty can be performed. Amniotic membrane transplantation for managing persistent epithelial defects and progressive stromal lesions has been reported to be useful.

Indications for TPK surgical management include:
- Large infiltrate extending or threatening to involve limbus
- Worsening on medical treatment
- Gross thinning or actual perforation.

Clinical pearls:
- Radial keratoneuritis is an early sign of amoebic keratitis and results from infiltration along corneal nerves. Infiltrates are present at mid stromal level extending toward the limbus, with no ulcer overlying these infiltrates.
- Long-term therapy is required because of the cysts that are present deep in the corneal.
- Stroma
- No single therapeutic agent that has shown good activity against both trophozoite and cystic forms, so a combination of PHMB (0.02%) and propamidine (0.1%) is most commonly used.
- Steroids are indicated only in cases with limbitis or scleritis, inflammatory complications, postkeratoplasty, indolent ulcer, deep vascularization, and severe pain.
- A gap of 3–6 months is recommended between complete resolution of infection on medical therapy and performing an optical keratoplasty.

9. Discuss management of nonhealing corneal ulcer. Describe current concepts in the management of nonhealing corneal ulcer.

Introduction

A corneal ulcer is termed nonhealing in case of:
- No response (worsening or static) to standard treatment even after 48 hours of treatment initiation in bacterial keratitis. Or
- No response (worsening or static) to standard treatment even after 7 days of treatment initiation in fungal keratitis.

Risk Factors

The various risk factors that could lead to a nonhealing corneal ulcer are summarized in **Table 15**.

TABLE 15: Risk factors for nonhealing corneal ulcer.

Ocular causes	Systemic causes

• *Persistent infection:*
  – Herpes zoster ophthalmicus
  – Herpes simplex keratitis
  – Lyme's disease
• Contact lens wear
• *Trauma to ciliary nerves (Iatrogenic):*
  – Laser, diathermy, cryotherapy
  – Post PK, post LIC
  – Post-refractive surgery
• *Topical drugs:*
  – Anesthetic agents
  – Timolol, betoxolol
  – Steroids
  – Diclofenac
• Ocular surface toxicity (chemical burns)
• *Chronic conjunctival inflammation:*
  – OCP
• Lid abnormalities—ectropion/entropion/trichiasis/lagophthalmos
• Tear film abnormalities—DED
• Tear outflow blocked—NLDO
• Orbit abnormalities—shallow orbits, proptosis
• Corneal dystrophies
• Persistent raised IOP
• External trauma
	• Diabetes
	• Leprosy
	• Vitamin A deficiency
	• Malnutrition
	• Collagen vascular diseases
	• Chronic alcoholism
	• *Nerve palsy:*
	  – Trigeminal nerve—neuralgia, palsy, tumor
	  – Facial nerve—palsy, acoustic neuroma, trauma
	  – Congenital causes—familial dysautonomia, Goldenhar's syndrome, Mobius syndrome
	• *Toxins:*
	  – Carbon disulphide exposure
	  – Hydrogen sulfide exposure

(IOP: intraocular pressure; LK: lamellar keratoplasty; NLDO: nasolacrimal duct obstruction; OCP: ocular cicatricial pemphigoid; PK: penetrating keratoplasty)

Treatment

Step-wise treatment of nonhealing corneal ulcer:
- Evaluate to look for precipitating causes (infection, drug toxicity, lid adnexal abnormalities, and toxins) and correct or remove them.
- Modify treatment (switch antimicrobial agents in atypical organisms, use nonepitheliotoxic drugs).
- Select the adequate treatment modality depending on the stage of the ulcer.

Pearl

Use of multiple topical drugs and preservatives is the common cause of indolent ulcers, giving a drug holiday for 24 hours and rescraping will help in definitive diagnosis.

10. Discuss perforated corneal ulcer.

Introduction

Perforated corneal ulcer is an ocular emergency condition that warrants urgent surgical intervention in order to salvage the integrity of globe as well as preserve the visual function. The varied etiology of this condition includes infectious keratitis, noninfectious keratitis, xerosis, chemical injury, and trauma.[1] Management of this condition needs to be tailored to the case. Small corneal perforations (<3 mm) are usually managed with glue and bandage contact lens.[1,2] Large corneal perforations, however, require either corneal patch graft or tectonic keratoplasty.[1] Any delay in the management of this condition may result in extrusion of ocular contents with permanent loss of the ocular integrity. Therefore, an appropriate and timely intervention is indispensable.

Etiopathogenesis

The causes of corneal ulcer leading to corneal perforation are infective keratitis, noninfectious causes (ocular surface disorder and autoimmune disorders), chemical injury, exposure keratopathy, trauma, etc. Infective keratitis is the most common cause implicated for perforated corneal ulcer.[3]

- *Infective keratitis:*
  - *Bacterial keratitis:* Bacterial keratitis is one the most common cause of perforated corneal ulcer. Most bacteria require a breach in corneal epithelium for further invasion into the corneal tissue. However, there are few organisms such as *Neisseria, Shigella, Haemophilus, Corynebacterium diphtheria,* and *Listeria* that penetrate intact corneal epithelium. Invasion of corneal tissue with these organisms leads to release of numerous cytokines that attracts inflammatory cells which release collagenase. This results in corneal stromal necrosis with further penetration of the organism into deeper tissue ultimately resulting in corneal perforation if not treated appropriately in time.[1] The organisms commonly implicated in corneal perforation due to bacterial keratitis include—*Pseudomonas, Staphylococcus* spp., *Streptococcus pneumoniae, Salmonella,* and *Moraxella*.[4,5]
  - *Fungal keratitis:* In developing countries, fungal keratitis still remains one of the important causes of infective keratitis. Though the course of fungal keratitis is slow, the poor efficacy and ocular penetration of the topical antifungal drugs result in progression. The rate of corneal perforation in fungal keratitis varies from 9 to 33% with *Fusarium solani* and *Aspergillus fumigatus* being the most common organism implicated.[5,6]
  - *Viral keratitis:* In developed countries, viral keratitis is an important cause of perforated corneal ulcer. Active viral replication and host immune response resulting in release of matrix metalloproteinases (MMPs) and collagenase result in stromal tissue necrosis and perforation. Also, recurrent episodes of viral keratitis result in corneal thinning that can predispose to corneal perforation.[1]
- *Noninfective keratitis*:
  - *Ocular surface disorder:* Severe dry eye disease can result in recurrent epithelial defects with poor healing of ocular surface resulting in increased risk of infective keratitis. Sjögren syndrome, vitamin A deficiency, Steven–Johnson syndrome, and mucous membrane pemphigoid are few ocular surface disorders with associated dry eye that can result in corneal perforation.[7-10]
  - *Autoimmune disorders:* Numerous collagen vascular disorders such as rheumatoid arthritis, systemic lupus erythematosus, Wegener granulomatosis, and sarcoidosis are associated with peripheral ulcerative keratitis (PUK)

which in severe cases can result in corneal perforation.[11] Malignant variant of Mooren's ulcer, an idiopathic variant of PUK, is associated with high corneal perforation rate up to 36%.[12,13]

- *Chemical injury:* Ocular chemical burn with alkali results in epithelial breakdown and stromal necrosis due to release of collagenase by the damaged corneal and conjunctival epithelial cells and neutrophils along with limbal ischemia and altered fibroblast response. Adequate and timely intervention can prevent this.
- *Exposure keratopathy:* Lagophthalmos leading to corneal exposure causes desiccation of corneal stromal tissue resulting in corneal thinning and perforation in some cases.
- Trauma.

Risk Factors

The risk factors associated with perforation in a case of corneal ulcer are as follows:[14]
- Delay in starting initial treatment
- Failure to start fortified antibiotics
- Lack of corneal vascularization
- Monotherapy with fluoroquinolones
- *Others:* Outdoor occupation, trauma with vegetable matter, illiteracy, excessive alcohol use, vision less than counting fingers at referral and central location of ulcer.

Clinical Features

Symptoms

- Sudden onset diminution of vision
- Severe ocular pain just before corneal perforation develops followed by some relief in symptoms after perforation develops.
- Sudden increase in watering from eyes.

Signs

- *Iris prolapse:* It is diagnostic of corneal perforation.
- *Positive Seidel's test:* 2% fluorescein is painted at the site of suspected corneal perforation and a bright yellow color of fluorescein is noted when it gets diluted with the leaking aqueous in case there is an underlying corneal perforation.
- *Pressure Seidel's test:* In case of a small or self-sealed corneal perforation, the Seidel's test may be negative and gentle pressure on the globe is necessary to confirm the presence of an underlying perforation.
- Radiating folds in the Descemet membrane is a sign of impending corneal perforation.

Work-up

History

A detailed history is imperative in these cases to reach the correct diagnosis. All the risk factors for corneal perforation as discussed above should be enquired for:
- Ocular trauma
- Ocular surgery
- Use of bandage contact lens
- Use of topical corticosteroids
- Dryness of eyes
- Any associated autoimmune disorder—rheumatoid arthritis, systemic lupus erythematosus, etc.

Clinical Examination

A detailed slit lamp examination should be done and the following points should be noted:
- *Size of corneal perforation:* Small corneal perforations (<3 mm) are amenable to corneal gluing while large corneal perforations require keratoplasty.
- Location of corneal perforation—central/peripheral
- Seidel's test

- *Pressure Seidel's test:* Performed in case Seidel's test is negative and an underlying small or self-sealed corneal perforation is suspected.
- Associated anterior segment inflammation.

Investigations

- *Ocular:*
  - *Corneal scraping:* A gentle corneal scraping should be done and sample sent for microbiologic assessment (microscopic assessment and culture sensitivity testing). Sample should be submitted for microscopic assessment with Gram stain, 10% KOH, and Calcofluor white. Specimen should be sent for culture in blood agar, Sabouraud dextrose agar, non-nutrient agar with *Escherichia coli* overlay, chocolate agar, and thioglycollate broth.
  - *Conjunctival swab:* In case of large corneal perforation with vitreous prolapse, corneal scraping may be difficult and may also increase the risk of suprachoroidal hemorrhage. In these cases, a conjunctival swab may be sent for microbiological assessment.
  - *Ultrasound B-scan:* B-scan ultrasound is done to rule out associated posterior segment pathology such as—endophthalmitis, retinal detachment, and choroidal detachment.
- *Systemic:* Collagen vascular disease needs to be ruled out, especially in cases of peripheral corneal ulcer. Rheumatoid arthritis is the most common collagen vascular disorder associated with corneal thinning and perforation. A proper evaluation of these cases in consult with a rheumatologist should be done.

Management

- *Nonsurgical management:*
  - *Treatment of infective keratitis:* Concentrated antibiotics (cefazolin 5% and tobramycin 1.3%) are started on hourly regimen after obtaining scraping specimen. Systemic antibiotics should be started for all cases of perforated corneal ulcer. The drugs are later modified based on the microbiologic reports.
  - *Topical cycloplegic:* Topical cycloplegics (homatropine 2% or atropine 1%) are given for pain relief and increasing the patient's comfort.
  - *Antiglaucoma medication:* Suppressing the aqueous production helps in wound healing and also prevents extrusion of intraocular contents.
  - *Anticollagenase drugs:* Drugs with anticollagenase action such as oral tetracycline and doxycycline are used in cases with corneal melting. These drugs act by chelating metallic ions which results in inhibition of MMP and prevent further collagenolysis and corneal perforation in cases with corneal melting.[15]
  - *Anti-inflammatory drugs:*
    - *Steroids:* Topical steroids can be used in cases of bacterial corneal ulcer where the organism implicated has been identified on microbiological assessment and appropriate antibiotics have been started for at least 48 hours.[16,17] Steroids help in controlling inflammation and preventing further damage to the cornea. Its benefit has been noted in cases with central corneal ulcer and presenting visual acuity finger counting close to face.[17] The steroid should be avoided in cases of post-traumatic and contact lens-induced keratitis as they may be fungal in nature.
    - Steroids should be used with caution in cases of viral necrotizing keratitis and should be prescribed in conjunction with topical and systemic antivirals.
    - *Steroid-sparing drugs:* Steroid-sparing agents such as cyclosporine are used in cases of severe noninfectious corneal ulcer. Both systemic and topical cyclosporine (1% or 2%) are used in cases with melting corneal ulcer such as Mooren's ulcer, associated severe dry eye and systemic autoimmune disease.[18,19] Cyclosporine is a specific T-cell inhibitor that modifies the cell-mediated immunity by inhibiting the release of IL-2 which is involved in recruiting activated T-cells.
- *Surgical management:*
  - *Corneal gluing:* The purpose of using tissue glue for corneal perforation is to urgently restore the tectonic integrity of the globe. Corneal perforation <3 mm in size is amenable to treatment with corneal glue. Also, the outcome of corneal gluing for central corneal perforation is better than peripheral perforation as glue adheres poorly to the adjacent conjunctiva. The two most commonly used tissue glues are synthetic (cyanoacrylate derivatives) and biologic (fibrin glue).[1]
    - *Cyanoacrylate glue:* The *n*-butyl monomer of cyanoacrylate has optimum adhesive strength and polymerization rate and is therefore used in management of corneal perforations <3 mm in size. Since cyanoacrylate is

nonbiodegradable, it induces significant inflammatory reaction, vascularization, foreign body reaction, and tissue necrosis.[2,20]
- *Fibrin glue:* It is biologic in nature and is therefore more biocompatible than cyanoacrylate glue. Fibrin glue is completely biodegradable and therefore induces minimal inflammatory reaction, vascularization, foreign body reaction, and tissue necrosis. The main disadvantage with fibrin glue is that it starts to degrade early and also has no bacteriostatic effect opposed to cyanoacrylate glue.[20]
- *Surgical technique:* Though corneal gluing can be performed on slit lamp, we prefer to perform the same under an operating microscope with aseptic precautions. The patient's eye is cleaned with betadine 5% followed by application of a surgical drape and speculum. A 2-mm trephine is used to cut a circular disc of drape which is adhered to a cotton-tipped applicator with the help of ointment. A drop of cyanoacrylate glue is then place over the circular disc of drape which is then applied to the site of perforation. It is important to keep the site of glue application absolutely dry and remove any debris present prior to glue application. De-epithelizing 1–2 mm of the surrounding corneal epithelium helps in better adherence of the glue. If leakage persists even after application of glue, augmentation can be done with application of another drop of glue around the previous site or the previous glue patch can be removed with re-application of glue. If the anterior chamber (AC) is flat, then air or viscoelastic should be used to form the AC prior to glue application. Direct contact of glue with iris tissue should be avoided as it induces severe anterior uveitis. At the end of procedure, a bandage contact lens is applied.[1]
- *Outcome:* It has been observed that >30% cases require a repeat application of glue to seal the corneal perforation and >50% cases require therapeutic keratoplasty for definitive management.[1,21]
- *Complications:* It is difficult to distinguish if the complications observed after application of glue are directly caused by glue or by the infective keratitis itself. The following complications are observed following application of glue:[20]
    - Cataract
    - Glaucoma
    - Corneal neovascularization
    - Giant papillary conjunctivitis
- *Amniotic membrane graft (AMG):* AMG has been described for sealing small corneal perforation (up to 3 mm).[22] Use of AMG for sealing the perforation site in corneal ulcer avoids the need for corneal graft in an acutely inflamed eye wherein the risk of graft failure and complication would be high. Several authors have reported a high success rate of AMG with fibrin sealant compared to AMG alone.[22-24] However, poor outcome was noted in cases with limbal involvement.[23]
- *Techniques:*
    - *Hyperdry AMG with fibrin glue:* Hyperdry AMG is obtained by consecutive treatment with infrared rays and microwave. It is then sterilized with gamma ray irradiation. A single layer of hyperdry AMG is then cut into the desired shape and size, and secured to the site of corneal perforation with the help of fibrin glue. Kitagawa et al. reported good results with this surgical technique.[25]
    - *Fibrin glue-assisted augmented AMG:* In this surgical technique, multiple layers (5–7 layers) of AMG are placed at the site of corneal perforation. Fibrin glue is used for adhering the layers of AMG to each other and 10-0 nylon is used for securing the AMG to the corneal surface. The size of AMG is designed to be 0.5 mm larger than the maximum dimension of corneal perforation. Kim et al. reported a success rate of 90% with this technique.[23]
- *Tenon patch graft:* Tenon patch graft is a good option for sealing corneal perforations that are not amenable to treatment with only glue. Corneal perforations with size 3–6 mm in size are ideal candidate for Tenon patch graft.
    - *Technique:* Peritomy is done at 4–5 mm from the limbus in the inferonasal or inferotemporal quadrant and the underlying Tenon capsule is then exposed. Tenon graft with size slightly larger than the size of corneal perforation is then obtained. The debris present at the host site corneal surface is cleared. The corneal epithelium of 2 mm zone around the site of perforation is gently removed with a 26-G needle. The surface is then dried with a Weck-Cell sponge. The Tenon patch graft is then placed over the perforation covering the iris and overlapping the edges of the corneal defect and sealed with the help of fibrin glue.[26] Cyanoacrylate glue may be applied to the edge of graft and later over the entire Tenon graft. Also, some authors prefer to suture the Tenon graft with 10-0 nylon suture to the corneal surface for better stability and support.[27] At this step it is essential to ensure that the AC is formed. In case of collapsed AC, reformation can be performed with air injection through a 30-G needle. Bandage contact lens is then placed over the cornea.[26]
    - *Outcome:* Korah et al. in his retrospective study of 28 cases reported an anatomical success rate of 74.1% with this procedure.[26] Most of the cases heal with formation of an adherent leukoma with formed AC.

The main advantage of this procedure is that it is independent of tissue availability, as is the case with corneal graft and AMG. Also, there is no antigenic sensitization and the patient can safely undergo a subsequent corneal graft without any increased risk of graft rejection.[26]
- *Complication:* The complications associated with Tenon patch graft are formation of corneal fistula, graft ectasia, and endophthalmitis.[27]
- *Conjunctival flap:* Conjunctival flaps have also been described for cases of perforated corneal ulcer though they are more commonly used for cases with severe corneal thinning and nonhealing/progressive ulceration.
- *Corneal transplantation:*
  - Patch graft
  - Therapeutic penetrating keratoplasty.

References

1. Jhanji V, Young AL, Mehta JS, Sharma N, Agarwal T, Vajpayee RB. Management of corneal perforation. Surv Ophthalmol. 2011;56(6):522-38.
2. Vote BJ, Elder MJ. Cyanoacrylate glue for corneal perforations: a description of a surgical technique and a review of the literature. Clin Experiment Ophthalmol. 2000;28(6):437-42.
3. Portnoy SL, Insler MS, Kaufman HE. Surgical management of corneal ulceration and perforation. Surv Ophthalmol. 1989;34(1):47-58.
4. Sharma N, Sachdev R, Jhanji V, Titiyal JS, Vajpayee RB. Therapeutic keratoplasty for microbial keratitis. Curr Opin Ophthalmol. 2010;21(4):293-300.
5. Sharma N, Jain M, Sehra SV, Maharana P, Agarwal T, Satpathy G, et al. Outcomes of therapeutic penetrating keratoplasty from a tertiary eye care centre in northern India. Cornea. 2014;33(2):114-8.
6. Lalitha P, Prajna NV, Kabra A, Mahadevan K, Srinivasan M. Risk factors for treatment outcome in fungal keratitis. Ophthalmology. 2006;113(4):526-30.
7. Cohen KL. Sterile corneal perforation after cataract surgery in Sjögren's syndrome. Br J Ophthalmol. 1982;66(3):179-82.
8. Krachmer JH, Laibson PR. Corneal thinning and perforation in Sjögren's syndrome. Am J Ophthalmol. 1974;78(6):917-20.
9. Gilbert C. The eye signs of vitamin A deficiency. Community Eye Health. 2013;26(84):66-7.
10. Md Noh UK, Then KY. Spontaneous bilateral corneal perforation in Stevens-Johnsons syndrome: a challenge in management. Malays J Med Sci. 2013;20(1):84-7.
11. Cao Y, Zhang W, Wu J, Zhang H, Zhou H. (2017). Peripheral ulcerative keratitis associated with autoimmune disease: Pathogenesis and Treatment. [online] Available from https://www.hindawi.com/journals/joph/2017/7298026/. [Last accessed July, 2022].
12. Young RD, Watson PG. Light and electron microscopy of corneal melting syndrome (Mooren's ulcer). Br J Ophthalmol. 1982;66(6):341-56.
13. Sangwan VS, Zafirakis P, Foster CS. Mooren's ulcer: current concepts in management. Indian J Ophthalmol. 1997;45(1):7.
14. Titiyal JS, Negi S, Anand A, Tandon R, Sharma N, Vajpayee RB. Risk factors for perforation in microbial corneal ulcers in north India. Br J Ophthalmol. 2006;90(6):686-9.
15. McElvanney AM. Doxycycline in the management of pseudomonas corneal melting: two case reports and a review of the literature. Eye Contact Lens. 2003;29(4):258-61.
16. Herretes S, Wang X, Reyes JMG. Topical corticosteroids as adjunctive therapy for bacterial keratitis. Cochrane Database Syst Rev. 2014;10(10):CD005430.
17. Srinivasan M, Mascarenhas J, Rajaraman R, Ravindran M, Lalitha P, Glidden DV, et al. Corticosteroids for bacterial keratitis: the steroids for corneal ulcers trial (SCUT). Arch Ophthalmol. 2012;130(2):143-50.
18. Tandon R, Chawla B, Verma K, Sharma N, Titiyal JS. Outcome of treatment of Mooren ulcer with topical cyclosporine a 2%. Cornea. 2008;27(8):859-61.
19. Stammen J, Althaus C, Sundmacher R. Mooren ulcer: 4 severe bilateral disease courses with systemic cyclosporin A therapy. Klin Monatsbl Augenheilkd. 1997;211(5):306-11.
20. Sharma A, Kaur R, Kumar S, Gupta P, Pandav S, Patnaik B, et al. Fibrin glue versus N-butyl-2-cyanoacrylate in corneal perforations. Ophthalmology. 2003;110(2):291-8.
21. Moorthy S, Jhanji V, Constantinou M, Beltz J, Graue-Hernandez EO, Vajpayee RB. Clinical experience with N-butyl cyanoacrylate tissue adhesive in corneal perforations secondary to herpetic keratitis. Cornea. 2010;29(9):971-5.
22. Hick S, Demers PE, Brunette I, La C, Mabon M, Duchesne B. Amniotic membrane transplantation and fibrin glue in the management of corneal ulcers and perforations: a review of 33 cases. Cornea. 2005;24(4):369-77.
23. Kim HK, Park HS. Fibrin glue-assisted augmented amniotic membrane transplantation for the treatment of large noninfectious corneal perforations. Cornea. 2009;28(2):170-6.
24. Rodríguez-Ares MT, Touriño R, López-Valladares MJ, Gude F. Multilayer amniotic membrane transplantation in the treatment of corneal perforations. Cornea. 2004;23(6):577-83.
25. Kitagawa K, Yanagisawa S, Watanabe K, Yunoki T, Hayashi A, Okabe M, et al. A hyperdry amniotic membrane patch using a tissue adhesive for corneal perforations and bleb leaks. Am J Ophthalmol. 2009;148(3):383-9.

26. Korah S, Selvin SST, Pradhan ZS, Jacob P, Kuriakose T. Tenons patch graft in the management of large corneal perforations. Cornea. 2016;35(5):696-9.
27. Maharana PK, Singhal D, Sahay P, Titiyal JS. Tenon patch graft for corneal fistula: a rare entity treated by a simple technique. BMJ Case Rep. 2017;2017:bcr2017222790.

Q 11. Describe the etiology, clinical features, approach, and management of herpes simplex virus keratitis.

Introduction

The herpes simplex virus (HSV) is a double-stranded DNA virus, which belongs to the *Herpesviridae* family of viruses. It is derived from the Greek word "herpes" which means "to creep or crawl." Humans are the only natural host and reservoir of HSV. There are two types of HSV namely HSV 1 transmitted by oropharyngeal secretions and HSV 2 transmitted by genital route.

Ocular infections are primarily caused by HSV type-1, and can range from epithelial keratitis to keratouveitis and retinitis. HSV keratitis is a leading cause of corneal blindness in the United States[1] and is highly ubiquitous. Studies examining the presence of HSV-1 DNA in the trigeminal ganglia have determined that at least 90%[2] of the world's population is infected with latent HSV-1 during their lifetime. HSV causes mucocutaneous infections in humans that are characterized by multiple recurrences, as the virus travels through sensory neurons to the nearest sensory ganglion and persists indefinitely in a latent state.

Pathophysiology

Herpes simplex virus is typically spread by direct contact, most often from virus shed into saliva or genital secretions. It can be acquired following contact with an active orolabial lesion. Asymptomatic individuals regularly shed HSV in their saliva, and therefore, HSV can also be acquired by contact with virus-laden saliva of asymptomatic patients. On infection, HSV binds to one or more cellular receptors and fuses with cell membrane. It enters the cell and nucleus where the transcription of viral DNA occurs. Both humoral and cellular immune mechanisms are involved in the pathophysiology.

After peripheral entry and primary infection, HSV travels in a retrograde fashion. The virus travels by axonal transport to neuronal cell bodies into the nucleus of the neuron on the superior cervical ganglia, the trigeminal ganglia, and the brainstem. Here, it resides during the entire lifespan of the host. Reactivation from latent state results in production of large amount of antisense RNA and cascade of events leading to production of viral polypeptides and intact infectious virus.

Factors causing reactivation are:[3]
- Fever
- Ultraviolet exposure
- Hormonal changes
- Psychological stress
- Ocular trauma
- Immunocompromised status such as HIV, diabetes mellitus, and transplant recipients
- Trigeminal nerve manipulation
- Surgical procedures such as laser assisted in situ keratomileusis (LASIK) and photorefractive keratectomy (PRK).

Clinical Features

Ocular herpes can present in three forms:
1. Congenital ocular herpes
2. Primary ocular herpes
3. Recurrent ocular herpes

Symptoms: A case of HSV keratitis can present with following symptoms:
- Foreign body sensation
- Extreme ocular pain
- Blurry vision
- Watery eyes
- Red eyes
- Photophobia.

Signs: Herpes simplex virus keratitis has multiple manifestations. The distinctive nature of these manifestations can be readily distinguished upon careful examination for involvement of the individual layers of the cornea (epithelium, stroma, and endothelium).

Herpes simplex virus keratitis can be simply classified based on anatomical localization of the principal site of corneal involvement.

HSV Keratitis: Classification[1]

Corneal layer	Nomenclature	Alternate terms
Epithelium	Infectious epithelial keratitis	• Dendritic epithelial ulcer • Geographic epithelial ulcer • Marginal ulcer
	Neurotrophic keratopathy	• Metaherpetic ulcer • Trophic ulcer
Stroma	HSV stromal keratitis without ulceration	• Non-necrotizing keratitis • Interstitial keratitis • Immune stromal keratitis
	HSV stromal keratitis with ulceration	Necrotizing keratitis
Endothelium	HSV endothelial keratitis	• Disciform keratitis • Diffuse keratitis • Linear keratitis

Infectious epithelial keratitis: It is caused by the presence of live virus. Patient presents with lacrimation, photophobia, irritation, and blurred vision occasionally.

Corneal lesions may manifest in various forms:

Punctate epithelial keratitis: The earliest epithelial lesions of HSV. Characterized by minute clear vesicles that correspond to the vesicular skin and mucosal eruptions. Patients generally do not present at this stage.

Dendritic ulcer: Vesicles coalesce to form a raised dendritic lesion (negative staining) which is clinically the precursor of the dendritic ulcer which is the most common presentation. Characterized by branching epithelial lesion with terminal bulbs and swollen epithelial borders that contain live virus. The dendritic pattern is due to the function of viral linear spread by contiguous cell to cell movement and represents the viral tract. Dendritic ulcers demonstrate a double-staining pattern:
- Along the length of the lesion—fluorescein stain
- Swollen epithelial cells and border—rose Bengal stain

The area over the dendritic ulceration is typically anesthetic.

Geographic ulcer: Occur due to enlargement and widening of dendritic ulcers which takes an amoeboid shape. They are true ulcers having swollen epithelial borders containing live virus. These ulcers have a relatively longer duration of symptoms and healing. They may be associated with previous use of topical corticosteroids.

Marginal ulcer: It is an uncommon manifestation of viral keratitis. It is essentially a dendritic ulcer present marginally, generally near a blood vessel. Its unique feature is its proximity to the limbus and intense inflammation. The typical presentation is of anterior stromal infiltrates underlying the ulcer and adjacent limbal injection. The etiopathogenesis involves both immune reaction and active viral infection. Immune reaction is more difficult to treat and may require topical corticosteroids. It is important to differentiate it from staphylococcal marginal keratitis.

Difference between herpes simplex virus marginal keratitis and staphylococcal marginal keratitis[1]

Characteristics	Staphylococcal marginal keratitis	HSV marginal keratitis
Cause	Immunologic response to staphylococcal antigen	Active virus
Associated blepharitis	Associated	None
Location	2, 4, 8, 10 o'clock meridians (point of contact of lid)	Any meridian
Epithelial defect	Usually absent	Present often dendritic
Infiltration	Infiltrate develops first followed by ulceration in late stages	Begins as an ulcer in which later infiltrate develops
Neovascularization	Absent	Usually present
Progression	Circumferentially	Centrally

(HSV: herpes simplex virus)

Sequelae of infectious epithelial keratitis:
- Complete resolution
- Dendritic epitheliopathy
- Stromal scarring
- Stromal disease—necrotizing or immune.

Neurotrophic epithelial keratopathy: It develops in patients with previous HSV epithelial keratitis due to damage to the Gasserian ganglion resulting in impaired corneal innervation and decreased tear secretion. It is exaggerated by chronic use of antivirals.

It presents as irregular corneal surface with loss of luster. There is presence of punctate epithelial erosions progressing to persistent epithelial defect. Neurotrophic ulcers are round to oval ulcers with rolled margins. Complications of neurotrophic keratopathy include: stromal scarring, neovascularization, corneal necrosis, perforation, and secondary bacterial infections.

Stromal Keratitis

Immune stromal keratitis: It is also known as interstitial keratitis and is a type 3 immune-mediated reaction associated with deposition of antigen–antibody complex in the stroma. Retained viral antigens in the stroma are the triggers for the immune reaction. The overlying epithelium is usually intact. It manifests as punctate stromal opacities, immune ring of Wessely, stromal neovascularization, or limbal vasculitis. Secondary lipid keratopathy may occur as a result of persistent inflammation.

Necrotizing stromal keratitis: It is caused due to direct viral invasion of the stroma and active viral replication. It occurs when topical steroids are administered without use of antiviral cover. The clinical features are of corneal necrosis, ulceration with dense infiltration of stroma. It may lead to corneal thinning and perforation.

Endotheliitis

Viral endotheliitis is caused by a type 4 cell-mediated hypersensitivity reaction to viral antigens by T lymphocytes (delayed-type hypersensitivity). It results in inflammatory reaction of the endothelium leading to stromal and epithelial edema, characterized by the presence of keratic precipitates (KPs), epithelial edema, and iritis.

Spectrum of endotheliitis: Disciform, diffuse, and linear

Features	Disciform	Diffuse	Linear
KPs	Disc-shaped distribution in central or paracentral area	Scattered KPs spread out over the entire endothelium	Line of KPs progressing from the limbus
Stroma	Disc-shaped area of edema	Stromal edema involving the entire cornea	Edema present peripheral to the line of KPs, extending into the limbus
Epithelium	Microcystic edema corresponding to severe stromal edema	Microcystic edema corresponding to severe stromal edema	Microcystic edema corresponding to severe stromal edema
Clinical course	Responds to topical corticosteroids	Treatment with topical and systemic corticosteroids and antivirals leads to resolution	• Aggressive treatment with systemic and topical antivirals and corticosteroids • Corneal decompensation is common

(KP: keratic precipitate)

Differential Diagnosis

Herpes zoster keratitis	Medicamentosa keratitis	Acanthamoeba keratitis	Others
• Thick ropy pseudodendrites • Elevated painted on appearance • Absence of terminal bulbs, minimal staining	• Chronic use of topical medication • Topical antibiotics, steroids • Contact lens solution • BAK preservative	• Elevated linear pseudodendrites • Radial keratoneuritis, microcysts • Ring-shaped stromal infiltrate	• Tyrosinemia • Rosacea • Trauma • Contact lens keratitis

(BAK: benzalkonium chloride)

Diagnosis

The diagnosis of HSV keratitis is done primarily on clinical examination but microbiological demonstration of the virus in culture and by staining helps making a definite diagnosis.

Cytologic examination: Tzanck smear is prepared by staining specimens obtained by corneal scraping, with Wright, Papanicolaou, or Giemsa stain. The characteristic finding is the presence of Cowdry type A intranuclear acidophilic inclusion bodies. In addition, multinucleated giant cells may also be seen. These staining techniques are rapid but not sensitive, thus, a negative result does not exclude HSV infection.

Viral culture: The virus is relatively easy to isolate from corneal scrapings by the inoculation of the rabbit cornea, the brains of suckling mice, the chorioallantoic membrane of embryonated hen's eggs, or a variety of tissue culture cells. Virus can be recovered readily from previously untreated dendritic ulcers.

The lesion is swabbed and placed in viral transport media or into viral monolayer tubes and sent to laboratory where carrier medium is inoculated into cultures. A typical cytopathic effect is noticed in 5–10 days and the virus recovery rate is higher if the specimen is taken within 2–3 days of appearance of lesion.[4]

Polymerase chain reaction (PCR): PCR is a highly sensitive tool to demonstrate herpes viral DNA. It is less responsive in patients with atypical lesions. In stromal keratitis, PCR may be negative, since the condition is due to the host immune response rather than direct viral infections. Dyes, such as rose Bengal and lissamine green, inhibit the detection of HSV DNA by PCR assay and thus may give false negative results.[5]

Enzyme linked immunosorbent assay (ELISA): ELISA and immunological tests such as immunofiltration test, latex agglutination assays can be used to demonstrate antiviral antibodies and viral antigen. Immunologic tests for the detection of ocular HSV are commercially available and can detect HSV antigen in cell culture and direct specimens within 5 hours. Along with PCR, ELISA has also been used to detect virus in tear collections.[6] ELISA has relatively low sensitivity and high specificity.

Treatment

Treatment of HSV ocular infections should be aimed at preserving the vision and reducing patient morbidity. Since herpes simplex infections are recurrent in nature, prevention of recurrences is extremely important in long-term management.

Management of Epithelial Keratitis

The mainstay of treatment for infectious epithelial keratitis is topical antiviral drugs. An adjuvant, often useful therapy is epithelial debridement, which reduces the viral load. This is performed by removal of the loose corneal epithelium with a dry, cotton-tipped applicator. The debrided epithelium can be sent for viral culture.

Topical antiviral drugs administered include 3% acyclovir ointment 5 times/day or 1% trifluridine solution 2 hourly when awake or ganciclovir gel 0.15% every 3 hours while awake. Topical antivirals are usually continued for 10–14 days. After 5–7 days, ganciclovir is usually tapered to three times a day for the duration of the treatment period, and trifluridine is usually tapered to five times a day for the rest of the treatment period. Epithelial lesions usually heal by 2 weeks as it takes 14 days for virus loaded basal epithelial cells to reach the surface and to shed off. Any epithelial keratitis persisting beyond 2 weeks with standard antiviral medication raises suspicion of epithelial toxicity or rarely antiviral resistance.

Supportive treatment with tear substitutes, prophylactic antibiotics, and cycloplegics can be added. Corticosteroids are not recommended in the treatment of infectious epithelial keratitis unless associated with significant stromal involvement.

Management of Neurotrophic Keratitis

The goals of treatment of neurotrophic keratitis are to avoid potentially toxic medications, prevent progression of corneal damage, and to promote epithelial healing. Therapeutic approaches include stopping of topical antiviral agents which are highly epitheliotoxic, and initiation of nonpreserved artificial tears and ointments. In cases of nonhealing ulcers, bandage contact lens (BCL) or amniotic membrane graft can be used. Other alternatives include a surgical tarsorrhaphy, botulinum toxin injection, or conjunctival flaps.

Management of Stromal Keratitis and Endotheliitis

Immune Stromal Keratitis

Immune stromal keratitis is the result of hypersensitivity reaction and hence topical steroids are the treatment of choice. Corticosteroids reduce severity of stromal inflammation, decrease the disease duration, and decrease resultant corneal scarring and neovascularization.

The dose of topical steroids is 0.1% dexamethasone or 1% prednisolone eye drops 4-6 times for severe disease to 0.12% prednisolone eye drops daily QID for less severe cases. Steroids are then tapered after 1 week depending upon the clinical response. It is recommended that topical antivirals should be administered along with corticosteroids with equal frequency. A mydriatic-cycloplegic can be added to decrease the ciliary spasm.

Necrotizing Stromal Keratitis

In mild cases of necrotizing stromal keratitis, topical corticosteroids are administered. In all cases, administration of topical corticosteroids is to be accompanied with topical antiviral drugs like 1% trifluridine or 3% acyclovir ointment. Topical corticosteroids have to be tapered very gradually over months usually 10 weeks to avoid reactivation of virus and rebound inflammation. Mydriatic cycloplegic drugs like 2% homatropine and 1% cyclopentolate are added to reduce ciliary spasm.

Oral antivirals are indicated in:
- Severe diffuse endotheliitis
- Herpetic iridocyclitis/trabeculitis
- Immunocompromised patients
- Prophylaxis in recurrent epithelial keratitis
- Prophylaxis for post PK patients with history of HSV keratitis
- Pediatric patients.

Summary of oral antiviral drugs used in HSV keratitis

Drug	Mechanism of action	Treatment dose	Prophylactic dose
Acyclovir	Activated by viral thymidine kinase to inhibit DNA polymerase	400 mg 5 times/day	400 mg BD usually for 1 year
Famciclovir	It is a prodrug that is converted by first-pass metabolism to the antiviral drug penciclovir which further inhibits DNA polymerase of susceptible viruses	500 mg BD	250 mg BD
Valacyclovir	Activated by viral thymidine kinase to inhibit DNA polymerase	1,000 mg TDS	500 mg OD

Herpetic Eye Disease Study (HEDS), done in USA, was a multiarmed set of five randomized placebo controlled trials designed to determine best treatments and prophylaxis of HSV keratitis and one epidemiologic study to investigate for risk factors of HSV.[7]

Summary of HEDS1

Group	Comparison	Results
HSV stromal keratitis (On topical trifluridine but not on steroids)	Group 1—Topical 1% prednisolone acetate Group 2—Placebo	Faster resolution with steroids Final visual acuity same
HSV stromal keratitis (On topical trifluridine and prednisolone 1%)	Group 1—Oral acyclovir 400 mg 5 times/day for 10 weeks Group 2—Placebo	No benefit of oral acyclovir
HSV iridocyclitis (On topical trifluridine and prednisolone 1%)	Group 1—Oral acyclovir 400 mg 5 times/day for 10 weeks Group 2—Placebo	Decrease in treatment failure rate with oral acyclovir

(HSV: herpes simplex virus)

Summary of HEDS2

Group	Comparison	Results
HSV epithelial keratitis trial (On topical trifluridine)	Group 1—Oral acyclovir 400 mg 5 times/day Group 2—Placebo	No added advantage
HSV acyclovir prevention trial (Past history of keratitis within 1 year)	Group 1—Oral acyclovir 400 mg BD for 1 year Group 2—Oral placebo	41% decrease in recurrence 50% decrease in more severe keratitis
HSV risk factors study	Risk factors evaluated	*Risk factors:* History of epithelial keratitis

Surgical Management

Surgical modalities employed in herpetic keratitis include conjunctival flap, amniotic membrane transplantation, surgical tarsorrhaphy, cyanoacrylate glue with BCL, and lamellar or penetrating keratoplasty. Keratoplasty in herpetic disease is indicated in cases of corneal perforation to maintain corneal integrity and for restoration of vision in cases of healed keratitis. Keratoplasty done in cases of herpetic eye disease usually have a high failure rate and the recurrence of herpetic infection has been reported in 12–19% cases.[7] It is important to differentiate postkeratoplasty graft rejection from viral reactivation. In cases of graft rejection, the inflammation is confined only to the donor cornea while in viral reactivation both host and donor cornea are involved. The KP's are typically seen on donor endothelium without affecting the host part in acute graft rejection while both host and graft are involved in case of viral reactivation. Also, epithelial rejection line and Khodadoust endothelial rejection line are typically seen in cases of graft rejection. The raised epithelial rejection line can sometimes be misdiagnosed as viral dendritic keratitis. In addition, a typical Khodadoust line may not be evident in all cases of endothelial graft rejection and can be misdiagnosed as viral keratouveitis. Thus, a definite distinction between graft rejection and viral reactivation is not always easy.

Treatment Summary

Lesion	Treatment
Infectious epithelial keratitis	• E/o Acyclovir 3% 5 time/day for 1 week followed by 3 times/day for 2 weeks • ± epithelial debridement
Neurotrophic keratitis	• Withdraw epitheliotoxic drugs • Use—Lubricants, BCL • Patching • Tarsorrhaphy • Amniotic membrane
Stromal keratitis	• E/o 3% Acyclovir 5 times/day for 1 week followed by 3 times/day for 3 weeks + • E/d Prednisolone acetate 1% 2–4 hourly followed by tapering over 6–8 weeks
Endothelial keratitis	• E/o 3% Acyclovir 5 times/day for 1 week followed by • 3 times/day for 3 weeks + • E/d Prednisolone acetate 1% 2–4 hourly followed by tapering over 6–8 weeks
Herpetic keratouveitis	• E/o 3% Acyclovir 5 times/day for 1 week followed by 3 times/day for 3 weeks + • E/d Prednisolone acetate 1% 2–4 hourly + (after the epithelium heals) followed by tapering over 6–8 weeks • E/d Homoatropine 2% 4 times/day + • Oral Acyclovir 400 mg 5 times/day 10 weeks + • Antiglaucoma drugs if needed

References

1. Holland EJ, Brilakis HS, Schwartz GS. Herpes simplex keratitis. In: Krachmer JH, Mannis MJ, Holland EJ (Eds). Cornea, 2nd edition. St. Louis: Mosby; 2004. pp. 1043-74.
2. Cohrs RJ, Randall J, Smith J, Gilden DH, Dabrowski C, van Der Keyl H, et al. Analysis of individual human trigeminal ganglia for latent herpes simplex virus type 1 and varicella-zoster virus nucleic acids using real-time PCR. J Virol. 2000;74(24):11464-71.
3. Pepose JS, Keadle TL, Morrison LA. Ocular herpes simplex: changing epidemiology, emerging disease patterns, and the potential of vaccine prevention and therapy. Am J Ophthalmol. 2006;141(3):547-57.
4. Shimeld C, Tullo AB, Easty DL, Thomsitt J. Isolation of herpes simplex virus from the cornea in chronic stromal keratitis. Br J Ophthalmol. 1982;66(10):643-7.
5. Seitzman GD, Cevallos V, Margolis TP. Rose bengal and lissamine green inhibit detection of herpes simplex virus by PCR. Am J Ophthalmol. 2006;141(4):756-8.
6. Satpathy G, Mishra AK, Tandon R, Sharma MK, Sharma A, Nayak N, et al. Evaluation of tear samples for herpes simplex virus 1 (HSV) detection in suspected cases of viral keratitis using PCR assay and conventional laboratory diagnostic tools. Br J Ophthalmol. 2011;95(3):415-8.
7. Oral acyclovir for herpes simplex virus eye disease: effect on prevention of epithelial keratitis and stromal keratitis. Herpetic Eye Disease Study Group. Arch Ophthalmol. 2000;118(8):1030-6.

12. Describe the etiology, clinical features, approach, and management of filamentary keratitis.

Introduction

Filamentary keratitis (FK) is a form of chronic and recurrent disorder of the ocular surface mainly involving the cornea and rarely, conjunctiva. It is characterized by the deposition of mucin filaments on the corneal surface.

Filamentary keratitis has been reported to be associated with several ocular surface disorders such as dry eye, keratoconjunctivitis, exposure keratitis, allergic conjunctivitis, postcataract surgery, brainstem injury, penetrating keratoplasty (PKP), ptosis, recurrent erosion, prolonged eye patch use, and large-angle strabismus.[1] FK is diagnosed clinically on slit-lamp biomicroscopic examination.

Pathophysiology

The majorly accepted composition of these filaments is a combination of degenerated epithelial cells with mucus. The composition of these filaments has been described by Tanioka et al.[2] Light microscopic analysis has shown that filaments contain a core of eosinophilic cells (corneal or conjunctival epithelium) with spindle-shaped cytoplasm and nuclei which are surrounded by basophilic fibers and areas including basophilic segments and polymorphic nucleic cells. Immunostaining demonstrated a central core of CK12-positive corneal epithelium surrounded by CK4- and CK13-positive conjunctival epithelium, peripheral mucin, deoxyribonucleic acid (DNA), and inflammatory cells. The mucin is positive for MUC1, MUC4, MUC5AC, and MUC16 and inflammatory cells are positive human leukocyte antigen–DR isotype (HLA-DR) and neutrophil elastase.

However, it has been shown earlier that these filaments are primarily composed of mucus with epithelial squamous cells, lipids, and foreign matter taken up secondarily.[3]

Several authors have described the theories leading to formation of the filaments in FK.

- *Zaidman theory:* The authors used transmission electron microscopy in a patient with brainstem disease to formulate this theory. It was seen that there is accumulation of inflammatory cells and fibroblasts below the basal epithelium with disruption of the epithelial basement membrane and Bowman's layer. This leads to epithelial basement membrane detachment due to the shearing force of eyelids. Then, the area of raised epithelium acts as a receptor for the mucus and the debris produced due to irregular corneal surface.[4]
- *Maudgal theory:* According to this theory, there are areas of focal degeneration of the corneal epithelial cells along with deposition of overlying mucus. This is followed by migration of surrounding epithelial cells into that area with focal defect. These cells are also covered by mucus, leading to the formation of a protuberance. This further gets elevated with the continued migration of epithelial cells forming a filament.[5]

Risk Factors/Associations

Various ocular and systemic associations have been reported with FK **(Table 16)**. The major ocular risk factors include dry eye with or without autoimmune diseases, meibomian gland dysfunction (MGD), and exposure keratitis. These conditions are associated with reduced tear secretion or decreased tear film breakup time (TFBUT) thereby leading to poor lubrication of epithelium and increased evaporation with tear film instability. This fragile and dried epithelium is often degenerated leading to focal defects and filament formation. These filaments are formed most commonly in the interpalpebral zone due to the shearing action of the eyelids.[6]

Other ocular surface diseases associated with FK include superior limbic keratoconjunctivitis, recurrent corneal erosions, herpes simplex keratitis, and neurotrophic keratopathy.[5,7]

Systemic diseases seen to be associated with FK include autoimmune diseases such as Sjögren's syndrome, psoriasis, and atopic dermatitis.[7] Brainstem injury may also be associated due to the exposure keratopathy and decreased blink rate. Seventh cranial nerve palsy leading to exposure keratopathy is also associated with FK. It has been described that the filaments seen in autoimmune diseases are located mainly at the limbus due to the rich capillary network leading to influx of lymphocytes, antibodies, and complement factors.[6]

Clinical Features

Symptoms: FK presents with symptoms of burning and foreign body sensation with mild ocular discomfort and pain. Other symptoms include photophobia, epiphora, and blepharospasm.

TABLE 16: Associations of filamentary keratitis.

Category	Examples
Ocular surface disease	• Keratoconjunctivitis sicca • Recurrent corneal erosions • Superior limbic keratoconjunctivitis • Prolonged patching
Infection	• Adenoviral keratitis • Herpes simplex keratitis
Systemic disease	• Cranial nerve palsy • Stevens–Johnson syndrome • Sjögren's syndrome • Psoriasis • Atopic dermatitis
Medication	• Diuretics • Diphenhydramine hydrochloride
Surgery	• Photorefractive keratectomy • Penetrating keratoplasty • Phototherapeutic keratectomy
Others	• Use of contact lenses • Extended patching of eyes

Signs: On slit-lamp examination, filaments are seen as gelatinous strands or protrusions attached to the corneal epithelium. These filaments can either be translucent or granular and may vary in shape from round to slender form.[8] The corneal stroma beneath these filaments is usually normal.[8,9] They can also elongate in size with each blinking and have a high rate of recurrence even after debridement.[n] These filaments stain positive with rose Bengal and fluorescein if there is an underlying epithelial defect while negative staining is seen in cases with elevated filaments.

The location of these filaments depends upon the underlying cause. In cases of dry eye and exposure, they are commonly located at the interpalpebral area while in cases of autoimmune diseases, they are located at the limbus. Filaments associated with ptosis and superior limbic keratoconjunctivitis are often located on the superior cornea while those secondary to PKP are located on the graft near a suture or at the graft–host interface.

Treatment

The initial step in the management of FK involves the management of the underlying cause. The treatment of FK is usually chronic and challenging.[9-13]

Topical Therapy

- *Tear supplements:* Initial management includes topical lubricants with application of ointments at night. High-viscosity tear substitutes may provide relief in severe cases but, at the same time, they may alter the tear film composition. It is always preferred to use preservative-free tear substitutes to prevent toxicity to the epithelium.
- *N-acetylcysteine:* The mainstay of treatment is the use of mucolytic agents like 10% N-acetylcysteine. This compound acts by decreasing the viscosity of the mucus in tear film. The ocular form is not commercially available and must be formulated. The major problem is—it has to be prepared without preservatives hence the self-life is just 7 days, thus the patient has to report every week.
- *Topical steroids:* Steroids can be used in cases of FK with severe dry eye and ocular inflammation. Although dramatic relief can be achieved, it should be used only in severe cases.
- *Topical sodium chloride:* Topical sodium chloride acts by reducing edema and obviates focal detachment in some patients.
- *Topical nonsteroidal anti-inflammatory drugs (NSAIDs):* Role of topical NSAID like diclofenac sodium, 0.1%, has been shown by Avisar et al. They have shown a greater symptomatic relief with topical diclofenac 0.1% as compared to topical 5% sodium chloride in cases of FK with secondary Sjögren's syndrome.

Bandage Contact Lenses

Bandage contact lenses have been used safely and effectively for FK. Complete disappearance of filaments has been reported by Bloomfield et al.[14] These lenses are always recommended along with the topical treatment mentioned above. A regular follow-up is essential to monitor for any contact lens-related complication. They should always be used only when lubricants fail. Other options such as succinylated collagen bandage lenses (SCBL) and amniotic membrane grafts have also been used successfully.[15]

Surgical Management

Surgical options for the management of FK include mechanical debridement of filaments and punctal occlusion.

- *Debridement of filaments:* Mechanical debridement of the filaments is only a temporary measure with a high rate of recurrence. They can be removed with a cotton-tip applicator or tying forceps if large.
- *Punctal occlusion:* It has been reported to be beneficial in cases of FK with severe dry eye by inhibiting the drainage of tears and thus providing symptomatic relief.[16,17] Punctual plugs can either be temporary which include collagen plugs or semipermanent including silicone plugs. Permanent punctual occlusion can be done using thermal or laser cautery.
- *Other options:* Other surgical procedures, which have been proven beneficial for FK, include ptosis surgery and botulinum injection.[18,19]

References

1. Lv H, Liu Z, Li X, Wang W. Effect of lacrimal plugs combined with deproteinized calf blood extract eye gel for filamentary keratitis. J Ocul Biol Dis Infor. 2010;3:134-40.
2. Tanioka H, Yokoi N, Komuro A, Shimamoto T, Kawasaki S, Matsuda A, et al. Investigation of the corneal filament in filamentary keratitis. Invest Ophthalmol Vis Sci. 2009;50(8):3696-702.
3. Wright P. Filamentary keratitis. Trans Ophthalmol Soc UK. 1975;95(2):260-6.
4. Zaidman GW, Geeraets R, Paylor RR, Ferry AP. The histopathology of filamentary keratitis. Arch Ophthalmol. 1985;103:1178-81.
5. Maudgal PC, Missotten L, Van Deuren H. Study of filamentary keratitis by replica technique. Albrecht Von Graefes Arch Klin Exp Ophthalmol. 1979;211(1):11-21.
6. Chen S, Ruan Y, Jin X. Investigation of the clinical features in filamentary keratitis in Hangzhou, east of China. Medicine (Baltimore). 2016;95(35):e4623.
7. Davis WG, Drewry RD, Wood TO. Filamentary keratitis and stromal neovascularization associated with brainstem injury. Am J Ophthalmol. 1980;90(4):489-91.
8. Tabery HM. Filamentary keratopathy: a non-contact photomicrographic in vivo study in the human cornea. Eur J Ophthalmol. 2003;13(7):599-605.
9. Hamilton W, Wood TO. Filamentary keratitis. Am J Ophthalmol. 1982;93(4):466-9.
10. Fraunfelder FT, Wright P, Tripathi RC. Corneal mucus plaques. Am J Ophthalmol. 1977;83(2):191-7.
11. Bloomfield SE, Gasset AR, Forstot SL, Brown SI. Treatment of filamentary keratitis with the soft contact lens. Am J Ophthalmol. 1973;76(6):978-80.
12. Hadassah J, Prakash D, Sehgal PK, Agarwal A, Bhuvaneshwari N. Clinical evaluation of succinylated collagen bandage lenses for ophthalmic applications. Ophthalmic Res. 2008;40(5):257-66.
13. Grinbaum A, Yassur I, Avni I. The beneficial effect of diclofenac sodium in the treatment of filamentary keratitis. Arch Ophthalmol. 2001;119(6):926-7.
14. Avisar R, Robinson A, Appel I, Yassur Y, Weinberger D. Diclofenac sodium, 0.1% (Voltaren Ophtha), versus sodium chloride, 5%, in the treatment of filamentary keratitis. Cornea. 2000;19(2):145-7.
15. Marsh P, Pflugfelder SC. Topical nonpreserved methylprednisolone therapy for keratoconjunctivitis sicca in Sjögren syndrome. Ophthalmology. 1999;106(4):811-6.
16. Ervin AM, Wojciechowski R, Schein O. Punctal occlusion for dry eye syndrome. Cochrane Database Syst Rev. 2010;(9):CD006775.
17. Diller R, Sant S. A case report and review of filamentary keratitis. Optometry. 2005;76(1):30-6.
18. Kakizaki H, Zako M, Mito H, Iwaki M. Filamentary keratitis improved by blepharoptosis surgery: two cases. Acta Ophthalmol Scand. 2003;81(6):669-71.
19. Gumus K, Lee S, Yen MT, Pflugfelder SC. Botulinum toxin injection for the management of refractory filamentary keratitis. Arch Ophthalmol. 2012;130(4):446-50.

 13. Discuss fungal keratitis.

Introduction

Mycotic keratitis is a leading cause of ocular morbidity in developing countries.[1-3] Fungal keratitis constitutes up to 50% of all microbial keratitis worldwide.[3-6] The commonly involved pathogens in tropical areas are filamentous fungi (*Aspergillus, Fusarium,* and *Curvularia*), while in temperate regions are *Candida* species (*C. albicans, C. parapsilosis*).[3]

The management and diagnosis of fungal keratitis are quite challenging. This may be due to the lack of early microbiological identification and limited efficacy and penetration of the antifungal agents.[3,7-9] In cases with failed medical management surgical interventions such as therapeutic keratoplasty (TKP), conjunctival flap, lamellar keratoplasty, or cryotherapy are required for control of infection and visual rehabilitation.[2,8,10,11]

Epidemiology

The incidence of fungal keratitis varies according to geography, climate, and occupation. In the developed countries, the incidence has been estimated to be as low as 6–20%.[12] However, in developing countries it is reported to be 50% of all microbial keratitis.[13]

Most commonly isolated fungal pathogens are the filamentous fungi worldwide with *Aspergillus* species (spp.) being the most common.[14] In India, the most commonly isolated organism in the south is *Fusarium* spp., while in the northern India is *Aspergillus* spp.[15,16]

It is more commonly seen in tropical areas with warm and humid climate. The most common age group is 21–50 years with males being more commonly affected as compared to females. A higher incidence has been reported during monsoon and early winter due to high humidity along with more frequent vegetative injuries during these seasons.[17]

Risk Factors

Various factors predisposing to fungal keratitis can be divided as ocular and systemic. The most common ocular risk factor is trauma with vegetative or organic matter.[16] Other ocular factors associated include contact lens wear, medications, and prior ocular surgery **(Box 1)**.

Etiopathogenesis

Fungal pathogens involved in infective keratitis can be classified into four—filamentous septated, filamentous nonseptated, yeasts, and others **(Box 2)**. These organisms can also be classified into four groups: *Moniliaceae* (nonpigmented filamentary fungi including *Fusarium* spp. and *Aspergillus spp.*); *Dematiaceae* (pigmented filamentary fungi including *Curvularia sp.* and *Lasiodiplodia spp.*); yeasts, including *Candida* spp., and other fungi.

Fungi are either saprophytic or pathogenic organisms. Many fungi associated with keratitis are saprophytic. These organisms often invade into the corneal stroma following epithelial defect that may be caused by various risk factors mentioned above. After the invasion, they proliferate and incite an inflammatory reaction, which leads to tissue necrosis. They can also penetrate through an intact Descemet's membrane (DM) gaining access into the anterior chamber from where it is often difficult to eradicate. Blood-borne growth inhibiting factors may not reach the avascular tissue such as the cornea, anterior chamber, and sclera, and hence the fungi continue to multiply and persist despite treatment.

BOX 1: Risk factors for the development of fungal keratitis.

Ocular factors:
- Trauma
- Chronic corneal inflammation:
  - Herpes simplex
  - Herpes zoster
  - Vernal allergic conjunctivitis
  - Ocular surface problems
  - Dry eye
  - Bullous keratopathy
  - Exposure keratopathy
  - Contact lens wear
- Drugs:
  - Corticosteroids
  - Anesthetics
- Corneal surgery:
  - Penetrating keratoplasty
  - Refractive surgery

Systemic factors:
- Diabetes mellitus
- HIV-positive patients
- Leprosy

Source: Adapted from Fungal Keratitis. In: Sharma N, Vajpayee RB (Eds). Corneal Ulcers: Diagnosis and Management, Chapter 16. New Delhi: Jaypee Brothers Medical Publishers; 2008.

BOX 2: Fungi causing human keratitis.

Septate
- *Nonpigmented:*
  - Fusarium: Solani, oxysporum, moniliforme, episphaesia, nivale
  - Aspergillus: Fumigatus, flavus
  - Acremonium (Cephalosporium)
  - Paecilomyces
  - Penicillium
- *Pigmented (dematiaceous)*
  - Curvularia: Senegalensis, verruculosa, pallescens
  - Lasiodiplodia: Theobromae
  - Alternaria
  - Cladosporium
  - Colletotrichum
  - Drechslera (Helminthosporium)

Nonseptated:
- Rhizopus (mucormycosis)

Yeast:
- Candida:
  - Albicans, Parapsilosis, Krusei, Tropicalis

Source: Adapted from Fungal Keratitis. In: Sharma N, Vajpayee RB (Eds). Corneal Ulcers: Diagnosis and Management, Chapter 16. New Delhi: Jaypee Brothers Medical Publishers; 2008.

Clinical Features

The clinical diagnosis of fungal keratitis is often challenging. It should be made on the basis of a careful evaluation of patient's history, examination, and laboratory investigations **(Box 2)**.

General Symptoms

A patient with fungal keratitis often presents with insidious onset of foreign body sensation with photophobia, gradually progressive pain, and diminution of vision. The patient gives a long duration of history of these symptoms, which are much less than the ocular signs.

General Signs

On slit-lamp examination, a fungal ulcer characteristically appears to have a dry texture with gray-white infiltrates and creamy raised exudates at the base. The characteristic findings include feathery margins (70%) with elevated areas and satellite lesions (10%).[15,18] Presence of a fixed hypopyon (no change in the position after 10 minutes of lying supine) is also a common feature seen in 45–66% cases.[17] Other features include an immune ring, deep stromal abscess, and an endothelial plaque[3] **(Figs. 1A and B and Box 3)**.

Candida keratitis often presents with a "collar button" configuration of infiltrates and *dematiaceous* fungi have a characteristic gray or brown pigmentation. This pigmentation is due to the alteration in melanin metabolism and indicates a more superficial infection with low virulence of the organism and less inflammatory reaction.[19]

Laboratory Diagnosis

The next step after clinical examination of a corneal ulcer is corneal scraping which plays an important role in diagnosis. Scraping should be taken from the base as well as the edge of the ulcer with the help of a surgical blade, Kimura's spatula, or a 26-gauge needle. Other important samples could be contact lenses and solutions used by the patient, any topical medication,

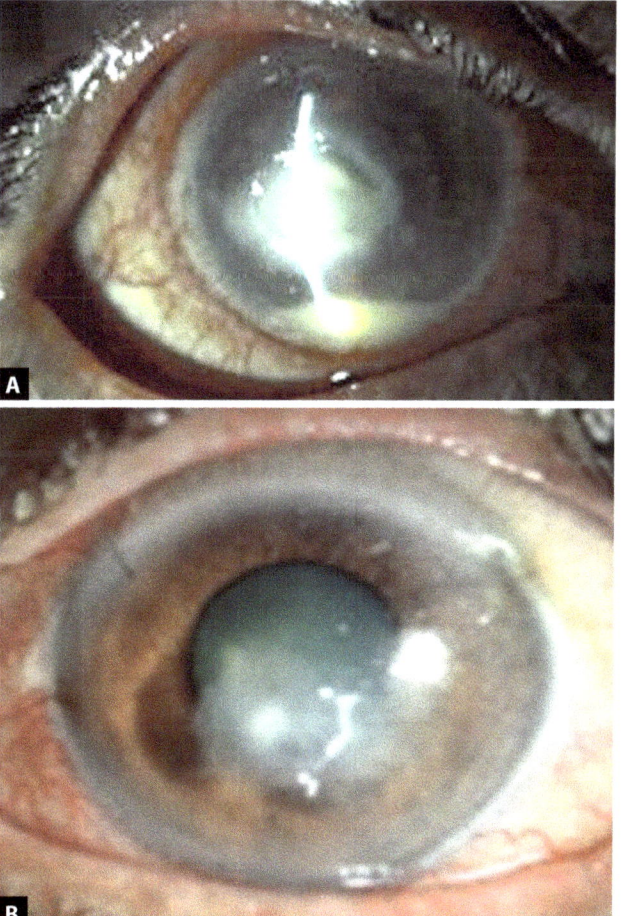

Figs. 1A and B: (A) A case of fungal keratitis following trauma with vegetative matter; (B) Resolving fungal keratitis on medical therapy.

> **BOX 3:** Clinical features of fungal keratitis.
>
> *Nonspecific:*
> - Conjunctival injection
> - Epithelial defect
> - Anterior chamber reaction
>
> *Specific:*
> - Dry look
> - Indolent course
> - Immune ring
> - Infiltrate
> - Feathery margins
> - Gray/brown pigmentation
> - Rough texture
> - Satellite lesions

or cosmetic agents. In cases with deep stromal abscesses without any epithelial defect, anterior chamber tap or corneal biopsy can be taken. The sample obtained should be sent for direct microscopy and culture examination.

Direct Microscopy

This includes 10% KOH wet mount preparation, which is rapid, cheap, and easily available and has a sensitivity of 72–90%.[20,21]

Other staining methods used are Gram stain (31–98% sensitive), Giemsa stain (27–87%), lactophenol cotton blue (70–80%), Grocott's methenamine-silver staining (89%), and calcofluor white stain (80–90% sensitive).[20-22]

Fungal Culture

Sabouraud dextrose agar (without cycloheximide) is commonly used for fungal culture. It should contain 50 µg/mL gentamicin and should be without cycloheximide as this inhibits saprophytic fungi. This is the gold standard method for diagnosis and takes around 2 weeks duration for the result.

Diagnosis of fungal keratitis is made if:
- Smear is positive for fungal elements.
- Fungus growth is positive in more than one medium if there is absence of fungus in smears.
- Fungus grows on a single medium in the presence of fungus in smears.
- Confluent growth at the inoculated site on a single solid medium.

The incidence of culture positivity is reported to be 52–68%.[4,15,18] Before declaring a culture negative for fungi, it is recommended to wait for at least a week. Increasing the humidity of the medium by placing the inoculated agar plates in plastic bags can enhance fungal growth.

Other Diagnostic Modalities

Polymerase Chain Reaction

This technique provides a rapid diagnosis with an early initiation of antifungal treatment. The result is obtained within 4 hours, which can make this technique a valuable adjunctive tool for the diagnosis of fungal keratitis.

Confocal Microscopy

In vivo confocal microscopy (IVCM) is emerging as a tool for early identification of fungal elements due to its property of providing optical sections with a better resolution and contrast. *Aspergillus* hyphae are seen as septate with a diameter of 5–10 µm and 200–400 µm long with dichotomous branching at 45° angle.[4] In contrast, *Fusarium* typically branches at a 90° angle.[23] These hyper-reflective elements must be differentiated from the basal corneal epithelial nerves, which have a more regular branching pattern. Stromal nerves, on the contrary, are much larger in diameter (25–50 µm). In addition, yeast such as *C. albicans* have round, budding bodies that may develop pseudohyphae. The structures are 10–40 µm in length and 5–10 µm in width.[24]

Confocal microscopy has a sensitivity of 94% and a specificity of 78% in patients with fungal keratitis.[25] IVCM is currently the only method that allows determination of the depth of infection which is an important prognostic factor. The main limitation is that it remains extremely user-dependent, as the testing requires a skilled operator, and interpretation requires an experienced viewer. Therefore, cornea cultures remain the gold standard and are required.

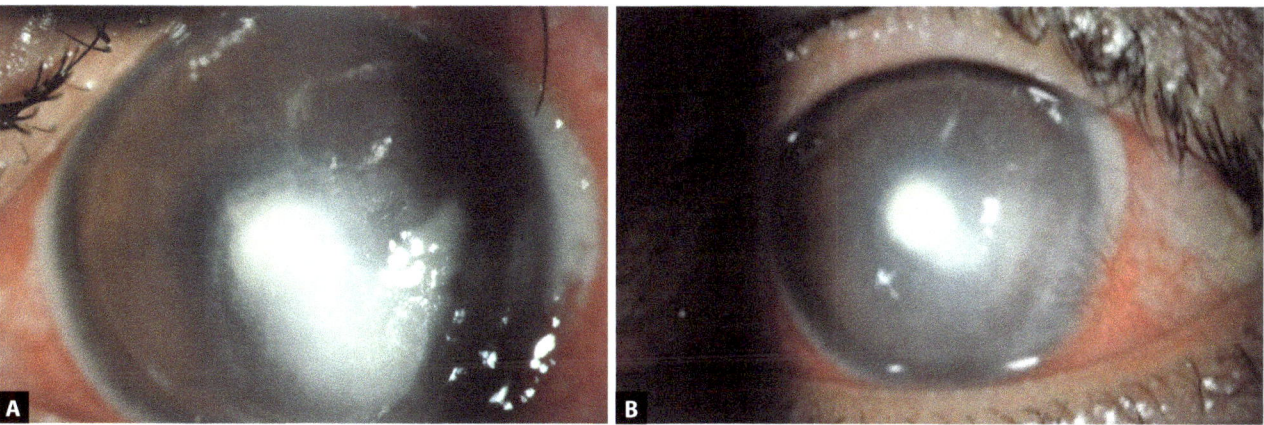

Figs. 2A and B: (A) A case of post-LASIK fungal keratitis with culture positive for *Fusarium* spp; (B) Resolving fungal keratitis on medical therapy. (LASIK: laser-assisted in situ keratomileusis)

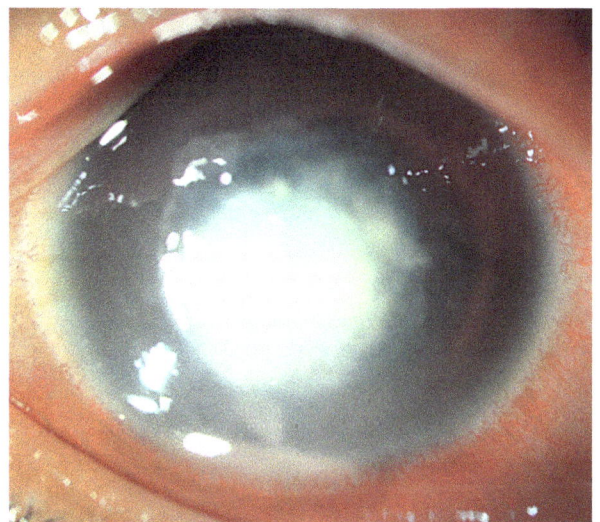

Fig. 3: A case of fungal keratitis showing feathery margins with a fixed hypopyon of 1 mm.

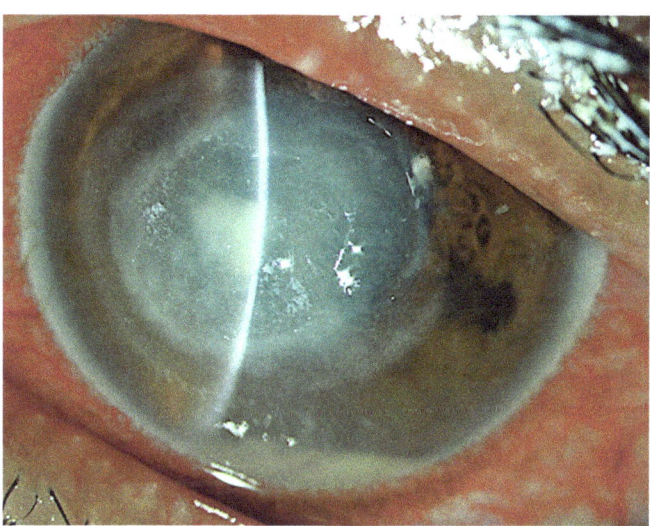

Fig. 4: A case of fungal keratitis showing a central endothelial plaque of 2 × 1.5 mm in size.

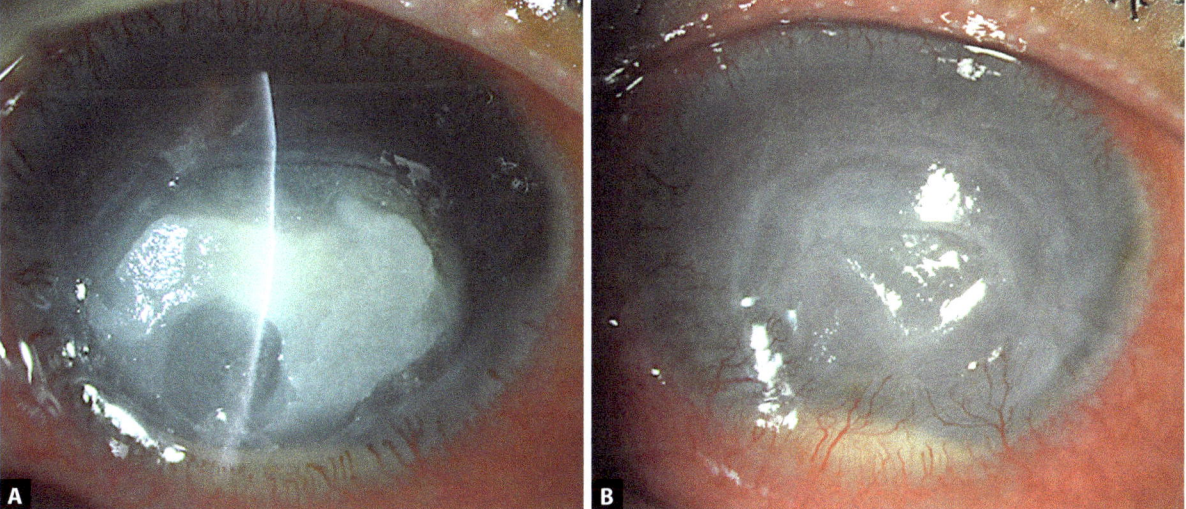

Figs. 5A and B: (A) A case of fungal keratitis showing overlying drug deposits; (B) Resolving fungal keratitis with central thinning after debridement of the drug deposits.

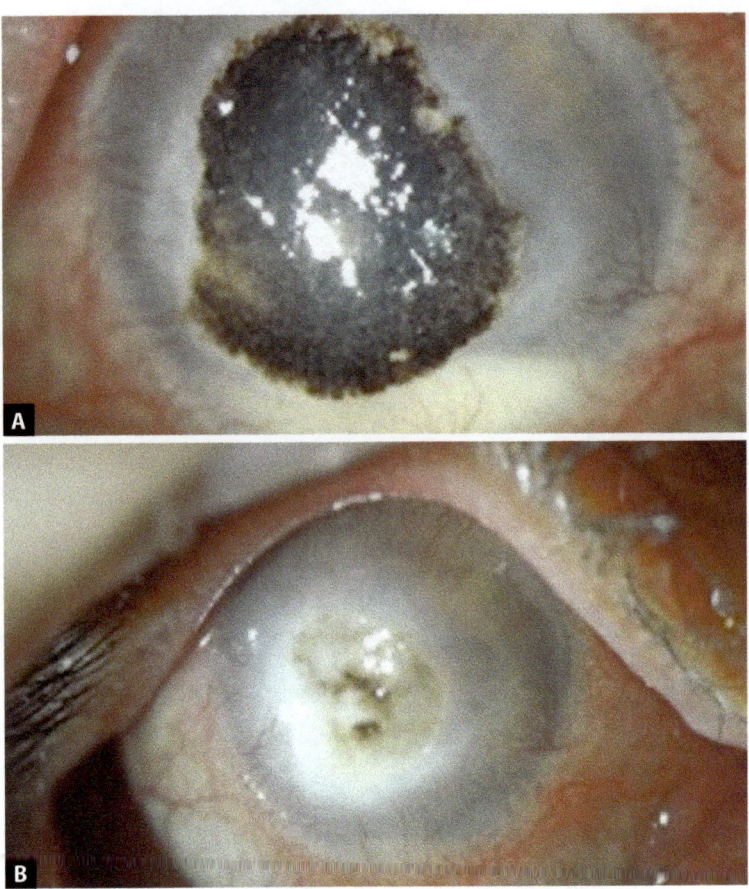

Figs. 6A and B: (A) A case of *Curvularia* keratitis showing central pigmented infiltrates; (B) Resolving *Curvularia* keratitis after epithelial debridement.

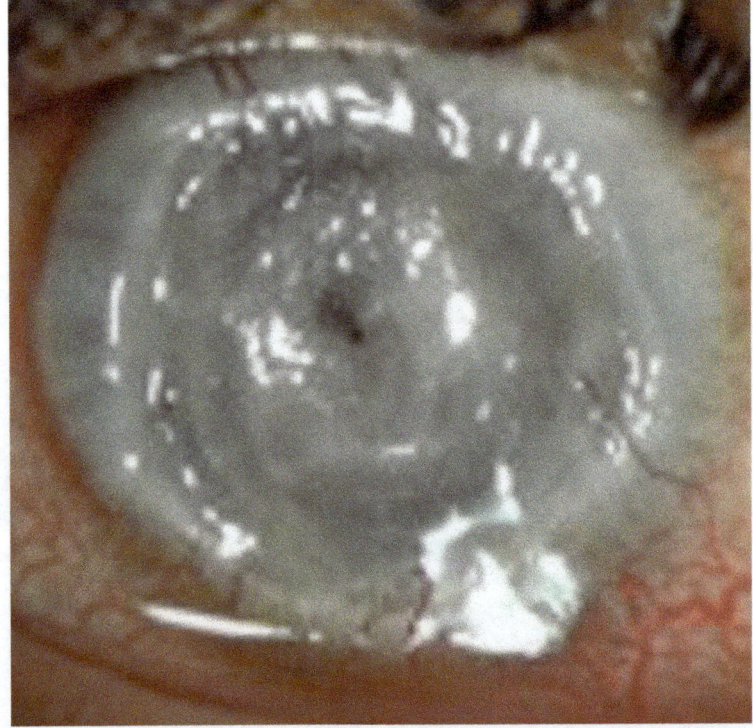

Fig. 7: A case of fungal keratitis showing central perforation and managed with therapeutic keratoplasty.

Management

The management options include medical or surgical intervention in cases not responding to medical therapy alone.

Medical Management

Antifungal drugs should be started once the corneal scraping sample is detected positive for fungal elements or fungal culture report is positive at 36–48 hours. It is not recommended to start antifungal treatment empirically on the basis of clinical examination.

Medical management includes either topical or systemic antifungal agents. The antifungal drugs can be broadly classified into different categories based on their molecular structure and mechanism of action. They are broadly classified as polyenes, azoles, pyrimidines, allylamines, echinocandins, heterocyclics, and others **(Table 17)**.

Topical Antifungal Agents

The initial drug of choice in fungal keratitis is 5% natamycin suspension.[26] It is the only United States Food and Drug Administration (US FDA)-approved topical antifungal drug for mycotic keratitis and is commercially available for ophthalmic use at a concentration of 5% (50 mg/mL). It is recommended to start topical natamycin 5% every 1 hour, for the first 48 hours and then 2 hourly during waking hours till epithelial healing, and then 4 hourly for 3 weeks. In addition, cycloplegics have to be prescribed in the form of topical homatropine 2% four times a day. We also recommend to start a broad-spectrum antibiotic such as a fluoroquinolone to prevent secondary bacterial infection. Antiglaucoma medication should be started in cases with high intraocular pressure (IOP).

These patients have to be examined twice daily to monitor the response of treatment. The frequency of topical natamycin can be decreased to 2 hourly once resolution starts and is continued till complete resolution. It is recommended to continue topical medication for at least 2 weeks after the resolution of infection.

If there is worsening even with topical natamycin other agents can be started according to the species isolated. Topical amphotericin B (AMB) 0.15% is preferred for yeast organisms.

A newer agent that can be used topically is voriconazole (VCZ). It is derived from fluconazole and acts by inhibition of cytochrome P450-dependent 14 alpha-sterol demethylase, an enzyme involved in the ergosterol biosynthesis.[27] It has a broad spectrum of action and can inhibit both yeast and filamentous fungi. The minimal inhibitory concentration of VCZ

TABLE 17: Common antifungals for medical therapy of fungal keratitis.

Drug	Mechanism	Spectrum of action	Routes of administration				
			Topical	Oral	Intravenous	Intrastromal	Intracameral
Polyenes	Binds to fungal cell membranes, altering membrane permeability	• Concentration-dependent killing • Fungicidal or fungistatic depending on the concentration • *In vivo efficacy best:* AUC/MIC ≥25 and/or C_{max}/MIC ≥10 • Optimal frequency for topical administration undetermined • *Recommended dosing:* Initial loading dose of one drop every half hour with a gradual reduction to 6–8 times a day • Do not penetrate intact epithelial barrier					
Amphotericin B		*Amphotericin:* First-line therapy for *Candida* species. Good to moderate activity against *Aspergillus, Fusarium* species	0.05–0.3% (0.15% commonly used)	NA	0.5–0.7 mg/kg		0.8–1.0 mg
Natamycin (pimaricin)		*Natamycin:* Good activity against most *Fusarium, Aspergillus,* less effective against *Candida* species; first-line treatment for fungal keratitis, 2% bioavailability	2.5–5%	Not available	Not available		

Contd...

Contd...

Drug	Mechanism	Spectrum of action	Routes of administration				
			Topical	Oral	Intravenous	Intrastromal	Intracameral
Azoles	Inhibitor of ergosterol biosynthesis of the fungal cell wall, through action on the cytochrome P-450-dependent enzyme. This leads to cell membrane destabilization and leakage	Concentration independent killing (time dependent) Mainly fungistatic; can be fungicidal at high concentrations or growth phase of the fungi *In vivo efficacy:* AUC/MIC >25 *Two classes:* 1. *Imidazoles* (clotrimazole, ketoconazole, miconazole). Do not penetrate intact cornea epithelium very well 2. *Triazoles* (fluconazole, itraconazole, voriconazole, and posaconazole). Good penetration of intact corneal epithelium					
Clotrimazole		*Clotrimazole:* Fungistatic Good activity against *Candida* and some *Aspergillus* species	1% topical 1% cream				
Econazole		*Econazole:* Effective against *Fusarium, Aspergillus,* and *Candida* species	0.02–2%	50–100 mg/day			
Ketoconazole		*Ketoconazole:* Effective against *Candida, Aspergillus,* limited effectiveness against *Fusarium* species	1–2%	200–400 mg/day			
Itraconazole		*Itraconazole: Aspergillus, Candida* species, not effective against *Fusarium*	1%	200–400 mg/day			
Fluconazole		*Fluconazole:* Effective against yeast, minimal activity against filamentous fungi	0.5–1%	100–400 mg/day			
Miconazole		*Miconazole:* Effective against *Paecilomyces, Scedosporium* species	1%		600–1,200/day		5 mg/0.5 mL
		Posaconazole: Limited information, has been used as savage rescue for *Fusarium, Scedosporium,* Spectrum similar to voriconazole		200 mg x3/day			
		Voriconazole: Fungicidal or fungistatic depending on concentration *Candida* species, *Aspergillus* species. non *Fusarium solani* species, *Scedosporium apiospermum*	1–2%	200–400 mg/day		5 mg/mL	50 mg/0.1 mL
Echinocandins	Blocks fungal cell wall beta-glucan synthesis	• Concentration-dependent killing • Fungicidal effective against yeasts, *Aspergillus* species; not effective against *Fusarium* species In vivo efficacy: best predicted by Cmax/MIC >10 or AUC/MIC >25					
Anidulafungin		Limited data					
Caspofungin				0.5%			
Micafungin				0.1%			

(AUC: area under the curve; MIC: minimum inhibitory concentration)
C_{max}/MIC = peak concentration over the MIC, >10; optimal dosing large infrequent doses, concentration-dependent antifungals (polyenes, allylamines). Natamycin is the only commercially available antifungal. All other ocular formulations are prepared extemporaneously.
%T>MIC percentage of the time above or near the MIC; optimal dosing smaller more frequent dosing. AUC/MIC = average concentration over 24 hours; optimal dosing; concentration over time.
Source: Adapted and modified from Groos EB Jr. Fungal keratitis. In: Miller D, Galor A, Alfonso EC (Eds). Cornea: Fundamentals of Cornea and External Disease, Chapter 80. St Louis, MO: Mosby; 1997.

(0.5 µg/mL) is less as compared to other imidazoles.[28] Topical VCZ 1% is preferred in cases of recalcitrant fungal keratitis, which are refractory to topical natamycin and AMB therapy.

The features indicating the response to treatment include reduction in pain, size of infiltrates and epithelial defect, disappearance of satellite lesions, rounding of feathery margins, and vascularization. The duration of treatment is longer as compared to bacterial keratitis and is usually around 4–6 weeks.

Systemic Antifungal Therapy

Oral antifungal therapy is recommended in cases of severe keratitis. Harrison described the grading of a corneal ulcer as mild, moderate, and severe on the basis of size and depth of ulcer, infiltrate density and extent, and scleral involvement.[29] Severe ulcers are defined as >5 mm in size and >50% depth with dense infiltrates deeper than mid-stroma with or without scleral involvement.[29] Other indications of oral therapy include scleral or limbal involvement, bilateral ulcers, endophthalmitis, pediatric cases, impending perforation or perforated corneal ulcer, recalcitrant mycotic keratitis, and post-keratoplasty cases.

Some of the most commonly used systemic antifungals are ketoconazole, itraconazole, fluconazole, and more recently VCZ.[30-32] Oral VCZ has been used as an adjunct to topical nontuberculous mycobacteria (NTM) in the treatment of severe and recalcitrant mycotic keratitis and is reported to have a high efficacy in such cases.[31,32]

It is important to evaluate liver function tests every 2 weeks after starting ketoconazole. The duration of systemic therapy is usually 6–8 weeks. Common side effects of ketoconazole reported are hyperglycemia/hypertension, infertility in young people, QT prolongation, anaphylaxis, adrenal insufficiency, gynecomastia, anorexia, hyperlipidemia, increased appetite, insomnia, nervousness, headache, dizziness, paresthesia, somnolence, photophobia, and orthostatic hypotension. Common adverse effects of oral VCZ include visual disturbances such as abnormal vision, transient visual hallucinations or confusion, color vision changes, and photophobia.

Posaconazole (PCZ) is a second-generation triazole similar to VCZ. It is a synthetic structural analog of ICZ and has a broad spectrum of action similar to VCZ with activity against most *Candida* spp. as well as fluconazole-resistant isolates. PCZ has been shown to be effective against mycotic keratitis resistant to common antifungals such as KCZ, FCZ, and VCZ. Altun et al. reported successful healing in two cases of mycotic keratitis with topical (4 mg/0.1mL) and oral PCZ (200 mg four times daily), which were not responding to conventional antifungal therapy (NTM, VCZ, fluconazole, and AMB).[33]

Targeted Drug Therapy

Intracameral therapy: Intracameral AMB may be a useful modality in the treatment of deep stromal keratitis with associated anterior chamber reaction and recalcitrant mycotic keratitis that is not responding to topical natamycin.[34] Dose for intracameral use is 5–10 µg/0.1 mL and can be repeated at an interval of 72 hours.

This route of administration allows adequate drug delivery into the anterior chamber and may also help to avoid surgical intervention in acute keratitis. VCZ can also be administered through intracameral route in a dose of 50 µg/0.1 mL. The advantage is that it has a broad-spectrum of action as compared to AMB. The proposed limitations of intracameral antifungals are breach of natural barriers of infection, deeper spread of infection, risk of iatrogenic spread to the site of injection, intraocular inflammation, lenticular damage, glaucoma, hyphema, and potential endothelial damage.

Intrastromal therapy (survey): Intrastromal antifungal injections have the same indications as described in intracameral. They are mainly indicated in deep stromal infections due to the poor penetration of topical agents such as natamycin. VCZ is the most commonly used antifungal agent for intrastromal delivery. The other antifungals include AMB and NTM. Intrastromal VCZ provides a depot of drug, close to the ulcerated area at a dose of 50 µg/0.1 mL in five divided doses, from where the drug is slowly released into the infected tissue. The method of intrastromal injection described by Prakash et al.[35] is as follows: 50 µg/0.1 mL of the reconstituted VCZ solution is loaded in a 1-mL tuberculin syringe with a 30-gauge needle. The needle is inserted obliquely into the cornea from the uninvolved, clear area to reach just flush to the ulcer at the mid-stromal level. Five divided doses are given around the ulcer to form a deposit of the drug around the circumference of the lesion. This is done in such a manner that the injected drug appeared to surround the ulcer along each meridian. In cases of suboptimal response, three such injections can be given 72 hours apart.[35] The major advantage is targeted drug delivery and also helps to avoid penetrating keratoplasty in deep stromal keratitis. The major limitation of this method may be a further spread of keratitis since performing any intervention through normal cornea in the presence of keratitis may lead to new foci of infection. There is also a definite risk of inadvertent anterior chamber entry while performing the procedure in a hazy cornea.[36]

Surgical Management

Tissue Adhesives

Cyanoacrylate glue can be used to treat small perforations (<3 mm), progressive stromal keratolysis, and thinned descemetoceles. The major advantage is that it provides tectonic support along with antibacterial action. However, it is known to be toxic to the corneal endothelium and incites stromal vascularization, which may later become a high-risk factor for optical keratoplasty later.

Patch Grafts

Patch graft is indicated in perforations of up to 5 mm diameter and is used to remove the visible margin of the infected area.

Therapeutic Keratoplasty

Therapeutic keratoplasty is indicated in cases not responding or worsening on medical treatment or in cases with impending perforation or large corneal perforation (>3 mm). It helps to maintain the integrity of globe as well as to control the infection.

The prognosis of TPK is poor in cases with involvement of limbus or sclera, endophthalmitis, and recurrent infection.

It is recommended to include a 1–1.5 mm clear zone of uninvolved cornea while host trephination to reduce the possibility of residual organisms peripheral to the ulcer. Interrupted sutures with slightly longer bites should be used to avoid cheese wiring if the edge of the recipient becomes involved. The anterior chamber should be irrigated to eliminate any organisms. The lens should be left intact to prevent involvement of posterior segment.

Any infected anterior segment structure should be removed and sent for both microbiology and pathology for culture and fixed section examination. An antifungal agent should be injected which includes AMB (5 µg/0.1 mL) or VCZ (50 µg/0.1 mL) in cases with suspected endophthalmitis.

At the end of the surgery both the donor and the host specimen should be sent for histopathological examination. Fungal hyphae on pathological examination are usually seen parallel to the stromal lamellae while if oriented perpendicularly are indicative of increased virulence and poor prognosis.[37,38]

After keratoplasty, it is recommended to continue the topical management along with systemic agents if needed till the histopathology report of the host specimen. If no organisms are detected at the edge of the specimen, antifungals could be stopped after 2 weeks. However, if the specimen is positive for fungal organisms the therapy should be continued for duration of at least 6–8 weeks. Topical corticosteroids may be used with antifungal cover only if the specimen is negative keeping in mind a risk of recurrence.

References

1. Jurkunas U, Behlau I, Colby K. Fungal keratitis: changing pathogens and risk factors. Cornea. 2009;28(6):638-43.
2. Said DG, Otri M, Miri A, Kailasanathan A, Khatib T, Dua HS. The challenge of fungal keratitis. Br J Ophthalmol. 2011;95(12):1623-4.
3. Thomas PA, Kaliamurthy J. Mycotic keratitis: epidemiology, diagnosis and management. Clin Microb Infect. 2013;19(3):210-20.
4. Leck AK, Thomas PA, Hagan M, Kaliamurthy J, Ackuaku E, John M, et al. Aetiology of suppurative corneal ulcers in Ghana and south India, and epidemiology of fungal keratitis. Br J Ophthalmol. 2002;86(11):1211-5.
5. Shokohi T, Nowroozpoor-Dailami K, Moaddel-Haghighi T. Fungal keratitis in patients with corneal ulcer in Sari, Northern Iran. Arch Iran Med. 2006;9(3):222-7.
6. Zhong WX, Xie LX, Shi WY, Sun SH. Spectrum of infection of fungal keratitis: analysis of 654 cases. Zhonghua Yi Xue Za Zhi. 2006;86(24):1681-5.
7. Iyer SA, Tuli SS, Wagoner RC. Fungal keratitis: emerging trends and treatment outcomes. Eye Contact Lens. 2006;32(6):267-71.
8. Rogers GM, Goins KM, Sutphin JE, Kitzmann AS, Wagoner MD. Outcomes of treatment of fungal keratitis at the University of Iowa Hospitals and Clinics: a 10-year retrospective analysis. Cornea. 2013;32(8):1131-6.
9. Miller D. Pharmacological treatment for infectious corneal ulcers. Exp Opin Pharmacother. 2013;14(5):543-60.
10. Ansari Z, Miller D, Galor A. Current thoughts in fungal keratitis: diagnosis and treatment. Curr Fung Infect Rep. 2013;7(3):209-18.
11. Ibrahim MM, Vanini R, Ibrahim FM, Fioriti LS, Furlan EM, Provinzano LM, et al. Epidemiologic aspects and clinical outcome of fungal keratitis in southeastern Brazil. Euro J Ophthalmol. 2009;19(3):355-61.
12. Thomas PA. Fungal infections of the cornea. Eye. 2003;17:852-62.
13. Srinivasan R, Kanungo R, Goyal JL. Spectrum of oculomycosis in South India. Acta Ophthalmol. 1991;69:744-9.
14. Foster CS. Fungal keratitis. Infect Dis Clin North Am. 1992;6:851-7.
15. Bharathi MJ, Ramakrishnan R, Vasu S, Meenakshi R, Palaniappan R. Epidemiological characteristics and laboratory diagnosis of fungal keratitis. A three-year study. Indian J Ophthalmol. 2003;51:315-21.
16. Chowdhary A, Singh K. Spectrum of fungal keratitis in North India. Cornea. 2005;24:8-15.

17. Hagan M, Wright E, Newman M, Dolin P, Johnson G. Causes of suppurative keratitis in Ghana. Br J Ophthalmol. 1995;79:1024-8.
18. Srinivasan M, Gonzales CA, George C. Epidemiology and aetiological diagnosis of corneal ulceration in Madurai, South India. Br J Ophthalmol. 1997;81:965-71.
19. Berger ST, Katsev DA, Mondino BJ, Pettit TH. Macroscopic pigmentation in dematiaceous fungal keratitis. Cornea. 1991;10:272-6.
20. Vajpayee RB, Angra SK, Sandramouli S, Honavar SG, Chhabra VK. Laboratory diagnosis of keratomycosis: comparative evaluation of direct microscopy and culture results. Ann Ophthalmol. 1993;25:68-71.
21. Garg P, Gopinathan U, Choudhary K, Rao GN. Keratomycosis: clinical and microbiologic experience with dematiaceous fungi. Ophthalmology. 2000;107:574-80.
22. Srinivasan M. Fungal keratitis. Curr Opin Ophthalmol. 2004;15:321-7.
23. Florakis GJ, Moazami G, Schubert H, Koester CJ, Auran JD. Scanning slit confocal microscopy of fungal keratitis. Arch Ophthalmol. 1997;115:1461-3.
24. Labbe A, Khammari C, Dupas B, Gabison E, Brasnu E, Labetoulle M. Contribution of in vivo confocal microscopy to the diagnosis and management of infectious keratitis. Ocul Surf. 2009;7:41-52.
25. Kanavi MR, Javadi M, Yazdani S. Sensitivity and specificity of confocal scan in the diagnosis of infectious keratitis. Cornea. 2007;26(7):782-6.
26. Prajna NV, John RK, Nirmalan PK, Lalitha P, Srinivasan M. A randomized clinical trial comparing 2% econazole and 5% natamycin for the treatment of fungal keratitis. Br J Ophthalmol. 2003;87:1235-7.
27. Jeu LA, Piacenti FJ, Lyakhovetskiy AG, Fung HB. Voriconazole. Clin Ther. 2003;25:1321-81.
28. Shah KB, Wu TG, Wilhelmus KR, Jones DB. Activity of voriconazole against corneal isolates of Scedosporium apiospermum. Cornea. 2003;22:33-6.
29. Harrison SM. Grading corneal ulcers. Ann Ophthalmol. 1975;7(4):537-9, 541-2.
30. Fitzsimons R, Peters AL. Miconazole and ketoconazole as a satisfactory first-line treatment for keratomycosis. Am J Ophthalmol. 1986;101(5):605-8.
31. Freda R. Use of oral voriconazole as adjunctive treatment of severe cornea fungal infection: case report. Arq Bras Oftalmol. 2006;69(3):431-4.
32. Jhanji V, Sharma N, Mannan R, Titiyal JS, Vajpayee RB. Management of tunnel fungal infection with voriconazole. J Cataract Refract Surg. 2007;33(5):915-7.
33. Altun A, Kurna SA, Sengor T, Altun G, Olcaysu OO, Aki SF, et al. Effectiveness of posaconazole in recalcitrant fungal keratitis resistant to conventional antifungal drugs. Case Rep Ophthalmol Med. 2014;2014:701653.
34. Sridhar MS, Sharma S, Gopinathan U, Rao GN. Anterior chamber tap: diagnostic and therapeutic indications in the management of ocular infections. Cornea. 2002; 21:718-22.
35. Prakash G, Sharma N, Goel M, Titiyal JS, Vajpayee RB. Evaluation of intrastromal injection of voriconazole as a therapeutic adjunctive for the management of deep recalcitrant fungal keratitis. Am J Ophthalmol. 2008;146(1):56-9.
36. Sharma N, Agarwal P, Sinha R, Titiyal JS, Velpandian T, Vajpayee RB. Evaluation of intrastromal voriconazole injection in recalcitrant deep fungal keratitis: case series. Br J Ophthalmol. 2011;95(12):1735-7.
37. Cristol SM, Alfonso EC, Guildford JH, Roussel TJ, Culbertson WW. Results of large penetrating keratoplasty in microbial keratitis. Cornea. 1996;15:571-6.
38. Killingsworth DW, Stern GA, Driebe WT, Knapp A, Dragon DM. Results of therapeutic penetrating keratoplasty. Ophthalmology. 1993;100:534-41.

8.5 Corneal Dystrophy

Sohini Mondal, Ritu Nagpal, Prafulla Kumar Maharana

 1. Highlight the new classification of corneal dystrophy.

The latest classification system of corneal dystrophy as proposed by the International Committee for Classification of Corneal Dystrophies (IC3D Revised classification-2015) is as follows:
- *Epithelial and subepithelial:*
    - Epithelial basement membrane dystrophy (EBMD)
    - Epithelial recurrent erosion dystrophy
    - Subepithelial mucinous corneal dystrophy
    - Meesmann corneal dystrophy
    - Lisch epithelial corneal dystrophy
    - Gelatinous drop-like corneal dystrophy (GDLD)
- *Epithelial and stromal [transforming growth factor beta 1 (TGF-β_1)]:*
    - Reis–Bücklers corneal dystrophy (RBCD)
    - Thiel–Behnke corneal dystrophy (TBCD)

- Lattice corneal dystrophy (LCD) type 1
- Granular corneal dystrophy (GCD) type 1
- GCD type 2
- *Stromal:*
    - Macular corneal dystrophy (MCD)
    - Schnyder corneal dystrophy (SCD)
    - Congenital stromal corneal dystrophy (CSCD)
    - Fleck corneal dystrophy (FCD)
    - Posterior amorphous corneal dystrophy (PACD)
    - Central cloudy dystrophy of Francois
    - Pre-Descemet corneal dystrophy (PDCD)
- *Endothelial:*
    - Fuchs endothelial corneal dystrophy (FECD)
    - Posterior polymorphous corneal dystrophy (PPCD)
    - Congenital hereditary endothelial dystrophy (CHED)
    - X-linked endothelial corneal dystrophy

The traditionally accepted International Committee for Classification of Corneal Dystrophies (IC3D) 2008 had certain limitations as they categorized corneal dystrophies anatomically based on their phenotypic appearance. They were solely assigned to a particular corneal layer that is most affected.

The Updated IC3D (2015) has made the following revisions:
- Considered multiple layers of involvement with primary cell of origin
- Excluded the acellular corneal layers—Bowman and Descemet membrane (DM)
- Included histopathological, electron microscopy, and confocal microscopy
- Added anterior segment optical coherence tomography wherever feasible
- Information on genetic mutation has been removed as it is rapidly changing
- Removed CHED autosomal dominant inheritance
- 10q23-24 dystrophy was no more considered a variant of TBCD
- Removed Grayson—Wilbrandt dystrophy

2. Describe stromal dystrophies with clinical features, histopathological changes, and special stains used for their identification and management.

The three major types of stromal corneal dystrophies are as follows: MCD, GCD, and LCD. The differentiating features between the major types of stromal corneal dystrophies are illustrated in **Table 1**.

Other less common types comprise SCD, CSCD, FCD, PACD, central cloudy dystrophy of Francois, and PDCD.

Macular Corneal Dystrophy

Macular corneal dystrophy is also known as:
- Groenouw corneal dystrophy type II
- Fehr spotted dystrophy

Inheritance pattern: Autosomal recessive

Genetics: Chromosome 16q22

Enzyme: Carbohydrate sulfotransferase 6 (CHST6)

Clinical Features

Symptoms

Cornea remains clear at birth and cloudiness appears at 3–9 years of life. Patient usually presents with slowly progressive diminution of vision with severe visual impairment between 10 and 30 years of age. Corneal sensitivity is reduced. Photophobia and painful recurrent erosions can rarely occur.

TABLE 1: Differentiating features between the major types of stromal corneal dystrophies.

Features	Granular dystrophy	Macular dystrophy	Lattice dystrophy
Age of onset • Deposit • Symptoms	 First decade Third decade	 First decade First decade	 First decade Second decade
Heredity	AD	AR	AD
Reduced vision	By fourth or fifth decade	First or second decade	By second or third decade
Erosions	Uncommon	Common	Variable
Opacities	• Discrete, sharp borders • Intervening stroma is clear • Subepithelial spots • Does not extend till the limbus	• Indistinct margins • Hazy intervening stroma • Extends to the limbus • Endothelium is affected	• Early • Refractile tiny lines and dots • Diffuse central haze • Limbal zone is clear except in advanced cases
Corneal thickness	Normal	Thinned	Normal
Histochemical stains	Masson's trichrome	Colloidal iron Alcian blue Periodic acid-Schiff	Congo red Periodic acid-Schiff
Materials accumulated	Hyaline	Glycosaminoglycans	Amyloid
Distinguishing clinical characteristics	Clear limbal zone	Opacities reach limbus Cornea is thinned unless decompensated	Lattice lines

Signs

Initially presents as central, superficial, irregular whitish fleck-like opacities that gradually progress and extend till limbus involving deep stroma and DM. Another characteristic feature is intervening stromal haze, which is absent in other stromal dystrophies such as granular and lattice dystrophy. The epithelium usually remains smooth without erosions. The cornea is much thinner than the normal, often associated with hypoesthesia. There is a thickening of DM along with endothelial guttae.

Histopathology

Product deposited: Extracellular and intracellular deposition of glycosaminoglycans (GAGs) which are unsulfated keratin sulfate in the endoplasmic reticulum.

Stain: The deposits composed of GAGs stain with alcian blue and colloidal iron.

Light microscopy: Epithelial thinning with degeneration of basal epithelial cells can be seen. Breaks in the Bowman's layer with diffuse accumulation of GAGs both intracellularly and extracellularly in the corneal stroma, beneath the epithelium and within keratocytes and endothelial cells are noted. Posterior corneal layers such as DM and endothelium are also involved.

Electron microscopy: Keratocytes and endothelial cells stain positive for GAGs.

Types of Macular Corneal Dystrophy

Macular corneal dystrophy is subdivided into three immunophenotypes: MCD types I, IA, and II—based on the reactivity of the patient's serum and corneal tissue to an antibody that recognizes sulfated keratan sulfate (KS) **(Table 2)**.
- *MCD type I:* Antigenic KS (AgKS) is undetectable in both serum and corneal tissue.
- *MCD type II:* AgKS is present in normal or subnormal levels in serum and is evident within the corneal stroma.
- *In MCD type IA:* AgKS is absent in the serum and in most of the cornea but can be detected in the keratocytes.

Management

Medical

Early stages can be managed with refraction and lubricants. Bandage contact lens may be advised if recurrent erosions occur.

Surgical

- Phototherapeutic keratectomy (PTK) might be an option in early stages; however, it is associated with increased chances of recurrence.

TABLE 2: Immunophenotypes of macular corneal dystrophy.

Type of MCD	AgKS in cornea	AgKS in serum
Type 1	Absent	Absent
Type 1a	Present	Absent
Type 2	Present	Present

(AgKS: antigenic keratan sulfate; MCD: macular corneal dystrophy)

TABLE 3: Deep anterior lamellar keratoplasty versus penetrating keratoplasty in macular corneal dystrophy.

Parameters	DALK in MCD	PKP in MCD
Points against	• Recurrence of pathology is higher • Endothelial dysfunction can compromise the graft survival postoperatively • Experienced surgeon	• Chances of graft rejection are higher • Chances of endothelial cell loss and glaucoma are higher
Points in favor	• Complications related to open-sky procedure can be minimized • Less chance of postoperative wound dehiscence • Graft can be replaced without the risk of getting into the high-risk category	• Recurrence of the pathology is less • Take care of the subclinical endothelial involvement part too

(DALK: deep anterior lamellar keratoplasty; MCD: macular corneal dystrophy; PKP: penetrating keratoplasty)

- Penetrating keratoplasty (PKP) is mandatory in cases of full-thickness corneal involvement.
- Deep anterior lamellar keratoplasty (DALK) is preferred in selected cases with noninvolvement of DM.

Over the last decade, there has been an ongoing controversy between performing deep lamellar keratoplasty and PKP in patients with MCD. The pros and cons of the individual procedure have been summarized in **Table 3**. Big-bubble DALK provides comparable visual outcome to PKP with no significant difference in best-corrected visual acuity and postoperative astigmatism. Moreover, there is no significant difference in graft survival rates.

Complications

Post-transplant recurrence rate is high in young age, male gender, and lamellar keratoplasty. Recurrence following PKP starts at the graft–host junction (GHJ) and progresses centrally, whereas in DALK, it usually commences with host bed opacification.

Schnyder Corneal Dystrophy

Schnyder corneal dystrophy is also known as:
- Crystalline stromal dystrophy
- Schnyder crystalline corneal dystrophy

Inheritance pattern: Autosomal dominant

Genetics: Chromosome 1p36, *UBIAD1* gene

Onset and progression: Onset is usually during second to third decade of life or as early as childhood in some cases with slow progression.

Clinical Features

Patient presents with diminution of visual acuity and glare. The disease is characterized by central comma-shaped subepithelial crystals which may progress to arcus lipoides in later stages as illustrated.

Histopathology

Stain: Oil Red O

Light microscopy: Intracellular and extracellular esterified, unesterified phospholipids, and cholesterol.

Polarized microscopy: Birefringent crystals of cholesterol in superficial stroma under polarized light.

Electron microscopy: Numerous electron-lucent spaces in cornea (dissolved cholesterol crystals)

Management

Lamellar keratoplasty is the surgery of choice depending on the depth of corneal involvement on anterior segment optical coherence tomography (AS-OCT).

Congenital Stromal Corneal Dystrophy

Congenital stromal corneal dystrophy is also known as congenital hereditary stromal dystrophy.
- *Inheritance pattern:* Autosomal dominant
- *Genetics:* Chromosome 12q21.33, *decorin* gene
- *Onset and progression:* This disease is congenital in nature with slow progression.

Clinical Features

Patient presents with moderate-to-severe vision loss. Slit-lamp examination reveals diffuse bilateral corneal clouding with flake-like opacities throughout stroma with increased stromal thickness.

Histopathology

- *Light microscopy:* Irregular placement of stromal lamellae with amorphous material
- *Confocal microscopy:* Increased reflectivity of anterior stroma
- *Electron microscopy:* Amorphous areas containing thin filaments randomly arranged in an electron-lucent ground substance separate lamellae of normal appearance. Accumulation of decorin in amorphous areas has also been noted.

Management

Lamellar keratoplasty is the surgery of choice depending on the depth of corneal involvement on AS-OCT.

Fleck Corneal Dystrophy

Fleck corneal dystrophy is also known as François-Neetens speckled corneal dystrophy.
- *Inheritance pattern:* Autosomal dominant
- *Genetics:* Chromosome 2q34, *PIKFYVE* gene
- *Onset and progression:* The disease might have congenital onset or present during the first year of life. It remains nonprogressive throughout life.

Clinical Features

Patient is generally asymptomatic. Dandruff-like opacities being sparsely scattered in stroma with intervening clear areas can be well appreciated on slit-lamp examination. The opacities might extend to the limbus in few cases. Unilateral presentation is not uncommon.

Histopathology

Stain: Alcian blue; colloidal iron; Sudan black, Oil Red O

Light microscopy: Swollen, vacuolated keratocytes containing GAGs and complex lipids

Confocal microscopy: Hyper-reflective dot-like material in the keratocyte nuclei.

Electron microscopy: Keratocytes show membrane-based inclusions with delicate granular material.

Management

There is no definitive management and patients do not require any surgical intervention. Refraction is the main modality of treatment.

Posterior Amorphous Corneal Dystrophy

Posterior amorphous corneal dystrophy is also known as posterior amorphous stromal dystrophy.
- *Inheritance pattern:* Autosomal dominant
- *Genetics:* Chromosome 12q21.33, KERA, and *decorin* gene
- *Onset and progression:* The disease usually presents in the first decade of life and is slowly progressive in nature.

Clinical Features

Patient is usually asymptomatic throughout life or may present with a slight blurring of vision. Diffuse gray-white sheet-like opacities are noted on slit-lamp examination in any layer of stroma (most prominent posteriorly). It may be associated with corneal thinning with flattening.

Histopathology

Stain: Colloidal iron

Light microscopy: Irregular posterior stromal lamellae with thin DM and focal attenuation of endothelial cells

Confocal microscopy: Microfolds and hyper-reflective layer in the posterior stroma

Electron microscopy: Disorganization of posterior stromal lamellae with abnormal keratocytes and orientation of collagen fibers.

Management

Patients generally do not require any form of surgical intervention. Refraction is the main modality for visual rehabilitation.

Central Cloudy Dystrophy of François

Inheritance pattern: Unknown

Genetics: None

Onset and progression: Disease onset is in the first decade of life and remains stationary throughout.

Clinical Features

Patients are usually asymptomatic. The disease is axially distributed, and is characterized by polygonal gray-white stromal opacities separated by linear areas of clear cornea that resemble posterior crocodile shagreen.

Histopathology

Stain: Colloidal iron, Alcian blue

Light microscopy: Faint undulating deep stroma and positive staining for GAGs

Confocal microscopy: Small highly refractile granules and deposits in the anterior stroma with multiple dark striae in the extracellular matrix

Electron microscopy: Extracellular vacuoles with fibrillogranular material and electron-dense deposits

Management

They never require any surgical treatment and refraction remains the mainstay for visual rehabilitation.

Pre-Descemet Corneal Dystrophy

Inheritance pattern: Unknown

Genetics: Isolated PDCD is unknown; PDCD associated with X-linked ichthyosis is chromosome Xp22.31 (*STS* gene)

Onset and progression: Onset is usually in the fourth decade of life and the disease is nonprogressive in nature.

Clinical Features

Patients are usually asymptomatic in nature. Focal, fine, polymorphic gray opacities can be appreciated on slit-lamp examination which may be central, annular, or diffusely located in deep stroma. In punctiform and polychromatic disease subtypes, the changes are uniform and polychromatic.

Histopathology

Light microscopy: Enlarged keratocytes in posterior stroma containing vacuoles and intracytoplasmic inclusions of lipid-like material

Confocal microscopy: Hyper-reflective dots anterior to DM

Electron microscopy: Intracellular vacuoles containing electron-dense material

Management

Surgical treatment is not necessary in these cases and refraction is the main modality of treatment.

Granular and Lattice Dystrophy

Kindly follow the discussion in subsequent Question.

 3. Discuss the transforming growth factor beta 1 (TGF-β$_1$)-related corneal dystrophies.

The various types of TGF-β$_1$ stromal corneal dystrophies are as follows:
- RBCD
- TBCD
- LCD type 1
- GCD type 1 (GCD-1)
- GCD type 2 (GCD-2).

Reis–Bücklers Corneal Dystrophy

Reis–Bücklers corneal dystrophy is also known as:
- GCD type 3 and (2)
- Superficial/atypical GCD

Inheritance pattern: Autosomal dominant

Genetics: Chromosome 5q31, TGF-β$_1$, and *BIGH3* gene

Onset and progression: The disease onset is during childhood.

Clinical Features

Vision remains impaired since childhood although recurrent corneal erosions may occur in first decade of life. Erosions associated with this disease form are generally more severe than TBCD. The disease is characterized by confluent, irregular, and geographic-like opacities at the level of Bowman's membrane and superficial stroma that might extend up to the limbus and deeper stroma.

Histopathology

Light microscopy: Bowman's layer is replaced by sheet-like layer of Masson's trichrome red deposits.

Confocal microscopy: Distinct deposits in epithelium and Bowman's membrane.

Electron microscopy: Subepithelial electron-dense rod or trapezoidal shaped bodies identical to that of GCD.

Immunohistochemistry: Rod-shaped bodies are immunopositive for TGF-β-induced protein (keratoepithelin) that is responsible for the cohesiveness of the cells.

Anterior Segment Optical Coherence Tomography

Prominent hyper-reflective material at the level of Bowman's membrane that is thickest at the center.

Management

Initial treatment is aimed at recurrent erosions with lubricants and bandage contact lens. Recurrence is common with superficial keratectomy and PTK when the depth of involvement is <160 and <100 μm, respectively.

Thiel–Behnke Corneal Dystrophy

Thiel–Behnke corneal dystrophy is also known as:
- Honeycomb-shaped corneal dystrophy
- Curly fiber corneal dystrophy

Inheritance pattern: Autosomal dominant

Genetics: Chromosome 5q31 and 10q24, TGF-$β_1$, and *BIGH3* gene

Onset and progression: The disease has a childhood onset.

Clinical Features

Vision is impaired since the first decade of life and is associated with recurrent corneal erosions, although they are less severe than RBCD. Initial signs are symmetrical, subepithelial, reticular (honeycomb) opacities with peripheral cornea typically uninvolved.

Histopathology

Light microscopy: Bowman's layer is replaced by a fibrocellular layer with pathognomonic "wavy saw tooth pattern."

Confocal microscopy: Distinct deposits in epithelium and Bowman's membrane.

Electron microscopy: Curly collagen fibers with a diameter of 9–15 nm are pathognomonic that distinguishes TBCD from RBCD.

Immunohistochemistry: Curly collagen fibers are immunopositive for keratoepithelin.

Anterior Segment Optical Coherence Tomography

Prominent hyper-reflective material at the level of Bowman's membrane extending into the epithelium.

Management

Initial treatment is aimed at recurrent erosions with lubricants and bandage contact lens. Surgical modality is decided based on the depth of involvement on AS-OCT:
- Superficial keratectomy is preferred when the depth of involvement is <160 μ whereas PTK is when the depth of involvement is <100 μ. However, recurrence remains one of the important drawbacks of the above-mentioned treatment modalities.

Lattice Corneal Dystrophy Type 1

Lattice corneal dystrophy is also known as:
- Classic LCD
- Biber-Haab-Dimmer

Inheritance pattern: Autosomal dominant

Genetics: Chromosome 5q31, *TGF-$β_1$* gene

Onset and progression: The disease onset is usually during the first and second decades of life. There occurs significant disease progression throughout life.

Clinical Features

Marked visual decrease occurs by fourth decade of life. Direct illumination of slit-lamp examination reveals glass-like branching lines in the stroma as depicted in **Figure 1**. Refractile lines, central subepithelial ovoid white dots, and diffuse stromal haze are best visualized on retroillumination as illustrated in **Figure 2**. DM and endothelium remain uninvolved. Ground-glass appearance of the stroma with the peripheral clear cornea is a typical feature accompanied by recurrent epithelial erosions. Development of diffuse central haze in the second to third decade may reduce vision sufficiently to necessitate surgical intervention.

Histopathology

Product: Amyloid

Stain: Congo red

Light microscopy: Deposition of amyloid heavily in the subepithelial and anterior stroma with distorted collagen lamellar structure.

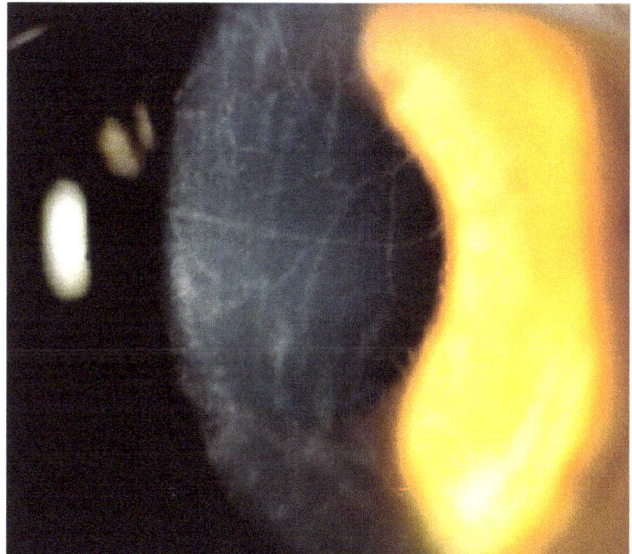

Fig. 1: Glass like branching refractile lines, central subepithelial ovoid white dots and diffuse stromal haze appreciated on slit lamp examination.

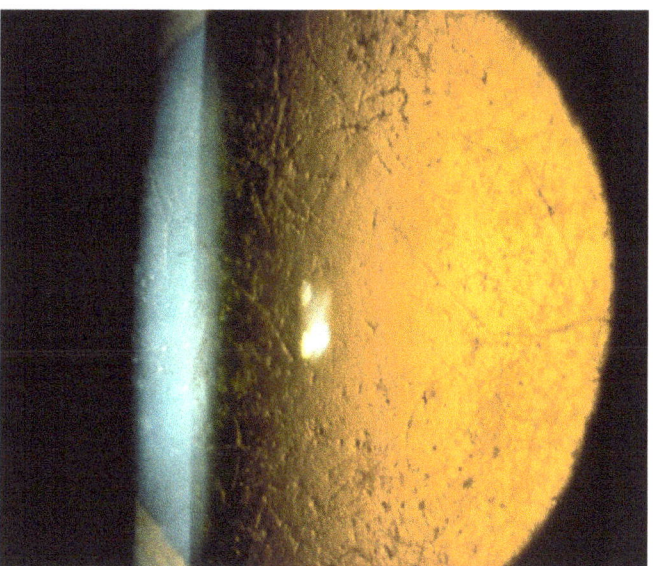

Fig. 2: Refractile lines or lattice lines best visualised on retro-illumination mode.

Polarized microscopy: Birefringence and red green dichorism under polarized light.

Confocal microscopy: Characteristic linear branching structures in stroma

Electron microscopy: Randomly arranged fine electrodense fibrils of 8–10 nm diameter. There are less number of keratocytes in the areas of amyloid deposition.

Management

Initial treatment is aimed at recurrent erosions with lubricants and bandage contact lens. Superficial keratectomy is preferred when the depth of involvement is <160 µ, whereas PTK is preferred when the depth of involvement is <100 µ.

Granular Corneal Dystrophy Type 1

Granular corneal dystrophy type 1 is also known as: corneal dystrophy Groenouw type 1.
- *Inheritance pattern:* Autosomal dominant
- *Genetics:* Chromosome 5q31, TGF-β_1 gene
- *Onset and progression:* This disease has a childhood onset and is slowly progressive in nature.

Clinical Features

Most patients maintain a fairly good vision of >20/200. Patients may initially complain of glare and photophobia alone. Crumb-like opacities in superficial cornea are pathognomonic of this dystrophy as depicted in **Figure 3**. On direct illumination, the opacities appear white whereas, on indirect illumination, they appear as small translucent dots with vacuoles resembling glassy splinters or crushed breadcrumbs. Recurrent erosions are seen frequently.

Histopathology

Product: Hyaline

Stain: Masson's trichrome

Light microscopy: Multiple stromal deposits of hyaline may extend from deep epithelium to DM.

Electron microscopy: Characteristic rod-shaped bodies in the corneal stroma

Confocal microscopy: Highly reflective granular material with irregular edges in the epithelium

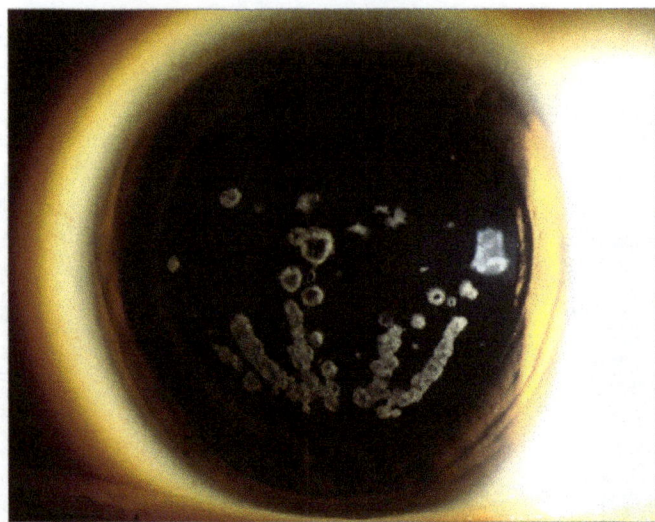

Fig. 3: On direct illumination the opacities appear white crumb like involving superficial cornea that are small, discrete and sharply demarcated.

Management

Initial treatment is aimed at recurrent erosions with lubricants and bandage contact lens. Superficial keratectomy is preferred when the depth of involvement is <160 μ, whereas PTK is preferred when depth of involvement is <100 μ.

Granular Corneal Dystrophy Type 2

Granular corneal dystrophy is also known as:
- Avellino dystrophy
- Combined granular-LCD

Inheritance pattern: Autosomal dominant

Genetics: Chromosome 5q31, TGF-β_1 gene

Onset and progression: Homozygous patients are known to have an earlier onset as early as 3 years of age. In heterozygotes, the presentation is usually delayed but presentation as early as 8 years has been noted in the previous studies. They are slowly progressive in nature with more rapid progression in homozygotes.

Clinical Features

Vision keeps on decreasing with age as the central visual axis gets affected. Symptoms such as pain and foreign body sensation are mostly attributable to epithelial erosions. On slit-lamp examination, one can appreciate stellate-shaped or snowflake- or icicle-like opacities between anterior and mid stroma. Dashed lines signifying lattice lines are also present, deeper than the snowflake opacities. Hyaloid deposits typical of granular and amyloid deposits typical of lattice dystrophy are seen as depicted in **Figure 4**. Dashed lines and translucent dot-like opacities are seen on retroillumination as illustrated in **Figure 5**.

Histopathology

Product: Hyaline and amyloid

Stain: Masson's trichrome and Congo red

Light microscopy: Opacities extend from basal epithelium to deep stroma and stain with Masson's trichrome and/or Congo red.

Electron microscopy: Rod-shaped bodies and randomly aligned fibrils of amyloid.

Confocal microscopy: Reflective breadcrumb-like round deposits with well-delineated borders present in the anterior stroma (similar to GCD type 1). Linear and branching deposits with changing reflectivity are also noted (similar to LCD type 1).

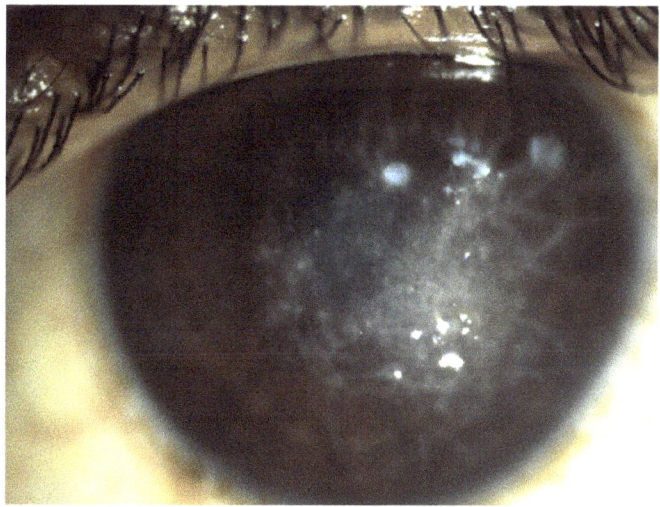

Fig. 4: Stellate shaped or snowflake like or icicle like opacities appear between anterior and mid stroma along with dash lines present deeper than snowflake opacities.

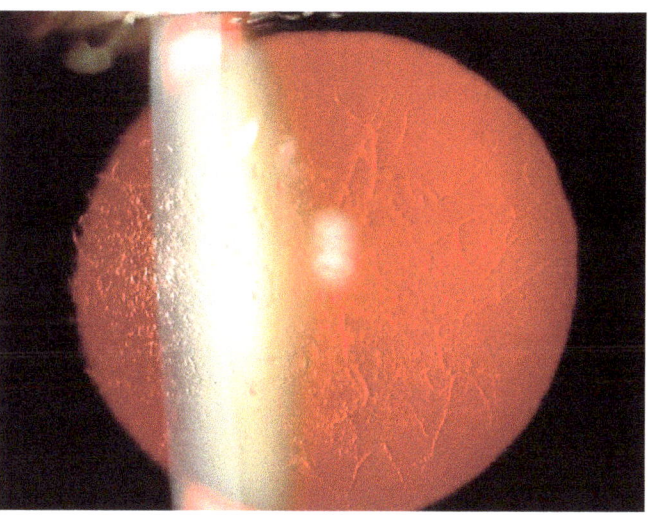

Fig. 5: Dash lines and tranlucent dot like opacities appreciate d on retro-illumination mode.

Management

Initial treatment is aimed at recurrent erosions with lubricants and bandage contact lens. Superficial keratectomy is preferred when the depth of involvement is <160 µ, whereas PTK is preferred when depth of involvement is <100 µ.

4. Discuss the differences between dystrophies and degenerations in eye.

Corneal Dystrophy

Corneal dystrophies are typically referred to as a group of inherited disorders that are usually bilateral, symmetric, slowly progressive, and not related to environmental or systemic factors.

Corneal Degeneration

These are tissue changes that cause deterioration and may impair function as a manifestation of a specific disease or simply from aging. They are usually unilateral, asymmetric, and often peripheral. Changes caused by inflammation, maturity, or systemic disease result in deposition, thinning, or vascularization of the corneal tissue.

The salient points of difference between these two categories of diseases are summarized in **Table 4**.

TABLE 4: Dystrophy versus degeneration.

Characteristics	Dystrophy	Degeneration
Laterality	Bilateral and symmetric	Unilateral and asymmetric
Location	Central	Peripheral
Heredity	Hereditary	Sporadic
Onset	Early age	Late age
Layer affected	Involves one layer to begin with	Multiple layers
Progression	Slow	Slow/fast
Vascularization	Avascular	Vascularized
Inflammation	Rare	Common
Associations	Rarely associated with systemic disease	Associated with systemic disease

5. Discuss the different clinically important corneal degenerations.

They are defined as a group of conditions in which the normal cells undergo some degenerative changes under the influence of age or some pathological condition.

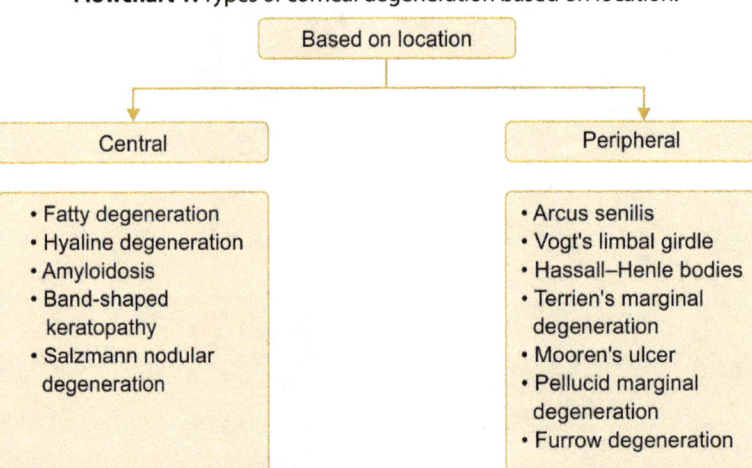

Flowchart 1: Types of corneal degeneration based on location.

Classification

- *Based on location:*
  - *Axial (Flowchart 1):*
    - Fatty degeneration
    - Hyaline degeneration
    - Amyloidosis
    - Band-shaped keratopathy
    - Salzmann's nodular degeneration (SND)
  - *Peripheral:*
    - Arcus senilis
    - Vogt limbal girdle
    - Hassall–Henle bodies
    - Terrien's marginal degeneration
    - Mooren's ulcer
    - Senile furrow degeneration
- *Depending on etiology:*
  - *Age-related:* Arcus senilis, Vogt limbal girdle, Hassall–Henle bodies
  - *Pathological:* Fatty degeneration, hyaline degeneration, amyloidosis, band-shaped keratopathy, Salzmann's nodular degeneration, Terrien's marginal degeneration

Arcus Senilis (Gerontoxon)

This is the most common peripheral corneal opacity occurring in elderly population due to annular stromal lipid deposition. Lipid in the form of cholesterol and cholesterol esters is initially deposited at DM and Bowman's membrane and then progresses into stroma in the form of hourglass appearance. A similar condition occurring in young individual is known as arcus juvenilis.

Signs

It starts in the superior and inferior quadrants and progresses circumferentially to form a 1-mm wide perilimbal ring. The annulus is wider in superior and inferior quadrants and is separated from the limbus by a clear zone known as lucid interval of Vogt.

Vogt's Limbal Girdle

It is composed of chalky white, fine granular hyaline deposits with elastotic degeneration at the level of Bowman's membrane.

Signs

It presents as symmetrical yellow-white crescentic limbal bands at 3 and 9 o' clock in the interpalpebral area.
- *Type 1:* Swiss cheese hole pattern with a lucid interval
- *Type 2:* More common and characterized by the absence of holes and lucid interval.

Hassall–Henle Bodies

These form the most common senile change occurring in the cornea. They are drop-like hyaline excrescences arising from the peripheral DM and projecting into the anterior chamber. In pathological conditions such as Fuchs, dystrophy, they become large and invade the central cornea known as corneal guttata.

Lipid Keratopathy

This condition is characterized by whitish or yellowish deposits of cholesterol and fatty acids. Initially, the deposits remain intracellular but may progress to become extracellular with stromal cell necrosis.
- *Primary:* Rare condition occurring in a naïve cornea not associated with vascularization
- *Secondary:* Commoner condition occurring in vascularized cornea secondary to keratitis or trauma

Treatment: Photocoagulation of the feeder vessels or keratoplasty in advanced cases

Hyaline Degeneration

This consists of hyaline spherules deposition in the superficial stroma.
- *Primary:* Bilateral condition associated with GCD
- *Secondary:* Unilateral condition occurring in diseased corneas such as keratitis or long-standing glaucoma. This is often complicated by recurrent erosions.

Treatment: Keratoplasty may be indicated.

Amyloidosis

This rare condition is characterized by deposition of subepithelial amyloid material which may be primary (in a healthy cornea) or secondary (in a diseased cornea).

Band-shaped Keratopathy (Calcific Degeneration)

It consists of deposition of calcium salts (hydroxyapatite) in subepithelium, Bowman's membrane, and superficial stroma. It can either be primary or secondary.

Etiology

- Ocular inflammation—chronic anterior uveitis, phthisis bulbi, silicone oil in anterior chamber
- Idiopathic/age-related
- Systemic or metabolic—hypercalcemia, hyperphosphatemia, chronic renal failure
- Chemicals (eye drops and irritants)
- Hereditary—familial.
  It presents as a band-shaped opacity with round holes within, located in the interpalpebral area (centripetal spread) with clear cornea between the margins of the band and the limbus (lucid interval).

Treatment

Ethylenediaminetetraacetic acid (EDTA) chelation (1.7%, 0.05 molar), PTK, treating the underlying condition.

Salzmann Nodular Degeneration

This condition is characterized by hyaline nodules located superficial to Bowman's membrane due to chronic corneal irritation and inflammation such as trachoma, dry eye, chronic blepharitis, and chronic allergic keratoconjunctivitis. This can be either primary or secondary. Primary SND is the more common form. Patient typically presents with ocular discomfort and elevated whitish or blue grey nodules usually located in the mid-periphery of the cornea.

Treatment: Lubricants in early stages; superficial keratectomy or lamellar keratoplasty depending on the depth of involvement in later stages.

Spheroidal Degeneration

Spheroidal degeneration is also known as climatic droplet/Labrador keratopathy.

Men are more affected than women as being outdoor worker, UV exposure is likely to be an etiological factor. This condition is typically characterized by amber-colored spheroidal granules at the level of Bowman's membrane and anterior stroma in the interpalpebral area.

Treatment: Sunglasses and lamellar keratoplasty in advanced cases.

6. Discuss spheroidal degeneration.

Introduction

Spheroidal degeneration is also known as Labrador keratopathy, Bietti nodular hyaline band-shaped keratopathy, climatic droplet keratopathy, Fisherman's keratopathy, and Eskimo's corneal degeneration.

It was first described by Bietti in 1955. It is a common degeneration of the cornea and/or conjunctiva, characterized by homogeneous, translucent, fine, golden yellow, spherules, or globules of varying size located in the superficial corneal stroma, Bowman's membrane, and subepithelium, and involves the epithelium in advanced cases. It can involve both the conjunctiva and the cornea.

Etiology/Risk Factors

- Increasing age
- Ultraviolet light
- Dry eye disease
- Malnutrition
- Microtrauma from sand particles
- Low humidity
- Extreme temperatures
- Keratitis
- LCD
- Glaucoma
- Welding burns.

Pathophysiology

- Accumulation of plasma proteins, possibly immunoglobulins and albumins, could diffuse into the cornea from the limbal circulation and are modified by UV exposure.
- These deposits include extracellular matrix and plasma proteins composed of sulfur-containing amino acids that could be secreted from corneal stroma or by fibroblasts, which can be associated with abnormal collagen. These proteins then precipitate due to UV radiation. Accumulation of advanced glycated end products has also been described.

Epidemiology

- Labrador communities located in Eastern Canada (between latitudes 55–56° north of the equator) showed the highest prevalence: UV light reflected from ice and snow.
- Low latitudes, around the equator: Sand and UV light exposure
- Men are affected more than women (7:3).

Symptoms

- Asymptomatic in majority of the cases.
- May experience reduced visual acuity (visual axis is involved).
- May experience pain, photophobia, and foreign body sensation (epithelial involvement).

Signs

- Presence of golden yellow globules at or beneath the corneal or conjunctival epithelium.
- Involvement of superficial corneal stroma, Bowman's membrane, subepithelium, and rarely epithelium is common in advanced cases. There can be stromal thinning, scarring with vascularization in these cases along with reduced corneal sensation.

Classification

Fraunfelder et al. classified into three basic forms:
1. *Primary corneal:* Lesions are located in the interpalpebral fissure. Progresses from periphery to center.
2. *Secondary corneal:* Lesions are located at the sites of previous pathology (trauma, neovascularization, inflammation).
3. *Conjunctival:* Lesions are located at 3 and 9 o'clock positions interpalpebrally due to its association with pinguecula.

Clinical Diagnosis

Grading system (Johnson and Ghosh) to describe the clinical features of spheroidal degeneration.
- *Trace:* A small number of lesions that are found in one eye or only one end of interpalpebral strips in each eye bilaterally.
- *Grade 1:* Lesions involving the interpalpebral cornea horizontally but not involving the central cornea
- *Grade 2:* Central corneal involvement without affecting visual acuity
- *Grade 3:* Central corneal involvement with a decline in visual acuity
- *Grade 4:* Grade 3 features with lesion elevation.

Clinical Staging System

- *Stage 1:* Spheroids confined to the corneal periphery. Vision is unaffected.
- *Stage 2:* Spheroids extending to the interpalpebral fissure. VA <6/60.
- *Stage 3:* Stage 2+ nodules/excavated area. VA is counting fingers or hand movements.

Histopathology

The deposits are composed of extracellular hyaline-like material and complex proteins including tryptophan, cysteine, and tyrosine involving the subepithelium, Bowman's membrane, and superficial stroma of the cornea. These deposits stain positively for fibrin. Bowman's membrane is often disrupted or absent locally in advanced stages. Usually, inflammatory cells are absent.

Under electronic microscopy, finely granular structures are collected on bands of collagen.

Differential Diagnosis

- Corneal amyloid degeneration
- GDLD
- Band-shaped keratopathy
- Climatic proteoglycan stromal keratopathy
- Primary lipoidal degeneration
- Salzmann nodular degeneration
- Limbal girdle of Vogt, type II.

Management

Prevention: Limited sun exposure (sunglasses)

General Treatment

- Asymptomatic patients do not require treatment.
- Lubricant eye drops if symptomatic and steroids if inflammation is present.
- Patients with central corneal involvement and reduced visual acuity, different treatments can be considered depending on the depth and density of the deposits such as superficial keratectomy, amniotic membrane graft, PTK, lamellar keratoplasty, or PKP in the most severe cases.

Complications

Elevated lesions may progress to complications such as:
- Epithelial defects
- Recurrent corneal erosions
- Sterile ulceration
- Superadded microbial keratitis.

Post-transplant Outcomes and Precautions

- Prior case studies reveal recurrence of spheroidal degeneration after 4 years of cornea transplant in patients who were continuously exposed to the aforementioned risk factors after keratoplasty.
- Disease starts in the periphery of the graft and gradually moves centrally.
- Advised to use protective sunglasses to avoid ocular UV exposure
- Adequate dietary intake of ascorbic acid to protect against UV radiation–induced oxidative stress.

 7. Write a short note on Fuchs endothelial corneal dystrophy (FECD).

This is also known as endoepithelial corneal dystrophy. This is the most common endothelial dystrophy seen in clinical practice.

Inheritance: Genetic basis is complex and variable due to incomplete penetrance.

Gene: COL8A2 encoding for alpha-2 chain of type VIII collagen.

Onset: Most cases are bilateral and asymmetric; begin in the fourth decade of life with female preponderance.

Course: Progressive.

Clinical Features

- *Stage of corneal guttae:* Patient is generally asymptomatic at this stage and on examination corneal guttae appears as dark spots on the posterior corneal surface on direct illumination and as "dew drops" on retroillumination of slit-lamp biomicroscopy. Corneal guttae start centrally and spread peripherally.
- *Stage of corneal stromal edema:* Patient presents with intermittent worsening of vision more so in the morning hours because of the increased epithelial/stromal edema after overnight eye closure. The corneal edema manifests in the posterior stroma to start with gradually progressing to microcystic epithelial edema and disruption of tear film.
- *Stage of corneal epithelial edema:* Patient presents with pain, photophobia, and watering due to epithelial erosions resulting from ruptured epithelial bullae. The epithelial microcystic changes coalesce to form epithelial bullae which may rupture on trivial trauma.
- *Stage of corneal scarring:* Patient presents with decreased vision associated with avascular subepithelial fibrosis which is best appreciated on tangential illumination.

Diagnosis

- *Specular microscopy:* Reveals decreased endothelial cell count with increased coefficient of variation (polymegathism) and decreased hexagonality (pleomorphism).
- *Confocal microscopy:* Apart from the above-mentioned features, endothelial cell drop outs with corneal guttae are appreciable.
- *Light microscopy:* Diffuse thickening and lamination of DM with hyaline excrescences. Reduction and degeneration of endothelial cells are also seen.

Differential Diagnosis

- *Hassall–Henle bodies:* Normal finding in elderly age group; not associated with vision loss or corneal edema
- *Focal guttae:* Seen in interstitial keratitis
- Macular dystrophy
- PPCD

- *Pseudoguttae:* Trauma, inflammation, infection
- *Central herpetiform keratitis:* Presence of keratic precipitates; responds to steroids
- *Chandler variant of iridocorneal endothelial (ICE) syndrome:* Typically unilateral.

Management

Medical
- Topical hypertonic saline, antiglaucoma, lubricants
- Desiccating measures such as hair dryer help in reducing corneal edema
- Bandage contact lens for recurrent erosions and epithelial bullae to alleviate the symptoms.

Surgical
- Endothelial keratoplasty such as Descemet stripping automated endothelial keratoplasty (DSAEK) or Descemet membrane endothelial keratoplasty (DMEK): In absence of significant stromal scarring and depending on the visual clarity.
- *PKP:* In the presence of significant stromal scarring.

 8. Write a short note on congenital hereditary endothelial dystrophy (CHED).

It is also known as Maumenee corneal dystrophy.

Inheritance: Autosomal recessive

Gene: Solute carrier family 4, sodium borate transporter, member 11 *(SLC4A11)*

Onset: Congenital *(Harboyan syndrome*—CHED with postlingual sensorineural hearing loss)

Symptoms: Blurry vision and corneal clouding often accompanied by to and fro movements of the eye (nystagmus). There is no tearing or photophobia.

Signs: Bilateral and asymmetric presentation with corneal clouding ranging from diffuse haze to ground-glass milky appearance with occasional focal gray spots. Endothelial cell count is significantly reduced such that the cornea is decompensated and thickened 2–3 times more than the normal limit.

Course: Relatively stationary with little or no progression.

Diagnosis: Often clinical. Other test to support the diagnosis may be:
- *Light microscopy:* Reveals thickened and laminated DM with multinucleated, sparse, atrophic endothelium. Defects in Bowman's layer with diffuse stromal and epithelial edema are also appreciable.

Differential diagnosis:
- Primary congenital glaucoma
- Anterior segment dysgenesis (Peters anomaly, Axenfeld anomaly)
- *Other corneal dystrophies:* Congenital hereditary stromal dystrophy, posterior polymorphous corneal dystrophy
- Mucopolysaccharidosis
- Birth trauma
- Congenital rubella syndrome.

Management

Medical: Refraction, topical hypertonic saline, and desiccating measures (blower).

Surgical: DSAEK is preferred over PKP depending on corneal clarity.

References

1. Weiss JS, Møller HU, Lisch W, Kinoshita S, Aldave AJ, Belin MW, et al. The IC3D classification of the corneal dystrophies. Cornea. 2008;27(Suppl 2):S1-83.

2. Weiss JS, Møller HU, Aldave AJ, Seitz B, Bredrup C, Kivelä T, et al. IC3D classification of corneal dystrophies—edition 2. Cornea. 2015;34(2):117-59.
3. Holland EJ, Brilakis HS, Schwartz GS. Herpes simplex keratitis. In: Krachmer JH, Mannis MJ, Holland EJ (Eds). Cornea, 2nd edition. St Louis, MO: Mosby; 2004. pp. 1043-74.
4. Liu NP, Smith CF, Bowling BL, Jonasson F, Klintworth GK. Macular corneal dystrophy types I and II are caused by distinct mutations in the *CHST6* gene in Iceland. Mol Vis. 2006;12:1148-52.
5. Kawashima M, Kawakita T, Den S, Shimmura S, Tsubota K, Shimazaki J. Comparison of deep lamellar keratoplasty and penetrating keratoplasty for lattice and macular corneal dystrophies. Am J Ophthalmol. 2006;142(2):304-9.

8.6 Fuchs Endothelial Corneal Dystrophy

Ritu Nagpal, Prafulla Kumar Maharana, Siddhi Goel

1. Discuss the etiology, clinical features, approach, and management of Fuchs endothelial corneal dystrophy (essay-type Question).

Introduction

Fuchs endothelial corneal dystrophy (FECD) was first described in 1910 by Austrian ophthalmologist Ernst Fuchs.[1] FECD is the most common corneal endothelial dystrophy seen in clinical practice. It is a progressive disease characterized by the loss of endothelial cells, thickening of Descemet's membrane, formation of guttae, and development of corneal edema resulting in a significant decrease in visual acuity. In a global survey of corneal transplantation and eye banking by Gain et al.,[2] FECD was the primary indication for all corneal transplantations performed worldwide, accounting for 39%, followed by keratoconus (27%), and infectious keratitis sequelae (20%).

Clinical Features

Fuchs endothelial corneal dystrophy is a slowly progressive disease affecting persons between fifth and seventh decade. The onset of the disease occurs around one decade earlier in Asian countries compared to the west. Females are affected more than males (corneal guttae 2.5 times and corneal edema 5.7 times more than males; overall ratio 4:1).[3]

Symptoms

A case of FECD can present with following symptoms depending on the stage of the disease:
- In the early stages, patients may be asymptomatic or complain of mild blurring of vision (initially in morning gradually improving as the day passes). Symptoms are more prominent in early waking hours as during sleep, the closure of eyelids and subsequent decreased tear film evaporation cause increased stress on the endothelial layer, which must accommodate the demand for regulating corneal water content. With decreased pump function, fluid is unable to effectively leave the cornea at night, leaving glare and blurriness of vision upon waking.
- As the disease progresses, patients complain of blurred vision due to stromal edema, glare, and colored haloes around lights (due to corneal edema).
- In late stages, patients complain of loss of vision, recurrent attacks of redness, and pain due to epithelial edema and rupture of bullae.
- Patients with advanced stages report loss of vision but without any pain or photophobia due to corneal scarring.

Signs

Clinical features depend on the stage of presentation.

Clinical Staging (Table 1)

- *Stage 1 (stage of corneal guttae):*
  - Patient is asymptomatic.
  - *Central corneal guttae:* They appear as tiny dark spots on the posterior corneal surface on direct illumination. Specular reflection also reveals dark spots and disruption of regular endothelial mosaic. In retroillumination, the guttae appear as dewdrops.

TABLE 1: Summary of clinical staging of Fuchs endothelial corneal dystrophy (FECD).			
Stage	Symptoms	Clinical features	Visual acuity
Stage 1	No symptoms	Few-to-moderate corneal guttae	Normal (6/6)
Stage 2	Mild-to-moderate loss of vision, no pain	Moderate-to-numerous corneal guttae, mild stromal edema	Mild-to-moderate reduction (6/6–6/24)
Stage 3	Moderate-to-severe vision loss, presence of pain	Confluent corneal guttae, moderate-to-severe corneal edema, epithelial bullae	Moderate-to-severe reduction (6/30–3/60)
Stage 4	Severe loss of vision, reduced pain	Subepithelial scarring, fewer epithelial bullae	Severe reduction (3/60 or worse)

- As the disease progresses, guttae spread peripherally and coalesce centrally. Endothelial pigment dusting is often present, this characteristically gives the appearance of "beaten metal appearance".
- As the disease progresses, the Descemet's membrane becomes thickened and irregular.
- *Stage 2 (stage of corneal stromal edema):*
  - Corneal edema initially appears in the posterior stroma, which is best seen with sclerotic scatter as a fine gray haze.
  - Vertical wrinkles appear in Descemet's membrane due to corneal stromal swelling.
  - Progressive stromal edema results in a ground-glass opacification with marked thickening of the central cornea.
- *Stage 3 (stage of corneal epithelial edema):*
  - Multiple epithelial microcysts are present that may coalesce to form bullae.
  - Rupture of bullae leads to epithelial erosions causing pain.
- *Stage 4 (stage of scarring):*
  - Avascular subepithelial fibrous scarring occurs between the epithelium and Bowman's membrane.
  - Peripheral superficial corneal neovascularization
  - Visual acuity is severely compromised and may be reduced to hand motions. At this stage, the patient is generally free of painful episodes due to scarring.

In 1979, Dr Jay Krachmer proposed a scale for grading of Fuchs dystrophy.[3] It is divided from grade 0–5 (**Box 1**). Limitations to the Krachmer grading scale include interobserver variability in grading as well as the development of stromal thickening or edema in stages other than grade 5. We, thus use the clinical staging in our cases.

Based on the time of onset of the disease, FECD is divided into two clinical subtypes: early onset and late-onset forms (**Table 2**). The early-onset form of FECD is rare (accounts for 1% of all FECD patients) and has been associated with autosomal

BOX 1: Krachmer grading scale.

Grade 0	No apparent disease 0–12 central guttae on each cornea
Grade 1	Definitive onset of disease >12 central nonconfluent guttae in at least one eye
Grade 2	1–2 mm zone of confluent central guttae
Grade 3	2–5 mm zone of confluent central guttae
Grade 4	>5 mm zone of confluent central guttae
Grade 5	>5 mm zone of confluent guttae with stromal or epithelial edema

TABLE 2: Early- and late-onset Fuchs endothelial corneal dystrophy (FECD).		
Parameters	Early FECD	Late FECD
ICD category	Category 1	Category 2/3
Genetics	Mutation in the gene for the α-2 chain of collagen VIII (COL8A2-Q455K) on chromosome 1 p34.3–p32.	AD, many with no inheritance pattern 13pTel-13q12.13/18q21.2-q21.32/possible SLC4A11
Onset	First decade	Fourth to fifth decade
Retroillumination	Fine, patchy distribution of corneal guttae	Coarse and distinct corneal guttae
Specular microscopy	Small, shallow guttae	Larger guttae
DM	Considerably thicker than late onset	–
Sex distribution	F = M	F > M

dominant mutations in the gene encoding the α-2 subunit of collagen 8[4,5] (COL8A2) on the *1p34.3-p32* gene locus. COL8A2 is an important structural component of Descemet's membrane. Patients with early-onset FECD can exhibit changes in the first decade of life, with continued progression over the next two to three decades. In contrast to late-onset FECD, in which there is a strong female predominance, men and women are equally affected in the early-onset form, a reflection of the autosomal dominant pattern of inheritance.

Late-onset FECD is more common than the early-onset form. Unlike early-onset FECD, a female predominance has been reported in late-onset FECD. Patients with late-onset FECD typically manifest changes by the fifth decade of life, with progression over the next two to three decades. Although the median age of onset for the late-onset form of FECD is at least four decades later than that of the early-onset form, both display a similar linear rate of disease progression, with advancement in clinical severity grade occurring on average every 5 years.

Differential Diagnosis

A case of FECD must be differentiated from following **(Table 3)**:
- Hassall–Henle bodies
- Aphakic or pseudophakic bullous keratopathy
- Congenital hereditary endothelial dystrophy (CHED)
- Iridocorneal endothelial syndrome (ICE)
- Posterior polymorphous corneal dystrophy (PPCD)
- X-linked endothelial corneal dystrophy (XECD)
- Secondary causes of endothelial dysfunction (anterior uveitis, herpes simplex keratitis, interstitial keratitis).

Investigations

Several technical devices are available to aid the slit-lamp based diagnosis. These may be helpful in determining the clinical stage and, therefore, determining the appropriate time for surgery. Due to their noninvasive nature, all examinations may be performed at all stages of the disease. These include:

Noncontact specular microscopy: Corneal endothelium in combination with the excrescences from Descemet's membrane is the key histological layer for diagnosis of FECD. Healthy corneal endothelial cells appear as a regular array of mainly hexagonal cells which exhibit bright cell bodies and dark cell borders. Parameters assessed can be divided into:

TABLE 3: Differential diagnosis of Fuchs endothelial corneal dystrophy (FECD).

Parameters	FECD	PPMD	CHED	ICE
Age of onset	40s to 50s	Teens to 20s	Birth to 10 years	Young adult
Laterality	Bilateral	Bilateral	Bilateral	Unilateral
Sex predilection	F > M	F = M	F = M	F > M
Heredity	AD	AD	AD	No inheritance pattern
Basic defect	Attenuation and reduced number of endothelial cells	Epithelialization of endothelium	Mutation of solute carrier family 4, sodium borate transporter member 11—SLC4A11	Abnormal proliferation of endothelium
Corneal findings	Guttae, stromal thickening, epithelial edema, subepithelial fibrosis	Vesicles, bands, diffuse opacities, plaques at Descemet's membrane	Marked corneal thickening and opacification, endothelium rarely visible	Fine, guttae-like changes, "hammered silver"
Other ocular abnormalities	Increased intraocular pressure, narrow angles	Iris atrophy/corectopia, broad peripheral synechiae, glaucoma 25%	Usually none	Iris atrophy, iris nodules, glaucoma in 80–100%
Progression	Progressive	Minimal	Progressive	Relentless
Specular microscopy	Pleomorphism, polymegathism, decreased endothelial cell count	Focal change, endothelial cells enlarged but count is usually normal	Not possible	Diffuse changes, ICE cell

(CHED: congenital hereditary endothelial dystrophy; ICE: iridocorneal endothelial syndrome; PPMD: posterior polymorphous dystrophy)

- *Qualitative parameters:*
  - Pleomorphism (variation in cell shape, indicates disruption in the regular hexagonal pattern of the endothelium)
  - Polymegathism (variation in cell size, indicates endothelial injury)
- *Quantitative parameters:*
  - Reduced endothelial cell density in mm^2
  - *Increased coefficient of variation (CV):* CV represents the degree of variation in the sizes of the endothelial cells (polymegathism); CV values between 0.22 and 0.31 are considered normal. CV values from 0.32 to 0.40 are elevated, and CV values above 0.40 are abnormal.
  - *Percentage of hexagonal cells (HEX):* In a healthy endothelium, more than 60% of the endothelial cells are hexagonal. In FECD it is <60%.

Corneal pachymetry: The pachymetry may range up to 1,100 μm in the late stage of FECD compared to normal thickness of 530 μm. A central corneal thickness greater than 640 μm usually indicates corneal edema. Measurement of central corneal thickness is important for diagnosis (in doubtful and early cases) and planning of treatment.

In vivo confocal microscopy (IVCM): IVCM is able to demonstrate microstructural changes that correlate well with histological studies. IVCM showed marked reduction of total nerve number and number of nerve branches in the sub-basal corneal nerve plexus with increasing stages of FECD compared to a control group.[6] In presence of corneal edema, confocal microscopy is the best technique for evaluation of corneal endothelium. IVCM can help to assess endothelial cell count and morphology in analogy to specular microscopy.

In addition, backscatter at the basal epithelial cell layer measured by IVCM predicts the need for endothelial keratoplasty (EK) after cataract surgery in patients with FECD. A cut-off of 1,894 scatter units[7] is taken as an indicator for need for a triple procedure.

Anterior segment optical coherence tomography (ASOCT): The advantage of anterior segment OCT is the possibility to measure corneal thickness layer by layer and not as overall thickness, therefore being able to better differentiate between stromal and epithelial edema. It also provides the details of anterior chamber in presence of an edematous cornea. In addition, corneal thickness and depth of scarring can also be detected.

Ultrasonography (USG): USG is done to rule out any posterior segment pathology before proceeding for keratoplasty.

Management

Medical Management

The medical management of FECD can be divided into symptomatic and causative therapy.

Symptomatic Therapy
- *Corneal edema:*
  - *Topical hypertonic saline solutions and ointments (sodium chloride 5% drops and 6% ointment):* They artificially raise the tear film osmolality and dehydrate the cornea by drawing fluid from the epithelium and anterior stroma. The toxic effects of hyperosmolar solutions for the ocular surface are considerably augmented if benzalkonium chloride is used as preservative. Therefore, hyperosmotic solutions without preservative should be preferred.
  - Dehydration of the cornea by a blow dryer in the morning or throughout the day can decrease the symptoms in early stages.
  - Cycloplegics and nonsteroidal anti-inflammatory agents are useful in diminishing corneal pain from bullous keratopathy.
  - *Reduction of intraocular pressure:* Use of intraocular pressure-lowering medications may help to reduce corneal edema in patients with elevated or even normal intraocular pressure.
- *Recurrent erosion:*
  - *Bandage contact lenses:* Use of therapeutic soft contact lenses help in relieving the pain from recurrent epithelial erosions. They also help in improving vision by decreasing irregular astigmatism in cases that have progressed to bullous keratopathy.
  - Anterior stromal puncture/amniotic membrane graft/photo-therapeutic keratectomy/conjunctival flaps (Gunderson flap) have been described for symptomatic relief of bullous keratopathy in cases where the visual prognosis is poor. However, these procedures are rarely required in FECD, as the visual potential is often good.

Causative Therapy

Because corneal endothelium does not divide in vivo, loss of endothelial cells seen in FECD is permanent. Given that apoptosis of endothelial cells is the main cause, different pathophysiological pathways for a possible medical therapeutic approach are been investigated.

One such class of drugs being studied are Rho kinase inhibitors. Various studies demonstrate inhibition of Rho-associated protein kinase (ROCK) enhances cell proliferation, promotes cell adhesion onto a substrate, and suppresses apoptosis of corneal endothelial cells (CECs). ROCK signaling has therefore attracted interest as a potential therapeutic target for these diseases. The administration of a ROCK inhibitor[8] in an eye drop form promoted corneal endothelial wound healing in a rabbit model in which the central corneal endothelium was damaged with a stainless steel cryoprobe (6 mm diameter). Two ROCK inhibitors, Y-27632 and Y-39983, enhanced the rate of wound healing and accelerated the recovery of corneal transparency. The promising responses to ROCK inhibitors appear to open up new therapeutic possibilities.

Surgical Management

Surgery in FECD is performed for advanced disease resulting in loss of daily function, low visual acuity, and/or pain secondary to epithelial bulla formation.

The different surgical options in a case of FECD are described below.

Endothelial keratoplasty: Currently, the treatment of choice. The different techniques of EK are as follows:
- Descemet's stripping endothelial keratoplasty (DSEK)—the donor tissue (consisting of DM-endothelium complex and posterior stroma) is prepared using manual technique.
- Descemet's stripping automated endothelial keratoplasty (DSAEK)—similar to DSEK except the donor tissue is prepared using a microkeratome.
- Descemet's membrane endothelial keratoplasty (DMEK)—donor tissue consists of only DM-endothelium complex and no stroma. Technically difficult than DSAEK but visual results are better than DSAEK.
- Predescemetic endothelial keratoplasty (PDEK)—donor tissue consists of DM-endothelium complex along with Dua's layer. Technically difficult than DSAEK but easier than DMEK due to increased graft thickness.

Advantages of EK are:
- Rapid visual rehabilitation
- No suture-related complications
- Decreased incidence of allograft rejection
- Intact globe, resistant to traumatic wound dehiscence
- Predictable corneal toricity, minimal topographic change
- Predictable, small hyperopic refractive shift (1.0–1.5 diopters)

Disadvantages of EK are:
- New procedure for the corneal surgeon
- Technically demanding, with a significant learning curve
- Potentially significant loss of donor endothelium during the transfer process (higher risk of primary graft failure)
- Incidence of dislocation (2–50%)
- Potential interface haze

Penetrating keratoplasty: A full-thickness graft is indicated in presence of corneal scarring or lack of skilled surgeon in lamellar keratoplasty.

Relative contraindications to EK are:
- Stromal scarring
- Keratoconus/ectasia
- Astigmatism >6Ds
- ACD < 2.8 mm
- PAS > 180°
- CCT > 800 μm
- Large peripheral iridectomy/posterior capsule rent/aphakia.

A study done by Moloney et al.[9] suggests that in Fuchs dystrophy with visual degradation due to central guttae, central 4 mm descemetorhexis without grafting is a viable procedure for visual rehabilitation. Careful patient selection is required, but with the advent of topical ripasudil as a salvage agent, a broader application of the surgery may be possible.

FECD with cataract: Senile cataract is commonly seen in cases of FECD due to the common age group of affection. It is often a dilemma to decide if cataract surgery alone is enough or the patient needs a triple procedure. Although there are no universal guidelines, most corneal surgeons follow the following approach:

- *Only cataract with IOL:*
  - Specular count >1,000 cells/mm^2
  - CCT <600 μm
  - Good corneal clarity to allow cataract surgery
- *Triple procedure:*
  - Specular count <800 cells/mm^2
  - CCT >640 μm
  - Backscatter at the basal epithelial cell layer measured by IVCM >1,894 scatter units[7]
  - Corneal clarity is not enough to allow cataract surgery.

In cases where the values of CCT and endothelial counts are in between, the decision is individualized and based on surgeons experience.

References

1. Fuchs E. Dystrophia epithelialis corneae. Albrecht Von Graefes Archiv Fur Klinische Und Experimentelle Ophthalmologie. 1910;76:478-508.
2. Gain P, Jullienne R, He Z, Aldossary M, Acquart S, Cognasse F, et al. Global survey of corneal transplantation and eye banking. JAMA Ophthalmol. 2016;134(2):167-73.
3. Krachmer JH, Purcell Jr JJ, Young CW, Bucher KD. Corneal endothelial dystrophy: a study of 64 families. Arch Ophthalmol. 1978;96:2036-39.
4. Eghrari AO, Gottsch JD. Fuchs' corneal dystrophy. Expert Rev Ophthalmol. 2010;5(2):147-59.
5. Liskova P, Prescott Q, Bhattacharya SS, Tuft SJ. British family with early-onset Fuchs' endothelial corneal dystrophy associated with p.L450W mutation in the *COL8A2* gene. Br J Ophthalmol. 2007;91(12):1717-8.
6. Bucher F, Adler W, Lehmann HC, Hos D, Steven P, Cursiefen C, et al. Corneal nerve alterations in different stages of Fuchs' endothelial corneal dystrophy: an in vivo confocal microscopy study. Graefes Arch Clin Exp Ophthalmol. 2014;252(7):1119-26.
7. van Cleynenbreugel H, Remeijer L, Hillenaar T. Cataract surgery in patients with Fuchs' endothelial corneal dystrophy: when to consider a triple procedure. Ophthalmology. 2014;121(2):445-53.
8. Okumura N, Kinoshita S, Koizumi N. Application of rho kinase inhibitors for the treatment of corneal endothelial diseases. J Ophthalmol. 2017;2017:2646904.
9. Moloney G, Petsoglou C, Ball M, Kerdraon Y, Höllhumer R, Spiteri N, et al. Descemetorhexis without grafting for Fuchs, endothelial dystrophy-supplementation with topical ripasudil. Cornea. 2017;36(6):642-8.

8.7 Keratoconus

Prafulla Kumar Maharana, Pranita Sahay

1. Discuss keratoconus (essay-type Question).

Introduction

Keratoconus (KC) is a disorder characterized by progressive corneal steepening (usually asymmetrical noninflammatory), most typically inferior to the center of the cornea, with eventual corneal thinning, induced myopia, and irregular astigmatism. It is the most common corneal ectatic disorder seen in clinical practice. Prevalence of KC is about 54.5 cases per 100,000.[1-3] KC is noted in people of all races with no significant gender predilection. KC usually occurs bilaterally. Unilateral cases have been described with incidence in the range of 2–4%.[1-3] The age of onset is usually around puberty. Progression of the disease is rapid till the age of 30 years and stops by the age of 40 years. KC is more prevalent in the Asian countries than in the West, compared to the western world Asian patients present at a younger age.

Etiology

Keratoconus is largely idiopathic but several ocular and systemic associations are seen. Ocular allergy is a common association in India.

- *Ocular associations:*
  - Floppy eyelid syndrome
  - Corneal granular dystrophy
  - Vernal keratoconjunctivitis (VKC)
  - Refractive surgery
  - Leber's congenital amaurosis
  - Cone-rod dystrophy
  - Trauma
- *Systemic associations:*
  - Down syndrome
  - Atopy-bronchial asthma, angioneurotic edema, Marfan syndrome
  - Mitral valve prolapse
  - Rosacea.

Clinical Features

Symptoms

A case of KC can present with following symptoms:
- Progressive visual blurring and/or distortion—due to associated irregular astigmatism. It may be associated with photophobia, glare, monocular diplopia, and ocular irritation.
- Frequent change of glasses—the irregular astigmatism is often difficult to correct with glasses hence the patient keeps on visiting different optometrist.
- Rarely a case may present with symptoms of associated disease such as recurrent attacks of itching, eye rubbing (VKC).

Signs

Following signs can be seen in a case of KC depending upon the stage of the disease:[1,4-7]
- *Mild cases:*
  - Scissoring of the red reflex on retinoscopy
  - *Charleux sign:* With a dilated pupil and a +6D lens positioned in front of the eye one can appreciate a dark reflex in the area of cone with a central bright reflex resembling a drop of honey or oil in the reflection of the red bottom from a direct ophthalmoscope.
- *Moderate-to-severe cases:*
  - *Corneal thinning:* Corneal thinning located outside the visual axis is a common sign preceding ectasia. It is most commonly seen inferiorly or inferotemporally.
  - *Corneal ectasia:* An eccentrically located ectatic protrusion of the cornea is noted in KC. The apex is usually seen inferior to a horizontal line passing through the pupillary axis.
  - *Corneal scarring:* Usually subepithelial scarring is seen **(Fig. 1)**.
  - *Fleischer's ring:* A partial or complete annular line of hemosiderin (iron deposits) is seen at the base of the cone. This ring is brown in color and best appreciated with the cobalt blue filter using a broad, oblique beam **(Fig. 2)**.
  - *Vogt's striae:* Fine vertical lines produced by compression of Descemet's membrane (DM), which tend to disappear when physical pressure is applied on the cornea digitally or by a gas permeable contact lens (CL). The lines are seen in the deep stroma and Descemet's membrane and are parallel to the axis of the cone.
  - *Prominent corneal nerves:* Increased visibility of corneal nerves results from the outward bowing and thinning of the ectatic cornea **(Fig. 3)**.
  - *Increased intensity of the corneal endothelial reflex:* An endothelial reflex may appear at the peak of the cone due to the increased concavity of the posterior corneal surface.
  - *Subepithelial fibrillary lines:* White subepithelial fibrillary lines in concentric bundles lying just inside the Fleischer's ring can be seen.[1]
  - *Corneal hyperesthesia:* It can be detected early in the course of the disease. Later the cone becomes relatively less sensitive.
- *Advanced stages:*
  - *Rizzuti phenomenon:* A bright focus of light is seen near nasal limbus when a penlight is projected on the temporal side of cornea or to the iris plane.

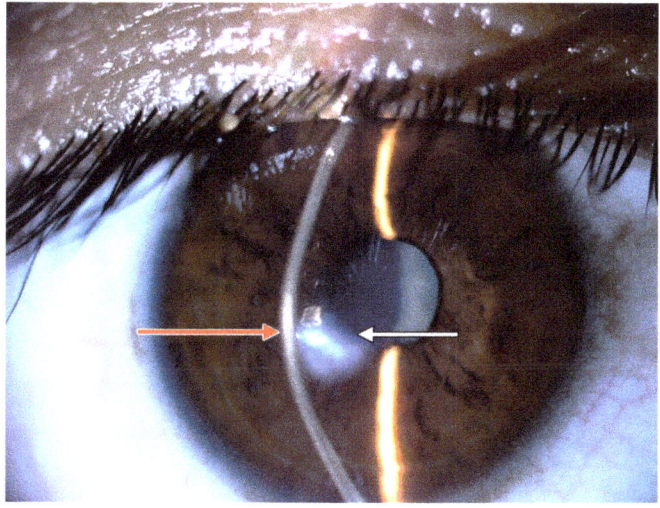

Fig. 1: A case of keratoconus with corneal ectasia and thinning (red arrow) and subepithelial scar (white arrow).

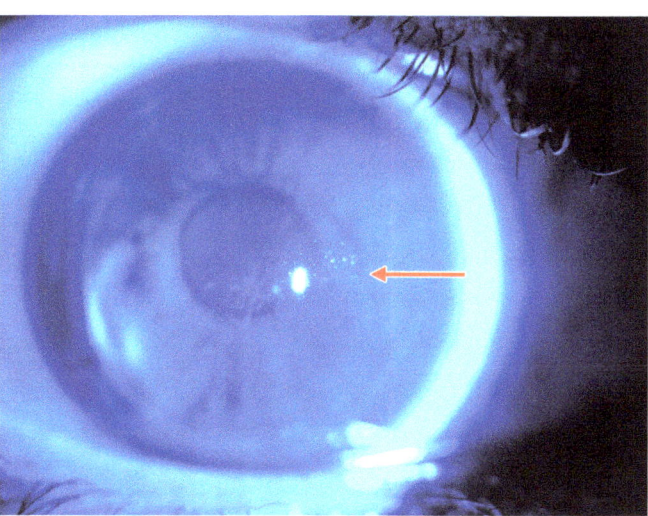

Fig. 2: Fleischer's ring as seen with cobalt blue filter on slit-lamp examination.

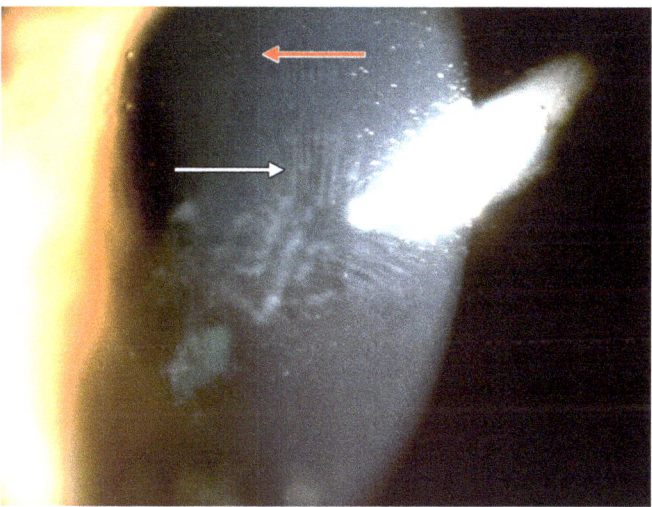

Fig. 3: Slit-lamp photograph showing Vogt's striae (white arrow) and prominent corneal nerve (red arrow).

- *Munson sign:* Anterior bowing of lower lid is seen on downward gaze of the patient.
- *Corneal hydrops:* Breaks in Descemet's membrane can lead to acute stromal edema causing sudden vision loss and significant pain **(Fig. 4)**.

Classification/Grading

Keratoconus is classified based on morphology, disease evolution, ocular signs, and index-based systems.
- *Morphological classification:*
  - *Nipple:* The cone has a diameter ≤5 mm, round morphology located in the central or paracentral cornea, more commonly in the inferonasal corneal quadrant. Correction with CLs is relatively easy.
  - *Oval:* The cone has a diameter >5 mm and a paracentral to peripheral location, more commonly in the inferotemporal quadrant. CL correction is relatively difficult.
  - *Globus:* The cone is located throughout 75% of the cornea. CL correction is a challenge in most of the cases.
- *Disease progression:* Amsler proposed the first KC classification based on the disease evolution **(Table 1)**.[2]

Differential Diagnosis

The differential diagnosis of KC has been described in **Table 2**.

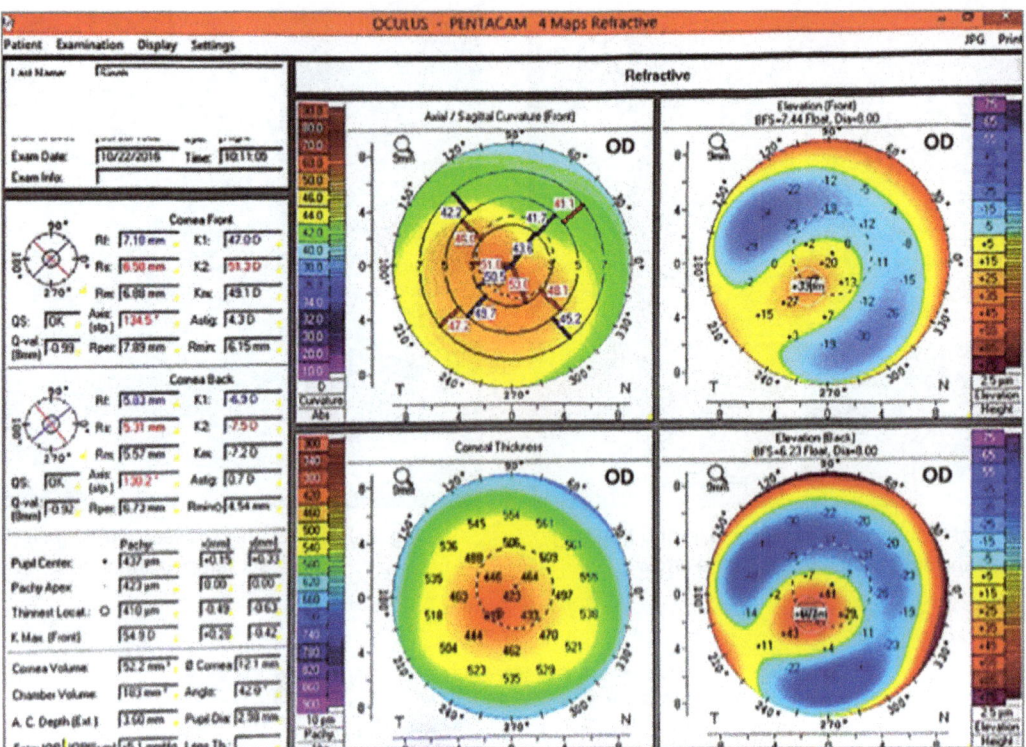

Fig. 4: Pentacam photograph of a case of keratoconus showing anterior ectasia, posterior ectasia, and decreased corneal thickness.

Stage	Description
1	• Eccentric corneal bulging • Myopia and/or astigmatism <5D • Corneal radius ≤48D • Vogt's striae • No central opacity
2	• Myopia and/or astigmatism >5D but <8D • Corneal radius ≤53D • No central opacity • Pachymetry ≥400 μ
3	• Myopia and/or astigmatism >8D but <10D • Corneal radius >53D • No central corneal opacity • Pachymetry 200–400 μ
4	• Refraction not possible • Corneal steepening >55.00D • Corneal scarring • Pachymetry <200 μ

TABLE 1: Amsler, Krumeich classification of keratoconus

Work-up

History

It is important to know whether the KC is progressive or not. In case of progression, the patient can be advised to undergo corneal collagen crosslinking (CXL). The best way to document progression is serial topography taking into consideration the change in keratometry. However, progressive deterioration of *best-corrected visual acuity* (BCVA), progressive decrease in corneal thickness, and a previously CL tolerant patient becoming CL intolerant are certain other clinical clues of KC progression. Following history must be recorded carefully:

- *Contact lens wear:* Its role in KC progression is controversial. A better BCVA with CL indicates good prognosis after keratoplasty.

TABLE 2: Differential diagnosis of keratoconus.

Characteristics	Keratoconus	PMD	Keratoglobus	TMD
Frequency	Most common	Less common	Rare	Rare
Laterality	Usually bilateral	Bilateral	Bilateral	Bilateral
Age at onset	Puberty	20–40 years	Usually at birth	Middle-aged to elderly
Thinning	Inferior paracentral	Inferior band 1–2 mm wide	Maximum in periphery	Superior cornea
CCT	Reduced	Usually normal	May be normal	Usually normal
Protrusion	Thinnest at apex	Superior to band of thinning	Generalized	Superior cornea
• Rizutti's phenomenon • Munson's sign	Present	Absent	Present	Absent
Fleischer ring	Present	Sometimes	None	Absent
Scarring	Common	Only after hydrops	Mild	Superior cornea with vascularization, lipid deposition, and inflammation
Vogt's striae	Common	Sometimes	Sometimes	Absent

- *Eye rubbing:* Mechanical epithelial trauma leads to release of cytokines that have a role in corneal weakening and ectasia.
- *Ocular surgery:* KC can occur secondary to ocular surgeries such as laser-assisted in-situ keratomileusis (LASIK), and radial keratotomy (RK). Hence, any past refractive surgery must be enquired. In few cases, a previous history of CXL may be there.
- *Past medical history:* KC can be associated with certain ocular and systemic disorders. A careful history must be taken to rule out these disorders.
- *Family history:* Between 6 and 18% of patients with KC have a positive family history.[1-3]

Examination

- *Visual acuity:* Uncorrected visual acuity (UCVA), BCVA, and refraction must be assessed in all cases.
- *Facial appearance/Orbit:* Look for sign of orbital fat atrophy/oculodigital phenomena suggestive of chronic eye rubbing.
- *Eyelid:* Look for signs of allergic conjunctivitis.
- *Conjunctiva:* Look for presence of papillae in tarsal conjunctiva. In India, KC is often associated with VKC or allergic conjunctivitis. Signs of VKC include papillae, Trantas dots (gelatinous thickening of limbus), limbal nodule, pigmentation, and ropy discharge.
- *Cornea:* Look for the various signs as described under signs.
- *Fundus examination:* Dilated fundus evaluation is essential for any concomitant fundus abnormality.

Investigations

Keratometry

Keratometry mires in KC are commonly steep, highly astigmatic, irregular, and often appear egg-shaped (rather than circular or oval). The disadvantages of keratometry in KC is that it provides information about central 3 mm of cornea only and is not useful in irregular astigmatism.

Pachymetry

Both ultrasonic and optical based principle (ASOCT) can be used to measure the pachymetry. Measurement of corneal thickness is useful for diagnosis, documentation of progression, and treatment (see treatment section).

Imaging in Keratoconus

The diagnosis of moderate-to-severe KC, clinically, is straightforward. The role of imaging in modern era is primarily in identifying mild and forme fruste KC (FFKC) which are known risk factors for post-LASIK ectasia, detecting progression of KC, especially when CXL is an option for arresting progression and to differentiate KC from other forms of corneal ectasia.[8] The different corneal imaging modalities commonly used are described below. Pentacam and spectral domain OCT are the most commonly performed imaging modalities for KC.

Placido-disc-based Imaging [Videokeratography (VKG)]

It provides qualitative contour information. In early cases, there will be an isolated area of smaller ring spacing and distortion. As the KC worsens, the cornea becomes steeper; the ring spacing decreases overall and becomes increasingly irregular. Its disadvantage is it does not give accurate information about posterior curvature (can not detect early KC) and corneal thickness.

Scanning slit-based Imaging (Orbscan)

It provides reliable data on anterior and posterior elevation, best-fit sphere, and corneal pachymetry map. However, the posterior curvature maps are based on assumptions and may not be 100% accurate.

Scheimpflug imaging (Pentacam/Oculyzer/Galilei)

It provides reliable measurement of anterior and posterior corneal elevation and accurate measurement of corneal thickness **(Fig. 4)**. It also covers significantly more of the cornea in periphery than was possible with earlier devices and thus, is extremely useful in proper diagnosis of peripheral diseases such as pellucid marginal corneal degeneration (PMCD). It is one of the useful tools for diagnosis of early KC. Different pentacam values that help in diagnosis of FFKC are summarized in **Table 3**.[9]

Anterior Segment Optical Coherence Tomography

Fourier-domain optical coherence tomography (OCT) can be used for examination and measurement of different layers. It can map the corneal epithelium thickness, facilitating early KC detection **(Table 4)**. In addition, it is extremely useful in assessing the depth of scar and hence, to decide upon the type of surgery. Another important use of ASOCT is in diagnosis and management of corneal hydrops as it can accurately show the area of DM tear and location of fluid pockets in the cornea. A new OCT classification for KC has been proposed based on structural corneal changes at the cone during the evolution of the disease. This classification is useful in advanced cases of KC in which the repeatability of corneal topography measurements is not reliable.[10]

Corneal Biomechanics in Keratoconus

The current concept for KC is that there is a focal area of weakening in corneal structure to begin with. Various environmental and other factors such as atopy, eye rubbing start a chronic cycle of biomechanical weakening that leads to localized thinning and steepening, which ultimately culminates in KC.[11,12] Thus, earliest changes in KC corneas can be detected by in-vivo assessment of corneal biomechanics. Currently, there are two commercially available devices for in vivo characterization of corneal biomechanics, i.e., ocular response analyzer (ORA); Reichert ophthalmic instruments (Buffalo, NY), and Corvis

TABLE 3: Pentacam parameters for diagnosis of early KC/FFKC.

Findings on the sagittal map:
- Central K-readings ≥48D
- SRAX ≥22°
- Superior–inferior difference (S–I) on the 5 mm circle ≥2.5D
- Inferior–Superior difference (I–S) ≥1.5D
- Corneal astigmatism ≥6D

Findings on the thickness map:
- Thinnest location < 470 μ
- Y-co-ordinate value of the thinnest location ≥ –500 μ
- Pachymetry apex – thickness at thinnest location ≥10 μ
- Superior–inferior at 5 mm circle ≥30 μ
- Difference in thickness between both eyes at thinnest locations ≥30 μ

Findings on the elevation maps:
- Isolated focal island of ectasia (BFS mode) on either surface
- Values ≥12 μ within the central 5 mm on the anterior elevation map (BFTE mode)
- Values ≥15 μ within the central 5 mm on the posterior elevation map (BFTE mode)

(BFS: best fit sphere; BFTE: best fit toric ellipsoid; KC/FFKC: keratoconus/forme fruste keratoconus; SRAX: skewed radial axis)

TABLE 4: Optical coherence tomography-based classification of keratoconus.		
Stage	**Classical features**	**Other features**
Stage 1	Thinning of epithelium and stromal layers at the cone	An annulus of thickened epithelium is seen surrounding the thin epithelium at the cone giving the characteristic "doughnut pattern"
Stage 2	Hyper-reflective anomalies at the Bowman's layer level with a thickened epithelium at the cone	Variable amount of stromal opacities
Stage 3	Posterior displacement of the hyper-reflective structures occurring at the Bowman's layer level with increased epithelial thickening and stromal thinning	Variable amount of stromal opacities
Stage 4	Pan-stromal scar	Thickened epithelium compensates for the stromal thinning
Stage 5	*Hydrops:* large intrastromal cysts communicating with anterior chamber through a tear in Descemet's membrane	*5a, acute onset:* Descemet's membrane rupture and dilaceration of collagen lamellae with large fluid-filled intrastromal cysts *5b, healing stage:* Total corneal scarring with a remaining aspect of Descemet's membrane rupture

ST (Oculus, Wetzlar, Germany). Although different studies have tried to evaluate biomechanical response, with majority on ORA, it is difficult to recommend precise guidelines. Various factors responsible for this are, wide variability in normative data among different population and overlap of parameters between normal and abnormal corneas.

From current evidence, it seems waveform-derived parameters that describe corneal deformation through specific waveform features such as width, peak area, height of the peaks, and radius of curvature at highest concavity or inverse concave radius in Corvis ST, are the parameters that may turn out to be useful in early cases of KC in future. The other major use of corneal biomechanics could be evaluation of biomechanical changes in KC with different management techniques such as CXL or keratoplasty. This may allow us to know the efficacy of the various procedures. Postoperative ORA assessments have shown that following deep anterior lamellar keratoplasty (DALK), corneas achieve biomechanical metrics similar to those of normal corneas while penetrating keratoplasty (PKP) treated corneas do not achieve the same. Similarly, experimental CXL studies have reported corneal stiffness increase of about 300% following CXL suggesting its efficacy in halting the progression.[11,12] However, as discussed earlier, changes in corneal stiffness could not be properly validated in in-vivo studies and further research is needed in this field.

Management

The treatment of KC management varies depending on the disease severity **(Flowchart 1)**. Early case is managed with spectacles, mild-to-moderate cases are managed with CLs, and severe cases can be treated with keratoplasty. Other surgical treatment options include intra-corneal rings segments, corneal cross-linking, intraocular lens implants, or a combination of these.

Nonsurgical Management

- *Spectacles:* Spectacles are normally used in early cases of KC only. As the disease progresses, irregular astigmatism develops and adequate visual acuity cannot be achieved with this type of visual correction.
- *Contact lens:* Different CLs used for treatment of KC are soft toric lenses, standard bicurved hard lenses, custom-back toric lenses, piggyback systems, hybrid lenses (made of combined hard lens with a soft skirt), scleral lenses, and mini-scleral lenses. Rigid gas permeable (RGP) lenses are the lenses of first choice for correcting the irregular astigmatism. The three-point touch fitting technique is the most popular technique. Piggyback systems consisting of the fitting a gas permeable on top of a soft CL improves the CL tolerance. The soft CL is used to improve wearing comfort and provide a more regular area for the gas permeable CLs to sit, whereas the gas permeable CL is primarily used for providing adequate visual acuity. Hybrid CLs (such as SoftPerm, Solotica, and Synergeyes) contain an RGP center with a soft skirt. New-generation hybrid CL provides higher oxygen permeability and greater strength of the RGP/hydrogel junction. Rose K lenses (Rose K, Rose K2 XL, and Rose K2 IC) are multicurve lenses with a small optical zone that snugly fits over the cone. Scleral lenses rest on the sclera and do not touch the cornea and limbus, leaving a clear area between the CL and the cornea. The advantages are good centration, stability, and improved visual acuity (VA).[2,3]

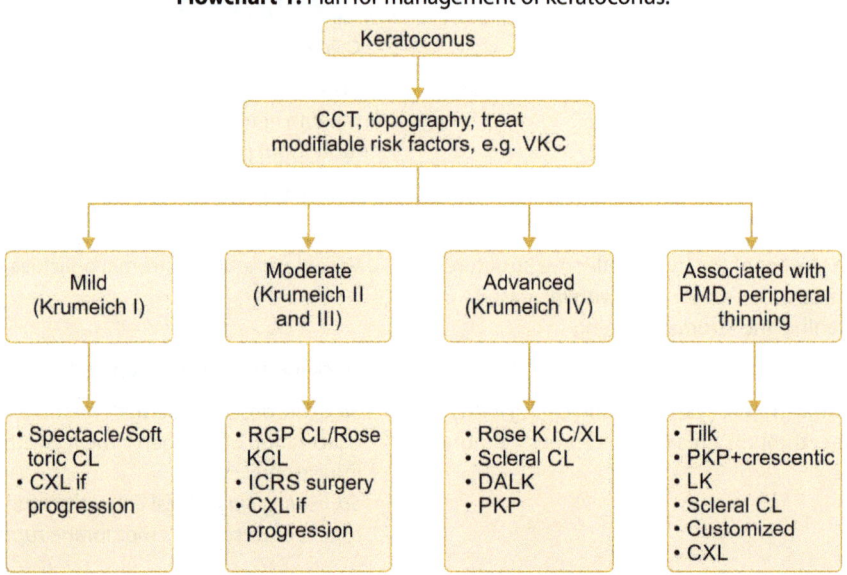

Flowchart 1: Plan for management of keratoconus.

(CCT: central corneal thickness; CL: contact lens; CXL: corneal collagen crosslinking; DALK: deep anterior lamellar keratoplasty; ICRS: intrastromal corneal ring segment; LK: lamellar keratoplasty; PKP: penetrating keratoplasty; PMD: pellucid marginal degeneration; RGP: rigid gas permeable; TILK: tuck in lamellar keratoplasty; VKC: vernal keratoconjunctivitis)

Surgical Management

Current surgical options include:
- *Corneal transplantation:* Penetrating keratoplasty, DALK
- *Intracorneal ring segment insert:* Intacs, Ferrara rings
- UV-A/riboflavin corneal cross-linkage (CXL)
- *Lenticular refractive surgery:* Refractive lens exchange with toric intraocular lenses, toric phakic intraocular lenses.

Penetrating keratoplasty (PKP): PKP in KC in comparison to other indications is considered a low-risk PKP in terms of graft rejection, graft survival, and postoperative complications. The success rate is 90–95%.

Deep anterior lamellar keratoplasty: DALK has several advantages over PKP. In KC, the corneal endothelium is usually healthy; with good cell counts even after cases of acute hydrops. Hence, DALK is the procedure of choice. The major disadvantage is corneal stromal rejection and migration of host keratocytes to replace donor keratocytes resulting in recurrence of the disease in graft. However, stromal rejection can never lead to graft failure and recurrence in graft is extremely rare.

The goal of DALK is to achieve a depth of dissection as close as possible to DM. Various agents have been used to create a plane of separation between DM and the deep stromal layers. These include air, fluid, viscoelastic, microkeratome, and a femtosecond laser. The common techniques of DALK are: Layer-by-layer manual dissection, air-assisted DALK (Archilla), big bubble DALK (Anwar), viscoelastic-assisted DALK (Melles NO et al.), hydrodelamination (Sugita), and femtosecond-assisted DALK.

Intracorneal ring segments (Intacs and Ferrara rings): The technique consists of the implantation of one or two polymethyl methacrylate segments in the corneal stroma to flatten the central cornea and improve visual acuity, CL tolerance and delay the need for corneal graft. It acts by its arc-shortening effect and is commonly used to treat mild-to-moderate cases of KC, as normal corneal transparency and a minimum corneal thickness of 450 μm at the site of the incision are required.

Three types of rings are available: Intacs which have a hexagonal cross-section and are placed more peripheral than Ferrara rings which are triangular/prismatic in shape. Recently, Intacs SK (SK-severe KC) has been introduced for use in more severe forms of corneal ectasia. It has two significant design modifications—a smaller inner diameter of 6.0 mm compared with 6.8 mm of the standard Intacs and an elliptical cross-section compared with a hexagonal cross-section of the standard Intacs.

The rings are inserted into the posterior stroma (about 75% of corneal depth at the incision site) in a quick daycare procedure performed under topical anesthesia. The circular intralamellar pockets for the rings are created either using a especially designed vacuum lamellar dissector or with the femtosecond laser. Intracorneal ring technology does not offer a cure for the condition but can very often produce a marked improvement in unaided and best-corrected visual acuity and allow eyes to be corrected with spectacles and/or soft rather than rigid lenses.

Corneal collagen crosslinking with riboflavin (C3R) or corneal cross-linkage (CXL): CXL using riboflavin (vitamin B_2)/ultraviolet A (UV-A) [370 nm] light is a therapeutic modality that can halt and stabilize the keratoconic process. It increases the corneal rigidity and biomechanical stability. The success rate varies between studies but overall 60–70% cases show some stabilization after CXL.[2,5] The procedure involves removing the corneal epithelium in a 6–7-mm diameter central zone followed by riboflavin 0.1% solution application and corneal radiation with UV-A light at 370 nm. UV-A light radiation activates riboflavin; generating reactive oxygen species that induce covalent bonds between collagen fibrils in the corneal stroma. The irradiation level at the corneal endothelium, lens, and retina is significantly smaller than the damage threshold. It has been recommended not to perform this technique in corneas thinner than 400 µm as toxic reactions could take place in the corneal endothelium. In such cases, hypotonic CXL have been tried with variable success.

CXL is largely safe except the risk of keratitis. No long-term problems in terms of loss of transparency of the cornea or lens and endothelial counts have been noted. In addition, this technique can successfully be used in combination with other surgical techniques, such as corneal rings segments.

A review of literature suggests reduction of Kmax in the range of 0.4–2.0D, stabilization of corneal thickness, one to two-line improvement in UCVA (although variable) at 1 year of CXL. The impact of CXL beyond 1 year is unpredictable as per the current evidence.[13]

Refractive lens exchange: Refractive lens exchange and toric phakic intraocular lens insertion may be of some benefit in correcting myopia and astigmatism in selected eyes with early and stable disease with good spectacle corrected visual acuity.

Key Points

- VKC is an important risk factor for KC in India.
- KC can present early in association with VKC.
- CXL is effective in halting the progression of KC.
- Most patients can be rehabilitated using RGP CLs.
- DALK is the surgical procedure of choice.

References

1. Krachmer JH, Feder RS, Belin MW. Keratoconus and related non-inflammatory corneal thinning disorders. Surv Ophthalmol. 1984;28:293-322.
2. Krachmer JH, Mannis MJ, Holland EJ (Eds). Cornea, 2nd edition, Volume 1. Philadelphia: Elsevier, Mosby; 2005. p. 955.
3. Maharana PK, Dubey A, Jhanji V, Sharma N, Das S, Vajpayee RB. Management of advanced corneal ectasias. Br J Ophthalmol. 2016;100(1):34-40.
4. Maharana PK, Agarwal K, Jhanji V, Vajpayee RB. Deep anterior lamellar keratoplasty for keratoconus: a review. Eye Contact Lens. 2014;40(6):382-9.
5. American Academy of Optometry. Keratoconus; 2008. pp. 1-13.
6. Espandar L, Meyer J. Keratoconus: overview and update on treatment. Middle East Afr J Ophthalmol. 2010;17:15-20.
7. Romero-Jiménez M, Santodomingo-Rubido J, Wolffsohn JS. Keratoconus: a review. Cont Lens Anterior Eye. 2010;33:157-66.
8. Matalia H, Swarup R. Imaging modalities in keratoconus. Indian J Ophthalmol. 2013;61:394-400.
9. Sinjab MM. Classifications and patterns of keratoconus and keratectasia. In: Quick Guide to the Management of Keratoconus. Springer, Berlin, Heidelberg; 2012.
10. Sandali O, El Sanharawi M, Temstet C, Hamiche T, Galan A, Ghouali W, et al. Fourier-domain optical coherence tomography imaging in keratoconus: a corneal structural classification. Ophthalmology. 2013;120(12):2403-12.
11. Ambrósio Jr R, Correia FF, Lopes B, Salomão MQ, Luz A, Dawson DG, et al. Corneal biomechanics in ectatic diseases: refractive surgery implications. Open Ophthalmol J. 2017;11:176-93.
12. Bao F, Geraghty B, Wang Q, Elsheikh A. Consideration of corneal biomechanics in the diagnosis and management of keratoconus: is it important? Eye Vis (Lond). 2016;3:18.
13. Kobashi H, Rong SS. Corneal collagen cross-linking for keratoconus: systematic review. Bio Med Res Int. 2017;2017:8145651.

8.8 Limbal Stem Cell Deficiency

Ritu Nagpal, Alisha Kishore, Prafulla Kumar Maharana

 1. Describe the etiology, pathogenesis, clinical features, work-up, and management of limbal stem cell deficiency (LSCD).

Introduction

Limbal stem cells are important for maintaining the stability of the ocular surface. These stem cells are located in the palisades of Vogt in the basal layer. These cells are pluripotent and help in the regeneration of the corneal epithelial cells. It also forms a barrier between the epithelium of the cornea and conjunctiva. Any condition affecting these stem cells results in a condition known as limbal stem cell deficiency. This results in loss of barrier function between the cornea and conjunctiva, and hence the conjunctival epithelium encroaches upon the cornea. This leads to loss of corneal transparency.[1,2]

XYZ hypothesis: It was given by Thoft and Friend in 1983 for the maintenance of corneal epithelium. According to it, the corneal epithelial cells which are lost from the surface (Z) are replaced by the cells from the periphery to the center of the cornea (X) and also from the basal layers to the surface of the epithelium (Y). Therefore to maintain homeostasis Z = X + Y.

Etiology

It can be hereditary or acquired. It can result from either the stem cell loss or the destruction of "niche" **(Table 1)**.[1-4]

Clinical Presentation

Symptoms

The clinical manifestation depends upon the severity and extent of the LSCD. It can be partial or total. The patient generally presents with the following symptoms:
- Recurrent episodes of pain, foreign body sensation, and redness
- Chronic redness of the eye
- Decrease of vision
- Photophobia
- Blepharospasm and watering
- Whitish patch in the eye.

Signs

The slit-lamp examination reveals the following:
- Dull and irregular corneal reflex
- Loss of limbal palisades of Vogt

TABLE 1: Causes of limbal stem cell deficiency.

	Limbal stem cell loss		Niche destruction	
Hereditary	Epidermal dysplasia		• Aniridia • Endocrine disorder leading to keratitis	
Acquired	Trauma	• Burns • Multiple surgeries • Radiation • Antimetabolites	Trauma	• Antimetabolites • Radiation
	Systemic conditions	• Stevens–Johnson syndrome (SJS) • Ocular cicatricial pemphigoid (OCP) • Vitamin A deficiency	Ocular conditions	• Postinfectious keratitis • Neurotrophic keratitis • Peripheral ulcerative keratitis • VKC • Contact lens use
	Idiopathic		Malignancy	

(VKC: vernal keratoconjunctivitis)

- Conjunctivalization of cornea—shows irregular and late stippled staining with fluorescein
- Vascularization resulting in fibrovascular pannus
- Recurrent epithelial defects
- Chronic keratitis
- Scarring
- Keratinization
- Calcification
- Corneal melt and perforation
- Subconjunctival fibrosis leads to symblepharon and forniceal shortening
- Abnormalities of the lid margins—posterior migration of mucocutaneous junction, irregularity of the lid margins, misdirected eyelashes, entropion, ectropion, and mechanical ptosis
- Periocular changes—suggestive of the etiology behind the LSCD.

Work-up

History

- Onset, progression, and duration of all the symptoms
- Ask relevant history to rule out any underlying etiology as listed in **Table 1**.
- Any endocrine disorder
- Recurrent episode of redness and pain
- History of chemical and thermal injury
- Antimetabolites use (mitomycin C, 5-fluorouracil)
- Previous history of surgery
- History of radiation
- Other mucosal involvement
- History of contact lens.

Examination

Visual acuity: Decreased due to loss of corneal clarity and later due to scar formation

Eyelid: Blister, scar formation, cicatrization in case of Stevens–Johnson syndrome (SJS), ocular cicatricial pemphigoid (OCP), burns

Conjunctiva: Subconjunctival fibrosis with symblepharon formation and forniceal shortening

Limbus: Loss of palisades of Vogt

Cornea: Dull corneal reflex, conjunctivalization of cornea, vascularization, pannus formation, keratitis, scarring, keratinization, persistent epithelial defect, and corneal perforation

Intraocular pressure: Look for any associated secondary glaucoma

Iris, anterior chamber, lens, and posterior segment details are generally not visible due to loss of corneal transparency. Hence, ultrasonography should be done to rule out any gross posterior segment abnormality.

Fellow eye: Look for any abnormality in the fellow eye

Classification

Holland–Mannis classification based on number of lost stem cells and conjunctival inflammation is extremely useful for grading, planning surgery, and prognostication of such cases **(Table 2)**.

TABLE 2: Holland–Mannis classification.

	Normal conjunctiva (Stage a)	Previously inflamed conjunctiva (Stage b)	Inflamed conjunctiva (Stage c)
Partial LSCD (Stage I)	Iatrogenic, CIN, contact lens	Chemical/thermal injury	Mild SJS, OCP, recent chemical injury
Total LSCD (Stage II)	Aniridia, severe contact lens	Severe chemical/thermal injury	Severe SJS, OCP, recent chemical injury

(CIN: conjunctival intraepithelial neoplasia; SJS: Stevens–Johnson syndrome; OCP: ocular cicatricial pemphigoid)

Investigations

Impression Cytology

It is the gold-standard test for LSCD. A nitrocellulose acetate filter paper is placed on the ocular surface which is able to remove the superficial layers. Immunohistological and molecular analysis is then done on these cells. The epithelial and goblet cells are evaluated. The presence of goblet cells on the corneal surface is indicative of conjunctivalization. But care should be taken as in thermal and chemical burns, there may be deficiency of goblet cells which can result in false-negative result. Cytokeratins are proteins which form intermediate filaments in epithelial cells and are unique for different epithelial cells. Immunocytochemistry on impression cytology specimens could identify these cytokeratins. Cytokeratin 3/12 is specific for corneal epithelium while 19 is for conjunctival epithelium. Recently cytokeratin 7, 13, mucin 1, and mucin 5AC have been found to be more specific than cytokeratin 19 for conjunctival epithelium.

In Vivo Laser Scanning Confocal Microscopy

It provides high-resolution images at the cellular level. In the normal cornea, the superficial cells have a dark cytoplasm with well-defined borders. The deeper epithelial cells appear smaller in size and they also have well-defined borders. The palisades of Vogt appear as hyper-reflective, double contour linear structures. The corneal epithelial cells in LSCD have less distinct borders and prominent nuclei. The size of basal epithelial cells also increases. Epithelial cells in the deeper layers become affected in more advanced stage of LSCD. In the late stage, epithelial cells show significant metaplasia and there is neovascularization. A combination of morphological changes in the corneal epithelium, and a significant reduction in both basal epithelial cell and sub-basal nerve density are the early signs of LSCD.

Ultrasonography

It is important for the evaluation of the posterior segment when it is not visible with the help of indirect ophthalmoscopy.

Systemic Work-up

Depending upon the underlying etiology suspected as discussed in **Table 1**, relevant investigations should be done.[2-4]

Management (Flowchart 1)

Aim

- *Stage 1:* Control the ocular surface inflammation in acute stage. If it is associated with any immune-mediated disease, then immunomodulator therapy should be used.
- *Stage 2:* Correct the adnexal abnormalities, make the surface suitable for survival of transplanted stem cells. Eyelid abnormality should be corrected prior to limbal stem cell transplantation. Limbal stem cells cannot survive in dry ocular surface; hence, it is important to treat dry eye disease prior to this procedure.
- *Stage 3:* Treat the LSCD. Before performing corneal transplantation, LSCD should be treated.
- *Stage 4:* Visual rehabilitation. Any of the procedures such as deep anterior lamellar keratoplasty (DALK), penetrating keratoplasty (PKP), or keratoprosthesis depending upon the patient's condition can be attempted to provide vision. Stage 3 and stage 4 can be combined together; however, the success rate may come down under such circumstances.

Acute Stage Management

- In the acute stage, it is important to control the inflammation as inflammation causes more damage to the stem cells than the primary injury.
- Medical management in the form of steroids is important to control the inflammation.
- Amniotic membrane graft has been proven to be very effective and its use within 2 weeks of disease such as SJS provides rapid healing.
- A newer approach, ProKera, is Food and Drug Administration (FDA) approved and consists of amniotic membrane with dual symblepharon ring. It reduces inflammation and promotes healing.

Chronic Stage Management

The management in the chronic stage depends upon the:
- *Degree of LSCD:* Partial or total
- *Laterality:* Unilateral or bilateral

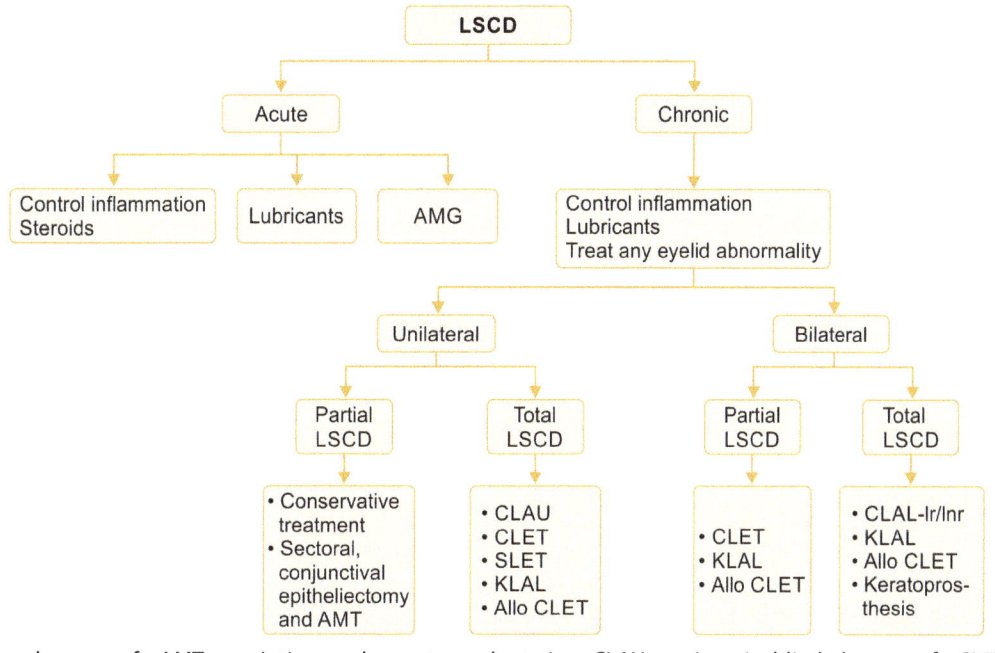

Flowchart 1: Management of limbal stem cell deficiency (LSCD).

(AMG: amniotic membrane graft; AMT: amniotic membrane transplantation; CLAU: conjunctival-limbal autograft; CLET: cultured limbal epithelial transplantation; SLET: simple limbal epithelial transplantation; KLAL: keratolimbal allograft; Allo-CLET: allogenic CLET; CLAL-lr/lnr: CLAL live relative/live nonrelative)

- Inflammation
- Presence of dry eye disease
- Extent of conjunctival disease
- Age and general health of the patient

Before considering any stem cell transplant procedure, following conditions should be treated:
- Control of inflammation
- *Ocular surface disorder:* Lubricants
- Adequate eyelid closure
- Elimination of keratinization and symblepharon.

Unilateral Partial Limbal Stem Cell Deficiency
- Partial LSCD not involving the visual axis may be managed conservatively with the help of anti-inflammatory drugs, lubricants, and bandage contact lens.
- Surgical management is required if there is involvement of the center of the visual axis. In partial LSCD, removal of conjunctival epithelium from the cornea and limbus followed by amniotic membrane transplantation is very helpful for reepithelialization.

Total Limbal Stem Cell Deficiency
- The management of total LSCD is surgical transplantation of limbal stem cells.
- The Cornea Society has given the nomenclature as:
  - *Based on the source of the donor:* Conjunctiva, limbus, and oral mucosa
  - *Based on the genetic source:* Autograft, allograft, cadaveric, living relative, living nonrelative
  - Based on the cell culture techniques used for donor tissue multiplication
- Before any transplantation procedure, the conjunctivalized pannus should be removed and hemostasis achieved.
- *Conjunctival-limbal autograft (CLAU):* Indicated in unilateral partial or total LSCD. 6–7 mm limbal arc length, partial thickness of conjunctival autograft along with limbus is taken from the fellow eye. Care should be taken while excision so as to avoid iatrogenic LSCD at the donor site.
- *Keratolimbal allograft (KLAL):* Indicated in case of unilateral LSCD who do not want any procedure in the fellow eye. Allogenic cadaveric limbal stem cells are transplanted. Immunosuppression is needed.

- *Conjunctival limbal allograft (CLAL):* It is also done in unilateral LSCD. The source of donor tissue can be cadaveric (c-CLAL), live relative (lr-CLAL) or a live nonrelative (lnr-CLAL). Immunosuppression is needed.
- *Cultured limbal epithelial transplantation (CLET):* In this limbal, tissue is taken in unilateral partial LSCD from the same eye and from the fellow eye in unilateral total LSCD. The limbal tissue is then cultured ex vivo to obtain a sheet of stem cells grown on the amniotic membrane graft. The advantage of this procedure is that a small amount of limbal tissue is taken therefore risk of iatrogenic LSCD is less. Also chance of rejection is less.
- *Cultivated oral mucosal epithelial transplantation (COMET):* Indicated in bilateral LSCD. In this, oral mucosal cells are excised and cultured to produce a sheet of epithelial cells. These are then transplanted later.
- *Simple limbal epithelial transplantation (SLET):* It has the advantage of both CLAU and CLET. In this, a 2 × 2 mm area of limbal tissue is excised and is divided into 10-15 small pieces. These are then placed onto the amniotic membrane over the recipient bed. These transplants are secured in place with fibrin glue and a bandage contact lens is applied.
- Keratoprosthesis can be used as an alternative to allograft transplantation so as to avoid immunosuppression. The Boston type 1 keratoprosthesis is used in eyes with LSCD which is due to nonimmunological disorders if there is adequate tear function. The osteo-odonto-keratoprosthesis and the Boston type 2 keratoprosthesis are preferred for total LSCD with no tear function.

References

1. Krachmer JH, Mannis MJ, Holland EJ (Eds). Cornea, 2nd edition, Volume 1. Philadelphia: Elsevier, Mosby; 2005. p. 955.
2. Dua HS, Saini JS, Azuara-Blanco A, Gupta P. Limbal stem cell deficiency: concept, aetiology, clinical presentation, diagnosis and management. Indian J Ophthalmol. 2000;48:83-92.
3. Lal I, Gupta N, Purushotham J, Sangwan VS. Limbal stem cell deficiency: current management. J Clin Ophthalmol Res. 2016; 4:3-12.
4. Sejpal K, Bakhtiari P, Deng SX. Presentation, diagnosis and management of limbal stem cell deficiency. Middle East Afr J Ophthalmol. 2013;20(1):5-10.

8.9 Corneal Transplantation

Aafreen Bari, Arpit Sharma, Ritu Nagpal

 1. Describe etiology, risk factors, pathogenesis, clinical features, and management of corneal graft rejection/approach to corneal allograft rejection.

Introduction

Corneal graft rejection is a specific immunologically mediated process in which a graft that has been clear for at least 2 weeks suddenly succumbs to graft edema in conjunction with anterior segment inflammatory signs. It was first described by Paufique et al. in 1948, by Maumenee (1951), and later elaborated by Khodadoust and Silverstein in 1969.

Immune rejection is the leading cause of graft failure, accounting for over half the cases of graft decompensation.

The highest incidence of rejection is seen within 2 months following surgery, and rejection after 2 years is unlikely.

According to Panda et al., 30% of eyes with penetrating keratoplasty experience at least one episode of rejection and about 5-7% lead to eventual graft failure.

Stromal immune rejection can occur in deep anterior lamellar keratoplasty (DALK), with an incidence of 1-24%; Descemet stripping endothelial keratoplasty (DSEK) has a mean endothelial rejection rate of 10% (range 0-45%), Descemet membrane endothelial keratoplasty (DMEK) has a very low rejection rate (mean of 1.9%, range 0-5.9%).

Etiology and Risk Factors

Several factors have been found to increase the risk of rejection in a case of corneal transplant, which have been enumerated in **Table 1**.

TABLE 1: Risk factors for corneal allograft rejection.		
Preoperative factors	**Intraoperative factors**	**Postoperative factors**
For penetrating keratoplasty: • Preoperative inflammation (including healed HSV keratitis, uveitis, etc.) • Corneal neovascularization (>2 quadrants, >2 mm in deep stroma) • Young recipient age • History of ocular surface disease (severe dry eye, severe chemical burns, radiation burns, ocular pemphigoid, Stevens-Johnson syndrome) • Prior ocular surgery (including PK in fellow eye) • Prior graft rejection • Prior use of glaucoma medications or surgery *For endothelial keratoplasty:* • African–American race • Pre-existing glaucoma • Steroid-responsive intraocular pressure	• Large graft, eccentric graft (proximity to limbal vessels) • Small graft (less endothelium) • Iris adhesion at graft-host junction (immune cells through iris vasculature get exposed to antigens) • Recent anterior segment surgery (associated inflammation brings more immune cells) • Anterior vitrectomy • Full thickness > lamellar graft	• Corneal epithelial breach • Exposed suture knots, loose suture (incite vascularization) • Postoperative uveitis • Postoperative glaucoma • Synechiae between iris and graft host junction

(HSV: herpes simplex virus; PK: penetrating keratoplasty)

Pathogenesis

Corneal allograft rejection occurs in three phases, as follows:[1-8]

1. *Afferent arm/Induction phase:*
   a. Sensitization of the host to donor antigens forms the "afferent" arm, also known as the induction phase of corneal allograft rejection **(Fig. 1)**. This allorecognition process is moderated by antigen-presenting cells (APCs) presenting donor antigens to naïve T-cells in draining lymph nodes. Two pathways are involved in the process of sensitization:
      i. *Direct pathway* constitutes a presentation of donor antigens to naïve T-cells directly by *donor* APCs through nonself major histocompatibility complex (MHC-II) recognition on their surface, resulting in the proliferation of direct alloreactive T effector cells **(Fig. 2)**.
      ii. *Indirect pathway* yields donor antigens to *host* APCs that travel the cornea, capture donor antigens, and transport them to draining lymph nodes, where antigen presentation occurs through recognition of self MHC-II by naïve T-cells.
2. *Priming:*
   a. Lymph nodes serve as the priming hub for naïve T-cell allosensitization and activation, which then drives the subsequent efferent arm.
   b. Following sensitization and activation of naïve T-cells, cytokines, and chemokines released induce proliferation and trafficking of these alloreactive T-cells to the cornea through expression of adhesion molecules.

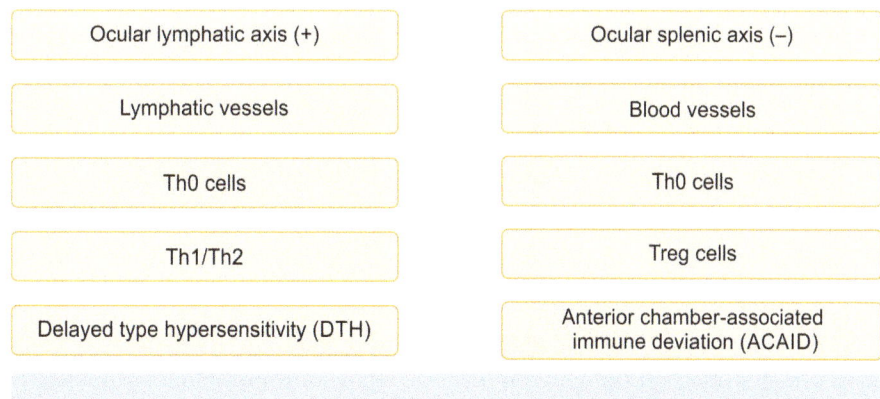

Fig. 1: Graft rejection (ocular lymphatic axis) versus tolerance (ocular splenic axis).

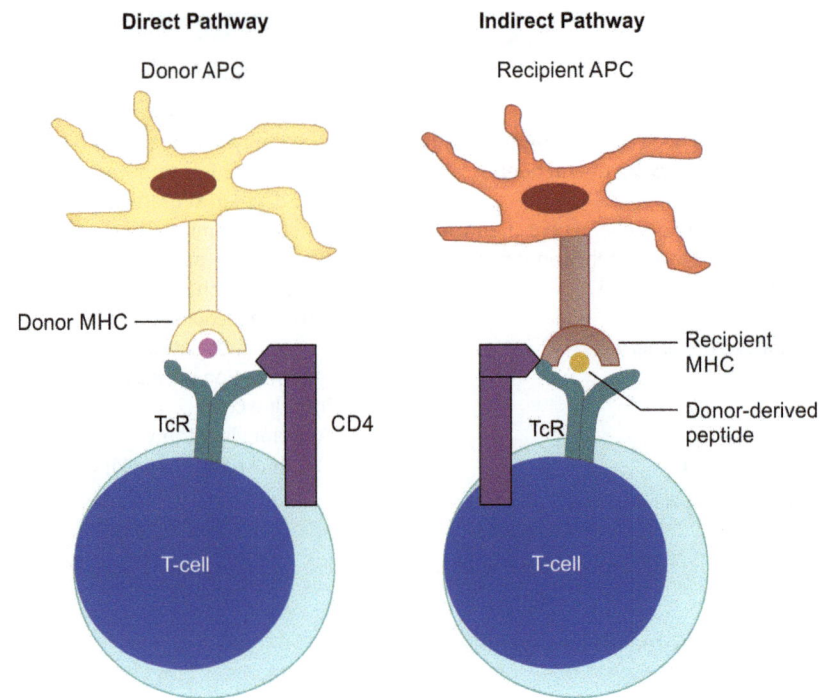

Fig. 2: Direct and indirect pathway for antigen presentation. (APC: antigen-presenting cells, MHC: major histocompatibility complex; TcR: T-cell receptor)

3. *Efferent Arm:*
    a. Immune-mediated damage to the graft begins with the release of cytokines secondary to the mechanical trauma of surgery, but in high-risk corneal transplantation, cytokines further induce the production of various early chemokines.
    b. Overexpression of chemokines monocyte chemotactic protein-1 (MCP-1), chemokine C-C motif ligand 2 (CCL2), regulated on activation normal T-cell expressed and secreted (RANTES; CCL5), macrophage inflammatory protein (MIP), MIP-1α (CCL3) and MIP-1β (CCL4) in acute graft rejection leads to additional recruitment of APCs and T-cells into the cornea.
    c. Once the graft and infiltrating leukocytes release late chemokines, guidance of alloreactive T-cells toward the graft begins. Alloreactive T-cells then migrate to the cornea where they recognize donor MHC antigens, and also induce the development of memory T-cells so that an immune response may be mounted against the same antigens upon reexposure as in the case of a re-graft.
    d. The primary cellular mediators of graft rejection are CD8+ CTL, and CD4+ T-helper (Th) lymphocytes, otherwise known as delayed type hypersensitivity (DTH) cells. Of the Th cells, Th1 cells, which secrete IL-2, IFN-gamma, and lymphotoxin, are largely considered to be the primary effector cells in corneal graft rejection.
    e. IL-2 provides positive feedback on T- and B-cell activation and proliferation. Interferon gamma (IFN-γ) ensures that macrophages are activated at the site of inflammation, and facilitates further expression of MHC-II antigens in the donor button.

Clinical Features

Symptoms

Though corneal allograft rejection is usually heralded by symptoms of Redness (R), Sensitivity to light (S), Vision loss (V), and Pain (P), some cases are identified on the basis of physical signs on routine follow-up visit, more often than not in operated Descemet stripping automated endothelial keratoplasty (DSAEK) cases. Therefore, the clinician should have a high index of suspicion, and the patient should be advised to come for follow-ups religiously.

Signs

Since allograft rejection is an immune-mediated inflammatory process, it shares the features of an inflammatory response: vascular dilation, vascular transudation, cellular infiltration, and tissue edema. The effects of these mechanisms are summarized in **Figure 3**.

Cornea and Conjunctiva

Vascular dilatation:
- Vascular dilation takes place within both conjunctival and uveal tissues
- Conjunctival vascular engorgement—diffuse congestion
- Deeper vascular engorgement—circumcorneal congestion
- Circumcorneal (ciliary) flush is the earliest sign of rejection reaction

Vascular transudation:
Anterior chamber flare indicates elevated levels of protein in the aqueous humor that has leaked from the uveal vasculature

A. Cellular infiltration
B. *Epithelium:* Epithelial rejection line
C. *Subepithelium:* Discrete subepithelial infiltrates
D. *Endothelium:* Keratic precipitates-scattered lesions/a linearly oriented wave of leukocytes migrating from the peripheral cornea toward the center also known as Khodadoust line (separates immunologically damaged endothelium from unaffected endothelium) is the hallmark of corneal allograft rejection

Tissue edema:
- Stromal and epithelial edema
- Often, there is associated edema of the stroma overlying the area that has been traversed by the advancing keratic precipitates

Fig. 3: Signs of corneal allograft rejection.

TABLE 2: Signs of corneal graft rejection depending upon the layer involved.

Rejection	Features
Epithelial rejection	• Epithelial rejection line (Krachmer's line) in graft from host-graft junction • Superficial epithelial infiltrates (Kaye's dots) • No KPs, No graft edema • Does not cause graft failure
Stromal rejection	• 6 weeks to 21 months postoperative • Subepithelial infiltrates on donor cornea • Responds well to steroids • In severe cases (rare), circumcorneal congestion, stromal patches of infiltrates, stromal edema near blood vessels, and rejection band away from vascularized part of graft may be seen
Endothelial rejection	• Endothelial rejection line (Khodadoust line) • Most symptomatic and devastating • KPs on graft endothelium • Minimum AC reaction • Seen in young patients, bilateral, and large grafts

(AC: anterior chamber; KP: keratic precipitates)

In particular, a few signs are seen depending on the layer involved, which are summarized in **Table 2**.

The diagnosis of immunologic graft failure is made if signs of rejection do not clear within 2 months of treatment.

Differential Diagnosis for Graft Rejection

It is of utmost importance to rule out the differentials before starting treatment since steroid treatment is notorious to cause flare-ups of some of these. **Table 3** lists the differentials of graft rejection.

Treatment

Treatment of graft rejection depends on the type of rejection; however, in all cases, corticosteroids are the mainstay of treatment.

An acute episode of corneal graft rejection should be treated aggressively with immunosuppression and adequate supportive therapy should be given.

Topical Corticosteroids

Topical corticosteroids are the mainstay of treatment in the management of acute graft rejection. Topical 1% prednisolone acetate is typically prescribed in acute graft rejection. A commonly prescribed regimen involves 1% prednisolone acetate every 1–2 hours for the first couple of weeks with gradual tapering over several months once response is seen.

TABLE 3: Differential diagnosis of corneal allograft rejection.

Condition	Features
Late graft failure	• Gradual onset of graft edema • Not associated with signs of inflammation such as AC cells or flare or KPs • No Khodadoust line or differential edema
Sterile/infectious endophthalmitis	• Inflammatory signs are severe • Presence of hypopyon • Presence of infiltrates in vitreous
Epithelial downgrowth	• Clumps of cells such as material in the AC • Cells larger than that of cells of inflammation • These cells do not respond to corticosteroid therapy • Argon laser will blanch the tissue confirming diagnosis • Associated with increased IOP unresponsive to medical therapy
Recurrent herpetic keratitis	• Both host (periphery) and donor cornea are affected • History of previous herpetic keratitis • Absence of K line • Responds to antiviral drugs

(AC: anterior chamber; IOP: intraocular pressure; KP: keratic precipitates)

Systemic Steroids

Oral and intravenous corticosteroids are equally effective when started within the first 8 days of rejection. High doses of oral steroids (60–80 mg) are given. Alternatively, intravenous dexamethasone, at a dose of 1 mg/kg, can be used for severe rejection. Reversibility of graft rejection is reported to be better with intravenous dexamethasone. Chronic systemic corticosteroid use is associated with complications such as osteoporosis, diabetes, and weight gain.

Intravenous (IV) Pulsed Corticosteroid Therapy: Following IV pulse methylprednisolone, transient lymphopenia is said to occur due to demarginalization of circulating lymphocytes, which affects T-lymphocytes to a greater extent than B-cells. The recommended intravenous pulse therapy dose of methylprednisolone is 500 mg in 150 mL of IV fluid. A single dose of intravenous steroid is advocated. Though the beneficial effect of additional doses of IV pulsed steroids is doubtful, up to 3 pulses may be given in case of persistence of signs and symptoms. Pulse therapy is effective in preventing subsequent rejection episodes, reducing the need for long-term oral steroids, and is beneficial when started within the first 8 days of rejection.

Calcineurin Inhibitors

Cyclosporine A (CsA) and tacrolimus have proven efficacious to varying degrees in the treatment of graft rejection as adjuvants to steroids. For patients in whom corticosteroids are contraindicated, topical CsA (0.5%) may provide an efficacious alternative for post-transplant maintenance of graft clarity and a low rejection rate. Tacrolimus, though having lesser clear graft survival rate than CsA and with no role in acute episodes, can be used as a steroid-sparing agent or in the prophylaxis of rejection.

Supportive Treatment

Antiglaucoma medications: Elevated intraocular pressure (IOP) is occasionally one of the earliest manifestations of rejection, and though infrequent, can be a sign of rejection. Corticosteroid therapy used to treat rejection can also cause rise in IOP, which needs to be lowered using antiglaucoma medications.

Cycloplegics can be given to relieve pain due to ciliary spasm.

In all cases of rejection, IOP should be monitored closely, especially when frequent corticosteroids are used. If necessary, elevated IOP should be controlled by topical medications to prevent glaucoma and to improve the chance of graft survival.

Treatment of Epithelial/Stromal Rejection

- *Epithelial or stromal rejection without endothelial involvement:* Usually does not progress to graft failure.
- Nonetheless, epithelial and stromal rejection should be aggressively treated, because they indicate host immunologic recognition of the graft and may precede a more severe endothelial rejection.
- Topical corticosteroids (e.g., dexamethasone 0.1%, prednisolone acetate 1%) are prescribed 4–6 times/day until the signs of rejection resolve, followed by a slow tapering of the topical medication.

- These patients should be followed closely to be certain that the signs of rejection are improving and that endothelial rejection has not developed.

Treatment of Endothelial Rejection
- Treatment of endothelial rejection must be more aggressive. Both topical and systemic steroids should be given.
- Topical corticosteroids should be used every hour while awake and as frequently as possible at night for 2–3 days, followed by every 2 hours while awake (Steroid ointment may be used at bedtime).
- Therapy should be continued until signs of rejection resolve and then tapered slowly over several weeks to a few months depending upon the patient's response to treatment.
- Therapy should be continued for at least 4 weeks in the absence of response before judging that the graft has failed.
- Other routes of administration of corticosteroids, e.g., subconjunctival, can be used in more severe endothelial rejections, in recurrent rejections, or if the patient is at high risk (e.g., alkali burns, patients with vascularized corneas).
- Pulsed steroids can be given as mentioned above.

Role of immunomodulators has been summarized in **Table 4**.

Newer modalities in treatment:
- *Tissue-cultured C3H corneal epithelial and endothelial cells:*
  - Administered orally in animal experiments
- *Antivascular endothelial growth factor (anti-VEGF):*
  - *Topical bevacizumab (2.5%, 25 mg/mL):*
    - Reduces the recurrence of neovascularization and thus helps increasing the frequency of graft survival in cases of high-risk corneal transplants.

TABLE 4: Immunomodulators of importance in corneal graft rejection.

Drug	Class	Mechanism of action	Dose in graft rejection	Adverse effects	Relevance
Azathioprine	Antimetabolite precursor of 6-mercaptopurine	Inhibits lymphocyte proliferation by blocking nucleotide synthesis	1–2 mg/kg/day orally	Pancytopenia, hepatocellular necrosis, increased risk of neoplasia	Of limited role due to its adverse effects
Cyclosporine	Calcineurin inhibitor	Binds cyclophilin blocks T-cell activation by preventing IL-2 transcription	*Topical:* 2% in castor oil/1% in artificial tears) 5 times/day with topical steroids *Systemic:* A target level between 130–170 mg/mL is aimed at	Nephrotoxicity, hypertension, hyperlipidemia, neurotoxicity, gingival hyperplasia, hirsutism	Rarely used nowadays, owing to the side effects
Tacrolimus (FK506)	Calcineurin inhibitor	Binds FK506 binding protein (FKBP); blocks T-cell activation by preventing IL-2 transcription	1 mg twice daily (target whole blood drug level 1–12 µg/L	Similar to cyclosporine; diabetes, and neurotoxicity; no gingival hyperplasia or hirsutism	
Sirolimus (Rapamycin)	mTOR inhibitor	Binds FKBP; blocks T-cell activation and B-cell differentiation by preventing response to IL-2	2–12 mg daily	Pancytopenia, insulin resistance, hyperlipidemia; not nephrotoxic	
Mycophenolate mofetil	Inosine monophosphate dehydrogenase inhibitor	Reversibly inhibits IMP dehydrogenase, preventing purine synthesis of B- and T-cells	1 g twice daily initially, tapered over 1 year	GI upset, pancytopenia, hypertension, hyperglycemia, Associated with invasive CMV infection	Most commonly used in management of graft rejection nowadays. As effective as CsA, with a favorable safety profile

(CMV: cytomegalovirus; CsA: cyclosporine A; GI: gastrointestinal; IL: interleukin; IMP: inosine monophosphate)

- *Selective glucocorticoid receptor agonists (SEGRAs):*
  - Activated glucocorticoid receptor (GR) can regulate gene expression via one of two pathways:
    1. The first (direct) pathway is called *transactivation* whereby the activated GR dimerizes, is translocated into the nucleus, and binds to specific sequences of deoxyribonucleic acid (DNA) called glucocorticoid response elements (GREs). Examples of glucocorticoid-responsive genes include those that encode anti-inflammatory proteins.
    2. The second (indirect) pathway is called *transrepression*, in which activated monomeric GR binds to other transcription factors such as NF-κB and AP-1 and prevents these from up-regulating the expression of their target genes. These target genes encode proteins for proinflammatory proteins.
  - Glucocorticoids activate GR to work through (at least) two signal transduction pathways.
  - SEGRA activates the glucocorticoid receptor (GR) in such a way that it only operates through one of the two main possible pathways.
  - Therefore, for specific inflammation-based diseases, SEGRAMs should more strongly transrepress than transactivate, or better yet solely transrepress and fail to transactivate. This should yield fewer side effects (ocular hypertension, glaucoma, etc.).
- *Gene therapy:* Acts by antiangiogenesis, immune response modulation, or antiapoptosis.
- *Monoclonal antibodies (MAB):*
  - Anti-CD3 and anti-CD6 MAB injected into the anterior chamber
  - Pan-T-cell antibody (CAMPATH-1H), → a strong T-cell-depleting agent, applied (systemically)
  - *Basiliximab, an anti-CD25 MAB:* Perioperative application of systemically administered MAB in combination with systemic CsA.
  - *Caution:*
    - First-dose anaphylactic reactions
    - Production of antibodies against the therapeutic antibody by the recipient
    - High cost.

Prevention

- *Preoperative (reducing the antigenic load of donor tissue):*
  - Use central corneal graft
  - Removal of the donor epithelium
  - Depletion of local macrophages by:
    - Pretreatment of the graft with hyperbaric oxygen
    - Use of heterologous antibody treated corneal button
    - Exposure to ultraviolet light
- Intraoperative factors—Meticulous surgical technique, including avoiding decentration of the recipient's bed cut, optimal suturing, and good graft-host apposition.
- Postoperative—Controlling or altering the host immune (steroids, immunomodulators). Steroids are started 6 times a day postoperatively, and gradually tapered over 2 years according to the clinical response. In high-risk cases, some surgeons advocate the continued use of steroids once a day indefinitely.

Conclusion

- Two factors, prevention and management, are of significant importance among all aspects of immunological graft rejection.
- Preventive aspects begin with the recipient selection, spread through donor antigenic activity, and end with meticulous surgery.
- Management of corneal graft rejection consists of early detection and aggressive therapy with corticosteroids.
- Addition of immunomodulators to the treatment regimen helps in faster and long-term recovery.

 2. Describe immunology of corneal allograft rejection.

- *Corneal immune privilege:*
  - The cornea is a uniquely avascular tissue (preventing direct access of the immune system to the cornea) and free of lymphatics (barring free transport of antigens and APCs to T-cell-rich secondary lymphoid organs).
  - Low constitutive expression of MHC-I and -II antigens in the cornea, limiting immunogenicity to foreign antigens.

- Even though dendritic cells are present in the cornea, they exist in an immature, inactivated state, maintaining immune quiescence in a healthy cornea.
- The cornea expresses many membrane-bound molecules that guard it from immune-mediated inflammation and induce apoptosis of immune effector cells [e.g., complement regulatory proteins (CRP), Fas ligand (FasL), MHC-Ib, and tumor necrosis factor (TNF)-related apoptosis-inducing ligand (TRAIL)].
- FasL (CD95L), a pro-apoptotic molecule expressed by the corneal epithelium and endothelium, serves to destroy polymorphonuclear neutrophils (PMNs) and effector T-cells that express its receptor Fas/CD95, promoting immune quiescence while protecting against immune-mediated graft rejection.
- The corneal epithelium, stroma, and cells of the ciliary body also express programmed death ligand-1 (PD-L1), which upon interaction with its cognate receptor (PD-1) on T-cells leads to inhibition of T-cell proliferative capacity, induction of apoptosis, and suppression of IFN-γ secretion, promoting graft survival.
- *Immune privilege in the anterior chamber:*
  - The anterior chamber is rich in soluble immunosuppressive factors such as TGF-β, α-melanocyte-stimulating hormone (α-MSH), calcitonin gene-related peptide (CGRP), CRP, somatostatin (SOM), indoleamine dioxygenase (IDO), vasointestinal peptide (VIP), and macrophage migration inhibitory factor (MIF), which inhibit T-cell and complement activation.
  - The induction of systemic tolerance is considered a deviation from the expected hypersensitivity immune response and is called anterior chamber-associated immune deviation (ACAID) **(Fig. 2)**. ACAID is an alloantigen-specific peripheral immune tolerance to antigens in the anterior chamber, which suppresses DTH response and maintains humoral immunity, promoting graft survival. Antigens within the anterior chamber are recognized and processed by F4/80+ APCs that orchestrate allotolerance by upregulating the expression of TGF-β with downregulation of the costimulatory molecule CD40/CD40L and interleukin-12 (IL-12).
- *Breach of ocular immune privilege:* Immune-mediated graft rejection is a complex interplay between lymphangiogenesis, hemangiogenesis, and inflammation, ultimately leading to loss of the privileged immune status **(Figs. 4 and 5)**.
- *Mechanism of corneal allograft rejection:* Refer to Pathogenesis of Corneal Allograft Rejection in Question 1.

3. Write a short note on high-risk keratoplasty.

Introduction

The Collaborative Corneal Transplantation Studies (CCTS) defined high-risk cornea as one with two or more quadrants of deep stromal vessels prior to surgery, or, one in which a prior graft has been rejected.

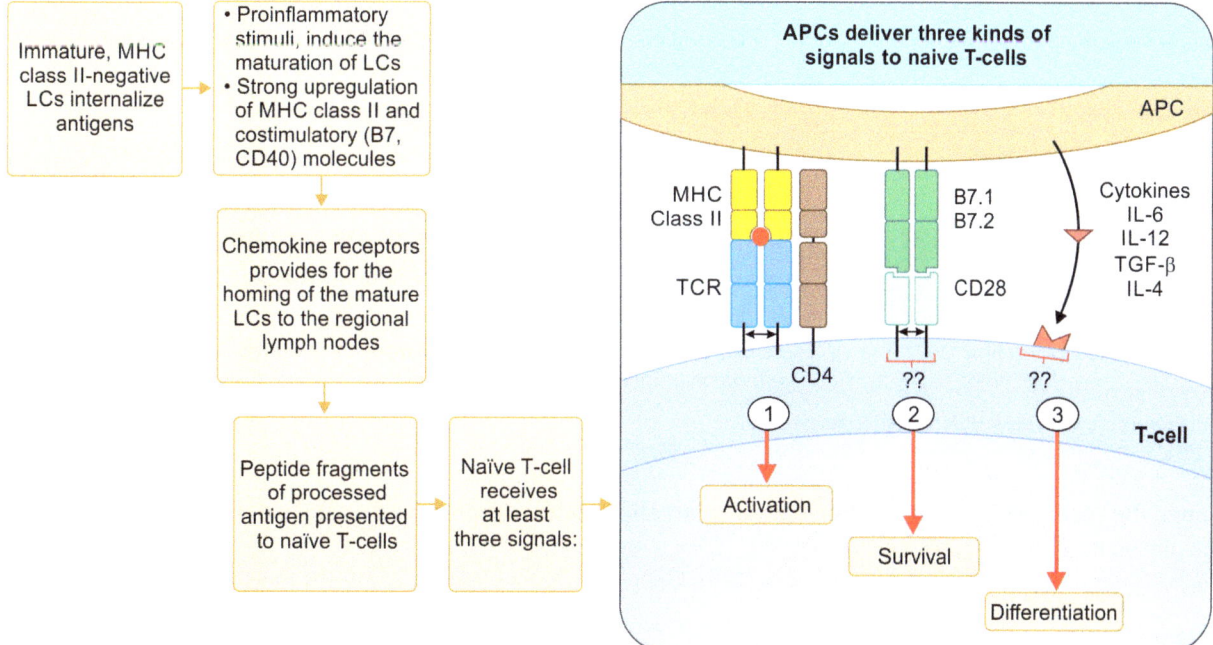

Fig. 4: T cell activation. (APC: antigen-presenting cells; LC: lethal concentration; IL: interleukin; MHC: major histocompatibility complex; TCR: T cell receptor; TGF: transforming growth factor)

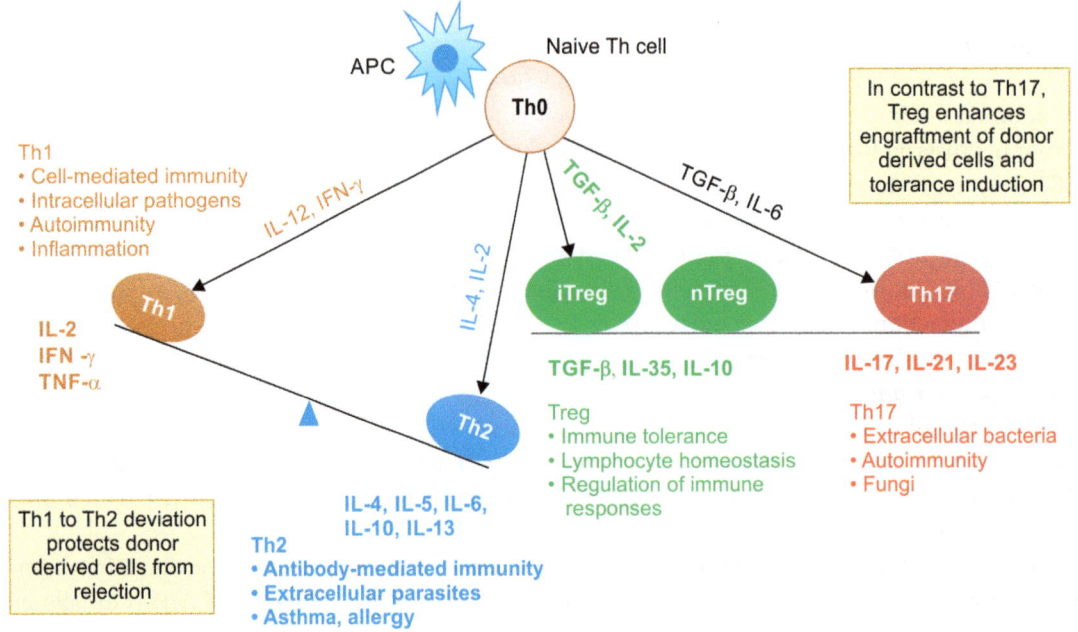

Fig. 5: T-cell differentiation (signal 3).[9] (IFN: interferon; IL: interleukin; TGF: transforming growth factor; Th: helper T-cells; TNF: tumor necrosis factor; Treg: regulatory T-cells)

TABLE 5: Frequently cited factors contributing to high risk for immunological rejection of corneal transplants and their putative mechanisms.

Risk factor	Probable mechanism leading to rejection
Allergic, inflammatory, or infectious cause of corneal opacity	• Accumulated immune cells and inflammatory mediators in the graft bed, with prior presence of neovascularization and neolymphangiogenesis • Less effective inherent immune-modulatory mechanisms
Regrafting	Prior alloimmune response present, with neovascularization and neolymphangiogenesis
Vascularized cornea/neolymphangiogenesis	Increased influx of innate and adaptive immune effectors, quicker and greater efflux of graft-derived alloantigens and APCs
Prior ocular surgery	• Increased presence of immune cells and inflammatory mediators in the graft bed • Loss of inherent immune-modulatory mechanisms
Glaucomatous eyes	Loss of inherent immune modulatory mechanisms
History of blood transfusion	Sensitization against allogeneic HLA
Large sized graft	Increased transfer of mature donor APCs
Lens status	Disordered anterior chamber immune-regulatory mechanisms
Surgical complications	Increased influx of innate and adaptive immune effectors, quicker and greater efflux of graft-derived alloantigens and APCs
Male-to-female transplantation	Female recipient immune response to male (H-Y) antigen, sex hormone receptor effects on immune response

(APC: antigen-presenting cells; HLA: human leukocyte cell)

Though the cornea is an ideal structure for transplantation with an impressive 2-year survival of 90%, the 2-year survival of grafts placed in high-risk corneas is <50%.

The CCTS reported a cumulative increase in the risk of rejection by a factor of 1.2 with every successive regraft.

Risk Factors

Table 5 describes the putative mechanisms contributing to corneal allograft rejection.

Management of High-risk Keratoplasty

The following pre-, intra-, and postoperative measures can be taken to reduce the risk of an allograft rejection in a high-risk corneal transplantation **(Fig. 6)**.[10-17]

- *Preoperative management:*
    - Elimination or reduction of host corneal stromal neovascularization by use of steroids, radiation, cystine, cryotherapy, sulfuric acid, dextran, conjunctival recession, and laser treatment using 577 nm yellow dye laser. A long-term efficacy is also achievable using fine needle diathermy before corneal grafting.
    - In patients with limbal stem cell deficiency, stem cell transplantation, either autologous or allogeneic, from limbal or oral mucosal cells should be performed before corneal grafting.
    - Preoperative use of corticosteroids 2 weeks prior to the procedure decreased the host bed neovascularization.
    - Topical dexamethasone (3–6 hourly), oral prednisolone (40–80 mg for 2–7 days), oral cyclosporine A (3–8 mg/kg), and single-dose intravenous methylprednisolone by have been used for this purpose.
- *Intraoperative considerations for high-risk corneal transplantation:*
    - *Choice of surgery:* Lamellar surgery is nowadays increasingly popular because of the reduced risk of immune rejection, better graft survival, rejection reversibility, visual and long-term surgical outcomes, and intraoperative or postoperative complications, in contrast to penetrating keratoplasty.
    - *Suturing technique:* In hot eyes (presence of infection and inflammation), the interrupted suture technique is more appropriate, as they have faster wound healing and sutures can be easily removed in cases of growth of new vessels or inflammation.
    - *Suture material:* 10–0 monofilament nylon is considered superior to other suture materials. The suture knot is usually rotated into and buried just beneath the corneal surface in the donor stroma, because placing the knot in the host's stroma may attract vessels.
- *Postoperative management:*
    - *Local therapies:*
        - *Steroids:* Corticosteroids represent the principal medication in the management of corneal transplantation. High-risk corneal allografts need to be more intensively treated and for a longer duration. Prednisolone acetate 1% or dexamethasone sodium phosphate 0.1% drops are given every 2 hours initially, slowly reduced over a period of 6 months to 1 year and a mild steroid, once daily, is maintained indefinitely.
        - *Topical immunomodulators:* Topical cyclosporine A and tacrolimus are being studied as prospective second-line treatment in patients with high-risk corneal grafts.
        - *Topical anti-VEGF:* Several anti-VEGF-A drugs have been evaluated for prevention and treatment of corneal neovascularization, and off-label use of topical bevacizumab has shown promising results in prevention of corneal neovascularization. Anti-VEGF agents have been used subconjunctivally and intrastromally as well, with better outcomes due to slower rate of release of drug and longer duration of action.
- *Systemic therapies:* Systemic immunosuppressants may be administered on a prophylactic basis in hazard ratio (HR) corneal grafts to inhibit or regress corneal lymph and hemangiogenesis and to prevent or reverse immune-mediated graft rejection **(Fig. 7)**.

Fig. 6: Goals of management.

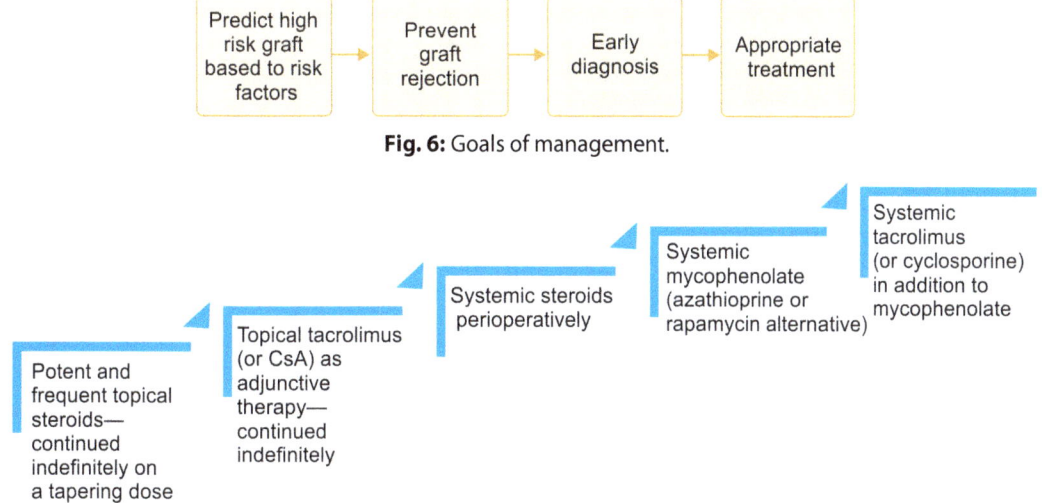

Fig. 7: Current stepwise prophylaxis for high-risk keratoplasty.[18]

- *Corticosteroids:* A short course of systemic corticosteroids may be used postoperatively in patients with HR corneal transplantation.
- *Cyclosporine A:* Oral CsA has long been employed for prevention of rejection in HR corneal transplantation, as a steroid sparing agent, though not many studies have been successful in proving its efficacy.
- *Tacrolimus (FK506):* In view of its potent immunosuppressive action, oral tacrolimus, according to some studies, can be an effective modality to prevent allograft rejection in HR corneal transplantation.
- *Mycophenolate mofetil (MMF):* MMF is another systemic immunosuppressive agent which has been used safely and effectively after solid organ transplantation. Though similar to CsA in terms of rejection episodes, and graft survival, MMF is a more attractive option due to its broad and safe therapeutic range.
- *Rapamycin (Sirolimus, Rapamune)* has also been shown to be similar in efficacy to MMF.

Novel strategies for immunomodulation in corneal transplantation:
- Regulatory T-cells (Tregs) and maturation-resistant tolerogenic dendritic cells (tolDCs) have been used in experimental models to induce tolerance and thus eliminate the use of immunosuppressive agents.
- A wide variety of polyclonal, monoclonal, and recombinant antibodies have been tested targeting immune cell determinant or costimulatory molecules, such as IL-1 blockade, leukocyte function antigen-1 (LFA-1), very late antigen-1 and 4 (VLA-1, VLA-4), CD40-CD154 pathway, CD28 and CD3 (CD80 and CD86).
- Promising results have also been shown by novel approaches to immunomodulate alloimmunity that have focused on morpholine oligonucleotides, cell-specific gene therapy, ribonucleic acid (RNA) interference, and anti-VEGF therapy.

4. Mention the recent advances in concepts and management pertaining to high-risk corneal transplantation.

- *Role of direct pathway:* While initially believed to be a phenomenon brought about exclusively by the *indirect pathway*, accumulated evidence indicates that both the *direct and indirect pathways* are implicated in the immune-mediated rejection of orthotopic corneal allografts, especially in high-risk corneal beds with higher immunogenicity and compromised immune privilege.
- *Role of human leukocyte antigen matching:* The CCTS did not report any advantage from human leukocyte antigen (HLA) class I or class II matching in corneal transplantation, while a modest benefit was detected from ABO antigen matching, but it was subsequently recognized that the serology-based tissue typing used in the study differed from molecular technique typing in 55% of the cases. Nonrandomized studies typically show a beneficial effect of HLA typing, and HLA matching is still performed in high-risk corneal transplantation at some centers.
- Outcome statistics from the past 5 years confirm that retransplantation following failure of one or more corneal allografts to the same eye is associated with high-risk for graft loss regardless of the primary corneal disease.
- Two or more preceding grafts in the contralateral eye have also been shown to be an independent risk factor for failure.
- Surgeon's experience, higher rate of surgeon follow-up, and graft diameter between 7.75 and 8.5 mm were all shown to have independent positive effects on corneal transplant survival.
- Recent studies also support a role for recipient polymorphisms of genes including thrombospondin-1, which are involved in the immune response and regulation of angiogenesis in the anterior eye, in determining rejection risk.

Recent Advances in Prevention of High-risk Corneal Allograft Rejection

- *Topical anti-VEGF:* Several anti-VEGF-A drugs have been evaluated for prevention and treatment of corneal neovascularization, and off-label use of topical bevacizumab has shown promising results in prevention of corneal neovascularization. Anti-VEGF agents have been used subconjunctivally and intrastromally as well, with better outcomes due to slower rate of release of drug and longer duration of action **(Table 9)**.
- *SEGRA:* Though similar to corticosteroids in terms of anti-inflammatory activity, SEGRAs lack the adverse effects of steroids such as steroid-induced glaucoma, posterior subcapsular cataract, and diabetes. Topical application of SEGRAs prolongs experimental corneal allograft survival following experimental keratoplasty. SEGRA compounds therefore might be of value as a future agent in corneal transplantation.
- *Monoclonal antibodies:* Though their application in clinical practice is limited by first-dose anaphylactic reactions, high costs, and production of antibodies against the therapeutic antibody by the recipient, monoclonal antibodies against CD3, CD6, CD25 (basiliximab), and pan-T-cell antibody (CAMPATH-1H) have shown potential in use in corneal transplantation for immunosuppression.[19-22]

Recent Advances in Management of High-risk Corneal Allograft Rejection

Standard management regimes have been explained in Question 1. Certain new concepts are as follows:[30-38]

- *Cyclosporine A:* Oral CsA has long been employed for prevention of rejection in HR corneal transplantation, as a steroid sparing agent, though not many studies have been successful in proving its efficacy.
- *Tacrolimus (FK506):* In view of its potent immunosuppressive action, oral tacrolimus, according to some studies, can be an effective modality to prevent allograft rejection in HR corneal transplantation.
- *Mycophenolate mofetil:* MMF is another systemic immunosuppressive agent which has been used safely and effectively after solid organ transplantation. Though similar to CsA in terms of rejection episodes, graft survival, MMF is a more attractive option due to its broad and safe therapeutic range.
- *Rapamycin (Sirolimus, Rapamune)* has also been shown to be similar in efficacy to MMF.

Q 5. Discuss lamellar keratoplasties and their role in corneal disorders. How would you decide which lamellar procedure would be appropriate for a patient?

Definition

- Replacement of diseased cornea with autologous or heterologous cornea is called keratoplasty.
- Either full thickness of the cornea also known as penetrating keratoplasty (PK) or a part of it also known as lamellar keratoplasty (LK) may be transplanted **(Fig. 8)**.

Types

Lamellar keratoplasty can be broadly divided into two categories:
1. *Replacement of epithelium and stroma (anterior lamellar):*
   a. Bowman's membrane transplant
   b. Superficial anterior lamellar keratoplasty (SALK), anterior lamellar therapeutic keratoplasty (ALTK)
   c. DALK
2. *Replacement of Descemet membrane (DM) (posterior lamellar or EK or PLK) can be:*
   a. DSAEK
   b. DMEK
   c. Pre-Descemet endothelial keratoplasty (PDEK).

Bowman's Layer Transplant

- *Bowman's layer:* Anterior-most compact collagen which provides biomechanical strength and shape to the anterior cornea.

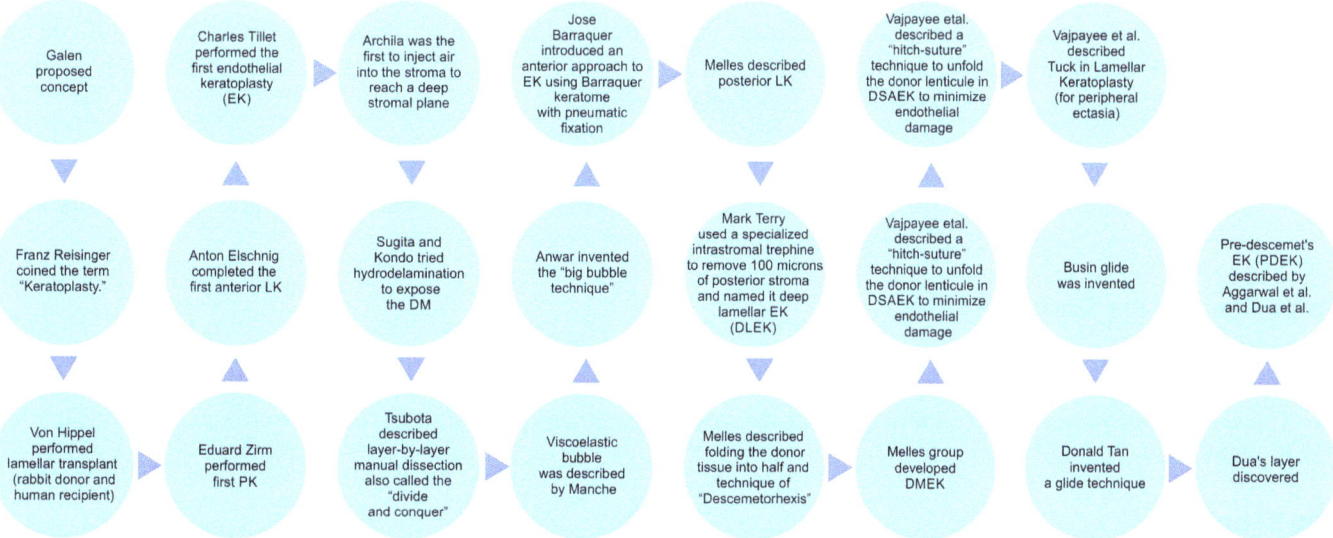

Fig. 8: Evolution of lamellar keratectomy.

- Bowman's layer thins and disrupts, weakening the cornea in ectasia, e.g., keratoconus. Replacing the Bowman's layer adds strength to the anterior cornea, restores shape (induces flattening), and arrests progression.
- Allows visual rehabilitation with contact lenses by improving fit and retention of the lens, which in turn delays the need for DALK/PK.
- The technique does not carry any risk of allograft rejection because no biological material is transplanted.
- *Procedure:* After removing the epithelium, air is injected in the donor cornea beneath the Bowman's layer to separate the anchoring fibrils to form the "Bowman's roll," which is immersed in 70% ethanol to remove remnant epithelial cells. The Bowman's layer can also be peeled off using forceps after creating a 360° edge using a needle.[39]
- Manual dissection or femtosecond laser is used to create a stromal pocket in recipient cornea in mid stroma and the roll (stained with trypan blue for better visualization) is placed in it using a special glide and then unrolled and covered with a scleral contact lens.
- This procedure leads to decrease in keratometry values, improved corneal thickness, and better tolerance of contact lens.
- The limitations are steep learning curve, risk of DM perforation (as high as 20%), and lack of adequate evidence in literature.

Superficial Anterior Lamellar Keratoplasty

- Superficial anterior lamellar keratoplasty is the replacement of the anterior corneal stroma. Pathologies located in the anterior third of the stroma (e.g., Reis-Buckler) and surface irregularity, astigmatism, and stromal thinning (keratoconus) can be managed by SALK.[40,41]
- Diseased stroma is removed and replaced by healthy stroma of similar thickness and an intact epithelium (A similar flap is cut in the donor's eye and punched to fit the diameter of the recipient bed, and the donor tissue is either glued or sutured in place). However, replacement of epithelium is not necessary.
- Both host and donor preparations are done using a microkeratome.
- Host dissection depth is usually up to 150–160 μ.
- Advantages are—in case of recurrence of the same dystrophy in the graft, replacement of the superficial graft can be easily done, smooth interface, no suture related problems, and early visual rehabilitation.
- Limitations are—need of microkeratome and donor-host graft size (diameter) mismatch, and irregular astigmatism.

Anterior Lamellar Therapeutic Keratoplasty

Very similar to SALK, except:
- Depth of host bed can be up to 200–250 μm.
- Sutures are used to secure donor attachment.

Deep Anterior Lamellar Keratoplasty

- Several stromal pathologies (stromal dystrophy, scars, ectasia, etc.) result in visual impairment due to an obstruction to the passage of light or distortion of focus, even though DM stays normal.
  - Stroma can be replaced with a full-thickness stromal button (often with donor epithelium) devoid of DM and endothelium, taken from a donor's eye.
  - This avoids the risk of graft failure due to endothelial rejection.
- *Challenges:*
  - Complete stromal removal, leaving behind only the host DM or DM with the pre-Descemet layer (PDL) (Dua's layer).
  - The button needs to be sutured in place, which introduces the major issues of post-DALK astigmatism and a prolonged recovery period requiring adjustment of astigmatism with selective suture removal.

Importance of Pre-Descemet Layer

- The bursting pressure of PDL is reported to be between 500 and 700 mm Hg; hence, it is likely that when the PDL is retained the eye has greater strength and does not rupture easily following trivial trauma, unlike PK.
- The surgical technique aims to induce a cleavage in the PDL or DM plane and the anterior stroma, e.g., Anwar's "big bubble (BB) technique".

Big Bubble

- Air is injected into the recipient stroma through a trephine cut of desired diameter (usually 7.5–8 mm).

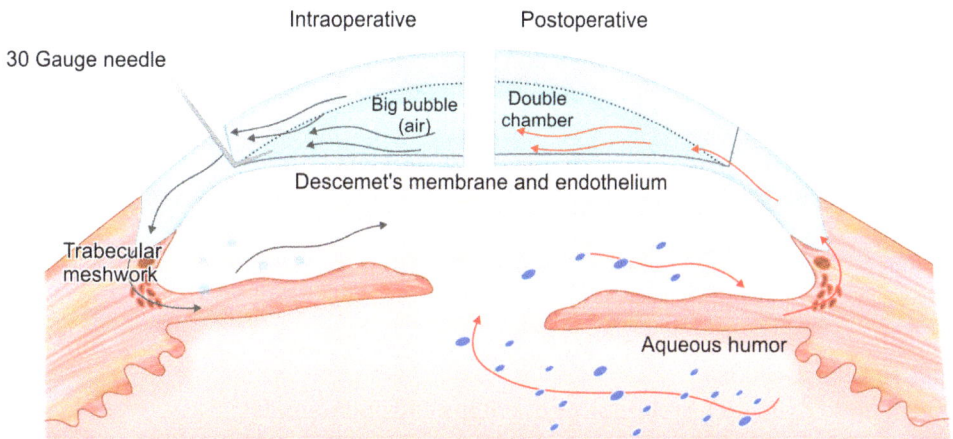

Fig. 9: Formation of double bubble while performing big bubble deep anterior lamellar keratoplasty.

- Most often (in 80% cases), the injected air follows a defined and reproducible path to reach the PDL plane, to produce a type-1 BB.[42-45]
- At times (12% cases), air accesses the plane between PDL and DM by passing through tiny fenestrations along the corneal periphery, central to the attachment of the DM. The BB so produced is the type-2 BB, where only the DM (without PDL) is exposed **(Fig. 9)**.
- Often a type-1 and type-2 BB (mixed BB) occur simultaneously with the former usually being complete and the Type-2 BB appearing as a smaller bubble.
- If pneumodissection does not yield a BB, a layer-by-layer dissection of the anterior stroma needs to be done till the PDL plane is reached. The dissection depth is very important with a residual stromal bed of <20 μ being ideal.

Femtosecond Laser in DALK (The Intrabubble Technique)

- Dissection of the stroma and precise channel formation for needle placement at predecided depth of 50 μ and 30° angle for BB formation can be achieved using femtosecond technology.[46-49]
- Matching donor and recipient edge using zig-zag cuts allow precise tissue apposition.

Endothelial Cell Loss

- *The endothelial loss after DALK is biphasic:* There is an early phase of rapid loss followed by a late phase of slow decline.
- DALK is, however, better than PK when it comes to endothelial cell counts.
- If there is an intraoperative perforation during the procedure, it leads to 25% reduction in endothelial cell counts.

Complications

- *Failure to separate DM/PDL by air or viscoelastic:* May require manual dissection
- *Intrastromal bubble with viscoelastic technique mimicking type-1 bubble:* Needle or cannula tip should be placed deep in stroma.
- *Perforation or bursting of DM/PDL:*
  - PDL perforation do not extend and DALK can be completed.
  - DM perforation (type-2 bubble) usually requires conversion to PK.[50,51]
- *Double AC:*
  - Break in DM through which aqueous can access the plane between DM and PDL (type-2 BB) or between PDL and posterior stroma (type-1 BB).
    - Management of the tear can be achieved by injection of air in the AC.
    - For type-2 component, air can be released by making tiny perforation over PDL.
- *Urrets-Zavalia syndrome:*
  - AC filled with air as part of lamellar procedure can result in a fixed dilated pupil.
  - *Can be prevented by:*
    - Preoperative inferior iridotomy
    - Wide dilation of the pupil

- Reducing the volume of air before the patient is taken off the operating table
- Checking IOP within an hour postoperative and releasing air from the AC if IOP is high (burping the bubble)
- Intravenous acetazolamide and/or mannitol can help if the pressure is not too high.
- *Interface wrinkling:*
  - Occurs due to mismatch between recipient DM and donor stromal button.
  - Oversize stromal button by 0.25–0.5 mm
- *Early suture loosening:*
  - As a result of shallow sutures (done sometimes to avoid damage to DM)
  - 80–90% suture depth should be aimed for.
- *Interface vascularization:*
  - Sign of possible stromal rejection
  - Aggressive topical steroids (+/– 2% cyclosporine eye drops and oral steroids)
  - Diathermy of vessel trunk at limbus
- *Epithelial rejection:*
  - Epithelial rejection does occur but does not lead to endothelial rejection.
  - Aggressive topical steroids

Endothelial Keratoplasty

- *Indications:*
  - Endothelial dysfunction (e.g., syndromes such as Fuchs endothelial dystrophy, posterior polymorphous dystrophy, iridocorneal endothelial syndrome, failed PK, pseudophakic, or aphakic bullous keratopathy, etc.) leading to stromal and epithelial edema, causing visual deterioration.[52-58]
  - No associated stromal scarring
- *Benefits:*
  - Maintains the structural integrity of the eye
  - Astigmatically neutral
  - Reduced risk of rejection (stromal and epithelial)

Endothelial Cell Loss

- Inherently associated with endothelial loss related to preparation, insertion, and attachment of the donor EK tissue.
- Up to 50% EC loss has been reported at 5-year postoperatively:
  - Select donors with good endothelial cell counts (at least 2,300 cells/mm^2).
  - Donors of 70 years of age or older are usually avoided.[59-64]

Descemet Stripping Endothelial Keratoplasty

- Donor tissues with high endothelial cell counts of 2,500–3,000 cells/mm^2 and from young donors are preferred.
- A large diameter scleral rim is required to mount the donor tissue on the artificial chamber.
- The graft can be harvested by manual dissection or by using microkeratome (DSAEK) or femtosecond laser. Stromal bed obtained using a microkeratome or a femtosecond laser is smoother than the manual dissection technique. Microkeratome gives a smoother surface, but inflammation is less with femtolaser. In microkeratome-assisted technique, decreased scleral rigidity from very young donors may lead to irregular dissections.
- Donor lenticule diameter should be at least 3 mm less than the recipient cornea diameter to prevent closure of the AC angle.
- The meniscus shape of the donor tissue where it is thinner in the center and thicker in the periphery leads to approximately 1.5 diopters of hyperopic shift postoperatively.

Creation of the Entry Wound

- Wound sizes ranging from 9 to 3 mm have been described.
- Smaller wound, with subsequent folding of the donor lenticule either in two unequal halves (Taco technique with forceps) or its rolling into a loose roll as with the Busin glide, enhances wound security and reduces induced astigmatism. The entry tunnel can be either corneal or sclera-corneal.

Descemetorhexis

- Usually carried out with the AC filled with balanced salt solution (BSS) by continuous irrigation. If carried out with viscoelastic filling the AC, as is often the case in phaco-DSEK, its thorough removal before insertion of the graft is important.
- Filling the AC with air, either during or after descemetorhexis, provides the best visualization of the DM.
- The diameter of the rhexis should preferably be larger than that of the graft lenticule.
- The area of DM to be removed is marked (on the epithelial surface) and scored with a reverse Sinskey hook.
- The membrane edge is gently lifted off with a "stripper" and the DM is peeled off by grasping the lifted edge and pulling or by stroking with a stripper.

Insertion of the Graft Lenticule

- It should be ensured that the AC maintainer is switched off during this step to ensure that the graft does not shoot out of the wound.
- Maneuvers used in folding of the tissue, its unfolding after insertion, and positioning are associated with stromal folds and loss of endothelial cells.
  - Donor endothelial cell loss can be up to 34–51% in the first 6 months.
  - The endothelial cell loss after DSEK is 53% at 5 years which then continues to reduce at 1% every year and that of PK is 69–75% at 5 years, which becomes statistically same for both at 10 years.
  - Primary graft failure rates vary from 6 to 45% using the folding technique and are as low as 2% using the TAN EndoGlide™ (Angiotech, Vancouver, Canada) technique.

Opening the Folded Graft in the Correct Orientation

- To ensure these an "S" or "F" mark with ink (in DSAEK), on the stromal surface can be used. These should be read in their correct orientation after unfolding the graft.
- A combination of stroking and irrigation maneuvers is used to unfold the graft and position it centrally.
- Finally, an air bubble is used to approximate the donor to the posterior corneal surface.
- A complete air fill without unduly raised pressure is desirable.
  - Intracameral air itself is associated with 10–20% loss of endothelial cells.
  - Air in the AC is maintained at 100% for at least 10 minutes, after which some air is burped to prevent pupillary block.
  - An inferior iridectomy performed intraoperatively or before surgery (with YAG laser) is desirable.
  - Assess the IOP within an hour after surgery and raised IOP can be controlled by burping the bubble.
- The patient is advised to lie flat on the back for a few hours, and the pressure checked again.
- Venting incisions can be made to drain the interface fluid and accelerate the adherence.
- Intraoperative anterior segment OCT can help confirm the opposition of the graft to host bed.

Complications[66-78]

- Small amounts of retained DM on the graft can interfere with graft attachment.
- Aphakic or pseudophakic eyes without a posterior capsule or even eyes with glaucoma drainage devices can be difficult candidates for air retention, but strict supine position or use of gases such as SF_6 can help.
- Donor detachment and dislocation are major complications requiring graft repositioning and rebubbling.
- *Graft failure:* If the attached graft fails to clear even after 2 weeks, it is known as primary graft failure (5% after DSEK).
  - Usually caused due to unhealthy donor epithelium or traumatic operative technique.
  - Incidence of primary graft failure is lower for automated dissection than the manual technique.
  - If the graft remains unattached, which may be due to retained DM, viscoelastic or interface fluid; it is termed as secondary graft failure.
  - Graft survival rates of 60–94% have been reported in long-term studies.
  - Endothelial graft rejection rates of 10% have been reported.
- Graft folds or wrinkles in the pupillary area can lead to reduced visual outcome, which may be an indication for a regraft.
- Interface scarring/haze and irregularity is another cause of postoperative reduced vision. Hence, it is very important to preoperatively rule out stromal scarring as it may persist postoperatively.

Prognosis

- Visual outcomes in terms of best corrected visual acuity (BCVA) are much better than that of PK because of reduced astigmatism due to the absence of sutures.

- DSEK induces a hyperopic shift of 1–2 diopters, which can impact on vision.
- The use of microkeratome in DSAEK procedure is beneficial in terms of decreased astigmatism, rapid visual recovery, and reduced rejection rate.
- In a post-DSAEK cornea, the posterior surface of the cornea is not parallel to the anterior surface of the DSAEK donor tissue. This leads to increase in the higher order aberrations of up to 25%.

F-DSAEK

- DSAEK in which femtosecond laser is used for graft preparation is called F-DSAEK.
- Visual outcomes are unsatisfactory due to following reasons:
  - Irregularity during tissue cutting
  - Laser-induced roughness due to deep ablation
  - It has been postulated that if the anterior surface of the cornea is depressed, as during F-DSAEK, persistent wrinkles form on the posterior surface of the graft.
  - There is also an element of interface scatter due to corneal collagen denaturation.

Ultrathin (UT) DSAEK

- These grafts are thinner than 130 µ and give a spherical equivalent similar to DSAEK, but with visual outcome comparable to DMEK.[74-78]
- Complication rate and ease of procedure are better with UT-DSAEK than with DMEK.

Descemet Membrane Endothelial Keratoplasty

- The indications for this procedure are the similar to DSEK.
- The donor tissue can be prepared by manual dissection, or by submerged cornea using backgrounds away (SCUBA) technique, where the dissection is mainly done after submerging the donor cornea under Optisol GS or BSS, enabling better visualization and easy handling of the tissue while dissecting [Pneumodissection has also been attempted (type-2 BB), but this can result in the formation of a Type-1 BB and provide PDEK tissue].[74-81]
- DMEK tissue always scrolls with the endothelial cell layer on the outside, and the scrolls can be very tight (cigar-shaped), double rolls, or loose folds.
- The "no-touch" technique is used for implantation and apposition of the DMEK graft, to reduce endothelial cell loss.
- The tissue is stained with trypan blue dye (for 2–3 min), and the scroll is aspirated into a glass tube from its wide end and injected into the eye through the narrow nozzle end by switching the syringe attachment. During injection, active irrigation of BSS into the AC should be stopped, and the eye should be soft (positive pressure can expel the scroll), soon after which the entry wound is stitched.
- *Moutsouris sign:* When placed anterior to the graft, the cannula can be moved under the roll of a correctly oriented scroll, turning the tip blue (Used to confirm graft orientation).
- After orienting the scroll (using mechanical tapping, fluidics, or air), the AC is made shallow and the cornea above the scroll is tapped with a blunt instrument.
- Once open and centered, an air bubble is injected between the tissue and iris to elevate the graft and oppose it to the posterior surface of the cornea from which the host diseased DM has been stripped off.
- Peripheral infolding can be flattened out with a *"bubble-bumping maneuver"* also known as *"Dapena maneuver"* where gentle taps on the outer surface of the cornea over the fold create an aqueous flow which leads to their disappearance.
- Finally, filling the AC completely with air for 20 minutes helps in graft fixation.

The differences between DSEK and DMEK are enumerated in **Table 6**.[81-89]

Pre-Descemet Endothelial Keratoplasty

The differences between PDEK and DMEK are enumerated in **Table 7**.
- Visual outcomes are similar for both PDEK and DMEK grafts.
- The donor tissue is prepared as follows:
  - A 30-gauge needle tip, bevel facing endothelium, is inserted intrastromally through the scleral rim of the sclerocorneal disc and advanced to mid-peripheral cornea.
  - Air is injected until a type-1 BB forms and extends to about 7–8 mm.

TABLE 6: Differences between Descemet stripping endothelial keratoplasty (DSEK) and Descemet membrane endothelial keratoplasty (DMEK).

	DSEK	DMEK
Visual outcomes (contrast visual acuity and aberrations)	Poorer (transplant of additional stroma and consequent hyperopic shift)	Better (only DM is grafted, with no hyperopic shift)
Postoperative graft detachment	Lower	Higher
Endothelial cell loss	Higher	Lower
Final visual acuity	Around 6/12	6/9 to 6/6
Donor age	Young donor age not a barrier but an advantage, due to a greater number of endothelial cells	Older (>50 years) donors preferred (as the DM is relatively firmly attached to the Dua's layer in young corneas)
Graft size	At least 3 mm less than the recipient cornea diameter (to prevent closure of the AC angle)	8–8.5 mm
Prognosis	Lower rate of primary graft failure	Higher rates of primary graft failure than DSEK (6–8%)

(AC: anterior chamber; DM: Descemet membrane)

TABLE 7: Difference between Descemet membrane endothelial keratoplasty (DMEK) and Pre-Descemet endothelial keratoplasty (PDEK).

	DMEK	PDEK
Graft constituents	Graft consisting of only DM-endothelium complex	Graft consisting of DM and PDL, the PDL being 10–13.6 µ thick
Amount of manipulation required during graft placement	More	Less (since PDEK graft scrolls less than a DMEK graft)
Donor tissue from very young patients	DM is relatively firmly attached to the Dua's layer in young donors' cornea, so older (>50 years) donors are preferred	Can be harvested, with associated higher endothelial cell counts
Endothelial cell loss during donor tissue preparation	Slightly more	Slightly less
Number of endothelial cells transplanted	More (larger sized graft)	Fewer cells, due to smaller size of graft

(DM: Descemet membrane; PDL: pre-Descemet layer)

- The donor tissue is then trephined with a 6–7.5 mm trephine depending on the size of the bubble (the graft scrolls with the endothelial side out).

The graft is transferred to the host AC after diseased endothelium is stripped off, unfolded, and centered by tapping and irrigation.

To decide upon the procedure to be used, it is necessary to pinpoint the layer of cornea that is pathological, and transplant that very layer.

Clinically, it can be detected on slit-lamp biomicroscopy, and confirmed by the following investigations:
- Anterior segment optical coherence tomography (ASOCT)
- Ultrasound biomicroscopy (UBM)
- Pentacam.

If the patient has been diagnosed with a pathology that is known to affect other layers (e.g., though macular corneal dystrophy primarily affects the stroma, it is known to extend down to the Descemet membrane and endothelium), treatment has to be modified accordingly.

Conclusion

- Lamellar corneal transplantation offers huge advantages and addresses the major risks associated with PK.
  - Endothelial rejection related graft failure is eliminated in DALK, and the eye is left stronger than after a PK on account of the retention of the PDL.
  - Graft–host junction weakness and induced astigmatism are almost totally eliminated in EK as the incision size is very small and need for sutures is minimal or not at all.

- Major disadvantage is of endothelial cell loss. Although there is around 6–9% endothelial cell loss at the cut edge after PK, surgical manipulation of the DM is minimal as compared to EK where the endothelial cell loss of up to 56% has been noted with 3 mm incisions.[90]

 6. Critically evaluate DSEK/DSAEK and DMEK. What are the causes of failure of a graft? How does DSAEK differ from DMEK surgically?

For details on DSAEK and DMEK, refer previous Question.
- The term "corneal graft failure" is used when the donor cornea fails to serve its purpose. It may be visual rehabilitation as in keratoplasty done for optical purposes or control the underlying infection as in therapeutic keratoplasty.
- Primary corneal graft failure is defined as corneal edema that never clears from the immediate postoperative period secondary to inherent deficiencies in the donor graft, surgical trauma, or improperly stored tissue.
- Secondary corneal graft failure is when the graft fails to serve its purpose due to an underlying secondary pathology. Most common causes are allograft rejection, glaucoma, infection, and surface problems.

The surgical differences between DSAEK and DMEK are enumerated in **Table 8**.

 7. Enumerate recent advances in endothelial keratoplasty.

- *Preloaded graft:* Folded DMEK grafts can be preloaded using transport medium in an intraocular lens (IOL) cartridge and stored up to 4 days with limited endothelial damage. This will simplify the surgery by reducing tissue wastage, cost, time, and logistical requirements.
- *PDEK:* Pre-Descemet endothelial keratoplasty is a newer variant of EK which involves the separation of pre-Descemet layer along with DM-endothelium complex as a donor lenticule. A reverse Sinskey's hook is used to perform descemetorhexis and scrape off the entire diseased endothelium with DM in the recipient eye. The donor graft is then injected into the AC and is unrolled using air and fluidics, with postoperative supine positioning.
- *DMET:* Since complete graft attachment is not essential for re-endothelialization to occur, a free-floating Descemet roll can be transplanted, with the edge of the graft sutured to the corneal incision to ensure a focal area of contact. Here, re-endothelialization may be dependent on a relatively healthy recipient peripheral endothelium, as well as contribution from the donor graft endothelial cells.
- *Descemetorhexis stripping without endothelial keratoplasty (DWEK)/Descemet stripping only (DSO)/descemetorhexis without grafting/descemetorhexis without graft placement:* In a patient with early Fuchs endothelial corneal dystrophy

TABLE 8: Surgical differences between DMEK and DSAEK.

	DMEK	DSAEK
Transplanted layers	Endothelium-Descemet membrane complex (stroma is not transplanted)	Endothelium-Descemet membrane complex along with stroma
Requirement of microkeratome	Not needed	Necessary
Learning curve	Steep	Less steep

(DMEK: Descemet membrane endothelial keratoplasty; DSAEK: Descemet stripping automated endothelial keratoplasty)

TABLE 9: Gene therapy in corneal graft survival: Antiangiogenic.

Target	Mechanism of action	Vector	Mode of delivery	Results
Neuropilin-2[23]	RNA interference	Plasmid	*In vivo*: Intrastromal	↓ Lymphangiogenesis
Flt23k[24]	VEGF intraceptor	Poly-lactic co-glycolic acid (PLGA) nanoparticle	Subconjunctival	↑ Graft survival ↓ Hemangiogenesis ↓ Lymphangiogenesis ↑ Graft survival
VEGFR1[25]	Alternative splicing	Vivo-morpholino	Subconjunctival	↓ Hemangiogenesis ↓ Lymphangiogenesis ↑ Graft survival

(RNA: ribonucleic acid; VEGF: vascular endothelial growth factor)

with central guttata and clear peripheral cornea with an endothelial cell count >1,000 cells/mm², the cornea is marked at the center of the pupil (prior to peribulbar block) in mesopic conditions to guide centration, following which the pupil is dilated. Intraoperative, under viscoelastic, a 4-mm diameter imprint centered on the previous mark is made to delimitate the descemetorhexis. Small side-to-side movements are performed using a reverse Sinskey hook at the edge of the imprint to create a small Descemet membrane tag, which is picked and propagated all around the mark to strip the central Descemet membrane, clearing the cornea of the guttae and allowing the peripheral endothelial cells to migrate to and repopulate the fresh area. Rho kinase (ROCK) inhibitors have also been used in conjugation, as salvage agents. The advantages of this procedure are no risk of immunologic graft rejection since no donor cornea is being transplanted, and no requirement of long-term corticosteroid use, eliminating its adverse effects.

- *Tissue-engineered endothelial keratoplasty:* Involves transplanting a thin layer (100 μm) of tissue-engineered human corneal stroma and DM seeded with human corneal endothelial cells, after exposing bare stroma as in the previous procedure. This is a potential optimal treatment for eyes with bullous keratopathy, by removing DM abnormalities and replacing it with a smooth basement membrane.

 8. Discuss the management of shallow anterior chamber after keratoplasty.

Background

- A shallow (or absent) anterior chamber can occur in early postoperative period (days 1–7), the intermediate postoperative period (days 7–30), and the late postoperative period (>30 days).
- A shallow anterior chamber is often associated with a soft eye, but it may also be present with normal or even elevated IOP.

TABLE 10: Gene therapy: Immune response modulation.

Target	Mechanism of action	Vector	Mode of delivery	Results
CTLA[26]	Inhibition of T-cell costimulation	Adenovirus	Ex vivo (donor): Organ-cultured	↓ T-cell activation
CTLA4Ig[27]	Inhibition of T-cell costimulation	Adenovirus	Ex vivo (donor): Organ-cultured	↑ Graft survival ↓ T-cell activation ↓ Th$_1$/Th$_2$/cytokines ↓ Anti-adenovirus antibodies ↑ Graft survival
CTLA4, IL-4[28]	Inhibition of T-cell costimulation	MIDGE (minimalistic immunologically defined gene expression)	Gene gun	Modest ↑ graft survival
IL-10, IL-12, IL-4[29]	Immunosuppression	Adenovirus	Ex vivo (donor): Organ-cultured	↑ Graft survival
TNF-R[30]	Immunosuppression	Adenovirus	Ex vivo (donor): Organ-cultured	Marginal ↑ graft survival
IDO (indoleamine 2,3-dioxygenase)[31]	Immunosuppression	Lentivirus	Ex vivo (donor): Organ-cultured	↑ Graft survival
T-cells, macrophages, DCs[32]	Immunosuppression	Chitosan-PLA nano-particles (RAPA loaded)	Topical	↑ Sustained graft survival by RAPA-loaded nanoparticles

TABLE 11: Gene therapy: Antiapoptosis.

Target	Mechanism of action	Vector	Mode of delivery	Results
P35, Bcl-xL[33]	Inhibition of apoptotic pathways	Lentivirus	Ex vivo (donor): Organ-cultured	↑ Survival of endothelial cells ↑ Retention of endothelial cell morphology
PD-L1 (programmed death ligand 1)[34]	Immunosuppression	Lentivirus	Ex vivo (donor): Organ-cultured	↑ Graft survival
Endothelial cells[35]	EGFP expression	CaP nanoparticles	In vitro	↓ Apoptosis

Evaluation

- A shallow anterior chamber can be detected with the help of a Pen torch or slit lamp evaluation **(Table 12)**. If ASOCT is done, it can also give extra information regarding the anterior segment details.[91-94]
- Fall in visual acuity (e.g., hypotonic maculopathy, choroidal detachment, etc.)
- Projection of rays can be inaccurate in choroidal detachment.
- Pupils size, shape, reaction (to), light, and accommodation (affected in presence of synechiae, relative afferent pupillary defect, etc.).
- Intraocular pressure (low in wound dehiscence, choroidal effusion, and high in malignant glaucoma and suprachoroidal hemorrhage).
- Presence of cell, flare, keratic precipitates, synechiae, hyphema, lens status, and corneal edema.
- Posterior segment evaluation (for hypotonic maculopathy, choroidal detachment, etc.).

Anterior Chamber Depth (ACD) Evaluation

- *Pen torch method:*
    - Shine a pen torch into the patient's eye from the temporal canthus such that the pen torch lies in the same plane of eye.
    - In the case of a deep anterior chamber, the iris lies flat and the whole iris will be illuminated.
    - In the case of a very shallow anterior chamber the iris lies forward, blocking some of the light and very little of the iris is illuminated.
    - Quantitative grading uses a four-point scale, derived from how much the iris is illuminated by the light of the pen torch (grade 1 ≤ one-third of the iris is illuminated, grade II = one-third to two-thirds, grade III ≥ two-thirds and grade IV = iris fully illuminated) (Vargas 1973)[91]
    - Qualitative grading can be used to describe the amount of shadow falling on the iris as shallow, medium or deep.[92]
- *Van Herrick's technique* **(Table 12)**[93]

TABLE 12: Van Herick's technique.

Van Herick's Grade	Ratio to limbal corneal section
Grade 1	<1:4
Grade 2	1:4
Grade 3	1:2
Grade 4	1:1 (or >1:1)

Differentials

- *Shallow anterior chamber with elevated IOP:*
    - Angle closure or pupillary block
    - Aqueous misdirection
- *Shallow anterior chamber with low IOP:*
    - Wound leak
    - Choroidal detachment
    - Trauma (can present with both high or low IOP)

Shallow Anterior Chamber with Elevated Intraocular Pressure

- *Angle-closure (pupillary block):*
    - Shallow anterior chamber, significant IOP elevation, and closure of the angle detected by gonioscopy.
        - Low or normal pressures may also be seen.[95]
    - In early postoperative period, air bubble behind the iris may cause pupillary block
        - Mydriasis and supine position of patient is helpful.
        - Excessive air can be removed intraoperatively.
        - Iridectomy should be done to prevent it—Posterior synechia or vitreous present in the iridectomy must be checked.
    - In late postoperative period, fibrin formation with formation of membranes can lead to pupillary block glaucoma, as well as damage to the endothelium leading to graft failure.[96]
        - Tissue plasminogen activator (TPA) can be used.[97,98]
    - Proper wound apposition, surgical iridoplasty/iridectomies, and use of mydriatics may prevent or lessen the risk for synechia formation.[99,100]
        - Use of mydriatics should be used judiciously, as wide dilations can lead to iris adhesion to the wound, or lead to permanent dilated pupils.[101]

- Medical management includes topical ocular pressure lowering agents, intravenous mannitol or acetazolamide, topical anti-inflammatory eye drops and/or systemic steroids.
- Once anterior synechia are observed postoperatively, close observation is adequate for small adhesions; however, synechia with >180° of angle involvement, and with evidence of early graft rejection/failure, necessitate surgical correction.[101,102]
- Chronic angle closure may have a much less dramatic presentation; however, gonioscopy readily determines the diagnosis.
- *Aqueous misdirection:*[103]
  - Most common in hyperopic eyes and in eyes with previous primary angle-closure glaucoma.
  - It is diagnosed when there is shallowing of the central anterior chamber in association with increased IOP and a normal posterior segment examination.
    - This condition is believed to be due to misdirection of aqueous humor flow posteriorly into the vitreous cavity, with an impermeable anterior hyaloid face.
      - Fluid buildup in the vitreous causes a forward force leading to anterior displacement of the lens-iris diaphragm.
  - It is usually treated with medical therapy, including topical atropine and aqueous humor suppressants, or surgically with disruption of the vitreous face.
    - Pseudophakic or aphakic eyes can be treated with Nd-YAG laser capsulotomy and disruption of the anterior hyaloid face.
    - Phakic patients are treated by cataract extraction with intraocular lens implantation, posterior capsulotomy, and vitrectomy.
      - In cases refractory to medical and laser therapy, surgical intervention to remove the vitreous can be done to increase aqueous flow into the anterior chamber.

Shallow Anterior Chamber with Low Intraocular Pressure

- *Wound leaks:*
  - Wound leak is usually associated with poor wound apposition between the graft and the host tissues.
    - More common with interrupted sutures then continuous suture.
    - Postoperative rise in IOP can cause wound dehiscence.
    - Wound construction, with the use of femtosecond laser, can lead to a decrease in wound leaks.[104-106]
  - A loose suture, wound tissue displacement, or poor wound closure may occur.
  - Seidel testing is helpful in detecting wound leaks.
    - This is performed by placing a fluorescein strip over the wound areas:
      - In the presence of leakage of fluid from the wound or suture track, the orange dye will be diluted and turn green.
      - To diagnose occult wound leaks, use of ultrasound biomicroscopy has been described by.
  - The treatment modality depends on the type and extent of leakage present.
    - If the wound dehiscence is large, especially if it is associated with a flattened anterior chamber or with iris prolapse, urgent resuturing of the wound is indicated.
      - The urgency is to avoid contamination that could lead to infection, as well as to avoid prolonged contact between the corneal endothelium and other structures, which may ultimately lead to endothelial cell death and graft failure.[5]
      - Delayed repair can also lead to persistent fistula and epithelial downgrowth.[106-108]
      - In addition, use of patching or bandage contact lens (BCL) may be helpful in the case of resuturing (for small leak postoperatively).
      - If the iris prolapse occurred with 24 hours, the tissue should be replaced using a blunt spatula and viscoelastic agents.
      - If the prolapsed tissue is over 24-hours old, with signs of necrosis, then it should be excised.
- *Choroidal detachment and hemorrhage:*
  - If the shallow chamber persists after ruling out wound leak and the IOP is very low, this may reflect choroidal detachment.
  - Another complication that can occur is a choroidal hemorrhage, which is usually accompanied by a sudden onset of pain and change in vision.
  - Risk factors include age, cardiovascular disease, hypertension, and glaucoma.[109,110]
  - Indirect ophthalmoscopy or B-scan ultrasonography can be used to confirm the diagnosis.
    - They present as domed shape elevations restricted by the vortex veins.

- Adequate treatment is warranted. In the case of a wound leak, proper repair is indicated. Otherwise, postoperative choroidal detachments are self-limiting.
- Treatment includes topical steroids.
- Since choroidal detachments can extend to the scleral spur and cause anterior displacement of the iris leading to angle closure and anterior synechia formation, if the detachment persists for over 3 days, then surgical drainage is indicated, with reformation of the anterior chamber.[63]
    - If a choroidal hemorrhage occurs, close follow-up is indicated, with possible surgical drainage.[110-112]
- *Trauma:*
    - Traumatic cyclodialysis cleft formation or wound dehiscence may be associated with hypotony and shallowing of the anterior chamber.
    - Pupillary block can occur following zonular dehiscence when the lens completely occludes the pupil, which prohibits the flow of aqueous humor from the ciliary body to the anterior chamber angle.
        - This results in a flat anterior chamber with a high posterior chamber IOP.

9. Discuss ocular graft-versus-host disease.

Definition

Graft-versus-host disease (GVHD) is a constellation of clinical symptoms caused by an *exaggerated donor-derived lymphocytic reaction to host antigens* following allogeneic hematopoietic stem cell transplantation **(Fig. 10)**.[113,114]

Background

- Currently, there are three different types of stem cell transplantation available:
    1. Autologous (self)
    2. Allogeneic (other individuals)
    3. Syngeneic (identical twins)[115]
- In allogeneic hematopoietic stem cell transplantation, donor stem cells are harvested from bone marrow, peripheral blood, or placental cord blood.
    - Approximately 40–60% of the recipients receiving this treatment may develop GVHD.[116-118]
    - It can be single organ or multi-organ.
    - Skin, gastrointestinal system, and liver are most commonly involved.
    - Ocular involvement is less frequent.

Classical Diagnostic Criteria (National Institutes of Health Consensus Criteria)

- *Acute GVHD:* If clinical manifestations occurred within the first 100 days after transplantation.[115,119]
- *Chronic GVHD:* If clinical manifestations occurred after the first 100 days after transplantation.[115,119]
- *Revised criteria (2005):* Acute and chronic GVHD based on *phenotype* rather than the temporal occurrence of the disease.[120]

Acute Graft-Versus-Host Disease

- Allogeneic hematopoietic stem cell transplantation is the most common cause.
- The risk factors include:
    - Female donor to male recipient
    - Older-aged recipient

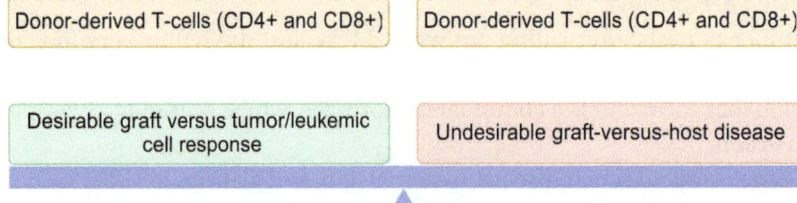

Fig. 10: Desirable versus undesirable graft-versus-host responses.

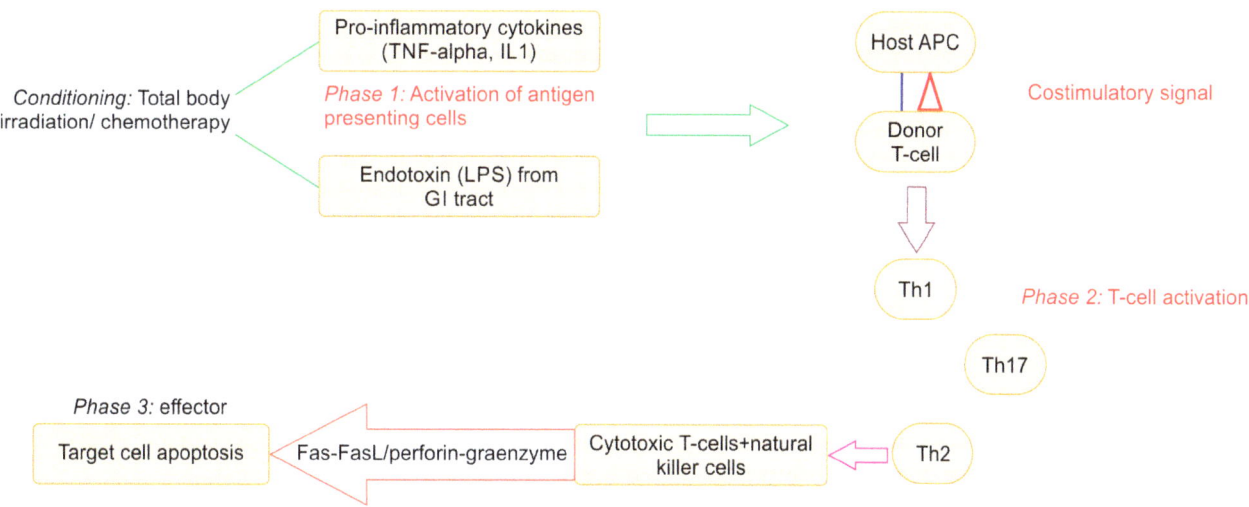

Fig. 11: Pathophysiology of acute graft-versus-host disease.
(APC: antigen-presenting cells; GI: gastrointestinal; IL: interleukin; LPS: lipopolysaccharide; TNF: tumor necrosis factor)

- Stem cells extracted from the peripheral blood
- Unrelated donor[115,119,121]
- Preconditioning of the recipient tissue through immunoablative chemotherapy and/or radiation prior to allogeneic hematopoietic stem cell transplantation.

Pathophysiology of Acute Graft-Versus-Host Disease (Fig. 11)

- Graft-versus-host disease occurs when donor T-cells respond to recipient tissue antigen mismatches between major histocompatibility antigens (found on chromosome 6p, also known as human leukocyte antigen region).[114,122]
- The incidence of GVHD is directly proportional to the degree of human leukocyte antigen mismatching.[114,122]
- Today, the majority of stem cell transplantation occurs with human leukocyte antigen matched unrelated donors; therefore, other genetic differences outside the human leukocyte antigen region or minor histocompatibility antigens contribute to GVHD.[114,122]
- *Acute GVHD occurs in three phases:*[113,114,121,123-125]
  1. Activation of antigen-presenting cells
  2. T-cell activation
  3. Cellular and inflammatory effector phase.

Chronic Graft-Versus-Host Disease

- At least one diagnostic feature should be observed in the skin, mucosa, musculoskeletal system, or the gastrointestinal tract.[116]
  - All mucosal surfaces may be involved, for example, ocular, oral, vaginal, and gastrointestinal.
- *Risk factor:*
  - Occurrence of acute form of GVHD.
  - Other risk factors are similar to those for the acute form.[116]

Pathophysiology of Chronic Graft-Versus-Host Disease

Aberrant recovery of the immune system after transplantation can cause a loss of normal function.
- Mimic autoimmune disorders such as scleroderma, Sjögren syndrome, and rheumatoid arthritis.[116]

Ocular Graft-Versus-Host Disease

- An umbrella term for conjunctival disease, keratoconjunctivitis sicca, and other ocular surface manifestations.[115,119]
- Its reported occurrence rate, varying between studies, is roughly 40–60% of patients receiving allogeneic hematopoietic stem cell transplantation.[119,126-130]
- Ocular involvement may be a precursor to systemic GVHD and is a poor prognostic factor for mortality.[130]

- *The risk factors:*
  - Preceding skin, oral mucosa, gastrointestinal tract, and liver involvement.[128,129]
  - In patients with moderate-to-severe systemic GVHD.[128]
  - Donor-recipient gender disparity is also a risk factor.
  - Diabetes mellitus[128]
- Ocular GVHD can present in acute and chronic forms.

Clinical Features

- The severity of acute ocular GVHD correlates with the severity of systemic disease.[115]
- Primarily manifests as keratoconjunctivitis sicca (may be the presenting sign of chronic ocular GVHD).[131]
  - Lacrimal glands are affected and infiltrated by lymphocytes along with conjunctival inflammation, cicatricial scarring, and meibomian gland dysfunction.[130]
  - The inner surfaces of the ductal areas of lacrimal glands and meibomian glands are composed of mucous membranes, which are frequently targeted by T-cells and inflammatory cells.[128]
  - Conjunctiva (conjunctiva-associated mucosal tissue) may mimic systemic mucosal membranes (mucosa-associated mucosal tissue) making it a target for inflammatory cell activity.[128]

Acute Ocular Graft-Versus-Host Disease

- *Mild conjunctival hyperemia in the presence of systemic GVHD:* Highly suggestive of ocular GVHD.
- *Conjunctival chemosis:* Rule out hyponatremia and hypoalbuminemia.[121]
- *Pseudomembranous conjunctivitis:* Marker of systemic involvement (one-third of these patients will also have corneal epithelial sloughing)[121]
- *Persistent corneal epitheliopathy:* Complication of severe dry eye disease and can subsequently lead to corneal ulceration (of infectious or noninfectious etiology).[1]
- *Severe dry eye disease:* However, this occurs more commonly in chronic GVHD.[119,121]
- The diagnosis can then be confirmed by conjunctival biopsy.

Chronic Ocular Graft-Versus-Host Disease

- Almost all components of the ocular surface may be affected:
  - Because of its autoimmune mimicry, there are no clinical signs or symptoms that are specific to chronic ocular GVHD.[132]
- Most common presentation of chronic GVHD is keratoconjunctivitis sicca along with conjunctival and lacrimal gland involvement (typically occurring 6–12 months after allogeneic hematopoietic stem cell transplantation).[119,126,130]
- Similar to dry eye disease, there may be punctate keratopathy and cicatricial conjunctivitis.[132]
- Dry eye disease is seen in 10–62% patients with systemic GVHD.[119,120,121,126,132]
  - The severity of dry eye is correlated with the severity of GVHD or may precede onset of systemic disease **(Table 13)**.[126]
- Meibomian gland dysfunction may occur in 45% of cases and may contribute to rapid tear breakup time, leading to ocular surface changes.[119]
- Frequent follow-ups with cultures and prophylactic antibiotics are important in such cases to prevent rapid progression to corneal perforation.[133]
- Conjunctival involvement occurs is considered a sign of severe chronic GVHD.[121]
  - Conjunctivitis may be the presenting sign (for classification, refer **Table 14**).[113]
  - These patients can also present with signs of sterile conjunctivitis such as chemosis, serosanguineous discharge, and less frequently corneal epithelial sloughing.[131]

TABLE 13: National Institutes of Health Organ Scoring in chronic graft-versus-host disease: eyes.

Score	Symptoms
0	No symptoms
1	Mild dry eye symptoms not affecting activities of daily living (requirement of lubricant eye drops 3 times per day)
2	Moderate dry eye symptoms partially affecting activities of daily living (requiring lubricant eye drops 3-6 times per day or punctal plugs), without new vision impairment due to KCS
3	Severe dry eye symptoms significantly affecting activities of daily living (special eyewear to relieve pain) or unable to work because of ocular symptoms or loss of vision due to KCS

TABLE 14: Classification of conjunctivitis in chronic graft-versus-host disease.[113]

Grade	Clinical feature
0	None
1	Subtle/mild hyperemia
2	Hyperemia + chemosis
3	Pseudomembranous conjunctivitis
4	Pseudomembranes + corneal epithelial sloughing

- Cicatricial conjunctivitis may manifest as palpebral or forniceal symblepharon, resulting in lid scarring and extensive altered lid anatomy.
- Although less frequent, involvement of the anterior chamber, vitreous, and choroid may also be possible during the course of chronic ocular GVHD.
    - The prevalence of uveitis in ocular GVHD has been reported approximately 2–4% and is thought to occur because of either the direct immune response of donor lymphocytes to host antigens or ischemic iridopathy related to localized necrosis.[134]
- Posterior segment findings in chronic GVHD include posterior scleritis, optic nerve edema, serous retinal detachment, central serous chorioretinopathy, microvascular retinopathy, and infectious retinitis such as cytomegalovirus retinitis (perhaps due to immunosuppression).[119,121]

Diagnostic Evaluation: National Institutes of Health (NIH) Consensus Development Project

- *Diagnostic signs and symptoms:* Clinical manifestations that establish the diagnosis of chronic GVHD without the need for further testing or evidence (not defined for eyes).[121]
- *Distinctive signs and symptoms:* Do not normally manifest in acute GVHD and are clinical manifestations that are not sufficient to establish a diagnosis of GVHD without further testing or involvement of additional organs.[116,135]
- *Other features or unclassified manifestations:* Nonspecific or uncommon features that are insufficient to establish a diagnosis of GVHD.[116,135]
- Common features are signs and symptoms that are found in both acute and chronic GVHD.[135]
- *Distinctive ocular manifestations of chronic graft-versus-host (defined by NIH diagnosing and staging working group):*
    - New-onset dry, gritty, or painful eyes
    - Cicatricial conjunctivitis
    - Keratoconjunctivitis sicca
    - Confluent areas of punctate keratopathy[116]
- *Unclassified manifestations:*
    - Photophobia
    - Periorbital hyperpigmentation
    - Blepharitis (erythema of the eyelids with edema).[116,135]
- Diagnosis of chronic GVHD requires at least one diagnostic clinical sign of chronic GVHD or the presence of at least one distinctive manifestation confirmed by pertinent biopsy or other relevant tests (e.g., laboratory tests or radiological findings) in the same or another organ.[116,126]
    - Ocular findings are distinctive signs that are not sufficient alone to establish a diagnosis of GVHD[126]
    - Diagnosis of ocular GVHD cannot be made in the absence of systemic GVHD.[128]

How is the dry eye defined?

International Chronic Ocular Graft-Versus-Host Disease Consensus Group

- Diagnostic criteria for dry eye include:[126]
    - *Ocular surface disease index:*
        - Quality-of-life questionnaire consisting of 12 questions
    - Schirmer test score (without anesthesia)
    - Corneal fluorescein staining
    - Conjunctival injection

Other tests:
- Tear film osmolarity[136,137]
- *Vital staining:* Lissamine green or rose Bengal dyes for conjunctival assessment and fluorescein dye for corneal assessment[115,127]
- *Conjunctival swabs or scrapes:* In cases of questionable etiology to rule out infectious causes.
- *Routine biopsy of the conjunctiva:* Considered nonbeneficial because of its invasive nature and potential for scarring
- *Impression cytology:* To assess for epithelial cell necrosis, goblet-cell loss, or squamous metaplasia[130,131]

Prevention of Graft-Versus-Host Disease

- Optimal human leukocyte-antigen matching[113]
- Prophylactic therapy targeted at donor T-cell depletion, interference of their activity, or inhibition of their proliferation[126,127,138]

Treatment of Established Graft-Versus-Host Disease

It has two components:[115,116,121]
1. Initial organ-specific therapy
2. Later systemic immunosuppression (if three or more organs are involved)

Treatment of Acute Graft-Versus-Host Disease

- Corticosteroid therapy is the criterion standard in first-line treatment because of its antilymphocyte, anti-inflammatory, and proapoptosis properties.[139]
- Response to steroid therapy is correlated with the severity of GVHD and with post-transplantation survival rate.[138]
  - Complete or partial remission may be seen in <50% of cases.
  - Steroid resistance can lead to a low 5-year survival rate.
- Steroid-dependent or refractory cases can be managed by:
  - *Extracorporeal photopheresis therapy:*[139]
    - White blood cells are separated out from serum, and exposed to 8-methoxypsoralen followed by ultraviolet A irradiation.
    - Induces T-cell destruction.
  - *Tumor necrosis factor blockade (infliximab and etanercept):*
    - Increases the risk of infections.[138]
  - Antithymocyte globulin
  - Monoclonal antibody (alemtuzumab, an anti-CD52 antibody)
  - Mesenchymal stem cells
  - Mechanistic target of rapamycin (mTOR) inhibitor (sirolimus)
  - Antimetabolite (pentostatin)

Treatment of Chronic Graft-Versus-Host Disease

- Corticosteroid therapy (such as methylprednisolone or prednisone) remains the mainstay.[138]
  - The duration of steroid therapy depends on the clinical response.
  - Often given in combination with other immunosuppressive.
- *Second-line therapy (with limited evidence):*[138]
  - Extracorporeal photopheresis
  - Calcineurin inhibitors
- Other immunosuppressive therapies are similar to acute GVHD.
- Supportive care with appropriate antimicrobial treatment and prophylaxis for comorbid bacterial, fungal, or viral infections as required.

Treatment of Ocular Graft-Versus-Host Disease

- There are currently no preventive therapies available for ocular GVHD[140]
- Treatment strategies for established ocular GVHD are described in **Table 15**.

TABLE 15: Treatment of ocular graft-versus-host disease.

Treatment strategies	Modalities
Ocular surface lubrication	• Preservative-free and phosphate-free artificial tears • Lubricating viscous ointment acetylcysteine (5–10%) ophthalmic solution • Oral muscarinic agonists such as pilocarpine or cevimeline
Tear preservation	• Punctal occlusion and collagen or silicone plugs (temporary) and thermal cauterization (permanent)
Prevention of tear evaporation (Meibomian gland dysfunction)	• Warm compresses + erythromycin ointment • Oral tetracyclines (doxycycline/minocycline) • Oral or topical azithromycin nutritional supplements (fish oil, flax-seed oil) • Thermal pulsation system
Inflammation reduction	• Topical cyclosporine A 0.05% or 0.1% topical corticosteroids • Anakinra (IL-1 receptor antagonist), topical • Tacrolimus (calcineurin inhibitor), topical • Tranilast, topical

Epithelial support	• Autologous serum tears (avoid in systemic inflammation/infection)
	• *Contact lenses:*
	  – Rigid gas permeable
	  – Silicone hydrogel
	  – Scleral lenses

Supportive care	• Moisture goggles • Humidifier • Topical antibiotics for infection prophylaxis
Surgical intervention	• Superficial epithelial debridement • Partial tarsorrhaphy • Sutureless amniotic membrane • Fornix reconstruction • Limbal stem cell transplantation • Penetrating keratoplasty

(IL: interleukin)

- Systemic immunosuppression for ocular GVHD is not generally desired because ocular sequelae do not necessarily respond to systemic therapy.[127,130]

Conclusion

- Graft-versus-host disease is a leading cause of increased mortality and morbidity in patients receiving allogeneic hematopoietic stem cell transplantation.
- Ocular involvement mainly occurs in chronic GVHD and does not, in general, cause permanent visual loss, but can decrease quality of life in its severest forms.[129]
- Management of GVHD should be tailored to individual cases.

 10. Discuss types and indications of keratoprosthesis.

Description

- Keratoprosthesis (KP) is an artificial cornea that is intended to replace the opacified corneal tissue and restore vision when severe bilateral corneal disease exists (e.g., prior failed cadaveric corneal transplant, chemical injury, or certain immunological condition).
- They are performed for bilateral corneal blindness not amenable to conventional penetrating keratoplasty often as a last resort.[141,142]
- The choice of keratoprosthesis (KP) depends on the underlying etiology, the anatomy of the ocular surface and the tear film status.

- Broadly speaking, keratoprostheses are categorized into:
  - *Type 1:* Ideal for eyes with normal lids, blink and tear film without an underlying immunological etiology (prototype is the Boston Type 1 KP).
  - *Type 2:* Severely dry or keratinized ocular surface with an underlying immunological disorder, associated with lid abnormalities.

Types of Keratoprosthesis/Design

- *The design of a KP consists of an optic and a haptic:*
  - The optic forms the central part of the KP responsible for viewing,
    - In most types, it is a cylinder made of polymethyl methacrylate (PMMA).
  - The haptic determines the type of the prosthesis, and this could be divided into:
    - Biocompatible—usually a PMMA skirt with the corneal graft as in the Boston Type 1 and 2 KP
    - Biointegrated—as in the Dacron mesh that forms the skirt around the PMMA optic in the Pintucci KP
    - Biological—tooth or the bone that forms an autologous biological tissue that supports the optical cylinder in the osteo-odonto and the osteo-KP, respectively.
- The supporting cover tissue adds to the KP complex and prevents the carrier graft desiccation.
  - *Type 1 KP:* BCL
  - *Type 2 KPs:* Skin and the buccal mucosa for the osteo and the osteo-odonto, and Pintucci KPs, respectively.
- Pediatric KP forms a separate entity and the Type 1 KP is performed in pediatric population to visually rehabilitate children with congenital bilateral corneal disorders not amenable to penetrating keratoplasty.
  - Type 2 KPs are usually not performed in the pediatric population.

Indications for Type 1 Keratoprosthesis

- *Good prognosis:*
  - Multiple failed grafts
  - Aniridia
  - Herpetic keratitis
  - Silicon oil-filled eyes
- *Guarded prognosis:*
  - Pediatric corneal conditions
  - Chemical injuries
- *Very guarded prognosis:*
  - Underlying immune conditions such as Stevens–Johnson syndrome (SJS)/ocular cicatricial pemphigoid (OCP)
  - Severe chemical injuries with severe forniceal shortening and lid abnormalities

Indications for Type 2 Keratoprosthesis

- The choice of KP in severe end-stage ocular surface disorders is preferably the modified osteo-odonto-keratoprosthesis (MOOKP).
  - In case of the patient being unsuitable for the same, the other Type 2 KP are chosen for the following:
    - SJS
    - OCP/mucous membrane pemphigoid
    - Severe chemical injuries
    - Severely keratinized surface
- The contraindications for KPs are tabulated in **Table 16.**

Preoperative Evaluation

- A detailed history taking to determine etiology, onset (to gauge extent of amblyopia—loss of vision before 5 years of age is considered as a poor indicator for visual recovery), and previous intraocular surgeries.
- Detailed ophthalmic evaluation including a B-scan with axial length measurement
- Perception of light and accurate projection of rays
- Intraocular pressure (digital tonometry)
- Ultrasound biomicroscopy/ASOCT to assess the anterior segment details in eyes with scarred opaque corneas

TABLE 16: Contraindications for keratoprosthesis procedures.

All KPs	MOOKP specific	Type 2 KP specific
Nil perception of light	Edentulous	Absent eyelids
Unrealistic expectation	Poor oral hygiene	
Advanced glaucoma	Unfit for general anesthesia	
Uncertainty about follow-up	<18 year old	
Poor prognosis (dense amblyopia, retinal pathology, etc.)		

- Adequacy of blink is confirmed (Type 1).
- Schirmer's I wetting is determined for adequacy of tears (Type 1).
- Patency of nasolacrimal duct is confirmed by means of syringing to rule out focus of infection (for Type 1, if puncta open for Type 2).
- Patients should have a detailed dental and oral mucosal evaluation with a spiral computed tomography scan to evaluate the canines preoperatively along with determining fitness for general anesthesia (for MOOKP).

Surgical Technique and Postoperative Care for Boston Type 1 Keratoprosthesis

- Decide on the type of KP to be ordered:
  - *Pseudophakic/aphakic:* Axial length to be specified for aphakic KP
  - Adult (8.5 mm backplate)/pediatric (7.0 mm backplate)
- An extra KP to be ordered as a standby
- Fresh therapeutic grade donor cornea is preferred to assemble the KP
- Local or general anesthesia as indicated.
- The recipient cornea is marked with the trephine as required.
- KP to be assembled before trephining the recipient.
  - Backplate of the KP measures 8.5 mm and hence the minimum donor graft size to be 8.5 mm.
    - The donor cornea is usually oversized by 0.5 mm.
  - The central 3 mm opening in the donor cornea is subsequently trephined.
  - The optic is placed on the adhesive strip upside down.
  - The donor graft is slid down the stem of the optic into its slot using a wrench.
  - The back-plate is slid in place.
  - The assembly is then locked with the titanium ring and checked for a snug fit.
- The recipient cornea is further trephined and removed. Any intraocular procedure as planned to be performed.
- The assembled KP is then sutured like in a PK using 16 interrupted 9-0 nylon sutures, preferably buried.
- A BCL is placed on the KP.[143]

Postoperative Regimen

- Fourth generation fluoroquinolone 4 times a day for a month, continued 2/day indefinitely.
- Topical vancomycin (14 mg/mL) 4 times a day for a month, continued 1/day indefinitely, for high-risk eyes.
- Topical steroids tapered to 2/day, indefinitely or discontinued after 6 months.
- Topical lubricants as required.
- BCL to be changed once in 3 months, application of 5% povidone-iodine in clinic at the time of BCL replacement.
- Follow-up every 3 months.[142]

Examination During Each Follow-up Visit

- *Change in refraction:*
  - A hyperopic shift could indicate an early leak.
  - A myopic shift could be indicative of raised IOP.
- Deposits on BCL, if any, to preferably be submitted for microbiological evaluation.
- To assess for air bubbles under the optic flange as well as immobile bubbles beneath the BCL.
  - Indicate early thinning of the carrier graft.

- The graft around the optic should be inspected for the presence of any infiltration.
- Slit-beam examination to assess for any irregularity in the carrier graft.
  - Presence of retroprosthetic membrane (RPM), if any.
  - Presence of loose sutures, if any, should be removed.
- Intraocular pressure is monitored by digital tonometry.
- 90D lens examination to document the optic disc and posterior pole findings.
- Following removal of the BCL for replacement, the graft should be stained with sterile fluorescein to look for the presence of any epithelial defect or leak.
- Use of 5% povidone-iodine in the eye is recommended at the time of BCL replacement.
- Humphrey visual field analysis once in 6 months.
- ASOCT to identify early graft thinning, periprosthetic tissue loss, RPM, and angle details once in 6 months.
- B-scan ultrasonography once in a year.

Boston Type 2 Keratoprosthesis

- The procedure is largely similar to the Boston Type 1 KP in terms of assembly and suturing. The differences include:
  - The anterior nub of the KP protrudes by 2 mm to accommodate the skin.
  - There is no separate titanium ring.
  - In the recipient, the entire conjunctival mucosa is removed from lid margin to lid margin.
  - Sphincterotomy is done to keep the pupil mid-dilated.
  - Following KP suturing, pars plana vitrectomy (PPV) is performed along with Ahmed glaucoma valve implantation in all eyes.
  - The lid margins are excised to completely be rid of hair follicles.

Postoperative Regimen

- Systemic and topical steroids to be tapered and stopped over a month.
- Topical antibiotic drops—fourth generation fluoroquinolone for 2 weeks.
- Topical antibiotic ointment at bedtime to be continued indefinitely.
- Meticulous cleaning over the KP for the first postoperative week to prevent skin overgrowth.
- Lid sutures are removed on day 10.
- Follow-up once every 3 months.

Modified Osteo-Odonto-Keratoprosthesis (Rome-Vienna Protocol)[144]

It consists of three stages (**Fig. 12**).

Postoperative Regimen

- Systemic and topical steroids and antibiotics are administered after every stage as warranted.
- Topical antibiotic ointment is continued once a day indefinitely.
- Topical lubricants are continued indefinitely.
- Follow-up once every 6 months, in addition, to evaluate the health of the oral mucosa and the lamina.

Stage 1 A: Eye is prepared for the procedure by removing the iris, doing a cryolens extraction and a limited anterior vitrectomy

Stage 1 B + C (1 month later):
- Canine tooth harvested and fashioned into osteo-odonto-alveolar lamina with the optical cylinder fixed
- The lamina is placed in the contralateral cheek subcutaneous pouch for it to develop its fibrovascular covering
- Buccal mucosa measuring 3 cm in diameter is harvested and draped over the ocular surface securing it to the 4 recti muscles

Stage 2 (3 months later):
- The lamina is removed from the subcutaneous pouch and prepared
- The mucosa over the ocular surface is reflected with an inferior hinge
- The central cornea is trephined as per the posterior diameter of the optical cylinder and the lamina is placed in the eye.
- The oral mucosa is reflected back over the lamina and sutured and a central opening is made in the mucosa for the cylinder to protrude through

Fig. 12: Modified osteo-odonto-keratoprosthesis (Rome-Vienna Protocol).[144]

Osteo-Keratoprosthesis

- The procedure is very similar to the MOOKP.
- The bone is harvested instead of the tooth from the tibia and the same is fashioned into an osteo-lamina, in which the optical cylinder is fixed.

Postoperative Regimen

- Systemic and topical steroids and antibiotics are administered after every stage as warranted.
- Topical antibiotic ointment is continued once a day indefinitely.
- Topical lubricants are continued indefinitely.
- Follow-up once every 6 months, in addition, to evaluate the health of the oral mucosa and the lamina.

Outcomes

The most common complications encountered are:
- Sterile melts
- Retroprosthetic membrane
- Glaucoma.

Sterile Melts

- In the presence of melt:
  - Assess the extent of associated thinning:
    - In mild cases, cyanoacrylate glue application to the area of thinning would suffice.
    - In moderate cases involving a few or more clock hours, a crescentic or annular lamellar graft can be used.
    - In the presence of extensive melts, associated with aqueous leak, it is best to replace the KP with a new one.
  - In addition, medical supportive measures include:
    - Topical medroxyprogesterone
    - Systemic doxycycline
    - Copious lubrication
    - Tarsorrhaphy in cases with frequent BCL displacements leading to graft desiccation.
- A similar process in the MOOKP/OKP is termed as laminar resorption.[145]
- A sterile inflammatory process that initiates the keratolysis could by virtue of proximity spill over into the vitreous leading to a sterile vitritis.[145]

Retroprosthetic Membrane

- Retroprosthetic membrane has been implicated as one of the causes for sterile corneal melts by virtue of preventing access of aqueous to the carrier graft.[146]
- Performing a total PPV reduces the rate of RPM formation.[147]
- An aphakic eye has a low rate of primary RPM formation due to lack of scaffold.
- Visually insignificant RPM's can be observed and monitored.
  - Visually significant RPM's can be addressed by means of neodymium:yttrium-aluminum-garnet laser membranotomy or a surgical membranectomy.

Glaucoma

- It is the most common comorbid factor with progressive decrease in vision post-KP.[142]
- In eyes with coexistent glaucoma before KP placement, glaucoma needs proactive and aggressive management.
  - It is recommended to simultaneously place a drainage implant in eyes with the Type 1 KP and MOOKP (according to stage of surgery).[148]

Endophthalmitis

- Noted in 9% of type 1 KP at 14.2 months mean follow-up[149] (10% of eyes with the MOOKP as well as the Boston Type 2 KP).
- Fungal etiology is noted in almost equal number of eyes as those with bacterial endophthalmitis.

Q 11. **(1) Critically evaluate organization of ideal blood bank with reference to maximize the needs of our region. (2) Planning an ideal eye bank at a tertiary ophthalmic hospital. (3) Eye banking and legislation. (4) How would you set up an eye bank?**

Composition

It is composed of three-tier organization structure **(Fig. 13)**.

Eye Retrieval Center (ERC)

- Eye Retrieval Center has to be affiliated to a registered eye bank (EB), and should provide the following services:
    - Public and professional *awareness* about eye donation
    - *Coordination* with donor families and hospital patients to motivate them eye donation
    - *Harvesting* corneal tissue (from the community and the hospital where they are based) along with collection of blood from the Cadaver, for serology
    - *Safe storage and transportation* of tissue to the parent eye bank.
    - All large hospitals in metros with mortality rate of >50 per month (1–2 per day) should be set up as donation/retrieval centers and linked to the nearest eye bank.

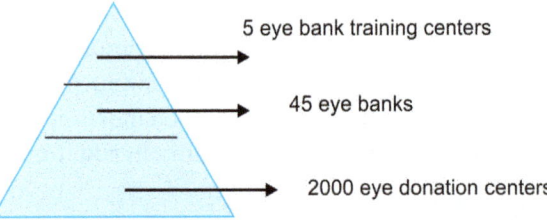

Fig. 13: Composition of eye banking system.

Eye Bank

- *Provides the following services:*
    - A round-the-clock *public response system* regarding eye donation queries over the telephone and conduct public awareness programs on eye donation.
    - *Coordinate* with donor families and hospital patients to motivate eye donation under the Hospital Cornea Retrieval Program (HCRP).
    - *Harvest* corneal tissues from cadavers/brain dead persons.
    - *Process*, preserve, and evaluate the collected tissue.
    - *Distribute* the corneal tissue in an equitable manner for keratoplasty.
    - *Ensure* safe transportation of tissue to the keratoplasty center.

Eye Bank Training Center

All of the eye bank functions plus training for all levels of personnel in eye banking and research.

Staff and Training

Eye Banking system should have at least the following personnel:
- *Board of Directors:*
    - All eye banks and eye bank training center (EBTC).
    - Ideally composed of medical professionals and other professionals who could contribute to the smooth functioning of the organization.
- *Executive Director/Eye Bank Manager:*
    - To be responsible for entire operations of the eye bank.
    - Maintain to compliance the policies of the Board or committee and wherever necessary shall consult the Medical Director (MD)/Eye Bank in-charge or other specialists for discharging the responsibilities.
- *Medical Director:*
    - Must be an ophthalmologist who has expertise in external eye diseases and corneal surgery.
    - MD shall oversee and provide advice on all medical aspects of eye bank operations.
    - Participate in training and supervision of technical staff with regard to tissue procurement, preservation, and evaluation (competency reviews).
- *Eye Bank Technician:*
    - Must be responsible for the entire activities of eye banking such as retrieval, processing, evaluation, documentation, distribution of tissue and maintenance of the laboratory, instruments, and equipment.

- Must be Higher Secondary or 12th pass qualified with Science or Higher Secondary education with experience in a diagnostic or similar lab or experience in operation theatre procedures.
- Must have undergone training and qualified from designated training centers for eye bank technicians.
- Training locations are defined in the Transplantation of Human Organs and Tissues Rules, 2014, as a, "registered, authorized, and functional eye bank or government medical college".
- *Training period:* 4–8 weeks
- Eye Donation Counselor (EDC):
  - EDC shall be responsible for counseling the families at hospitals and coordinate with eye bank and hospital for retrieval of cornea.
  - Must also be responsible for awareness campaigns regarding eye donation, both within the hospital and outside the hospital.
  - *On job training period:* 1 month in local language.

Facilities and Equipment

- *Refrigerator:*
  - Each eye bank laboratory shall have a refrigerator with a device, internal or external for continuously recording temperature.
  - Current temperature shall be monitored and recorded daily.
  - The continuous temperature device shall be calibrated against a reference thermometer as defined by the appropriate regulatory agency at least once a year.
  - It must contain clearly defined and labeled areas for all tissues stored (i.e., surgical tissue awaiting distribution/released, quarantined tissue, tissue rejected, tissue for research), and defined areas for nontissue items (e.g., reagents).
- *Laminar airflow hood:*
  - A high-efficiency particulate air (HEPA)-filtered biohazard safety cabinet shall be cleaned before and after each use and at regularly scheduled intervals to prevent cross-contamination.
  - The laminar air flow hood must meet ISO Class 5 standards or documented annually to have <25 colony forming units per 90 mm settle plate per 1-hour exposure.
  - Calibration, including settle-plate air culturing, must be performed annually.
- *Slit lamp:*
  - Each eye bank must have routine access to a functioning slit lamp with the ability to accurately and adequately evaluate donor corneas.
  - Maintenance, calibration, and cleaning should be as per the manufacturer's recommendations.
- *Specular microscope:*
  - Each eye bank laboratory shall have a specular microscope to capture an image of donor cornea endothelium and calculating endothelial cell density.
  - Maintenance, calibration, and cleaning should be as per the manufacturer's recommendations.
- *Recovery instruments:*
  - *Corneal excision set:*
    - Drapes, torch, loupe
    - Disposable syringes (5 mL^{-1}, 10 mL^{-1}) with disposable needles (21 G and spinal needle) with two test tubes or plain vials to collect blood sample.
    - Conjunctival scissors
    - Corneal scissors (right and left)
    - Fixation forceps
    - Iris forceps
    - Spring or wire speculum
    - Bard Parker handle with sterile surgical blade (no. 11 or 15).
  - *Enucleation set:*
    - Same as corneal excision set, except for
    - Enucleating spoon
    - Strabismus scissor

- *Eye Bank Laboratory:*
  - The laboratory shall be a separate area with limited access in which activities directly related to eye tissue processing are carried out.
  - The laboratory shall have a sink with a drain and running water and a dedicated hand-washing sink.
  - Appropriate documentation of regular laboratory cleaning schedules shall be retained for a minimum of three years.

Standard Operating Procedures Manual

- Eye Banks shall document in their Standard Operating Procedures (SOP) Manual details of all critical processes that affect safety and quality of tissues and ensure that they are carried out under controlled conditions, as appropriate to the particular process being performed.
- Its validation shall be based on the following:
  - *Performance* of specific tests, trials, or procedures
  - *Risk* assessment for potential effect on safety and quality
  - Previously *published* studies
  - *Retrospective* evaluation of the eye bank's own data

Bio-Hazardous Waste Disposal

Human tissue and waste items shall be disposed of in such a manner as to minimize any hazard to eye bank personnel and the environment and comply with applicable regulations.

Consent Documentation

Consent shall be obtained in writing (by a signed consent form), as determined by local or national legislation (including, *Transplantation of Human Organs Act 1994, 2014 Rules*).[150,151]

Donor Serologic Testing

- A blood sample from the donor must be tested. This sample may be either:
  - A postmortem sample drawn as soon as practicable after the time of death, or at the time of tissue recovery, or
  - A premortem sample drawn within 7 days prior to death.
- *Minimum Testing:* Blood (serum or plasma) must test nonreactive to the following required infectious diseases:
  - *Human immunodeficiency virus types 1 and 2:* Anti-HIV-1, anti-HIV-2
  - *Hepatitis C virus (HCV):* Anti-HCV
  - *Hepatitis B virus (HBV):* HBsAg
  - Syphilis
  - COVID-19
- *Plasma dilution/hemodilution*
  - The testing of plasma or serum samples shall take into account any factors which may cause dilution sufficient to alter tests results.
  - A pretransfusion/infusion sample shall be obtained and tested.
  - The eye bank shall use an algorithm for calculating the effect of plasma dilution on the donor sample and demonstrate that it is less than the designated limit.

Donor Screening[152]

Tissue from donors with the following is potentially hazardous to eye bank personnel and harvesting eyes should be strictly avoided.
- Active viral hepatitis
- Acquired immunodeficiency syndrome (AIDS) of HIV
- Active viral encephalitis or encephalitis of unknown origin
- Creutzfeldt–Jakob disease
- Suspected rabies and persons who, within the past 6 months, were bitten by an animal suspected to be infected with rabies.

Contraindications for Transplantation

Conditions with potential risk of transmission of local or systemic communicable disease from donor to recipient:

- Death with progressive neurodegenerative disease of unknown etiology, including but not limited to the following:
  - Amyotrophic lateral sclerosis
  - Multiple sclerosis
  - Huntington's chorea
  - Alzheimer's disease
  - Dementia (exceptions include dementia due to CVA, brain tumor, head trauma, or medication or drug-induced)
  - Myasthenia gravis
  - Parkinson's syndrome
  - Parkinson's like disease
  - Creutzfeldt–Jakob disease
  - Chronic idiopathic demyelinating polyneuropathy
- Death of unknown cause and likelihood of exclusionary criteria as outlined in this list.
- Active meningitis (viremia, bacteremia, and tubercular) or viral encephalitis of unknown origin.
- Progressive encephalopathy (including but not limited to subacute sclerosing panencephalitis, and progressive multifocal leukoencephalopathy)
- Active septicemia at the time of death.
  - Clinical evidence of infection; and
  - Two or more of the following systemic features:
    - Temperature of > 38 °C (100.4 °F)
    - WBC >12,000 cells/mm^3, <4,000 cells/mm^3, or >10% immature (band) forms
  - Positive (premortem) blood cultures
- The following are examples of specific exclusions for systemic viral disease (viremia) which is active at the time of death:
  - Active chikungunya or active dengue fever
  - Active H1N1 influenza, COVID-19 infection
  - Active viral hepatitis, hepatitis B surface antigen positive, or hepatitis C seropositive donors
  - Congenital rubella
  - Reye's syndrome
  - Suspected rabies
  - Active miliary tuberculosis
  - HTLV-I or HTLV-II infection
  - HIV seropositive donors
  - Active syphilis or seropositive for syphilis (should be confirmed with FTA)
  - Leprosy

Conditions with potential risk of transmission of noncommunicable disease from donor to recipient

- *Intrinsic eye disease:*
  - Active ocular or intraocular inflammation conjunctivitis, scleritis, iritis, uveitis, vitreitis choroiditis, keratitis, and retinitis (at the time of death).
  - Retinoblastoma.
  - Malignant tumors of the anterior ocular segment.
  - Known adenocarcinoma in the eye of primary or metastatic origin.
- Snake bites specific for neurotoxins

Conditions that will affect graft outcome

- *NOT suitable for PKP or ALK:*
  - Superficial disorders of the conjunctiva or corneal surface involving the central optical area of the corneal button
  - Prior surgery, local eye disease, disorder, or pathology which compromises the corneal stroma
- *NOT suitable for PKP or EK:*
  - Local eye disease, disorder, or pathology affecting the posterior stroma or corneal endothelium
  - Endothelial density below 2,000 cells per square millimeter
- *Therapeutic/tectonic tissue:* Tissue not suitable for optical use may be used for therapeutic or tectonic use.
- *Sclera tissue for transplantation:* Medical exclusionary criteria are the same, except that tissue with local eye disease, disorder, or pathology affecting only the cornea (listed above) is acceptable for use.

- *Behavioral/history, laboratory and medical exclusion criteria:*
  - HIV or high risk for HIV corneas from persons meeting any of the following criteria should not be offered for transplantation:
    - Men who have had sex with other men in the preceding 5 years (homosexual behavior).
    - Persons who report nonmedical intravenous, intramuscular, or subcutaneous injection of drugs in the preceding 5 years (IV drug abuse).
    - Persons with hemophilia or related clotting disorders who have received human-derived clotting factor concentrate.
    - Men and women who have engaged in sex for money or drugs in the preceding 5 years (commercial sex workers).
    - Persons who have had sex in the preceding 12 months with any person or with a person known or suspected to have HIV infection.
    - Persons who have been exposed in the preceding 12 months to known or suspected HIV-infected blood through percutaneous inoculation or through contact with an open wound, or mucous membrane.

Interval between Death, Enucleation, Excision, and Preservation

- If ambient temperature is hot (e.g., summer weather), then eyes must be preserved or refrigerated within 6 hours of death.
- If ambient temperature is not hot (e.g., winter weather), then eyes must be preserved or cooled within 8 hours of death.
- If ocular area including eyes, or the entire body, or enucleated eyes are continuously cooled within the above constraints of 6 or 8 hours, respectively, then tissue can be preserved up to 12 hours from time of death.

Recovery Procedures

- Retrieval procedure could be either enucleation of the whole globe or corneoscleral rim excision.
- The retrieval procedures should be documented in detail.
- All eye bank technicians should take universal precautions during the retrieval process.
- Donor's personal and medical history or medical records if available should be collected.
- A detailed gross physical examination to rule out possible contraindications should be carried out.

Tissue Processing

Processing must be performed in:
- A laminar air flow hood which meets ISO Class 5 standards,
- An accredited operating room, or
- Another environment documented annually to have <25 colony-forming units per 90 mm settle plate per 1-hour exposure.

Gross Examination

The corneal-scleral segment shall be initially examined grossly for clarity, epithelial defects, foreign objects and contamination, and scleral color, e.g., jaundice.

Slit-lamp Examination

The cornea shall be examined for epithelial and stromal pathology and in particular endothelial disease and documented on the donor records.

Specular Examination

Determination of endothelial cell density via specular microscopy shall be a standard method of corneal tissue evaluation for all eye banks.

Storage of Tissue

- All surgical tissue shall be stored in quarantine until results of HIV, HbsAg, HCV, syphilis and any other relevant donor screening tests have been recorded as nonreactive.
- All tissue shall be stored aseptically at a temperature appropriate to the method of preservation used.
- Eye bank shall use approved corneal storage medium (such as MK, Optisol GS, EUSOL, etc.) from a reliable source.

Packaging

The eye bank shall use a packaging method that will maintain a cool temperature while in transit, i.e., packaged with wet ice/gel packs.

Transport

Transport procedures shall take account of the factors such as time in transit, temperature conditions, and tracking of the shipment from distributing eye bank to the consignee.

Distribution

- Eye banks shall establish and document a system of eye tissue distribution that is applicable to their service area.
- Distribution of donor tissue should follow the priority norms as per the cornea distribution algorithm prescribed by National Organ and Tissue Transplant Organization (NOTTO) **(Table 17)**.
- Tissue for transplantation shall only be distributed to registered ophthalmologist/institutes and to other eye banks.
- The eye bank shall ensure anonymity of the donor to any individual or institution receiving tissue for surgical use.

Recipient Follow-up Information

The distributing eye bank shall request from the transplanting surgeon postoperative outcome and recipient follow-up information concerning possible adverse reactions on all eye tissue used for transplantation. This information shall include the following:
- Recipient's name
- Date of birth (or year of birth if a precise date of birth is unknown) or age
- Diagnosis, i.e., indication for transplant
- Name of surgeon receiving/transplanting tissue
- Date of surgery
- Location of surgery.

Adverse Reactions

- The eye bank shall establish a procedure for investigating, documenting, and reporting on all adverse reaction notifications.
- The Medical Director shall receive and review such reports on each adverse reaction and authorize a response to the transplanting surgeon.

Tissue Labelling

Each corneal or scleral tissue container shall be clearly and indelibly labeled to include at least the information here:
- Name of source eye bank
- Tissue identification number. There must be unique identification number for each ocular tissue or fraction there of that is distributed for surgical use.
- Type of tissue
- Date and time of donor's death
- Date and time of cornea/scleral preservation
- Preservation date for scleral tissue and long-term preserved tissue

TABLE 17: Cornea allocation criteria.[153]

Category	Eligibility
Emergency (E)	• Patients requiring emergency therapeutic keratoplasty • Pediatric keratoplasty for children <10 years
Top priority (TP)	• Bilaterally blind patients (BCVA ≤3/60 in better eye) • Patients with progressive corneal disease suitable for endothelial keratoplasty
Priority (P)	Bilateral corneal disease with better eye BCVA ≤6/60
General (G)	Patients >10 years of age with unilateral corneal blindness

- A statement that the tissue is intended for single patient application only and that it is not to be considered sterile and culturing or reculturing is recommended.
- Type of preservation medium.

Quality Assurance

- The eye bank shall have a formally established quality assurance program (hereafter called quality system) that defines and documents a series of systematic processes that shall to be followed by all those working in the organization.
- The eye bank shall define and document how the requirements for quality will be met.

Legislative Aspect

- Each eye bank unit should be registered under 1994 Transplantation of Human Organs Act/2014 THOTA Rules and also should undergo the accreditation appraisal.
- *The application form for getting registered is the form 15 in THOTA 2014 rules which also mentions the prescribed fee.*
- They should perform their activities as prescribed in the applicable law like 1994 Transplantation of Human Organs Act/2014 THOTA Rules until the registration is completed.
- Eye Retrieval Centres need not apply for a THOTA Registration.

Accreditation

- After registration the eye bank units should offer themselves for appraisal by an Accreditation Authority (AA) within 1 year.
- Accreditation will include evaluation of the following:
  - Demonstrate compliance with medical standards
  - Demonstrate compliance of all requirements during site inspection
  - Demonstrate proficiency in all aspects of eye banking, viz. procuring, processing, and distributing corneal tissue
- In cases of noncompliance a reasonable time period will be given to rectify deficiencies and satisfy accreditation requirements
- If the eye bank does not meet the standards within the deadline it may not receive accreditation as an eye bank and may be redesignated as an ERC.

Accreditation Authority

This shall be a body comprising nominees by Government of India, State Government, any other nominated by National Programme for Control of Blindness and Visual Impairment (NPCBVI) and Eye Bank Association of India (EBAI).

 12. Discuss: (1) Corneal preservation. (2) Disease screening and donor cornea preservation. (3a) Enumerate the various short-term and intermediate-term methods for corneal preservation. (3b) What are their main constituents? (3c) Advantages and disadvantages of these media. (4) Eye banking and corneal preservation techniques.

Donor Cornea Evaluation

- Gross examination
- Slit-lamp examination
- Specular microscopy.

Corneal Evaluation

Gross evaluation:
- In situ examination of cornea
- Torch-light examination
- Any epithelial defects, edema, any abnormal shape of cornea, corneal scars, discharge, and conjunctivitis
- Evidence of any intraocular surgery
- *Prerequisites:*
  - Slit-lamp evaluation—viewing chamber
  - Endothelial side up
  - Allow the cornea stored in media reach room temperature (but not >1 hour)

Epithelium

- Intact/not intact
- Haze—none/mild/mild-moderate/moderate-severe/severe
- Exposure keratitis—none/mild/mild-moderate/moderate-severe/severe
- Site—central/paracentral/peripheral/mid-peripheral/diffuse/band exposure
- Sloughing—absent/present (central/paracentral/peripheral/mid-peripheral/diffuse/band exposure)
- Debris—yes/no

Stroma

- Clear and compact—clear only/compact only/clear and compact/neither
- Edema—none/mild/mild-moderate/moderate/moderate-severe/severe
- Location—central/paracentral/peripheral/mid-peripheral/diffuse/band
- Arcus—none/mild/mild-moderate/moderate/moderate-severe/severe (diameter of clear zone)
- Opacity—surgical scar/LASIK/other/none
- Infiltrate—yes/no
- Stria—yes/no (relative number of stria)

Descemet Membrane

- Folds—none/mild/mild-moderate/moderate/moderate-severe/severe
- Relative number of fold—few/few-several/several/several-numerous/numerous
- Defects—none/Descemet tear/defect at IOL scar
- Grading of DM folds **(Fig. 14)**

Endothelium

- Stress lines—yes/no
- Location—central/paracentral/peripheral/mid-peripheral/diffuse/band
- Relative number of folds
- Defects—yes/no
- Cell dropout—few/few-several/several/several-numerous/numerous
- Location—central/paracentral/peripheral/mid-peripheral/diffuse/band
- Polymegathism—none/mild/mild-moderate/moderate/moderate-severe/severe
- Pleomorphism—none/mild/mild-moderate/moderate/moderate-severe/severe

Specular Microscopy

- Cell density (CD)—number of endothelial cells/sq mm
- Coefficient of variation of cell area (CV)
- Percentage of hexagonal cells

Cell Density

- *Excellent:* Cell density of >3,000 cells/mm^2
- *Very good:* Cell density of 2,500–3,000 cells/mm^2
- *Good:* Cell density of 2,000–2,500 cells/mm^2

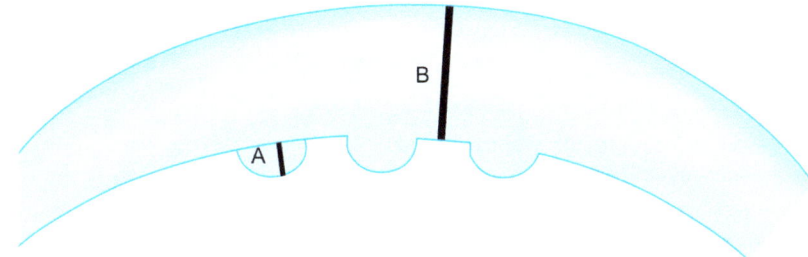

Fig. 14: Grading of DM folds. (A = height of fold above baseline; B = height of thickness of cornea, A/B x 100 = percentage, clear = no fold, trace = 0–10%, mild = 11–15%, moderate = 16–25%, and severe = >25%).

- *Fair:* Cell density of 1,500–2,000 cells/mm^2
- *Poor:* Cell density of 1,200–1,500 cells/mm^2

Coefficient of Variation of Cell Area (CV)
- *Normal range:* 0.20–0.30
- Higher the CV (wide variety in cell sizes) higher polymegathism
- Lower the CV more stable the cornea.

Percentage of Hexagonal Cells (6A)
- Represents the shape factor of cells (pleomorphism)
- Irregular cell shapes in traumatized endothelium
- 6A is calculated as number of hexagonal cells/number of cells entered
- Higher the 6A—more stable the cornea >50% hexagonality is desirable.

Grading of Donor Eyes

Grading has been summarized in **Table 18**.

Preservation

Criteria for the "Ideal" Corneal Preservation Method
- Maintains endothelial viability
- Maintains a clear, thin cornea during preservation
- Allows unlimited preservation time
- Provides cost-effectiveness
- Ensures sterility
- Allows transportation of donor tissue.

Types
- Short-term storage (24–96 hours)
- Intermediate storage (~2 weeks)
- Long-term storage (>1 month).

Short-term Storage Method
- *Moist chamber method:*
  - Whole globe in metal holder in a sealed chamber with gauze moistened by saline or antimicrobial solution.
  - Storage—24 hours, 4°C.
  - *Advantage:* Simple, inexpensive, easily transportable
  - *Disadvantage:* 25–30% decrease in endothelial viability due to accumulation of toxic metabolites in aqueous.
- *MK media (McCarey and Kaufman):*
  - Stores the corneoscleral button

TABLE 18: Grading of donor eyes.				
Grade	Descemet folds	Corneal thickness	Stromal haze	Specular count
Excellent (A+)	None	Nil	Nil	>3,000 cells/sqmm
Very good (A)	None	>10%	Nil	>3,000 cells/sqmm
Good (B+)	Peripheral Descemet fold or few paracentral/central folds that disappear completely on pressure	10–25%	Nil	>2,000–3,000 cells/sqmm
Fair (B)	Moderate peripheral Descemet fold/few central Descemet fold/that disappear partially on pressure	25–33%	Mild	>1,500–2,000 cells/sqmm
NSFS (B−)	Descemet folds reaching center which persists even with increase in pressure	33–50%	++	<1,500 cells/sqmm

- Storage time 23 days at 4°C
- *Composition:*
    - Tissue-culture *medium (TC 199)*
    - 5% dextran
    - Antibiotics—gentamicin, penicillin (100 µg/mL) polymyxin
    - HEPES as buffer
    - pH 7.4 and osmolarity 290 mOsm
- *Advantages:*
    - Protective effect on the endothelium compared to moist chamber.
    - Dextran—osmotic agent, keep the cornea in dehydrated stage.
- Modified MK medium:
    - *Composition:* Basic MK medium with steroid and reduced glutathione (0.92 g/L)
    - *Advantages:*
        - Steroids stabilize lysosome and reduce oxidative damage
        - Glutathione acts as antioxidant.

Intermediate Storage Media

- K-SOL:
    - Basic MK medium enriched with chondroitin sulfate
    - Storage time—10 days
    - *Composition:*
        - Base medium—TC-199
        - Chondroitin sulfate 2.5%
        - HEPES as buffer
        - Antibiotic—gentamicin (100 µg/mL)
    - *Disadvantage:* Increased osmotic flow causing cornea to swell
- DEXSOL:
    - *Composition:*
        - Base medium—MEM
        - Chondroitin sulfate *1.35%* (lower then K-Sol)
        - HEPES buffer
        - Dextran 1 %
        - Antibiotic—gentamicin
        - Sodium bicarbonate, sodium pyruvate—antioxidants, nonessential amino acid
- Chondroitin sulfate enriched optisol media:
    - Storage time—14 days at 2–6 °C
    - *Composition:*
        - Base medium-TC 199 and MEM (minimum essential medium)
        - Chondroitin sulfate (2.5%)—dextran 1%
        - HEPES buffer
        - Antibiotic—gentamicin (Optisol GS—Gentamycin and streptomycin)
        - Sodium bicarbonate, sodium pyruvate—antioxidants, nonessential amino acid—ascorbic acid, vitamin B_{12}, ATP
    - *Advantage:*
        - Chondroitin sulfate acts as an antioxidant and reduces endothelial cell loss by 6%.
        - Dextran—dehydrating effect
- CORNISOL:
    - Storage time—14 days at 2–8°C
    - *Composition:*
        - Chondroitin sulfate
        - Recombinant human insulin (enhances metabolism, conserve phospholipid)
        - Dextran
        - Stabilized L-glutamine
        - ATP precursors, vitamins, trace elements

- Gentamicin, streptomycin
- pH indicator
- *Advantages:*
  - Microscopic evaluation without transferring tissue to viewing chamber
  - Enhances endothelial and epithelial cell preservation—reduces corneal thickness and folds
  - pH color indicator helps in detection of unacceptable deviation in pH
- *EUSOL-C:*
  - Storage time—14 days at 2–6°C
  - *Composition:*
    - Dextran
    - Sodium pyruvate, glucose, amino acid, mineral salts, and vitamins
    - Gentamicin
    - HEPES bicarbonate
    - Phenol red (pH indicator)
  - *Advantages:*
    - pH indicator—rapid visualization of pH variations
    - Optically clear vial bottom allows to evaluate cornea.

Long-term Storage Method

- *Organ culture method:*
  - Cornea is incubated in tissue culture medium at 30–37°C
  - Storage time—5–7 weeks
  - Retains active metabolism
  - *Composition:*
    - Media–Eagle's MEM
    - Eagle's salt without L-glutamine
    - Decomplemented calf serum—1.5% chondroitin sulfate
  - *Disadvantage:* Risk of contamination
- *Cryopreservation:*
  - Corneoscleral rim passed through varying concentration of dimethyl sulfoxide 7.5%
  - Frozen up to –80°C and stored at –160°C
  - *Storage time-indefinite:*
    - *Disadvantages:*
      - Expensive instrument
      - Careful temperature monitoring
- *Glycerine:*
  - Colorless, odorless, and viscous fluid
  - Antibacterial, antifungal, and antiviral properties
  - *Composition:*
    - 100% glycerine
  - Storage up to 1 year at room temperature
  - Used for patch grafts, and lamellar keratoplasty
  - Endothelium is not viable.

13. A 76-year-old man underwent cataract surgery for Grade 4 nuclear sclerosis. There was incomplete recovery followed by diminution of vision 6 weeks after surgery. Discuss the causes for diminution of vision and management in brief.

Background[154]

- 8.5% of cataract surgeries in India have BCVA <6/60.
- Most common causes are ocular comorbidity (41.4%), operative complications (31.2%), long-term complications (18.7%), and refractive error (8.8%).

Cornea and Conjunctiva

History

- With background of advanced and Grade 4 nuclear sclerosis, poor gain of vision followed by further deterioration, following details must be sought:
    - Flashes, floaters, or field loss (vitreous hemorrhage, retinal detachment, and intermediate uveitis)
    - Metamorphopsia [epiretinal membrane, age-related macular degeneration (ARMD), and vitreomacular traction (VMT)]
    - Glare or seeing color halos (raised IOP and corneal edema)
    - Redness, pain, and fever (endophthalmitis—late onset or metastatic)
    - Trauma (IOL dislocation, retinal detachment, etc.)
    - Seeing edge of lens (IOL dislocation)
    - Details of cataract surgery (complicated-corneal decompensation, and retinal detachment)
    - *Past history:*
        - History suggestive of ocular comorbidities (early morning worsening of vision—Fuchs endothelial dystrophy, diabetes/RVOs/Uveitis—macular edema, pseudoexfoliative glaucoma—IOL dislocation, capsular phimosis)
        - History of glaucoma or retinal surgery
    - *Medication history:*
        - *Topical:*
            - PG analog—macular edema, dorzolamide—corneal decompensation, steroid-PCO, raised IOP
        - *Systemic:*
            - Niacin, rosiglitazone, fingolimod-macular edema.

Examination

- BCVA, IOP, and pupillary reflex
- Evaluate the fellow eye
- Slit-lamp biomicroscopy
- Indirect ophthalmoscopy/USG for posterior segment evaluation.

Differential

Following differentials can be considered:

Posterior capsular opacification:

- Sometimes associated with Elschnig's pearls, this is the most frequent late complication from cataract surgery.[155]
- Incidence varies from 14 to 60%[155]
- *Mechanism:* Proliferation and migration, or growth of residual lens epithelial cells left on the anterior capsule after cataract surgery.
- *Risk factors:* Myopes, diabetes, uveitis, previous vitrectomy and patients with greater amounts of posterior subcapsular or cortical cataracts.[155]
- *Treatment:*
    - Determine if the patient's best corrected vision has become problematic
    - YAG laser capsulotomy needed in up to 20% of patients.[155,156]
        - Retinal complication concerns such as lattice, holes, and weak spots should be addressed prior to proceeding with laser due to risk of retinal detachment.

Glaucoma:

- Often associated with corneal edema, if acute rise of IOP.
- *Mechanism:*[157]
    - *Distortion of anterior chamber:* Internal white ridge protruding into the anterior chamber as an inverted snowbank along the ridge of the corneal incision[158]
    - *Inflammation and hemorrhage:*[157]
        - *Uveitis Glaucoma Hyphema (UGH) syndrome:* Rubbing of the lens implant on the iris
        - *Swan syndrome:* Neovascularization of internal corneal wound
    - *Pigment dispersion:*[157] Single piece lens inappropriately placed in sulcus.
    - Vitreous filling the anterior chamber[157]

- Peripheral anterior synechiae and/or trabecular damage:[157] Excessive inflammation postsurgery
- *Neodymium:* YAG laser posterior capsulotomy:[157]
    - Unknown mechanism
- Lens particle glaucoma[157]
■ *Risk factors:*[157] Preexisting glaucoma and steroid response
■ *Treatment:*[157]
- Medical (topical/oral) and/or surgical management (trabeculectomy) depending on etiology and response.
- Diode cyclophotocoagulation may be spared for those with advanced disease with poor vision.

Corneal decompensation:
■ Present with gradual worsening of their vision, particularly in the morning[159]
■ Look for corneal edema (epithelial, stromal, and endothelial), endothelial folds/microcysts/bullae, stromal haze/scar, corneal neovascularization, and increased corneal thickness
■ Examine other eye for central/confluent guttae (Fuchs), endothelial vascular changes (PPCD), iris changes, and endothelial hammered silver/beaten bronze appearance (ICE syndrome)
■ *Risk factors:*[159]
- Short axial length, shallow anterior chamber, and longer phacoemulsification time
- Preexisting endothelial dysfunction
- Advanced age
- Insertion of anterior chamber intraocular lens (ACIOL)
- Pre-existing glaucoma, presence of glaucoma drainage devices
- Systemic conditions (diabetes and chronic obstructive pulmonary disease)
■ *Mechanism:*[159]
- The endothelial cells continuously pumping fluid out of the corneal stroma.
- Damage to the endothelial cells will adversely affect corneal transparency when aqueous entering the cornea outweighs the pumping capacity of the remaining viable endothelial cells.
- At least, 700 cells/mm^2 are needed to maintain corneal transparency.
■ *Treatment:*
- *Medical therapy:*
    - Hypertonic saline drops and ointment (sodium chloride 5%) are the first-line treatment.
        - These drops create a hypertonic tear film, drawing water out of the cornea.
    - Ruptured epithelial bullae should be with antibiotic and lubricating drops, and use of BCL for symptomatic relief.
- *Surgery:*
    - Corneal transplantation is the definitive treatment.
    - It can be done in the form of PK, DMEK, or DSAEK.[4,5]
    - Other surgical options for symptomatic relief:[160,161]
        - *CXL with riboflavin and ultraviolet A:* Induce stromal compaction with thinning and less water influx into the cornea and consequently less fluid in the subepithelial space (bullae formation).[6]
        - *Amniotic membrane transplant (AMT):* Contains various growth factors and protease inhibitors which promote epithelial cells migration and adhesion to the underlying basement membrane.[7]
        - *Anterior stromal puncture (ASP):*
            1. Increases the formation of various extracellular matrix proteins that increase the adhesion of the epithelial cells to the underlying stroma.
            2. It also induces subepithelial fibrosis which acts as physical barrier limiting fluid migration to the subepithelial space.
        - *Phototherapeutic keratectomy (PTK):*
            1. Decreases pain perception by ablations the subepithelial nerve plexus.
            2. It also strengthens the adhesions between the epithelial cells and underlying stroma.

Pseudophakic cystoid macular edema (Irvine-Gass Syndrome):
■ Occurs following 2% of uncomplicated procedures.[162,163]
■ Presents with blurry vision, central scotoma, metamorphopsia, and mild photophobia.
■ On slit-lamp biomicroscopy—retinal thickening and loss of the foveolar depression, cystic changes (appreciable on red-free).

- FF shows retinal telangiectasis, capillary dilatation, and leakage from perifoveal capillaries in the early phase frames, and perifoveal hyperfluorescent spots classically described as a "petaloid" pattern in late phase frames (cystic spaces).
- Optical coherence tomography (OCT) shows loss of the foveal depression, retinal thickening, and cystic hyporeflective areas within the macula.
- Optical coherence tomography angiography (OCTA) shows disruption of parafoveal capillary arcade and cystoid spaces in the deep capillary plexus.
- *Mechanism:*
  - Inflammatory mediators are upregulated in the aqueous and vitreous humors after surgical manipulation.
  - Inflammation breaks down the blood aqueous and blood retinal barrier, which leads to increased vascular permeability.[162]
  - Transudate accumulates in the outer plexiform and inner nuclear layers to create cystic spaces that coalesce to form larger pockets of fluid.[163]
- *Risk factors:*
  - Complicated cataract surgery (vitreous loss, vitreous wick, iris trauma, posterior capsular rupture, and iris-fixated/anterior chamber IOL)
  - Diabetic macular edema
  - Uveitis
  - Antiglaucoma medication (PG analogs, timolol)
- *Treatment:*
  - *NSAIDs (cyclooxygenase 2-inhibition):*[164]
    - FDA approved for postoperative inflammation, although not for cystoid macular edema (CME)—Ketorolac 0.4%, diclofenac 0.1%, bromfenac 0.09%, and nepafenac 0.1%.
  - *Corticosteroids (phospholipase A2 inhibition):*[165-171]
    - Topical often given in combination with NSAIDs
    - *Periocular if refractory to topical treatment:* Refractory (to topical and periocular corticosteroids) pseudophakic CME, can be treated with 4 mg of intravitreal triamcinolone or drug delivery system (Ozurdex, Yutiq, etc.)
    - Others with limited evidence (anti-VEGF, carbonic anhydrase inhibitor and other immunomodulators, e.g., subcutaneous interferon-alpha and intravitreal infliximab)
    - Neodymium: YAG laser anterior vitreolysis to release vitreous incarceration.
    - PPV may be considered for vitreoretinal traction, and/or if the CME is unresponsive to other treatments (to reduce concentration of inflammatory mediators and growth factors).

Retinal detachment:
- *Often caused by small, pinpoint retinal holes at the vitreous base* and may be difficult to detect.
  - Majority being found in the superotemporal quadrant
- *Risk factors:*
  - *Younger age (under 60 years):* An almost 6 times higher risk
  - *Myopia with axial length greater than or equal to 25 mm:* Six-fold increase in the incidence of pseudophakic RDs in individuals with axial length greater than or equal to 25 mm.
  - History of RD in the fellow eye
  - *Unplanned disruption of the posterior capsule:* A five-fold rise in pseudophakic RDs has been reported in cases complicated by the posterior capsular tear.[173]
  - There is conflicting evidence regarding the association between YAG (yttrium-aluminum-garnet) laser capsulotomy, and pseudophakic RDs.[174]
  - Operated eye stands a five times higher risk of developing retinal detachment following surgery compared to the nonoperated eye.[175-177]
    - If within 6 months after surgery, about 90% of that risk can be attributed to the surgery.
    - Once 2–5 years pass, this risk stabilizes at about 70%, but after 5 years, you still have an attributable risk that is significantly above 50%.
- *Mechanism:*
  - The exact mechanism of retinal break formation in pseudophakic RDs remains unclear.
  - *Theories:*
    - Development of posterior vitreous detachment (PVD) or rapid progression of preexisting PVD.

- Loss of dampening effect of the posterior protuberance of the crystalline lens, forward movement of the vitreous body, and traction on the peripheral retina after vitreous incarceration in the wound likely modify kinetics of the vitreous base.[172]
- Changes in the biochemical microenvironment of the vitreous and retina in pseudophakic eyes are known to occur as a result of lens cortical fibers leaking into the vitreous during cataract surgery.
- Retinal break formation following laser capsulotomy could be due to rupture of the anterior vitreous face or acoustic trauma to the vitreous body by waves, which alters the dynamics of the vitreous body, with resultant retinal tear formation.[172]

- *Treatment:*
  - *Pneumatic retinopexy:*
    - Ideal cases for pneumatic retinopexy include phakic eyes with a superiorly located single tear not exceeding 1 clock hour; or multiple superior retinal breaks dispersed within 1 clock hour; absence of advanced grade (C and D) proliferative vitreoretinopathy (PVR); absence of lattice degeneration in other areas; and absence of uncontrolled glaucoma.
    - Anatomical success rate of pneumatic retinopexy in pseudophakic RDs is at least 60%.[178-180]
  - *Scleral buckling and vitrectomy:*
    - Anatomical success rates is 81% following SB, 91% after PPV, and 97% for the combined technique of PPV with SB after a single surgery.[181,182]
    - *PPV advantages:*
      - Removing posterior capsular opacity
      - Clearing vitreous debris
      - Detecting unseen breaks
      - Releasing vitreous traction
      - Removing gliogenic cells
    - *Limitations:*
      - Inadequate endotamponade to inferior breaks in the absence of an FDA-approved heavy tamponade
      - Difficulties in postoperative positioning
      - Moisture globules forming on the posterior surface of the IOL during air–fluid exchange, may significantly limit visibility of the retina

Endophthalmitis:
- In India, incidence of clinical acute post-cataract endophthalmitis was from 0.04 to 0.15%.[183-189]
- *Risk factors:*
  - *Preoperative:*
    - Immune compromise/HIV, diabetes mellitus
    - Chronic blepharitis
    - Infection of the lacrimal drainage system
    - Contaminated eye drops
    - Contact lens wear
    - Contralateral ocular prosthesis
  - *Intraoperative:*
    - Prolonged surgery
    - Secondary IOL
    - Posterior capsular rupture, vitreous loss
    - Contaminated irrigating solution
    - Clear corneal incision
    - Concurrent nasolacrimal duct surgery
  - *Postoperative:*
    - Wound leak
    - Vitreous incarceration
- *Treatment:*
  - Seidel test for potential wound leak
  - *Obtain intraocular specimen:*
    - 30-gauge needle for AC-tap (optional)

- 25- or 23-gauge needle for vitreous tap
- Small gauge PPV
- *Intravitreal injection:*
  - Vancomycin 1 mg/0.1 cc (for coverage of gram-positive organisms)
  - Ceftazidime 2.25 mg/0.1 cc or Amikacin 0.4 mg/0.1 cc (for gram-negative organisms)
  - Dexamethasone 0.4 mg/0.1
- *Endophthalmitis vitrectomy study (EVS):*[190] EVS endophthalmitis patients after ECCE, scleral tunnel phacoemulsification, or secondary IOL.
- *EVS primary results:*
  - Patients with light perception LP vision fare better with initial PPV.
  - When patients presented with hand motion (HM) or better vision, equal visual acuity outcomes were achieved in the vitrectomy and vitreous tap groups.
  - There was no apparent benefit from the use of EVS systemic antibiotics (amikacin and ceftazidime) compared to controls (no IV antibiotics).
- *EVS secondary results:* Patients with diabetes mellitus and vision better than LP achieved better visual outcomes with initial vitrectomy surgery (not statistically significant).
- *Prophylaxis with intracameral antibiotic:*
  - *Vancomycin:* Caution with hemorrhagic occlusive retinal vasculitis[191]
  - *Cefuroxime: ESCRS Endophthalmitis Study*—nearly 5-fold decrease in incidence of postoperative endophthalmitis[192]
  - Moxifloxacin (routine intracameral moxifloxacin prophylaxis reduced the overall endophthalmitis rate by 3.5-fold:[193] Not FDA approved- caution TASS[194]

Refractive surprise:
- 96% achieve within 1.00 D of target outcome.[195-198]
- *Causes of poor refractive outcome include:*
  - *Inaccurate axial length measurement:*
    - Poor fixation
    - Oil-filled eye
    - Staphyloma
  - *Inaccurate keratometry readings:*
    - Dry eye
    - Corneal dystrophy and degenerations
    - Contact lens related corneal warpage
    - Prior refractive surgery
  - Wrong IOL selection
  - Transcription errors
- *Primary prevention:*
  - *Accurate preoperative measurements:*
    - *Normal Ks 41–47:* Intereye difference <0.9D
    - *Axial length:* Intereye difference <0.7 mm
  - Appropriate IOL formula
- *Diagnosis:*
  - Subjective refraction
  - Dilated examination
  - Recheck history and surgical records
  - Repeat biometry, keratometry, and macular OCT
  - Error in effective lens position if none of the above
- *Treatment:*
  - Patients who are asymptomatic and satisfied with visual outcomes after surgery may simply be observed.
  - If patients are amenable to wearing glasses, spectacle correction should be the first option.
  - Contact lenses may be preferable in cases of anisometropia, high astigmatism, or in patients accustomed to wearing contact lenses.
  - *Surgical options:*
    - *Keratorefractive surgery:* Error <2D, no corneal pathology, no glare/halos/contrast sensitivity

- *IOL exchange:* Error >2D, known source of error, visual phenomenon in premium IOLs
- *IOL rotation:*
  - Cylindrical error due to improper placement of toric IOL
  - <1-2 month from initial surgery
- *Piggyback IOL:* Hyperopic surprise, zonulopathy, or posterior capsular tear

Decentered IOL:
- Subluxated IOLs involve such extreme decentration that the IOL optic covers only a small fraction of the pupillary space.
- Luxation involves total dislocation of the IOL into the posterior segment.
- Patients may complain of decreased vision, edge glare, diplopia, streaks of light, haloes, photosensitivity, and ghost images.
- Risk factors:
  - Posterior capsular rupture
  - *Zonular weakness:*
    - Pseudoexfoliation syndrome and trauma
    - Prior vitreoretinal surgery
    - Connective tissue disorders.
  - Improper fixation within the capsular bag and instability of the IOL–capsular bag complex
  - *Capsular contraction syndrome:*
    - Small capsulorhexis
    - Silicone-plate IOL
  - *Capsular fusion:* An eccentric capsulorhexis may allow one of its edges to be more peripheral than the optic in one area, with fusion developing, producing decentration away from the area of contact.

ACIOL decentration:
- In patients with ACIOL decentration, slit-lamp examination and gonioscopy may reveal iris tuck, which can cause uveal inflammation.
- The eye may be red and tender.
- A peaked or oval pupil can be found.
- Inappropriate ACIOL size may cause a mobile lens.
- ACIOL malposition may produce ongoing mechanical trauma to the cornea, iris, ciliary body, or anterior chamber angle.
- Chronic inflammation may lead to corneal endothelial cell loss, CME, glaucoma, microhyphema, and pain.

Posterior chamber intraocular lens (PCIOL) decentration:
- Visual acuity can be compromised by optical aberrations and refractive changes. Slit-lamp examination usually does not reveal evidence of inflammation unless contact of a portion of the IOL with the cornea or vitreous prolapse is present.
- Corneal edema from IOL or vitreous touch can be found. In these cases, CME may be a complication.
- Vitreous traction can increase the risk of a retinal detachment, while vitreous to the wound can be implicated in endophthalmitis.

IOL dislocation:
- The posterior capsule usually has an obvious defect.
- Zonular dialysis may be present.
- The IOL may be freely mobile in the vitreous cavity; it may be in apparent contact with the retina; or it may have one haptic attached to the posterior capsule, iris, or ciliary body.
- *Complications:* Rhegmatogenous retinal detachment, glaucoma, cystoid macular edema, bullous keratopathy, and uveitis
- *Treatment:*
  - *Observation:* In the absence of symptoms and no evidence of inflammatory sequelae
  - *Miotics:* If symptoms from a decentered PCIOL are infrequent and limited to evening, due to a dilated pupil, these patients may be treated conservatively by using a topical miotic such as pilocarpine 0.5–1% qhs.
  - *IOL reposition:* An IOL may become decentered due to either insufficient zonular support or to irregular fibrosis of the posterior capsule. In the case of inadequate support, early in the postoperative period the surgeon may attempt to rotate the IOL surgically where there is clinical evidence of sufficient capsule and zonules to support the implant. A helpful maneuver is the bounce test where the optic is pushed gently toward each haptic to ensure spontaneous

recentration. In some cases, repositioning may be supplemented by the use of transiris IOL fixation (McCannel) suture.
- *IOL explantation:* Certain circumstances warrant removal of an IOL without secondary IOL implantation. This is determined on an individual basis and taking into account the patient's expectation.
- *IOL exchange:* The most common indications for removal or exchange of a modern posterior chamber lens (PCL) are wrong IOL power and malposition. Deformation of the implant due to irregular capsular fibrosis may make simple rotation insufficient to properly center of the IOL. The IOL may be exchanged for an ACIOL, a sulcus-fixated IOL with or without McCannel sutures, a trans-sclerally sutured PCIOL, or a posterior iris-claw IOL.

References

1. Hjortdal J, Pedersen IB, Bak-nielsen S, Ivarsen A. Graft rejection and graft failure after penetrating keratoplasty or posterior lamellar keratoplasty for Fuchs endothelial dystrophy. Cornea. 2013;32(5):e60-3.
2. Bartels MC, Doxiadis II, Colen TP, Beekhuis WH. Long-term outcome in high-risk corneal transplantation and the influence of HLA-A and HLA-B matching. Cornea. 2003;22(6):552-6.
3. Griffith TS, Brunner T, Fletcher SM, Green DR, Ferguson TA. Fas ligand-induced apoptosis as a mechanism of immune privilege. Science. 1995;270:1189-92.
4. Streilein JW, Okamoto S, Sano Y, Taylor AW. Neural control of ocular immune privilege. Ann NY Acad Sci. 2000;917:297-306.
5. Illigens BM, Yamada A, Fedoseyeva EV, Anosova N, Boisgerault F, Valujskikh A, et al. The relative contribution of direct and indirect antigen recognition pathways to the alloresponse and graft rejection depends upon the nature of the transplant. Hum Immunol. 2002;63:912-25.
6. Liu Y, Hamrah P, Zhang Q, Taylor AW, Dana MR. Draining lymph nodes of corneal transplant hosts exhibit evidence for donor major histocompatibility complex (MHC) class II-positive dendritic cells derived from MHC class II-negative grafts. J Exp Med. 2002; 195:259-68.
7. He YG, Niederkorn JY. Depletion of donor-derived Langerhans cells promotes corneal allograft survival. Cornea. 1996;15:82-9.
8. Huq S, Liu Y, Benichou G, Dana MR. Relevance of the direct pathway of sensitization in corneal transplantation is dictated by the graft bed microenvironment. J Immunol. 2004;173:4464-9.
9. Ardjomand N, McAlister JC, Rogers NJ, Tan PH, George AJ, Larkin DF. Modulation of costimulation by CD28 and CD154 alters the kinetics and cellular characteristics of corneal allograft reject ion. Invest Ophthalmol Vis Sci. 2003;44:3899-905.
10. Li XY, D'Orazio LT, Niederkorn JY. Role of Th1 and Th2 cells in anterior chamber-associated immune deviation. Immunology. 1996;89:34-40.
11. Krachmer J, Mannis M, Holland E. Cornea, 2nd edition. Elsevier Mosby; 2005. pp. 1284-314.
12. Guilbert E, Bullet J, Sandali O, Basli E, Laroche L, Borderie VM. Long-term rejection incidence and reversibility after penetrating and lamellar keratoplasty. Am J Ophthalmol. 2013;155(3):560-69.e2.
13. Price MO, Jordan CS, Moore G, Price Jr FW. Graft rejection episodes after Descemet stripping with endothelial keratoplasty: part two: the statistical analysis of probability and risk factors. Br J Ophthalmol. 2009;93:391-5.
14. Panda A, Vanathi M, Kumar A, Dash Y, Priya S. Corneal graft rejection. Surv Ophthalmol. 2007;52:375-96.
15. Reinhart WJ, Musch DC, Jacobs DS, Lee WB, Kaufman SC, Shtein RM. Deep anterior lamellar keratoplasty as an alternative to penetrating keratoplasty a report by the American Academy of Ophthalmology. Ophthalmology. 2011;118:209-18.
16. Lee WB, Jacobs DS, Musch DC, Kaufman SC, Reinhart WJ, Shtein RM. Descemet's stripping endothelial keratoplasty: safety and outcomes: a report by the American Academy of Ophthalmology. Ophthalmology. 2009;116:1818-30.
17. Deng SX, Lee WB, Hammersmith KM, Kuo AN, Li JY, Shen JF, et al. Descemet membrane endothelial keratoplasty—safety and outcomes: a report by the American Academy of Ophthalmology. Ophthalmology. 2018;125:295-310.
18. Jabbehdari S, Rafii AB, Yazdanpanah G, Hamrah P, Holland EJ, Djalilian AR. Update on the management of high-risk penetrating keratoplasty. Curr Ophthalmol Reports. 2017;5(1):38-48.
19. Gerstenblith AT, Rabinowitz MP. The Wills Eye Manual, Office and Emergency Room Diagnosis and Treatment of Eye Disease. Lippincott Williams & Wilkins; 2012.
20. Reidy JJ, Gebhardt BM, Kaufman HE. The collagen shield: a new vehicle for delivery of cyclosporin A to the eye. Cornea. 1990;9(3):196-9.
21. Bhatti N, Qidwai U, Hussain M, Kazi A. Efficacy of topical bevacizumab in high-risk corneal transplant survival. Pak J Med Sci. 2013;29(2):519-22.
22. Pleyer U, Yang J, Knapp S. Effects of a selective glucocorticoid receptor agonist on experimental keratoplasty. Graefe's Arch Clin Exp Ophthalmol. 2005;243:450-55.
23. Tang XL, Sun JF, Wang XY, Du LL, Liu P. Blocking neuropilin-2 enhances corneal allograft survival by selectively inhibiting lymphangiogenesis on vascularized beds. Mol Vis. 2010;16:2354-61.
24. Cho YK, Uehara H, Young JR, Tyagi P, Kompella UB, Zhang X, et al. Flt23k nanoparticles offer additive benefit in graft survival and anti-angiogenic effects when combined with triamcinolone. Invest Ophthalmol Vis Sci. 2012;53(4):2328-36.
25. Cho YK, Zhang X, Uehara H, Young JR, Archer B, Ambati B. Vascular endothelial growth factor receptor 1 morpholino increases graft survival in a murine penetrating keratoplasty model. Invest Ophthalmol Vis Sci. 2012;53(13):8458-71.

26. Comer RM, King WJ, Ardjomand N, Theoharis S, George AJ, Larkin DF. Effect of administration of CTLA4-Ig as protein or cDNA on corneal allograft survival. Invest Ophthalmol Vis Sci. 2002;43(4):1095-103.
27. Gong N, Pleyer U, Yang J, Vogt K, Hill M, Anegon I, et al. Influence of local and systemic *CTLA4Ig* gene transfer on corneal allograft survival. Gene Med. 2006;8(4):459-67.
28. König Merediz SA, Zhang EP, Wittig B, Hoffmann F. Ballistic transfer of minimalistic immunologically defined expression constructs for IL4 and CTLA4 into the corneal epithelium in mice after orthotopic corneal allograft transplantation. Graefes Arch Clin Exp Ophthalmol. 2000;238(8):701-7.
29. Gong N, Pleyer U, Volk HD, Ritter T. Effects of local and systemic viral interleukin-10 gene transfer on corneal allograft survival. Gene Ther. 2007;14(6):484-90.
30. Rayner SA, Larkin DF, George AJ. TNF receptor secretion after ex vivo adenoviral gene transfer to cornea and effect on in vivo graft survival. Invest Ophthalmol Vis Sci. 2001;42(7):1568-73.
31. Beutelspacher SC, Pillai R, Watson MP, Tan PH, Tsang J, McClure MO. Function of indoleamine 2,3-dioxygenase in corneal allograft rejection and prolongation of allograft survival by over-expression. Eur J Immunol. 2006;36(3):690-700.
32. Yuan XB, Yuan YB, Jiang W, Liu J, Tian EJ, Shun HM, et al. Preparation of rapamycin-loaded chitosan/PLA nanoparticles for immunosuppression in corneal transplantation. Int J Pharm. 2008;349(1-2):241-8.
33. Fuchsluger TA, Jurkunas U, Kazlauskas A, Dana R. Anti-apoptotic gene therapy prolongs survival of corneal endothelial cells during storage. Gene Ther. 2011;18(8):778-87.
34. Nosov M, Wilk M, Morcos M, Cregg M, O'Flynn L, Treacy O, et al. Role of lentivirus-mediated overexpression of programmed death-ligand 1 on corneal allograft survival. Am J Transplant. 2012;12(5):1313-22.
35. Hu J, Kovtun A, Tomaszewski A, Singer BB, Seitz B, Epple M, et al. A new tool for the transfection of corneal endothelial cells: calcium phosphate nanoparticles. Acta Biomater. 2012;8(3):1156-63.
36. Ippoliti G, Fronterre A. Usefulness of CD3 or CD6 anti-T monoclonal antibodies in the treatment of acute corneal graft rejection. Transplant Proc. 1989;21:3133-4.
37. Newman DK, Isaacs JD, Watson PG, Meyer PA, Hale G, Waldmann H. Prevention of immune-mediated corneal graft destruction with the anti-lymphocyte monoclonal antibody, CAMPATH-1H. Eye. 1995;9:564-9.
38. Schmitz K, Hitzer S, Behrens-Baumann W. Immune suppression by combination therapy with basiliximab and cyclosporin in high risk keratoplasty. A pilot study. Ophthalmology. 2002;99:38-45.
39. van Dijk K, Parker J, Tong CM, Ham L, Lie JT, Groeneveld-van Beek EA, et al. Midstromal isolated bowman layer graft for reduction of advanced keratoconus: a technique to postpone penetrating or deep anterior lamellar keratoplasty. JAMA Ophthalmol. 2014;132:495-501.
40. Ganger A, Tandon R, Vanathi M, Sagar P. Superficial anterior lamellar keratoplasty (SALK) for trauma-induced post refractive surgery corneal opacity. J Ophthalmic Vis Res. 2016;11:326-8.
41. Yoo SH, Kymionis GD, Koreishi A, Ide T, Goldman D, Karp CL, et al. Femtosecond laser-assisted sutureless anterior lamellar keratoplasty. Ophthalmology. 2008;115:1303-7.
42. AlTaan SL, Mohammed I, Said DG, Dua HS. Air pressure changes in the creation and bursting of the type-1 big bubble in deep anterior lamellar keratoplasty: an *ex vivo* study. Eye. 2018;32:146-51.
43. Zaki AA, Elalfy MS, Said DG, Dua HS. Deep anterior lamellar keratoplasty-triple procedure: a useful clinical application of the pre-Descemet's layer (Dua's layer). Eye. 2015;29:323-6.
44. Dua HS, Faraj LA, Kenawy MB, AlTaan S, Elalfy MS, Katamish T, et al. Dynamics of big bubble formation in deep anterior lamellar keratoplasty by the big bubble technique: *in vitro* studies. Acta Ophthalmol. 2018;96:69-76.
45. Goweida MB. Intraoperative review of different bubble types formed during pneumodissection (big-bubble) deep anterior lamellar keratoplasty. Cornea. 2015;34:621-4.
46. Buzzonetti L, Laborante A, Petrocelli G. Standardized big-bubble technique in deep anterior lamellar keratoplasty assisted by the femtosecond laser. J Cataract Refract Surg. 2010;36:1631-6.
47. Buzzonetti L, Petrocelli G, Valente P. Femtosecond laser and big-bubble deep anterior lamellar keratoplasty: a new chance. J Ophthalmol. 2012;2012:264590.
48. Farid M, Steinert RF. Deep anterior lamellar keratoplasty performed with the femtosecond laser zigzag incision for the treatment of stromal corneal pathology and ectatic disease. J Cataract Refract Surg. 2009;35:809-13.
49. Shetty R, Nagaraja H, Veluri H, Shivanna Y, Kugar T, Nujits R, et al. Sutureless femtosecond anterior lamellar keratoplasty: a 1-year follow-up study. Indian J Ophthalmol. 2014;62:923-6.
50. Leccisotti A. Descemet's membrane perforation during deep anterior lamellar keratoplasty: prognosis. J Cataract Refract Surg. 2007;33:825-9.
51. Singh NP, Said DG, Dua HS. Lamellar keratoplasty techniques. Indian J Ophthalmol. 2018;66:1239-50.
52. Terry MA, Chen ES, Shamie N, Hoar KL, Friend DJ. Endothelial cell loss after Descemet's stripping endothelial keratoplasty in a large prospective series. Ophthalmology. 2008;115:488-96.
53. Ratanasit A, Gorovoy MS. Long-term results of Descemet stripping automated endothelial keratoplasty. Cornea. 2011;30:1414-8.
54. Sugar J, Montoya M, Dontchev M, Tanner JP, Beck R, Gal R, et al. Donor risk factors for graft failure in the cornea donor study. Cornea. 2009;28:981-5.

55. Terry MA, Ousley PJ. Small-incision deep lamellar endothelial keratoplasty (DLEK): six-month results in the first prospective clinical study. Cornea. 2005;24:59-65.
56. Ang M, Saroj L, Htoon HM, Kiew S, Mehta JS, Tan D, et al. Comparison of a donor insertion device to sheets glide in Descemet stripping endothelial keratoplasty: 3-year outcomes. Am J Ophthalmol. 2014;157:1163-9.e3.
57. Patel SV. Graft survival and endothelial outcomes in the new era of endothelial keratoplasty. Exp Eye Res. 2012;95:40-7.
58. Price MO, Calhoun P, Kollman C, Price Jr FW, Lass JH. Descemet stripping endothelial keratoplasty: ten-year endothelial cell loss compared with penetrating keratoplasty. Ophthalmology. 2016;123:1421-7.
59. Mearza AA, Qureshi MA, Rostron CK. Experience and 12-month results of Descemet-stripping endothelial keratoplasty (DSEK) with a small-incision technique. Cornea. 2007;26:279-83.
60. Tsubota K, Laing RA, Chiba K, Kenyon KR. Effects of air and irrigating solutions on the corneal endothelium. Cornea. 1988;7:115-21.
61. Eiferman RA, Wilkins EL. The effect of air on human corneal endothelium. Am J Ophthalmol. 1981;92:328-31.
62. Hesse M, Kuerten D, Walter P, Plange N, Johnen S, Fuest M, et al. The effect of air, SF_6 and C_3F_8 on immortalized human corneal endothelial cells. Acta Ophthalmol. 2017;95:e284-90.
63. Hong A, Caldwell MC, Kuo AN, Afshari NA. Air bubble-associated endothelial trauma in Descemet stripping automated endothelial keratoplasty. Am J Ophthalmol. 2009;148:256-9.
64. Lee WB, Jacobs DS, Musch DC, Kaufman SC, Reinhart WJ, Shtein RM, et al. Descemet's stripping endothelial keratoplasty: safety and outcomes: s report by the American Academy of Ophthalmology. Ophthalmology. 2009;116:1818-30.
65. Suh LH, Yoo SH, Deobhakta A, Donaldson KE, Alfonso EC, Culbertson WW, et al. Complications of Descemet's stripping with automated endothelial keratoplasty: survey of 118 eyes at one institute. Ophthalmology. 2008;115:1517-24.
66. Fajgenbaum MA, Hollick EJ. Modeling endothelial cell loss after Descemet stripping endothelial keratoplasty: data from 5 years of follow-up. Cornea. 2017;36:553-60.
67. Patel CR, Ritterband DC, Knoll F, Wu E, Seedor JA, Koplin RS. Long-term graft survival rates in Descemet's stripping endothelial keratoplasty. Invest Ophthalmol Vis Sci. 2012;53:48.
68. Bahar I, Kaiserman I, McAllum P, Slomovic A, Rootman D. Comparison of posterior lamellar keratoplasty techniques to penetrating keratoplasty. Ophthalmology. 2008;115:1525-33.
69. Jun B, Kuo AN, Afshari NA, Carlson AN, Kim T. Refractive change after Descemet stripping automated endothelial keratoplasty surgery and its correlation with graft thickness and diameter. Cornea. 2009;28:19-23.
70. Terry MA, Shamie N, Chen ES, Phillips PM, Shah AK, Hoar KL, et al. Endothelial keratoplasty for Fuchs' dystrophy with cataract: complications and clinical results with the new triple procedure. Ophthalmology. 2009;116:631-9.
71. Tomida D, Yamaguchi T, Ogawa A, Hirayama Y, Shimazaki-Den S, Satake Y, et al. Effects of corneal irregular astigmatism on visual acuity after conventional and femtosecond laser-assisted Descemet's stripping automated endothelial keratoplasty. Jpn J Ophthalmol. 2015;59:216-22.
72. Yamaguchi T, Ohnuma K, Tomida D, Konomi K, Satake Y, Negishi K, et al. The contribution of the posterior surface to the corneal aberrations in eyes after keratoplasty. Invest Ophthalmol Vis Sci. 2011;52:6222-9.
73. Rossi M, Mistò R, Gatto C, Garimoldi P, Campanelli M, D'Amato Tóthová J, et al. Protective effects of deswelling on stromal collagen denaturation after a corneal femtosecond laser cut. Invest Ophthalmol Vis Sci. 2013;54:4148-57.
74. Busin M, Madi S, Santorum P, Scorcia V, Beltz J. Ultrathin Descemet's stripping automated endothelial keratoplasty with the microkeratome double-pass technique: two-year outcomes. Ophthalmology. 2013;120:1186-94.
75. Busin M, Albé E. Does thickness matter: ultrathin Descemet stripping automated endothelial keratoplasty. Curr Opin Ophthalmol. 2014;25:312-8.
76. Dickman MM, Kruit PJ, Remeijer L, van Rooij J, Van der Lelij A, Wijdh RH, et al. A randomized multicenter clinical trial of ultrathin Descemet stripping automated endothelial keratoplasty (DSAEK) versus DSAEK. Ophthalmology. 2016;123:2276-84.
77. Melles GR. Posterior lamellar keratoplasty: DLEK to DSEK to DMEK. Cornea. 2006;25:879-81.
78. Letko E, Price DA, Lindoso EM, Price MO, Price Jr FW. Secondary graft failure and repeat endothelial keratoplasty after Descemet's stripping automated endothelial keratoplasty. Ophthalmology. 2011;118:310-4.
79. Laaser K, Bachmann BO, Horn FK, Schlötzer-Schrehardt U, Cursiefen C, Kruse FE, et al. Donor tissue culture conditions and outcome after Descemet membrane endothelial keratoplasty. Am J Ophthalmol. 2011;151:1007-18.e2.
80. Price MO, Giebel AW, Fairchild KM, Price Jr FW. Descemet's membrane endothelial keratoplasty: prospective multicenter study of visual and refractive outcomes and endothelial survival. Ophthalmology. 2009;116:2361-8.
81. Dapena I, Moutsouris K, Droutsas K, Ham L, van Dijk K, Melles GR, et al. Standardized "no-touch" technique for Descemet membrane endothelial keratoplasty. Arch Ophthalmol. 2011;129:88-94.
82. Bennett A, Mahmoud S, Drury D, Cavanagh HD, McCulley JP, Petroll WM, et al. Impact of donor age on corneal endothelium-Descemet membrane layer scroll formation. Eye Contact Lens. 2015;41:236-9.
83. Feng MT, Price MO, Miller JM, Price Jr FW. Air reinjection and endothelial cell density in Descemet membrane endothelial keratoplasty: five-year follow-up. J Cataract Refract Surg. 2014;40:1116-21.
84. Guerra FP, Anshu A, Price MO, Giebel AW, Price FW. Descemet's membrane endothelial keratoplasty: prospective study of 1-year visual outcomes, graft survival, and endothelial cell loss. Ophthalmology. 2011;118:2368-73.
85. Dua HS, Faraj LA, Said DG, Gray T, Lowe J. Human corneal anatomy redefined: a novel pre-Descemet's layer (Dua's layer). Ophthalmology. 2013;120:1778-85.

86. Agarwal A, Dua HS, Narang P, Kumar DA, Agarwal A, Jacob S, et al. Pre-Descemet's endothelial keratoplasty (PDEK). Br J Ophthalmol. 2014;98:1181-5.
87. Dua HS, Termote K, Kenawy MB, Said DG, Jayaswal R, Nubile M, et al. Scrolling characteristics of pre-Descemet endothelial keratoplasty tissue: an ex vivo study. Am J Ophthalmol. 2016;166:84-90.
88. Altaan SL, Gupta A, Sidney LE, Elalfy MS, Agarwal A, Dua HS, et al. Endothelial cell loss following tissue harvesting by pneumodissection for endothelial keratoplasty: an *ex vivo* study. Br J Ophthalmol. 2015;99:710-3.
89. Terry MA, Saad HA, Shamie N, Shah AK. Peripheral endothelial cell damage after trephination of donor tissue. Cornea. 2009;28: 1149-52.
90. Terry MA, Saad HA, Shamie N, Chen ES, Phillips PM, Friend DJ, et al. Endothelial keratoplasty: the influence of insertion techniques and incision size on donor endothelial survival. Cornea. 2009;28:24-31.
91. Vargas E, Drance SM. Anterior chamber depth in angle closure glaucoma: clinical methods of depth determination in people with and without the disease. Arch Ophthalmol. 1973;90(6):438-9.
92. He M, Huang W, Friedman DS, Wu C, Zheng Y, Foster PJ. Slit lamp-simulated oblique flashlight test in the detection of narrow angles in Chinese eyes: the Liwan eye study. Invest Ophthalmol Vis Sci. 2007;48(12):5459-63.
93. Van Herick W, Shaffer RN, Schwartz A. Estimation of width of angle of anterior chamber. Incidence and significance of the narrow angle. Am J Ophthalmol. 1969;68:626-9.
94. Smith RJ. A new method of estimating the depth of the anterior chamber. Br J Ophthalmol. 1979;63(4):215-20.
95. Greenlee EC, Kwon YH. Graft failure: III. Glaucoma escalation after penetrating keratoplasty. Int Ophthalmol. 2008;28:191-207.
96. Starck T, Hopp L, Held KS, Marouf LM, Ree RW. Low-dose intraocular tissue plasminogen activator treatment for traumatic total hyphema, postcataract, and penetrating keratoplasty fibrinous membranes. J Cataract Refract Surg. 1995;21:219-24.
97. Snyder RW, Sherman MD, Allinson RW. Intracameral tissue plasminogen activator for treatment of excessive fibrin response after penetrating keratoplasty. Am J Ophthalmol. 1990;109:483-4.
98. Heidemann DG, Williams GA, Blumenkranz MS. Tissue plasminogen activator and penetrating keratoplasty. Ophthalmic Surg. 1990;21:364-5.
99. Fukuda R, Usui T, Tomidokoro A, Mishima K, Matagi N, Miyai T, et al. Noninvasive observations of peripheral angle in eyes after penetrating keratoplasty using anterior segment Fourier-domain optical coherence tomography. Cornea. 2012;31:259-63.
100. Yenerel NM, Kucumen RB, Gorgun E. The complementary benefit of anterior segment optical coherence tomography in penetrating keratoplasty. Clin Ophthalmol. 2013;7:1515-23.
101. Karadag O, Kugu S, Erdogan G, Kandemir B, Ozdil SL, Dogan OK. Incidence of and risk factors for increased intraocular pressure after penetrating keratoplasty. Cornea. 2010;29:278-82.
102. Inoue K, Amano S, Oshika T, Tsuru T. Risk factors for corneal graft failure and rejection in penetrating keratoplasty. Acta Ophthalmol Scand. 2001;79:251-5.
103. Shahid H, Salmon JF. Malignant glaucoma: a review of the modern literature. J Ophthalmol. 2012;2012:852659.
104. Meyer JJ, McGhee CN. Incidence, severity and outcomes of traumatic wound dehiscence following penetrating and deep anterior lamellar keratoplasty. Br J Ophthalmol. 2016;100(10):1412-5.
105. Gunasekaran S, Sharma N, Titiyal JS. Management of traumatic wound dehiscence of a functional graft 34 years after penetrating keratoplasty. BMJ Case Rep. 2014;2014:bcr2014205903.
106. Foroutan A, Tabatabaei SA, Behrouz MJ, Zarei R, Soleimani M. Spontaneous wound dehiscence after penetrating keratoplasty. Int J Ophthalmol. 2014;7:905-8.
107. Eye Bank Association of America (2015). Eye Banking Statistical Report. Available from www.restoresight.org/wp-content/uploads/2016/03/2015-Statistical-Report.pdf. [Last accessed July, 2016].
108. Ma JF, Rapuano CJ, Hammersmith KM, Nagra PK, Dai Y, Azari AA. Outcomes of wound dehiscence post-penetrating keratoplasty. Cornea. 2016;35:778-83.
109. Park Y, Kim MH, Won JY, Kim HS, Park YH. Vitreoretinal complications after penetrating keratoplasty. Retina. 2016;36(11):2110-5.
110. Duncker GI, Rochels R. Delayed suprachoroidal hemorrhage after penetrating keratoplasty. Int Ophthalmol. 1995;19:173-6.
111. Shi W, Liu M, Gao H, Li S, Xie L. Perioperative treatment and prognostic factors for penetrating keratoplasty in acanthamoeba keratitis unresponsive to medical treatment. Graefes Arch Clin Exp Ophthalmol. 2009;247:1383-8.
112. Wagoner MD, Al-Swailem SA, Sutphin JE, Zimmerman MB. Bacterial keratitis after penetrating keratoplasty: incidence, microbiological profile, graft survival, and visual outcome. Ophthalmology. 2007;114:1073-9.
113. Shikari H, Antin JH, Dana R. Ocular graft-versus-host disease: a review. Surv Ophthalmol. 2013;58:233-51.
114. Choi SW, Levine JE, Ferrara JL. Pathogenesis and management of graft-versus-host disease. Immunol Allergy Clin North Am. 2010;30:75-101.
115. Espana EM, Shah S, Santhiago MR, Singh AD. Graft versus host disease: clinical evaluation, diagnosis and management. Graefes Arch Clin Exp Ophthalmol. 2013;251:1257-66.
116. Filipovich AH, Weisdorf D, Pavletic S, Socie G, Wingard JR, Lee SJ. National Institutes of Health Consensus Development Project on criteria for clinical trials in chronic graft-versus-host disease: I. Diagnosis and staging working group report. Biol Blood Marrow Transplant. 2005;11:945-56.
117. Sung AD, Chao NJ. Acute graft-versus-host disease: are we close to bringing the bench to the bedside? Best Pract Res Clin Haematol. 2013;26:285-92.

118. Magenau J, Runaas L, Reddy P. Advances in understanding the pathogenesis of graft-versus-host disease. Br J Haematol. 2016;173:190-205.
119. Hessen M, Akpek EK. Ocular graft-versus-host disease. Curr Opin Allergy Clin Immunol. 2012;12:540-7.
120. Filipovich AH, Weisdorf D, Pavletic S, Socie G, Wingard JR, Lee SJ. National Institutes of Health Consensus Development Project on criteria for clinical trials in chronic graft-versus-host disease: I. Diagnosis and staging working group report. Biol Blood Marrow Transplant. 2005;11:945-56.
121. Nassar A, Tabbara KF, Aljurf M. Ocular manifestations of graft-versus-host disease. Saudi J Ophthalmol. 2013;27:215-22.
122. Magenau J, Runaas L, Reddy P. Advances in understanding the pathogenesis of graft-versus-host disease. Br J Haematol. 2016;173:190-205.
123. Sung AD, Chao NJ. Acute graft-versus-host disease: are we close to bringing the bench to the bedside? Best Pract Res Clin Haematol. 2013;26:285-92.
124. Qian L, Wu Z, Shen J. Advances in the treatment of acute graft-versus-host disease. J Cell Mol Med. 2013;17:966-75.
125. Ferrara JL, Reddy P. Pathophysiology of graft-versus-host disease. Semin Hematol. 2006;43:3-10.
126. Ogawa Y, Kim SK, Dana R, Clayton J, Jain S, Rosenblatt MI. International chronic ocular graft-vs-host-disease (GVHD) consensus group: proposed diagnostic criteria for chronic GVHD (part I). Sci Rep. 2013;3:3419.
127. Dietrich-Ntoukas T, Cursiefen C, Westekemper H, Eberwein P, Reinhard T, Bertz H. Diagnosis and treatment of ocular chronic graft-versus-host disease: report from the German-Austrian-Swiss Consensus Conference on clinical practice in chronic GVHD. Cornea. 2012;31:299-310.
128. Na KS, Yoo YS, Mok JW, Lee JW, Joo CK. Incidence and risk factors for ocular GVHD after allogeneic hematopoietic stem cell transplantation. Bone Marrow Transplant. 2015;50:1459-64.
129. Wang JC, Teichman JC, Mustafa M, Donnell H, Broady R, Yeung SN. Risk factors for the development of ocular graft-versus-host disease (GVHD) dry eye syndrome in patients with chronic GVHD. Br J Ophthalmol. 2015;99:1514-8.
130. Townley JR, Dana R, Jacobs DS. Keratoconjunctivitis sicca manifestations in ocular graft versus host disease: pathogenesis, presentation, prevention, and treatment. Semin Ophthalmol. 2011;26:251-60.
131. Balasubramaniam SC, Raja H, Nau CB, Shen JF, Schornack MM. Ocular graft-versus-host disease: a review. Eye Contact Lens. 2015;41:256-61.
132. Jacobs R, Tran U, Chen H, Kassim A, Engelhardt BG, Greer JP, et al. Prevalence and risk factors associated with development of ocular GVHD defined by NIH consensus criteria. Bone Marrow Transplant. 2012;47:1470-3.
133. Stevenson W, Shikari H, Saboo US, Amparo F, Dana R. Bilateral corneal ulceration in ocular graft-versus-host disease. Clin Ophthalmol. 2013;7:2153-8.
134. Hettinga YM, Verdonck LF, Fijnheer R, Rijkers GT, Rothova A. Anterior uveitis: a manifestation of graft-versus-host disease. Ophthalmology. 2007;114:794-7.
135. Jagasia MH, Greinix HT, Arora M, Williams KM, Wolff D, Cowen EW. National Institutes of Health Consensus Development Project on criteria for clinical trials in chronic graft-versus-host disease: I. The 2014 Diagnosis and Staging Working Group report. Biol Blood Marrow Transplant. 2015;21:389e1-401.e1.
136. Schargus M, Meyer-ter-Vehn T, Menrath J, Grigoleit GU, Geerling G. Correlation between tear film osmolarity and the disease score of the International Chronic Ocular Graft-Versus-Host-Disease Consensus Group in hematopoietic stem cell transplantation patients. Cornea. 2015;34:911-6.
137. Na KS, Yoo YS, Hwang KY, Mok JW, Joo CK. Tear osmolarity and ocular surface parameters as diagnostic markers of ocular graft-versus-host disease. Am J Ophthalmol. 2015;160:143-9.e1.
138. Garnett C, Apperley JF, Pavl J. Treatment and management of graft-versus-host disease: improving response and survival. Ther Adv Hematol. 2013;4:366-78.
139. Bredeson C, Rumble RB, Varela NP, Kuruvilla J, Kouroukis CT. Extracorporeal photopheresis in the management of graft-versus-host disease. Curr Oncol. 2014;21:e310-25.
140. Na KS, Kim MS. Allogeneic serum eye drops for the treatment of dry eye patients with chronic graft-versus-host disease. J Ocul Pharmacol Ther. 2012;28:479-83.
141. Khan B, Dudenhoefer EJ, Dohlman CH. Keratoprosthesis: an update. Curr Opin Ophthalmol. 2001;12:282-7.
142. Saeed HN, Shanbhag S, Chodosh J. The Boston keratoprosthesis. Curr Opin Ophthalmol. 2017;28:390-6.
143. Dohlman CH, Mona HD, Graney J. The Boston keratoprosthesis: a new threadless design. Digit J Ophthalmol. 2007;13:3.
144. Hille K, Grabner G, Liu C, Colliardo P, Falcinelli G, Taloni M, et al. Standards for modified osteoodontokeratoprosthesis (OOKP) surgery according to Strampelli and Falcinelli: The Rome-Vienna protocol. Cornea. 2005;24:895-908.
145. Iyer G, Srinivasan B, Agarwal S, Rachapalle SR. Laminar resorption in modified osteo-odonto-keratoprosthesis procedure: a cause for concern. Am J Ophthalmol. 2014;158:263-900.
146. Chan CC, LoVerde L, Qiang J, Nordlund ML, Holland EJ. Incidence, risk factors, and surgical management of Boston type 1 keratoprosthesis corneal melts, leaks, and extrusions. Cornea. 2016;35:1049-56
147. Perez VL, Leung EH, Berrocal AM, Albini TA, Parel JM, Amescua G, et al. Impact of total pars plana vitrectomy on postoperative complications in aphakic, snap-on, type 1 Boston keratoprosthesis. Ophthalmology. 2017;124:1504-9.
148. Iyer G, Srinivasan B, Agarwal S, Shetty R, Krishnamoorthy S, Balekudaru S, et al. Glaucoma in modified osteo-odonto-keratoprosthesis eyes: role of additional stage 1A and Ahmed glaucoma drainage device-technique and timing. Am J Ophthalmol. 2015;159:482-900.

149. Aldave AJ, Sangwan VS, Basu S, Basak SK, Hovakimyan A, Gevorgyan O, et al. International results with the Boston type keratoprosthesis. Ophthalmology. 2012;119:1530-8.
150. Transplantation of Human Organs and Tissues Rules, 2014. Ministry of Health and Family Welfare, 27 March, 2014, New Delhi.
151. Transplantation of Human Organs and Tissues Act, 1994. Ministry of Law, Justice and Company Affairs (Legislative Department), 11 July, 1994, New Delhi.
152. Standards of Eye Banking in India 2009, National Program for Control of Blindness, Directorate General of Health Services, Ministry of Health and Family Welfare, Government of India, New Delhi. 2009. Available from http://npcb.nic.in/writereaddata/mainlinkfile/file176.pdf.
153. Allocation criteria for corneas. (2020). Available from https://notto.gov.in/WriteReadData/Portal/News/389_1_29082016Final CorneaAllocationPolicy.pdf.
154. Vemparala R, Gupta P. National Programme for Control of Blindness (NPCB) in the 12th Five year plan: an overview. DJO. 2017;27:290-2.
155. Raj SM, Vasavada AR, Johar SRK, Vasavada VA, Vasavada VA. Post-operative capsular opacification: a review. Int J Biomed Sci. 2007;3:237-50.
156. Ernest PH, Obasawa M, Kurosaka H, Nakamura K. Posterior capsule opacification and neodymium: YAG capsulotomy rates with AcrySof acrylic and PhacoFlex II silicone intraocular lenses. J Cataract Refract Surg. 2003;29:1546-50.
157. Chapter 26. In: Allingham RR, Shields MB Damji KF, Safranov G (Eds). Shields' Textbook of Glaucoma. Philadelphia: Lippincott Williams & Wilkins; 2005.
158. Kirsch RE, Levine O, Singer JA. Ridge at internal edge of cataract incision. Arch Ophthalmol. 1976;94(12):2098-104.
159. Narayanan R, Gaster RN, Kenney MC. Pseudophakic corneal edema: a review of mechanisms and treatments. Cornea. 2006;25(9):993-1004.
160. Khan MS, Basit I, Ishaq M, Shakoor T, Yaqub A, Intisar R. Corneal collagen cross linking (CXL) in treatment of pseudophakic bullous keratopathy. Pak J Med Sci. 2016;32(4):965.
161. Pires RT, Tseng SC, Prabhasawat P, Puangsricharern V, Maskin SL, Kim JC, et al. Amniotic membrane transplantation for symptomatic bullous keratopathy. Arch Ophthalmol. 1999;117(10):1291-7.
162. Benitah NR, Arroyo JG. Pseudophakic cystoid macular edema. Int Ophthalmol Clin. 2010;50(1):139-53.
163. Flach AI. The incidence, pathogenesis and treatment of cystoid macular edema following cataract surgery. Trans Am Ophthalmol Soc. 1998;96:557-634.
164. Gamache DA, Graff G, Brady MT, Spellman JM, Yanni JM. Nepafenac, a unique nonsteroidal prodrug with potential utility in the treatment of trauma-induced ocular inflammation: I. Assessment of anti-inflammatory efficacy. Inflammation. 2000;24(4):357-70.
165. Wittpenn JR, Silverstein S, Heier J, Kenyon KR, Hunkeler JD, Earl M, et al. A randomized, masked comparison of topical ketorolac 0.4% plus steroid vs steroid alone in low-risk cataract surgery patients. Am J Ophthalmol. 2008;146(4):554-60.
166. Randazzo A, Vinciguerra P. Chronic macular edema medical treatment in Irvine-Gass syndrome: case report. Eur J Ophthalmol. 2010;20(2):462-5.
167. Benhamou N, Massin P, Haouchine B, Audren F, Tadayoni R, Gaudric A. Intravitreal triamcinolone for refractory pseudophakic macular edema. Am J Ophthalmol. 2003;135(2):246-249.
168. Conway MD, Canakis C, Livir-Rallatos C, Peyman GA. Intravitreal triamcinolone acetonide for refractory chronic pseudophakic cystoid macular edema. J Cataract Refract Surg. 2003;29(1):27-33.
169. Jonas JB, Kreissig I, Degenring RF. Intravitreal triamcinolone acetonide for pseudophakic cystoid macular edema. Am J Ophthalmol. 2003;136(2):384-6.
170. Ahmadabadi HF, Mohammadi M, Beheshtnejad H, Mirshahi A. Effect of intravitreal triamcinolone acetonide injection on central macular thickness in diabetic patients having phacoemulsification. J Cataract Refract Surg. 2010;36(6):917-22.
171. London NJ, Chiang A, Haller JA. The dexamethasone drug delivery system: indications and evidence. Adv Ther. 2011;28(5):351-66.
172. Lois N, Wong D. Pseudophakic retinal detachment. Surv Ophthalmol. 2003;48(5):467-87.
173. Day AC, Donachie HJ, Sparrow JM, Johnston RL. United Kingdom National Ophthalmology Database Study of cataract surgery: report 3: pseudophakic retinal detachment. Ophthalmology. 2016;123:1711-5.
174. Grzybowski A, Kanclerz P. Does Nd:YAG capsulotomy increase the risk of retinal detachment? Asia Pac J Ophthalmol (Phila). 2018;7(5):339-44.
175. Boberg-Ans G, Henning V, Villumsen J, Cour ML. Long-term incidence of rhegmatogenous retinal detachment and survival in a defined population undergoing standardized phacoemulsification surgery. Acta Ophthalmol Scand. 2006;84:613-18.
176. Solborg Bjerrum S, Mikkelsen KL, Cour ML. Epidemiology of 411,140 cataract operations performed in public hospitals and private hospitals/clinics in Denmark between 2004 and 2012. Acta Ophthalmol. 2015;93:16-23.
177. Daien V, Pape AL, Heve D, Carriere I, Villain M. Incidence, risk factors, and impact of age on retinal detachment after cataract surgery in France: a national population study. Ophthalmology. 2015;122:2179-85.
178. Tornambe PE, Hilton GF, Brinton DA, Flood TP, Green S, Grizzard WS, et al. Pneumatic retinopexy. A two-year follow-up study of the multicenter clinical trial comparing pneumatic retinopexy with scleral buckling. Ophthalmology. 1991;98(7):1115-23.10.
179. Grizzard WS, Hilton GF, Hammer ME, Taren D, Brinton DA. Pneumatic retinopexy failures. Cause, prevention, timing, and management. Ophthalmology. 1995;102(6):929-36.11.
180. Eter N, Böker T, Spitznas M. Long-term results of pneumatic retinopexy. Graefe's Arch Clin Exp Ophthalmol. 2000;238(8):677-81.

181. Arya AV, Emerson JW, Engelbert M, Hagedorn CL, Adelman RA. Surgical management of pseudophakic retinal detachments. A meta-analysis. Ophthalmology. 2006;113(10):1724-33.13.
182. Brazitikos PD, Androudi S, Christen WG, Stangos NT. Primary pars plana vitrectomy versus scleral buckle surgery for the treatment of pseudophakic retinal detachment. A randomized clinical trial. Retina. 2005;25(8):957-64.
183. Jambulingam M, Parameswaran SK, Lysa S, Selvaraj M, Madhavan HN. A study on the incidence, microbiological analysis and investigations on the source of infection of postoperative infectious endophthalmitis in a tertiary care ophthalmic hospital: an 8-year study. Indian J Ophthalmol. 2010;58:297-302.
184. Das T, Hussain A, Naduvilath T, Sharma S, Jalali S, Majji AB. Case control analyses of acute endophthalmitis after cataract surgery in South India associated with technique, patient care, and socioeconomic status. J Ophthalmol. 2012;2012:298459.
185. Narang S, Gupta A, Gupta V, Dogra MR, Ram J, Pandav SS, et al. Fungal endophthalmitis following cataract surgery: clinical presentation, microbiological spectrum, and outcome. Am J Ophthalmol. 2001;132:609-17.
186. Chakrabarti A, Shivaprakash MR, Singh R, Tarai B, George VK, Fomda BA, et al. Fungal endophthalmitis: fourteen years' experience from a center in India. Retina. 2008;28:1400-7.
187. Ravindran RD, Venkatesh R, Chang DF, Sengupta S, Gyatsho J, Talwar B. Incidence of post-cataract endophthalmitis at Aravind Eye Hospital: outcomes of more than 42,000 consecutive cases using standardized sterilization and prophylaxis protocols. J Cataract Refract Surg. 2009;35:629-36.
188. Gupta A, Gupta V, Gupta A, Dogra MR, Pandav SS, Ray P, et al. Spectrum and clinical profile of post cataract surgery endophthalmitis in North India. Indian J Ophthalmol. 2003;51:139-45.
189. Anand AR, Therese KL, Madhavan HN. Spectrum of aetiological agents of postoperative endophthalmitis and antibiotic susceptibility of bacterial isolates. Indian J Ophthalmol. 2000;48:123-8.
190. Endophthalmitis Vitrectomy Study Group. Results of the Endophthalmitis Vitrectomy Study. A randomized trial of immediate vitrectomy and of intravenous antibiotics for the treatment of postoperative bacterial endophthalmitis. Arch Ophthalmol. 1995;113:1479-96.
191. Witkin AJ, Chang DF, Jumper JM, Charles S, Eliott D, Hoffman RS, et al. Vancomycin-associated hemorrhagic occlusive retinal vasculitis. Ophthalmology. 2017;124(5):583-95.
192. ESCRS, Endophthalmitis Study Group. Prophylaxis of postoperative endophthalmitis following cataract surgery: results of the ESCRS multicenter study and identification of risk factors. J Cataract Refract Surg. 2007;33:978-88.
193. Haripriya A, Chang DF, Ravindran RD. Endophthalmitis reduction with intracameral moxifloxacin prophylaxis: analysis of 600,000 surgeries. Ophthalmology. 2017;124(6):768-75.
194. Park CY, Lee JK, Chuck RS. Toxic anterior segment syndrome-an updated review. BMC Ophthalmol. 2018;18(1):276.
195. Lagrasta JM, Allemann N, Scapucin L, Moeller CT, Ohkawara LE, Melo LA, et al. Clinical results in phacoemulsification using the SRK/T formula. Arq Bras Oftalmol. 2009;72(2):189-93.
196. Cooke DL, Cooke TL. Comparison of 9 intraocular lens power calculation formulas. J Cataract Refract Surg. 2016;42(8):1157-64.
197. Kane JX, Van Heerden A, Atik A, Petsoglou C. Accuracy of 3 new methods for intraocular lens power selection. J Cataract Refract Surg. 2017;43(3):333-9.
198. Aristodemou P, Knox Cartwright NE, Sparrow JM, Johnston RL. Formula choice: Hoffer Q, Holladay 1, or SRK/T and refractive outcomes in 8108 eyes after cataract surgery with biometry by partial coherence interferometry. J Cataract Refract Surg. 2011; 37(1):63-71.

8.10 Keratomalacia

Ritu Nagpal, Archita Singh, Prafulla Kumar Maharana

 1. Write a short note on keratomalacia.

Introduction

Keratomalacia refers to corneal melting in children with severe vitamin A deficiency. Hypovitaminosis A has a varied ocular presentation depending upon the severity of vitamin deficiency.[1] These include night blindness, Bitot's spots, conjunctival xerosis, corneal ulceration ("keratomalacia"), and corneal scarring. Out of which keratomalacia is one of the major causes of ocular morbidity and blindness among the pediatric age group, especially in the developing world.[2,3] It is a potentially blinding condition with asymmetrical bilateral presentation. Keratomalacia is one the most important preventable cause of nutritional blindness which should be recognized early and managed aggressively. The age group at risk is typically between 2 and 6 years, though it has also been seen in infants younger than 6 months particularly due to improper weaning practices.[4,5]

Etiology[1,6-13]

It is a form of nutritional blindness attributed to deficiency of fat-soluble vitamin, vitamin A. Various factors attributing to this deficiency may be decreased intake, malabsorption, impaired metabolism, and other systemic associations. In a developing country like ours, poor dietary intake is the major cause.

The contributing factors are as listed here.
- *Impaired dietary intake:*
  - Low socioeconomic group
  - Inadequate and improper breastfeeding practices
  - Incorrect weaning practices
  - Ignorance and poor knowledge regarding nutritional requirements of the newborns
- *Malabsorption:*
  - Intestinal parasitic infestations
  - Congenital short bowel
  - Cystic fibrosis
  - Impaired hepatic storage and metabolism
- *Systemic associations:*
  - Failure to thrive
  - Preterm and low birth weight babies
  - Postmeasles sequelae
  - Protein energy malnutrition.

Clinical Features[14,15]

Symptoms

Keratomalacia is one of the most severe manifestation of vitamin A deficiency. It has a reported percentage of about 8–27.3%.[16]

It can present with following symptoms which are usually as narrated by the parent(s)/care-giver(s):
- Redness and watering
- Failure to open eyes in bright light
- White reflex (whitish discoloration of the corneas)
- Purulent discharge with or without matting of eyelashes
- *Systemically:* Irritability, failure to feed, and poor general condition.

Signs

The presentation of keratomalacia is characterized by unilateral/bilateral ocular involvement which may be symmetrical or asymmetrical. Typical presentation includes punched out corneal ulcers usually in the inferior half of the cornea, mostly inferonasal quadrant. Hypopyon (collection of sterile infiltrates in anterior chamber) is usually present. They are rapidly progressive ulcers which may progress to full-thickness perforated ulcers with prolapse of the uveal tissue. Secondary infections are common.

If adequately treated superficial ulcers usually heal with maculo-leucomatous corneal scars. Deep ulcers are associated with uveal tissue prolapse and heal as adherent leucomas and anterior staphylomas with or without secondary glaucoma.

Classification/Grading[17]

The ocular manifestation of vitamin A deficiency or xerophthalmia as described by the WHO Expert group has been listed in **Table 1**. They were first classified in 1976 and later modified.

TABLE 1: Classification of xerophthalmia (WHO Expert Group).

Stage	Description
XN	Night blindness
X1A	Conjunctival xerosis
X1B	Bitot's spots
X2	Corneal xerosis
X3A	Keratomalacia. Corneal ulceration <1/3 corneal surface
X3B	Keratomalacia. Corneal ulceration ≥1/3 corneal surface
XS	Corneal scars
XF	Xerophthalmic fundus

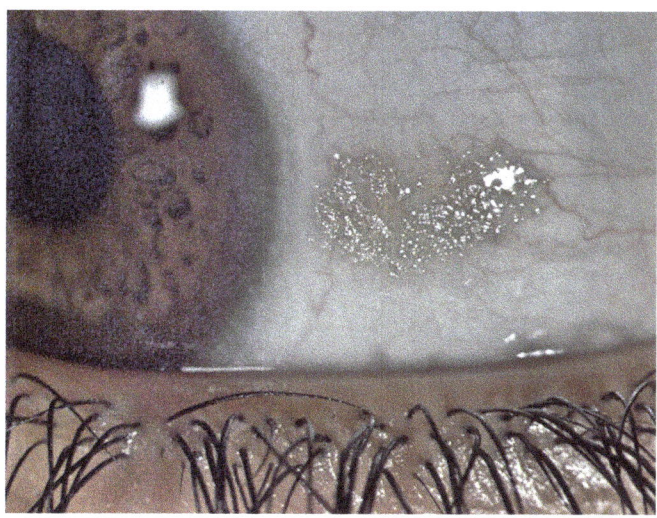

Fig. 1: Slit-lamp biomicroscopy clinical picture of left eye showing Bitot's spots in the temporal aspect of the palpebral conjunctiva.

Ocular manifestations of xerophthalmia have been briefly discussed here.[17]
- *Night blindness (XN):* Impaired dark adaptation has been seen in children in early stages of vitamin A deficiency. It is mainly due to the interruption of the visual cycle as there is a failure in synthesis and metabolism of the rhodopsin pigment thus disrupting normal functioning of the rods. It responds within 1–2 days of administration of oral high-dose vitamin A.
- *Conjunctival xerosis (X1A):* Xerosis typically involves the epithelial surface. It is due to dryness of the conjunctiva and generalized keratinization. It is recognized by areas of wrinkling and pigmentation.
- *Bitot's spots (X1B):* More commonly seen in the temporal part of the palpebral conjunctiva followed by nasal quadrant. They appear to be foamy collections in the exposed part of the conjunctiva and formed as a result of desquamated and keratinized epithelium that heaps up **(Fig. 1)**. *Corynebacterium xerosis* is considered responsible for the foamy appearance. They are more commonly seen in males.

  They tend to resolve early in younger children usually within 2–5 days of administration of vitamin A therapeutic dose, maximum up to 2 weeks.[18]
- *Corneal xerosis (X2):* It refers to dryness of corneal surface characterized by superficial punctate staining particularly in inferior half of the cornea. It tends to improve within 2–5 days of administration of vitamin A therapeutic dose, maximum up to 2 weeks.[18]
- *Keratomalacia (X3A/3B):* Refers to corneal melting due to sterile necrosis. The stroma becomes edematous and begins to melt. There are variable reasons described for this, most accepted is activation of collagenases and other enzymes.

  It may or may not be preceded by the above-mentioned stages in cases of young children. It is an ocular emergency and requires prompt intervention from both the ophthalmologist and pediatrician.
- *Corneal scars (XS):* It occurs as a sequelae of corneal involvement. The scarring may range from superficial nebulomacular scars to deep leucomatous corneal scars. In cases of deep ulcers, they may present as adherent leucomas and anterior staphylomas **(Fig. 2)**.
- *Xerophthalmic fundus (XF):* Characterized by whitish retinal lesions. There may be associated constriction of visual fields.

Differential Diagnosis

The diagnosis of keratomalacia is mostly clinical. It is particularly important to differentiate keratomalacia from infective keratitis. Keratomalacia though is a sterile melt of the cornea, secondary infections are commonly seen. As a result, clear differentiation between keratomalacia and other causes of infective keratitis is difficult.

But for children presenting with postkeratomalacia corneal scarring differentials can be:
- Healed infective keratitis
- Anterior segment dysgenesis
- Congenital hereditary endothelial dystrophy
- Congenital glaucoma.

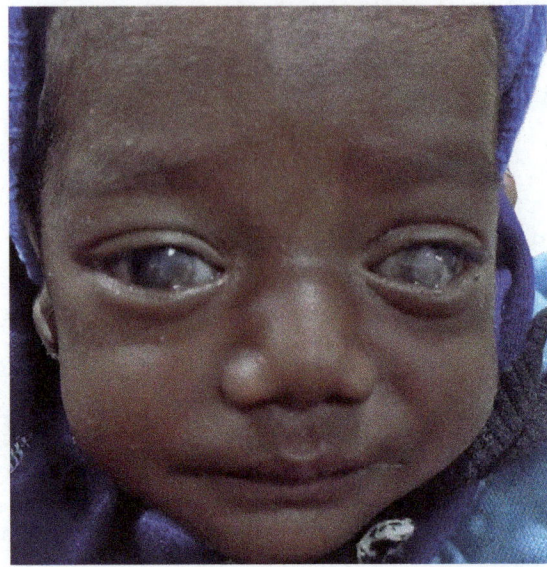

Fig. 2: Clinical photograph of a child with bilateral healed corneal opacities following healed keratomalacia.

Work-up

History

A descriptive history is important in cases of keratomalacia to identify the clinical condition. Preferably history should be taken from the parents.

Following history must be recorded carefully:
- *Perinatal history*—low birth weight, intrauterine growth restriction (IUGR), failure to thrive, recurrent pneumonia, and gastroenteritis
- *General well-being*—poor weight gain, low level of activity, poor feeding, and irritability
- *Feeding practices*—whether colostrum was administered, exclusive breastfeeding, top feeding, bottle-feeding, and improper weaning
- *Immunization*—immunization of the child especially measles vaccine
- *Past medical history*—previous history of measles, and recurrent gastroenteritis
- *Systemic association*—malabsorption syndromes, and cystic fibrosis
- *Socio-economic status*—low socio-economic status is usually associated with decreased dietary intake, poor hygiene, and less awareness about infant-feeding practices.

Examination

Systemic Examination
- Look for generalized signs of protein-energy malnutrition
- Weight of the infant
- General awareness and reflexes
- Signs of respiratory tract infections or gut infestations
- Rule out other systemic associations.

Ocular Examination
- Examination under anesthesia is preferred. Both the eyes should be examined in detail.
- Corneal scrapping for staining and culture is preferred so as to confirm associated infections.
- Examination is done to assess the degree and extent of corneal involvement, whether perforated, any evidence of uveal tissue prolapse.

Investigations
- *Corneal smear and culture sensitivity:* Evaluation of the corneal scraping to look for evidence of superadded infection.

- *Ultrasonography:* B-scan of the eye to assess for any pathology in the posterior segment, optic nerve head status, and chorioretinal thickness.
- *Visual evoked potential:* To assess the optic nerve function and visual function.
- *Serum retinol levels:* The normal level of serum retinol is about 0.30–0.80 mg/L. WHO has defined low serum retinol levels as serum level below <0.30 mg/L. Xerophthalmic manifestations become prominent at serum levels below 0.70 mg/L and become more severe with serum retinol values below 0.3 mg/L.

The above-mentioned prevalence rates in **Table 2** indicate the significance and severity of the vitamin A deficiency as a health problem in a community or population group.

Management

The treatment of keratomalacia depends on the severity at presentation and general well-being of the child. Supplementation of therapeutic dosages of vitamin A is of utmost importance and may be accompanied with or without surgical intervention (**Flowchart 1**).

Medical Management

- Therapeutic high doses of vitamin A as recommended based upon the age are given at 0, 1, and 14 days. The dosages are as tabulated in **Table 3**.

TABLE 2: Assessment of prevalence in the community.[17]

Criteria	Prevalence in risk population (6 months to 6 years)
Night blindness	>1%
Bitot's spots	>0.5%
Corneal xerosis	>0.01%
Keratomalacia	>0.05%
Serum retinol (<10 µg/dL)	>5%

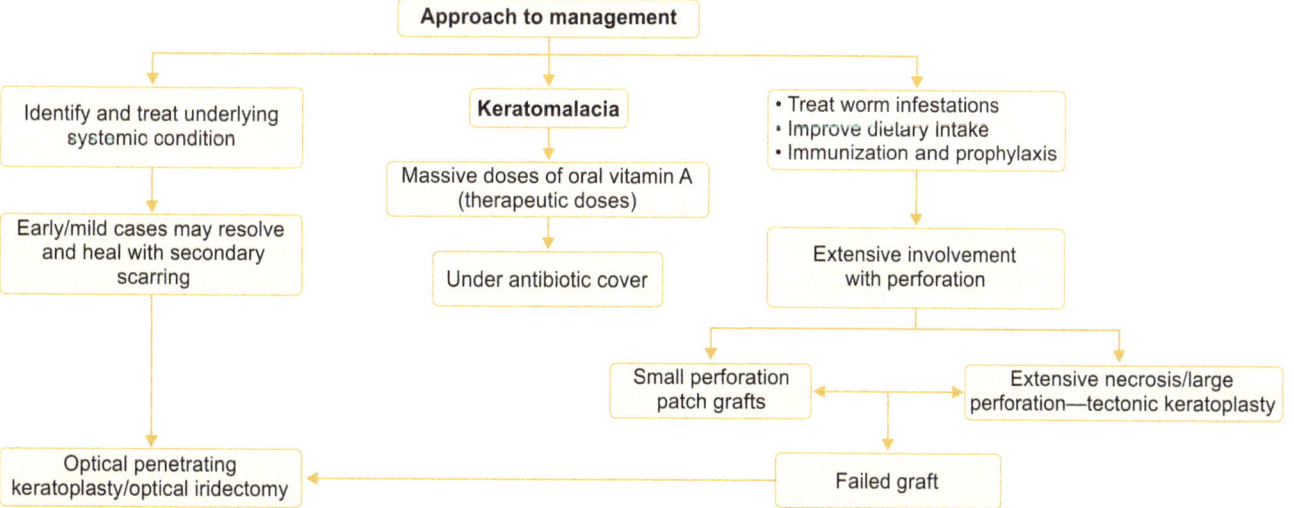

Flowchart 1: Approach to keratomalacia: Points to remember during management.

TABLE 3: Recommended doses of oral vitamin A for cases with xerophthalmia.

Age	Dose of oral vitamin A	Schedule
<6 months	50,000 IU	0, 1, 14 days
6–11 months (<8 kg)	100,000 IU	0, 1, 14 days
12 months or more	200,000 IU	0, 1, 14 days

- Intramuscular injections (water-miscible formulations) are advised in children wherein oral intake is not possible or absorption may be low such as severe malabsorption, gut inflammation/gastroenteritis and vomiting.
- Evaluate the child for any other underlying systemic disorder or condition which tends to cause a decreased utilization of vitamin A hence deficiency.
  These systemic disorders should then be dealt with accordingly.
- Treat for underlying protein-energy malnutrition as it further tends to worsen keratomalacia.
- *Antibiotic therapy:* As most of these cases have secondary infection:
  - Topical fortified broad-spectrum antibiotics
  - Oral/systemic antibiotics depending upon the severity of infection.

Surgical Management[16,19-23]

Surgical interventions are required in severe cases of keratomalacia where massive doses of vitamin A alone are not suffice. The available surgical options include:
- Tectonic keratoplasty (TKP)
- Patch grafts
- Optical penetrating keratoplasty
- Optical iridectomy.

Tectonic Keratoplasty

Children presenting with keratomalacia with associated corneal perforation require a corneal transplant in the acute stage of the disease. This is required so as to maintain the integrity of the globe. Usually, large size grafts are required as extensive corneal melting is present in most of the cases.

Tectonic keratoplasty in these children is challenging and is subjected to the fitness for general anesthesia due to high degree of associated systemic morbidity. Also, the success rate of tectonic procedure is limited with high risk of graft failure requiring regrafts.

Patch Grafts

Patch grafts may be done in cases with small paracentral perforations. This procedure is of particular importance as the complications associated with patch grafts tend to lower when compared to tectonic full-thickness keratoplasty.

Also, they may be planned for a full-thickness optical keratoplasty at a later stage.

Optical Penetrating Keratoplasty

Full-thickness keratoplasty is considered for post-keratomalacia scarring for the purpose of visual rehabilitation.

Optical Iridectomy

Optical iridectomy may be considered in cases with small paracentral scars usually in the superior quadrant. The preferred site for iridectomy is the inferonasal quadrant.

> *Problems faced during keratoplasty in keratomalacia*
> - Risk of general anesthesia
> - Low scleral rigidity
> - High vitreous up-thrust
> - Need for larger grafts
> - Difficult trephination
> - Cheese wiring of sutures due to extensive edema and involvement
> - Need for removal of crystalline lens/spontaneous extrusion
> - Postoperative high risk of poor wound healing, secondary glaucoma, graft dehiscence, graft infection, graft rejection, and failure of the grafts

Prevention

Vitamin A deficiency is a preventable cause of blindness. Prevention is possible by appropriately considering the following:
- *Dietary supplementation:* Neonates should be adequately breastfed. It is important to provide supplementation to the breastfeeding mothers. Food rich in vitamin A includes β-carotene-rich green leafy vegetables, carrots, sweet potatoes, and cantaloupe and food rich in retinoids includes fish and eggs.

- *Implementation in national immunization schedule:* For children, as per the national immunization schedule, vitamin A oral first dose is given at 9 months of age, second at 16 months, and then every 6 months 5 doses are given. The first dose is of 1 lakh IU and thereafter 2 lakh IU is given orally.
- Consider *aggressive management* of protein-energy malnutrition and measles along with supplementing vitamin A as they tend to enhance ocular manifestations.
- *Identify and treat underlying systemic* associations such as malabsorption syndromes.

Key Points

- Keratomalacia is one of the most common cause of bilateral blindness among pediatric population of our country.
- It is a preventable cause of blindness.
- Massive doses of oral vitamin A is the first line of management.
- Keratoplasty has poor outcomes, both anatomical and functional.
- Children with severe keratomalacia have poor visual prognosis.

References

1. Sommer A. Xerophthalmia and vitamin A status. Prog Retin Eye Res. 1998;17(1):9-31.
2. Rahi JS, Sripathi S, Gilbert CE, Foster A. Childhood blindness due to vitamin A deficiency in India: regional variations. Arch Dis Child. 1995;72:330-3.
3. Sommer A, Sugana T. Corneal xerophthalmia and keratomalacia. Arch Ophthalmol. 1982;100:404-11.
4. Oomen HA. Clinical epidemiology of xerophthalmia in man. Am J Clin Nutr. 1969;22:1098-105.
5. Rahmathullah L, Raj MS, Chandravathi TS. Aetiology of severe vitamin A deficiency in children. Natl Med J India. 1997; 10:62-5.
6. Cella W, Urbano AP, Vinhadelli WS, Donatti M, Rocha EM. Xerophthalmia secondary to short bowel syndrome. J Pediatr Ophthalmol Strabismus. 2002;39(2):125-7.
7. Whitcher JP, Srinivasan M, Upadhyay MP. Corneal blindness: a global perspective. Bull World Health Organ. 2001;79(3):214-21.
8. Ansari EA, Sahni K, Etherington C, Morton A, Conway SP, Moya E, et al. Ocular signs and symptoms and vitamin A status in patients with cystic fibrosis treated with daily vitamin A supplements. Br J Ophthalmol. 1999;83(6):688-91.
9. Brooks Jr HL, Driebe Jr WT, Schemmer GG. Xerophthalmia and cystic fibrosis. Arch Ophthalmol. 1990;108(3):354-7.
10. Muniz-Junqueira MI, Queiroz EF. Relationship between protein-energy malnutrition, vitamin A, and parasitoses in living in Brasilia. Rev Soc Bras Med Trop. 2002;35(2):133-41.
11. Payne LG, Koski KG, Ortega-Barria E, Scott ME. Benefit of vitamin A supplementation on ascaris reinfection is less evident in stunted children. J Nutr. 2007;137(6):1455-9.
12. Suchdev PS, Davis SM, Bartoces M, Ruth LJ, Worrell CM, Kanyi H, et al. Soil-transmitted helminth infection and nutritional status among urban slum children in Kenya. Am J Trop Med Hyg. 2014;90(2):299-305.
13. Moreira DS, Rocha GM. Toxocara canis: impact of preweaning nutritional deprivation on the pathogenesis of pneumonia in the mouse. Exp Parasitol. 2005;110(4):349-52.
14. Vitamin A deficiency and xerophthalmia. Report of a joint WHO/USAID meeting. Geneva: World Health Organization; 1976. WHO Technical Report Series, No. 590. [online] Available from http://whqlibdoc.who.int/trs/WHO_TRS_590.pdf [Last accessed July, 2022].
15. McLaren DS, Kraemer K. (2012). Manual on Vitamin A Deficiency Disorders (VADD), third edition. Basel: Sight and Life Press. [online] Available from https://sightandlife.org/wp-content/uploads/2017/05/SightandLife_vitamin_a_deficiency_disorders_VADD_Manual.pdf [Last accessed July, 2022].
16. Vajpayee RB, Vanathi M, Tandon R, Sharma N, Titiyal JS. Keratoplasty for keratomalacia in preschool children. Br J Ophthalmol. 2003;87(5):538-42.
17. Control of vitamin A deficiency and xerophthalmia. Report of a joint WHO/UNICEF/USAID/Helen Keller International/IVACG meeting. Geneva: World Health Organization; 1982. WHO Technical Report Series, No. 672. Available from http://whqlibdoc.who.int/trs/WHO_TRS_672.pdf [Last accessed July, 2022].
18. Sommer A. Vitamin A Deficiency and its Consequences. A Field Guide to their Detection and Control, 3rd edition. World Health Organization; 1995.
19. Ben-Sira E, Ticho U, Yasur Y. Surgical treatment of active keratomalacia by "covering graft". Isr J Med Sci. 1972;8:1209-10.
20. Singh G, Malik SR. Therapeutic penetrating keratoplasty in keratomalacia. Br J Ophthalmol. 1973;57:638-40.
21. Vanathi M, Panda A, Vengayil S. Pediatric keratoplasty. Surv Ophthalmol. 2009;54:245-71.
22. Dada T, Sharma N, Vajpayee RB. Indications for pediatric keratoplasty in India. Cornea. 1999;18:296-8.
23. Sharma N, Prakash G, Titiyal JS, Tandon R, Vajpayee RB. Pediatric keratoplasty in India: indications and outcomes. Cornea. 2007;26:810-3.

8.11 Shield Ulcer

Pranita Sahay

Q 1. Write a short note on shield ulcer.

Introduction

Vernal keratoconjunctivitis (VKC), also known as spring catarrh, is a chronic allergic condition of the ocular surface seen more commonly in young males living in a dry and hot climate.[1] It is characterized by symptoms of intense itching, photophobia, foreign body sensation, congestion, and watering. Its three clinical variants include palpebral, bulbar, and mixed form. Shield ulcer occurs as a complication to VKC and is more commonly seen in the palpebral variant. Its reported incidence in cases of VKC varies from 3 to 11% and is characterized by its typical superior location, oval-shaped epithelial defect, and indolent course.[1,2] This condition has acquired its name from its shape which is similar to the shields used by warriors. The damage to the corneal epithelium by mechanical trauma with papillae and the released toxins result in this condition and also retard the process of reepithelialization.[3] Judicious management of this condition at an early stage can prevent further complications such as secondary corneal infections, perforation, severe corneal scarring, and neovascularization.

Etiology

The two proposed hypotheses for the pathogenesis of shield ulcer are as follows:
1. *Mechanical theory:* The papillae located in the superior tarsal conjunctiva result in constant mechanical damage to the corneal epithelium. The location of shield ulcer in superior aspect of the cornea is explained by this hypothesis.
2. *Toxin theory:* Various toxic inflammatory mediators released by mast cells and eosinophils cause corneal epithelial damage. The major basic protein (MBP), a toxic protein derived from activated eosinophils, plays an important role in this process.

The initial damage to the corneal epithelium is in the form of punctuate erosions which is followed by coarse epitheliopathy and macroerosions. The epithelial damage extending up to the Bowman's layer leads to the formation of shield ulcer.

Clinical Features

Symptoms

A case of shield ulcer presents with:
- Severe photophobia
- Pain
- Redness
- Watering
- Intense itching
- Diminution of vision.

Signs

The characteristic features of shield ulcer are as follows:
- Indolent course
- Superior location—more common (can be located elsewhere as well)
- Oval or hexagonal shape
- Well-defined edge
- *Base of the ulcer:*
  - Transparent in grade 1 shield ulcer
  - Translucent or opaque with yellow/white deposits in grade 2 shield ulcer
  - Elevated plaque above the adjacent normal epithelium in grade 3 shield ulcer.

TABLE 1: Clinical grading of shield ulcer (by Cameron).

Grade	Clinical description
1	Transparent ulcer base
2	Translucent ulcer base with or without opaque white or yellow deposits
3	Elevated plaque

Classification/Grading

Cameron graded shield ulcer based on its clinical appearance **(Table 1)**.[3] Grade 1 shield ulcer is characterized by a transparent base. Grade 2 ulcers have a translucent ulcer base with or without yellow–white deposits. Grade 3 ulcers have an elevated plaque.

Differential Diagnosis

- Infective keratitis
- Neurotrophic ulcer

Work-up

History

The patient gives a history of chronic ocular irritation, foreign body sensation, itching, watering, and photophobia with seasonal aggravation of these symptoms.

Examination

On examination, the ulcer is usually hexagonal or oval in shape located in the superior half of the cornea. Its edges are well-defined and have a transparent base in stage 1. Grayish white deposits are noted at its base in stage 2 ulcer while an elevated plaque is noted in stage 3 ulcer.

Investigations

The diagnosis of shield ulcer is based on clinical examination. However, in cases where secondary infective keratitis is suspected corneal scraping is performed and sample is evaluated for microscopic examination (Gram stain and 10% potassium hydroxide (KOH) wet mount) as well as culture sensitivity testing (blood agar and Sabouraud dextrose agar).

Management

The goal while treating any case of shield ulcer is as follows:[4]
- *Promote rapid re-epithelialization:* This is achieved by medical management of VKC to reduce the inflammatory mediators released in these cases.
- *Prevent mechanical trauma to ulcer by the papillae:* This is done by medical management and control of VKC with amniotic membrane transplant to cover and protect the ulcer site.
- *Provide a healthy environment for the epithelium to heal:* Debridement of the corneal plaque is done to remove the toxic inflammatory mediators along with amniotic membrane graft to prevent further exposure of the ulcer site. The treatment algorithm for the management of shield ulcer has been highlighted in **Flowchart 1**.

Nonsurgical Management

Grade 1 ulcers, those with clear base and margin, respond well to medical therapy alone. These cases are given the following treatment:
- *Preservative-free antibiotic (preferably a 4th generation fluoroquinolone):* It is added to avoid secondary infective keratitis.
- *Mast cell stabilizers:* It inhibits degranulation of mast cells and thereby the release of inflammatory mediators. The drugs that belong to this class include sodium cromoglycate (QID), lodoxamide (QID), nedocromil (BD), and pemirolast (QID).
- *Antihistaminic:* Emedastine and levocabastine (0.05%) are topical H_1 receptor antagonist used for controlling signs and symptoms of VKC.
- *Dual action drug:* It acts both as an H_1 receptor blocker and mast-cell stabilizer. Olopatadine, epinastine, ketotifen, and azelastine belong to this class of drug. It is used in BD dosing. Among all these, olopatadine (0.1%) is the most commonly

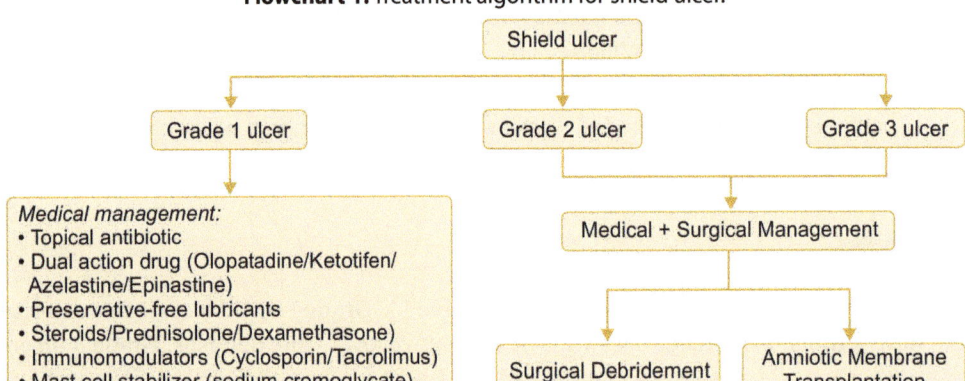

Flowchart 1: Treatment algorithm for shield ulcer.

used medication. In addition to its H_1 receptor blocking and mast cell stabilizer activity, it also inhibits the release of tumor necrosis factor alpha (TNF-α) and other cytokines released by the conjunctival epithelial cells. Therefore it is more effective in controlling the allergic inflammatory process when compared to other antiallergic medication. It also decreases the goblet cell density in the conjunctiva and thereby the mucoid discharge.

- *Corticosteroids:* This is the mainstay of treatment in cases of active VKC with shield ulcer. However, judicious use of this medication is recommended as its prolonged use can result in steroid-induced glaucoma, cataract and also increased susceptibility to viral and fungal infections. The drugs that are commonly used include prednisolone phosphate, loteprednol etabonate, fluorometholone, and rimexolone. Also, supratarsal injection of corticosteroids (dexamethasone sodium succinate, triamcinolone acetonide, and hydrocortisone sodium succinate) is given in cases of refractory VKC, although it results in only temporary cessation of symptoms.
- *Immunomodulators:* Cyclosporine A, a calcineurin inhibitor, is the most commonly used agent for immunomodulation in cases of active VKC. It acts on both cell-mediated and humoral immune response. It blocks the proliferation of Th2 lymphocyte and IL-2 production. Also, it inhibits the release of histamine by reducing IL-5 production.[5] Cyclosporine 2% is recommended when treating cases of shield ulcer in QID dosing which is later reduced to cyclosporine 0.05% BD dose after healing of ulcer occurs. Any recurrence of shield ulcer is managed by increasing the strength of cyclosporine.[6,7] It is not only effective as a steroid-sparing agent but also works well in recalcitrant cases of shield ulcer not responding to topical steroids.[6] Transient ocular irritation is noted after instillation of this medication.

    Topical tacrolimus, a calcineurin inhibitor, is also used for immunomodulation in cases of VKC and shield ulcer. Like cyclosporine A, tacrolimus also acts via inhibition of T-cell activation that reduces the IL2 production. It also reduces the histamine release.[8] Few long-term studies have shown that tacrolimus 0.1% alone, without topical steroids, can promptly heal corneal epitheliopathy and shield ulcers.[9] Transient burning sensation is the most common ocular adverse effect noted with this drug.[10]
- *Lubricants:* Frequent preservative free-lubricants are used to aid epithelial healing as well as dilute the inflammatory mediators in cases of VKC.
- *Antimetabolite:* Use of mitomycin C has also been described in VKC, though its role still remains controversial. It decreases the fibroblast proliferation, mucous secretion, hyperemia, and limbal edema in cases of severe VKC refractory to topical steroids.[11,12] It is used as mitomycin C 0.01% TDS for 2 weeks. Long-term studies are, however, needed to assess its adverse effect on the ocular surface.

Surgical Management

Grade 2 and 3 ulcers usually require a combination therapy of both medical and surgical management for rapid recovery. An immunofluorescence study has demonstrated the presence of eosinophilic granule MBP in the inflammatory debris recovered from the inflammatory debris of patients with shield ulcer.[13,14] It stimulates the release of histamine, activates neutrophils, and also prevents reepithelialization. Therefore, surgical debridement of the debris deposited at the base of shield ulcer is essential to aid rapid healing of shield ulcer.

- *Surgical debridement:* The procedure is performed under topical anesthesia for adults while children may require general anesthesia. Under aseptic conditions, an eyelid speculum is placed and a 15 no. blade or a crescent surgical blade is used to scrape the base of the ulcer under slit-lamp or microscope-guided examination. The thick plaque is first removed following which a firm crusty layer adherent to the underlying cornea, often noted in grade 3 shield ulcer, is then removed.[14,15] Superficial keratectomy may be required in cases where dense adhesion is noted between the plaque and cornea and no surgical plane for dissection is noted. Some authors have also described the use of excimer laser phototherapeutic keratectomy for smoothening of ocular surface and removal of residual inflammatory deposit.[16]

- *Amniotic membrane transplantation:* Prevention of further exposure to inflammatory mediators is pertinent to help rapid healing of the ulcer. The entire corneal surface is covered with an amniotic membrane with epithelium side down and stromal side up. The edges of amniotic membrane are sutured with interrupted 8-0 vicryl suture at a distance of 2–3 mm from the limbus. Some authors prefer to apply a bandage contact lens after this, though it is not absolutely necessary.[4,14,15,17] The basement membrane of the amniotic membrane provides a scaffold for migration of the corneal epithelium. Also, it reinforces the adhesion of basal epithelial cells, promotes differentiation of the epithelial cells, and prevents epithelial apoptosis. In addition, it provides multiple growth factors (basic fibroblast growth factor, hepatocyte growth factor, and transforming growth factor-β) which help in epithelial healing.[17]

Studies have shown that corneal plaques that were treated, only medical management required longer time to re-epithelize compared to eyes that were primarily treated with surgical debridement and amniotic membrane transplantation.[3]

Complications

Microbial Keratitis

All cases of shield ulcer whether they undergo medical or surgical treatment undergo reepithelialization; however, the duration of healing is much prolonged in grade 2 and 3 ulcers that are treated with medical management only. The prolonged time for re-epithelialization as well as the use of steroids that alter the natural microbial flora of eye increases the risk of microbial keratitis. Both fungal and bacterial keratitis have been reported in cases of shield ulcer.[18,19]

Corneal Perforation

Severe VKC with shield ulcer not treated appropriately in time may also result in devastating complication such as corneal perforation.[20]

Corneal Scarring

The ulcer heals with eventual corneal scar formation that may interfere with the best-corrected visual acuity of the patient.[21]

Glaucoma and Cataract

The long-term use of steroid in these eyes to control the inflammation can result in secondary glaucoma as well as steroid induced cataract, both of which further compromise the patients best-corrected visual acuity. The patient may require surgery for both these conditions on follow-up.[4]

Limbal Stem Cell Deficiency

Chronic ongoing inflammation in cases of severe VKC can lead to damage of the limbal stem cells by the toxic mediators. This results in partial or total limbal stem cell deficiency in these cases resulting in diffuse corneal haze and vascularization.[4]

Conclusion

Shield ulcer is a rare complication of VKC, which if managed appropriately can result in rapid healing. Often a combination of both medical and surgical management is required for optimal outcomes.

Key Points

- Primary cause is chemical instead of mechanical.
- Steroids and Lubricants are the treatment of choice.
- AMG is useful in cases with plaque formation.
- Superior quadrant of corneal location is characterictic but can occur in any quadrant.
- Most cases resolve with formation of a nebulo-macular opacity.

Key Points

- Primary cause is chemical instead of mechanical.
- Steroids and Lubricants are the treatment of choice.
- AMG is useful in cases with plaque formation.

- Superior quadrant of corneal location is characterictic but can occur in any quadrant.
- Most cases resolve with formation of a nebulo-macular opacity.

References

1. Kumar S. Vernal keratoconjunctivitis: a major review. Acta Ophthalmol. 2009;87(2):133-47.
2. Neumann E, Gutmann MJ, Blumenkrantz N, Michaelson IC. A review of four hundred cases of vernal conjunctivitis. Am J Ophthalmol. 1959;47(2):166-72.
3. Cameron JA. Shield ulcers and plaques of the cornea in vernal keratoconjunctivitis. Ophthalmology. 1995;102(6):985-93.
4. Reddy JC, Basu S, Saboo US, Murthy SI, Vaddavalli PK, Sangwan VS. Management, clinical outcomes, and complications of shield ulcers in vernal keratoconjunctivitis. Am J Ophthalmol. 2013;155(3):550-9.e1.
5. Farrell AM, Antrobus P, Simpson D, Powell S, Chapel HM, Ferry BL. A rapid flow cytometric assay to detect CD4+ and CD8+ T-helper (Th) 0, Th1 and Th2 cells in whole blood and its application to study cytokine levels in atopic dermatitis before and after cyclosporin therapy. Br J Dermatol. 2001;144(1):24-33.
6. Cetinkaya A, Akova YA, Dursun D, Pelit A. Topical cyclosporine in the management of shield ulcers. Cornea. 2004;23(2):194-200.
7. Ebihara N, Ohashi Y, Uchio E, Okamoto S, Kumagai N, Shoji J, et al. A large prospective observational study of novel cyclosporine 0.1% aqueous ophthalmic solution in the treatment of severe allergic conjunctivitis. J Ocul Pharmacol Ther. 2009;25(4):365-72.
8. Vichyanond P, Kosrirukvongs P. Use of cyclosporine A and tacrolimus in treatment of vernal keratoconjunctivitis. Curr Allergy Asthma Rep. 2013;13(3):308-14.
9. Miyazaki D, Fukushima A, Ohashi Y, Ebihara N, Uchio E, Okamoto S, et al. Steroid-sparing effect of 0.1% tacrolimus eye drop for treatment of shield ulcer and corneal epitheliopathy in refractory allergic ocular diseases. Ophthalmology. 2017;124(3):287-94.
10. Fukushima A, Ohashi Y, Ebihara N, Uchio E, Okamoto S, Kumagai N, et al. Therapeutic effects of 0.1% tacrolimus eye drops for refractory allergic ocular diseases with proliferative lesion or corneal involvement. Br J Ophthalmol. 2014;98(8):1023-7.
11. Jain AK, Sukhija J. Low dose mitomycin-C in severe vernal keratoconjunctivitis: a randomized prospective double blind study. Indian J Ophthalmol. 2006;54(2):111-6.
12. Akpek EK, Hasiripi H, Christen WG, Kalayci D. A randomized trial of low-dose, topical mitomycin-C in the treatment of severe vernal keratoconjunctivitis. Ophthalmology. 2000;107(2):263-9.
13. Trocmé SD, Kephart GM, Bourne WM, Buckley RJ, Gleich GJ. Eosinophil granule major basic protein deposition in corneal ulcers associated with vernal keratoconjunctivitis. Am J Ophthalmol. 1993;115(5):640-3.
14. Solomon A, Zamir E, Levartovsky S, Frucht-Pery J. Surgical management of corneal plaques in vernal keratoconjunctivitis: a clinicopathologic study. Cornea. 2004;23(6):608-12.
15. Lin HY, Yeh PT, Shiao CS, Hu FR. Surgical management and immunohistochemical study of corneal plaques in vernal keratoconjunctivitis. J Formos Med Assoc. 2013;112(9):569-73.
16. Cameron JA, Antonios SR, Badr IA. Excimer laser phototherapeutic keratectomy for shield ulcers and corneal plaques in vernal keratoconjunctivitis. J Refract Surg. 1995;11(1):31-5.
17. Sridhar MS, Sangwan VS, Bansal AK, Rao GN. Amniotic membrane transplantation in the management of shield ulcers of vernal keratoconjunctivitis. Ophthalmology. 2001;108(7):1218-22.
18. Jain V, Mhatre K, Nair AG, Shome D, Natarajan S. Aspergillus keratitis in vernal shield ulcer: a case report and review. Int Ophthalmol. 2010;30(6):641-4.
19. Gedik S, Akova YA, Gür S. Secondary bacterial keratitis associated with shield ulcer caused by vernal conjunctivitis. Cornea. 2006;25(8):974-6.
20. Buckley RJ. Vernal keratopathy and its management. Trans Ophthalmol Soc UK. 1981;101(Pt. 2):234-8.
21. Solomon A. Corneal complications of vernal keratoconjunctivitis. Curr Opin Allergy Clin Immunol. 2015;15(5):489-94.

8.12 Toxic Anterior Segment Syndrome

Pranita Sahay, Prafulla Kumar Maharana

 1. Write a short note on toxic anterior segment syndrome.

Introduction

Toxic anterior segment syndrome (TASS) is an acute, sterile, postoperative inflammatory condition of the anterior segment characterized by limbus-to-limbus corneal edema and fibrinous reaction in anterior chamber.[1] The term TASS was coined by Monson et al. in 1992.[1] The incidence of TASS postcataract surgery has been reported to be 0.22–0.8%.[2,3] It occurs most commonly after cataract surgery, though it can occur after any surgery of the anterior segment.[1,4-6] Acute inflammation of the anterior segment is thought to occur due to substances that enter the eye during or immediately after the surgery and cause damage to the intraocular structures. The greatest concern with this entity is that it tends to occur in clusters, which needs to be thoroughly investigated to prevent such complications in other patients.

Etiology

Corneal endothelium is extremely sensitive to any substance that enters the eye. Various factors implicated in causing TASS are described in **Box 1**.

Intraocular Irrigating Solution

Intraocular irrigating solutions such as balanced salt solution (BSS) are most commonly implicated in cases of TASS. Incorrect ionic composition, osmolarity, and pH of the solution can lead to intraocular inflammation and endothelial cell damage.[7] Also, medications such as epinephrine and antibiotic (gentamicin/vancomycin) added to the irrigating solution can add to the problem. It is important to ensure that there is no contamination of the solution with bacterial endotoxins. Such contamination of BSS can result in cluster cases of TASS, as was noted in United States of America in 2005 wherein 112 cases of TASS occurred due to endotoxin contamination of BSS.[8]

> **BOX 1:** Factors implicated in etiology of toxic anterior segment syndrome (TASS).
>
> *Intraocular irrigating solutions:*
> Incomplete chemical composition
> Incorrect pH
> Incorrect osmolality
> Preservatives or additives (e.g., antibiotics, dilating medications)
>
> *Intraocular medications:*
> Epinephrine
> Pilocarpine
> Trypan blue
> Antibiotics
> Lidocaine
>
> *Ophthalmic viscoelastic device*—denatured OVD
>
> *Ophthalmic instrument contaminants:*
> Detergent residues (soaps, enzymatic cleaners)
> Bacterial lipopolysaccharides or other endotoxin residues
> Metal ion residues (copper and iron)
> Denatured OVDs
>
> *Intraocular lenses:*
> Polishing compounds
> Cleaning and sterilizing compounds
>
> (OVD: ophthalmic viscoelastic device)

Intraocular Drugs and Preservatives

Various drugs used intraocularly for ocular anesthesia, mydriasis, and miosis can directly or indirectly lead to TASS due to either the drug itself or its preservative/stabilizing agent.

Epinephrine

Epinephrine contains bisulfite and metabisulfite as stabilizing agents to keep it in the reduced state. Even these stabilizing agents are implicated in causing inflammatory damage to the endothelial cell as well as other structures of the anterior segment.[9,10] So, it is advisable to use these medications without these stabilizing agents.

Pilocarpine

Use of intracameral pilocarpine has also been implicated as a cause for TASS.

Trypan Blue

Use of generic trypan blue 0.06% has been associated with acute anterior segment inflammatory reaction in few cases. Cell culture studies have revealed generic trypan blue dye to be twice as toxic as proprietary trypan blue.[11,12]

Antibiotics

Various intraocular antibiotics are used by ophthalmologists to reduce the risk of postoperative endophthalmitis. Most commonly used agents are cefuroxime, vancomycin, and moxifloxacin. Anterior segment inflammation may be caused by the drug itself, its preservatives, abnormal pH, or osmolality.[13] Cefuroxime 1 mg/0.1 mL and preservative-free moxifloxacin 500 µg/0.1 mL are relatively safe if used in appropriate dose.

Anesthetic Agents

Intracameral lidocaine 2% is used by many surgeons to supplement topical anesthesia. Preservative-free lidocaine used at a concentration higher than 2% has been known to cause TASS. Therefore, it is important to use intracameral lidocaine which is not only preservative free but also of correct dose.[14]

Ophthalmic Viscoelastic Devices

Ophthalmic viscoelastic devices (OVDs) if retained in large amount in the anterior chamber can induce ocular inflammation. Also, denatured OVD present in reusable cannulas, tips, and handpiece that have not been adequately flushed postsurgical use can induce severe inflammatory reaction when injected into the patient's eye. The denatured OVD is the site for retaining detergent and enzymes while cleaning these instruments further increasing the risk of TASS.[15-17] Therefore, it is important to flush all reusable cannulas and tips immediately after use.

Cleaning and Sterilization of Instruments

Residue of detergents and enzymes used for cleaning of instruments may result in TASS. The ultrasound bath used for cleaning of bath is a source for contamination with gram-negative organism. Though these organisms are inactivated during autoclaving the released endotoxin remains stable and can induce severe inflammatory reaction.[18]

Clinical Features

Symptoms

Patients with TASS usually present within 12–48 hours of surgery with complaints of blurred vision. Pain is usually absent in these cases.

Signs

The clinical features of TASS are as follows:
- *Diffuse corneal edema:* It is classically described as "limbus-to-limbus" corneal edema. The diffuse corneal edema represents widespread corneal endothelial cell damage.
- *Fibrinous reaction in anterior chamber:* This occurs due to widespread breakdown of the blood–aqueous barrier.
- *Hypopyon:* It may result due to settling down of the inflammatory cells in the lower part of anterior chamber.
- *Iris stromal thinning with or without fixed and dilated pupil:* Inflammatory damage to the iris tissue may result in the above changes.
- *Secondary glaucoma:* Inflammatory damage to the trabecular meshwork may result in secondary glaucoma.
- Posterior segment remains uninvolved.

Differential Diagnosis

Endophthalmitis is the most important differential diagnosis of TASS.[19,20] Therefore, it is important to make a proper diagnosis to initiate appropriate treatment in time. The differentiating features between endophthalmitis and TASS have been illustrated in **Table 1**.

Work-up

History

The patient usually gives history of recent ocular surgery (within 1–3 days). The primary complaint of the patient is blurred vision or mild diminution of vision. Pain is usually absent.

Examination

On examination the following features are observed:
- Mild reduction of visual acuity
- Raised intraocular pressure
- "Limbus-to-limbus" corneal edema
- Anterior chamber reaction—fibrinous membrane, hypopyon
- Absence of vitritis
- Fixed dilated pupil with iris stromal thinning in late stage.

Investigations

In the presence of severe corneal edema, clinical assessment of posterior segment may become difficult. Ultrasound B scan may be performed to rule out presence of vitritis. In the presence of vitritis, vitreous tap may be performed and sample is subjected to microscopic examination and culture-sensitivity testing.

Management

As prevention is better than cure, it is essential that the entire surgical team is aware of factors that can lead to this condition and thereby take preventive measures to prevent its occurrence. Staff involved in cleaning and sterilization of instruments

TABLE 1: Differentiating features of endophthalmitis and toxic anterior segment syndrome (TASS).

Clinical features	Endophthalmitis	TASS
Pathology	Infective etiology	Sterile inflammatory reaction to toxic agents used during surgery
Onset	3–7 days after surgery	1–3 days after surgery
Occurrence in clusters	Sporadic	Presents in outbreaks
Visual acuity	Severe diminution of vision	Mild-to-moderate diminution of vision
Elevated IOP	Uncommon	Common
Pain	Present (25% have no pain)	None or mild to moderate
Lid swelling	Present	Usually absent
Conjunctival chemosis and congestion	Present	Absent
Corneal edema	Mild edema	Limbus to limbus corneal edema
Anterior chamber reaction	• Cells are usually 3+ • Fibrinous reaction is variable	• Cells are 1+ to 3+ • Fibrinous reaction is present
Hypopyon	Present	Present
Pupil	Circular, reactive	Mydriasis, anisocoria (usually observed in late stage)
Vitritis	Present	Absent
Vitreous tap	Positive cultures	Sterile
Response to steroids	Poor	Good
Response to antibiotics	Good	Poor
Prognosis	Poor	Usually good

(IOP: intraocular pressure)

should take special care to avoid any toxic residues over the instrument. Also, those involved in preparation of drugs for intracameral use should be aware of the appropriate concentration of the drugs. The use of reusable instruments should be minimal.[18]

Medical Management

Treatment with topical steroid remains the mainstay for treatment of TASS. Prednisolone acetate 1% is used 1 hourly for the first 3–4 days followed by gradual tapering. Use of intraocular steroids and anterior chamber wash, though have been tried by some researchers, its definite role has yet not been proven. Also, anterior chamber wash itself increases the risk of infection.

Surgical Management

Surgical management in the form of endothelial or penetrating keratoplasty is required for cases with persistent corneal edema despite maximum treatment.

Complications

The following complications can occur post TASS:[21]
- Persistence of corneal edema due to endothelial decompensation.
- Secondary glaucoma—resulting from trabecular meshwork damage and peripheral anterior synechiae formation due to severe inflammation.
- Fixed dilated pupil—resulting from damage to the iris stromal tissue due to severe inflammation.

Prognosis

The prognosis of patients with TASS depends upon the severity of the condition and promptness in diagnosis and management. Patients with mild inflammation show good response to steroid therapy with rapid clearing of the cornea (days to weeks). Patients with moderate inflammation take a longer time for the cornea to clear (weeks to months) with slight residual corneal edema. Patients with severe TASS result in permanent damage like persistent corneal edema requiring corneal transplant.[22] Secondary glaucoma in these cases is usually resistant to medical therapy and requires surgical management such as trabeculectomy or shunt surgery.

Key Points

- TASS is an inflammatory phenomena.
- Exact cause is difficult to find.
- Good OT sterilization and cleaning practices often avoids TASS.
- Treatment of choice is steroids.
- Any inflammation in the post-operative period of cataract surgery, endophthalmitis must be ruled out.

References

1. Monson MC, Mamalis N, Olson RJ. Toxic anterior segment inflammation following cataract surgery. J Cataract Refract Surg. 1992;18(2):184-9.
2. Sengupta S, Chang DF, Gandhi R, Kenia H, Venkatesh R. Incidence and long-term outcomes of toxic anterior segment syndrome at Aravind Eye Hospital. J Cataract Refract Surg. 2011;37(9):1673-8.
3. Ozcelik ND, Eltutar K, Bilgin B. Toxic anterior segment syndrome after uncomplicated cataract surgery. Eur J Ophthalmol. 2010;20(1):106-14.
4. Cetinkaya S, Dadaci Z, Aksoy H, Acir NO, Yener HI, Kadioglu E. Toxic anterior-segment syndrome (TASS). Clin Ophthalmol Auckl NZ. 2014;8:2065-9.
5. Sevimli N, Karadag R, Cakici O, Bayramlar H, Okumus S, Sari U. Toxic anterior segment syndrome following deep anterior lamellar keratoplasty. Arq Bras Oftalmol. 2016;79(5):330-2.
6. Maier P, Birnbaum F, Böhringer D, Reinhard T. Toxic anterior segment syndrome following penetrating keratoplasty. Arch Ophthalmol. 2008;126(12):1677-81.
7. Parikh CH, Edelhauser HF. Ocular surgical pharmacology: corneal endothelial safety and toxicity. Curr Opin Ophthalmol. 2003;14(4):178-85.
8. Kutty PK, Forster TS, Wood-Koob C, Thayer N, Nelson RB, Berke SJ, et al. Multistate outbreak of toxic anterior segment syndrome, 2005. J Cataract Refract Surg. 2008;34(4):585-90.
9. Bodnar Z, Clouser S, Mamalis N. Toxic anterior segment syndrome: update on the most common causes. J Cataract Refract Surg. 2012;38(11):1902-10.
10. Myers WG, Edelhauser HF. Shortage of bisulfite-free preservative-free epinephrine for intracameral use. J Cataract Refract Surg. 2011;37(3):611.
11. Matsou A, Tzamalis A, Chalvatzis N, Mataftsi A, Tsinopoulos I, Brazitikos P. Generic trypan blue as possible cause of a cluster of toxic anterior segment syndrome cases after uneventful cataract surgery. J Cataract Refract Surg. 2017;43(6):848-52.
12. Buzard K, Zhang J-R, Thumann G, Stripecke R, Sunalp M. Two cases of toxic anterior segment syndrome from generic trypan blue. J Cataract Refract Surg. 2010;36(12):2195-9.
13. Braga-Mele R, Chang DF, Henderson BA, Mamalis N, Talley-Rostov A, Vasavada A. Intracameral antibiotics: safety, efficacy, and preparation. J Cataract Refract Surg. 2014;40(12):2134-42.
14. Bielory BP, Shariff A, Hussain RM, Bermudez-Magner JA, Dubovy SR, Donaldson KE. Toxic anterior segment syndrome: inadvertent administration of intracameral lidocaine 1% and phenylephrine 2.5% preserved with 10% benzalkonium chloride during cataract surgery. Cornea. 2017;36(5):621-4.
15. Altıntaş AK, Ciritoğlu MY, Beyazyıldız Ö, Can ÇÜ, Polat S. Toxic anterior segment syndrome outbreak after cataract surgery triggered by viscoelastic substance. Middle East Afr J Ophthalmol. 2017;24(1):43-7.
16. Althomali TA. Viscoelastic substance in prefilled syringe as an etiology of toxic anterior segment syndrome. Cutan Ocul Toxicol. 2016;35(3):237-41.
17. Kim JH. Intraocular inflammation of denatured viscoelastic substance in cases of cataract extraction and lens implantation. J Cataract Refract Surg. 1987;13(5):537-42.
18. Cutler Peck CM, Brubaker J, Clouser S, Danford C, Edelhauser HE, Mamalis N. Toxic anterior segment syndrome: common causes. J Cataract Refract Surg. 2010;36(7):1073-80.
19. Mamalis N, Edelhauser HF, Dawson DG, Chew J, LeBoyer RM, Werner L. Toxic anterior segment syndrome. J Cataract Refract Surg. 2006;32(2):324-33.
20. Lee MH, Cugley D, Atik A, Ang GS. Endophthalmitis or toxic anterior segment syndrome. Clin Exp Optom. 2017;100(1):94-5.
21. Mamalis N, Edelhauser HF, Dawson DG, Chew J, LeBoyer RM, Werner L. Toxic anterior segment syndrome. J Cataract Refract Surg. 2006;32(2):324-33.
22. Kaur M, Titiyal JS, Falera R, Arora T, Sharma N. Outcomes of descemet stripping automated endothelial keratoplasty in toxic anterior segment syndrome after phacoemulsification. Cornea. 2017;36(1):17-20.

8.13 Ectatic Disorders of the Cornea

Nagesh BN, Dhwni Shahanand, Vineeta Pai

 1. Describe peripheral corneal thinning disorders and their management.

Peripheral corneal thinning disorders are characterized by thinning of peripheral corneal stroma within 1–2 mm from the limbus. Peripheral thinning may affect vision by inducing irregular astigmatism or by centripetal progression of the disease process and finally involving the visual axis. Peripheral corneal thinning disorders are not well defined and include varied groups of disorders with different underlying causes.

Pellucid marginal degeneration (PMD) is a painless, progressive, often bilateral, noninflammatory, peripheral ectatic disorder characterized by 1–2 mm zone of thinning in the inferior cornea. The area of thinning is 1–2 mm away from the limbus and mostly extends from 4 to 8 o'clock position. Maximum corneal ectasia occurs superior to the area of thinning. Vision loss is mainly due to high, irregular, against-the-rule astigmatism.

Terrien's marginal degeneration (TMD) is a painless, asymmetric, bilateral peripheral corneal thinning disorder that affects the superior cornea initially. Vascularization and lipid deposition are classical features, even though the condition is predominantly noninflammatory and nonulcerative. Slow, circumferential progression can lead to irregular against the rule astigmatism.

Senile furrow degeneration is characterized by shallow thinning of peripheral cornea between arcus senilis and limbus. It is usually seen in the elderly and visually insignificant.

Dellen are saucer-like depressions that occur due to desiccation of tear film in a localized area of cornea adjacent to conjunctival elevation at the limbus. Pterygium, limbal tumors, filtering blebs, chemosis, thyroid ophthalmopathy, subconjunctival hemorrhages, and rigid gas permeable (RGP) lenses, after cataract surgery, have been noted to cause dellen formation.

Peripheral ulcerative keratitis (PUK) (Mooren's ulcer) is a crescent-shaped, ulcerative destruction of the peripheral cornea with the involvement of adjacent sclera. Thinning can lead to perforation sometimes and can be often due to underlying systemic connective tissue disorders such as rheumatoid arthritis. Mooren's ulcer is essentially an idiopathic form of PUK with painful ulceration with overhanging edges **(Table 1)**.

TABLE 1: Differential diagnosis of peripheral corneal thinning disorders.

	Pellucid marginal degeneration	**Terrien's marginal degeneration**	**Mooren's ulcer**	**Furrow degeneration**
Age at onset	10–50 years	35–60 years	After 50 years	Elderly
Eye involved	Bilateral	Bilateral	Unilateral or bilateral	Bilateral
Gender	No gender predisposition	Male preponderance	Male preponderance	No gender predisposition
Astigmatism	Common	Common	Sometimes	None
Area of thinning	Inferior cornea 1–2 mm from limbus	Starts superiorly and can extend circumferentially	Within palpebral fissure but can extend	Within arcus
Inflammation	Absent	Rare	Typical; worse in bilateral type	Absent
Epithelial defect	Absent	Usually none	Typical	Absent
Vascularization	Absent	Crosses areas of thinning	Peripheral edge of thinning	Absent
Lipid deposition	Absent	Common; central to thinning	Not acutely	Corneal arcus
Perforation	Hydrops more common	Unusual	Common in bilateral ulcer	Never

Other causes of peripheral corneal thinning are as follows:
- *Postsurgical peripheral corneal melts*—following surgeries for pterygium, limbal dermoid, ocular surface squamous neoplasia (OSSN), etc.
- *Catarrhal marginal ulcer*—hypersensitivity to staphylococcal antigens leading to peripheral ulceration
- *Miscellaneous conditions* such as exposure keratopathy, keratoconjunctivitis sicca, and neurotrophic ulcers.

Management

Ocular Investigations

- *Corneal topography:* Pentacam, Orbscan, Galilei dual Scheimpflug, etc.
  Pellucid marginal degeneration will have asymmetric, against-the-rule astigmatism and inferior peripheral steepening covering an island of relatively flat cornea giving a typical crab-claw appearance. Thinning of the peripheral cornea can be noted. TMD will have asymmetric, but with the rule of astigmatism it will have superior steepening and thinning. All others can show irregular astigmatism.
- *Anterior segment optical coherence tomography (ASOCT):* It can detect peripheral corneal thinning in all these disorders. PMD can show beer belly appearance in vertical scans. Scarring at different levels of stroma is appreciated and so is Descemet's membrane (DM) scarring of healed hydrops. Detection of previous perforations and corneo-iridic adhesions helps in planning surgery appropriately.
- *Ultrasound biomicroscopy (UBM):* It can give valuable information about iris (peripheral anterior synechiae) and other anterior segment structures [intraocular lens (IOL)] if visibility is compromised by scarred cornea.
- *Corneal scraping:* If there is active ulceration, corneal scraping should be sent for microbiological assessment [Gram stain, potassium hydroxide (KOH), culture] to rule out infectious causes.

Systemic Investigations

Systemic investigations should include tests to detect systemic association in cases of PUK or Mooren's ulcer. Complete hemogram, erythrocyte sedimentation rate (ESR), antinuclear antibody (ANA) antigen, rheumatoid factor (RF) antigen, serum angiotensin-converting enzyme (ACE) levels, cytoplasmic antineutrophil cytoplasmic antibody (c-ANCA), hepatitis B surface antigen (HBsAg), etc.

Treatment can be conservative or surgical.

Conservative Management

Conservative management includes the following:

- Topical and systemic antibiotics in case of active ulcers such as PUK or Mooren's ulcer depending on corneal scraping reports
- Systemic collagenase inhibitors such as tetracycline to reduce corneal melt
- Topical and systemic steroids if there is no active infection
- Immunosuppressive therapy with cyclophosphamide, methotrexate, cyclosporine, etc. can be tried in PUK and Mooren's ulcer.
- Copious lubrication of cornea in case of dellen and furrow degeneration with irregular cornea
- Visual rehabilitation by spectacles helps only in the early stages of ectasias.
- Large-diameter RGP lenses can give good vision albeit poor long-term acceptance.
- Hybrid lenses have shown good visual gain and comfortable fitting in long-term use.
- Scleral lenses give the best possible visual rehabilitation and long-term tolerance.
- PROSE lens—a customized scleral lens developed by Boston group has shown promising results in peripheral ectasias.

Surgical Management

Indications

- Tectonic support—in patients with descemetocele or frank perforation
- Arresting progression of ectasia—in cases of PMD, TMD
- Visual rehabilitation—in patients with high, irregular astigmatism not improving with glasses or contact lens.

Surgical Techniques

Tissue adhesives—for small perforations of <2–3 mm or impending perforations in peripheral corneas in case of PUK, Mooren's ulcer, marginal keratitis, etc. Cyanoacrylic glue with or without a scaffold (small drape) is used to plug the hole till the perforation heals.

Amniotic membrane grafting (AMG): Amniotic membrane overlay can be used in early sterile melts post-pterygium excision or OSSN excision. Multilayer AMG can be used to give tectonic support and to prevent corneal transplantation in small perforations or impending perforations in the peripheral cornea.

Corneal collagen cross-linking with riboflavin (C3R): Various studies have proven the beneficial effects of C3R in arresting progression of ectasia and reducing astigmatism in PMD.

Intracorneal ring segments have been shown to improve uncorrected visual acuity (UCVA) and reduce corneal refractive power and astigmatism in patients with PMD. At least 450 μm of corneal thickness is needed at 6–9 mm diameter zone for the implantation of ring segments.

Peripheral lamellar keratoplasty: It is used to treat significant corneal thinning in cases of PMD, TMD, and PUK. Crescentic-shaped grafts are fashioned without DM and endothelium and sutured onto the peripheral area of thinning after removing epithelium. Tight compressive sutures with smaller graft sizes can also be used to flatten the central cornea.

Tuck-in lamellar keratoplasty (TILK): It is done in patients with coexisting keratoconus and PMD. In TILK, a central full-thickness graft without DM and endothelium and a peripheral 2–3 mm partial-thickness flange is sutured on to a host bed with peripheral flange buried into a groove created in stroma in thinned out peripheral cornea. Similar technique of peripheral corneal strengthening by tucking flange of donor tissue in peripheral cornea can be employed in full-thickness grafts also. It also helps in better graft–host apposition and reduces postkeratoplasty astigmatism.

Staged procedures: Initial peripheral crescentic lamellar keratoplasty is done to provide tectonic support, followed by central lamellar or penetrating keratoplasty (PK) at a later stage for visual rehabilitation.

Large-diameter keratoplasty: 9–10 mm diameter corneal grafts are done to remove peripheral thinned cornea for better graft–host approximation and lesser astigmatism but at the cost of increased risk of rejection and glaucoma. Endothelial keratoplasty after rejection of graft helps in long-term survival of such grafts.

2. **Discuss the etiology, pathogenesis, work-up, differential diagnosis, and management of keratoconus.**

Keratoconus is a condition in which noninflammatory thinning and protrusion of stroma propels the cornea to assume a conical shape. Although asymmetrical during presentation, keratoconus is mostly a bilateral disease. Maximum protrusion happens just below and nasal to the center of the cornea resulting in severe irregular astigmatism and significant vision loss.

Etiology

According to recent studies, eye rubbing is the single most important etiological factor responsible for keratoconus. Other causes can be long-term contact lens use, and collagen abnormalities are also implicated in the development of keratoconus. Several ocular and systemic diseases or syndromes are associated with the development of keratoconus **(Table 2)**.

TABLE 2: Few important systemic and ocular associations of keratoconus.

Systemic associations	Ocular associations
Down syndrome	Vernal keratoconjunctivitis
Ehlers–Danlos syndrome	Retinitis pigmentosa
Osteogenesis imperfecta	Leber's congenital amaurosis
Mitral valve prolapse	Retinopathy of prematurity
Floppy eyelid syndrome	Aniridia
Albinism	Fuchs' dystrophy
Congenital hip dysplasia	Granular and lattice dystrophy
Apert's and Crouzon's syndrome	Essential iris atrophy

Pathogenesis

Microtrauma to the Bowman's layer caused by eye rubbing and long-term contact lens use can lead to the downward proliferation of epithelial cells into stroma and projection of connective tissue anteriorly into epithelium causing Z-shaped interruptions in Bowman's layer. These epithelial cells produce interleukin-1, which disperses into stroma and acts on keratocytes whose cell membrane shows four times the normal interleukin-1 binding receptor because of upregulation. This interleukin-1 triggers apoptosis of stromal keratocytes. There is increased concentration of degradative lysosomal enzymes such as acid esterase, acid phosphatase, cathepsin B and G, and some matrix metalloproteinases. This results in increased destruction of intercellular matrix in stroma and reduced production of collagen and matrix leading progressive thinning of cornea. Pleomorphism and polymegathism of endothelial cells occur due to stretching of DM.

Clinical Work-up

History

Detailed history of onset of blurring of vision, any doubling of images, or shadowing is elicited. History of use of glasses and or contact lens is noted. Any frequent change in glass power or intolerance to contact lens wear is noted. A detailed history of associated allergic eye disorders, atopy, frequent eye rubbing, recurrent redness, and whitish discoloration along the limbus is elicited. Any history of ectatic disorder in a sibling or other family member should be noted. Frequent prone position during sleep is noted. A history of prolonged use of steroid therapy is noted. Any history suggestive of associated ocular and systemic conditions should be noted.

Visual Acuity

Mild to marked impairment can be expected according to the stage of the disorder. UCVA, best spectacle-corrected visual acuity, and contact lens trial with best contact lens-corrected visual acuity and the tolerance are all evaluated.

Retinoscopy

High irregular myopic astigmatism with scissoring reflex on retinoscopy is very typical in established keratoconus.

Direct Ophthalmoscopy

"Oil droplet" sign of Charleux is seen as a dark reflex at the region of the base of the cone in keratoconus.

Slit-lamp Biomicroscopy

Slit-lamp biomicroscopy reveals characteristic signs in keratoconus—thinning of the cornea, Fleischer's ring at the base of the cone in the corneal basal epithelium, prominent corneal nerves, deep stromal stress lines—Vogt's striae, and corneal scarring. To look for papillary reaction in lids, limbal follicles, and other signs of associated allergic eye diseases.

Other Signs of Keratoconus

Rizzuti's sign and Munson's sign are noted.

Corneal Hydrops

It results from stromal imbibition of aqueous through ruptures in DM at the apex of the cone. The edema may persist for weeks or months, diminishing gradually and eventually being replaced by deep stromal scarring.

Corneal pseudocysts or intrastromal clefts can be found in association with hydrops in keratoconus. Stromal neovascularization is common and can affect future graft survival.

Keratometry

The inability to superimpose central keratometric rings suggests irregular corneal astigmatism, a hallmark of keratoconus. Inferior corneal steepening is an early sign of keratoconus. A value of 47.2 D or greater is suggestive of keratoconus.

Fundus Evaluation

Fundus evaluation is done to look for signs of associated ocular conditions such as retinitis pigmentosa or any glaucomatous changes of disc due to long-term steroid use for allergic eye disease.

Anterior segment optical coherence tomography is done in cases of scarred cornea to assess the involvement of DM.

Corneal Topography

Corneal topography is done for keratometry, elevation, and thickness analysis. Pentacam, Orbscan-2, Galilei Dual Scheimpflug, etc. give comparable and repeatable measurements of the above parameters. There are various topographical criteria for the diagnosis of keratoconus. Steep keratometry, eccentric steepening, thinning of cornea corresponding to steepening, inferior–superior asymmetry, high irregular astigmatism, skewing of principle axis, and significant posterior elevation above the base curve are few of the topographical signs to look for in the diagnosis of keratoconus.

Differential Diagnosis

Keratoconus should be differentiated from other noninflammatory ectatic disorders such as keratoglobus, PMD, TMD, and posterior keratoconus **(Table 3)**.

TABLE 3: Differential diagnosis of keratoconus.

	Keratoconus	Keratoglobus	PMD	TMD
Age of onset	Second decade (puberty)	First decade	Second to fifth decade	Middle age to elderly
Frequency	Most common	Rare	Less common	Rare
Thinning	Central and paracentral cornea	Entire cornea involved	Inferior periphery	Superior periphery
Hereditary	At times	None	None	None
Corneal scarring	Common	Rare	Only after hydrops	In involved region
Maximum steepening	At the area of thinning	Entire cornea is steep	Superior to band of thinning	At the region of thinning
Iron line	Fleischer ring	None	Sometimes	Sometimes

Management

Arresting Progression of Keratoconus

Arresting progression of keratoconus is an important step in the management of keratoconus detected early and should be the first step in the management of a newly diagnosed keratoconus. By arresting progression, the need for keratoplasty in the future can be alleviated. Global Consensus on Keratoconus and Ectatic Diseases 2015 criteria for progressive keratoconus are two or more of the following over a period of 6 months:
- Steepening of the anterior corneal surface: Cornea apex power >1 D from baseline
- Steepest keratometry >1 D increase from baseline
- Flattest keratometry >1 D increase from baseline
- Mean keratometry >0.75 D increase
- Manifest spherical equivalent >0.5 D increase from baseline
- Thinning/increase in the rate of corneal thickness change >2% decrease from baseline.

There is only one surgery proven beyond doubt for arresting the progression of keratoconus, i.e., *corneal collagen crosslinking with riboflavin* [C3R/corneal cross-linking (CXL)/KXL].

In C3R, the cornea is soaked with 0.1% riboflavin (vitamin B2) solution followed by exposure to ultraviolet (UV)-A radiation with a total dose of 5.4 J/cm^2. UV radiation induces oxygen-free radical generation, which in turn activates lysyl oxidase (LOX) enzyme responsible for cross-linking between collagen fibers. C3R increases the overall strength of the cornea by 329% and prevents further ectasia. Should be done in all patients with recognized progression in keratoconus if thickness allows. CXL is also advocated in children younger than 18 years, with severe vernal keratoconjunctivitis (VKC) or atopy, syndromic associations such as Down syndrome, and collagen vascular disorders even without documented progression by few authors.

Visual Rehabilitation

Glasses

Glasses give good vision in early cases. A better option for children who cannot use contact lenses for various reasons. Irregular astigmatism in keratoconus can cause shadowing and doubling of images with glasses in moderate to advanced keratoconus. Vision is also suboptimal in eccentric cones.

Contact Lens

Contact lens is the mainstay of visual rehabilitation in patients with keratoconus as they completely replace the anterior refractive surface of the cornea and negates the effect of ectasia. Various types of lenses have been tried in keratoconus with varied results.

Conventional Hydrogel Lens

Conventional hydrogel lens can be used in early cones with little astigmatism, but drapes the cornea and molds to the shape of it. So not useful in astigmatism >2 D.

- *Silicone hydrogels:* Useful in early cones and astigmatism up to 5 D, has higher modulus, and so less drape
- *Torics:* In patients of early cones with regular astigmatism
- *Soft keratoconic designs:* Thicker centrally to mask irregular astigmatism, used in early to moderate cones
- *RGP multicurve:* In early to moderate cones. Individual lens parameters can be modified to enhance fit.
- *Aspheric RGP:* In moderate cases. Decentration can cause visual disturbances.
- *RGP keratoconic design:* Can add toric surfaces and can be customizable; used in moderate to advanced cones
- *Mini-sclerals, sclerals, and PROSE treatment:* In advanced cones, these lenses vault the apex and also prevent scarring and can add toric surfaces.
- *Hybrids and piggybacks:* In moderate to advanced cases, they give the comfort of soft lenses and vision of hard lenses. Higher *Dk* material is recommended.

Intracorneal Ring Segments (ICRS: INTACS, Keraring)

These are spacers implanted in the stroma of the cornea at 5–7 mm diameter area and at a depth of 70–80% thickness. They induce arc-shortening effect and reduce the height of the cones. Used either in combination with cross-linking or individually, they help in:

- Arresting the progression of keratoconus
- Reducing the overall power of the corneal surface by flattening
- Centralizing the eccentric cone and reducing irregular astigmatism
- Reducing the inferior peripheral lift of RGP lenses and restoring tolerance in these patients
- Reducing or postponing the need for keratoplasty in these patients.

Topography-guided Photorefractive Keratectomy

Topography-guided photorefractive keratectomy (TPRK) is a refractive procedure often combined with cross linking to reduce irregular astigmatism and to improve visual distortions with glasses in patients with early to moderate cones. The maximum ablation advocated is 50 μm and the procedure must aim at regularizing the surface and reducing irregularity rather than complete correction of refractive power. Some amount of superficial scarring can be seen after TPRK.

Phakic toric IOLs [implantable collamer lens (ICL)/implantable phakic contact lens (IPCL)] for correction of refractive error can be attempted in mild to moderate cones, which are stable topographically and/or underwent C3R for arresting progression. Patients who are intolerant to contact lens can also try phakic IOL implantation. Can correct astigmatism up to 4 D in the corneal plane and spherical power up to 20D. Vision is inferior to RGP lenses as irregular cornea remains in front of the lens but better than glasses due to the magnifying effect of phakic IOLs. Usual complications or phakic IOLs can happen in keratoconus patients also.

Anatomical Restoration

Anatomical restoration in the form of corneal transplantation should be reserved for advanced cases of keratoconus who cannot be fitted with contact lens and/or intolerant to it.

Penetrating keratoplasty is the traditional surgery of choice with 5-year graft survival rate of >90%. Graft and host cut can be kept the same to reduce postoperative myopia and flatten the cornea. Deep stromal scarring or involvement of DM or nonresolving hydrops is the main indication for PK. Risk of rejection is present though uncommon in keratoconus.

Anterior lamellar therapeutic keratoplasty (ALTK) is a microkeratome-assisted procedure in which the microkeratome of the required thickness (250–350 μm) is passed over both host cornea and donor cornea. The donor corneal button is placed on the host bed and sutured to provide tectonic support to the recipient cornea. Since both dissections in the host and donor corneas are done by microkeratome, the approximating surfaces are smooth and result in minimal or no interface haze. A minimum pachymetry of 450 μm is necessary for this procedure as perforation of the host cornea can occur as a complication.

Deep anterior lamellar keratoplasty (DALK) is the treatment of choice if there is no scarring involving DM. Dissection is done using air or viscoelastic substance to remove the entire stroma till DM or Dua's layer. Also gives a smooth interface and better flattening than ALTK. Perforation of DM can happen during surgery.

Lamellar keratoplasty reduces the risk of graft rejection, leads to early tapering of steroids, and reduces all complications associated with their use. Suture removal and visual rehabilitation with contact lens postsurgery can be done earlier than PK.

Tuck-in lamellar or penetrating keratoplasty (TILK/TIPK) can be done in patients with coexisting keratoconus and PMD or other peripheral-thinning disorder.

 3. Describe the optical principles and application of corneal topography. Discuss concepts of management of keratoconus.

Corneal topography refers to the computerized, video-assisted technique that provides detailed information about the shape of the cornea. Present-day technology provides a complete three-dimensional structure of the cornea with cross-sectional images and is hence referred to as corneal tomography systems.

Currently available tomographers use one or combinations of the following working principles.

Placido Disc Principle

It Works on the principle of reflection. The anterior surface of the cornea acts as a convex mirror and the size of the image formed is based on the curvature of the mirror (cornea). The steeper cornea produces a smaller image and the flatter cornea produces a larger image of the same object located at the same distance from the cornea.

The basic unit of a topography system consists of three parts:
1. *A projection device:* A placido disc system projects 8–32 concentric and numbered rings onto the cornea. The specified ring in different instruments covers different parts of the cornea.
2. *Video camera:* The reflected images of the projected objects (such as rings) are captured using charge-coupled device (CCD) camera. The precision and accuracy of the device are dependent on focusing, decentration, shadows or artifacts, and proper acquisition of images from the camera.
3. *Computer:* The acquired images are digitized and algorithms are used to determine the radius of curvature of the innermost ring. The radius of curvature of the next ring is calculated using the knowledge of the distance between two rings in the projected placido disc. Dioptric power is calculated using the following formula:

$$\text{Dioptric power} = \frac{\text{Refractive index of the cornea} - \text{Refractive index of air}}{\text{Radius of curvature in meters}}$$

The computer also generates the topographic map of the cornea based on analysis of all the points of assessment captured by the camera.

Slit-scanning Corneal Tomography System

It uses scanning slits that step over the corneal surface to acquire topographic information. In this principle, similar to slit lamp, an edge point on the corneal surface is triangulated by mathematically intersecting the diffuse reflected camera edge ray with the calibrated slit-beam surface. The two slit beams are at 45° angle to either side of the instrument axis. Twenty slit-beam images are captured from each direction with an overlap in the central 7 mm corneal area. This can capture accurately the posterior surface of the cornea along with the anterior surface and calculate the thickness of the cornea at different points.

Scheimpflug Imaging Principle

This is based on a geometric rule describing the orientation of the plane of focus of an optical system when the lens plane is not parallel to the image plane. An oblique tangent can be drawn from the image, object, and lens plane and the point of intersection is Scheimpflug point, where the image is in the best focus.

Optical Coherence Tomography-based Corneal Tomography

Optical coherence tomography-based corneal tomography is a method of cross-sectional scanning based on reflection and scattering of light from structures of the cornea. OCT works on the principle of low-coherence interferometry. A light is split into two beams, a reference beam and the reflected beam from eye structures. The delay in the back-reflected beam and its intensity are analyzed by superimposing it on the reference beam to know the depth at which the reflection has happened and thereby mapping the structures of the eye.

Digital Rasterstereography-based Topography System

Digital rasterstereography-based topography system uses a calibrated grid, which is projected onto the corneal surface stained with fluorescein dye and the diffuse reflection is recorded at two separate known angles.

Laser Holographic Interferometry

Laser holographic interferometry uses the optical technique of light-wave interference fringes as projection device **(Table 4)**.

TABLE 4: Currently available topographers and their working principles.

Commonly available topographers	Topographic principles
Tomey TMS-4M, EyeSys Desktop, CA-200F Corneal Analyzer	Placido disc/cone-based topography
Pentacam, Galilei G6, Sirius, Oculyzer, TMS-5, Preciso	Dual-Scheimpflug and placido disc imaging
Orbscan IIz	Dual horizontal slit scan and placido dick imaging
PAR corneal topography	Rasterstereography
Artemis 3	Very-high-frequency (VHF) ultrasound with ARC scanning
Visante Omni, SS-1000 Casia	Rotating optical coherence tomography and placido disc imaging
RTVue-100, 3D OCT 2000, Cirrus HD-OCT 5000	Spectral domain OCT
IOLMaster 700	Swept source OCT and placido disc imaging
Cornea lens analysis system (CLAS II)	Laser holographic interferometry

(OCT: optical coherence tomography)

Applications of Topography Systems

- Indispensable tool in the management of corneal ectasias:
  - Early diagnosis of corneal ectasias such as keratoconus, PMD, TMD, and keratoglobus
  - To determine progression by serial scans
  - To assess stabilization after treatments such as C3R
  - Contact lens fitting
- Helps in contact lens fitting in difficult cases such as advanced keratoconus and scarred corneas with irregular astigmatism
- Helps in orthokeratology
- *Prior to any keratorefractive surgery:*
  - For accurate measurements of corneal power
  - Prior to topography-guided ablation procedures
  - For the detection of forme fruste keratoconus (FFKC) as keratorefractive surgery is contraindicated in such conditions
  - To detect complications such as irregular ablation, decentration of ablation, etc.
  - Early diagnosis of post-LASIK ectasia
- *Following keratoplasty:*
  - Topography-guided removal of tight sutures to reduce astigmatism
  - Postkeratoplasty contact lens fitting
- Accurate IOL power calculation
- Latest topography systems give valuable information about the anterior chamber depth (ACD) and can be used to assess ACD prior to phakic IOL implantation.

Management of Keratoconus

Refer to Question 2.

 4. Corneal topography changes in keratoconus. How do you grade the severity of keratoconus?

Topography is an indispensable tool in the diagnosis and management of keratoconus.

The topographical changes in keratoconus are:
- *Keratometry:* Cornea becomes steep due to ectasia and the keratometric power increases. According to Rabinowitz–Mc Donnel criteria central keratometry (K_{max}) reading >47.2 D is indicative of keratoconus and >48.7 D is diagnostic of keratoconus. The difference between maximum keratometric values between two eyes if >1.9 D is also suggestive of keratoconus.
- *Skewing of radial axis:* >20° deviation of principal radial axis beyond the center is indicative of keratoconus.

- *Inferior–superior asymmetry (I–S ratio):* Because the maximum ectasia happens below and nasal to the center of the cornea, there is difference of keratometric power in the principle meridian. If the inferior keratometric power is greater by >1.4 D than superior, it is keratoconus suspect and >1.9 D is diagnostic of keratoconus.
- *Astigmatism:* Irregular astigmatism of asymmetric bow tie pattern is also a strong indicator of keratoconus. Astigmatism >2.5 D should raise suspicion of keratoconus.
- *Pachymetry:* Reduced thickness corresponding to the apex of cone is characteristic of keratoconus. It is difficult to predict at what thickness the ectasia occurs and what is the cutoff for the diagnosis of keratoconus. It is widely agreed that thickness <470 µm should raise alarms, especially if it corresponds to steep keratometry. Also, the difference between the thinnest pachymetry of >10 µm between both eyes needs evaluation.
- *Anterior and posterior elevation* above the base curve in elevation-based tomography charts may not be diagnostic of keratoconus per se, but helpful in the early detection of eyes having the risk of developing keratoconus. Both anterior and posterior elevations are increased in keratoconus. Anterior elevation >15 µm and posterior elevation >20 µm in Pentacam strongly suggests a diagnosis of keratoconus.

More often than not, any individual parameters above can lead to a false-negative or false-positive diagnosis of keratoconus. Certain indices are devised which incorporate two or more of these parameters for a more accurate diagnosis of keratoconus.

KISA index: KISA% index is usually applied to the axial map. It uses four indices on the topography.

$$\text{KISA\%} = \frac{(K) \times (\text{I-S}) \times (\text{AST}) \times (\text{SRAX}) \times 100}{100}$$

where K is the central keratometric value in excess of 47.2 D (i.e., $K - 47.2$), if value is ≤47.2, it is replaced by 1.

I–S is the inferior–superior asymmetry—difference between keratometry between superior and inferior cornea along vertical principle axis

AST is the difference between Sim K1 and SimK2.

SRAX is calculated from 180—the angle between two steep axis above and below the horizontal meridian (smaller of the two angles).

KISA% >100% is considered highly suggestive of keratoconus

Other indices devised are given in **Table 5.**

TABLE 5: Various indices for the diagnosis of keratoconus.

Rabinowitz and Mc Donnel	K-value and I–S value	47.2 D and 1.4 D	Diagnosis is performed based on the central keratometry and the inferior–superior asymmetry in keratometric power
Maeda et al.	KPI and KCI%	0.23 and 0%	KPI is derived from eight quantitative video keratography indexes KCI% is derived from KPI and other four indexes
Smolek and Klyce	KSI	0.25	Keratoconus detection and the level of severity are assessed using an artificial intelligent system
Schwiegerling and Greivenkamp	Z3	0.00233	Diagnosis is performed based on videokeratoscopic height data decomposed into orthogonal Zernike polynomials
Rabinowitz and Rasheed	KISA%	100%	Diagnosis is derived from K-value, I–S value, AST, and SRAX
Mc Mahon et al.	KSS	0.5	Diagnosis is performed based on slit-lamp findings, corneal topography, corneal power, and higher-order first corneal surface wavefront root mean square error
Mahmoud et al.	CLMI	>0.45	Diagnosis based on detecting the presence or absence of keratoconic patterns and determining the location and magnitude of the curvature of the cone

(CLMI: Cone Location and Magnitude Index; I–S: inferior–superior asymmetry; KCI: keratoconus index; KPI: keratoconus prediction index; KSI: keratoconus severity index; KSS: keratoconus severity score; SRAX: skewed radial axes)

Grading Severity of Keratoconus

Several grading systems have been devised to determine the severity of keratoconus.

Based on the Severity of Curvature
- Mild <45 D in both meridians
- Moderate 45–52 D in both meridians

- Advanced >52 D in both meridians
- Severe >62 D in both meridians

Based on Shape of Cone
- Nipple cone—small diameter (<5 mm), easiest to fit with contact lens
- Oval cone—large diameter (>5 mm)
- Globus cone—largest diameter (>6 mm), most difficult to fit with contact lens

Rabinowits–McDonnel Grading
- Keratoconus suspect—Maximum K >47.2 D
  Difference of K between two eyes <1.9
  I–S >1.4 D
- Keratoconus—Maximum K >48.7
  Difference of K between two eyes >1.9
  I–S >1.9

The Massachusetts Eye and Ear Infirmary Keratoconus Classification

The Massachusetts Eye and Ear Infirmary (MEEI) classification takes into account history, ocular and systemic association, clinical findings, as well as topographic features in grading severity of keratoconus. It can also be used in ruling out FFKC prior to keratorefractive surgery if advanced topographers are not available.

		Score			Score		
Kod-Kos	≥1.9	0			0	≤1.9	Kos-Kod
	>1.9	1			1	≤1.9	
Kod	<47.2	0			0	<47.2	Kod
	47.2–48.7	1			1	<47.2–48.7	
	>48.7	2			2	>48.7	
ISod	<1.4	0			0	>1.4	ISod
	1.4–1.9	1			1	>1.4–1.9	
	>1.9	2			2	>1.9	
≥2 Findings on hx (atopy, down), FH and exam (Fleisher, Vogt, Munson, nerves, scarring)	No	0			0	No	≥2 Findings on hx hx (atopy, down), FH and exam (feisher, Vogt, munson, nerves, scarring
	Yes	2			2	Yes	
Corneal hydrops (by exam or hx) OD	No	0			0	No	Corneal hydrops (by exam or hx) OS
	Yes	2			2	Yes	
		Total score	OD	OS	Total score		

Socre	Diagnosis
(Zero)	Normal
(1–3)	Suspect
(4–5)	Early KC
(6–9)	Advanced KC

Diagnosis: _____ OD   Diagnosis: OS

Amsler–Krumeich Keratoconus Classification

- *Stage I—eccentric steepening:*
  - Myopia and astigmatism <5.00 D
  - Mean central K readings <48.00 D
- *Stage II—myopia and astigmatism 5.00-8.00 D:*
  - Mean central K readings <53.00 D
  - Absence of scarring
  - Minimum corneal thickness >400 μm
- *Stage III—myopia and astigmatism 8.00-10.00 D:*
  - Mean central K readings >53.00 D
  - Minimum corneal thickness 300-400 μm
  - Absence of scarring
- *Stage IV—refraction not measurable:*
  - Mean central K reading >55.00 D
  - Central corneal scarring
  - Minimum corneal thickness 200 μm.

The Belin ABCD Grading System

This is a relatively newer keratoconus staging system that incorporates anterior and posterior curvature, thinnest pachymetry values, and distance visual acuity. This better reflects the anatomical changes seen in keratoconus.
- Criteria A and ARC (3.0 mm zone)—anterior radius of curvature. Average curvature in the 3.0 mm zone centered on the thinnest location of the cornea.
- Criteria B and PRC (3.0 mm zone)—posterior radius of curvature in the 3.0 mm zone. Average curvature in the 3.0 mm zone centered on the thinnest location of the cornea.
- Criteria C and thinnest pachymetry in microns
- Criteria D and DCVA—distance best corrected visual acuity—should be input manually
  Scarring— (-) clear cornea, no scarring
  (+) scarring present but iris details are visible.
  (++) scarring present, iris details are obscured **(Table 6)**.

TABLE 6: ABCD classification of keratoconus.

ABCD criteria	A	B	C	D		Scarring
	ARC (3 mm zone)	PRC (3 mm zone)	Thinnest pachymetry	BDVA		
Stage 0	>7.25 mm (<46.5 D)	>5.90 mm (<57.25 D)	>490	= 20/20 (= 1.0)		–
Stage 1	>7.05 mm (<48 D)	>5.70 mm (<59.25 D)	>450	<20/20 (<1.0)		–, +, ++
Stage 2	>6.15 mm (<53 D)	>5.15 mm (<65.5 D)	>400	<20/40 (<0.5)		–, +, ++
Stage 3	>6.15 mm (<55 D)	>4.95 mm (<68.5 D)	>300	<20/100 (<0.2)		–, +, ++
Stage 4	<6.15 mm (>55 D)	<4.95 mm (>68.5 D)	<300	<20/400 (<0.05)		–, +, ++

(ARC: anterior radius of curvature; BDVA: best corrected distant visual acuity; PRC: posterior radius of curvature)

 5. Discuss posterior keratoconus.

First described by Butler, posterior keratoconus is a rare, nonprogressive and noninflammatory condition characterized by increased posterior corneal curvature, which may or may not be accompanied by overlying stromal opacity.

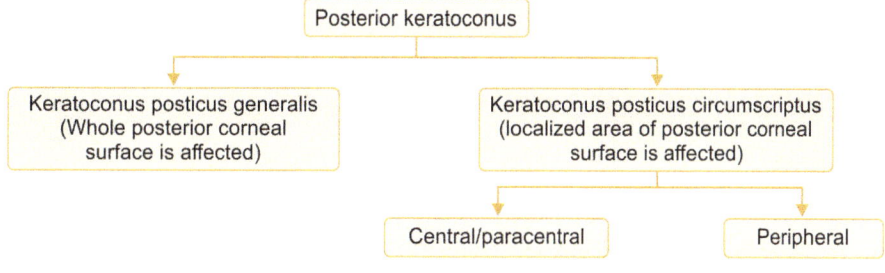

Congenital, unilateral, and sporadic form of posterior keratoconus is more common. Other type is acquired, bilateral, and familial and may be associated with systemic features.

Risk Factors

Congenital form—no associated risk factors

Acquired—trauma, which may lead to disruption of the inner corneal layers.

Pathology

- Abnormalities in DM—disorganized and widely spread collagen with abnormal banding and multilamellar configuration
- Occasional guttae on the endothelium
- Bowman's layer—replaced by randomly arranged collagen and fibroblasts
- Abnormalities in basal epithelial cells may be present.

Pathophysiology

Several hypotheses have been proposed:
- Posterior keratoconus is a part of cleavage abnormalities such as a mild form of Peter's anomaly.

> Inadequate separation forces during the embryological period of iridocorneal development
>
> Delayed separation of the lens from the surface ectoderm
>
> Iridocorneal adhesions or pigment remnants on the endothelium surrounding the lesion

- Posterior keratoconus is a mesenchymal dysgenesis.

> Delayed separation of primitive lens or iris tissue
>
> Altered migration of mesenchyme across the anterior chamber
>
> Altered corneal development in center, which prevents proper migration of the stromal cells

Acquired cases—trauma leading to the destruction of inner corneal layers leading to damage to the DM and endothelium and resultant remodeling may lead to posterior keratoconus. Lastly, familial cases are autosomal dominant and are associated with syndromic features.

Clinical Features

Symptoms

- Diminution of vision since childhood
- Strabismus
- Corneal opacity (may present at an earlier age).

Signs

- Corneal thinning with posterior excavation
- Absence of the DM in the area of excavation along with pigment deposition around the lesion
- Stromal opacity
- Clinically normal appearance of the anterior corneal surface.

Associated Ocular Features

Associated ocular features are endothelial guttae, embryotoxon, anterior keratoconus, microcornea, DM tears, iridocorneal adhesions, cataract (anterior polar, anterior subcapsular), and anterior lenticonus.

Systemic features commonly associated with familial cases are webbing of neck, cleft lips or palate, hypothyroidism, and mental retardation.

Investigations

Corneal Topography

Placido-based topographers do not pick up posterior keratoconus well as they map only the anterior surface of the cornea and extrapolate the posterior surface for calculation of corneal power. But when combined with scanning slit technique of mapping the cornea like in Orbscan, it can detect posterior keratoconus more reliably. However, Scheimpflug imaging with posterior curvature mapping and elevation mapping is more sensitive for the diagnosis of posterior keratoconus.

Distinct topographic patterns were identified.
- Generalized posterior keratoconus showed uniform corneal steepening.
- Localized central and paracentral posterior keratoconus showed corneal steepening, and localized peripheral posterior keratoconus showed corneal flattening overlying the area of corneal change.
- The changes in central and paracentral posterior keratoconus appear to progress with an increase in patient age.
- Unilateral disease may have more amblyogenic potential.

Pachymetry

There is localized thinning of the corneal thickness in the area of posterior keratoconus.

ASOCT/UBM—localized excavation of posterior corneal surface, with the absence of DM in that area. Stromal thinning and enhanced reflectivity are due to stromal opacity.

Differential Diagnosis

- Keratoconus, especially FFKC, is usually progressive.
- PMD—progressive, late onset, and classical crab-claw appearance on topography
- Peter's anomaly can be confused, especially in the mild forms—with other associated ocular features.
- Corneal scar can be ruled out by ASOCT and the absence of posterior excavation.

Management

Refractive correction may present with anisometropia. Correction can be done with spectacles or contact lenses.

Amblyopia management is usually unilateral and present from a very early age. Sensory deprivation or anisometropic amblyopia. After refractive correction, occlusion therapy may be useful.

Surgical management—in case of a small scar in pupillary axis, optical iridectomy may be attempted. Keratoplasty in case of dense corneal scars may be beneficial. PK or rotational autograft is advisable.

If iridocorneal adhesions are present management for glaucoma is crucial.

Prognosis

- In mild cases, the prognosis is usually very good.
- Since it is nonprogressive, chances of worsening are not there.
- Early diagnosis and amblyopia management are the mainstay of the treatment.

 6. Discuss the changes in topography in cases of corneal ectasia.

Corneal ectasia is a noninflammatory condition, the hallmark of which is progressive corneal steepening and thinning.

Types of corneal ectasia include the following:
- Keratoconus
- PMD
- TMD
- Keratoglobus
- Post-LASIK ectasia
- Wound ectasia after PK.

The most important diagnostic tool for the diagnosis of corneal ectasia is corneal topography. Commonly used topographers can be widely divided into:
- Reflection-based corneal topography such as a Placido-based system
- Scanning slit tomography such as Orbscan
- Scheimpflug tomography such as Pentacam
  Pentacam provides detailed information regarding the structure of the cornea and also the density of the tissue.
- *Keratoconus*—refers to Question 2 for topographical changes in keratoconus.
- *PMD* is a bilateral, progressive, corneal ectasia with thinning located 1–2 mm from the limbus along with corneal protrusion above the area of thinning. It can be confused with inferior keratoconus. On slit lamp, findings such as band-like thinning inferiorly and protrusion right above the thinning are observed in PMD. Vogt's striae and Fleischer's ring are characteristically absent.
  - The classic topographic finding for PMD is a "Butterfly" shape, or a crab-claw appearance or a Pincer Grasp appearance on the sagittal curvature map which is characterized by steepening of the anterior corneal curvature in the inferior corneal periphery and flattening of the cornea in the vertical meridian.
  - The thinnest pachymetry is located in the area just above the steepest point and not coinciding with the steepest point.
  - The anterior and posterior elevation areas are located in the periphery in the area of steepest keratometry.
  - Because of similar sagittal topographic features, inferior keratoconus is generally confused with PMD.
  - The deviation indices from Belin Ambrosio Enhanced Ectasia Display are lower in case of PMD as compared to keratoconus.
  - The corneal densitometry values in 6–10 and 10–12 mm zones are higher in PMCD as compared to keratoconus.
- *Postkerato-refractive surgery ectasia:* Corneal ectasia is a serious complication of refractive surgery. It is progressive, symmetric, inferior corneal steepening with a rapid increase in myopia, irregular astigmatism, and corneal aberrations, followed by a consequent loss of best-corrected visual acuity that may require corneal transplantation.

Topographic findings are as follows:
  - Crab-claw/pellucid-like (most common 65.9%)
  - Isolated steep cone
  - Asymmetric bow-tie with inferior steepening
  - The progressive thinning, i.e., decrease in pachymetry values postrefractive surgery may be diagnostic of postrefractive surgery ectasia.

Apart from the keratometry findings, elevation data are very important in the diagnosis of the post-LASIK ectasia. The positive anterior and posterior elevation values at the area of steepening are suggestive of ectasia in the history of a patient with refractive surgery.
- *Keratoglobus* is also a progressive condition of the cornea characterized by generalized thinning and globular protrusion of the cornea. Clinically, it is characterized by progressive diminution of vision due to irregular corneal topography, diffuse thinning of cornea from limbus to limbus, and absence of Vogt's striae and Fleischer's ring. Extreme thinning has a risk of perforation.

  Topographically, these patients have irregular astigmatism with irregular distribution of power of the cornea, along with peripheral arc of steepening resulting in flattening of arching of the bow-tie configuration. The pachymetry values show generalized thinning of corneal pachymetry up to one-fifth of the normal corneal thickness. The corneal diameter (white to white measurement) in these patients is normal and is useful to differentiate these patients from patients with buphthalmos.
- *TMD:* It is also an uncommon but peripheral thinning disorder of cornea which is progressive, noninflammatory, unilateral, or asymmetrical in bilateral cases in nature.

  Corneal thinning can be localized or involve extensive proportions of the peripheral cornea. Degeneration typically begins superiorly with mild, punctuate subepithelial and/or anterior stromal opacities and leaves a clear area between the opacities and the limbus. Opacification is followed by the development of a peripheral, superficial, and fine vascular pannus, which progresses over the years to include subepithelial opacity at the advancing edge, without the overlying edge (characteristic of Mooren's ulcer). The thinning spreads circumferentially, rarely involves the inferior limbus, and leaves the epithelium intact. The central wall is steep, and the peripheral wall slopes gradually. A yellow line of lipid deposits appears at the leading edge of the pannus (central edge of the furrow). Vessels traverse the furrow and pass beyond it. Spontaneous perforation is rare, although perforation can occur easily with minor trauma. Spontaneous ruptures in DM can result in interlamellar fluid or even a corneal cyst.

Diagnosis of this condition is mostly clinical and no diagnostic tests are needed for this disease. However, topography, if done, shows high against-the-rule or oblique astigmatism from the progressive flattening of the vertical meridian. Differentiating TMD from PMD, TMD more commonly involves superior limbus and rarely involves the inferior limbus, whereas its vice-a-versa in PMD. The presence of peripheral corneal opacities and vascularization is an important differentiating feature.

 7. Discuss corneal cross-linking—principle, indication, technique, and different protocols.

Corneal cross-linking is an established method for the treatment of keratoconus and other corneal ectasias. CXL has been proven to strengthen the corneal structure, and hence inhibiting the progression of keratoconus.

Principle

Corneal stroma is formed of collagen and the inter- and intrafibrillar collagen covalent bonds are a major factor determining the strength and stiffness of the connective tissue. LOX enzyme catalyzes the formation of covalent bonds between lysine or hydroxylysine groups from the C-terminus of one molecule to the N-terminus of an adjacent collagen fiber by oxidative process. Advanced glycation end-products (AGEs) generated in patients with diabetes mellitus also mediate cross-linking between collagen fibers by nonenzymatic glycation of proteins. Keratoconus has been linked to an overall reduction in LOX-mediated cross-links.

In CXL, the cornea is presoaked with 0.1% riboflavin solution till riboflavin percolates into the anterior chamber. Riboflavin acts as a photosensitizer and helps in the absorption of UV radiation in the corneal stroma. After soaking with riboflavin, the cornea is irradiated with UV-A radiation (370 nm) with the fluence ranging between 3 and 30 mW/cm^2. This UV-A radiation generates reactive oxygen species from the diffused oxygen in the stroma. These oxygen-free radicals activate LOX enzyme which in turn catalyzes the formation of intra- and interfibrillar covalent bond formation in collagen leading to increased stiffness of corneal stroma. By increasing stiffness, CXL prevents the progression of ectasia and stabilized the shape and topography of the cornea.

Indications for Corneal Cross-linking

The main indication for CXL is divided into:
- *Corneal ectasias*—to prevent the progression of corneal ectasias
- Keratoconus (most common indication)
- PMD
- Postrefractive ectasias.

Combined Treatments

- With LASIK (LASIK-Xtra)
- With Relex-SMILE (SMILE-Xtra)
- With Intracorneal ring segments (ICRS).

Others

- Infectious keratitis (most effective for bacterial ulcers, moderately effective for fungal ulcers, not effective for acanthamoeba)
- Bullous keratopathy (for symptomatic relief)
- Burns (to prevent corneal melts).

Technique (Dresden Protocol)

- CXL should be performed under sterile conditions in an operating theater or minor procedure room with all aseptic precautions.
- Epithelium is debrided to help in better penetration of riboflavin into the stroma.
- Riboflavin solution, 0.1% in 20% dextran, is then applied to the cornea every 2 minute for 30 minutes. The saturation of the cornea with riboflavin and its presence in the anterior chamber is ensured by slit-lamp examination.

- Prior to the treatment, ultrasound pachymetry should be performed at the thinnest point of the deepithelialized cornea to ensure a minimal corneal thickness of 400 µm.
- Riboflavin saturation ensures the formation of free radicals, whereas riboflavin shielding ensures the protection of deeper ocular structures such as the corneal endothelium.
- UV-A irradiation is performed using a duly calibrated optical system (Koehler type illumination) consisting of an array of seven UV-A diodes with a potentiometer in series to allow for regulation of voltage.
- Irradiance is performed for 30 minutes using 3 mW/cm^2, corresponding to a total surface dose of 5.4 J/cm^2.
- After the treatment, one drop of topical antibiotic is instilled and a bandage contact lens is placed until complete re-epithelialization.
- The patients are instructed to instill topical antibiotics four times daily until contact lens removal on the third or fourth postoperative day. Topical steroids in a tapering dose along with copius lubricants are prescribed.

Various Protocols for Corneal Cross-linking

Accelerated Corneal Cross-linking

The increased surgical time for Dresden protocol was one of the major drawbacks of the procedure. According to Bunsen–Roscoe Law of reciprocity, the effect of photochemical or photobiological reaction is directly proportional to total irradiation dose, irrespective of the time span over which the dose is administered. Thus, the same effect of UV-A radiation can be achieved by applying higher intensity radiation for shorter duration. Various intensity and time combinations such as 9 mW for 10 minutes, or 15 mW for 6 minutes, or 18 mW for 5 minutes or 30 mW for 3 minutes have been tried. The most widely studied and accepted protocol with the best results are with 9 mW for 10 minutes.

Advantages: The overall duration of the treatment is reduced significantly.

Disadvantage: Chances of recurrence/decreased effect of treatment.

Pulsed Corneal Cross-linking

The basis of cross-linking lies in type I and type II photodynamic reactions. Type II reaction mediates the cross-link formation via reactive oxygen species. It has been hypothesized that more rapid depletion of the oxygen with accelerated protocols leads to reduced efficacy. Pulsed delivery of UV-A radiation with predetermined on–off duration enables better diffusion of oxygen into stroma and hence better effect of cross-linking. However, the rate of oxygen depletion and restoration of normal tissue levels of oxygen has to be determined to define an ideal pulsing approach.

Corneal Cross-linking without Removal of the Epithelium (Epi-ON CXL)

A cross-linking procedure without epithelial removal would likely be less painful than one with the large diameter epithelial removal and would be ideal if it efficiently stabilizes keratectasia.
- Several substances (benzalkonium chloride as a preservative with riboflavin) have been used with varied success to loosen the tight junctions of the epithelial layer and thus increase the penetration of riboflavin.
- Partial grid-pattern epithelial removal (as opposed to complete debridement) allows some riboflavin penetration, but uptake is limited and irregular, which may affect the efficacy of the cross-linking process.
- Iontophoresis in which application of the electric current forces hypo-osmolar riboflavin to enter the corneal stroma and hence enhances the penetration of the riboflavin through an intact epithelium (transepithelial) has also been tried.

Cross-linking Protocol Modifications for Thinner Corneas

The normal pachymetry cutoff for a patient undergoing cross-linking is 400 µm. However, a few modifications in the protocol have been proposed for patients with thinner corneas.

Hypo-osmolar riboflavin leads to corneal stroma hydration and hence grants the cornea eligible for cross-linking. However, owing to lower concentration of corneal stroma due to hydration, the effect is not predictable and uniform.

Customized pachymetry-guided epithelial debridement—by preserving the epithelium on the thinnest part of the cone. The effect is limited to 150 µm and hence not highly effective.

Contact lens-assisted corneal cross-linking (CA-CXL)—use of contact lens soaked in riboflavin over thin corneas to enhance the thickness by 100 µm (contact lens should be UV light permeable).

SMILE lenticule—placing lenticule removed during refractive procedure such as SMILE temporarily on the thin corneas to increase the thickness of the area of irradiation.

Adapted fluence: This is the most promising of all modifications of protocols for thin corneas as it allows the constant energy (3 mW) to be delivered for customized irradiation time based on the thickness of the cornea, eliminating the use of variable factors, and promising more predictable results.

Various other modifications in the CXL are as follows:

Combination of Treatments
- Topo-guided PRK with CXL is used to regularize corneal surface in cases of early keratoconus for better compliance and tolerability to glasses and contact lens.
- LASIK/SMILE Xtra–CXL is combined with keratorefractive procedure in cases of preclinical or keratoconus suspects undergoing refractive correction.
- CXL with INTACS is used in cases with contact lens intolerance or in patients showing continued progression after undergoing CXL.

Customized Corneal Cross-linking

It is an emerging concept. Use of nonincisional, nonablative treatment approach involving high-fluency irradiation to induce subsequent flattening and refractive correction. UV-A irradiation is delivered by advanced pupil tracking technology to deliver customized treatment.

Possible advances include the development of a nomogram for astigmatic correction, the addition of supplemental oxygen to enhance the efficacy of epithelium on approach, and topography-guided treatment patterns.

8. How will you suspect, investigate, and treat a case of preclinical keratoconus?

Preclinical keratoconus is a term used to categorize eyes showing features of early keratoconus on topography before they show any clinical signs visible on detailed slit-lamp examination.

Keratoconus is an absolute contraindication for keratorefractive surgery. Detection of preclinical keratoconus is useful in patients undergoing keratorefractive surgery to prevent the occurrence of iatrogenic ecstasies after surgery.

Nomenclature

Forme Fruste Keratoconus

The fellow eye of a clinically manifest keratoconus that has no clinical findings of any sort except for certain topographical changes

Keratoconus Suspect

As per Rabinowitz definition, an eye with no slit-lamp findings or scissoring on retinoscopy but only abnormal AB/SRAX (asymmetric bow tie with skewed radial axis) on videokeratography (VKG) irrespective of the status of fellow eye (after excluding contact lens-related warping).

Subclinical Keratoconus

Fellow eye with a clinically manifest keratoconus with (1) no clinical findings—keratometric, retinoscopic, or biomicroscopic, (2) I-S asymmetry and/or bow-tie SRAX on placido disc-based VKG, and (3) no history of contact lens wear/surgery or trauma.

Suspecting a Pre-clinical Keratoconus

High suspicion for preclinical keratoconus should be in the following cases:
- Contralateral eye of patients with unilateral clinically manifest keratoconus
- Eyes of first-degree relatives with clinical keratoconus
- Prospective patients for refractive surgery
- Patients with unexplained irregular astigmatism or higher order aberrations
- Patients with frequently changing refractive error
- Patients with high astigmatism (>2.5 D) with active allergy or history of eye rubbing.

Diagnosis

Preclinical keratoconus can be diagnosed by various methods such as:
- Placido-based VKG
- Elevation-based topography
- Corneal biomechanics
- Wavefront aberrations.

Placido-based Videokeratography

- A central K >47.2 D but <48.4 and I–S asymmetry >1.4 D but <2 D indicate subclinical keratoconus.
- KISA index of 60–100% indicates subclinical keratoconus and >100% indicates clinically manifest keratoconus. (KISA% = $(K) \times (I–S) \times (AST) \times (SRAX) \times 100/300$, where K is central keratometry, I–S is the difference between the five superior and five inferior points at 3 mm from the center at 30° interval, AST is astigmatism, and SRAX is skewing of the radial axis)
- The Rabinowitz system, the Made–Klyce system, and the later developed neural network system were the three most widely used diagnostic systems based on VKG to define normal cornea, subclinical keratoconus (or keratoconus suspect), and clinically manifest keratoconus.
- CLMI—Cone Location and Magnitude Index—may also be useful.

Disadvantage: Poor repeatability, surface irregularities such as dry eyes affect quality of image, and complex calculations

Elevation-based Topography (Slit Scanning/Scheimpflug)

The most important advantage was being able to utilize the posterior corneal surface mapping, which had higher sensitivity and specificity in detecting keratoconus in early stages of keratoconus. However, posterior elevation alone may not be capable of accurately diagnosing subclinical keratoconus; hence, the posterior elevation should be combined with other parameters such as cornea curvature, cornea power, anterior elevation, and thickness to achieve a better effect.

Belin/Ambrosio-enhanced ectasia display (BAD): Belin/Ambrosio-enhanced ectasia display is a comprehensive display, which enables a global view of the tomographic structure of the cornea, through combination of elevation and pachymetric data. BAD combines nine different tomographic parameters in a unified screening tool. The display implements deviation of normality values for the following parameters individually.
- Anterior elevation at the thinnest point
- Posterior elevation at the thinnest point
- Change in anterior elevation
- Change in posterior elevation
- Corneal thickness at the thinnest point
- Location of the thinnest point
- Pachymetric progression
- Ambrósio Relational Thickness
- K_{max}

A final "D" is calculated based on a regression analysis that weights differently each parameter **(Table 7)**.

TABLE 7: Belin/Ambrosio-enhanced ectasia total deviation value (D value).

BAD "D" value	Inference
D <1.6 SD	Normal range
1.6 < D > 2.6	Keratoconus suspect
D >2.6	Keratoconus

(BAD: Belin/Ambrosio-enhanced ectasia display)

Belin/Ambrosio-enhanced ectasia display—D value has a sensitivity of 81% and a specificity of 73% in differentiating keratoconus suspect from normal population.

Disadvantages of elevation-based topographers:
- Scanning slit and Scheimpflug systems cannot be compared.
- Elevation details alone are not diagnostic.

Corneal Biomechanics–Ocular Response Analyzer and Corvis ST

Keratoconus eyes have a significantly lower central corneal thickness (CCT), corneal hysteresis, and corneal resistant factor (CRF) than normal eyes. In the low corneal central thickness groups (500 and 540 μm), corneal hysteresis achieves 91% of sensitivity for both cornea thickness groups to distinguish FFKC and normal eyes. But for CRF it is only 81 and 87% sensitivity. Corneal biomechanics from Corvis ST when combined with tomography values of Pentacam gives a sensitivity of 99% in detecting preclinical keratoconus.

Wavefront Aberrations

An index made up of two lower-order aberrations (defocus and astigmatism) detects keratoconus as effective as curvature characteristics such as I–S value, steepest radial axes, and surface asymmetry index.

Vertical coma is the most important higher-order aberration which differentiates between subclinical keratoconus and normal eyes. However, it alone is not sufficient to diagnose subclinical keratoconus, but if combined with I–S value and pachymetry changes may increase the specificity of the higher-order aberrations.

Epithelial Thickness Mapping (RT Vue ASOCT and MS-31)

Hypothesis that epithelial changes can mask very early changes in the surface topography making the diagnosis of preclinical keratoconus difficult. However, the presence of an epithelial doughnut pattern with epithelial thinning over the cone and surrounded by annulus of epithelial thickening could be an early indicator of the presence of underlying stromal cone.

Management of a Patient with Preclinical Keratoconus

- Determination of the risk factors
- Establish the progression of disease
- Treatment of progression and visual rehabilitation.

Determination of Risk Factors

As per Shetty et al. there is a risk factor scoring system based on the prevalence of the risk factor and the patients can be classified as low, moderate, or high risk **(Table 8)**.

TABLE 8: Risk factors for progression of keratoconus.

Risk factor	Levels	Score
Age (years)	<20	2
	20–30	1
	>30	0
Rubbing of eyes	Active	2
	Past	1
	Absent	0
Atopic eye disease	Active	2
	Past	1
	Absent	0
Frequent change of glasses	Present	2
	Absent	0
Others	Pregnancy	2
	Down syndrome	2
	Connective tissue disorder	1
	Retinitis pigmentosa	1
	Leber's congenital amaurosis	1

Score >8: high risk of progression; 6–8: Moderate risk of progression; <6: Low risk of progression.

The patients who fall under the high-risk category need not wait for documented progression in a clinically manifest keratoconus for cross-linking. However, patients in low- to moderate-risk category or subclinical keratoconus can wait for documented progression.

There are studies proving lower levels of serum vitamin D3 in patients with keratoconus compared to the age-matched individuals with healthy corneas. Hence, supplementation of vitamin D3 if found deficient might be useful as well.

Establish the Progression of the Disease

In case of preclinical keratoconus, it is imperative to establish the progressive nature of the disease by serial topography. According to the Global Consensus on Keratoconus and Ectatic Diseases 2015, the criteria for progressive keratoconus—any two or more over a period of 6 months.

- Steepening of the anterior corneal surface: Cornea apex power >1 D from baseline
- Steepest keratometry >1 D increase from baseline
- Flattest keratometry >1 D increase from baseline
- Mean keratometry >0.75 D increase
- Manifest spherical equivalent >0.5 D increase from baseline
- Thinning/increase in rate of corneal thickness change >2% decrease from baseline.

Management of Preclinical Keratoconus

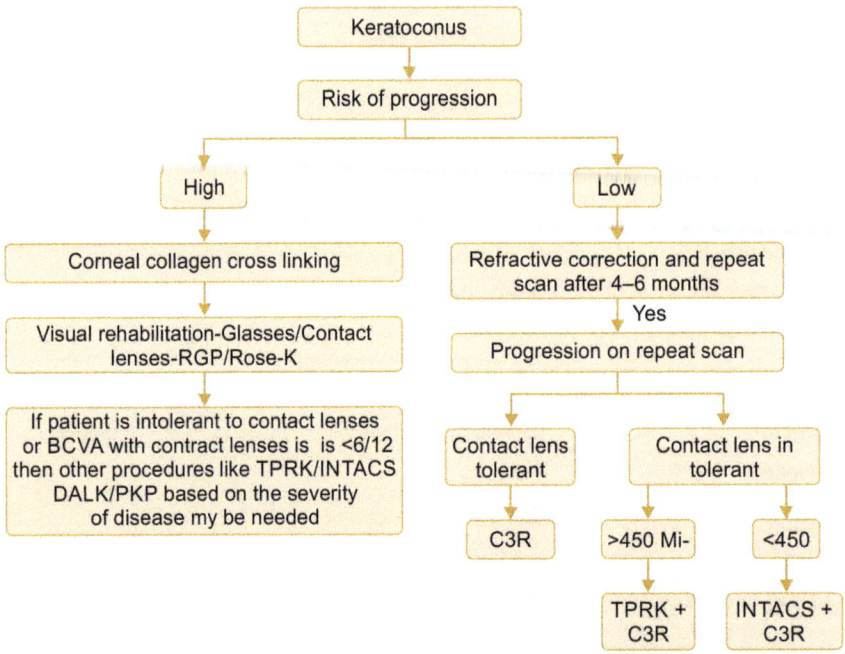

(C3R: corneal collagen cross-linking with riboflavin; DALK: deep anterior lamellar keratoplasty; PKP: penetrating keratoplasty; RGP: rigid gas permeable; TPRK: topography-guided photorefractive keratotomy)

 9. A 25-year-old woman presents with inability to correct her vision completely with glasses. Her keratometric values are 48 D at 95°/52 D at 185° (OD), 50 D at 65°/55 D at 155°. What is your plausible diagnosis and discuss the important steps in further confirming your diagnosis and factors influencing her management?

Provisional diagnosis—corneal ectatic disorder, most probably keratoconus.

To confirm the diagnosis, a detailed history taking with retinoscopy, slit-lamp examination, pachymetry, and corneal topography are imperative.

The most common corneal ectatic diseases of the cornea are keratoconus, PMD, keratoglobus, and keratoconus being the most common.

Can refer question 2 for investigations, differential diagnosis, and treatment of keratoconus.

10. Explain the principles of contact lens fitting in keratoconus.

Contact lens is one of the most important nonsurgical method of visual rehabilitation in eyes with keratoconus. Keratoconus can give quality vision in most eyes with keratoconus irrespective of severity. Contact lens forms a new refractive surface over cornea completely negating the structural irregularities of keratoconus. Contact lenses are indicated when good functional vision is not attained by glasses and patient is not satisfied with glasses because of shadowing, ghost images, and diplopia.

Permeability and Transmissibility

Dk is the expression for oxygen permeability—it is the physical property of a contact lens, defined as the rate of oxygen flow under specified conditions through unit area of contact lens material of unit thickness when subjected to unit pressure differences.

Dk/t is used to denote oxygen transmissibility of a specific lens, which is a measure of oxygen permeability as a function of lens thickness.
- D = coefficient for oxygen diffusion in the lens material
- k = solubility coefficient of oxygen of the material
- t = time

Increased oxygen transmissibility is important as cornea depends on atmospheric diffusion for its oxygen needs and the lack of it can cause hypoxia and can affect all layers of cornea. Oxygen transmissibility depends on various factors such as material of lens, thickness, water content, etc. Higher the Dk/t number, higher the oxygen transmissibility.

Preliminary Assessment

- Rule out certain syndromic associations with lower IQ which limits patients from taking good care of the contact lens and the eyes by themselves.
- Assess patients ability and motivation to take good care of lenses and their eyes. Avoid prescribing lenses to school children.
- Patients should be explained about the advantages and disadvantages of contact lens over spectacles.

Fitting Considerations

- After taking full history and symptoms, the preliminary examination should include age, occupation, and motivation. Any history of previous contact lens intolerance or allergies should be noted.
- Detailed slit-lamp evaluation is done. Any allergic eye disease is treated sufficiently before advising contact lens.
- Dry eyes should be treated prior to prescribing lenses and the treatment should continue with contact lens use.
- Topography is helpful guide for a better fitting and should be utilized whenever available.
  - Cone position shape and size
  - Corneal radius of curvature (central and steepest)
  - Corneal toricity/astigmatism
- Subjective and objective refraction (autorefraction) is helpful before fitting.
- Keratoconus progression should be arrested with CXL, preferably prior to contact lens fitting for better stability and long-term comfort.

Lens Fitting

Good lens fitting is important in giving patient comfort, tolerability, and best possible vision is case of rigid gas permeable contact lens.

There are three types of contact lens fitting:
1. *Apical bearing:* Lens bears heavily on corneal apex. It provides good vision but may result in corneal abrasions and scarring.
2. *Apical clearance:* The back surface of the lens vaults over apex of the cone. There is lesser risk of corneal scarring. It causes variable vision due to uncorrected astigmatism.
3. *Three-point touch:* Lens rests lightly against the cone apex (feathery touch) and also has bearing on nasal and temporal side in mid periphery, which is used to distribute the weight of the lens evenly over cornea. It provides stable fitting and good vision.

Fitting Algorithm

- When selecting lens, choose the correct base curve using corneal topography; start with the base curve equivalent to the steeper of the two keratometer readings. But trial and error method give best results.
- Allow the lens to settle for about 20 minutes before evaluating the fluorescence pattern. Also assess movement of lens with blinking of lids.
- Examine the central area, the mid peripheral area, and the periphery.
- Evaluate the lens in the central position. Once you have judged the fit, alter the fit as necessary (e.g., flattens, if pooling) until you obtain gentle apical touch and the three-point touch. There should be minimal bearing (touch) at the apex of the cone, as well as an area of bearing between the periphery of the lens and the intermediate zone of the cornea. Small edge lift must be present for smoother and adequate tear exchange. Lens should move up to 1–2 mm with each blink and not more.
- The lens should be ordered in mid-high Dk material after an over-refraction has been undertaken.
- Trial lenses can be prescribed for 2–4 weeks before actual, more expensive lens purchase from patient.

Types of Lenses for Keratoconus Patients

Soft Hydrogel Lenses

Though comfortable, they are not of much use in keratoconus as they drape around cornea and cannot maintain their shape for correction of refractive error.

Silicone Hydrogels

Silicone hydrogel has higher modulus of elasticity and reduced drape over cornea due to combination of hydrophilic hydrogel and hydrophobic silicone. It is useful in early cones and astigmatism up to 5 D and also has higher water content and higher Dk/t values (NovaKono, KeraSoft IC).

Soft Torics

Soft Torics is useful in patients of early cones with regular astigmatism (Clarity XR Toric).

Soft Keratoconic Designs

These lenses are thicker centrally than conventional soft lenses to mask irregular astigmatism. They have excellent comfort, centration over visual axis, and support of corneal epithelium. They correct mild to moderate amounts of irregular astigmatism and are used in early to moderate cones (KeraSoft IC).

Rigid Gas Permeable Lens with Single and Multicurve Design

Rigid gas permeable lens with single and multicurve design is used in early to moderate cones. Central steeper curves and peripheral flatter curve give best fitting solution. Individual lens parameters can be modified to enhance the fit (Soper cone lenses—bicurve design, McGuire cone lenses with multicurve design.)

Aspheric Rigid Gas Permeable Lense

Aspheric RGP lenses can be used in moderate cases. Decentration can cause visual disturbances (Rose K 2).

Rigid Gas Permeable Keratoconic Design

Rigid gas permeable keratoconic design can add toric surfaces and can be customizable. It is used in moderate to advanced cones (Rose-K KC and IC)

Mini-scleral and Scleral Lenses

Mini-scleral and scleral lenses can be used in advanced cones, these lenses rest on conjunctiva and sclera. They vault the apex with apical clearance fit and also prevent scarring. They can add toric surfaces (mini-scleral—custom stable lenses, scleral—PROSE lenses).

Hybrids and Piggybacks

Hybrids and piggybacks can be used in moderate to advanced cases who are intolerable to regular RGP lenses. Hybrid lenses have central RGP lens material for better vision and peripheral soft skirt for better comfort. Higher *Dk* material is recommended. In piggy back lenses, eye is fitted with large diameter soft lenses and then an RGP lens is fitted over it for good vision. Soft lenses can have groves in them to hold the RGP better (hybrid lenses—ClearKone, UltraHealth, piggyback system—Flexlens).

11. Discuss prominent corneal nerve and thickened corneal nerve.

Cornea is the most densely innervated structure in the human body and corneal nerves are responsible for the sensations of touch, pain, and temperature and play an important role in the blink reflex, wound healing, and tear production and secretion.

- Nerve supply of cornea is derived from long ciliary nerves, which is a branch of nasociliary nerve which in turn is a branch of ophthalmic division of trigeminal nerve.
- These long ciliary nerves enter the eye around optic nerve and travel forward in suprachoroidal space.
- They emerge out by piercing the sclera at a short distance from limbus and divide dichotomously and connect each other and with conjunctival nerves to form *pericorneal or limbal plexus*.
- 60 to 80 trunks of myelinated nerve fibers from this plexus enter the cornea at various levels (e.g., sclera, episclera, and conjunctiva). These nerves lose perineurium and myelin sheath after travelling 1–2 mm in cornea, branch dichotomously, and form *stromal plexus*.
- Most of these nerves pass anteriorly and form *subepithelial plexus*.
- Nerve fibers enter through pores in Bowman's layer, lose their Schwann's sheath, divide into multiple filaments, and form *intraepithelial or sub-basal plexus*.
- Hence, innervation is extensive near the center of cornea, least in periphery. Central stroma, DM, and endothelium have no innervation.
- Autonomic innervation may travel along with these nerve fibers, although it is believed to be scarce (sympathetic) or unknown (parasympathetic).

In normal eyes, corneal nerves are not visualized by slit-lamp biomicroscopy because:
- Lack of perineurium and myelin sheath around the nerves
- Nerves organize in parallel to collagen lamellae reducing the scatter of light
- The slender nature of nerve fascicles and filaments

The Increased visibility of corneal nerves, however, is recognized in some ocular and systemic diseases. Secondary thickening of corneal nerves caused by nerve regeneration or regional inflammation can be seen in corneal diseases such as anterior keratoconus, Fuchs' corneal dystrophy, and failed graft. The visibility itself, however, is mild and localized.

Conversely, prominent corneal nerves over the entire cornea are thought to be associated with systemic diseases such as multiple endocrine neoplasia, neurofibromatosis, and leprosy. Among these, it is generally accepted that multiple endocrine neoplasia type 2B consistently shows the most prominent corneal nerve in both corneas.

Grading of Corneal Nerves by Kinoshita et al.

- Grade 0—nerves are not visible.
- Grade 1—fine nerves visible on slit-lamp examination but not on any photographs
- Grade 2—fine nerves visible on both slit lamp and slit image photographs, but not scleral scattering
- Grade 3—nerves visible by slit lamp, slit image, and scleral scatter
- Grade 4—prominent nerves visible by all three methods.

Systemic Conditions with Prominent Corneal Nerves

- Multiple endocrine neoplasia type 2B
- Refsum disease
- Hereditary ichthyosis
- Neurofibromatosis type 1

- Leprosy
- Primary amyloidosis.

Ocular Conditions with Enlarged Corneal Nerves

- Keratoconus
- Fuchs' corneal endothelial dystrophy
- Reis–Bückler's corneal dystrophy
- Acanthamoeba keratitis
- Corneal graft failure
- Congenital glaucoma.

References

1. Lohchab M, Prakash G, Arora T, Maharana P, Jhanji V, Sharma N, et al. Surgical management of peripheral corneal thinning disorders. Surv Ophthalmol. 2019;64(1):67-78.
2. Rabinowitz YS. Keratoconus. Surv Ophthalmol. 1998;42:297-319.
3. Krachmer JH, Mannis MJ, Holland EJ. Cornea: Fundamentals, Diagnosis and Management, 4th edition. New York, NY: Elsevier Inc.; 2011. pp. 820-43.
4. Maharana PK, Dubey A, Jhanji V, Sharma N, Das S, Vajpayee RB. Management of advanced corneal ectasias. Br J Ophthalmol. 2016; 100(1):34-40.
5. Belin MW, Ambrosio R. Scheimpflug imaging for keratoconus and ectatic disease. Indian J Ophthalmol. 2013;61:401-6.
6. Matalia H, Swarup R. Imaging modalities in keratoconus. Indian J Ophthalmol. 2013;61:394-400.
7. Parker JS, van Dijk K, Melles GR. Treatment options for advanced keratoconus: a review. Surv Ophthalmol. 2015;60(5):459-80.
8. Shetty R, Kaweri L, Pahuja N, Nagaraja H, Wadia K, Jayadev C, et al. Current review and a simplified "five-point management algorithm" for keratoconus. Indian J Ophthalmol. 2015;63:46-53.
9. Silas MR, Hilkert SM, Reidy JJ, Farooq AV. Posterior keratoconus. Br J Ophthalmol. 2018;102(7):863-7.
10. Krachmer JH, Rodrigues MM. Posterior keratoconus. Arch Ophthalmol. 1978;96(10):1867-73.
11. Masiwa LE, Moodley V. A review of corneal imaging methods for the early diagnosis of pre-clinical keratoconus. J Optom. 2020;13(4):269-75.
12. Huseynli S, Abdulaliyeva F. Evaluation of Scheimpflug tomography parameters in subclinical keratoconus, clinical keratoconus and normal caucasian eyes. Turk J Ophthalmol. 2018;48(3):99-108.
13. Shi Y. Strategies for improving the early diagnosis of keratoconus. Clin Optom (Auckl). 2016;8:13-21.
14. McKay TB, Priyadarsini S, Karamichos D. Mechanisms of collagen crosslinking in diabetes and keratoconus. Cells. 2019;8(10):1239.
15. Sinha R, Gupta N, Sharma N, Gupta R, Titiyal JS. Management of keratoconus: a review. Indian J Ophthalmol. 2010;58(4):353-8.
16. Sachdev G, Sachdev M. Recent advances in corneal collagen crosslinking. Indian J Ophthalmol. 2017;65(9):787-96.
17. Jankov MR, Jovanovic V, Nikolic L, Lake JC, Kymionis G, Coskunseven E. Corneal collagen cross-linking. Middle East Afr J Ophthalmol. 2010;17(1):21-7.
18. Cummings AB, McQuaid R, Mrochen M. Newer protocols and future in collagen cross-linking. Indian J Ophthalmol. 2013;61(8):425-7.
19. Gausson A, Morris J. The Contact Lens Manual: A Practical Guide to Fitting, 4th edition.
20. Lekhanont K, Sontichai V, Bunnapradist P. Prominent corneal nerves, conjunctival neuromas, and dry eye in a patient without MEN2B. Can J Ophthalmol. 2019;54(6):e313-7.
21. Kriszt A, Losonczy G, Berta A, Takács L. Presence of Fleischer ring and prominent corneal nerves in keratoconus relatives and normal controls. Int J Ophthalmol. 2015;8(5):922-7.
22. Kinoshita S, Tanaka F, Ohashi Y, Ikeda M, Takai S. Incidence of prominent corneal nerves in multiple endocrine neoplasia type 2A. Am J Ophthalmol. 1991;111(3):307-11.

Cataract and Refractive Surgery

9.1.1 Preoperative Laboratory Testing for Cataract Surgery

Archita Singh, Ritu Nagpal, Prafulla Kumar Maharana

 1. Discuss work-up for cataract surgery.

Introduction

Cataract surgery is the most common ophthalmic surgery performed worldwide by the ophthalmologist. The aim of cataract surgery has shifted from restoration of visual acuity to providing perfect refractive outcomes in terms of both distance and near visual acuity. The goal at present is to improve the quality of life and also the quality of visual acuity for patients undergoing surgery for cataract.

A patient before being taken up for a cataract surgery should undergo in detail not only a thorough work-up for intraocular lens (IOL) power calculation and IOL selection but also be evaluated systemically to ensure effective and favorable outcomes. There are certain guidelines and parameters which should be kept in mind while planning a patient for cataract surgery to ensure both safety and efficacy.

NICE Guidelines for Cataract Surgery

Cataract has been known to affect the quality of life significantly and can sometimes be severely disabling. The *National Institute for Health and Care Excellence issued guidelines for cataract surgery in adults* in 2017 referred to as the *NICE Guidelines*.[1] These are as described here.

Informing your Patients

It emphasizes the need for both a detailed verbal and written communication about the cataract surgery, which should be in a format that is understandable and as per the requirements of the patient and/or the relatives.

Information to Provide When Referred for Cataract
- About the cataract and its impact on quality of visual acuity
- The need for surgical intervention, benefits of surgery, and its results
- Preoperative procedure, intraoperative events and postoperative period of recovery, and visual rehabilitation.

Information Before Surgery
- Preoperative work-up and post of refractive outcomes (options for IOLs)
- Anesthesia considerations
- Routine to follow on the day of cataract surgery
- Intraoperative events or risks based upon individual case scenario and systemic comorbidities
- Outcomes in cases with preexisting ocular morbidities or previous ocular surgeries
- What to expect intraoperatively and on the day of surgery
- Postoperative complications.

Information on the Day of the Surgery
- Patients should always be informed about their position in wait list for surgery
- Before surgery reemphasis the procedure being performed and the possible duration
- After the surgery inform about visual quality to expect, any significant intraoperative events, signs and symptoms to notice, ocular hygiene and medications, follow-up visit and doctor information, and precautions and restrictions.

Information on Follow-up
- Next follow-up visits
- Clinical condition and schedule for medications
- Precautions and restrictions
- Managing of other ocular comorbidities
- Scheduling surgery for another eye
- Provision for refractive correction.

Systemic Work-up

Before taking up the patient for cataract surgery ensure stabilization of systemic comorbidities and adequate control so as to ensure safety profile.

Literature review suggests that there seems to be no significant benefit of routine preoperative laboratory testing in preventing cataract surgery-related adverse events.[2] Cataract surgery though associated with a low-risk profile, it is of importance to recognize the potential at-risk population to prevent eventful intraoperative and postoperative period.

It has been advised that preoperative tests should be taken up when history or systemic symptom/sign is suggestive of a medical condition requiring evaluation.[3]

The routine evaluation includes:
- Complete blood picture
- Serum electrolytes, blood urea, and creatinine
- Fasting blood sugars
- Electrocardiography (ECG).

These investigations may be carried out for any cataract surgery in an elderly patient to identify systemic comorbidity. This is of prime importance in developing country like ours as not all patients have access to medical care/evaluation and ophthalmic intervention might be the first medical contact.

Special consideration in patients who have an underlying systemic association or give history suggestive of one should undergo following tests as tabulated in **Table 1**.

It is important to remember that the systemic evaluation might not prevent or be directly related to cataract surgery-related adverse event but help prevent any preventable undesirable events during cataract surgery.

There are certain systemic associations which may have significant ocular effects thus may change postoperative results. These include:
- *Diabetes mellitus:* Risk of increase of diabetic macular edema (DME)
- *Hypertension:* Periocular hemorrhage, subconjunctival hemorrhage
- *Benign prostatic hypertrophy (BPH):* Intraoperative floppy iris syndrome (IFIS) leading to postoperative increased inflammation and postoperative rise of intraocular pressure
- *Patient on blood thinners:* Retrobulbar hemorrhage related to peribulbar blocks.

Ophthalmic Work-up

A detailed ocular history and evaluation is of utmost importance. Goals should be to:
- Identify the grade of cataract and its visual impact with or without associated lenticular abnormalities
- Assess for visual potential
- Screen for ocular comorbidities (glaucoma, retinal and macular pathologies, and corneal dystrophies)
- Plan for appropriate cataract surgery
- Calculated properly for IOL power so as to achieve good refractive outcomes
- Decide for appropriate IOLs.

TABLE 1: Medical condition-specific laboratory tests for patients with special situations.	
Medical comorbidity	*Laboratory investigations and special advice*
Diabetes Mellitus*	• Fasting blood sugar (<140 mg/dL)[4] • Postparandial blood sugar (<180 mg/dL)[4] • Glycosylated hemoglobin (HbA1c <7.1) • Rule out infection elsewhere (diabetic foot, ulceration, etc.) • Systemic clearance from a specialist
Hypertension[#]	• Blood pressure control (<140/90 mm Hg) • Systemic clearance from a specialist
Cardiac morbidity[5] (CAD, stenting, pacemaker in situ, prosthetic heart valves)	• Blood pressure control (<140/90 mm Hg) • ECG, ECHO, serum electrolytes • Stop clopidogrel for 5–7 days in those on combination therapy (to prevent iatrogenic hemorrhage) • Continue warfarin if INR <2.4 and surgery performed under topical anesthesia • "Bridging anticoagulation"—Shift from warfarin to LMWH (Heparin) in case risk of hemorrhage when under local anesthesia (peribulbar block) • Systemic clearance from a specialist
Chronic kidney disease[6]	• Blood urea and creatinine (<2 mg/dL) • Serum electrolytes • Dialysis—Plan heparin free dialysis one day prior to surgery • Systemic clearance from a specialist
Dementia, mental illness, subnormal intelligence	• Routine investigations for general anesthesia • Systemic clearance from a specialist
Pulmonary conditions	• COPD/Asthma: Pulmonary function tests • Tuberculosis: Chest X-ray/CT Chest—rule out active infection • Systemic clearance from a specialist
Benign prostate hypertrophy	• No specific investigations • Explain risks of intraoperative floppy iris pertaining to medication • Rule out any active urinary tract infections
HIV or hepatitis B positive	• Rule out secondary or super-added infections • CD4 counts, viral load assessment • Complete blood picture • Systemic clearance from a specialist

*Continue all medications with breakfast if patient not fasting as in routine cataract surgery. Omit if patient is fasting due to need for general anesthesia.
#Continue disease specific medications on the day of surgery.
(CAD: computer-aided diagnosis; COPD: chronic obstructive pulmonary disease; ECG: electrocardiogram; ECHO: echocardiogram; HIV: human immunodeficiency virus; LMWH: low-molecular-weight heparin)

Preoperative Biometry

Calculation of biometric data includes measurement of the axial length (AL) and keratometry (KM).

Axial Length

- It refers to the measurement of distance between the anterior surface of the cornea and the retinal pigment epithelial layer.
- Techniques for measurement include:
  - Applanation methods
  - Optical methods
- Currently as per the NICE guidelines optical biometry is preferred.[1]

Applanation methods:

- The most frequently used is the ultrasound based *direct contact method* using a 10 MHz probe. Higher frequency offers better resolution of the underlying structures.
- *Immersion scan* is assessment of AL under water bath using an Ossoinig shell. It is considered better and more accurate in aphakic patients.[7,8] It overestimates AL by 0.25–0.33 mm as compared to direct contact method.[9]
- *Points to remember while measuring AL:*
  - Ensure sterilization of A-scan probe
  - Proper calibration of the instruments

- Low gain settings preferred for accurate readings
- Always hold the probe parallel to the visual axis
- Check for the normal four spike pattern before documenting readings
- Aim to obtain consistent readings. Repeat measurements in cases where there exists a difference between both eyes of more than 0.3 mm.
- *Special considerations for:*
  - *Silicon oil-filled eyes:* Multiply the measured AL by 0.71 to account for change in speed of sound waves in oil-filled eyes as compared to phakic eyes
  - *Pathological myopia:* Erroneous readings due to posterior staphyloma therefore optical method of measurement preferred over the contact methods.

Optical methods:
- Preferred method in view of improved accuracy for measurement of AL
- It is a noncontact procedure based upon principle of partial coherence interferometry (IOL master) and optical coherence reflectometry (Lenstar)
- Particularly useful in silicon oil-filled eyes, high myopia, and postrefractive surgery patients.

Keratometry
- It involves measurement of radius of curvature of the anterior corneal surface across a fixed chord length in the central optical zone.
- The measurements can be made using automated keratometers, manual keratometers, or optical biometers.
- Need to repeat the keratometry readings arises when keratometry of either eye is less than 40D or more than 47D, difference between both eyes >1D or the cylinder does not correlate with cylinder on refraction.
- Corneal topography should be considered in cases of excessively steep or flat corneas, irregular corneas, and past history of keratorefractive procedure, Operated corneal transplant and significant astigmatism.[1]

IOL Power Calculations
- IOL power for eyes with AL between 22 and 24.5 mm is calculated using the SRK-formula.
  IOL power = A – 2.5 AL – 0.9 KM

Axial length	Modification of A-constant
<20 mm	A + 1.5
20–21 mm	A + 1
21–22 mm	A + 0.5
22–24.5 mm	A
24.5–26 mm	A – 1
>26 mm	A – 1.5

- Modified SRK-II for eyes with AL outside the limit as mentioned above.
- The *NICE Guidelines*[1] mention the various IOL formulas to be used depending upon the AL of the patients. These are as follows:
  - If AL <22 mm, use Haigis or Hoffer Q.
  - If AL is between 22.00 and 26.00 mm, use Barrett Universal II if available or SRK/T.
  - If AL >26.00 mm, use Haigis or SRK/T.

Special situations:
- *Previous corneal refractive procedure:*
  - Explain the patient regarding variable postoperative outcomes.
  - Patients who have undergone a previous keratorefractive procedure IOL power calculation using conventional biometry or single method of estimation does not suffice. Detailed evaluation with assessment of both anterior and posterior corneal curvature is necessary.
  - While calculating, optical biometry is recommended with corneal topography for keratometry measurements.

- *Silicon oil-filled eyes:*
  - Optical biometry is the preferred modality.
  - In cases where optical methods are unable to assess the AL, ultrasound-based AL can be estimated with a correction factor of 0.71.
  - The velocity of sound in the vitreous cavity is 1532 m/s[22] and through silicon oil (*viscosity of 1000 centistokes) is 987 m/s[22]. Thus, there is a delay in transmission of sound impulse through the vitreous cavity. This results in an overestimation of the AL when this factor is not taken into consideration.

Assess for Visual Potential

Visual assessment is essential to know the outcomes postsurgery and also to counsel and explain the patients about risks of poor visual gain in difficult situations.
- *Laser interferometry:* For assessment in cases where visual outcomes are doubtful and the degree of cataract fails to corroborate with the presenting vision.
- *Visual evoked response:* Particularly in those cases with dense cataract associated with other ocular morbidities which may prevent adequate visual gain postoperatively such as post-traumatic, uveitic, postvitreoretinal surgery, and childhood cataracts.
- *Applanation tonometry and Humphrey visual fields:* Those with preexisting glaucoma and IOP rise.

Assess for Other Comorbidities

- *Endothelial cell health:* Specular microscopy and central corneal thickness. In cases with endothelial corneal dystrophies, pseudoexfoliation, glaucoma, operated keratoplasties, previous multiple anterior, or posterior segment surgeries.
- *Assessment of the macula:* Optical coherence tomography:
  - In patients with diabetes and uveitis for preexisting macular edema
  - In high/pathological myopia to assess for foveal thinning
  - Look for macular scarring and features of age-related macular degeneration.

Key Points

- Cataract surgery is the most common surgery by ophthalmologists worldwide.
- Preoperative patient counseling is of utmost importance.
- Systemic stability should be confirmed before posting for surgery to prevent risk.
- Preoperative work-up should be done thoroughly in terms of visual assessment and biometry to ensure favorable visual outcomes.

References

1. National Institute for Health and Care Excellence, 2017. Cataracts in adults: management. (NICE) Guidelines [NG77]. Available from https://www.nice.org.uk/guidance/ng77 [Last accessed July, 2022].
2. Keay L, Lindsley K, Tielsch J, Katz J, Schein O. Routine preoperative medical testing for cataract surgery. Cochrane Database Syst Rev. 2012;3:CD007293.
3. American Academy of Ophthalmology, 2014. Routine preoperative laboratory testing for patients scheduled for cataract surgery. Available from https://www.aao.org/clinical-statement/routine-preoperative-laboratory-testing-patients-s [Last accessed July, 2022].
4. Guidelines for the Management of Cataract in India: A VISION 2020: The Right to Sight INDIA Publication. Available from https://www.sightsaversindia.in/reports/2014/06/guidelines-management-cataract-india/[Last accessed July, 2022].
5. Davies BR. Combined aspirin and clopidogrel in cataract surgical patients: a new risk factor for ocular haemorrhage? Br J Ophthalmol. 2004;88(9):1226-7.
6. Fleisher LA, Fleischmann KE, Auerbach AD, Barnason SA, Beckman JA, Bozkurt B, et al. 2014 ACC/AHA guideline on perioperative cardiovascular evaluation and management of patients undergoing noncardiac surgery: executive summary: a report of the American College of Cardiology/American Heart Association Task Force on Practice Guidelines. Circulation. 2014;130(24):2215-45.
7. Shammas HJF. A comparison of immersion and contact techniques for axial length measurements. Am Intra-Ocular Implant Soc J. 1984;10:444-7.
8. Schelenz J, Kammann J. Comparison of contact and immersion techniques for axial measurement and implant power calculation. J Cataract Refract Surg. 1989;15:425-8.
9. Kenneth J, Hoffer MD. FACS. Biometry. J Emmetropia. 2011;2:210-6.

9.1.2 Congenital Cataract

Chirakshi Dhull, Ritu Nagpal, Prafulla Kumar Maharana

Q 1. Discuss the various aspects of pediatric cataract.

Introduction

Pediatric cataract is a leading cause of childhood blindness. Untreated cataracts, especially in children, lead to tremendous social, economic, and emotional burden to the child, family, and society. Blindness related to pediatric cataract can be treated with early identification and appropriate management. There are significant advances in knowledge and technology, which have improved outcomes of these patients. Favorable outcomes depend not only on effective surgery but also on meticulous postoperative care and visual rehabilitation including glasses and amblyopia treatment.

Epidemiology

Pediatric cataract is a treatable leading cause of childhood blindness. The incidence is from 1.8 to 3.6/10,000 per year and the prevalence is about 1.03 per 10,000 children (0.32–22.9/10,000). There is no difference in the prevalence based on gender or laterality.[1]

Genetics

Congenital cataract is hereditary in 8.3–25% of the cases, with 75% being autosomal dominant in inheritance.[2,3] Autosomal-dominant cataracts have varying amount of penetrance. Crystallin and connexin gene mutations are the most commonly described in nonsyndromic inherited cataracts.

Etiology

Table 1 depicts the causes of pediatric cataract.[4]

TABLE 1: Bilateral and unilateral cataract.

Bilateral cataracts	Unilateral cataracts
• Idiopathic	• Idiopathic
• Hereditary cataracts (autosomal dominant)	• Ocular anomalies:
• *Genetic and metabolic diseases:*	– Persistent fetal vasculature (PFV)
– Down syndrome	– Anterior segment dysgenesis
– Lowe syndrome	– Posterior lenticonus
– Galactosemia	– Posterior pole tumors
– Marfan syndrome	• Traumatic (rule out child abuse)
– Trisomy 13–15	• Rubella (rarely)
– Hypoglycemia	• Asymmetric bilateral cataract
– Alport syndrome	
– Myotonic dystrophy	
– Fabry disease	
– Hypoparathyroidism	
• *Maternal infection:*	
– Rubella	
– Cytomegalovirus	
– Varicella	
– Syphilis	
– Toxoplasmosis	
• *Ocular anomalies:*	
– Aniridia	
– Anterior segment dysgenesis syndrome	
– Corticosteroids	

History Taking

Usually first complaint is white reflex noticed by the parents or the caretaker. The parent may also complain of abnormal movements, child not looking at light, squinting of eyes, or abnormal size of the eye. A detailed history is taken that includes asking about age of onset and duration of symptoms. A significant family history should be noted. Prenatal and birth history should also be noted.

The older children may present with difficulty in viewing distant object, teacher may notice child not being able to read blackboard, or the parent noticing child bringing things very close to face and viewing television at a close distance. In case of trauma, the mode of injury should be enquired, which helps to ascertain the severity of the injury.

Any significant systemic comorbidities should also be elicited.

Systemic Examination

Children with cataract often present with systemic illness and syndromic features. The systemic examination may show dysmorphic features, e.g., mongoloid slant (Down's syndrome), associated hearing or cardiac involvement (congenital rubella syndrome), abnormal head circumference, etc.

Ocular Examination

Visual Acuity Assessment

The most challenging and difficult part is the visual acuity assessment. First, we look for fixation. Central fixation suggests that the fovea is the fixing point, steady suggests that there is no component of nystagmus, and maintained suggests that there is no squint. Specialized tests have been developed to record the visual acuity in preverbal children. The test which can be used in infants is visual evoked response and Teller Acuity Cards. In children 1–2 years of age, the screening test for young children and retards (STYCAR) and Cardiff acuity test can be done. In children 2–3 years of age, coin test and LEA Symbol Test can be done. In children 3–5 years of age, Lippman's HOTV test and Letter test can be done. In children older than 5 years, Tumbling E, Landolt broken ring, Snellen chart, and LogMAR chart can be used.[5]

Screening for Cataract

The child is most comfortable in the mother's lap. After assessing the visual acuity, pupillary response and distant direct examinations are done to look for anterior segment abnormalities. The red reflex screening with direct ophthalmoscope kept at 30 cm and focused on each pupil separately (Bruckner test) helps in the identification of lenticular opacity.

Refractive Errors

The child at birth is mildly hyperopic. The refraction of a child under 5 years is essentially done under strong cycloplegia preferably under atropine 1%.

Nystagmus and Head Position

Nystagmus develops because the child is not able to maintain fixation. Rarely the child might acquire a head position that helps the child to get maximum vision with a minimum amplitude of nystagmus (null position).

Pediatric Cataract Morphology

Table 2 shows the pediatric cataract morphology.[5,6]

TABLE 2: Morphology of cataract.

Whole lens	Central	Anterior	Posterior	Miscellaneous

• Total
• Congenital Morgagnian
• Membranous
	• Lamellar
	• Central pulverulent
	• Ant egg
	• Nuclear
	• Oil droplet
	• Cortical
	• Coronary
		• *Anterior polar:*
		  – Dot like
		  – Plaque like
		  – Anterior pyramidal
		• Anterior subcapsular
		• Anterior lenticonus
			• Mittendorf dots
			• Posterior cortical
			• Posterior subcapsular
			• Posterior lenticonus
				• Punctate lens opacities
				• Sutural
				• Coralliform
				• Wedge shaped
				• Persistent hyperplastic primary vitreous

Investigations

Ultrasonography helps us rule out retinal detachment, fundal coloboma, and retinoblastoma.[7] Ultrasonography in a case of unilateral cataract can diagnose a persistent fetal vasculature (PFV).[8] Magnetic resonance imaging (MRI) and color Doppler may be used in cases of doubt. X-ray is done in cases of traumatic cataract, and computed tomography (CT) scan is performed to localize an intraocular foreign body. Specific investigations can be performed for suspected disease.

Timing of the Surgery

The critical period of eye development ranges from 2 to 6 months of age. In visually nonsignificant opacities (blue dot cataract or small posterior polar cataract), the child can be observed at regular intervals. Surgery is advised in visually significant opacities, i.e., >3 mm central opacity. Unilateral cataracts should be operated as early as possible before 6 weeks of age and bilateral cataracts should be operated before 8 weeks of age.[9]

Preoperative Evaluation

Examination Under Anesthesia

Examination under anesthesia is carried out to record essential parameters for intraocular lens (IOL) power calculation.

Biometry

Axial Length

Predicting axial length (AL) growth and hence the myopic shift is difficult after pediatric cataract surgery. AL first increases rapidly up to 6 months (0.46 mm/month), then has a relatively slower (infantile phase) growth (0.15 mm/month) till 18 months, followed by a slow (juvenile phase) growth (0.10 mm/month).[10] AL measurement is done using ultrasound A scan with contact or immersion method with the latter being more accurate.

Keratometry

Keratometry values are obtained using a handheld Auto Keratometer in children. Keratometry also steeply reduces in the first 6 months (−0.40 D/month), −0.14 D/month in the next 6 months, and −0.08 D/month in the second year reaching the adult range at about 3 years of age.[10]

Optical biometry can also be used in older children.

Intraocular Lens Power Calculation

Predicting accurate power for the child's eye is difficult. The IOL can be implanted in eyes with AL >17 mm and corneal diameter >10 mm.[5] Various studies have devised different formula for IOL power calculation. Dahan et al. suggested undercorrection of 20% in children younger than 2 years and 10% in children 2–8 years of age.[11] According to Prost, 20% undercorrection between 1 and 2 years of age, 15% undercorrection between 2 and 4 years, and 10% between 4 and 8 years of age are adequate.[12] Enyedi's postoperative target refraction can be used for IOL power calculation according to age (age in years + postoperative refraction = 7).[13]

According to our experience, Enyedi's formula is closest to correct IOL implantation in Indian eyes.

Ultrasound Biomicroscopy

Ultrasound biomicroscopy is a noninvasive imaging technique that helps in identifying anterior PFV, posterior capsular defect, and posterior polar cataract preoperatively. It also helps us in post-traumatic cases to look for cyclodialysis, subluxation, foreign body localization in anterior segment, and rupture of posterior capsule.

Choice of Intraocular Lens

Hydrophobic acrylic lens with square edges inhibits migration of lens epithelial cells (LECs) and reduces posterior capsule opacification (PCO) formation and is hence preferred in pediatric age group.[14] Multifocal IOLs can also been used preferably in older children.[15]

Surgery

The main aim of the treatment is to clear the visual axis followed by postoperative visual rehabilitation with minimum associated complications. In the bag, IOL implantation is the standard of care in children. Superior incision with two side ports is preferred which allows the wound to be protected by the eyelid. Preservative-free adrenaline (1:100,000) is injected for pupillary dilation. Trypan blue dye (0.06%) under air stains the capsule. Then a nick is given on the anterior capsule with the help of cystitome. Further capsulorhexis is completed with the help of utrata or microincision capsulorhexis forceps through 2.2 mm or microvitreoretinal (MVR) entry, respectively. Gentle multiquadrant hydrodissection is done, followed by bimanual lens aspiration to remove the lens matter. Posterior capsulotomy is a must for all patients younger than 6 years of age. Vitrectomy can be deferred after 5 years of age. In children, older than 8 years posterior capsulorhexis is required mainly in children (with mentally retardation or with nystagmus) who may not cooperate for laser capsulotomy on a slit lamp.[16] Posterior continuous curvilinear capsulorhexis (PCCC) can be done manually (preferred) or with vitrectomy cutter. For manual PCCC, the cystitome is used to give nick over the posterior capsule sideways and posterior capsulorhexis is completed using microincision capsulorhexis forceps. Anterior vitrectomy breaks the scaffold for migration of lens epithelial cells thus preventing visual axis opacification (VAO) formation. A careful IOL insertion is of utmost importance after opening posterior capsule. After making a 2.75 mm entry wound, IOL is inserted by pushing the leading haptic against the back surface of anterior capsule and then pushing down the trailing haptic followed by tucking of the trailing haptic into the bag. This is a safe method and results in no complications related to faulty IOL implantation.[17]

Intraocular lens (IOL) can be implanted in sulcus where in the bag implantation is not possible. Optic capture can also be helpful in cases of capsulorhexis run off. Peripheral iridectomy should be done in patients with aphakia. Peripheral iridectomy can also be considered in younger children <6 months of age or in those with complicated cataracts depending on presentation. The surgical incisions need to be sutured using 10-0 monofilament nylon for safety.

Postoperative Treatment

Patients are prescribed topical steroids (prednisolone acetate 1% six times per day) and cycloplegics (preferably homatropine 2%) postoperatively. Similar results for safety and efficacy have been observed for difluprednate 0.05% four times a day in children aged 0–3 years undergoing cataract surgery.[18] Topical steroids should be tapered over 6–8 weeks. Examination under anesthesia is advised during the postoperative period for 1 and 3 months thereafter.

Visual Rehabilitation and Amblyopia Therapy

Surgery is immediately followed by prescription of glasses and amblyopia therapy. The suture removal and repeat refraction are done at 1 month postoperatively and again at 3 months. The parent must ensure that the child wears the prescribed glasses and occlusion therapy (for unilateral or asymmetrical cases). Contact lens are more suitable in children with unilateral aphakia. In younger children, glasses are prescribed for near vision. In school-going children, executive bifocal glasses with near add are prescribed after correcting for distance.

In children younger than 12 months of age occlusion is given where both eyes are occluded depending on age (a 6-month-old child is given occlusion half of the waking hours per day in alternate eyes). A child older than 1 year is given occlusion in the better eye more than in the worse eye (a 3-year-old child is given full time occlusion for 3 days in better eye and 1 day in the worse eye). The worse eye is occluded to avoid development of occlusion amblyopia in the better eye. Patients are followed up every 4–6 weeks initially and every 3 months thereafter to see for response of treatment. Occlusion is gradually tapered off once the desired effect is achieved.

Complications

Major complications include VAO, secondary glaucoma, inflammation, and retinal detachment. VAO is the most common complication after pediatric cataract surgery with or without IOL surgery and may cause visual deprivation amblyopia. In older and cooperative children, yttrium aluminum garnet (YAG) capsulotomy can be tried. In a thick VAO, posterior capsulotomy combined with anterior vitrectomy may be required.

Glaucoma following cataract surgery is observed in 10–25% of children. Younger age at surgery and presence of microphthalmia are high risk factors.[19] Intraocular pressure may be controlled on medication or may require surgical intervention.

Postoperative reaction is seen more commonly in uveitic cataract. Appropriate use of steroids, cycloplegics, and systemic immunosuppressants may reduce this complication.

Retinal detachment is rare but more common in eyes with PFV.[20]

Improvement in surgical techniques and frequent use of topical steroids and cycloplegics in the postoperative period have significantly decreased the complications.[21]

References

1. Sheeladevi S, Lawrenson JG, Fielder AR, Suttle CM. Global prevalence of childhood cataract: a systematic review. Eye Lond Engl. 2016;30(9):1160-9.
2. Santana A, Waiswo M. The genetic and molecular basis of congenital cataract. Arq Bras Oftalmol. 2011;74(2):136-42.
3. Francis PJ, Moore AT. Genetics of childhood cataract. Curr Opin Ophthalmol. 2004;15(1):10-5.
4. Khokhar SK, Pillay G, Dhull C, Agarwal E, Mahabir M, Aggarwal P. Pediatric cataract. Indian J Ophthalmol. 2017;65:1340-9.
5. Gole G. Visual acuity assessment in children. Clin Exp Ophthalmol. 1989;17(1):1-2.
6. Amaya L, Taylor D, Russell-Eggitt I, Nischal KK, Lengyel D. The morphology and natural history of childhood cataracts. Surv Ophthalmol. 2003;48(2):125-44.
7. Kaya A. Preoperative usage of ultrasound biomicroscopy in pediatric cataract. Arq Bras Oftalmol. 2016;79(1):62.
8. Khokhar S, Tejwani LK, Kumar G, Kushmesh R. Approach to cataract with persistent hyperplastic primary vitreous. J Cataract Refract Surg. 2011;37(8):1382-5.
9. Vasavada AR, Nihalani BR. Pediatric cataract surgery. Curr Opin Ophthalmol. 2006;17(1):54-61.
10. Capozzi P, Morini C, Piga S, Cuttini M, Vadalà P. Corneal curvature and axial length values in children with congenital/infantile cataract in the first 42 months of life. Investig Opthalmol Vis Sci. 2008;49(11):4774.
11. Dahan E, Drusedau MUH. Choice of lens and dioptric power in pediatric pseudophakia. J Cataract Refract Surg. 1997;23:618-23.
12. Prost E. IOL calculations in cataract operations in children. Klin Oczna. 2004;106(4-5):691-4.
13. Enyedi LB, Peterseim MW, Freedman SF, Buckley EG. Refractive changes after pediatric intraocular lens implantation. Am J Ophthalmol. 1998;126(6):772-81.
14. Ness PJ, Werner L, Maddula S, Davis D, Zaugg B, Stringham J, et al. Pathology of 219 human cadaver eyes with 1-piece or 3-piece hydrophobic acrylic intraocular lenses: capsular bag opacification and sites of square-edged barrier breach. J Cataract Refract Surg. 2011;37(5):923-30.
15. Wilson ME, Johnson WJ, Trivedi RH. Primary multifocal intraocular lens implantation for teenage-onset bilateral cataracts: visual results a decade after surgery in 3 siblings. J AAPOS. 2013;17(6):623-5.
16. Lin AA, Buckley EG. Update on pediatric cataract surgery and intraocular lens implantation. Curr Opin Ophthalmol. 2010;21(1):55-9.
17. Khokhar S, Sharma R, Patil B, Sinha G, Nayak B, Kinkhabwala RA. A safe technique for in-the-bag intraocular lens implantation in pediatric cataract surgery. Eur J Ophthalmol. 2015;25(1):57-9.
18. Kaur S, Sukhija J. Difluprednate versus prednisolone acetate for inflammation following cataract surgery in pediatric patients: a randomized safety and efficacy study. Eye Lond Engl. 2017;31(3):506.
19. Baden C, Shija F, Lewallen S, Courtright P, Hall A. Glaucoma after pediatric cataract surgery in a population with limited access to care. J AAPOS. 2013;17(2):158-62.
20. Gasper C, Trivedi RH, Wilson ME. Complications of pediatric cataract surgery. Dev Ophthalmol. 2016;57:69-84.
21. Phatak S, Lowder C, Pavesio C. Controversies in intraocular lens implantation in pediatric uveitis. J Ophthalmic Inflamm Infect. 2016;6(1):12.

9.1.3 Traumatic Cataract

Manthan Chaniyara

 1. Write a short note on traumatic cataract.

Introduction

Ocular trauma leading to the damage of various ocular structures is not uncommon. It still remains the most common cause for acquired monocular blindness in children. Ocular injuries represent roughly 8–14% of total injuries in children. Trauma leads to cataract formation seen in 5–10% of all ocular trauma cases. Both mechanical (both open and closed globe injury) and nonmechanical (radiation, electrical shock, etc.) ocular trauma can lead to cataract formation.[1-3]

Trauma may lead to cataract formation at any age. Ocular injury is most commonly seen in the age group of 6–10 years. Males are more commonly affected. Various types of traumas such as road traffic accident, sports-related trauma, gunshot injury, firecracker injury, injury by animal tail or horn, fish hook injury, bow and arrow injury, hammer and chisel injury, and others may result in cataract formation.[4]

Mechanism for Cataract Development

Both blunt and penetrating ocular injury may result in the development of cataract. After trauma, cataract may develop immediately or after several months. Pathophysiology of the cataract development in mechanical ocular injury is complex. Different mechanisms responsible for the development of cataract are as:
- Coup injury
- Counter coup injury
- Equatorial expansion
- Direct capsular rupture.

All these types of injuries lead to the damage of lens capsule and lens epithelial barrier mechanism. Lens capsule and lens epithelial cells have an important role in maintaining the lens transparency by controlling the lens hydration. Disturbance of these barrier mechanisms facilitates the water and ions movement across the lens capsule.

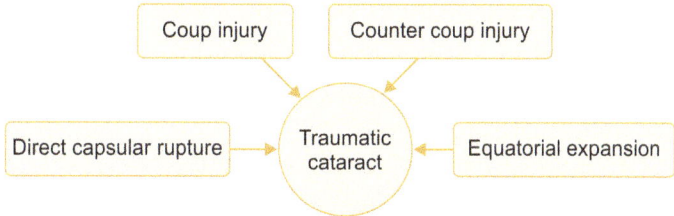

Direct injury to the lens capsule is known as coup injury and indirect injury due to shock waves is known as a counter coup injury. Both types of injuries may lead to focal or diffuse and stationary or progressive cataract formation by disturbing the anterior or posterior lens capsule. Blunt trauma may cause anteroposterior compression leading to equatorial expansion resulting in lens capsular rupture causing cataract formation or zonular dehiscence which results in lens subluxation or dislocation. To understand the nature of the forces leading to capsular tear, Por and Chee have proposed that the combined equatorial stretching–pulling force on the zonules, along with backward push of the lens due to anteroposterior forces, leads to capsular tear. Similarly, stronger anatomical attachments of the Wieger's ligament at the midperipheral posterior capsule leave the central weaker area vulnerable to anteroposterior forces.

Penetrating injuries directly lead to rupture of anterior and/or posterior capsule resulting in rapid hydration of the lens matter and the development of cataract.[5-10]

Morphological Classification

- Total intumescent white cataract
- Partially absorbed cataract
- Membranous cataract
- Early and late rosette cataract
- Discrete opacity.

In total intumescent white cataract, the capsules are intact, there is no clear lens matter between the capsule and the nucleus with increased intralenticular pressure. Partially absorbed and membranous cataract may result due to rupture of the lens capsule. In partially absorbed cataract, there is still some lens matter between the anterior and the posterior capsule that is separating them from each other, while in membranous cataract both the anterior and the posterior capsules along with organized lens matter are fused with each other, and it is not possible to separate them. Rosette cataract appears as feathery lines of opacity along with suture lines more commonly seen in the posterior cortex. Clinically late rosette cataract has shorter suture extension and is more compact as compare to early rosette.[11]

Investigation

A number of ocular comorbidities such as lens capsular defect, vitreous hemorrhage, retinal detachment, and retained foreign body can be associated with traumatic cataract. Various preoperative investigations are very important for optimal outcome in such cases. They are also important for the determination of the prognosis.
- B-scan ultrasonography
- Ultrasonic biomicroscopy (UBM)
- X-ray or computed tomography (CT) scan
- Ocular biometry
- Visual evoked response.

In most cases of ocular trauma, posterior segment evaluation by indirect ophthalmoscopy or by slit lamp biomicroscopy is difficult due to media haze resulted due to associated hyphema, traumatic miosis, cataract development, or vitreous hemorrhage. In these cases, B-scan can be used for the evaluation of the posterior segment. Ultrasound B-scan is a sensitive, noninvasive, and rapid way of assessing intraocular damage caused by blunt or penetrating eye injuries.[12]

Ultrasonic biomicroscopy is used for the diagnosis of preexisting posterior capsular defect, zonular dehiscence, or foreign body embedded in the ciliary body region. UBM is found to be superior for the determination of the posterior capsular defect as compared to anterior segment optical coherence tomography and Scheimpflug imaging.[13]

X-ray and CT scan are useful in case of the metallic foreign body. Scanning in both sagittal and coronal planes with thin cuts (1.0–1.5 mm) through the orbit is done for the localization of the foreign body.[14]

Ocular biometry including axial length and keratometry is done in long-standing traumatic cases for intraocular lens (IOL) power calculation.

Preoperative Evaluation

In case of severe blunt trauma, systemic status of the patient must be evaluated. Patient must be systematically stabilized before any ocular intervention. In acute trauma cases one should evaluate the extent of open globe injury before dealing with the lenticular damage. Open globe injury must be repaired first.

A thorough lenticular examination should be done before any surgical intervention. One should look for zonular dehiscence, preexisting capsular defect, and morphology of the cataract for optimal outcome. Traumatic cataract, especially secondary to blunt trauma, is more likely to be associated with capsular defect or zonular dehiscence.

Traumatic cataract cases are associated with more inflammation. Post-traumatic inflammation may be due to ruptured lens capsule and traumatic iritis. Proper preoperative control of this inflammation should be done.

Traumatic cataract may be associated with secondary glaucoma due to inflammation, hyphema, lens induced, or secondary to angle recession. Intraocular pressure control prior to ocular surgery is necessary.

When to Operate?

In open globe injury with acute-onset cataract formation recommendation is to close the globe first and control the inflammation and lens aspiration with IOL implantation done in the second-stage procedure. However, in some cases of acute trauma lens aspiration is done during primary globe repair with or without IOL implantation. Indications for early lens aspiration include the following:
- Lens-induced glaucoma
- Ruptured anterior lens capsule with lens matter in the anterior chamber touching the endothelium
- Dislocated lens with lens endothelial touch
- Media haze because of cataract hampering the posterior segment visualization for the management of posterior segment morbidity
- Child in amblyopic age group.

Surgical Management

Management of traumatic cataract can be done either through anterior limbal approach or through posterior pars plana approach. Anterior approach is the preferred approach. Anterior approach is used in case of nondislocated lens with intact posterior capsule. For cataract with ruptured posterior capsule or posterior dislocation of lens, posterior pars plana approach is used for optimal management.[15]

A number of factors can affect the surgical removal of cataract, IOL implantation, and final visual outcome in case of traumatic cataract.[16] The factors are:
- Subluxation or dislocation
- Ruptured capsule
- Hardness of lens
- Morphology of cataract
- Posterior segment pathology
- Iris anatomy
- Glaucoma.

Traumatic cataract without subluxation and with intact lens capsule can be managed using standard surgical technique that are used in routine senile or congenital cases. However, the presence of glaucoma iris damage should be taken under consideration while planning the surgery. Minimum manipulation during surgery should be done to minimize the risk of extension of any occult zonular dialysis.

Traumatic cataract secondary to penetrating or blunt trauma may be associated with capsular rupture. In case of open globe injury with lens capsular defect, globe repair with primary cataract surgery is preferred. In cases without open globe, one may delay the surgery. In cases with preexisting capsular rupture, surgical approach depends upon the hardness of the nucleus and the presence of zonular dehiscence. In cases of hard nucleus, it is better to go ahead with either extracapsular cataract extraction or intracapsular cataract extraction depending upon the zonular status.

In cases of subluxated lens, management depends upon the degree of zonular dehiscence and hardness of the nucleus. Anterior approach is preferred when risk of lens dislocation is minimum. Intraoperative standard protocol of subluxated cataract management is followed. Capsular tension ring, modified capsular tension ring, or capsular tension segment is used depending upon the degree of zonular dehiscence. In cases of large posterior capsular defect or posterior dislocated lens, pars plana approach is used. Ultrasonic fragmentation of the dislocated lens is used in cases with hard nucleus.[17]

Intraocular lens placement in case of traumatic cataract depends upon the patient's age, posterior capsular status, and presence of zonular dehiscence. Acute open globe injury which required primary lens removal is generally left aphakic in the primary surgery. IOL is put in the second-stage procedure. In patients with intact posterior capsule, posterior chamber IOL implantation is preferred. In cases of in adequate capsular support, IOL placement is done either in the form of anterior chamber IOL or by scleral fixation of IOL.

References

1. Scribano PV, Nance M, Reilly P, Sing RF, Selbst SM. Paediatric nonpowder firearm injuries: outcomes in an urban paediatric setting. Paediatrics. 1997;100:e-5.
2. Takvam JA, Midelfart A. Survey of eye injuries in Norwegian children. Acta Ophthalmol (Copenh). 1993;71:500-5.
3. Tsurimaki Y. Traumatic cataract. Current encyclopedia of ophthalmology. Tokyo: Nakayama-Shoten; 1993. pp. 175-80.
4. Strahlman E, Elman M, Daub E, Baker S. Causes of paediatric eye injuries: a population-based study. Arch Ophthalmol. 1990;108: 603-6.
5. Wolter JR. Coup-contrecoup mechanism of ocular injuries. Am J Ophthalmol. 1963;56:785-96.
6. Weidenthal DT, Schepens CL. Peripheral fundus changes associated with ocular contusion. Am J Ophthalmol. 1966;62:465-77.
7. Por YM, Chee SP. Implantation of foldable intraocular lens with anterior optic capture in isolated posterior capsule rupture. J Cataract Refract Surg. 2006;32:707-8.
8. Campanella PC, Aminlari A, DeMaio R. Traumatic cataract and Wieger's ligament. Ophthalmic Surg Lasers. 1997;28:422-3.
9. Michael R, Bron AJ. The ageing lens and cataract: a model of normal and pathological ageing. Philos Trans R Soc Lond B Biol Sci. 2011;366:1278-92.
10. Bhat SP. The ocular lens epithelium. Biosci Rep. 2001;21:537-63.
11. Shah MA, Shah SM, Shah SB, Patel CG, Patel UA. Morphology of traumatic cataract: does it play a role in final visual outcome? BMJ Open. 2011;1(1):e000060.
12. Shazlee MK, Ali M, Ahmed MS, Hussain A, Hameed K, Lutfi IA, et al. Diagnostic accuracy of ultrasound B scan using 10 MHz linear probe in ocular trauma: results from a high burden country. Pak J Med Sci. 2016;32(2):385-8.
13. Tabatabaei A, Hasanlou N, Kheirkhah A, Mansouri M, Faghihi H, Jafari H, et al. Accuracy of 3 imaging modalities for evaluation of the posterior lens capsule in traumatic cataract. J Cataract Refract Surg. 2014;40(7):1092-6.
14. Yeh S, Colyer MH, Weichel ED. Current trends in the management of intraocular foreign bodies. Curr Opin Ophthalmol. 2008;19(3):225-33.
15. Kwitko MR, Kwitko GM. Management of traumatic cataract. Curr Opin Ophthalmol. 1990;1:25-7.
16. Lamkin JC, Azar DT, Mead MD, Volpe NJ. Simultaneous corneal laceration repair, cataract removal, and posterior chamber intraocular lens implantation. Am J Ophthalmol. 1992;113:626-31.
17. Zaidman GW. The surgical management of dislocated traumatic cataracts. Am J Ophthalmol. 1985;5:583-85.

9.1.4 Nondilating Pupil

Chirakshi Dhull, Ritu Nagpal, Prafulla Kumar Maharana

1. Write a short note on nondilating pupil.

Small pupil during cataract surgery is generally due to fibrosis or hyalinization. Cataract surgery in small pupil remains challenging and complications are more common in this scenario.

Causes include uveitis, diabetes, pseudoexfoliation, glaucoma, senile miosis, use of alpha-1 antagonists, etc.

Complications include increased risk of iris damage, bleeding, iris prolapse from one or more wounds, anterior capsule damage, incomplete evacuation of the cortical material, and difficulties with placing and aligning the intraocular lens (IOL) in the bag.[1,2]

Patients with intraoperative floppy iris syndrome (IFIS) may experience progressive pupillary constriction and greater chances of iris prolapse from the wound.

Techniques for Management of Iris

- *Preoperatively:*
  - Use of mydriatics, especially phenylephrine 10% preoperatively, can lead to greater dilatation.
  - For IFIS use of atropine 1% preoperatively helps in maintaining greater pupillary dilatation intraoperatively.
  - Nonsteroidal anti-inflammatory drugs (NSAIDs) such as flurbiprofen sodium 0.03% helps in avoiding intraoperative pupillary constriction.
- *Intraoperative:*
  - Injection of epinephrine 1:10,000 at the beginning of surgery.
  - Viscoadaptive agents, e.g., Healon 5 (AMO), can be used to maintain greater dilatation intraoperatively.
  - Release of posterior synechiae if that is the cause of small pupil using visco cannula or Sinskey hook.
  - Special surgical instruments, e.g., pupil dilating hooks[3] and expansion rings, e.g., iris hooks, Malyugin ring (microsurgical technology),[4,5] Graether's ring,[6] etc. **(Table 1 and Figs. 1 to 3)**.

TABLE 1: Special surgical instruments.

Pupil dilators	Material	Tips/special considerations
Iris hooks	NYLON (disposable), previously titanium	• Check for anterior bend • Locking system • Tip of the hook • Sharpness • Angulation: U and not V • Use the locking peg to manipulate **(Fig. 1)**
Malyugin ring	Polypropylene	• Placed through 2.2 mm with injector • Provides eight points fixation for 6.25 or 7.00 mm pupil • Made of four circular scrolls to engage the pupillary margin **(Figs. 2A and B)**
Graether's ring	Silicone	• Injected and removed through 2.75 incision • Provides 6.3 mm dilatation • Easy to use • Cost is a limiting factor **(Figs. 3A to D)**
Morcher's pupil expander ring type 5S	PMMA	• Expands pupil 300° with even tension • Can be implanted with forceps/injector
Perfect pupil	Polyurethane	• 7 mm diameter • 315° circle is made

(PMMA: polymethylmethacrylate)

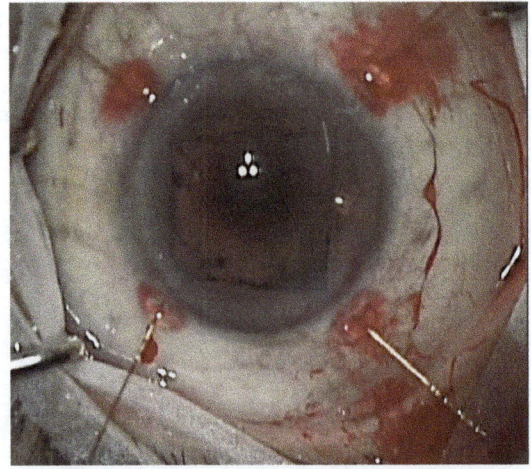

Fig. 1: Flexible nylon iris hooks (Grieshaber, Alcon) being used to dilate pupil in a uveitic patient.

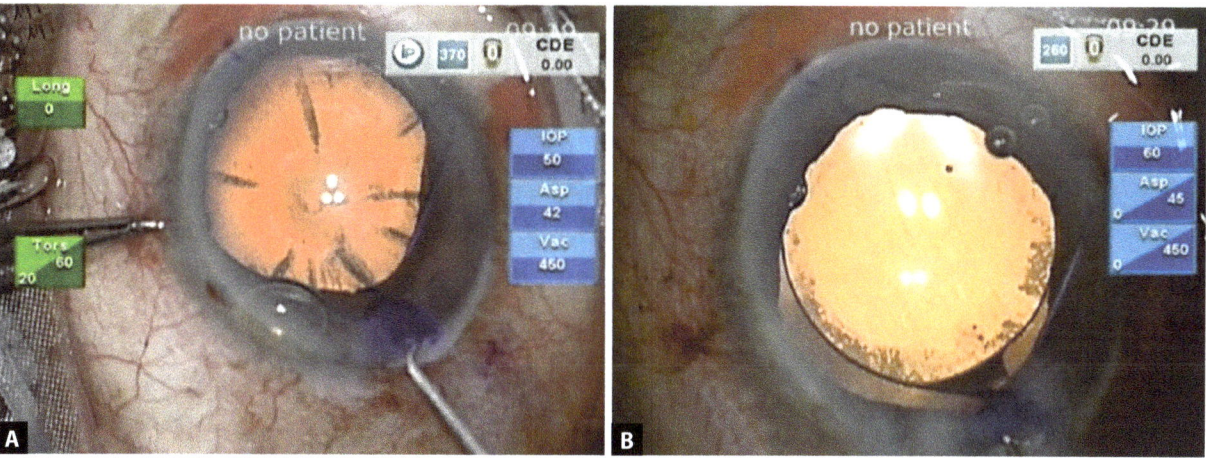

Figs. 2A and B: Malyugin ring. (A) Malyugin ring placed before the start of capsulorhexis. (B) Pupil dilatation nearly 6.5 mm maintained till the end of uneventful surgery.

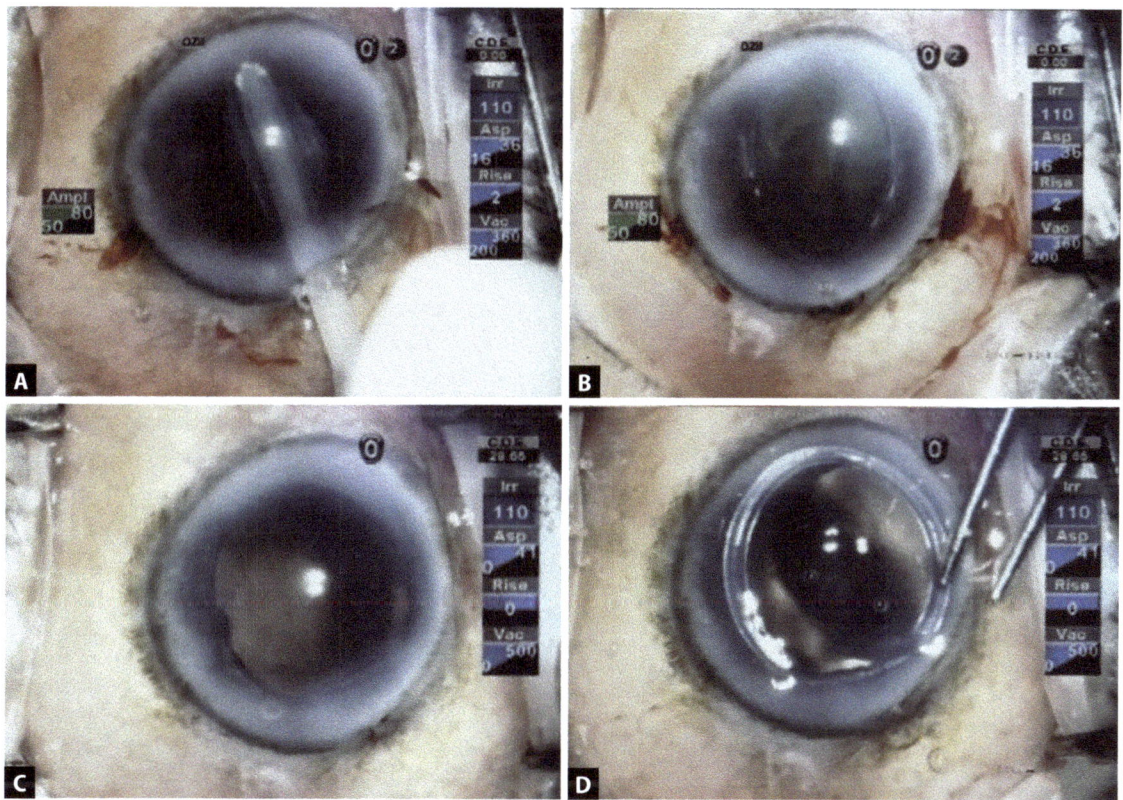

Figs. 3A to D: Graether ring. (A) Insertion of ring using inserter through 2.75 mm incision. (B) Ring opens smoothly covering almost entire pupil. (C) Intraocular lens (IOL) in bag, pupillary dilatation maintained up to 6.3 mm throughout surgery. (D) Easy removal without any trauma to iris.

- Iris sphincterotomies or iridectomy may also be used **(Table 2)**.
- Peeling of pupillary membrane may result in pupillary dilatation up to 5 mm and may help in avoiding use of any extra instrument **(Fig. 4)**.[7]

Role of Fluidics

Lower bottle height/IOP can reduce billowing of iris and iatrogenic iris damage. Greater bottle height/IOP has its own advantage, especially if bimanual technique is used. It reduces surgical time as it allows greater flow rates and faster emulsification. Hence, a balance has to be established between the two.

TABLE 2: Iris surgery.		
Surgery	**Procedure**	**Salient features**
Proximal sphincterotomy	• Grasp a small segment of superior sphincter and cut • Reposition iris	• Causes permanently enlarged oval pupil • Useful in glaucoma patients undergoing cataract
Sector iridectomy	Make mid-iris iridectomy followed by sphincterotomy	• Causes glare postoperative • Can be repaired with straight or loop sutures
Multiple sphincterotomies	6–8 equally placed sphincterotomies can be made using microincision scissors or rappazzo scissors	• Permanent pupil dilatation • Useful in uveitic cases • Use cycles of cycloplegics, miotics to prevent synechiae formation

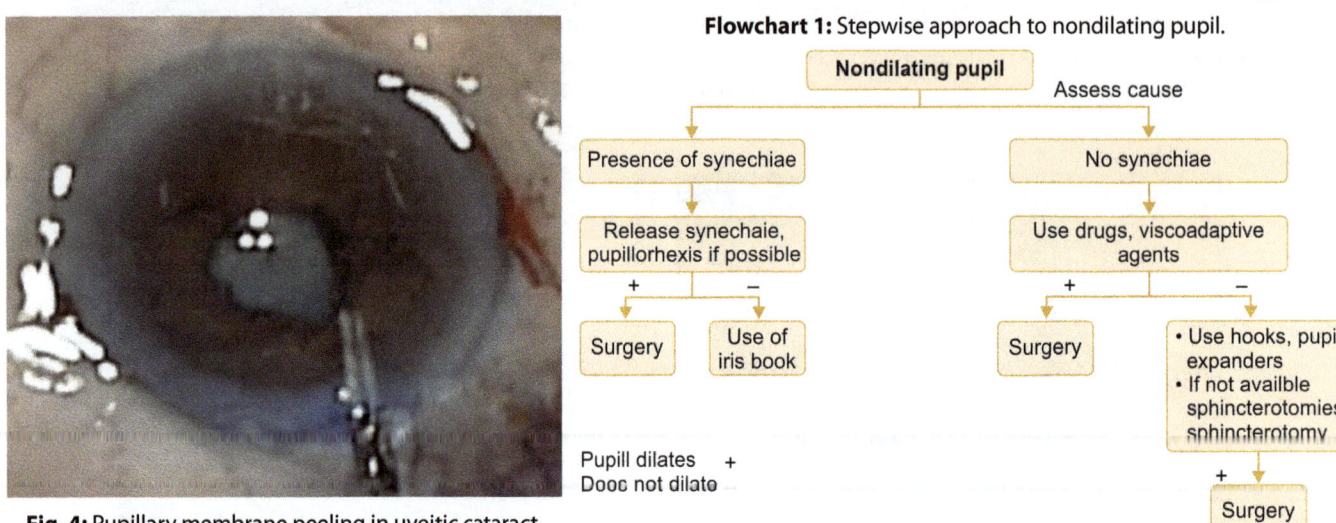

Fig. 4: Pupillary membrane peeling in uveitic cataract.

Flowchart 1: Stepwise approach to nondilating pupil.

Role of Bimanual Technique

- Bimanual microincision phacoemulsification is advantageous in soft to moderate nucleus
- Small incision leads to less iris prolapse
- Better control
- Irrigation is anterior to iris which prevents billowing
- Can use irrigation cannula for iris manipulation
- Better for removal of subincisional cortex as well
- Ideal for IFIS.

Conclusion

With improvement in technology, cataract surgery in small pupil is no longer associated with multiple inadvertent complications. Safety and efficacy of such surgery is improved.

Surgeons can now use a step-by-step approach to enlarge the pupil to a safe diameter **(Flowchart 1)**. With this approach, desirable outcomes can be achieved.

References

1. Bartlett JD, Miller KM. Phacoemulsification techniques for patients with small pupils. Compr Ophthalmol Update. 2003;4:171-6.
2. Malyugin B. Complications of small-pupil cataract surgery. Cataract Refr Surg Today Europe. 2013;26-30.
3. Nichmain LD. Enlarging the pupil for cataract extraction using flexible nylon iris retractors. J Cataract Refract Surg. 1993;19:795-6.
4. Agarwal A, Malyugin B, Kumar DA, Jacob S, Agarwal A, Laks L. Modified Malyugin ring iris expansion technique in small-pupil cataract surgery with posterior capsule defect. J Cataract Refract Surg. 2008;34(5):724-6.
5. Jacob S. The Malyugin ring. EuroTimes. 2013;18:34.
6. Graether JM. Graether pupil expander for managing the small pupil during surgery. J Cataract Refract Surg. 1996;22(5):530-5.
7. Osher RH. Pupillary membranectomy [videotape]. Audiovisual J Cataract Implant Surg. 1994;20:192-6.

9.1.5 Uveitis and Cataract Surgery

Tejaswini V, Ritu Nagpal

 1. Approach to a patient with uveitis undergoing cataract surgery.

Introduction

Majority of cases of chronic uveitis present with complicated cataract. Management of such cataracts is quite challenging for an ophthalmologist. Its incidence varies from 57% in pars planitis to 78% in Fuchs heterochromic iridocyclitis.[1] Performing cataract surgery in such cases has intraoperative challenges such as poor visibility due to band keratopathy, small pupils, posterior synechiae, pupillary membranes, bleeding from abnormal iris vessels, and unusual anterior capsules as well as risk of postoperative complications such as severe inflammation, hypotony, maculopathy, and phthisis bulbi.

With improved understanding of the disease processes, immunosuppressive agents have been employed during the perioperative period to tackle the inflammation in these eyes. Development of minimally invasive surgical techniques, availability of biocompatible intraocular lens (IOL) material, improved surgical training in performing complicated cataract surgeries, and with anticipatory management of complications, the outcomes of surgery in these patients looks quite promising at present.

Preoperative Evaluation

- A detailed history regarding onset, duration, and the recurrent nature of the disease is noted. Symptoms of redness, pain, photophobia, watering, duration of diminution of vision, field loss, and floaters. It is important to note the time of last attack of redness and pain and the number of attacks in a year.
- History of preexisting systemic comorbidities is noted.
- Previous and ongoing treatment, both topical and oral, for the ocular as well as the systemic condition is noted.
- Any known systemic/drug allergies are noted.
- General systemic examination for anemia, lymphadenopathy, hepatomegaly, splenomegaly, mouth/skin ulcers, rheumatoid arthritis, and skin diseases.
- Best-corrected visual acuity, near vision, and projection of rays from each quadrant are noted.
- Pupillary reactions, both direct and consensual, are carefully checked for presence of any afferent pupillary defect which gives an idea about optic nerve damage and retinal involvement.
- Intraocular pressure (IOL) by applanation tonometry is done and any secondary glaucoma is to be treated.
- Detailed slit-lamp examination should be done. Look for band-shaped keratopathy, corneal opacity, pigments, and keratic precipitates on corneal endothelium.
- Grade the anterior chamber cells and flare as per the standardization of uveitis nomenclature (SUN) classification. A laser flare meter can be used to quantify it.
- Presence of iris bombe, iris nodules, neovascularization of iris, pupillary membrane, peripheral anterior synechiae, and posterior synechiae are noted.
- Angle anatomy noted by doing gonioscopy.
- Density of cataract graded and documented.
- Dilated fundus examination is done to note the presence of vitritis, optic nerve atrophy and cupping, macular edema and ischemia, preexisting active lesions in retina and choroid.
- In presence of dense cataract which obscures view of fundus, B-scan ultrasonography should be done to rule out retinal detachment. Optical coherence tomography may be done for picking up macular atrophy, macular edema, or hole. A fundus fluorescein angiogram may also demonstrate macular ischemia or edema, retinal ischemia, active posterior segment disease, and active disc leakage.

Indications of Cataract Surgery[2]

- Visually significant cataract
- Phacoantigenic uveitis
- Cataract that obscures the view of fundus for assessment and further treatment of posterior segment pathology.
- Dense cataract in cases posted for posterior segment surgery.

Patient Selection

- Appropriate patient selection is important prior to surgery. Eyes in which visual loss is mainly attributable to cataract formation is most likely to benefit from cataract surgery. The outcome of surgery depends upon several factors, namely the uveitic diagnosis, proper perioperative management, and meticulous surgery.
- Diseases that spare the posterior segment generally have a better prognosis.
- Pediatric patients, especially those with juvenile idiopathic arthritis, have poorer outcomes and have a tendency of recurrent membrane formation postsurgery.

Preoperative Control of Inflammation

- This is a vital step in management of patients with uveitic cataracts.
- A general dictum of at least 3 months quiescent period is accepted to reduce the risk of postoperative cystoid macular edema.
- Patients with Behcet's disease require a minimum of 6 months of inactivity.
- Topical and systemic corticosteroids are used to control inflammation.[3] Oral steroids are started at 1 mg/kg/day starting 3 days preoperatively, tapering the steroid dose according to the amount of inflammation over the subsequent month postoperatively.
- Alternatively, if there are no contraindications, such as documented steroid response or infectious uveitis, a posterior sub-Tenon's injection of depot steroid, such as triamcinolone acetonide 40 mg/1 mL may be given, especially in patients where high doses of oral steroid are contraindicated and in diabetics.
- Topical prednisolone acetate 1% 2 hourly is administered 2 days prior to surgery, together with an oral and topical nonsteroidal anti-inflammatory agent.
- Intravitreal injection of preservative-free triamcinolone acetonide 4 mg in 0.1 mL at the conclusion of cataract surgery can be given to decrease the risk of postoperative macular edema.[4]
- Side effects from long-term treatment with systemic corticosteroids such as weight gain, acne, anxiety, mood changes, necrosis of head of the femur,[5] pancreatitis, suppression of adrenals, hypertension, diabetes mellitus, and psychosis. Children below the age of 15 years are especially prone to growth retardation.[6]
- Immunomodulatory agents are useful when inflammation is not controlled even after high dose of corticosteroids for 1 month, control of inflammation requires >10 mg of steroids daily or development of potential side effects which require stopping or tapering of steroids.
- The choice of immunomodulatory drugs depends on many different factors such as tolerance of the drug by the patient, control of inflammation, route of administration, side effect profile, general systemic condition of the patient, and the cost of the treatment.

High-Risk Surgical Cases

- Eyes with chronic hypotony
- Seclusio papillae with normal IOL
- Nonresponding chronic uveitis
- Choroidal effusion and thickened choroid on B-scan ultrasonography
- Ciliary body atrophy diagnosed on ultrasound biomicroscopy (UBM).

Patient Counseling

- Visual prognosis should be explained depending on the preoperative evaluation and a realistic outcome should be presented to the patient.
- General risks involved in any intraocular surgery like infection are explained.
- Patients should be made aware of the possibility of intraoperative complications and extended surgical time.
- Young patients should be explained regarding loss of accommodation post IOL implantation and the need for using reading glasses.
- Expected postoperative complications, need for resurgeries, need for follow-up, and the course of visual rehabilitation are explained.

Surgical Technique[7-12]

Choice of surgery: Cataract removal by phacoemulsification is safer for the uveitic cataract as it has lesser chances of inciting inflammation.

Posture: Patients with ankylosing spondylitis with a fixed flexion of the cervical spine are best postured in the Trendelenburg position, whereby their lower limbs are elevated above the level of the head. Additional pillows can be placed below the head to attain this position.

Surgical challenges: These include small pupil, shallow anterior chamber, posterior synechiae, peripheral anterior synechiae, pupillary membranes, and zonulolysis. Complications that may arise from these problems include an undersized or incomplete capsulorhexis, iris prolapse, increased risk of posterior capsular rent, increased risk of intraoperative zonular dehiscence, and increased postoperative inflammation.

Anesthesia: It is better to operate under peribulbar block with adequate analgesia and akinesia in adults and under general anesthesia in pediatric population.

Incision: Adequately sized main incision should be made in order to prevent iris prolapse in eyes with small or stretched pupils.

Pupil enlargement: Agents used are:
- Diluted adrenaline (1:1,000 0.5 mL adrenaline in 500 mL)
- Viscoadaptive viscoelastic such as Healon 5 (sodium hyaluronate 2.3%) which can physically roll open the pupil.

Synechiolysis and Removal of Pupillary Membrane

Peripheral anterior synechiae (PAS) should be released before the posterior synechiae.
- They are separated by injecting viscoelastic and using tip of the viscoelastic cannula to sweep the iris away from the peripheral cornea and in PAS and from lens capsule in case of posterior synechiae.
- In cases with a central membrane, a 26-gauge needle is used to make a nick in the membrane and release it from the anterior capsule and thus stretch the pupil.

Expansion: Often, once the pupillary membrane has been removed, the pupil begins to widen with viscoelastic.
- In cases where the pupil fails to dilate, it may be stretched using a pair of angled Kuglen hooks introduced through the main incision, used in a manner to latch around the pupil edge, pulling the iris in opposite directions. This is then repeated in a direction perpendicular to the initial stretch.
- Multiple sphincterotomies by means of intraocular scissors or vitrectomy probe, avoiding damage to the anterior lens capsule.
- Beehler pupil dilator (2 or 3 pronged) to mechanically stretch the pupil in a single injector system.
- Pupil retainers
- Disposable iris hooks are easy to place through multiple limbal entries.
- Malyugin ring (Microsurgical Technologies, Redmond, WA, USA) can be injected into the anterior chamber through a 2.2 mm incision and maneuvered to expand and maintain the pupil open at a 6 or 7 mm diameter.

Continuous Circular Capsulorhexis

Creating the ideal capsulorhexis is important in preventing posterior capsule opacification. It should be centered, overlapping the edge of the optic at all times, but not too small to prevent capsular phimosis. The capsulotomy can be initiated with a 26-gauge bent cystitome and modified vitreoretinal forceps can be then inserted from the side port to complete the rhexis.

Nucleus Management

Trauma to iris should be avoided at all times. The safest technique is the vertical chop technique. Chopping of fragments is done within the pupillary aperture with the phaco tip kept in view.

Irrigation and Aspiration

Thorough cortical cleanup is to be done so as not to leave any residual lens fragments or cortical remnants.

Intraocular Lens Implantation

- Safe to implant IOL in all inflammation-controlled cases including those of juvenile idiopathic arthritis.
- Most biocompatible IOL for the anterior chamber and the capsular bag is a single-piece, square-edged acrylic (either hydrophilic or hydrophobic) IOL.[13]

- Greater incidence of posterior capsular opacification, postoperative cystoid macular edema, synechiae formation, and pupillary membranes in silicone IOLs.
- In eyes with chronic uncontrolled uveitis, IOL implant should be deferred.
- Removal of viscoelastic from under the IOL and pressing the optic against the posterior capsule is an important step in reducing the incidence of posterior capsular opacification.

Surgery in Pediatric Cases[14,15]

- Surgery in children is technically difficult with increased incidence of postoperative inflammation.
- Issues of postoperative amblyopia therapy and visual rehabilitation.
- Current consensus is to place IOL in pediatric complicated cataracts which were previously thought to be a contraindication.
- However, careful monitoring for potential side effects and timely intervention to treat them should be done.

Complications

Intraoperative Complications

- *Zonulolysis:* Insertion of a plain capsular tension ring (CTR) or a modified Cionni CTR ensures that the IOL remains centered. Failure to use a CTR in the presence of weak zonules may result in capsular phimosis.
- *Retained lens fragments:* At the end of phacoemulsification, a gentle shake should be done whilst aspirating to ensure no nuclear fragments are inadvertently left behind. Any retained soft lens material or nuclear fragment should be removed surgically as soon as possible.

Early Postoperative Complications

- *Excessive postoperative inflammation and cystoid macular edema:* The incidence of cystoid macular edema in uveitic patients following phacoemulsification ranges from 12 to 59%.[6] If preoperative prophylactic oral steroids are ineffective in controlling the uveitis, the dose of oral steroids may be sharply increased. If no prophylactic oral steroids had been given, the patient should be given an oral pulse of steroids or injection of periocular steroids or an intravitreal injection of triamcinolone acetonide if this had not been given intraoperatively.
- Posterior synechiae
- Pupillary or ciliary membrane formation
- Transient rise in IOL
- *Hypotony:* Wound leak should be ruled out. Increase the anti-inflammatory therapy topically and systemically. In severe cases, vitrectomy and trimming of ciliary body traction membranes and silicone oil filling may be needed if UBM shows the presence of ciliary body detachment secondary to tractional membranes.
- *Recurrence of uveitis:* Recurrence rate following intraocular surgery has been reported to be as high as 51%. Stepping up the immunosuppression for the long term may be necessary to prevent further recurrences.

Late Postoperative Complications

Posterior capsular opacification: Most common complication following any type of cataract surgery in the late postoperative period.

Preventive measures include:
- Circular well-centered capsulorhexis which is smaller than the optic size
- Acrylic IOL with a square-edged optic design
- Meticulous removal of viscoelastic from within the capsular bag
- Ensuring the optic is stuck on to the posterior capsule at the conclusion of surgery
- Control of postoperative inflammation.

Explanting an IOL:[16] Indications for explant include:
- Formation of perilental membrane
- Chronic low-grade inflammation not responding to anti-inflammatory treatment
- Cyclitic membrane resulting in hypotony and maculopathy.

References

1. Velilla S, Dios E, Herreras JM, Calonge M. Fuchs' heterochromic iridocyclitis: a review of 26 cases. Ocul Immunol Inflamm. 2001;9(3):169-75.

2. Baheti U, Siddique SS, Foster CS. Cataract surgery in patients with history of uveitis. Saudi J Ophthalmol. 2012;26(1):55-60.
3. Jabs DA, Rosenbaum JT. Guidelines for the use of immunosuppressive drugs in patients with ocular inflammatory disorders: recommendations of an expert panel. Am J Ophthalmol. 2001;131(5):679.
4. Alkawas AA, Hamdy AM, Shahien EA. Intraoperative intravitreal injection of triamcinolone acetonide for cataract extraction in patients with uveitis. Ocul Immunol Inflamm. 2010;18(5):402-7.
5. Dada T, Dhawan M, Garg S, Nair S, Mandal S. Safety and efficacy of intraoperative intravitreal injection of triamcinolone acetonide injection after phacoemulsification in cases of uveitic cataract. J Cataract Refract Surg. 2007;33(9):1613-8.
6. Polito C, La Manna A, Papale MR, Villani G. Delayed pubertal growth spurt and normal adult height attainment in boys receiving long-term alternate-day prednisone therapy. Clin Pediatr (Phila). 1999;38(5):279-85.
7. Estafanous MF, Lowder CY, Meisler DM, Chauhan R. Phacoemulsification cataract extraction and posterior chamber lens implantation in patients with uveitis. Am J Ophthalmol. 2001;131(5):620-5.
8. Kawaguchi T, Mochizuki M, Miyata K, Miyata N. Phacoemulsification cataract extraction and intraocular lens implantation in patients with uveitis. J Cataract Refract Surg. 2007;33(2):305-9.
9. Ram J, Gupta A, Kumar S, Kaushik S, Gupta N, Severia S. Phacoemulsification with intraocular lens implantation in patients with uveitis. J Cataract Refract Surg. 2010;36(8):1283-8.
10. Rahman I, Jones NP. Long-term results of cataract extraction with intraocular lens implantation in patients with uveitis. Eye (Lond). 2005;19(2):191-7.
11. Rojas B, Foster CS. Cataract surgery in patients with uveitis. Curr Opin Ophthalmol. 1996;7(1):11-16.
12. Foster CS, Fong LP, Singh G. Cataract surgery and intraocular lens implantation in patients with uveitis. Ophthalmology. 1989;96(3):281-8.
13. Abela-Formanek C, Amon M, Schauersberger J, Kruger A, Nepp J, Schild G. Results of hydrophilic acrylic, hydrophobic acrylic, and silicone intraocular lenses in uveitic eyes with cataract: comparison to a control group. J Cataract Refract Surg. 2002;28(7):1141-52.
14. BenEzra D, Cohen E. Cataract surgery in children with chronic uveitis. Ophthalmology. 2000;107(7):1255-60.
15. Zaborowski AG, Quinn AG, Gibbon CE, Banerjee S, Dick AD. Cataract surgery with primary intraocular lens implantation in children with chronic uveitis. Arch Ophthalmol. 2008;126(4):583.
16. Adán A, Gris O, Pelegrin L, Torras J, Corretger X. Explantation of intraocular lenses in children with juvenile idiopathic arthritis-associated uveitis. J Cataract Refract Surg. 2009;35(3):603-5.

9.1.6 Ectopia Lentis

Pulak Agrawal, Manasi Tripathi

1. Discuss ectopia lentis.

Definition

Partial displacement of the lens from the patellar fossa due to loss of zonular support.

History

- The term "ectopia lentis" was coined by Stellwag in 1856.
- Term "ectopia" is a latin word which means "outside".

Etiology

There are number of factors which may lead to subluxation of lens. They may be broadly classified into:
- Traumatic
- Hereditary
- Associated with other ocular diseases
- Postprocedural.

Table 1 enumerates the most important causes in each of the categories.

Classification

There are few classification systems for subluxated lenses.
Clarke gave one of them which goes as given below.

TABLE 1: Causes of ectopia lentis.	
Traumatic	It constitutes around 50% of the cases of subluxation
Hereditary	• Marfan syndrome • Weill–Marchesani syndrome • Ehlers–Danlos syndrome • Stickler syndrome • Crouzon syndrome • Homocystinuria • Hyperlysinemia • Sulfite oxidase deficiency • Isolated ectopia lentis • Ectopia lentis et pupillae
Associated with other ocular diseases	• High myopia • Buphthalmos • Megalocornea • Aniridia, uveal coloboma • Uveitis, anterior uveal tumors • Mature/hypermature cataract • Pseudoexfoliation • Eales disease • Retinitis pigmentosa • Retinal detachment
Postprocedural	• Post trabeculectomy • Post DLCP • Post cyclocryo

(DLCP: diode laser cyclophotocoagulation)

Clarke Classification of Congenital Dislocation of Lens[1]

Simple	There is a defective zonule and ciliary body, and apart from the dislocation of the lens, the eye is grossly normal
Associated with anomalies of ocular dimension	For example, ectopia with axial myopia, microphthalmos, or buphthalmos
Associated with anomalies of ocular structure	For example, persistent pupillary membrane, corectopia, aniridia, polycoria, coloboma of iris, choroid, or lens, and megalocornea
Associated with congenital anomalies elsewhere in the body	For example, dwarfism or arachnodactyly

Classification Based on Degree of Subluxation

Hoffman[2] classified degree of subluxation based on slit-lamp examination under dilated pupil conditions:

Minimal to mild	The lens edge uncovers 0–25% of the dilated pupil
Moderate	The lens edge uncovers 25–50% of the dilated pupil
Severe	The lens edge uncovers >50% of the dilated pupil

Few conditions that deserve special mention are given here.

Traumatic Subluxation
- Usually due to blunt trauma.
- Males are more disposed to it.
- Associated with other signs of blunt trauma (seven rings of trauma).
- Can also have associated cataract with it (rosette cataract).
- There can be vitreous in anterior chamber (AC) which may lead to difficulties during cataract extraction.
- Chances of glaucoma are also high due to angle recession.

Marfan Syndrome
Genetics:
- Fibrillin-1 gene (FBN1) mutation

- Chromosome 15
- Autosomal dominant inheritance.

Diagnosis: Diagnosis is made by following the 2010 revised Ghent's nosology.[3]

Ocular manifestations:[4]
- Crystalline lens disorders (most commonly superotemporal lens subluxation)
- Premature cataracts
- Myopia
- Retinal detachment
- Strabismus
- Glaucoma
- Megalocornea, flatter corneas.

Homocystinuria

Genetics:
- Cystathionine b-synthase deficiency
- Chromosome 21
- Autosomal recessive disorder.

Ocular and clinical features:
- Should be considered in patients with attention-deficit/hyperactivity disorder (ADHD) and developmental delay.
- They increase the chance of thromboembolic phenomenon.
- Patients also manifest mental retardation.
- Myopia and lens subluxation and prominent ocular features.

Microspherophakia[5]

- Lenticular abnormality resulting from nutritional deficiency due to defects in the tunica vasculosa lentis at 5–6 months of embryonic life.
- This arrests the development of secondary lens fibers as a result of which the existing zonules are weak and lack tension.
- Homozygous mutation to the *LTBP2* gene.
- *Common associations:* Large myopic refractive errors, cataract and glaucoma secondary to pupil block, and angle-closure mechanisms
- Weill–Marchesani is a common cause of microspherophakia.

Ectopia et Pupillae

- It is a rare congenital inherited disorder characterized by lenticular and pupillary ectopia.
- Neuroectodermal, mesodermal, and mechanical developmental defects have been postulated.
- A neuroectodermal defect results in hypoplasia or absence of the posterior pigment epithelium layer and dilator muscle of the iris.
- Localized dilator muscle hypoplasia allows the pupil to be drawn to the opposite meridian, resulting in pupillary ectopia, and poor dilatation.
- Marked stretching of the iris and deficiency of the posterior pigmented layer—transillumination effect.
- The localized iris abnormality is accompanied by a corresponding zonular defect resulting in ectopia lentis.

Features:
- Bilateral ectopia of the lens and pupils
- Small poorly dilating elliptical or slit-like pupils
- Iridodonesis
- Iris transillumination
- Enlarged corneal diameter
- Microspherophakia
- Persistent pupillary membranes
- Iridohyaloid adhesions
- Anterior uveitis
- Elevated intraocular pressure, cataract, and retinal detachment.

Work-up

- Chief complaints
- Duration
- History of trauma
- Family history
- Associated systemic illness.

Systemic Evaluation

- Delayed developmental milestones
- *Musculoskeletal:* Height, US:LS (upper segment:lower segment) ratio, armspan
- *Cardiac status:* Murmurs
- *Others:* IQ, ADHD.

Ocular Examination

- Visual acuity (distant and near)
- Nystagmus
- Strabismus
- AC depth
- Vitreous in AC
- Angle
- Iridodonesis
- Pupil
- Phacodonesis
- Lens
- Retina.

Signs of Loose or Broken Zonules

Preoperative

- Phacodonesis/iridodonesis
- Presence of vitreous in the anterior chamber
- Irregular anterior chamber
- Exfoliation of the lens.

Postoperative

- Radial folds when puncturing the anterior capsule
- Excessive movement of the lens during capsulorrhexis and hydro procedures
- Difficulty in nuclear rotation
- Posterior displacement of the lens on starting infusion
- Vitreous herniation around the lens.

Management

It is mainly surgical.

Up to 3 clock hours	• CTR (capsular tension ring) with IOL implantation • Larger-sized IOL can be used with haptics being used to stretch the bag
>3–6 clock hours	Modified CTR with single loop (cionni) with IOL implantation[6]
>6–9 clock hours	Modified CTR with double loop/cionni or CTR with CTS (capsular tension segment) with IOL implantation in the bag
>9 clock hours	ICCE or intralenticular aspiration with ACIOL or scleral fixated IOL in the same or different sitting
Microspherophakia	ICCE with ACIOL or lens aspiration with CTR with CTS fixed to sclera and IOL implantation in the bag can be done[7]

(ACIOL: anterior chamber intraocular lens, ICCE: intracapsular cataract extraction; IOL: intraocular lens)

Important points while operating:
- Incision should be in the direction of intact zonules.
- Continuous curvilinear capsulorhexis (CCC) should be done using forceps, while starting in direction opposite the intact zonules which gives countertraction.
- Good hydrodissection and delineation should be done.
- Keep bag inflated.
- Capsular or iris hooks (as many required) should be used to support capsule. It also keeps the vitreous away (trampoline effect).
- Cohesive/dispersive ophthalmic viscosurgical device (OVD) should be used as and when required. Viscoat can be used to keep the vitreous away from the wound. It also helps to prevent vitreous coming in the phaco probe.
- Nucleus can also be expressed out of the bag to avoid pressure on the bag.
- Parameters—low infusion, vacuum, and flow.
- Irrigation/aspiration (IA)—tip should move tangentially and not radially while taking the cortical fibers.
- Preferably bimanual IA should be used, as more controlled vacuum can be given.
- Avoid vitrectomy till late.
- Proper docking of the prolene and 26G needles to avoid PCR and trauma to cornea, iris, and angles.
- Ensure tight incisions and close stable chamber.

References

1. Clarke CC. Ectopia lentis: a pathologic and clinical study. Arch Ophthalmol. 1939;21(1):124-53.
2. Hoffman RS, Snyder ME, Devgan U, Allen QB, Yeoh R, Braga-Mele R, et al. Management of the subluxated crystalline lens. J Cataract Refract Surg. 2013;39(12):1904-15.
3. Loeys BL, Dietz HC, Braverman AC, Callewaert BL, De Backer J, Devereux RB, et al. The revised Ghent nosology for the Marfan syndrome. J Med Genet. 2010;47(7):476-85.
4. Nahum Y, Spierer A. Ocular features of Marfan syndrome: diagnosis and management. Isr Med Assoc J. 2008;10(3):179.
5. Chan RT-Y, Collin HB. Microspherophakia. Clin Exp Optom. 2002;85(5):294-9.
6. Vasavada AR, Praveen MR, Vasavada VA, Yeh R-Y, Srivastava S, Koul A, et al. Cionni ring and in-the-bag intraocular lens implantation for subluxated lenses: a prospective case series. Am J Ophthalmol. 2012;153(6):1144-53.
7. Khokhar S, Gupta S, Kumar G, Rowe N. Capsular tension segment in a case of microspherophakia. Contact Lens Anterior Eye. 2012;35(5):230-2.

9.2 Refractive Surgery

Luci Kaweri, Namrata Bhuta, Payal Pandit

Corneal Refractive Surgery

 1. (a) How will you work-up a case for laser-assisted in situ keratomileusis (LASIK) surgery?
(b) What are the modalities available and which one is preferred and why?

Work-up in a Case of LASIK

It includes (**Flowchart 1**):
- *Detailed history:* A complete ocular history is vital to determine the outcome of refractive procedure and should begin with documenting the patient's reason for undergoing refractive surgery. When done for job requirements, the details of the same, and whether or not it includes a refractive surgery to get 20/20 vision should be confirmed. Other details that should be included are:
  - *Ocular herpes simplex virus (HSV):* Excimer laser can induce recurrence.
  - *Prior refractive surgery:* This can be done in cases with hyperopic shift after radial keratotomy (RK) but is associated with significantly higher risks of complications.
  - *Strabismus:* There can be recurrence of strabismus post-LASIK and continued need of prismatic glasses. Patients with strong fixation preference for their dominant eye may have difficulty with monovision.

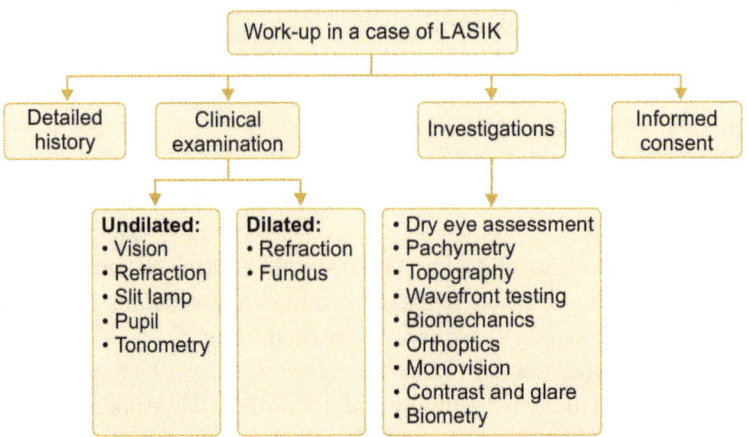

Flowchart 1: Laser-assisted in situ keratomileusis (LASIK) work-up.

- *Monocular patients:* All the risks of the procedure should be explained in detail to avoid any potential complication, although the risk is relatively low.
- *Contact lenses (CTLs), dry eyes and presbyopia:* Soft spherical CTL wearers should be asked to refrain from lens use for at least 2 weeks, 3 weeks for soft toric lenses, 3 weeks for extended wear lenses and at least 6 weeks plus 2 weeks per decade of wear for rigid gas-permeable CTLs (The Abott Medical Optics recommendation). LASIK is known to increase the severity of preexistent dry eye. Presbyopic patients should be given a trial of monovision CTLs before procedure, to assess adjustability postprocedure.
- *Pregnancy and lactation:* Physiological changes may result in less than optimal result.
- *Participation in high-risk activities:* Involvement in high-risk activities such as martial arts and contact sports may cause injury to the flap.
- *Medicines:* Drugs such as Tretinoin (Retin A) and Antihistaminics can cause severe dryness, Sumatriptan can alter corneal wound healing. Cordarone (Amiodarone) and hydroxychloroquine should be discontinued 1 month prior to LASIK and alternative medications should be considered, to avoid future corneal deposits. Topical steroids should be discontinued 1 week, and oral steroid 1 month, before LASIK to allow for optimal healing.
- *Comorbidities:* Medical conditions such as diabetes, active autoimmune diseases, and immunodeficiency states (HIV) alter wound healing, thereby affecting the outcome.
- Clinical examination:
  - *Visual acuity:* Uncorrected and best-corrected distance and near vision should be documented.
  - *Refraction:* Both manifest and cycloplegic refraction should be done. Cases of latent ciliary hypertonus should be ruled out.
  - *Pupil examination:* Large mesopic pupil size increases the risk of glare, halos and night vision complaints.
  - *Slit-lamp examination:* Special attention should be given to the health of the tear film and lid margin. Corneal assessment should negate the presence of any anterior membrane dystrophy, stromal scarring or vascularization. LASIK should be avoided in ectatic disorders such as keratoconus, pellucid, or Terrien's degeneration. Descemet membrane haze or corneal guttata should be ruled out. Cornea-based procedures for refractive correction should be avoided in presence of cataractous lens.
  - *Fundus examination:* A complete dilated fundus examination is a must as these cases are at risk of floaters and retinal detachment due to the increased length of the myopic eye.
  - *Tonometry:* Preoperative intraocular hypertension must be identified and evaluated. There is significant underestimation postoperatively as a result of altered corneal curvature and thickness.
- Investigations:
  - *Dry eye testing:* Schirmer's test to determine aqueous deficiency, tear break-up time (TBUT) to determine quality of tear film. In case of abnormality, dry eye should be treated first and ocular surface stabilized before performing refractive procedure. Tear film osmolarity (TearLab), tear film inflammation (InflammaDry), Lissamine green staining of the cornea, and conjunctiva are the other tests for dry eye assessment.
  - *Pachymetry:* Helps the surgeon to determine the final residual stromal bed (RSB) thickness.
  - *Corneal topography:* Topography helps to find a variety of corneal abnormalities that are associated with poor outcomes with LASIK, such as keratoconus, forme fruste keratoconus, and pellucid marginal degeneration.

- *Wavefront testing:* It is a useful screening device, since patients with severe wavefront abnormalities may not be ideal candidates for conventional refractive surgery. Wavefront-guided (WFG) and wavefront-optimized treatments can be planned based on these measurements. Wavefront-adjusted manifest refraction (WAMR) is the most effective technique for refractive planning. The wavefront map is first obtained and then the manifest refraction is refined from the wavefront refraction.
- *Corneal biomechanics:* If available, corneal biomechanics should be assessed in all cases. Poor corneal strength may increase the chance of ectasia, especially when treated for higher refractive errors.
- *Orthoptics:* Accurate assessment of latent strabismus is a must as it may manifest postprocedure.
- *Monovision testing:* This is important in patient >40 years of age who have adjusted well to CTL trial of monovision. Determination of ocular dominance is done preoperatively. Simplest technique to do so is the sighting test whereby the patient is asked to fix on a large letter of the Snellen chart while viewing through a half inch aperture at arm's length.
- *Contrast and glare assessment:* A baseline assessment would help in postoperative comparison.
- *Biometry:* Documentation preoperative and on postoperative visits will be helpful in unusual case of progressive axial myopia. This would also aid in post refractive intraocular lens power calculation whenever the patient needs cataract surgery in future.

- *Informed consent:* Before signing the consent, a detailed interaction between the patient and the surgeon is needed to ensure all the probable risks and complications have been well understood. Patients >40 years of age should be informed about the need for near vision glasses. Appropriate selection, education, and evaluation of the prospective patient for refractive surgery are key elements in obtaining satisfactory outcomes.

Available Modalities of LASIK

These include:
- *Conventional LASIK:* Treats lower-order, or spherocylindrical, aberrations such as myopia, hyperopia, and astigmatism.
- *Wavefront-guided:* It creates ablation profiles that are customized for individual patients. In addition to addressing higher-order aberrations (HOAs), WFG treatments can correct the lower-order aberrations (LOAs) of spherical error and astigmatism.
- *Wavefront-optimized:* Wavefront-optimized lasers do not use patient-specific wavefront data. Instead, they adjust the ablation profile of conventional treatments to create a more prolate shape with the additional peripheral ablation in the myopic patient, thereby reducing spherical aberration; however, they have no effect on other HOAs.
- *Topography-guided:* Topography-guided systems use corneal topography data to create ablation profiles that treat existing corneal shape irregularities and optimize corneal curvature.

Which one is preferred and why?
Preferred options depend on surgeon's expertise and availability of machines.

Wavefront-guided ablation is beneficial compared with wavefront-optimized ablation for patients with significant preoperative HOAs. However, it may be not be suitable for all patients, especially in multifocal intraocular lenses (IOLs) and highly irregular corneas or in eyes with small pupils.

Topography-guided ablations have gained popularity in treatment of corneas with irregular surfaces, such as those with small or decentered optical zones from prior excimer ablations, LASIK flap complications, or post-RK corneal irregularities. It shows excellent outcomes even for routine laser vision correction (LVC) cases in previously unoperated eyes.

 2. Describe LASIK surgery and its complications.

Laser-assisted in situ keratomileusis (LASIK) is a cornea-based refractive surgery performed to correct spherocylindrical ametropia. It was first described by Ioannis Pallikaris in 1990 using excimer laser for the refractive correction after the creation of the corneal flap.

Evolution of LASIK

The techniques and technology have been consistently refined. Customized wavefront corrections and wavefront-optimized corrections were introduced. The excimer lasers now include eye trackers, iris registration and eye identification as well as adjustments for centroid shift and cyclorotation of the eye. Algorithms are available for bitoric ablations for mixed astigmatism, bioptic correction for high myopia and hyperopic astigmatism. Zernike and Fourier transformations have been used to reconstruct and refine the wavefront map. Customized zone techniques reduced the depth of ablations and elliptical flaps better conform to the shape of the cornea.

LASIK Work-up

Refer to Answer 1 for details.

Preoperative Planning

- A manifest, cycloplegic, and wavefront refraction should be obtained in all patients. Wavefront adjusted manifest refraction (WAMR) is the most effective technique for planning.
- Age-appropriate adjustments should be done for spherical components (<25 years benefit from extra 0.25-0.5D minus sphere, >45 years would be best under-corrected by 0.25D)
- *Coupling:* Patients with >2D of minus cylinder will experience a coupling effect due to treatment of astigmatism. This will increase their spherical myopia correction by 0.12-0.25 per 1D of myopic cylinder.
- Monovision correction should only be done if the patient has successfully used or trialed CTLs for monovision for 24 hours a day for 2 weeks.
- Residual stromal bed thickness should not be <250-325 microns.
- Novice surgeons should begin with flap size of 8.8-9 mm and slowly decrease it to 8.5 mm to allow faster healing, less dry eyes, and to preserve the integrity of cornea.
- Horizontal elliptical flaps are preferred since they are better anatomic match for the cornea and have less chances of rotation and flap striae, unlike rounded flaps.
- Superior positioning of pockets is advantageous as they are covered by lids and are visually insignificant.

Surgical Steps [Using Femtosecond (FS) Laser for Flap]

- Preoperative antibiotic prophylaxis should be given.
- Check for calibration of the machine as per manufacturers recommendations.
- Single use disposable instruments should be used and sterility should be maintained throughout.
- Time out should be carried out and all safety checks regarding patient identification, eye/eyes to be operated, refractive error, and flap size must be confirmed.
- Clean and drape the eye under all aseptic precautions after betadine cleaning.
- Topical anesthetic eyedrop to be applied only minutes before the procedure to avoid corneal exposure.
- Iris registration ensures that the treatment is applied to the correct eye of the correct patient and nullifies the effect of cyclorotation and centroid shift.
- Docking
- Refining the flap position
- Creation of LASIK flap and side cuts
- Lifting the flap
- Laser ablation
- Flap replacement and alignment
- Epithelial trauma during the procedure should be avoided at all steps.

Advantages of femtosecond over microkeratome flaps:
- Consistency of flap thickness eliminates the risk of very thin flaps causing striae and free flaps.
- Uniform planar profile as opposed to meniscus flap profile (thin center) in microkeratome.
- The more vertical side cut allows more precise realignment thereby reducing the risk of epithelial ingrowth.

Postoperative Care

Flap position should be confirmed on slit lamp before sending the patient home. Instruction should be given to avoid touching and rubbing the eye. Antibiotic, topical steroids, and preservative-free lubricant eye drops are generally given as per surgeons' protocol.

Future:
- *LASIK Xtra:* The LASIK Xtra technique involves the application of the riboflavin/saline solution to stromal bed for 45-60 seconds. The stromal bed is then irrigated and flap replaced and smoothened. High-fluence (30 mW/cm^2) pulsed ultraviolet (UV) light is then applied for 45 seconds. This technique reduces the chances of ectasia by strengthening the cornea.

- *Refractive lenticular extraction (ReLEx) small-incision lenticule extraction (SMILE):* ReLEx is a procedure that is performed with only the FS laser which creates the interface for the corneal flap as well as the interface for a corneal lenticule, which is extracted and flap replaced. SMILE is a refinement of this technique in which the lenticule is removed through a small incision.

Complications of LASIK

The safety profile of LASIK has improved significantly over the last decade. These complications include **(Flowchart 2)**:

Perioperative Complications

- *Anesthesia related:* Excessive use of topical anesthesia before LASIK surgery can result in superficial punctate keratopathy (SPK) and frank epithelial defects. Placing a drop of anesthetic on the superior and inferior bulbar conjunctiva rather than directly on the cornea reduces the incidence of SPK. Frank epithelial defects may require the use of a bandage soft CTL.
- *Conjunctival lesions:* Repeated suction loss during LASIK can cause conjunctival chemosis. Excessive chemosis will in turn inhibit development of adequate suction. In such cases, it is advisable to postpone the procedure. Raised conjunctival lesions such as nevi or conjunctival scars may also lead to pseudo suction. Positioning the ring, in a way that, its opening does not overlap with the pathology, can avert this problem.
- *Inadequate exposure* by the drapes or eyelid speculum can cause blockage of microkeratome head progression producing an incomplete flap.

Intraoperative Complications

Femtosecond Flap-related

- *Suction loss:* Can occur in deep-set eyes, prominent brow, narrow palpebral fissure, significantly flat keratometric power, excessive eyelid squeezing, and a patient's inability to maintain fixation and follow instructions. Most common reason is excessive torqueing of the suction ring on the laser cone and movement of the patient's head when docked.
  - *Clinical:*
    - Loss of meniscus will be visible on the screen.
    - Loss of suction will be felt.
    - Movement of patient's head
    - Vertical gas breakthrough
  - *Management:* Depends on the stage of lamellar cut when it occurs—
    - *The raster stage before side cut:* Repeat with the same diameter and pocket disabled using the same cone.
    - *During side cut:* Skip this step and perform side cut with 0.5 mm smaller diameter.

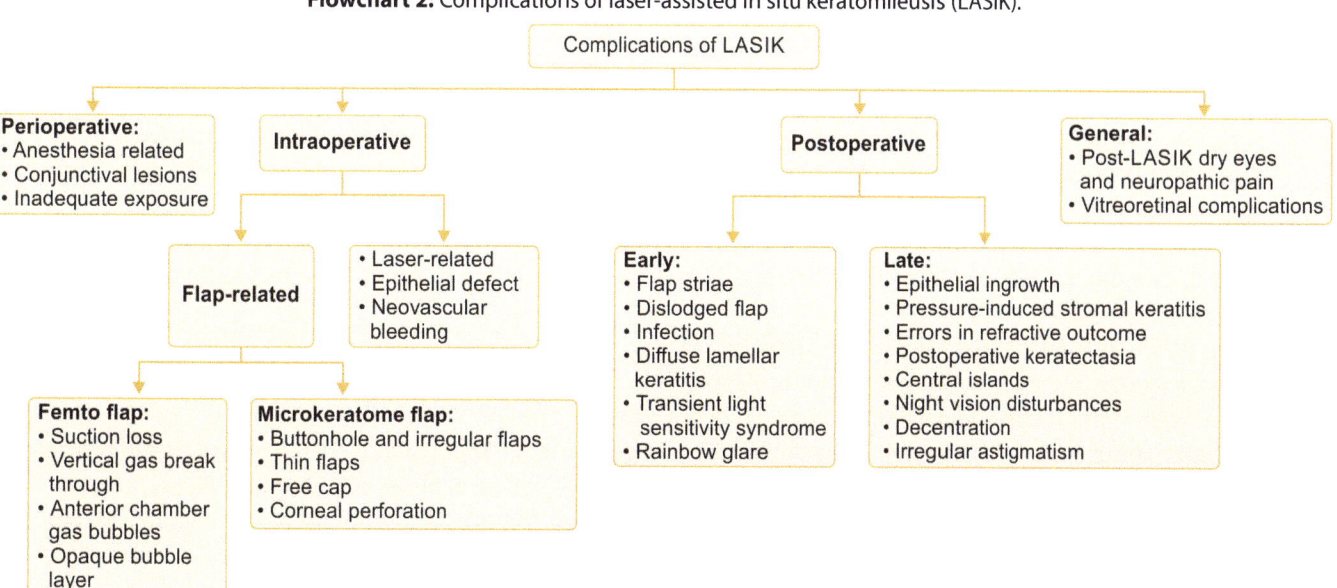

Flowchart 2: Complications of laser-assisted in situ keratomileusis (LASIK).

Other option is wait for 1–3 months and perform advanced surface ablations.
- *Prevention:*
  - Ensure adequate suction before initiating laser.
  - During docking, keep the plane of the suction ring perpendicular to the line of descent on the laser cone.
  - Encourage patients to remain steady.
- *Vertical gas breakthrough:*
  - *Clinical:* In presence of a break or a scar in the anterior stroma, gas can escape through the break and accumulate on the anterior corneal surface, blocking the laser pulses and resulting in an incomplete flap. The gas breakthrough will appear as a round clear spot on top of the gray lamellar flap plane.
  - *Management:*
    - <1 mm → proceed with smooth dissection
    - >1 mm → switch to photorefractive keratectomy (PRK) and consider using topical mitomycin
  - *Prevention:* Screen for stromal scars prior to procedure and counsel for PRK. Recent (<2 years, larger (>1 mm), and deeper (>20% corneal thickness) have more chances of breakthrough.
- *Anterior chamber (AC) gas bubbles:*
  - *Clinical:* Occurs when the edge of the flap is close to the limbus or if there are blood vessels in the peripheral cornea. The bubbles can affect tracking in certain lasers by causing the infrared tracker to calculate a displaced center of the distorted pupil.
  - *Management:* Wait for the bubbles to resorb, or proceed with the excimer correction with manual fixation and centration after turning off the eye tracker.
  - *Prevention:*
    - Reduce the flap size by 0.5 mm in smaller corneas.
    - Advise PRK in patients with significant peripheral corneal blood vessels.
- *Opaque bubble layer:*
  - *Clinical:* Occurs in the corneal stroma, when the gas bubbles are not allowed to pass uniformly through the lamellar interface, into the pocket and then outside the treatment area. It results in adhesions in the lamellar interface, making flap lifting and eye tracking difficult. Attempts to break larger or more coalescent adhesions may result in flap tears.
  - *Management:*
    - Can be reduced by gently rubbing the stromal bed with a smooth instrument such as the neck of cannula.
    - Can wait for 10–30 minutes for the OBL to be absorbed and then proceed.
  - *Prevention:*
    - The key is to create a good meniscus (halfway between the edge of the cone and the edge of the flap) during the docking process.
    - "Soft docking" that is slow lifting of the laser cone after applanation to increase the size of the meniscus until only the minimum amount of applanation is being applied is also useful.

Microkeratome Flap-related

- *Buttonhole and irregular flaps:* Occurs in absence of adequate suction. Increased risk is suggested in cases with steep corneal keratometry readings (>50 diopters).
  - *Clinical:* The defect in the center of the flap is seen immediately after the microkeratome has completed the reverse pass. The stromal bed has a clear area in the center about 2–3 mm in size that is slightly elevated, representing the uncut area of the cornea where the epithelium is still present.
  - *Management:* If identified immediately, the flap should not be lifted. If the flap has been lifted, it should be replaced and then refloated into position. The eye should be allowed to heal for at least 3 months before planning another refractive procedure.
  - *Prevention:* Ensure adequate suction and a perfect blade.
- *Thin flaps:* Occur due to considerable standard deviation in the average cut thickness. The Hansatome generally cuts 40 microns thinner than the depth indicated on the depth plate.
  - *Clinical:* Thin flaps they tend to roll along the distal cut edge. Flaps of 100 μm or more do not demonstrate this pattern. Once a very thin flap has healed, a hazy area with irregular striae will form in the center of the cornea.
  - *Management:* Replace the flap and allow it to heal for 3 months. The procedure can then be repeated with a deeper plate.
  - *Prevention:* Ensure adequate suction and a perfect blade.

- *Free cap:* Occurs in preoperative very flat keratometry (<41D) or in cases of thin flaps due to inadequate pressure.
  - *Clinical:* Free caps are circular and completely separated from the stromal bed. May have irregular edges and will fold onto itself when thin.
  - *Management:* In case of low preoperative keratometry readings, free cap should be placed on a drop of balanced salt solution in the antidesiccation chamber with epithelial side down. This can be replaced with proper alignment after finishing the ablation.
  - *Prevention:* In flat corneas, use the Hansatome or a larger microkeratome head (9.5 mm ring).
- *Corneal perforation:* It is the most feared and rare complication. It occurs when the depth plate is not properly screwed into the microkeratome head.
  - *Management:* Suturing the corneal incision and immediate referral for further management if needed.
  - *Prevention:* Staff should be well trained for correct assembly and this should always be crosschecked by the surgeon before the procedure.

Laser-related Complications

The most preventable complication is incorrect laser programming. The most insidious programming problems occur with prescription transposition errors. If the pupil tracker is offset then this will be carried out to the iris registration adjustments. On rare occasions, the excimer laser will actually fail in the middle of a procedure.
- *Clinical:* This will result in unexpected postoperative residual refractive error.
- *Management:* In case of laser failure, the flap should be replaced and the patient taken from the surgical room. The percentage of the correction performed should be recorded, in case all data are lost from the laser. The laser company should be called to determine the cause of the failure. Often, with company guidance, steps can be taken that return the laser to full function. Most excimer lasers have the procedure in memory so the patient can be brought into the room and the procedure continued from the previous point with no detrimental effect on the outcome. Patient reassurance during this phase is critical to maintain confidence.
- *Prevention:* Always check and double check all programming prior to performing LASIK. Iris registration ensures that the correct eye of the correct patient is being treated.

Epithelial Defect

Intraoperative epithelial defects significantly increase with older age, preoperative corneal thickness, and maintenance of suction ring vacuum during the reverse pass of the microkeratome. It occurs more in the second eye during bilateral procedure.
- *Clinical:* This is seen as irregular areas along the epithelial surface. This can be less than 1 mm or as large as the entire corneal flap. This occurs more on the superior edge where the epithelium is less adherent.
- *Management:* Use bandage CTL if the defect is >3 mm. Start a prophylactic antibiotic and observe daily for any evidence of infection.
- *Prevention:* Avoid ocular surface drying and toxicity from topical medication.

Neovascular Bleeding During LASIK

- *Clinical:* It occurs immediately after the keratectomy along the superior flap edge. It may be self-limiting, lasting for less than a minute, or persist for several minutes, depending on the size of the vessels cut and the coagulation status of the patient.
- *Management:* The suction ring can be left in place and downward pressure from it can tamponade some of the bleeding vessels. The flap is lifted and the bleeding vessels can be dried with a dry Murocel spear. If there is continued bleeding that could extend into the ablation area, dry rectangles of instrument wipe cut in 2 × 4 mm segments are placed on the area of bleeding. This sponge allows the ablation to be performed without further interruption. The sponges can be removed and the flap replaced with copious irrigation to make sure there is no further bleeding underneath the flap. The same sponges, which have been soaked in iopidine (apraclonidine hydrochloride), are placed over the areas of bleeding. Iopidine is used, as it is an alpha-2 agonist with a vasoconstrictive effect without the pupillary dilation that occurs with phenylephrine. The sponges are left in place for approximately 1 minute while the flap is adhering to the stromal bed.
- *Prevention:* Use a smaller suction ring in cases with neovascularization. Pretreatment with Alphagan (brimonidine tartrate) has been suggested to reduce the incidence.

Postoperative Complications

Early Postoperative Complications

- *Flap striae:* Incidence has reduced with FS laser. Sources are misalignment of the corneal flap after flap replacement, movement of the corneal flap during the first postoperative day, and the "tenting effect" of the corneal flap over the ablated stromal bed.
  - *Clinical:* Striae are oriented horizontally with a nasal hinge, vertically with superior hinge and oblique in displaced flaps. Can be easily localized using retroillumination through a dilated pupil and by using fluorescein staining **(Table 1)**.
  - *Management:* Early identification and treatment improves prognosis. Treatment is indicated in cases where striae extend through the visual axis, cause a decrease in best-corrected visual acuity (BCVA) or diplopia, or induce regular or irregular astigmatism. Treatment includes the stretch and smooth technique, flap hydration with hypotonic saline epithelial debridement, flap applanation, phototherapeutic keratectomy (PTK), and flap suturing.
  - *Prevention:* Prevention consists of intraoperative attention to the repositioning of the flap, with minimal manipulation. Postoperatively, patients are instructed to avoid rubbing or squeezing the eye. Patients wear eye protection 24 hours a day for the first week to prevent any eye trauma while the flaps are healing. Use of FS laser and elliptical flaps have reduced the incidence.
- *Dislodged flap:* Flap subluxation or dehiscence occurs when the flap is completely separated from the stromal bed.
  - *Clinical:* This is seen in first 24 hours. Nasal flap is found rolled onto the nasal conjunctiva and superiorly hinged flaps are seen 4–5 mm onto the nasal conjunctiva. Flap has striae and folds, epithelium can be seen growing over it and vision may reduce significantly (<20/200) due to edema.
  - *Management:* Urgent intervention is needed. Use lubrication and eye patch prior to treatment to improve discomfort. Flap can be unrolled and smoothed out at surgical center. The stromal side of the flap and the stromal bed must be thoroughly cleaned of all debris and mucus. The epithelium growing over the area of the exposed stroma should also be removed. The flap is then replaced and allowed to adhere to the stromal bed for at least 5 minutes because of the edematous state. The flap striae should then be treated as described above. Finally, a bandage CTLs should be placed on the eye to safeguard against a repeat dislodgement of the flap. When managed properly, the outcome should not be compromised by flap dislodgement.
  - *Prevention:* Advise adequate precautions for the first postoperative day. 4 hours sleep immediately after going home postprocedure allows eyes to heal. Patients should be warned not to touch or rub their eyes. Sunglasses or clear eye shields should be worn whenever possible even at night.
- *Infection:*
  - *Incidence:* 0–1.5%
    - Causative organisms vary from Gram-positive bacteria to atypical mycobacteria, fungal and viral pathogens.
  - *Donnenfeld proposed classification:*
    - Early onset (within 2 weeks of surgery) → *Staphylococcus* and *Streptococcus*
    - Late onset (2 weeks to 3 months) → Fungi, *Nocardia* and atypical *Mycobacteria*
  - *Clinical:* Bacterial keratitis presents within 72 hours as an acute onset of symptoms. The infiltrate is usually seen at the flap or at the flap interface, is generally single and localized, about 1–2 mm in size, white/gray in color, with hazy indistinct margins. If located on the surface of the cornea, it may be slightly elevated and associated with an epithelial defect. If allowed to progress without treatment, it will slowly increase in size like an early corneal ulcer. Inflammation

TABLE 1: Classification of flap striae.

	Probst classification of flap striae		
	Grade 1	Grade 2	Grade 3
Flap	Fine parallel lines	Fine parallel lines or basket weave pattern	Large parallel or basket weave pattern
Identification	Difficult	Obvious	Obvious
Visual axis involvement	No	Yes	Yes
UCVA or BCVA	No reduction	Reduced to 20/25–20/40	Worse than 20/40
Refractive error induced	None	Less than 1D astigmatism	1D or more of astigmatism
Complaints	Nil	Diplopia	Blur, diplopia, and glare
Treatment	Not needed	Needed	Needed

(BCVA: best-corrected visual acuity; UCVA: uncorrected visual acuity)

of the cornea with surrounding interface keratitis, conjunctival injection, and an AC reaction may all occur if the infection persists.

Reactivation of herpes simplex and zoster viral infections has also been reported after LASIK, and presents with corneal dendrites in the postoperative period. Fungal infections after LASIK have a delayed onset and have been related to prolonged topical steroid use.

- *Treatment:* Immediate treatment is warranted. Culture of the infiltrate helps in identifying the organism early.

  Early-onset infections → topical fourth-generation fluoroquinolones should be started alternating with fortified vancomycin 25 mg/mL every 30 minutes. Topical steroids should be reduced or discontinued. Patient should be followed up daily.

  Late-onset infections → topical fourth-generation fluoroquinolones should be alternated with topical amikacin 35 mg/mL every 30 minutes. Oral doxycycline 100 mg twice daily can be added, and topical steroids should be discontinued.

  Corneal epithelial dendrites that occur in any postoperative LASIK patient, particularly those with a past history of herpes simplex keratitis or herpes zoster, should be treated immediately with the appropriate topical and oral antiviral therapy.

- *Prevention:* Preoperative prophylaxis: Blepharitis should be treated aggressively prior to the procedure. Betadine lid scrubs and antibiotic drops [polymyxin B sulfate and trimethoprim ophthalmic solution for methicillin-resistant *Staphylococcus aureus* (MRSA)] should be used before and after LASIK. If a patient has a past history of herpes simplex, the risk of reactivation should be discussed with the patient. If proceeding with the procedure, a prophylactic course of oral antiviral is recommended 1 week prior to and 4 weeks after the LASIK procedure.

Intraoperative: Prevention of epithelial defects during and after LASIK should greatly reduce or eliminate the risk of a superficial bacterial corneal infection. Infection at the flap interface is avoided by preventing contamination of the instruments used to treat the interface.

Microkeratome heads should be sterilized for each patient. New sterile blades to be used for each patient. Disposable instruments such as microkeratomes or cannulas ensure the sterility of that step of the procedure. Sterile BSS is used for interface irrigation.

- **Diffuse lamellar keratitis (DLK):** Also known as Sands of Sahara, Sands, nonspecific diffuse keratitis, and LASIK interface keratitis. It is more common in FS LASIK compared to microkeratome. Etiology is unknown. Have been associated with ocular inflammation, ocular trauma, cleaning solutions, talc from gloves, meibomian gland secretions, microkeratome oil, rust on instruments, blade debris, iodine skin cleaners, and carboxymethylcellulose lubrication drops.
  - *Clinical:* Presentation varies depending on the grade of DLK **(Table 2)**
  - *Prevention:*
    - Avoid epithelial defects whenever possible
    - Avoid proliferation of gram-negative bacteria by maintaining dry environment (reservoirs of autoclave to be drained, instruments to be washed and dried daily)
    - Topical steroids to be used in postoperative period to suppress any subclinical inflammation.

TABLE 2: Grading of diffuse lamellar keratitis (DLK).

	Grade 1	Grade 2	Grade 3	Grade 4
Presentation • Color • Interface (1–7 days) • Inflammation • Visual acuity	• Focal • White to gray • Granular material • Absent • Normal	• Diffuse • White to gray • Granular material • Absent • Normal	• Diffuse, confluent • White to gray • Granular material • Slight conjunctival injection • No anterior chamber reaction • Reduced	• Diffuse, confluent • White to gray • Granular material • Intense central inflammation • Slight conjunctival injection • No anterior chamber reaction • Markedly reduced
Treatment • Interface irrigation • Topical steroids • Follow-up	• Not required • Hourly • Every 2–3 days	• Required • Hourly • Daily	• Required • Hourly • Daily	• Required • Hourly • Daily
Prognosis	Excellent	Excellent	Excellent	Reduced vision due to residual interface haze, stromal thinning and persistent striae
Stabilization	1 week	1–2 weeks	Several weeks	

- *Transient light sensitivity syndrome (TLSS):* Unusual photosensitivity seen 2–6 weeks after FS LASIK may be due to pulse energy. Vision is unaffected, no findings on slit lamp but steroid therapy helps.
- *Rainbow glare:* It occurs due to diffraction of light from the grating pattern created on the back surface of the flap by FS laser. Topical steroids can be tried postoperatively, but usually patients neuroadapt in few months. It can be prevented by using new lasers with high frequencies (60 kHz) and with their proper maintenance.

Late Postoperative Complications

- *Epithelial ingrowth:* Risk factors include anterior basement dystrophy, history of recurrent erosions, postoperative epithelial defects, repeat LASIK, flap slippage within 24 hours, and microperforations.
  - *Clinical:* Classification of epithelial ingrowth based on the grade **(Table 3)**
  - *Management:* Generally, the flap is lifted and the epithelial ingrowth removed from the stromal bed and the stromal side of the flap. Ease of removal depends on the duration of ingrowth. Epithelial bed can be cleaned using alcohol and PTK of approximately 10 microns. Suturing of the flap and fibrin glue has been used to prevent recurrences.
  - *Prevention:* It is safer to perform PRK in high risk cases.
- *Pressure-induced stromal keratitis (PISK):* Title is actually a misnomer since it is not actually keratitis but a steroid response manifesting with rapid rise in intraocular pressure (IOP) and fluid accumulation in the interface.
  - *Clinical:* The amount of fluid present may be relatively small, resulting in diffuse haziness in the interface and overlying stroma without an obvious fluid layer, or it may be pronounced resulting in a visible fluid cleft separating the anterior flap from the posterior residual bed. It is important to differentiate this condition from DLK stage III, and initiate an appropriate treatment strategy.
  - *Management:* Establish true IOP by measuring peripheral cornea. Antiglaucoma medications along with stoppage of steroid use are sufficient.
  - *Prevention:* Follow-up cases with chronic high frequency steroids (>2 weeks) post-LASIK.
- *Errors in refractive outcome:* Undercorrections are noted immediately and regressions occurs over next several months.
  - *Clinical:* Patient will be unable to function without glasses or contacts if undercorrections and regressions are significant and bilateral. They may also complain of night glare.
  - *Management:* Prescribe temporary glasses or CTLs. Recorrection can be attempted after refractive stability which usually takes approximately 1 month for each diopter treated. Surface ablation or lifting of the original corneal flaps are preferred techniques for enhancement.
  - *Prevention:* Cycloplegic refraction should be done in all cases during preoperative refraction. Operating room environment should be tightly controlled as low humidity and high temperatures are associated with overcorrections.
- *Postoperative keratectasia:* Usually occurs 1–12 months post-LASIK.
  - *Clinical:* Usually seen in corrections over 8D. Ectasia is usually associated with regression of the refractive effect, loss of uncorrected visual acuity (UCVA), BCVA, and irregular astigmatism. Topography demonstrates irregular astigmatism often with inferior steepening of the cornea. Orbscan topography will demonstrate posterior corneal ectasia on the posterior float map with a deep orange to red color in the central area of the cornea, with maximum thinning in the same area of the pachymetry map. Risk factors for post-LASIK ectasia include abnormal topography, RSB thickness, age, and preoperative corneal thickness. An ectasis risk score system helps to identify those at more risk.

TABLE 3: Classification of epithelial ingrowth.

	Probst/Machat epithelial ingrowth classification		
Grade	*1*	*2*	*3*
- Growth - Thickness - Size - Color - Detection - Demarcation - Flap changes - Progression	- Thin - 1–2 cells thick - ≤2 mm of flap edge - Transparent - Difficult - Well-delineated white line - No - Nonprogressive	- Thick - Discrete cells evident within nest - 2 mm from flap edge - Translucent - Easily seen - No demarcation lines - Edges rolled or gray - No flap edge melting or erosion - Progressive	- Pronounced - Several cells thick - ≥2 mm from flap edge - Opaque - Obvious - White geographic areas of necrotic epithelial cells with no demarcation line - Margins rolled with thicker whitish gray appearance - Progressive
Treatment	Not required	Nonurgent treatment within 2–3 weeks	Urgent treatment needed with close follow-ups

- *Management:* Corneal crosslinking (CXL) is needed to prevent progression. Some patients might need Intacs or corneal transplant to get functional vision.
- *Prevention:* Avoid LASIK in high-risk cases. Calculate RSB appropriately and not <250 microns should be left.
- *Central islands:* Occurred with broad beam lasers and are rare now because of use of scanning spot and rotating beam laser delivery systems.
  - *Clinical:* A central island has been defined as an area of higher refractive power of >1.5D and 2.5 mm or more in diameter or 3.0D and 1.5 mm in diameter. Postoperative monocular diplopia, visual distortions, and myopia are the main symptoms associated with central islands. Eyes with central islands may also have reduced BCVA, often in the 20/25 or 20/30 range. Unlike central islands observed with PRK, the topographical abnormalities observed with LASIK do not resolve over time. Topographically, a central island appears as a central steepening, appearing as red or a lighter shade of blue-green, 2–3 mm in diameter, relative to the surrounding area, which is notably a darker green or more typically blue. The difference in the diopter height of the island compared to the peripheral cornea can range from 3 to 8 D.
  - *Management:* Customized wavefront laser correction can be utilized to identify and treat patients with central islands. Corneal videokeratography also allows the identification of central islands. In this case, central islands are treated by using the Munnerlyn formula [depth of ablation = diameter^2 × diopter correction (height of the island)/3]. Computerized videokeratography is used to measure the diameter of the central island, and the height of the island is then calculated by noting the diopter color change between surrounding ablation and the peak of the island.
  - *Prevention:* The new generation of scanning excimer lasers has effectively eliminated the risk of central islands for standard refractive correction with the excimer laser. However, in the rare circumstance that a central accumulation of stromal hydration is noted during the excimer ablation, this can be removed by wiping the stromal bed during the ablation. Central islands may still occur when performing large (>50 μm) PTK treatments for corneal scars or haze. For these types of treatments, the addition of a small myopic correction of 1-2D will eliminate the risk for a postoperative central island.
- *Night vision disturbances: halos and glare:* Incidence has reduced after FS lasers.
  - *Clinical:* Halos occur when the optical zone of the laser treatment is smaller than the mesopic pupil size. Glare occurs because of the optical aberrations of the optical system that are magnified when the pupil dilates at night.
  - *Management:* Symptoms generally abate over 3–6 months. Over the recovery phase, the treatment of dry eyes and any residual refractive error or monovision often improves the symptoms. Turning on the car dome light when driving, 0.125% pilocarpine drops just before night driving and Alphagan (brimonidine) have recently been found to be useful.
  - *Prevention:* Pupillometry should be performed in all LASIK patients preoperatively to identify those with pupils >7 mm in dim light. The most accepted treatment is to adjust the blend zone of the treatment correction to cover the measured pupil size.
- *Decentration:* Incidence has reduced after the availability of eye trackers. This is seen in cases with large angle kappa.
  - *Clinical:* There may be an undercorrection or induced astigmatism. Presenting complaints include diplopia, halos, reduction in BCVA and UCVA. Diagnosis is confirmed topographically.
  - *Management:* Various techniques described for the treatment of decentrations include masking techniques to expand the ablation zone, transepithelial ablation opposite to the decentered ablation, or simply correction of the residual refraction with an expanded zone. Spectacle correction will correct any induced astigmatism, but CTLs will provide better improvement in the quality of the vision. The best improvement will be with rigid gas permeable CTLs. Alphagan drops can be helpful to minimize pupillary dilation at night, which should reduce night vision symptoms.
  - *Prevention:* Decentrations are avoided by appropriate centration of the laser ablation. Generally, the laser ablation should be centered on the center of the pupil. If the fixation is off the center of the pupil, the laser ablation should then be placed between one-half and one-third the distance from the center of the pupil to the visual axis.
- *Irregular astigmatism:* Refers to irregularities in the corneal surface identified on corneal topography that does not follow the regular "bow-tie" pattern of astigmatism.
  - *Clinical:* Usually occurs in association with flap complication, grade 4 DLK, flap striae, a decentered ablation or an asymmetrical healing response of the cornea. Patients complain of reduced UCVA, blurred vision, diplopia and glare at night. Irregular astigmatism is often associated with a reduced BCVA. Topography will demonstrate the areas of asymmetrical elevation or depression of the cornea within the visual axis.
  - *Management:* Persistent irregular astigmatism or irregular astigmatism that occurs alone is difficult to treat with the current laser systems. CTLs offer the best method for the correction of irregular astigmatism. Soft CTLs will provide up to a 50% improvement in the vision, while hard CTLs can offer full improvement if the patient is agreeable to their use.

- *Prevention:* Presence of irregular astigmatism is a contraindication for standard LVC. Prior to using the excimer laser, the quality of the laser beam should be tested to ensure that there are no irregularities of the beam. The LASIK technique should be performed in a manner that allows even application of the laser treatment to avoid irregular astigmatism.

Post-LASIK Dry Eyes and Neuropathic Pain

These occur due to the creation of a temporary neurotrophic cornea by severing the corneal nerves during the creation of the LASIK flap. There is decreased corneal sensation with decreased feedback to the lacrimal gland with reduced tear production. Confocal microscopy has demonstrated that the number of stromal nerve fiber bundles decreases by 90% immediately after LASIK. Hypoesthetic post-LASIK corneas can be a source of persistent pain and can be long-lasting. This is consistent with denervation sensitivity. Microneuromata that develop at the proximal ends of axotomized afferents and along regenerating axons would be expected to evoke spontaneous pain. During the first year after LASIK, the nerve fiber bundles gradually return, although by 1 year their number remains less than half of that before LASIK. Patients can present with severe debilitating pain with hardly any signs of vital dye stain on the cornea.

- *Management:* Assessment is same as done for classic dry eye patients. Frequent nonpreserved artificial tears are suggested to ensure good healing of cornea. Punctal plugs are used if symptoms persist. Frequency of lubricant drops and need of ointment at night depend on the severity of the symptoms. Steroids should be used in presence of inflammatory component and/or allergy. Scleral CTLs could be of help if everything else fails. Environmental controls for dry eyes, including a bedroom humidifier and protective sunglasses, may also be useful for patients who have chronic dry eye problems. Continuous reassurances and encouragement that the corneal signs and symptoms are resolving slowly are absolutely necessary.
- *Prevention:* Any patient with preexisting or suspected dry eyes should not be treated till quality of ocular surface improves. Other procedures such as PRK or LASEK (laser assisted sub-epithelial keratomileusis) which may preserve more of the corneal sensation should be considered in these cases. During the LASIK procedure, every effort should be made to preserve the epithelium, as epithelial defects will prolong healing and exacerbate the post-LASIK dry eye symptoms.

Vitreoretinal Complications after LASIK

There has been a theoretical risk of increased occurrence of retinal detachment after LASIK due to the alteration of anterior retina by the suction ring. Other complications noted to occur at a low frequency after LASIK include lattice degeneration (0.3%), posterior vitreous detachment (0.1%), macular hemorrhage (0.1%), retinal tear without retinal detachment (0.1%), and choroidal neovascularization (0.1%).

3. Discuss SMILE refractive surgery: indications, intraoperative and postoperative complications, and their management.

Small-incision lenticule extraction is the most recent iteration of refractive lenticule extraction (ReLEx) procedure using the VisuMax FS system, a proprietary technology of Carl Zeiss Meditec AG. It is an all-in-one laser refractive procedure which involves the incision of the posterior surface of the lenticule, followed by the anterior surface, which extends beyond the diameter of the posterior cut.

Current Technique and Instrumentation

The technique can be divided in two parts:
1. *Femtosecond laser application:* After setting up the parameters in the machine, docking is performed, followed by laser cuts: (a) The posterior plane cut, (b) the lenticule edge cut, (c) the anterior plane cut, and (d) the entrance wound cut. The time required for this step is twice of LASIK flap.
2. *Lenticule extraction:* Immediately after the FS cuts are completed, the lenticule is not freely extractable, as there are micro-bridges between the interfaces. The surgeon breaks those micro-bridges by bluntly dissecting in the plane between the lenticule and the stromal cap and that between the lenticule and the stromal bed, to free the lenticule from its surroundings. The lenticule is then retrieved and removed from the pocket. Surgical steps include:
   - Sterile field with routine disinfection and draping of the upper half of the face
   - Placement of eyelid speculum
   - The patient is instructed to fixate on the light at all times.

- The hook end of the Seibel's spatula or Chansue ReLEx dissector (CRD) is used to break the entrance wound open.
- A small pocket (1 × 2 mm) is made with the hook. The most distal part of the hook should be parallel to the corneal surface to ensure that the pocket is located anterior to the surface.
- The edge of the lenticule is then located by rotating the CRD so that the tip of the hook is pointed down toward the center of the eyeball. The tip is then pressed down and pushed across centripetally in tangential direction.
- The dissecting end of CRD is used to separate the anterior plane followed by the posterior plane.
- The patient is then asked to look down and the lenticule forceps is used to pull the lenticule from the stromal pocket.
- The pocket may be irrigated to wash out debris or foreign bodies such as epithelial cells.

Indications

- Myopia from –1D to –8D and myopic astigmatism up to 3D.
- Prerequisites include stable refraction within ±0.5D for at least 1 year, mesopic pupil size <7 mm, RSB >250 microns, central corneal thickness >475 microns, and expected post-procedure keratometry between 35D and 47D.

Complications of SMILE

Complications of SMILE are as listed in **Table 4**.

TABLE 4: Complications of small-incision lenticule extraction.

Intraoperative	Postoperative
- Suction loss	- Haze, grade 0.5–1
- Decentration of treatment	- Dry surface day 1
- Minor tear at the incision	- Epithelial islands at incision
- Cap perforation	- Fiber in interface
- Abrasions at the incision	- Infiltrates/keratitis
- Lenticule extraction difficulties	- Monocular ghost images
- Central abrasion	- Interface inflammation
- Major tear	- Irregular astigmatism
- Residual lenticule remnant at the interface	- Postoperative ectasia

Management

- *Intraoperative:*
  - *Suction loss during the procedure*: It occurs due to the patient squeezing the eyes or moving suddenly, fluid ingress between the suction ports of the contact glass and the cornea, gas bubble migration and subsequent compressive forces against the contact glass.

    Management: Depending on stage of suction loss, VisuMax automatically goes into a specific mode.
    - If suction loss occurs during the first pass (i.e., the pass which defines the posterior surface of the lenticule), the machine does not allow to complete the procedure and asks to convert into femto-LASIK. SMILE can be attempted again but at a different depth.
    - If suction loss occurs during laser firing, the procedure can be completed in the same session after redocking of the contact glass. The main challenge here is to retain the same centration. Using the same contact glass, it helps to match the footprints of the previous attempt.
  - *Decentration of the treatment*: Asking the patient to focus on the central light might minimize this.
  - *Incision tear or cap perforation during the SMILE procedure:* With the trend toward using smaller and smaller incision (1.5 mm), the chances of corneal cap tears at the incision edges have increased.

    Management: If tears are small and outside the pupillary area, there are no adverse outcomes other than a small scar. If the tear is large, align the anterior surface properly and put a bandage CTL. For prevention, it is better that surgeon only attempts to use an incision size commensurate with their experience and surgical dexterity.
  - *Tearing of the lenticule during the extraction process and subsequent retention of some lenticule tissue within the cornea:* Tearing of the lenticule can occur if it is a thin lenticule or the laser separation is not optimal (because of severe opaque bubble layer or corneal opacities or a fiber or other foreign matter between the contact glass and the cornea). In this case, while attempting the separation, the lenticule gets torn. A surgeon can also inadvertently leave some lenticule tags behind, especially at the edges. If some portion of the lenticule remains behind, it can result in irregular astigmatism and an unacceptable outcome.

Management: To prevent this from happening, it is best to do a complete separation in the first instance. It is best to use the spatula to completely separate the lenticule from both surfaces, along the entire circumference. It is best not to attempt to partially separate the lenticule and then grasp the lenticule with forceps and then pull or tug at the unseparated portions. This increases the risk of lenticule tearing and of tags being left behind. When the surgeon is in doubt about the lenticule tearing or of tags being left behind, it is best to uncurl the lenticule on the epithelial surface of the cornea after removing it and check to see if its size matches the original edge of the laser separation along its entire diameter.
- *Opaque bubble layer leading to difficult extraction of the lenticule:* It is characterized by accumulation and transient opacification of cavitation bubbles in intrastromal interface.

  Management: Wait for OBL to disappear or gently massage out from interface.
- *Lenticule adherence to the cap:* It results in a difficult extraction procedure. Lenticule mis-dissection can occur wherein the posterior plane is dissected before anterior plane. Intraoperative signs include:
  - *Meniscus sign* [Meniscus-shaped gap between the inner ring (diameter of lenticule cut) and the lenticule edge created by slightly pushing the lenticule edge away from the surgeon during creation of the posterior lamellar channel]. Meniscus sign clearly visible during posterior plane dissection and can act as a guide to identify the correct plane of dissection.
  - *Shimmer sign:* Bright reflex observed around the dissecting instrument. Reflex is not visible during dissection of anterior plane and helps to identify the correct plane of dissection.
  - *White ring sign:* Light reflex from the lenticular side cut. Position of the white ring relative to the instrument is useful in identifying the dissection plane, as the white ring is posterior to the instrument during anterior plane dissection and anterior to the instrument during posterior plane dissection

  Management: Sinskey hook-assisted dissection, modified strippers, and Y-shaped tip instruments can be used. There is increased likelihood of irregular interface, cap and side-cut tears, retained lenticule, and epithelial defects.
- *Epithelial defects:*

  Management: Frequent instillation of artificial tears. Bandage CTL can be used in large defects.
- **Postoperative complications:**
  - *Epithelial ingrowth:* Sometimes epithelial ingrowth can be observed, after SMILE. Unlike with LASIK, where ablation of the hinge can result in a path for the epithelium to encroach under the flap, in SMILE, it is usually an isolated nest of cells. They can either be left alone, if the nest is silent, or it can be scraped off by entering with an epithelial scraper from the original incision.
  - *Irregular astigmatism consequent to decentration:* Incorrect docking can result in decentration of the treatment and consequent irregular astigmatism and/or induction of aberrations.
  - *Corneal scarring:* In some cases, a fine scarring is observed at the cap edge or the lenticule edge. However, this is outside the pupillary zone and is visually nonsignificant.
  - *Interface haze:* It can occur several months after the procedure. In the majority of cases, it is not visually significant. Since the haze is sometimes related to ease of dissection, some surgeons increase and prolong their steroid regimen in cases of difficult dissection.
  - *Bowman's layer micro-distortions:* This may occur due to a geometrical mismatch between the undersurface of the cap and the stromal bed after lenticule removal, particularly after highly myopic SMILE. In the majority of cases these microfolds are smoothed out by the epithelium as time goes by. If desired, an early intervention with pressurized flushing of the pocket can be attempted.
  - *Sterile keratitis:* This is extremely rare. Severe inflammation after the procedure has been seen in cases where energy settings of the laser were too high, or in cases with large peri-incisional epithelial abrasion or intraoperative epithelial slough off or in presence of residual debris in pocket.
  - *Infection:* Best managed with topical medication, pocket flushing, and drug injection into the interface.
  - *Ectasia:* Occurrence is less in comparison to LASIK. Combining SMILE with crosslinking in borderline cases also reduces the chances.

4. Discuss SMILE in refractive surgery: advantages and disadvantages over conventional LASIK surgery.

Refer to Answer 3.

Advantages of SMILE

- *More accurate and repeatable tissue removal:* Intrastromal lenticule procedures may have advantages over LASIK and PRK because the potential errors associated with excimer laser ablation such as stromal dehydration, laser fluence projection and reflection losses, and other environmental factors are avoided. Also, the cutting time in SMILE is always the same, and it is independent from the refraction. Tissue removal is defined only by the accuracy of the FS laser, a device that is not affected by any changes in environmental conditions.
- *Greater biomechanical strength:* The two characteristics of the SMILE treatment, the absence of a flap and stromal tissue removal from within the stroma, mean that the anterior-most stromal lamellae remain intact postoperatively, except for in the region of the small incision. Because the anterior corneal stroma is the strongest part of the stroma, SMILE leaves the cornea with greater biomechanical strength than LASIK and PRK. Also, there is also the possibility of treating thinner corneas with SMILE.
- *Allows larger optical zone:* The superior tensile strength provided by preserving the stronger anterior stroma in SMILE allows larger optical zones, thus improving spherical aberration control and, hence, optical quality. This is achieved while leaving the cornea stronger than LASIK leaves the stroma.
- *Reduction in postoperative dry eye:* The cornea is one of the most densely innervated peripheral tissues in humans, with the majority of the nerve bundles within the anterior stroma. These anterior nerves are cut by the microkeratome or FS laser in LASIK and by the ablation in PRK, which results in dry eye symptoms. On the other hand, the anterior stromal nerve plexus is disrupted significantly less with SMILE.
- *Suitable for most patients:* The lack of a flap would be of significant advantage in patients who play contact sports, such as boxing, soccer, and martial arts.
- *Higher stability:* SMILE has also shown higher stability in high myopia and thus would be a preferred choice for high myopia.

Disadvantages

Small-incision lenticule extraction is not a preferred choice in cases with:
- Corneal opacity or dystrophy
- For cases of high wavefront aberrations or eyes with topographic irregularities
- Large difference between the pupil center and the visual axis.

5. Explain customized excimer laser corneal ablation.

Customized excimer laser corneal ablation includes WFG ablation and topography-guided refractive surgery.

Need for Customized Procedures

The human eye is an imperfect optical system. It consists of two types of aberrations. The LOAs which include defocus and astigmatism, and the HOAs which include large number of complex elements, most significant being coma, trefoil, and spherical aberrations. The LOAs in the eye are associated with the quantity of vision whereas the HOAs are associated with the quality of vision. The conventional excimer laser ablations that were initially used in clinical practice were based on the Munnerlyn formula. Their main aim was to correct the refractive error or the LOA. However, in doing so, these conventional ablation profiles lead to induction of large amount of HOA, in turn affecting quality of vision. This led to the development of different sophisticated ablation profiles over time to try and address the deficiencies of their predecessors.

Indications

- *Wavefront-guided procedure:* Normal corneas with significant HOAs.
- *Topography-guided procedure:* Irregular astigmatism, scarring, and ectasia, transplanted corneas, post-refractive surgery complications such as flap complications, small optical zones, decentered ablations, post-LASIK ectasia, and complications from RK.

Technique

- *Wavefront-guided procedure* is designed to correct the HOAs of the entire eye, measured preoperatively. Several wavefront mapping systems and WFG lasers are available commercially. Wavefront mapping systems are unique to the specific WFG laser used. Calibration should be performed according to the manufacturer's specifications. For WFG ablations, the wavefront maps are taken with the patient sitting up at an aberrometer under scotopic conditions; the mapping results are then applied to the cornea in the laser suite with the patient lying down under the operating microscope. Some systems require pupillary dilation to capture wavefront data. The wavefront refraction indicated on wavefront analysis is then compared with the manifest refraction. If the difference between them exceeds 0.75 D, the manifest refraction and the wavefront analysis may need to be repeated. The data are either electronically transferred to the laser or downloaded to a portable drive and then transferred to the laser. Unlike conventional or wavefront-optimized excimer laser treatment, in which the manifest or cycloplegic refraction is used to program the laser, WFG laser treatment uses programmed wavefront data to create a custom ablation pattern.

- *Topography-guided laser treatment:* Topography-based ablation profiles are designed by converting a height map of the cornea using a Zernike or Fourier matrix. The topography method and instrument used are dependent upon the make of the excimer laser and which topography unit its accompanying proprietary software will interface. Platforms used include Nidek Advanced Vision Excimer Laser Platform, topography-guided customized ablation treatment (TCAT, ALLEGRETTO platform, Alcon), CRS Master (Carl Zeiss Meditec, Jena, Germany), and corneal interactive programmed topographic ablation (CIPTA, iVis Suite).

Treatment methods, surgical technique, and ablation design vary by platform and surgeon. However, as a basic rule, topography-based ablation profile addresses the spherocylindrical refractive error in addition to irregularities in corneal elevation. Each treatment is based on the individual "true" (as opposed to mathematically modeled) preoperative corneal shape acquired through diagnostic equipment, often requiring multiple measurements to obtain a high-quality and reproducible map. After capture of the topographical data and importation into a software package with the refraction and corneal thickness, algorithms seek to combine treatment of corneal elevation irregularities with an ablation that maintains the aspheric shape of the cornea while minimizing the amount of tissue to be ablated. Simply stated, the topography is analyzed by software that calculates the difference between the actual cornea and the target asphere, and the difference is then ablated. Most software offers the customization of treatment parameters—for instance optical and transition zones, target asphericity, manifest or cycloplegic refraction, and centration on the corneal apex or the pupil—for surgical planning with simulated treatment profiles.

Comparison of Topography-Guided Versus Wavefront-Guided Customized Ablation

- Topography-guided ablations are particularly applicable in cases where corneal irregularities prevent reliable wavefront analysis, such as corneal scars, lens opacities.
- Even in cases where wavefront is available, it is superior in cases with problems due to irregular corneal surface.
- In cases of an increased angle kappa, topography-guided ablations centered on the corneal vertex better approximate the visual axis than WFG ablations centered on the entrance pupil.
- Topography-guided customized ablation also compares favorably to WFG customized ablation for primary treatments.

6. What is wavefront-guided ablation?

A traditional conventional excimer laser treatment corrects for spherical and cylindrical refractive errors, which are considered lower-order optical aberrations. In comparison, a WFG treatment considers measured LOAs and HOAs to create a more precise ablation profile in an attempt to obtain better postoperative quality of vision.

Methods of Wavefront Testing

A wavefront sensor or aberrometer measures and reconstructs the composite refractive monochromatic aberrations of the eye, based upon principles of ray tracing or interferometry. Wavefront sensors can be categorized as utilizing outgoing reflection aberrometry (Hartmann–Shack sensor), ingoing retinal imaging aberrometry (Tscherning aberroscope, sequential ray tracing aberrometry), ingoing adjustable refractometry (spatially resolved refractometer), and double pass aberrometry (slit skiascopy).

Technique

Refer to Answer 5

Limitations of Wavefront-guided LASIK

- Wavefront measurements are limited by the pupil and therefore peripheral measurements are not taken into consideration.
- Eyes undergo pupil centroid shift causing visual quality deterioration.

- Opacities in the cornea, lens, and vitreous can lead to flawed data. Opacities can lead to light scattering, which can influence the measurements provided by the aberrometer. Highly aberrated eyes can have a similar effect as well.

7. Critically discuss recent advances in keratorefractive procedures.

See Answer of Question 9

8. Discuss the changing scenario in diverse refractive procedures.

See Answer of Question 9

9. What are newer advances in refractive surgery?

Recent Advances in Keratorefractive Procedures

- Conventional LASIK has been replaced by *WFG and topography-guided customized ablation techniques.* (Refer Answer 5)
- *Small-incision lenticule extraction:* Refer to Answer 3.
- *Corneal crosslinking plus refractive procedures:* Iatrogenic keratectasia is a rare but serious complication of refractive surgery. Risk factors for post-LASIK ectasia include preoperative high myopia or hyperopia, thin corneas and patients with abnormal topography (such as forme fruste keratoconus). In order to prevent the development of iatrogenic keratectasia, simultaneous CXL and refractive surgery is currently performed in many countries worldwide.

  Corneal crosslinking was first performed in combination with LASIK (LASIK Xtra, a term introduced by Avedro, Inc., Waltham, MA, USA) before subsequently being used in PRK (PRK Xtra) and SMILE (SMILE Xtra). The initial purpose of CXL was to treat keratoconus and iatrogenic ectasia though currently its uses are expanded to include ectasia prophylaxis and infectious keratitis treatment.

Mechanism of Action

Corneal crosslinking uses the combined action of riboflavin and ultraviolet-A (UV-A) to cause photopolymerization of corneal collagen fibers, enhancing corneal biomechanical strength through the formation of new covalent bonds.

Complications

- Corneal haze and scarring
- Infective keratitis
- Sterile infiltrates
- Delayed epithelial healing
- Excessive corneal flattening with hyperopic shift.

Procedure

- *LASIK Xtra:* The LASIK Xtra protocol recommended by Avedro is as follows:
  - The LASIK flap is created and laser ablation is done.
  - With the flap left open, 0.22% riboflavin is applied onto the underlying stromal bed and allowed to soak for 45–120 seconds.
  - The stromal bed is irrigated to remove the riboflavin solution and the corneal flap is repositioned.
  - UV-A irradiation through the closed corneal flap is performed at 30 mW/cm^2 for 45-90s, 1.4–5.4 J/cm^2 delivered in total.
- *PRK Xtra:*
  - Transepithelial PRK photoablation is performed without the creation of a corneal flap.
  - 0.1% riboflavin with hydroxypropyl methylcellulose is applied for 90 seconds and subsequently rinsed off with a chilled balanced salt solution.
  - UV-A irradiation of 30 mW/cm^2 is performed for 90 seconds (total energy 2.7 J/cm^2)
  - 0.02% mitomycin C (MMC) is applied for 20 seconds and subsequently rinsed off.
  - Bandage CTL application.

- *SMILE Xtra:*
  - SMILE is performed following the standard protocol.
  - 0.25% riboflavin in saline is injected into the interface and left to diffuse for 60 seconds, after which it is rinsed off with saline.
  - UV-A irradiation of 45 mW/cm^2 for 75 seconds (total energy 3.4 J/cm^2) is performed.
- *Presbyopic LASIK:* Excimer laser is used to create a multifocal cornea by using following ablation pattern:
  - A small, central steep zone ablation, in which the central portion of the cornea is used for near vision and the midperiphery is used for distance vision.
  - An inferior near-zone ablation
  - An inferiorly decentered hyperopic ablation
  - A central distance ablation with an intermediate/near midperipheral ablation.
- *IntraCOR or corneal intrastromal FS laser treatment:* In this procedure, the FS laser makes concentric rings within the stroma, starting in the center with a ring diameter of 1.8 mm, and proceeding with subsequent rings toward the periphery. The formation of these rings produces a localized biomechanical change that reshapes the cornea to create multifocality. The procedure is typically performed only in the nondominant eye. Studies have demonstrated that this procedure can benefit patients with hyperopic presbyopia (+0.50D to +1.25D), as the treatment causes an increase in the corneal true net power as well as a potential gain of 4–5 lines of near vision.
- *Corneal inlays:* Corneal inlays improve near vision by several different mechanisms: changing corneal curvature, increasing depth of field via a small central aperture, or changing the refractive index of the cornea. Few commercially available inlays include the KAMRA corneal inlay (AcuFocus Inc, Irvine, CA), the Flexivue Microlens (Presbia, Dublin, Ireland), and the Raindrop Near Vision Inlay (Revision Optics, Lake Forest, CA). All currently available inlays are implanted only in the nondominant eye, which should have a stable refractive spherical equivalent of –1.00 to 0.00D at the time of surgery. The inlay is typically placed in a corneal pocket created by a FS laser, allowing for better centration, lower risk of corneal striae, and minimal impact on the peripheral corneal nerve innervation. The inlay must be centered on the visual axis, as even a slightly decentered placement can significantly affect the visual outcome.

Recent Advances in Lens-based Procedures

- *Advances in phakic IOL:* The EVO implantable collamer lens (ICL Model V4c; STAAR Surgical) is a single-piece posterior chamber (PC) phakic refractive IOL designed with a central port to eliminate the need for iridotomy or iridectomy that was required by earlier ICL models. The central port functions by allowing sufficient aqueous flow from the PC to the AC to maintain the normal physiology of the anterior segment of the eye. It is designed with a central convex/concave optical zone diameter of 4.9–5.8 mm and a 360 μm central port.

  The EVO ICL Model V5 (EVO+) includes a larger optical zone diameter of 5.0–6.1 mm. The EVO lens is produced from collamer, a proprietary hydroxyethyl methacrylate/porcine-collagen-based biocompatible polymer material and an ultraviolet absorbing chromophore.

  Advantages:
  - Reduced risk of cataract due to central port design. The 0.36 mm central port incorporated in the design of EVO provides sufficient aqueous flow to maintain normal fluid dynamics in the eye and improves the circulation of aqueous around the crystalline lens, which may reduce the incidence of cataract formation in comparison to earlier ICL models without the central port.
  - The risk of elevated IOP may also be reduced by the central port design.
  - Optical studies have demonstrated that the presence of the central port does not compromise the optical quality of the image as measured by modulation transfer function (MTF), wavefront aberrometry, or adaptive optics simulation.
- *Refractive lens exchange (RLE):* RLE is well-tolerated and effective for the correction of moderate-to-severe myopia and hyperopia. Monofocal, toric, multifocal, and accommodative IOLs are all used based on patient needs and expectations. The safety of the procedure is enhanced through the introduction of microincision cataract surgery (MICS) and the introduction of lenses that can be inserted through 1.8 mm incisions. Because RLE causes loss of accommodation, multifocal and accommodating lenses should be preferred along with this procedure.
  - *Multifocal IOLs:* Multifocal, multifocal toric lenses, accommodating lenses, or monofocal lens with monovision are various options that the surgeon can provide patients undergoing RLE to achieve spectacle/CTL independence after surgery. Multifocal IOLs provide a wide range of vision by correcting near, intermediate and distance visual acuity by distributing light into different foci for the same.

- *Accommodative IOLs:* Accommodating lenses are fashioned on the basis of normal physiological mechanism of accommodation. Most of these accommodative lenses are based on the principle of changing the axial position of the IOL. These lenses are either of the single optic or the dual optic variety. Eyeonics Crystalens (Eyeonics, Inc., Aliso Viejo, CA, USA) is a single optic silicone lens with hinges on its side plates.

  Synchrony AIOL (Visiogen, Inc.) is a dual-optic based accommodating silicone IOL. The anterior IOL component has a higher plus power in addition of that required for emmetropia. The posterior IOL component has a minus power to return the eye to emmetropia. Upon ciliary muscle contraction, the distance between the anterior and posterior component of the optic decreases and the anterior IOL component provides for near vision.

- *Monofocal IOL with monovision:* Monovision works on the principle of blur suppression and is mediated by the central nervous system. Using this approach, the dominant eye is completely corrected for distance and the nondominant eye is corrected for near. This approach after RLE can be used for offering spectacle independence to patients where multifocal or accommodative IOL cannot be implanted. A preoperative trial can also be given to the patient by using CTLs or high-powered trial lens in spectacle frame. Thus, if tolerated well by the patient, this can turn out to be a cost-effective approach in patients in whom multifocal IOLs are contraindicated or not available in extended range.

- *Smart IOL Medennium, Inc. (Irvine, California):* The concept behind the Smart IOL is to fill the entire capsular bag so that the ciliary muscle may resume control of lens shape alteration. This hydrophobic acrylic IOL, customized with precise optical specifications such as power and anterior and posterior curvatures, has unique thermoplastic properties that allow it to be reconfigured into a thin rod. After it is implanted through a phaco incision, the Smart IOL warms to body temperature and transforms back into its originally designed configuration.

- *Light Adjustable Lens Calhoun Vision, Inc.:* The power of the light adjustable lens (LAL) can be noninvasively adjusted and fine-tuned by applying UV light at 365 nm after the lens is implanted in the eye. Postoperatively, homogeneously distributed photosensitive macromers in the lens are irradiated with spatially distributed UV light to cause selective polymerization. Diffusion of the unirradiated macromers to the irradiated region then induces changes to the lens' shape and/or refractive index and produces a predictable power change. Correction of myopia, hyperopia, and astigmatism of up to 2.00D is reportedly possible. After the desired refractive state is achieved, the lens is photo-locked to consume any remaining, unreacted macromer and stabilize the refractive power.

 10. Explain astigmatic and refractive corneal surgeries.

The refractive apparatus of the eye essentially consists of the cornea, the AC, the lens, and the vitreous. These elements constitute two functional groups, the corneal system and the lens system. Astigmatism arises when one or both of the two refractive media—the cornea and the lens—have a different curvature, and therefore a different refractive power—in two meridians. Two currently established surgical methods for the correction of refractive error are refractive corneal surgery and refractive lens surgery. Excimer laser techniques and incisional procedures are used in refractive corneal surgery; phakic intraocular lenses (PIOLs) and RLE are used in lens surgery.

Refractive Corneal Surgery

Refractive surgical techniques used for myopia can be adapted to correct astigmatism alone or simultaneously as follows:
- *Incisional refractive procedures:*
  - *Astigmatic keratotomy:* It refers to making transverse or arcuate cuts in mid periphery perpendicular to the steepest corneal meridian. Can treat astigmatism up to 4–6D. Types are:
    - *Transverse keratotomy:* These are usually done in pairs along the steepest meridian and extend for 3 mm. A second pair may be added to the same meridian for greater effect. Since these are tangential to a given optical zone size, incremental flattening power decreases accordingly as the incisions are lengthened.
    - *Arcuate keratotomy (AK):* AK is an incisional surgical procedure in which arcuate incisions of approximately 95% depth are made in the steep meridians of the midperipheral cornea at the 7–9 mm optical zone. It has coupling ration of 1. For AK, the amount of cylinder correction is increased by increasing the length or depth of the incision, using multiple incisions, or reducing the optical zone. Older patient age is associated with increased effect of astigmatism incisions.
  - *Limbal relaxing incisions (LRIs):* Can treat up to –1 to –2D astigmatism. Produces less glare and discomfort and heals faster compared to AK. Optical quality of the cornea is preserved by making incisions at the limbus.

Instruments: The instruments used in AKs and LRIs are similar. Adjustable diamond blades are more often used in AKs. Preset diamond blades are more often used in LRI surgical procedures, although adjustable blades may be used. The FS laser has been adapted to create peripheral arcuate incisions. These incisions may be titratable, as only part of the incision may be opened initially, followed by a larger area later if there is a need for greater astigmatic correction.

Surgical techniques: Accurate determination of the steep meridian is essential. There are various nomograms available. Examples are J Gills, D Koch, R Lindstrom, S Thorton, L Nichamin, and E Donnenfeld. Among these, the nomograms by Nichamin and Donnenfeld are more popular and commonly used. In Nichamin Nomogram (also known as "NAPA"—Nichamin Age and Pachymetry Adjusted Nomogram), astigmatism is considered to be with-the-rule if the steep axis (plus cylinder) is between 45 and 135°. In against-the-rule astigmatism, steep axis is considered to fall between 0 and 44, and 136 and 180°. The patient's age with the amount of preoperative cylinder to be corrected is considered and then an incision is made as per the suggested arc length. Paired incisions are preferred to optimize symmetric corneal flattening and they are expressed in degrees of arc rather than length of the incision as the relative length of incision may vary according to corneal diameter.

Outcomes: The outcome of AK and LRI surgery depends on several variables, including patient age; the distance separating the incision pairs (optical zone); and the length, depth, and number of incisions. The Astigmatism Reduction Clinical Trial (ARC-T) of AK, which used a 7 mm optical zone and varying arc lengths, showed a reduction in astigmatism of 1.6 ± 1.1D in patients with preoperative, naturally occurring astigmatism of 2.8 ± 1.2 D. Other studies of AKs have shown a final UCVA of 20/40 in 65–80% of eyes. Overcorrections have been reported in 4–20% of patients. One study on LRI showed an absolute change in refractive astigmatism of 1.72 ± 0.81D after LRIs in patients with mixed astigmatism. Astigmatism was decreased by 0.91 D, or 44%, in another series of LRIs in 22 eyes of 13 patients. Incisions in the horizontal meridian have been reported to cause approximately twice as much astigmatic correction as those in the vertical meridian.

- *Laser ablation corneal refractive procedures:*
  - Surface treatment techniques include*:*
    - Photorefractive keratectomy
    - Laser-subepithelial keratomileusis (LASEK)
    - Epi-LASIK.

In these three types of procedure, corneal tissue is ablated with an excimer laser just below the corneal epithelium. Before ablation, the corneal epithelium is removed by a mechanical or chemical method or with a laser (as in PRK), with an alcohol solution (as in LASEK), or else it is separated from the underlying tissue with a microkeratome (as in epi-LASIK). The advantage of epi-LASIK over LASEK is that the epithelium can be peeled off as a complete sheet without the use of alcohol. Several epi-keratomes have been developed for the epithelial dissection, which will allow the creation of epithelial sheet.

  - Lamellar treatment technique*:*
    - LASIK
    - Customized LASIK (C-LASIK).

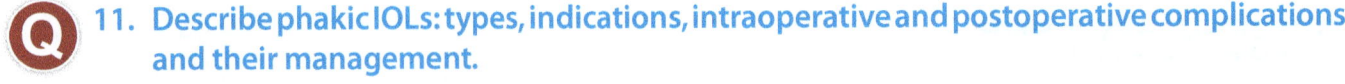

11. Describe phakic IOLs: types, indications, intraoperative and postoperative complications, and their management.

See Answer of Question 13

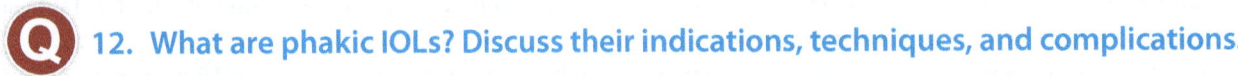

12. What are phakic IOLs? Discuss their indications, techniques, and complications.

See Answer of Question 13

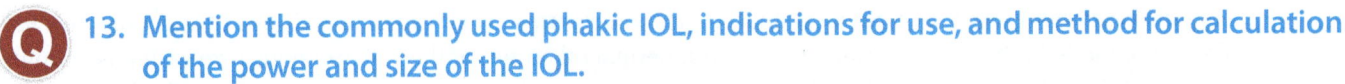

13. Mention the commonly used phakic IOL, indications for use, and method for calculation of the power and size of the IOL.

Phakic intraocular lenses are clear implantable lenses that are surgically placed either in AC or PC without removing the natural lens, enabling light to focus on the retina for improved UCVA. It is a reversible refractive procedure that preserves accommodative function.

Indications of Phakic Intraocular Lenses

- Correction of myopia or myopic astigmatism beyond the range of LVC
- Stable keratoconus
- Post-corneal transplant for residual refractive error
- To correct residual refractive error in pseudophakic eyes, i.e., piggyback lens
- To correct residual refractive error post-LVC
- To correct high anisometropia in amblyopic children noncompliant with traditional medical treatment.

Types of Phakic Intraocular Lenses (Table 5)

- Anterior chamber angle-fixated PIOL
- Anterior chamber iris-fixated PIOL
- Posterior chamber PIOL.

Method of calculation

Prerequisites:
- Age >21 years
- Stable refraction (<0.5D change for 1 year)
- Clear crystalline lens
- Ametropia not appropriate for excimer laser surgery
- Unsatisfactory vision with CTLs or spectacles
- Appropriate pupil size for the specified PIOL
- Adequate anterior chamber depth (ACD)
- Minimum endothelial cell count (ECC) specified for each PIOL
- No ocular pathology such as compromised corneal endothelium, iritis, iris atrophy, rubeosis iridis, cataract, glaucoma, and retinal disorders.

Ancillary testing:
- Specular microscopy or confocal microscopy to evaluate ECC and morphology looking for polymegathism and pleomorphism.
- Anterior chamber depth measurement by ultrasound, anterior-segment optical coherence tomography (AS-OCT), optical biometry, or Scheimpflug imaging.

TABLE 5: Types of phakic intraocular lenses (IOLs).

Type	Material	Power
Angle-supported anterior chamber:		
• Kelman	• PMMA haptic • Silicon optic	−8 to −20
• AcrySof	Hydrophobic acrylic	−6 to −16.5
Iris claw anterior chamber:		
• Verisyse/Artisan	PMMA single piece	• Myopia −3 to −23.5 • Hyperopia +1 to +12
• Veriflex/Artiflex	• PMMA haptics • Polysiloxane optic	• Myopia −2 to −14.5 • Toric −1 to −13.5
Posterior chamber:		
• Implantable collamer lens (ICL)	Collamer	• Myopia −3 to −23 • Hyperopia +3 to +22 • Toric: +1 to +6
• Phakic refractive lens (PRL)	Silicone	• Myopia −3 to −20 • Hyperopia +3 to +15

(PMMA: polymethylmethacrylate)

- Sulcus-to-sulcus (STS) distance by high-frequency ultrasound. Other methods such as AS-OCT, slit-beam topography, or Scheimpflug imaging can also be used to estimate the STS distance by measuring the WTW diameter and adding 0.5 mm to it.

Intraocular lens power calculation and selection: For refractive phakic iris-claw IOLs and angle-supported IOLs, the patient's refraction, keratometry at the corneal apex, and adjusted ultrasound central ACD are used. Based on this formula, the manufacturers provide nomograms or software to calculate the required PIOL power.

For PC PIOLs for calculating PIOL power, most users use the patient's refraction at the 12.0 mm spectacle plane or the vertex refraction, the corneal keratometric dioptric power at its apex, and adjusted ultrasound central ACD. The overall diameter depends on the ACD and should provide perfect stability, with no unnecessary compression forces on the angle that could damage the angle structures.

Surgical Technique

- *Surgical technique for anterior chamber phakic IOL:*
  - The surgeon can choose between topical, sub-Tenon, retrobulbar, or general anesthesia
  - Corneal incision and the creation of the tunnel of approximately 3.0 mm in a superior position, in a temporal position, or along the corneal axis of greatest curvature.
  - The IOL is loaded into the Monarch II or III injector (Alcon) with the anterior optic surface facing upward.
  - The exit channel from the cartridge is positioned halfway along the pupil to exploit the deepest area of the AC and to prevent the exiting IOL moving into contact with the crystalline lens.
  - When the distal loops reach the angle, the cartridge must be withdrawn as the injection of the IOL continues.
  - The proximal loops are still outside the incision; these are inserted one at a time and positioned at the angle.
  - Removal of viscoelastic
  - Closing the corneal incision with suture
- *Surgical technique for iris fixated PIOL:*
  - Most surgeons induce pupillary miosis before they initiate iris-fixated PIOL implantation, both to protect the crystalline lens and to make the iris easier to manipulate.
  - The long axis of the PIOL is ultimately oriented perpendicular to the axis of the incision.
  - A side port incision is made approximately 2–3 clock-hours on either side of the center of the incision; thus, a 12 O'clock incision requires side port incisions near the 10 and 2 O'clock meridians.
  - The "claw" haptics are fixated to the iris in a process called enclavation.
  - After the PIOL has been carefully centered over the pupil, it is stabilized with a forceps while a specially designed enclavation needle is introduced through one of the side port incisions, and a small amount of iris is brought up into the claw haptic. This procedure is repeated on the other side.
  - Iridectomy should be performed at the end of the implantation procedure and prior to completing the suture. Alternatively, a neodymium-doped yttrium aluminum garnet (Nd:YAG) laser iridotomy can be performed prior to the operation and is useful for avoiding a pupillary blockage.
  - If adjustment of the PIOL position becomes necessary after fixation, the iris must be released before the PIOL is moved.
- *Surgical technique for posterior chamber PIOL:*
  - Using a modified McPherson forceps with long, blunt, curved tips, the ICL is grasped and checked under the operating microscope.
  - The ICL has two tiny holes on the footplates (distal right and proximal left) that allow correct anterior–posterior orientation.
  - The cartridge is filled with ophthalmic viscosurgical device (OVD) and ICL is loaded with dome up.
  - A piece of soft material, the Staar foam tip, is positioned to protect the ICL from contact with the plunger of the shooter.
  - Broad pharmacological mydriasis is essential for uneventful implantation.
  - The ICL can be inserted through a sub-3.0 mm incision with one or two paracenteses to enable easier implantation of the haptics in the ciliary sulcus.
  - The AC is filled with a cohesive low-viscous OVD to protect the corneal endothelium and crystalline lens from surgical trauma.
  - The cartridge is inserted bevel down, and the ICL is carefully injected. The optic zone is considered to be a "no touch zone" during the maneuvers.
  - Finally, the haptics are gently pushed under the iris with a blunt spatula.

- Complete extraction of the OVD is mandatory to prevent postoperative ocular hypertension.
- Finally, the wound is hydrated.

Complications

Intraoperative Complications

These occur due to:
- The surgeon's inexperience
- Incorrect evaluation of the anatomical values of the eye to be operated
- Error in the choice of the IOL
- Due to an inappropriate surgical technique.

General intraoperative complications of phakic IOLs can be summarized as follows:
- Damage to the crystalline lens
- Damage to the corneal endothelium
- Iris prolapse
- Damage to the iris angle and/or choroidal bleeding
- Inverted insertion of the IOL.

Management: During the corneal incision, careful attention must be paid to the position of the knife tip to avoid contact with the iris or the anterior capsule of the crystalline lens. Damage to the crystalline lens and the corneal endothelium are often due to an insufficient ACD. The viscoelastic has to be injected in sufficient quantity to avoid this. The right IOP is essential to avoid the consequences of excessive vitreous pressure, which could cause the iris to collapse and provoke choroidal hemorrhage during surgery.

Specific to AC iris fixated PIOL:
- *Difficulty maintaining the ACD:* This may be due to—
  - An increase in the incision width and its corneoscleral position with respect to the scleral tunnel will increase the risk of losing ACD or iris prolapse during the delicate enclavation phase of the operation.
  - External factors such as the posterior thrust following retro- or peribulbar anesthesia may increase this problem.
  - Internal factors may include the excessive quantity of the viscoelastic substance introduced into the AC.

  Management: These complications can be avoided and resolved with the following:
  - Peribulbar anesthesia associated with mannitol administered in the preoperative (to reduce the vitreous push) or general anesthesia that will eliminate any posterior push
  - Partially suture the incision prior to enclavation
- The release of the IOL from its injector may prove to be difficult and there may be a risk of minor trauma caused by the instrument to the anterior surface of the crystalline lens or endothelium.
- *Bleeding:* This may be observed following iridectomy or may be caused by unexpected movements during enclavation. Injecting some viscoelastic into the area where the bleeding has taken place may be sufficient to stop the hemorrhage.
- *Difficulties with enclaving:* For this maneuver, the choice of the appropriate instruments is very important. The quantity of iris tissue caught during the enclavation procedure is important—too little will increase the risk of the IOL detaching in the postoperative while too much will increase the risk of decentering the lens and also lead to the ovalization of the pupil. This should all be managed on the basis of the iris thickness.
- *Decentration of the IOL:* This occurs when the enclavation is asymmetric. The amount of iris tissue caught should be the same on both sides of the IOL. The loop that is more difficult to manage (usually in the nasal position) is positioned first. Once it has been inserted, the temporal loop is inserted in a symmetrical position. The surgeon should then inject viscoelastic above the IOL and check the centration of the lens on the pupil. The final and definitive control of the position of the optic disc is then performed once the viscoelastic has been removed. Insufficient miosis makes enclavation more difficult as the iris will lose some of its tension in the site of enclavation.

Specific to posterior chamber PIOL: The intraoperative complications are largely due to sudden or incorrect technical maneuvers.
- *Damage to the IOL:* The collamer material used in the production of the lens is very delicate and sensitive to the conditions of its surroundings. If it is removed from its aqueous ambience, it will stiffen and be more vulnerable to rupture. The procedures of insertion in the cartridge and the exit of the loops, the manipulations, or the capture of the loops inside the cartridge must be performed very carefully to avoid damage to the IOL.

- *ICL upside-down:* With the old loading technique, the lens was positioned inside the cartridge and then pushed out. This maneuver could cause the lens to flip over. With the new loading method, the ICL is pulled when inside the cartridge using crocodile-type forceps. This prevents the lens from flipping over as it exits. If the lens actually does flip over, the surgeon should never attempt to flip it back inside the AC as such a maneuver is associated with a high risk of touching and damaging the crystalline lens and/or the corneal endothelium. The ideal solution is to extract the lens completely and repeat the implantation procedure.

Postoperative Complications
- *Loss of corneal endothelial cells*
- *Pupil ovalization or iris retraction:* It is a specific complication of AC PIOLs. The position of haptics in the sclerocorneal angle and their size might lead to mild deformation of the iridosclerocorneal architecture, resulting in iris retraction and pupil ovalization.

    Management: Topical use of miotic agents should be considered in the early postoperative phase if pupil ovalization associated with glare is detected. Minor pupil ovalization requires observation only, but gross ovalization indicates entrapment of the iris root and ovalization may become irreversible if the PIOL is not explanted promptly. In contrast to AC PIOLs, no cases of pupil ovalization or iris retraction have been reported to date with PC PIOLs.

- *Optical quality, glare, halos:* AC PIOLs are positioned in front of the pupil, with edge effects as a potential source of optical aberrations. Furthermore, the relationship between pupil size and the center of the PIOL optic is a crucial factor that should be evaluated preoperatively. If the scotopic pupil size is significantly larger than the optic of the PIOL, one should be very cautious about implanting a PIOL because it will probably result in postoperative glare and subjective discomfort. In PC PIOL, a small optic diameter (ICL up to 5.5 mm; PRL up to 5.0 mm) and decentration of PC PIOLs in relation to the pupil size, can result in glare and haloes, especially at night.

    Management: To avoid this complication, a preoperative mesopic pupil larger than 5.0 mm should be considered a limitation.

- *Chronic inflammation or uveitis:* As AC PIOLs are positioned directly in front of the iris, chronic inflammation and development of pigment dispersion are possible as pupil movement can induce some friction with the PIOL.
- *Intraocular pressure elevation/pupillary block glaucoma:* Acute pupillary block glaucoma can occur with angle-supported and other PIOLs. Due to the position of the PC PIOL, the iris may be pushed forward and cause acute pupillary block glaucoma, especially in hyperopic eyes.

    Management: A preoperative iridotomy using a laser or an intraoperative surgical iridectomy should be done to prevent acute pupillary block glaucoma.

- *Phakic intraocular lens rotation:* Rotation of an AC PIOL might occur because of undersizing. For PC PIOLs, it is mandatory to properly measure the white-to-white (WTW) distance to choose a PIOL with sufficient length to prevent decentration or rotation.
- *Cataractogenesis:* As the position of AC PIOLs is away from the lens, the formation of cataract is less significant than with a PC PIOL. The size of PC PIOL is very important as this determines the vault. Low vault increases risk of cataract formation.
- *Vitreoretinal and other complications*

 14. Describe refractive surgery for patients not suitable for LASIK.

Patients not suitable for LASIK may be considered for PIOL or RLE provided they meet all the prerequisites for these procedures.
- Phakic intraocular lens: Refer to Answer 13
- Refractive lens exchange: Refer to Answer 9

 15. Write critical note on selection of patient for refractive surgery.

Refractive surgery is performed on seemingly normal eyes with refractive error. So, the main challenge for the refractive surgeons is to select the right patient, the right procedure, and to achieve the desired outcome.

The selection criteria can be divided into three parts:
1. Basic selection criteria for surgical procedure
2. Contraindications
3. Role of personality.

Basic Selection Criteria for Surgical Procedure

Basic selection criteria should include:
- *Patient motivation:* It may be based on occupational requirements, desire for improved cosmetic appearance, recreational needs, and CTL intolerance. The patient should understand clearly that the surgical procedure greatly reduces dependence on optical aids but might not eliminate it completely.
- *Age:* Minimum age is 18 years and no upper limit as per Food and Drug Administration (FDA), but some surgeons are comfortable doing it at the age of 14 years also because of ease of retreatments. Refraction has to be stable for at least 1 year before the procedure.
- *Refractive error:* The optimal range varies from procedure to procedure.
- *Corneal thickness:* Customary target is RSB of 250 microns but there is no substantive scientific evidence to support the same. Many surgeons prefer a lower limit of 275 or 300 microns RSB. During preoperative planning, the surgeon should keep in mind that optical pachymetry maps in topographers may be lower when compared to ultrasonic pachymetry. Abnormally thick corneas (>620 µm) raise suspicion of endothelial dysfunction and warrant endothelial specular microscopy.
- *Corneal topography:* Normal topography is a prerequisite. Eyes with forme fruste keratoconus, early keratoconus, or pellucid marginal degeneration must be identified and LASIK should be avoided in them in view of ectasia risk. Surface ablation can be done in cases with mild topographical irregularities.
- *Keratometry:* In general, a postoperative minimum value of 34D and a maximum value of 50D set the limits after surgery, and must be calculated before surgery. Beyond these values, optical quality can be degraded. Multiple videokeratographic methods utilize simulated keratometry to screen for keratoconus. One such method, the Rabinowitz I–S ratio, describes an I–S threshold of 1.9 for clinical keratoconus-like patterns, and I–S values of 1.4–1.9 as the range for detecting keratoconus suspect-like patterns.
- *Pupil size:* Patients with large pupil diameter of 7.5–8 mm under mesopic conditions are at greater risk of optical aberrations.

Contraindications

These are given in **Table 6**.

Role of Personality

The role of personality cannot be stressed enough in patients undergoing refractive surgery. Patients with extremely high expectations should be carefully vetted. Anxious patients obsessed with complete independence from glasses should be thoroughly counseled. They should be clearly explained about the risks and benefits of each procedure. Patients with unrealistic expectations should be explained that this surgery is being done with purpose of reducing the dependence on glasses and having a refractive surgery does not mean complete independence from glasses.

TABLE 6: Contraindications for refractive surgery.

Absolute		Relative	
Systemic:	Ocular:	Systemic:	Ocular:
• Systemic lupus erythematosus	• Steven–Johnson syndrome	• Controlled diabetes	• Monocularity
• Rheumatoid arthritis	• Sjogren syndrome	• Contact sports	• Mild-to-moderate dry eyes
• Ocular cicatricial pemphigoid	• Keratoconus		• Congenital dystrophies and scars
• Collagen vascular disorders	• Other ectatic disorders		• Herpetic eye disease
• Uncontrolled diabetes			• Glaucoma with nerve damage
• Pregnancy			• Strabismus, amblyopia

16. What are the causes of dry eye post-LASIK surgery? How will you manage it?

Dry eye following LASIK is the most common problem faced by refractive surgeons, while dealing with patients postoperatively. This side effect has been the prime contributor of patient dissatisfaction after LASIK and causes frustration for both patients and surgeons.

Causes of Dry Eye Post-LASIK

- Preexisting dry eyes
- Long-term use of CTLs, previous blepharoplasty, lagophthalmos, diabetes mellitus, and Asian ancestry
- Higher refractive error correction
- Suction time and diameter of the ablation zone
- *Hinge location:* Few studies have shown that dry eyes are more common in superior hinge than nasal hinge.
- More in microkeratome in comparison to FS laser. May be due to damage of conjunctival goblet cells damage by suction pressure, decreased sensitivity due to trauma to perilimbal conjunctival nerves and thicker flaps.
- Reduced corneal sensation and blink reflex
- Altered tear film stability due to change in corneal curvature
- Inflammation
- Toxic effect of drugs
  Causes can also be classified based on presenting signs as shown in **Flowchart 3**.

Management of Dry Eyes Post-LASIK

Evaluation

- Evaluation of dry eyes post-LASIK is similar to classic dry eye evaluation. The Schirmer's test remains the mainstay in the clinical diagnosis of dry eye despite its inaccuracy (with only 25% sensitivity and 90% specificity). The ocular protection index (OPI) is calculated by measuring the TBUT and interblink interval (IBI) and dividing TBUT by the IBI; a score >1 predicts a better protected ocular surface. Additional examinations include tear osmolarity, tear mucin measurement, goblet cell count, tear lysozyme measurement, and lactoferrin measurement, but these tests are rarely done in clinical practice.
- Prior to surgery, LASIK candidates should undergo a detailed evaluation of the external ocular surface. The Ocular Surface Disease Index (OSDI) questionnaire helps in collecting a detailed preoperative information regarding dry eye symptoms and signs. The refractive surgeon must look for the signs of dry eye syndrome, including conjunctival injection, punctate keratitis, reduced tear meniscus, tear film debris, abnormal TBUT, and abnormal Schirmer testing.
- A trial of dry eye treatment is needed before performing LASIK surgery in patients with mild-to-moderate dry eye. Severe dry eye patients should not be considered as potential candidates for LASIK.

Treatment

- Artificial tears are the key treatment of the post-LASIK dry eye, especially the preservative-free type. Postoperatively, all patients undergoing LASIK should be started on preservative-free artificial tears for a time period at the discretion of the surgeon.
- Topical cyclosporine A 0.05% (Restasis) may also be effective for treating LASIK-induced dryness, inflammation, and neurotrophic epitheliopathy. Likewise, it is extremely beneficial in patients with preexisting dry eye who are considering LASIK surgery. Tacrolimus is another immunosuppressive agent, but its efficacy in post-LASIK dry eye has still not been established.

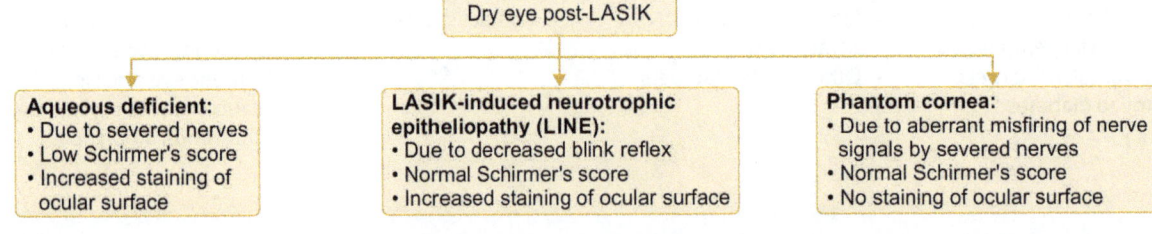

Flowchart 3: Dry eyes post-laser-assisted in situ keratomileusis (LASIK).

- A promising novel medication for dry eye treatment is the Diquafosol ophthalmic solution 3%, which stimulates fluid secretion from conjunctival epithelial cells and mucin secretion from the conjunctival goblet cells.
- For refractory dry eyes post-LASIK, autologous serum drops or punctal plugs can be tried. Punctal plugs are a safe, effective, and reversible method of preserving aqueous and artificial tears on the ocular surface in order to reduce the signs and symptoms of dry eye. In post-LASIK patients, punctal occlusion was shown to improve both UCVA and functional visual acuity. In addition, it also reduces LOAs and HOAs by changing the curvature, surface tension, volume, and dynamics of the tear film.
- Additional treatments that can benefit in post-LASIK ocular dryness include nutritional supplements, such as omega-3 essential fatty acids, and eye-warming devices.
- Finally, in cases where additional factors are contributing to the dryness, such as meibomian gland dysfunction or anterior blepharitis, treatment should include lid hygiene with scrubs and hot compresses and topical azithromycin or oral doxycycline.
- Many biologic molecules such as lubricin (proteoglycan-4), recombinant human nerve growth factor, tumor necrosis factor-α-stimulated gene/protein-6, interleukin-1 receptor antagonist, antitumor necrosis factor-α therapy, and anti-interleukin-17 are still in experimental stages as potential treatments for post-LASIK dry eye.

 17. Discuss corneal ring segments—indications and complications.

Intracorneal ring segments (ICRS) are PMMA (polymethylmethacrylate) devices, which are implanted at 70–80% depth of the cornea, with an aim to alter the corneal geometry and improve the refractive property of the cornea. Colin first proposed the use of ICRS implantation for the management of keratoconus in 2000. Commonly used models include:
- Intacs Addition Technology, Inc. (Fremont, CA, USA)
- Ferrara Ring Segment (Ferrara Ophthalmics, Belo Horizonte, Brazil)
- Keraring (Mediphacos, Belo Horizonte, Brazil)
- MyoRing (DIOPTEX GmBh, Linz, Austria).

Mechanism of Action

Intracorneal ring segments act as spacer elements between the collagen fibers of the corneal tissue inducing shortening of the arc length and causing central flattening of the cornea. Various theoretical models based on finite element analysis have proved that the flattening observed after ICRS implantation is directly proportional to the thickness of the implanted segment and inversely proportional to the corneal diameter of the implantation site; this means that the thicker and the smaller the ICRS diameter, the higher the corneal flattening effect. However, the keratoconic cornea disobeys the norms of the normal cornea, thereby increasing the unpredictability of the ICRS effect.

Indications

- Low myopia
- Keratoconus
- Irregular astigmatism after penetrating keratoplasty (PK)
- Corneal ectasia after excimer laser
- Irregular astigmatism after RK
- Pellucid marginal degeneration
- Post-trauma corneal surface irregularities.

Surgical planning: For selection of the ICRS size and position, the surgeon must consider refraction, keratometry, and corneal thickness. Implant manufacturers usually suggest a nomogram to be followed for the implantation of the ICRS. Various surgeons have proposed their own nomograms as well. While some nomograms have suggested the steepest keratometric axis as the most suitable site to place vertical incision, others consider the axis of coma as their preferable guide for implantation. Furthermore, the asymmetry of segments may provide more astigmatic effect. Therefore, in cases of central cones, using two symmetrical segment rings is likely to produce maximum flattening effect. In oval cones, however, asymmetrical ring segments or even single ring segment placed inferiorly according to the topographic profile may induce greater regularization. In cases of post-LASIK ectasia, single inferior ring segment appears to be the best option. In patients with pellucid marginal degeneration, the location of ICRS implantation is still debated.

Surgical technique: The surgical procedure is carried out under sterile conditions and topical anesthesia.
- *Manual dissection:* The procedure is centered on the corneal reflex of the microscope light, and a circular marker is used to create two concentric circles on the cornea. Using a diamond knife set to a depth chosen by the surgeon, a radial corneal incision is created between the two marked circles at the periphery of the cone and on its steep axis. A corneal spreader is then used to facilitate insertion of the double metallic arcuate guide, rotated to dissect two intrastromal channels around the cone area. Vacuum may be used to create the channels. The channel diameter depends on the type of ring selected. The two PMMA segments are implanted around the center of the cone in the clockwise and counterclockwise tunnels. In most cases, no suture is placed in the incision. A therapeutic bandage lens is placed at the conclusion of the procedure, and the patient is treated with a topical antibiotic/steroid combination and artificial tears for 2 weeks.
- *Femtosecond laser-assisted dissection:* Centration is based on the microscope corneal light reflex. The parameters used for tunnel and incision creation are inner diameter, outer diameter, and incision length and depth. The tunnel is created with the aid of an infrared, neodymium glass FS laser (ultrafast 10–15 second) with a wavelength of 1,053 nm. The laser beam of 3 μm diameter spot size is optically focused at a specific predetermined intrastromal depth by computer scanners, which give a focus (dissection) range between 90 and 400 μm from the corneal anterior surface. This beam generates cavitations, microbubbles of carbon dioxide, and water vapor by photodisruption, and the interconnecting series of these bubbles forms a dissection plane. The laser is scanned by computer-controlled mirrors with an accuracy of approximately 1 μm. A disposable suction ring is applied to hold the eye in position. The creation of the intrastromal tunnel with the FS laser is completed within 15 seconds with no manipulation of the cornea.
- *Combined:* Combined procedures that have been performed so far include:
  - Keraring/CXL
  - Intacs/transepithelial CXL
  - ICRS/PRK/PTK/CXL
  - Intacs/MyoRing
  - ICRS/miscellaneous.

Complications

- *Using the manual technique of tunnel creation:*
  - *Intraoperative:* Epithelial defects at the keratotomy site, anterior and posterior perforations during channel creation, extension of the incision toward the central visual axis or toward the limbus, shallow placement of the ICRS segments.
  - *Immediate postoperative:* Infectious keratitis, persistent incisional gaping, decentration, stromal thinning, cornea stromal edema around the incision and channel, extrusion of the implant, migration, undercorrection, overcorrection, intrastromal deposits.
  - *Late postoperative:* Glare, night halos, chronic pain caused by direct contact between the segment and a corneal nerve, persistent inflammation, persistent fluctuation of vision, neovascularization at the site of the incision.
- *Using FS laser:* Decentration, incomplete channel creation, and segment migration.

18. What is conductive keratoplasty? What are the mechanism, indication, and advantages and disadvantages of conductive keratoplasty?

Conductive keratoplasty (CK) is a noninvasive procedure that delivers radiofrequency current (350 kHz) directly into the corneal stroma. CK uses the electrical properties of corneal tissue to generate heat in the cornea. The resistance of stromal tissue to the current flow generates gentle and controlled collagen heating and causes optimal collagen shrinkage when temperature reaches 65°C. This produces a cylindrical footprint that extends approximately to 80% of the depth of the peripheral cornea.

Mechanism of Action

- *Collagen shrinkage:* Collagen, the principal component of corneal tissue, is present as chains, wound in triple helices. Covalent bonds hold the polypeptide chains together in the spiral, triple-helix configuration, whereas hydrogen bonds give a particular shape to the polypeptide molecules. Slight heating breaks the hydrogen bonds so that the polypeptide segments are free to form different configurations. However, these realignments are temporary, and the molecules can revert back to normal configuration upon rehydration. Additional heating breaks the covalent bonds of the collagen backbone. These bonds can be restored upon cooling, but the final orientation is usually different from the original.

Finally, when collagen is subjected to very high temperatures, it is reduced to gelatin, a mixture of polypeptides that solidifies into an amorphous structure upon cooling. The change in collagen structure caused by heat is known as denaturation (shrinkage) of the collagen and changes in the mechanical behavior of the tissue. In hyperopia treatment procedures, the desired mechanical change is peripheral corneal flattening and the resulting central corneal steepening.

- *Influence of temperature and time:* Collagen denaturation depends not only on the temperature to which it is subjected, but also to the duration of exposure to the elevated temperature. Thermokeratoplasty is a dynamic (not steady-state) heating process, and the state of collagen while undergoing thermokeratoplasty can be inferred, but not exactly defined, through steady-state temperature studies. The effect of CK is determined generally by three criteria: (1) number of spot applications, (2) number of rings of applications, and (3) diameter of application rings.

Rings of eight evenly spaced spots can be placed at 6 mm, 7 mm, and 8 mm. In addition, a second ring of eight spots can be placed at 7 mm. Thus, treatments consist of 8, 16, 24, or 32 spots. Using a single ring of eight spots at a 7 mm diameter gives an expected correction of 0.75–0.875 D. Adding a second ring at a 6 mm diameter gives a correction of 1.0–1.625 D. Adding a third ring at 8 mm gives 1.75–2.25 D. Finally, adding eight spots at the 7 mm diameter gives an expected correction of 2.375–3.00 D **(Fig. 1)**.

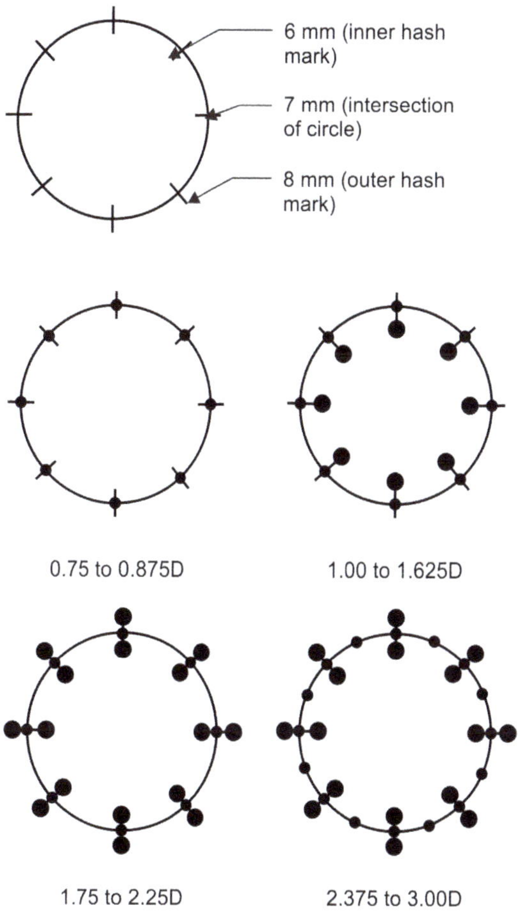

Fig. 1: Conductive keratoplasty.

Advantage Over Laser Thermal Keratoplasty

- Footprints of CK are deeper, homogeneous, and cylindrical than those created by LTK. Therefore, CK shows mild-to-moderate regression rates compared with LTK (laser thermokeratoplasty).
- It has a more controlled delivery system and causes less thermal damage to the surrounding collagen lamellae compared with LTK.
- Low to moderate hyperopic patients who are not suitable for excimer laser surgery may be candidates for thermal techniques, CK in particular.

Advantage Over Laser Ablation Technique

- They take place outside the optical zone
- Avoid flap-related complications
- Preserve the integrity of the cornea
- Cheaper and easier to perform
- Monovision CK has been shown to be successful for the management of presbyopia.

Advantages Over PIOL

Conductive keratoplasty can be used to treat hyperopia and astigmatism of <1.00D whereas PIOLs are available only from +1.00D for sphere and astigmatism.

Disadvantages of CK

- Not very effective for treatment of high levels of hyperopia
- Recent advances in laser ablation surgery including FS flap and WFG treatments have enhanced their potential of achieving greater accuracy and predictability as compared with CK.
- Development of multifocal and accommodative IOLs provides a wider spectrum of addressing hyperopia and/or presbyopia.

Q 19. (a) Enumerate keratorefractive surgeries. (b) Describe intraoperative and postoperative complications of LASIK and their management.

Keratorefractive surgeries include:
- *Incisional procedures:*
  - Radial keratotomy
  - Arcuate keratotomy
  - Limbal relaxing incisions
  - Opposite clear corneal incision (CCI)
- *Surface ablation:*
  - Photorefractive keratotomy
  - Laser subepithelial keratomileusis
  - Epithelial LASIK
- *Intrastromal ablation:*
  - Laser-assisted in situ keratomileusis
  - Customized LASIK
  - Presbyopic LASIK
- *Refractive lenticule extraction:*
  - Femtosecond lenticule extraction (FLEX)
  - Small-incision lenticule extraction
- *Corneal shrinkage procedures:*
  - Thermal laser keratoplasty
  - Conductive keratoplasty
- *Corneal implants:*
  - Onlays and inlays
  - Intrastromal corneal ring segments
- *Corneal tissue modeling:*
  - Orthokeratology.

For (b) part answer, refer to Answer 2.

Q 20. What is femtosecond laser?

Principle

The FS laser is a near-infrared laser, with a wavelength of 1,053 nm with ultrashort pulse duration of 10–15 seconds.

Mechanism of Action

Femtosecond laser such as Nd:YAG laser works by producing photodisruption or photoionization of the optically transparent tissue such as the cornea. It is a solid-state Nd:glass laser which is based on the principle of photoionization (laser-induced optical breakdown), producing a rapidly expanding cloud of free electrons and ionized molecules (plasma), at a focal point. Small volumes of tissue are vaporized with the formation of cavitation gas bubbles consisting of carbon dioxide and water, which then dissipate into the surrounding tissues. The 1,053 nm laser wavelength has a diameter of 0.001 mm, and can be focused to a <1.8 micrometer with ultrashort pulses. Due to the production of such concentrated and focused energy, there is minimal trauma to surrounding tissue and minimum heat generation.

Femtosecond Laser Refractive Platforms

The first ophthalmic FS laser system was designed by Dr Juhsaz in collaboration with Dr Kurtz at the University of Michigan in the early 1990s. There are currently five FDA-approved FS laser platforms [IntraLase FS (Abbott Medical Optics Inc., CA, USA), FemTec 2010 (Technolas Perfect Vision, MO, USA), Femto LDV (Ziemer Ophthalmic Systems AG, Port, Switzerland), VisuMax (Carl Zeiss Meditec AG, Jena, Germany), and WaveLight FS200 (Alcon, Fortworth, TX, USA)] for use in corneal refractive surgery. Of these, the IntraLase FS laser was the first commercially available FS laser.

The different FS laser platforms differ in available applications, pulse energy and frequency, applanation surface (flat or curved), and laser delivery pattern (raster/zigzag or centrifugal/spiral).

Comparison of Various FS Laser Platforms

Table 7 shows the comparison of various FS laser platforms.

Applications of FS Laser in Refractive Surgery

- *Laser-assisted in situ keratomileusis:* Femtosecond laser gained popularity in the field of refractive surgery after researchers proved its ability in producing LASIK flaps. The FS laser pulses, when applied adjacent to each other in a raster pattern, result in a cleavage plane to create the lamellar cut. More pulses are then applied in a peripheral circular pattern to create vertical side cuts, thus creating a LASIK flap.

    The FS-assisted flap creation is a critical step in LASIK surgery, with advantages when compared to microkeratome-related flap. Although modern microkeratome-related flap complications are very uncommon, the introduction of the FS laser has improved the safety, precision, and reproducibility of flap creation. With the use of FS laser, the surgeons have a greater choice for adjustment of flap diameter, hinge size, location, and depth as well as side cut angle and thickness of the flap. Thinner flaps can be fashioned in patients with high myopia, who need higher ablation.

    Femtosecond laser flaps are planar in architecture as opposed to most microkeratome flaps. Microkeratome flaps show large variability in their thickness profile which could affect the predictability of excimer laser stromal photoablation as stromal anatomy, hydration, and ultraviolet absorbance vary with corneal depth.

    Loss of suction during FS laser LASIK flap creation is easier to handle and the suction ring may be reapplied. Studies have shown FS laser to be safe and the visual and refractive outcomes of FS laser LASIK are equivalent to microkeratome LASIK.
- *FLEX and SMILE:* Carl Zeiss Meditec introduced a new approach called FLEX for refractive surgery to correct myopia and myopic astigmatism. This new innovation uses a FS laser alone, compared with other procedures that require both excimer and FS laser. FLEX involves making two cuts (posterior and anterior) in the cornea that intersect in the periphery, creating a lenticule, which is ultimately removed through a 3–5 mm incision. However, with further advances in FS surgery, this lenticule can be now be pulled out of 2 mm incision, popularly called the SMILE surgery. This procedure involves creating one or two small incisions through which the lenticule interfaces can be separated thus eliminating the need to create a flap. Therefore, this procedure will only cut a small proportion of anterior corneal nerves and cause less dryness.
- *ICRS implantation:* FS laser technology can also be used to create channels for the implantation of ICRS in patients with keratoconus. Intrastromal corneal ring segments are inserted in intrastromal channels at 75% depth of the thinnest

TABLE 7: Comparison of different laser platforms.

Laser platform	iFS advanced femtosecond laser	Femto LDV	VICTUS femtosecond laser platform	Wave light FS200 femtosecond laser	Visu max femtosecond system
Company	Johnson and Johnson	Ziemer Ophthalmics	Bausch and Lomb	Alcon Novartis	Carl Zeiss Meditec, Inc.
Laser type	Amplifier	Oscillator	Amplifier	Oscillator–amplifier	Fiber optic amplifier
Wavelength	1,053	1,045	1,053	1,045	1,043
Laser pattern	Segmental				
Centration	Computer	Manual	Manual	Computer	Manual
Visualization of surgery	Visual and virtual	Virtual	Visual	Visual and virtual	Visual
Mobile	No	Yes	No	No	No
Suction	Single syringe	Single built in	Single built in	Dual built in	Single built in on limbus
Applanation surface	Planar	Planar		Modified planar	Curved
Additional procedures	AK wedge, LK, PKP bioscopy, pocket ICRS	LK, PKP, ICRS pocket		AK, LK, PKP, ICRS	FLEX SMILE

(AK: arcuate keratotomy; FLEX: femtosecond lenticule extraction; FS: femtosecond; ICRS: intracorneal ring segments; LK: lamellar keratoplasty; PKP: penetrating keratoplasty; SMILE: small-incision lenticule extraction)

pachymetry. This results in an arc shortening effect and redistribution of corneal peripheral lamellae to produce flattening of the central cornea. Their effect is proportional to the thickness of the implant and inversely proportional to the implant diameter. Compared to the manual technique, a FS laser makes tunnel creation faster, easier, and more reproducible and offers accurate tunnel dimensions (width, diameter, and depth). With mechanical dissectors, segment depth may be shallower at positions further from the incision but depth is consistent throughout when using a FS laser.

- *Presbyopic refractive surgery:* One of the most recent developments in the ophthalmologic application of the FS laser is its use in the correction of presbyopia. The intrastromal correction of presbyopia (IntraCOR procedure) has been pioneered by Ruiz using the Technolas 520 FS laser platform. Intracorneal inlays are available with different mechanisms including refractive intracorneal inlays, which have an annular refractive zone for near vision, whereas other intracorneal inlays have no refractive power and work by increasing the curvature in the center of the pupil; in addition, pinhole intracorneal inlays enable near vision by taking advantage of the pinhole effect. Intracorneal inlays are inserted in the nondominant eye either under a LASIK flap or into a stromal pocket created by a FS laser. FS laser-assisted intracorneal pocket creation could increase the precision of the inlay position by customization of depth and length of the tunnel.

Disadvantages of Femtosecond Laser

- Suction loss
- Opaque bubble gas layer
- Vertical gas breakthrough
- Bubbles in the anterior chamber
- Transient light sensitivity syndrome.

21. Discuss the surgical procedures to manage corneal astigmatism with or without cataract surgery.

Surgical procedures to manage corneal astigmatism:

With cataract surgery: Phacoemulsification eliminates the lenticular component of astigmatism. To eliminate the corneal component, the surgeon must determine the amount and meridian of corneal astigmatism and factor in the surgically induced astigmatism (SIA) that will be generated by the cataract incision. The prevalence of preoperative astigmatism in cataract patients has been reported to be 86.6%, of which 35–40% of the cataract patients have astigmatism <1.0D and 19–22% have astigmatism <1.5D. While preexisting astigmatism of 0.5D does not need correction, resultant astigmatism should be <0.75D in patients seeking spectacle independence after cataract surgery, especially with multifocal IOLs. Following intraoperative techniques are used to correct astigmatism during cataract surgery. These can be done either manually or with FS assistance.

- *Clear corneal incision on the steepest meridian:* The incision on the steep meridian has been reported to correct astigmatism of 0.85 ± 0.75D. It works best for with-the-rule astigmatism. A CCI flattens the meridian in which it is placed, with a coupling effect that steepens the perpendicular meridian 90° away. For a 3.2 mm wide incision, the resultant SIA is approximately 0.5D. Incisions of <2.4 mm wide, as used in microcoaxial or bimanual phacoemulsification, may induce smaller degrees of SIA. The flattening due to the incision would be seen to a maximum extent in the superior incision and least when the incision is temporal. Consequently, when placing a cataract incision on the steep meridian, the surgeon can predict an approximate 0.25–0.75D correction of preexisting corneal astigmatism, which is ideal for patients with less than 1D of corneal astigmatism.
- *Paired opposite corneal incisions at the steepest meridian:* Performing an additional CCI opposite (180°) to the first CCI enhances the flattening effect. When compared to the single CCI, paired opposite clear corneal incisions (POCCIs) (3.2 mm incision) have been documented providing an enhanced effect of 1.66 ± 0.5D and 1.33 ± 0.9D for correcting preexisting corneal astigmatism during cataract surgery using POCCIs of 3.2 mm.
- *Corneal/limbal relaxing incisions:* Corneal relaxing incisions/LRIs flatten the cornea in the incised meridian; therefore, they are created on the steepest meridian. Additionally, these incisions produce a coupling effect on the meridian 90° away. Although relaxing incisions can be performed manually employing inexpensive instrumentation, the efficacy of reducing astigmatism is limited to low keratometric astigmatism. This type of incision can be single or paired and can potentially correct up to 1.5D of astigmatism. LRIs maintain a coupling ratio of 1:1 which means that the amount of flattening that occurs in the incised meridian is equal to the steepening that results 90° away; and therefore, there is little change in sphero-equivalent, obviating the need to make any change in the IOL power.

The clinical application of the FS laser for creating relaxing incisions of precise length, depth, and radius presumably improves clinical outcomes. With integrated optical coherence tomography/Scheimpflug imaging, the depth of the incision can be controlled accurately, which allows making precise incisions at a depth equivalent to 85–90% of the corneal thickness. While some surgeons choose to open the incisions at the time of surgery, it can be done up to a month later, in the office, depending on visual acuity, refraction, and topography.

- *Toric IOL implantation:* Toric IOL implantation can correct preexisting astigmatism as low as 0.75D and is the method of choice for correcting high levels of astigmatism. In addition, it is considered the most predictable method to correct astigmatism in cataract surgery. However, they are not suitable for cases with irregular astigmatism or zonular instability. In addition, toric IOL implantation should be avoided in patients with severe dry eye, not responding to treatment.

Without cataract surgery: Refractive surgical techniques used for myopia can be adapted to correct astigmatism alone or simultaneously as follows:

- *Incisional refractive procedures (repeated):*
  - *Astigmatic keratotomy:* It refers to making transverse or arcuate cuts in mid-periphery perpendicular to the steepest corneal meridian. It can treat astigmatism up to 4–6D. Types:
    - *Transverse keratotomy:* These are usually done in pairs along the steepest meridian and extend for 3 mm. A second pair may be added to the same meridian for greater effect. Since these are tangential to a given optical zone size, incremental flattening power decreases accordingly as the incisions are lengthened.
    - *Arcuate keratotomy:* AK is an incisional surgical procedure in which arcuate incisions of approximately 95% depth are made in the steep meridians of the midperipheral cornea at the 7–9 mm optical zone. It has coupling ration of 1. For AK, the amount of cylinder correction is increased by increasing the length or depth of the incision, using multiple incisions, or reducing the optical zone. Older patient age is associated with increased effect of astigmatism incisions.
  - *Limbal relaxing incisions:* These can treat up to –1 to –2D astigmatism. These produce less glare and discomfort and heal faster compared to AK. Optical quality of the cornea is preserved by making incisions at the limbus.

Instruments: The instruments used in AKs and LRIs are similar. Adjustable diamond blades are more often used in AKs. Preset diamond blades are more often used in LRI surgical procedures, although adjustable blades may be used. The FS laser has been adapted to create peripheral arcuate incisions. These incisions may be titratable, as only part of the incision may be opened initially, followed by a larger area later if there is a need for greater astigmatic correction.

Surgical techniques: Accurate determination of the steep meridian is essential. There are various nomograms available. Examples are J Gills, D Koch, R Lindstrom, S Thorton, L Nichamin, and E Donnenfeld. Among these, the nomograms by Nichamin and Donnenfeld are more popular and commonly used. In Nichamin Nomogram (also known as "NAPA"—Nichamin Age and Pachymetry Adjusted Nomogram), astigmatism is considered to be with-the-rule if the steep axis (plus cylinder) is between 45 and 135°. In against-the-rule astigmatism, steep axis is considered to fall between 0 and 44, and 136 and 180°. The patient's age with the amount of preoperative cylinder to be corrected is considered and then an incision is made as per the suggested arc length. Paired incisions are preferred to optimize symmetric corneal flattening and they are expressed in degrees of arc rather than length of the incision as the relative length of incision may vary according to corneal diameter.

Outcomes: The outcome of AK and LRI surgery depends on several variables, including patient age; the distance separating the incision pairs (optical zone); and the length, depth, and number of incisions. The ARC-T of AK, which used a 7 mm optical zone and varying arc lengths, showed a reduction in astigmatism of 1.6±1.1D in patients with preoperative, naturally occurring astigmatism of 2.8±1.2D. Other studies of AKs have shown a final UCVA of 20/40 in 65–80% of eyes. Overcorrections have been reported in 4–20% of patients. One study on LRI showed an absolute change in refractive astigmatism of 1.72±0.81D after LRIs in patients with mixed astigmatism. Astigmatism was decreased by 0.91D, or 44%, in another series of LRIs in 22 eyes of 13 patients. Incisions in the horizontal meridian have been reported to cause approximately twice as much astigmatic correction as those in the vertical meridian.

- *Laser ablation corneal refractive procedures:*
  - *Surface treatment techniques include:*
    - Photorefractive keratectomy
    - Laser-subepithelial keratomileusis
    - Epi-LASIK.

In these three types of procedure, corneal tissue is ablated with an excimer laser just below the corneal epithelium. Before ablation, the corneal epithelium is removed by a mechanical or chemical method or with a laser (as in PRK), with an alcohol solution (as in LASEK), or else it is separated from the underlying tissue with a microkeratome (as in epi-LASIK). After ablation, the corneal epithelium is put back in place. The advantage of epi-LASIK over LASEK is that the epithelium can be peeled off as a complete sheet without the use of alcohol. Several epi-keratomes have been developed for the epithelial dissection, which will allow the creation of epithelial sheet.

- *Lamellar treatment technique:*
  - LASIK
  - Customized LASIK.

22. What are the recent advances in management of postoperative astigmatism?

Traditional methods of managing postkeratoplasty astigmatism include:
- Suture removal
- Relaxing incision/compression sutures
- Wedge resection
- Regraft.

Recent advances in the management include:
- Toric ICL
- Refractive lens exchange/toric IOL/femto incisions
- Laser refractive surgery.

CHAPTER 10: Ocular Trauma

10.1 Eyelid Trauma

Adarsh Shashni, Anushka Agarwala

Q 1. Discuss management of eyelid trauma.

Introduction

Eyelids are fold of skin that not only covers the eye and protect it from injuries but also gives shape to the face. Any eyelid trauma, therefore, requires meticulous evaluation and appropriate surgical repair for better cosmetic outcome.

Preoperative Evaluation

History

- Careful history about the cause and duration of injury is important for characterization of the type (blunt or penetrating) and extent of trauma.
- Gathered history can raise suspicion of any foreign body in cases of trauma caused by projectile mechanism or may raise suspicion of underlying orbital fracture in cases of blunt trauma.
- A decrease in vision may be associated with either ocular injury or optic neuropathy.

General Examination

- Patients with ocular adnexal trauma should be evaluated systemically as these patients often have other significant injury.
- This is specially seen in patients with road traffic accidents or falls.
- Systemic stabilization of these patients is of paramount importance.

Ocular Examination

- Once determined that patient is systemically stable, priority should be given to preserve the vision.
- Visual acuity and pupillary reflex assessment should be done to rule out any ocular or optic nerve injury.
- Anterior and posterior segment examination—for type of injury (open globe or closed globe injuries).
- Ocular motility examination for any extraocular muscle injury or paresis.
- Any proptosis (indication orbital hematoma) or enophthalmos (indicative of orbital floor fracture) should be ruled out.
- These cases should be managed accordingly.

Eyelid Examination

Eyelid trauma should be assessed for characterization into the following types:
- Based on nature of injury, eyelid trauma can be broadly classified into blunt or penetrating type.
- Blunt trauma includes bruise, abrasions and ecchymosis, or hematoma formation.
- *Penetrating trauma:*
  - Full-thickness or partial thickness
  - Eyelid laceration whether involving eyelid margin or not

- Involvement of medial or lateral canthus
- With or without canalicular injury
- With or without tissue defect
- If any infection is present, wound repair may be delayed.

Investigation

- Involves blood investigation including complete hemogram, liver, and renal function test including serum electrolytes.
- Orbital and head imaging in the form of computed tomography for ruling out any orbital fracture or intracranial injury.

Timing of Surgery

- Wound repair should be done as early as possible.
- However surgical procedure may be delayed 48–72 hours post-trauma if patient is systemically unstable or has active wound infection.

Management of Eyelid Laceration

General Consideration

- Adequate wound cleaning should be done to wash out any dirt or foreign matter.
- This should be followed by assessment of extent of injury.
- Surgery can be done under local or general anesthesia after patient individualization.
- Wound closure or repair is to be done in layers and according to anatomical alignment.
- Anatomical landmark includes the eyebrow, eyelid crease, and eyelid margin including the eyelash line, gray line, and puncta.
- Wound exploration to be done only if there is radiological confirmed or suspected foreign body.
- Wound closure should have maximum horizontal and minimum vertical tension.
- Any nonviable necrotic tissue should be debrided.

Repair of Nonmarginal Eyelid Laceration

- *Superficial laceration:*
  - These include laceration involving skin and underlying orbicularis muscle.
  - Eyelid skin should be closed by 6-0 nylon and orbicularis with 6-0 Vicryl.
  - Superficial eyelid laceration with tissue defect may be managed by advancement or rotation flaps after undermining the adjacent eyelid skin.
  - Large tissue defects can be managed with skin grafting.
- *Deep laceration:*
  - These cases include breach of orbital septum with orbital fat prolapse, involvement of levator aponeurosis, and the full-thickness injury involving the conjunctiva.
  - Repair of such injuries requires layer by layer closure of the wound with 6-0 Vicryl and conjunctival closure should be done with 8-0 Vicryl with knots facing toward the skin side to avoid any ocular irritation and keratopathy.
  - Skin sutures can be removed after 1 week.

Repair of Eyelid Laceration Involving the Eyelid Margin

- *Eyelid defect less than 1/3rd of the horizontal eyelid dimension:*
  - Minimum tissue sacrifice should be done.
  - These cases can be managed by direct closure of the defect.
  - Wound margins should be freshened to remove any slough or necrotic tissue.
  - Pouting sutures to be placed to avoid postoperative notching.
  - Pouting suture includes three vertical mattress sutures one from the gray line, one from the posterior lash line, and one posterior to gray line.
  - The outer bite of the vertical mattress suture is 3 mm and inner bite is 1 mm from either wound margin.
  - These sutures should be tightened sufficiently so as to get pouting or eversion of the wound.

- Skin sutures can be removed after 1 week.
- Eyelid margin sutures can be removed after 10–14 days.

■ *Eyelid defect of 1/3rd to 1/2 of the horizontal eyelid dimension:*
- These can be managed by direct closure assisted with canthotomy (splitting the Y of lateral canthal tendon) along with cantholysis (incising the superior or inferior crus of the lateral canthal tendon depending upon the eyelid involved).
- Those having larger defect can be managed by Tenzel semicircular flap. After doing a canthotomy a semicircular flap of skin and orbicularis of vertical diameter 22 mm and horizontal diameter of 18 mm in continuation with canthotomy incision is made such that the arch of the flap is inferiorly for upper eyelid defect and superiorly for lower eyelid defect. Once the flap is undermined, the eyelid wound is closed as done in direct closure with mobilization of the flap.

■ *Eyelid defect more than 1/2 of the horizontal eyelid dimension:*
- *Cutler Beard bridge technique:* This two-stage procedure is primarily described for upper eyelid defects. In first stage, after measuring the defect, a full-thickness incision along the curve and 4 mm from the lower eyelid margin is given. Care is taken that the incision is along the contour of the eyelid margin so as to avoid damage to the eyelid marginal arcade which may result in necrosis of the eyelid. Then two full-thickness vertical incisions extending inferiorly are given according to the height of the defect so as to create an inverted U-shaped flap of full-thickness lower eyelid. This flap is then mobilized to the upper eyelid and closed in layers. In second stage the eyelids are separated (usually after 2 months). Care is taken that the cut given in oblique fashion (in cross-section) so as to get at least 2 mm or more of conjunctiva which is then closed with the skin with uninterrupted 8-0 Vicryl sutures. This is done to avoid rubbing of the keratinized skin tissue onto the ocular surface. For lower eyelid a reverse Cutler Beard procedure can be done.
- *Hughes tarsoconjunctival flap technique:* This procedure was originally described for lower eyelid. In stage one a partial thickness lamellar tarsoconjunctival flap is mobilized from the upper eyelid 4 mm from the upper eyelid margin of size according to the lower eyelid defect and sutured in layers with the help of 6-0 Vicryl suture and the bare area of mobilized tarsoconjunctival flap is covered by advancing the adjacent lower eyelid skin-orbicularis flap or skin grafting can be done for larger defects. In second stage eyelids are separated (after 2 months). With similar technique as in Cutler Beard procedure. For upper eyelid reverse Hughes procedure can be done.
- *Mustarde Cheek rotation:* This procedure is done for lower eyelid defect of >75% of eyelid horizontal length. A large myocutaneous cheek flap with arc facing superiorly is created in the form of inverted triangle. The medial side of the triangle should be nearly vertical. This is a single-stage procedure.

Repair of Canalicular Laceration

- After cleaning the wound, the first step is to identify the cut ends of the canaliculi.
- The lateral end can be identified by simply probing the system from the puncta.
- The medial end can be identified by direct visualization as the canalicular mucosa as it has a white glistening surface. Other methods include injecting methylene blue dye, diluted fluorescein, viscoelastic substance, or injecting air after creating a localized pool of saline through the opposite puncta (if the system is intact). A pigtail probe can be used but can damage the normal canalicular system.
- Once the system is identified a monocanalicular silicon stent can be passed from puncta. The medial canthal tendon is identified and sutured using 4-0 proline or suture and the eyelid is closed in layers.
- In cases of bicanalicular injury if the cut ends are identified a bicanalicular silicon stent can be placed which are passed through the nasolacrimal duct into the nasal cavity and tied to each other. If cut ends of canaliculi are not identified, primary wound repair should be done with further tissue manipulation. These patients will have epiphora in the postoperative period and can be managed by conjunctivodacryocystorhinostomy.
- These stents are removed after 3 months following the procedure.

Repair of Lateral Canthal Injury

- This includes identifying lateral canthal tendons proximal and distal end and suturing them with 6-0 Vicryl suture.
- If the distal end is not seen then proximal end can be sutured to the lateral orbital wall periosteum approximately 5 mm from orbital rim with the help of 4-0 Prolene or a 5-0 nylon in the form of horizontal mattress.

10.2 Penetrating Ocular Trauma

Tejaswini V, Anushka Agarwala

  1. Discuss management of penetrating ocular trauma.

Introduction

Ocular trauma is a major cause of ocular morbidity and is a leading cause of monocular visual loss. Children and young adults are particularly prone to ocular injuries which add on to the overall disability burden in the community. The setting in which trauma occurs can vary and a detailed assessment is mandatory in every case.

Cases of ocular trauma which concur with polytrauma presenting to the emergency should be quickly assessed and a management protocol formulated.

Initial Assessment

- Assessment of the systemic status and mental orientation of the patient.
- Monitoring of vital signs.
- Brief counseling of the ailing patient and providing comfort to the relatives.
- Special attention should be given to medico legal cases to avoid litigation.

Detailed History

Proper documentation is critical for treatment, research, legal purposes, and in cases of referral.
- A detailed history of mode of injury, duration since injury, and treatment sought if any is noted.
- History of projectile vomiting, headache, and loss of consciousness for any duration should be enquired.
- Symptoms of ocular pain, redness, irritation, blurring of vision, and loss of visual fields are noted.
- Preexisting systemic comorbidities
- Current medications
- Drug allergies
- Prior surgeries
- History of any complications during anesthesia
- Tetanus immunization status
- Time when the patient last ate or drank.

Classification of the Ocular Injury

A standardized classification given by Birmingham Eye Trauma Terminology (BETT) provides a clear definition for all injury types and places each injury type within the framework of a comprehensive system **(Flowchart 1)**.[1]

Type
- Rupture
- Penetrating
- Intraocular foreign body
- Perforating
- Mixed.

Grade
- ≥20/40
- 20/50 to 20/100
- 19/100 to 5/200
- 4/200 to light perception
- Nil perception of light.

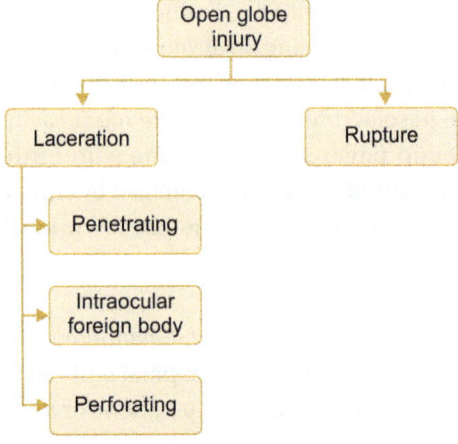

Flowchart 1: BETT classification of open globe.

(BETT: Birmingham Eye Trauma Terminology)

Pupil

- Positive, relative afferent pupillary defect (APD) in injured eye
- Negative, relative APD in injured eye.

Zone

- Cornea and limbus
- Limbus to 5 mm posterior into sclera
- Posterior to 5 mm from the limbus.

Prognostication of the Injury

The Ocular Trauma Score (OTS) has been developed to prognosticate the ocular injuries (**Table 1**). It uses a limited number of variables and enables the ophthalmologist a 77% chance to predict the final functional outcome of the ocular injury within one visual category.[2] Early prognostication helps the ophthalmologist to counsel the patient and give a realistic idea of the condition and to take appropriate management decisions.[3-5]

- Sum of raw points is calculated.
- Conversion of raw points into OTS and likelihood of final visual categories is given.

Designing a Management Strategy

Flowchart 2 depicts the management strategy.

Ophthalmologic Evaluation

External Inspection

Inspect the head, scalp, face, periorbital tissues, and eyelids under bright illumination for:

- Lacerations
- Ecchymoses
- Obvious protruding foreign bodies
- Lid and periorbital edema
- Ptosis
- Presence/absence of enophthalmos
- Gross prolapse of intraocular contents.

Palpation

Palpate the scalp, face, and periorbital soft tissue for:

- Orbital wall blowout fractures
- Crepitus

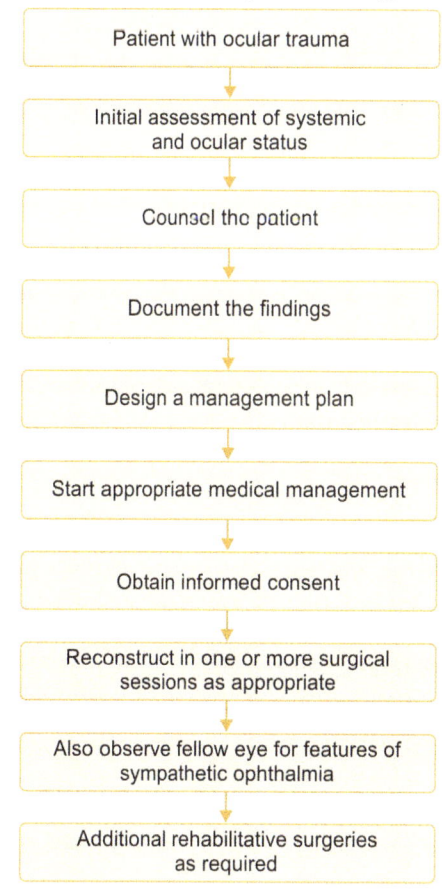

Flowchart 2: Management strategy.

TABLE 1: Calculating the ocular trauma score.

Variables used	Raw points
Initial vision	
NLP	60
LP/HM	70
1/200–19/200	80
20/200–20/50	90
>20/40	100
Rupture	−23
Endophthalmitis	−17
Perforating injury	−14
Retinal detachment	−11
Afferent pupillary defect	−10

(LP/HM: light perception/hand motion; NLP: no light perception)

- Rim deformities
- Infraorbital hypoesthesia.

Visual Acuity

As discussed earlier, the presenting visual acuity is a crucial prognostic indicator in cases of ocular trauma. Visual acuity is measured in each eye separately. Care should be taken, particularly in children to ensure that the patient does not cheat or inadvertently use the fellow eye.

- Illiterate charts (E chart, Landolt C chart) should be used for patients unable to read.
- For preschool children, Allen cards, HOTV letters can be used.
- In infants, fixation and smooth pursuit can be assessed by using colorful targets or a torch light.
- Perception of light and projection of rays are checked using light source from an indirect ophthalmoscope and documented.
- Rapid assessment of the patient's peripheral visual field can provide additional information about the eye's overall visual function.
- Field abnormalities may indicate optic nerve damage or retinal injury.

Pupillary Reactions

Both direct and consensual pupillary reflexes are noted. The presence of APD indicates optic nerve damage or significant retinal damage and has prognostic significance.

Motility

Assessment of ocular motility is important in cases of known or suspected cranial nerve and orbital fractures.

Intraocular Pressure

Intraocular pressure (IOP) is assessed digitally in a gentle manner in frank open globe injuries. Hypotony is noted usually. However, absence of hypotony does not rule out the possibility of an open globe wound. Low IOP is also noted in ciliary body injury or retinal detachment.

Slit Lamp Examination

Conjunctiva

- Note conjunctival lacerations.
- In cases of hemorrhagic chemosis, check for an underlying scleral wound.
- Foreign bodies if any are noted.

Cornea

- Perforations in the cornea and their extent and location are noted. It is a good practice to diagrammatically document the same in the patient's cards. In case of doubt whether the wound is full-thickness or not, fluorescein dye staining is done and a Seidel's testing is done under blue filter in the slit lamp which demonstrates an aqueous leak in cases of full-thickness injury.
- Deeply seated foreign bodies in the corneal stroma and entering into the anterior chamber (AC) are should be removed in the operating room.

Sclera

Scleral perforation can occur in isolation or in continuity with a corneal perforation. In cases of isolated scleral perforation, conjunctiva overlying the wound may remain intact and chemosis is noted for which an exploratory surgery will be performed.

Anterior Chamber

- Cells, flare, red blood cells, pigments, hypopyon, hyphema, and intraocular foreign bodies in the AC are noted.
- Deeper AC is noted in cases of scleral rupture.
- Shallow chamber can be seen in corneal or corneoscleral perforations with uveal tissue prolapse into the wound.

Iris and Angle
Examine for:
- Iris defects or tears
- Iris holes
- Embedded foreign bodies in the iris and angle.

Vitreous

Examine for retrolental cells, vitritis, and vitreous exudates in suspected cases of intraocular foreign body with endophthalmitis.

Crystalline Lens
Examine for:
- Breach in the anterior capsule or posterior capsule of lens
- Sectoral or total cataract
- Intralenticular foreign body.[6]

Fundus Examination

If the media permits and the integrity of the ocular structures is maintained, a detailed fundus examination by indirect ophthalmoscopy should be done in a cooperative patient.

Imaging

Ultrasonography

It can be done gently in small wounds where the risk of expulsion of intraocular contents is minimal.[7] It is used to detect:
- Retinal detachment
- Choroidal detachment
- Posterior vitreous detachment
- Vitreous hemorrhage and opacities
- Choroidal and scleral ruptures
- Intraocular foreign bodies.

X-ray Orbit

It is used as a screening tool for orbital fracture and intraocular/intraorbital retained foreign body.

Computed Tomography
- Axial and coronal sections of the entire orbit with 1.5 mm cuts are done to look for retained intraocular foreign bodies.[8]
- Ideal study to rule out orbital fractures.

Photodocumentation
- Superior to sketches
- Can document the course of the injury and its clinical implications.
- Useful as evidence in lawsuit and litigation
- For education and research.

Surgical Management

Goals in the management of corneal/scleral injury include:
- Maintaining the integrity of the globe.
- Prevention of further injury and exposure to infectious agents.
- Visual rehabilitation as a secondary goal.

General anesthesia is preferred in majority of cases of penetrating ocular trauma. Cases of small intraocular foreign body with maintained globe integrity can be done under peribulbar block.

Closure of Corneal Wounds[9]

Self-sealed Corneal Wounds

In small self-sealed corneal wounds of 2 mm or less with no other intraocular tissue at the wound, no foreign material is present in the wound and a negative Seidel's test, suturing is not required and a bandage contact lens can placed for a period of 2 weeks to allow healing.

For larger self-sealed lacerations, we can do:
- Routine surgical repair
- Cyanoacrylate tissue glue with bandage contact lens.

Corneal Lacerations with Flaps

- Corneal lacerations with displaced flaps have to be repositioned and secured with sutures passing partial thickness through the surrounding stroma.
- Cases with epithelial growth underneath the flap have to be debrided before suturing and adequate irrigation of the bed and under surface of the flap should be done.

Full-thickness Nonself-sealing Corneal Wounds

The most preferred suturing method to appose the wound edges is interrupted suturing using 10-0 nylon. Suture passes should be approximately 1.5–2 mm total in length, i.e., 0.75–1 mm on either side at 85–90% depth of the corneal thickness. Longer passes may be required in cases of edematous corneal wound edges.

In vertical lacerations, the suture entry and exit sites should be equidistant from the wound margins so that the corneal suture is centered over the wound. In beveled or shelved lacerations, suture is centered on the posterior aspect of the wound margin.

Running Sutures

- Quicker procedure
- Can lead to large zone of compression and thus excessive flattening of the cornea and misalignment of wound edges.

Rowsey–Hay's Technique of Corneal Suturing

A Fleringa ring or a hinge spring of a safety pin is held over the cornea and its refection is examined under illumination which should be circular ideally. The ring appears oval or distorted in cases of astigmatism which guides the surgeon to tighten or loosen the sutures.

Stellate Wounds

Require a combination of sutures and tissue adhesive or a patch graft for a proper closure.

Loss of Fragments

- Small defects can be closed with sutures.
- Tissue loss of >5 mm requires a corneal patch graft.

Closure of Scleral Wounds[10,11]

Full-thickness scleral wounds are apposed with interrupted sutures using 6-0 Vicryl.
- Peritomy is done to ensure adequate exposure and Tenon's capsule is retracted posteriorly.
- The scleral wound is closed by interrupted sutures from anterior to posterior, allowing the periorbita to support the globe till the apposition is complete.
- Any prolapsed tissue through the wound should be gently reposited. Vitreous should be amputated ideally with a vitrectomy probe. Unnecessary traction on vitreous is to be avoided.
- A "close as you go" strategy should be adopted for more posterior wounds. Leaving the last tied suture ends longer allows rotation of globe for adequate exposure of the posterior part of the wound.
- In cases where the scleral wound extends through or under an extraocular muscle, an assistant can retract the muscle gently using a muscle hook to aid in exposure. For more exposure, the muscle can be temporarily disinserted so as to allow the suturing.

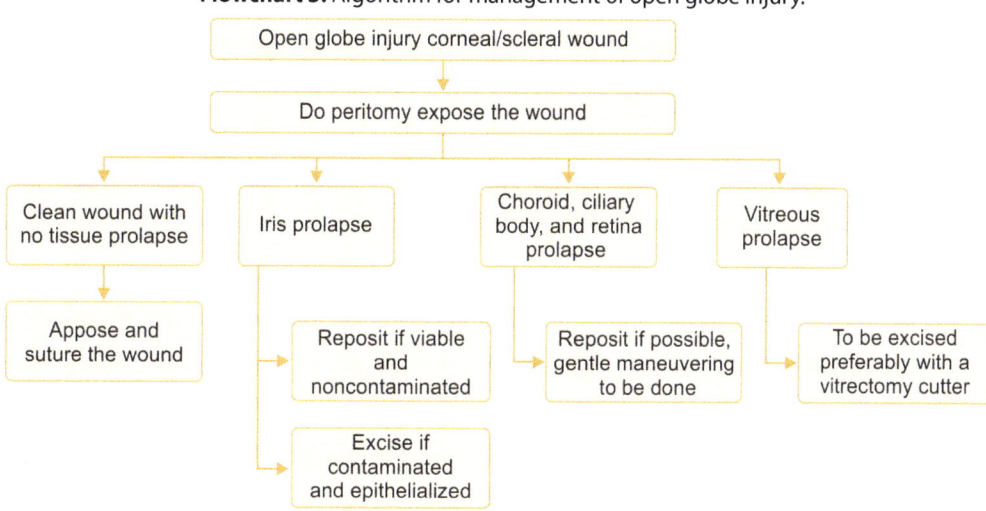

Flowchart 3: Algorithm for management of open globe injury.

Closure of Corneoscleral Wounds

- Major landmark in these is the limbus and so that is the area to be apposed first.
- This is followed by the repair of the corneal aspect and then the scleral aspect of the wound adhering to the principles already discussed **(Flowchart 3)**.

Post-traumatic Endophthalmitis[12-14]

Endophthalmitis following penetrating eye injuries has a relatively poor prognosis due to the underlying eye trauma and the frequency of more virulent organisms such as *Bacillus* species.

Risk factors for infection include:
- Retained intraocular foreign body
- A rural injury setting
- Delay in primary wound closure
- Disruption of the crystalline lens.

Recognition of early clinical signs of endophthalmitis, such as hypopyon, vitritis, or retinal periphlebitis, is important and early treatment is recommended. Comprehensive prophylactic antibiotic treatment at the time of injury repair combined with timely vitrectomy and injection of intravitreal antibiotics may significantly improve visual acuity outcomes following penetrating injuries. Vitrectomy is also warranted in the setting of retained intraocular foreign bodies and traumatic retinal detachment.[12]

Conclusion

Each case of trauma is unique and the ophthalmologist should treat the eye and the patient as a whole. Proper classification and prognostication of penetrating ocular trauma should be done. Appropriate imaging is to be done and documentation should be clear. Primary closure of the wound is to be done followed by reconstructive surgeries.

References

1. Kuhn F, Morris R, Witherspoon CD, Heimann K, Jeffers JB, Treister G. A standardized classification of ocular trauma. Ophthalmology. 1996;103(2):240-3.
2. Pieramici DJ, Sternberg Jr P, Aaberg Sr TM, Bridges Jr WZ, Capone Jr A, Cardillo JA. A system for classifying mechanical injuries of the eye (globe). The Ocular Trauma Classification Group. Am J Ophthalmol. 1997;123:820-31.
3. de Juan E, Sternberg P, Michels R. Penetrating ocular injuries: types of injuries and visual results. Ophthalmology. 1983;90:1318-22.
4. Hutton WL, Fuller DG. Factors influencing final visual results in severely injured eyes. Am J Ophthalmol. 1984;97:715-22.
5. Esmali B, Elner SG, Schork A, Elner VM. Visual outcome and ocular survival after penetrating trauma. Ophthalmology. 1995;102:393-400.
6. Mieler WF, Ellis MK, Williams DF, Han DP. Retained intraocular foreign bodies and endophthalmitis. Ophthalmology. 1990;97(11):1532.
7. Kwong JS, Munk PL, Lin DT, Vellet AD, Levin M, Buckley AR. Real-time ultra-sonography in ocular trauma. Am J Radiol. 1992;158:179-82.

8. Joseph DP, Pieramici DJ, Beauchamp NJ. Computed tomography (CT) in the diagnosis and prognosis of open globe injuries. Ophthalmology. 2000;107:1899-906.
9. Beatty RF, Beatty RL. The repair of corneal and corneoscleral lacerations. Semin Ophthalmol. 1994;9:165-76.
10. Hamill MB. Management of scleral perforation. In: Krachmer JH, Mannis MJ, Holland EJ (Eds). Cornea, Surgery of the Cornea and Conjunctiva. St. Louis: Mosby; 1997.
11. Navon SE. Management of the ruptured globe. Int Ophthalmol Clin. 1995;35:71-91.
12. Liggett PE, Gauderman WJ, Moreira CM, Barlow W, Green RL, Ryan SJ. Pars plana vitrectomy for acute retinal detachment in penetrating ocular injuries. Arch Ophthalmol. 1990;108:1724-8.
13. Cebulla CM, Flynn Jr HW. Endophthalmitis after open globe injuries. Am J Ophthalmol. 2009;147:567-8.
14. Zhang Y, Zhang MN, Jiang CH, Yao Y, Zhang K. Endophthalmitis following open globe injury. Br J Ophthalmol. 2010;94(1):111.

10.3 Acute Chemical Injury

Mohamed Ibrahime Asif, Ritika Mukhija, Pranita Sahay

Q 1. Discuss acute chemical injury.

Introduction

Ocular chemical injuries are true ophthalmic emergencies due to the potential for permanent corneal and intraocular damage leading to visual impairment or even blindness. The visual prognosis is usually poor in these cases and the physical loss of the eye is not uncommon.[1] Recently, the prognosis is partly improved due to workplace protection, better understanding of inflammatory, and healing response with targeted medical and surgical management.

Epidemiology

Ocular trauma from chemical causes is relatively common and it constitutes 11.5–22.1% of the traumatic ocular injuries,[2] a majority of which occur in young males because of exposure in the industrial accidents. Since alkali is common in domestic and industrial cleaning products, alkali injuries are typically more common than acid injuries to the eye.[1] In terms of severity, the majority of chemical injuries are classified as mild and fortunately severe injuries are relatively rare.[1,3,4]

Etiology

Chemical burns can be caused by acids, bases, oxidants, solvents, reducing agents, and alkylating agents. They can also be caused by chemical weapons such as mustard gas or urticants such as phosgene oxide. A few common acids and alkalis responsible for acute chemical burns are described below.

Acids

- *Sulfuric acid:* Most common acid responsible for injury which is commonly used in inverter batteries, fertilizers, dye manufacturing, explosives, and petroleum refining.
- *Nitric acid:* It is also a strong acid used in the manufacturing of fertilizers, rocket propellants, and nylon products. It leads to a yellowish corneal opacity.
- *Chromic acid:* It is used in electroplating, ceramic glazes, and wood preservation and causes brownish discoloration of conjunctiva, often simulating chronic conjunctivitis.
- *Hydrofluoric acid:* Though a weak acid, gives the most reactive anion. It acts like alkali saponifying lipids, causing deep rapid penetration, extensive ischemia, and calcific plaques in corneal stroma. It is used in etching glass, semiconductor production, and rust removal.

Alkali

- *Ammonia:* It is a common cause of alkali injury, and is found in fertilizers, refrigerants, and cleaning solutions. It combines with water to form ammonium hydroxide with very rapid penetration.
- *Sodium hydroxide (lye):* It is a common constituent of drain cleaners. It has rapid penetration like ammonia.
- *Potassium hydroxide (caustic potash):* It causes similar injury like lye.
- *Magnesium hydroxide:* It is a constituent in fireworks which results in combined chemical and thermal injury.

- *Calcium hydroxide (lime)*: It is the most common cause of chemical injury in workplace. It is a constituent of plaster, mortar, cement, and whitewash. Though it has poor penetration, the toxicity is increased by retained particulate matter causing prolonged severe damage.

Risk Factors

Certain occupations: Chemical burns account for 3–4% of occupational injuries.

Noncompliance with health and safety regulations such as inadequate or inappropriate use of protective eyewear and clothing.

Pathogenesis

Change in tissue pH following chemical injury → pH-dependent chemical alterations → tissue damage.[1]

Though pH was regarded as a major factor for damage, other factors that influence this process are temperature, impact force, amount and concentration of chemical, dissociation coefficient, redox-potential, and specific reactivity with the ocular tissues (pK values).[5]

- *Alkali:* On contact, they dissociate into cations and hydroxyl ions. The former is responsible for penetration while the latter saponifies the membranes resulting in cell disruption and death. Cations react with the carboxyl groups of stromal collagen and glycosaminoglycans (GAGs) resulting in loss of stromal clarity.[1,6]
- *Acids:* Hydrogen ions cause damage by pH alteration while the anion causes precipitation and denaturation of proteins in the corneal epithelium and anterior stroma.[6] Precipitation offers physical barrier against further ingress.[6,7] However, if acid succeeds in penetrating stroma, damage is similar to alkali injury. Alterations include precipitation of extracellular GAGs, corneal opacification, damage to trabecular meshwork and other anterior chamber structures, and reduced ascorbate levels.[1,6] Low ascorbate levels due to ciliary body damage are related to subsequent retarded collagen synthesis. Due to limited buffering capacity of cornea both acid and alkali injury cause change in osmolality leading to cellular dysfunction. Both acid and alkali may cause vascular damage leading to ischemic insult.

Clinical Features

The clinical course following an acute chemical injury can be characterized in three stages:[8]
1. *Acute stage (immediate to 1 week):* Representing the immediate effects of the injury.
   a. *Ocular surface epithelium:* There may be a central corneal abrasion with an intact limbus or the limbus may be partially or totally involved. Varying areas of the conjunctiva too may be involved. Limbal and conjunctival involvement are more common in the inferior half. Fluorescein staining is helpful in determining the extent of abrasion.
   b. *Limbal ischemia:* Presents as sectors of blanched or pale limbus with associated necrosis and hemorrhage. Injured blood vessels appear as dark columns of blood with no visible flow.
   c. *Corneal stroma:* It may be hazy or opaque and thick with folds or striae secondary to endothelial involvement. Corneal sensations may be impaired.
   d. *Anterior chamber:* The iris may show injection, hemorrhage, necrosis, and pigment dispersion. The pupil response may be sluggish or absent. The lens may be intumescent and ciliary body damage can manifest as hypotony. Clogging of the trabecular meshwork with inflammatory debris can result in raised pressure.
2. *Early reparative (intermediate) stage (1–3 weeks):* Representing the host healing response. If some limbal or conjunctival epithelium survives reepithelialization commences. The cornea may be covered by corneal or conjunctival epithelium. If no epithelium survives, the ocular surface is covered by a centripetally advancing fibrovascular pannus. Recanalization of some of the damaged blood vessels may lead to further hemorrhages. Inflammatory cell infiltration occurs and can later lead to stromal melts and ulceration.
3. *Late reparative stage (>3 weeks):* Representing changes associated with repair, regeneration or lack thereof. In the late stage of moderate to severe burns, the cornea is covered by a fibrovascular pannus. Superficial and deep vascularization, stromal ulceration, and persistent epithelial defects can lead to a descemetocele and perforation. Loss of nerves may lead to a neurotrophic state with repeated healing and breakdown of the surface.
   a. Conjunctival repair may lead to symblepharon, subepithelial fibrosis with progressive contracture leading to forniceal shortening and lid margin deformities such as entropion, trichiasis, and lagophthalmos with exposure. Tear film abnormalities due to loss of goblet cells (mucin) and obstruction of orifices of the lacrimal or accessory lacrimal ductules (aqueous) may manifest. This can lead to keratinization of the cornea and conjunctiva. Cicatricial stenosis or occlusion of the lacrimal puncta may occur and offset a "dry eye" state.

b. Retrocorneal or cyclitic membranes and fibrosis of the ciliary body can lead to persistent hypotony and phthisis. On the other hand, scarring in the drainage angle and peripheral anterior synechiae can lead to intractable glaucoma.

Sequelae

Lids	• Posterior displacement of meibomian orifices • Trichiasis • Ectropion • Entropion • Lagophthalmos
Ocular surface	• Dry eye • Loss of goblet cells • Damage to lacrimal system • Corneal melt • Corneal opacity/scarring • Corneal neovascularization • Intraocular inflammation • LSCD • Recurrent erosions • Persistent epithelial defects • Symblepharon/ankyloblepharon • Microbial keratitis
IOP	• Secondary glaucoma
Intraocular structures	• Iris ischemia • Fixed dilated pupil • Ciliary body shutdown • Cataract • Retinal detachment • Phthisis bulbi

(IOP: intraocular pressure; LSCD: limbal stem cell deficiency)

Classification

Roper-Hall Classification 1965 of Chemical Injuries[9]

Grade	Prognosis	Corneal appearance	Limbal ischemia
I	Good	Epithelial damage	None
II	Good	Haze but iris details are visible	<1/3
III	Guarded	Total epithelial loss with haze that obscures iris details	1/3 to 1/2
IV	Poor	Cornea opaque with iris and pupil obscured	>1/2

Dua Classification 2001 of Chemical Injuries[10]

Grade	Prognosis	Clock hours of limbal involvement	Conjunctival involvement	Analog scale*
I	Very good	0	0%	0/0%
II	Good	≥3	<30%	0.1–3/1–29.9%
III	Good	>3–6	>30–50%	3.1–6/31–50%
IV	Good to guarded	>6–9	>50–75%	6.1–6/51–75%
V	Guarded to poor	>9–<12	75–100%	9.1–11.9/75.1–99.9%
VI	Very poor	12	100%	12/100%

*The analog scale records accurately the limbal involvement in clock hours of affected limbus/percentage of conjunctival involvement. While calculating the percentage of conjunctival involvement, only involvement of bulbar conjunctiva, up to and including the conjunctival fornices, is considered.

Management

The primary goals of treatment are as follows:
- Restoring intact epithelium
- Control inflammation
- Aid in the reparative process
- Prevention of complications.

Emergency/Immediate Treatment

It should be done within few minutes of injury aiming to minimize the ingress of chemical agent into anterior chamber and to remove a potential reservoir for ongoing injury. It involves prompt irrigation with any available neutral irrigation fluid and the removal of residual chemical debris from the eye. The most important intervention to reduce the severity is copious irrigation.[11,12] It should be continued until pH neutralization is achieved (minimum of 30 minutes is recommended). pH should be measured from cul-de-sac 5–10 minutes after completion of irrigation and further irrigation is done if required till pH approaches normal level. The pH of both eyes should be tested even in apparent unilateral injury to avoid unrecognized injury. Topical anesthetic drops should be applied to reduce pain and blepharospasm during irrigation. Eyelid speculum or Morgan lens (sclera irrigating lens) may be used to keep the eyes open while irrigation.

After irrigation, thorough examination should be carried out by double eversion of eyelids to examine the fornices. Any particulate matter should be removed. Chuna particles should be removed with cotton-tipped applicator.

Aqueous humor replacement: External irrigation is of limited use once chemicals have reached anterior chamber. Paracentesis and subsequent chamber reformation with buffered phosphate solution can lower aqueous pH in animal models.[13] However, this is not a part of routine practice and it is still controversial.

Medical Management

A retrospective study showed that intensive therapy with a combination of topical steroids, antibiotics, ascorbate and citrate, atropine, and oral vitamin C was most effective in treatment of patients with Roper-Hall grade III injuries with reference to time to reepithelialize and visual acuity.[14] Conversely in grades I and II intensive therapy delayed healing due to drug toxicity and inhibition of reepithelialization by steroids.

- *Preservative-free broad-spectrum antibiotics:* Any epithelial defect warrants the use of topical antibiotic for prophylaxis. The choice of antibiotic must take into consideration the likelihood of microbial contamination at the time of injury. Generally, a broad-spectrum antibiotic is preferred.
- *Topical cycloplegics:* Agents such as cyclopentolate or atropine reduces ciliary spasm and thereby decreases pain and the risk of posterior synechiae. Phenylephrine and other adrenergic drugs should be avoided as vasoconstriction may exacerbate limbal ischemia.
- *Antiglaucoma agents:* Collagen shrinkage after a chemical injury will lead to contraction of cornea and sclera leading to acute elevated intraocular pressure (IOP).[15] Inflammatory or direct damage to the trabecular meshwork and posterior synechiae due to inflammation can impede aqueous outflow, resulting in subacute and chronic elevation in IOP.[16] So, an aqueous suppressant such as oral acetazolamide or topical beta-blocker is the drug of choice in this scenario.
- *Drugs to control inflammation:*
  - *Topical corticosteroids:* There is controversy regarding its use and timing of use. It has the advantage of suppressing inflammatory cells and collagenase inhibition, however, they suppress keratocyte migration and collagen production causing corneal thinning. Risk of sterile ulceration in the first week is relatively modest but increases as the corneal repair process becomes established around day 14.[1] Steroids should be used in the initial 10 days after injury as it does not appear to have an adverse effect on outcome[17] and then it is rapidly tapered after 10 days if the epithelium is not intact, as it slows repair process.
  - *Progestational steroids:* Medroxyprogesterone acetate 1% can be used instead of corticosteroids.
  - *Topical nonsteroidal anti-inflammatory drugs (NSAIDs):* These drugs should be cautiously used due to possibility of corneal melting in conjunction with epithelial defects.
  - *Vascular endothelial growth factor (VEGF) inhibitors:* Local bevacizumab has shown to exhibit both anti-neovascularization and anti-inflammatory properties.[15] Importantly, studies have shown increased levels of VEGF within 6 hours following chemical burn, suggesting early initiation of treatment may diminish neovascularization cascade.[18] However, theoretically it can aggravate scleral ischemia and necrosis, so currently must be viewed with caution.

- *Drugs to support repair and minimize ulceration:*
  - *Ascorbate:* The scorbutic state following a chemical injury has the potential to compromise stromal repair (collagen synthesis).[19] Topical or systemic supplementation has been demonstrated to reduce the incidence of corneal thinning and ulceration. So early supplementation is absolutely critical.
  - Dose—Oral ascorbate 2 g/day (500 mg four times per day), Topical 10% sodium ascorbate solution instilled hourly.
  - *Tetracycline:* Its efficacy in reducing collagenase activity and corneal ulceration has been demonstrated in alkali injuries.[1] It does by inhibition of gene expression of neutrophil collagenase, inhibition of $\alpha 1$ antitrypsin degradation, and scavenging of reactive oxygen species.[20] It also inhibits matrix metalloproteinases through chelation of zinc.
  - Dose—doxycycline 100 mg twice daily/tetracycline 250 mg four times per day.
  - *Citrate:* In contrast to ascorbate, citrate is effective in both preventing and retarding the progression of corneal ulcers.[21] It chelates extracellular calcium and diminishes the activity of neutrophils by reducing membrane and intracellular calcium levels.[1] It also has an inhibitory effect on collagenase.[22] Because citrate and ascorbate reduce corneal ulceration via different mechanisms, their combined use offers therapeutic advantage over citrate alone.[21] Citrate has greater effect than ascorbate and its topical route is superior to the systemic route.
  - Dose—10% sodium citrate drops made in artificial tears instilled hourly.
- *Drugs to promote reepithelialization:*
  - *Preservative-free tear substitutes:* They promote reepithelialization, ameliorate persistent epitheliopathy, decrease the risk of recurrent erosions, and accelerate visual rehabilitation by washing out inflammatory cells and hydrating the ocular surface.[23] Temporary or permanent punctual occlusion may also augment its function.
  - *Autologous serum eye drops (20–40%):* Both peripheral blood serum and umbilical cord serum are effective in ocular surface restoration after moderate to severe chemical burns owing to various growth factors (Dua classification grades III to V).[24,25]
  - Fibronectin[26] has shown a favorable effect in animal models.
  - *Epidermal growth factor:* Favorably influences epithelial migration in human studies. However, recurrent erosions have been seen after discontinuation.
  - *Retinoic acid:* It is theoretically useful in promoting goblet cell recovery, tear film stabilization, and improved ocular surface wetting.

Early Surgical Intervention

- *Debridement:* Careful excision of all necrotic tissues should be carried out, as it acts as a store for inflammatory mediators that elicit a neutrophil response and further hasten ulceration.
- *Symblepharon lysis:* Prevention of symblepharon formation should be considered if the conjunctiva is involved. Procedures such as lysis using glass rod, inserting symblepharon ring, and lining with amniotic membrane or a sutured plastic drape[23] help in maintaining the fornices.
- *Tenon advancement:* It helps to reestablish limbal circulation and reduce the risk of immediate anterior segment necrosis and aseptic ulceration when total loss of limbal vasculature occurs following severe chemical burn.[23]

Intermediate Surgical Intervention

- *Amniotic membrane transplant (AMT):* Several studies have showed a beneficial effect in grades II and III chemical burns. Amniotic membrane facilitates epithelialization, reduces inflammation, and prevents symblepharon formation, vascularization, and scarring. It also provides fast and dramatic relief from pain and photophobia. However, there were no overall differences in final visual acuity, corneal clarity, symblepharon formation with or without AMT.[27]
- *Tenoplasty flaps:* Involves rotating vascularized pedicle of tenon capsule over cornea. This is an alternative method of promoting epithelialization and preventing ulceration.
- *Conjunctival flaps:* Should generally be avoided as simple conjunctiva causes excessive vascularization and are not effective in sealing leaks.
- *Oral mucosal epithelial cell transplantation:* Cultivated oral mucosal epithelial cell transplantation (COMET) promotes reepithelialization and stabilizes the ocular surface.[28] Oral mucosal biopsy harvests epithelial cells which are then cultivated on amniotic membrane and transplanted on the ocular surface. Long-term immunosuppression is not needed. Further reconstructive surgeries may be required such as keratoplasty.
- *Tissue glue:* It offers a means of preserving the integrity of globe in cases of impending or a small perforation. It is usually accompanied with bandage contact lens for comfort.

Intermediate/Late Surgical Intervention

- *Conjunctival transplantation:* It is used for reconstructing forniceal shortening or cicatricial fibrosis. It has an added advantage over other mucosa that it provides compatible tissue with a basement membrane.[23] It is a useful procedure only in unilateral cases.
- *Buccal and nasal mucosa transplantation:* They are useful when both eyes are involved. It is usually obtained from posterior aspect of the lower lip or from nasal septum and lower or middle turbinates. Nasal mucosa provides additional intraepithelial mucous cells.[23]

Late Surgical Intervention

- *Limbal stem cell transplant:* This might be required especially in high-grade chemical injuries with extensive perilimbal ischemia. Sources for limbal stem cell transplants range from conjunctival autografts, living related, and cadaveric donors, to ex-vivo culture-expanded limbal epithelium.
- *Corneal transplantation:* Penetrating keratoplasty or deep anterior lamellar keratoplasty can be done as a rehabilitative procedure. The decision of keratoplasty is made after considering the status of the limbus. In severe injury, limbo-keratoplasty as a single-stage procedure or combination of normal-sized graft (8 mm) with limbal stem cell transplant before transplant or during transplant should be considered. All these procedures should be delayed for 18 months to 2 years because keratoplasty in acute inflammatory stage is fraught with a high failure rate.
- *Glaucoma surgery:* Required for secondary glaucoma recalcitrant to maximal medical therapy. This leads to extensive scarring of perilimbal and bulbar conjunctiva with foreshortening of fornices. Cyclodiode ablation of ciliary body may be considered.

The End-stage Eye

- *Keratoprosthesis:* It is the last resort for patients with severely damaged eyes who are poor candidates for or have failed keratoplasty.
- *Evisceration or enucleation:* For a painful, blind eye in which all treatment options have been exhausted.

References

1. Wagoner MD. Chemical injuries of the eye: current concepts in pathophysiology and therapy. Surv Ophthalmol. 1997;41(4):275-313.
2. Clare G, Suleman H, Bunce C, Dua H. Amniotic membrane transplantation for acute ocular burns. Cochrane Database Syst Rev. 2012;9:CD009379.
3. Morgan SJ. Chemical burns of the eye: causes and management. Br J Ophthalmol. 1987;71(11):854-7.
4. Beare JD. Eye injuries from assault with chemicals. Br J Ophthalmol. 1990;74(9):514-8.
5. Schrage NF, Langefeld S, Zschocke J, Kuckelkorn R, Redbrake C, Reim M. Eye burns: an emergency and continuing problem. Burns. 2000;26(8):689-99.
6. Kuckelkorn R, Schrage N, Keller G, Redbrake C. Emergency treatment of chemical and thermal eye burns. Acta Ophthalmol. 2002;80(1):4-10.
7. Fish R, Davidson RS. Management of ocular thermal and chemical injuries, including amniotic membrane therapy. Curr Opin Ophthalmol. 2010;21(4):317-21.
8. McCulley JP. Chemical injuries. In: Smolin G, Thoft RA (Eds). The Cornea: Scientific Foundation and Clinical Practice, 2nd edition. Boston: Little, Brown and Co.; 1987. pp. 527-42.
9. Roper-Hall MJ. Thermal and chemical burns. Trans Ophthalmol Soc UK. 1965;85:631-53.
10. Dua HS, King AJ, Joseph A. A new classification of ocular surface burns. Br J Ophthalmol. 2001;85(11):1379-83.
11. Ikeda N, Hayasaka S, Hayasaka Y, Watanabe K. Alkali burns of the eye: effect of immediate copious irrigation with tap water on their severity. Ophthalmologica. 2006;220(4):225-8.
12. Burns FR, Paterson CA. Prompt irrigation of chemical eye injuries may avert severe damage. Occup Health Saf. 1989;58(4):33-6.
13. Paterson CA, Pfister RR, Levinson RA. Aqueous humor pH changes after experimental alkali burns. Am J Ophthalmol. 1975;79(3):414-9.
14. Brodovsky SC, McCarty CA, Snibson G, Loughnan M, Sullivan L, Daniell M, et al. Management of alkali burns: an 11-year retrospective review. Ophthalmology. 2000;107(10):1829-35.
15. Paterson CA, Pfister RR. Intraocular pressure changes after alkali burns. Arch Ophthalmol. 1974;91(3):211-8.
16. Pfister RR, Friend J, Dohlman CH. The anterior segments of rabbits after alkali burns. Arch Ophthalmol. 1971;86(2):189-93.
17. Donshik PC, Berman MB, Dohlman CH, Gage J, Rose J. Effect of topical corticosteroids on ulceration in alkali-burned corneas. Arch Ophthalmol. 1978;96(11):2117-20.
18. Hosseini H, Nowroozzadeh MH, Salouti R, Nejabat M. Anti-VEGF therapy with bevacizumab for anterior segment eye disease. Cornea. 2012;31(3):322-34.
19. Levinson RA, Paterson CA, Pfister RR. Ascorbic acid prevents corneal ulceration and perforation following experimental alkali burns. Invest Ophthalmol Vis Sci. 1976;15(12):986-93.

20. Ralph RA. Tetracyclines and the treatment of corneal stromal ulceration: a review. Cornea. 2000;19(3):274-7.
21. Pfister RR, Haddox JL, Yuille-Barr D. The combined effect of citrate/ascorbate treatment in alkali-injured rabbit eyes. Cornea. 1991;10(2):100-4.
22. Pfister RR, Nicolaro ML, Paterson CA. Sodium citrate reduces the incidence of corneal ulcerations and perforations in extreme alkali-burned eyes?acetylcysteine and ascorbate have no favorable effect. Invest Ophthalmol Vis Sci. 1981;21(3):486-90.
23. Merle H, Gérard M, Schrage N. Brûlures oculaires. J Fr Ophtalmol. 2008;31(7):723-34.
24. Sharma N, Goel M, Velpandian T, Titiyal JS, Tandon R, Vajpayee RB. Evaluation of umbilical cord serum therapy in acute ocular chemical burns. Invest Ophthalmol Vis Sci. 2011;52(2):1087-92.
25. Sharma N, Lathi SS, Sehra SV, Agarwal T, Sinha R, Titiyal JS, et al. Comparison of umbilical cord serum and amniotic membrane transplantation in acute ocular chemical burns. Br J Ophthalmol. 2015;99(5):669-73.
26. Nishida T, Nakagawa S, Nishibayashi C, Tanaka H, Manabe R. Fibronectin enhancement of corneal epithelial wound healing of rabbits in vivo. Arch Ophthalmol. 1984;102(3):455-6.
27. Tandon R, Gupta N, Kalaivani M, Sharma N, Titiyal JS, Vajpayee RB. Amniotic membrane transplantation as an adjunct to medical therapy in acute ocular burns. Br J Ophthalmol. 2011;95(2):199-204.
28. Ma DH, Kuo MT, Tsai YJ, Chen HJ, Chen XL, Wang SF, et al. Transplantation of cultivated oral mucosal epithelial cells for severe corneal burn. Eye. 2009;23(6):1442.

10.4 Blunt Ocular Trauma

Shreyas Temkar, Pranita Sahay

1. Write a short note on traumatic hyphema.

Introduction

Traumatic hyphema is defined as the presence of blood within the aqueous fluid of the anterior chamber produced after a projectile strikes the eye. The most common cause of hyphema is blunt trauma.[1] It occurs most commonly in young males.

Pathophysiology

The choroid and the iris contain a rich complex of vessels. The most common source of bleeding is a tear at the anterior aspect of the ciliary body. Hyphema has been postulated to occur by two different mechanisms. Blunt trauma causes anteroposterior compression followed by equatorial expansion. This sudden dynamic shift leads to stress on anterior chamber angle structures with resultant rupture of iris stromal and/or ciliary body vessels releasing blood into the anterior chamber. Other postulated mechanism is due to rapid raise in intraocular pressure (IOP) caused by compressive force leading to rupture of fragile vessels of the iris from sphincter or angle. The most frequently ruptured vessels are the major arterial circle of the iris and its branches, the recurrent choroidal arteries, and the veins crossing the suprachoroidal space between the ciliary body and episcleral venous plexus.[2,3]

Clinical Features

History

Recent history of (H/o) ocular trauma:
- Mechanism of injury
- Presence of protective eyewear
- Time of injury
- *Visual compromise:*
  - At the time injury
  - Deteriorating over time—suggestive of rebleeding
- Usage of anticoagulants
- H/o sickle cell disease or trait
- H/o bleeding disorders.

Symptoms
- Blurry vision
- Pain

- Photophobia
- Headache.

Signs

- Check for ocular integrity—rule out ruptured globe
- Decreased visual acuity
- Pupillary examination—traumatic mydriasis, sphincter tears
- Raised IOP
- Gonioscopy—to evaluate the angle and trabecular meshwork, rule out angle recession, iridodialysis, cyclodialysis
- Fundoscopy—to rule out retinal breaks.

Investigations

- B-scan ultrasound—if fundus is not visible
- Ultrasonic biomicroscopy—evaluate anterior segment, rule out lens capsule rupture, intraocular foreign body
- CT scan of orbits and head—suspected orbital fracture or intraocular foreign body.

Grading of Hyphema

Grading	Hyphema	Incidence
Grade 0	No visible layering, but red blood cells within the anterior chamber (microhyphema)	
Grade I	Layered blood occupying less than one-third of the anterior chamber	58%
Grade II	Blood filling one-third to one-half of the anterior chamber	20%
Grade III	Layered blood filling one-half to less than total of the anterior chamber	14%
Grade IV	Total filling of the anterior chamber with blood	8%

If the anterior chamber is completely filled with bright red blood it is called a total hyphema. If the anterior chamber is filled with dark red-black blood it is called a *blackball or eight-ball hyphema*. The black color is suggestive of impaired aqueous circulation and decreased oxygen concentration. This distinction is important because an eight-ball hyphema is more likely to cause pupillary block and secondary angle closure.

Complications

Raised IOP: Elevated IOP (>22 mm Hg) may be anticipated in approximately 32% of all patients with hyphema.[3] Raised IOP is more commonly associated with near total or total hyphemas. Cases with rebleeding have a more than 50% chance of having elevated IOP.

Various mechanisms have been postulated to cause IOP raise in patients with hyphema. Acute glaucoma is caused by occlusion of trabecular meshwork by red blood cells (RBCs) and inflammatory cells and pupillary block due to the clot. Delayed glaucoma is caused by circulating ghost cells (dehemoglobinized RBCs), trabecular meshwork—fibrosis, damage to trabecular meshwork endothelium by siderotic changes, peripheral anterior synechiae, and angle recession glaucoma.

Rebleeding: The major concern after a traumatic hyphema is rebleeding. The incidence of rebleed is higher with higher grades of hyphema. It is usually seen to occur between 2 and 7 days after trauma. It has been hypothesized to occur due clot lysis and clot retraction causing stretch on traumatized vessels. Rebleed can cause raised IOP and corneal blood staining. A significant reduction of vision (<20/200), an initial hyphema of more than one-third of the anterior chamber, and elevated IOP at presentation are significant risk factors for secondary bleeding.[4]

Corneal blood staining: The combination of elevated IOP, endothelial dysfunction, and anterior chamber blood predisposes the eye to corneal blood staining. RBCs within anterior chamber release hemoglobin and penetrate posterior corneal stroma, where it is absorbed by keratocytes and converted to hemosiderin. Endothelial degeneration is a common accompaniment of this process.[5] It starts centrally as yellow granular discoloration and slowly spreads peripherally.

Optic atrophy: This can be caused by either due to elevated IOP or from traumatic optic neuropathy.

Management

Earlier management strategies in hyphema included hospitalization, bedrest, bilateral patching, sedation and topical, and systemic steroids. Now most of the cases are managed on outpatient basis with ambulation. Noncompliance to treatment, patients with bleeding disorders, severe ocular injuries, significantly raised IOP, sickle cell trait/disease, and suspected cases of child abuse require hospitalization. Based on the available evidence, following treatment regimen can be adopted in the management of patients with traumatic hyphema:

- *General measures:*
  - *Patch and shield:* Improves patient comfort in an injured eye and also prevents chances of further trauma to the eye (including during sleeping).
  - *Head end elevation:* Helps for the bleed to settle down which in turn helps to keep pupillary axis clear.
  - *Systemic anticoagulants and antiplatelets:* These agents may increase the risk of persistence of hyphema or chances of rebleed. Decision regarding temporary cessation of these drugs can be taken in consultation of the treating physician.
  - *Preference of analgesics:* Nonsteroidal anti-inflammatory drugs can increase the risk of rebleed secondary to their antiplatelet effect. In patients requiring analgesia drugs like paracetamol should be preferred.
- *Medical management:*
  - *Topical mydriatics and cycloplegics:* These agents improve patient comfort by relieving ciliary spasm, keep pupil mobile/dilated and prevent synechiae formation.
  - *Corticosteroids:* Topical corticosteroids help to prevent rebleed by stabilizing blood–ocular barrier. They also help to decrease associated inflammation. The role of oral steroids in the management of hyphema is controversial. They may be used in patients who are at high risk of rebleed.
  - *Antiglaucoma medications:* Various combinations of topical and oral antiglaucoma medications can be given to control IOP. Acetazolamide is avoided in patients with blood disorders like sickle cell anemia.
  - *Antifibrinolytic agents:* These drugs have been shown to reduce incidence of rebleed in cases of traumatic hyphema. Systemic agents used include aminocaproic acid and tranexamic acid. Topical aminocaproic acid has been shown to be equally effective to its systemic counterpart with no systemic side effects.[6]
- *Surgical management:* Most patients of traumatic hyphema can be managed by medical management. Only a small proportion of patients will require surgical intervention. Following are the indications for surgical intervention in patients with hyphema:[7]
  - Microscopic corneal blood staining
  - Total hyphema with IOP ≥50 mm Hg or more for 5 days (to prevent optic nerve damage)
  - Hyphema that are initially total and do not resolve below 50% at 6 days with IOP ≥25 mm Hg (to prevent corneal blood staining)
  - Hyphema that remain unresolved for 9 days (to prevent peripheral anterior synechiae).

References

1. Spoor TC, Kwitko GM, O'Grady JM, Ramocki JM. Traumatic hyphema in an urban population. Am J Ophthalmol. 1990;109:23-7.
2. Wilson II FM. Traumatic hyphema: pathogenesis and management. Ophthalmology. 1980;87:910.
3. Bansal S, Gunasekeran DV, Ang B, Lee J, Khandelwal R, Sullivan P, et al. Controversies in the pathophysiology and management of hyphema. Surv Ophthalmol. 2016;61(3):297-308.
4. Lawrence T, Wilison D, Harvey J. The incidence of secondary hemorrhage after traumatic hyphema. Ann Ophthalmol. 1990;22:276.
5. Gottsch JD, Messner EP, McNair DS, Font RL. Corneal blood staining: an animal model. Ophthalmology. 1986;93:797.
6. Crouch Jr ER, Williams PB, Gray MK, Crouch ER, Chames M. Topical aminocaproic acid in the treatment of traumatic hyphema. Arch Ophthalmol. 1997;115(9):1106-12.
7. Read J. Traumatic hyphema: surgical vs medical management. Ann Ophthalmol. 1975;7(5):659-62, 664-6, 668-70.

Systemic Disorders and Eye

Athul S Puthalath, Devesh Kumawat, Pranita Sahay

Q 1. Enumerate the pregnancy-induced ocular problems.

Pregnancy causes major changes in all systems of the body, including the eye. Pregnancy affects eyes in three main ways: physiologic ocular changes, pathologic ocular changes, and effects on preexisting ocular diseases.

1. *Physiologic ocular changes:*
   a. *External eye:* The most frequent physiological change is an increase in pigmentation around the eyes. Darkening of face is seen, known as pregnancy mask, chloasma, or melasma, and is due to increased estrogen, progesterone, and melanocyte-stimulating hormone. Unilateral ptosis may be seen as a result of fluid accumulation and hormonal effect on levator aponeurosis; it resolves postpartum. Dry eye is also seen, with an increased secretion of lysozyme. Conjunctival capillaries decrease in number along with a granularity of conjunctival venules, which are reversible after delivery.
   b. *Cornea:* Corneal curvature and thickness increase during pregnancy, secondary to concomitant stromal edema. Corneal sensitivity decreases during pregnancy. Krukenberg's spindles are also seen, which tend to disappear postpartum.
   c. *Intraocular pressure (IOP):* IOP tends to decrease during pregnancy in both normal and glaucoma patients. Many mechanisms have been proposed which include increased aqueous outflow, lower episcleral venous pressure due to decreased systemic vascular resistance, lower scleral rigidity as a result of increased tissue elasticity, and general acidosis during pregnancy.
   d. *Lens:* Myopic shift is seen due to an increase in lens curvature. Transient accommodation insufficiency may also be seen sometimes.
   e. *Visual field:* Since pituitary gland shows physiological growth during pregnancy, bitemporal field contractions are seen occasionally in cases of abnormal anatomical relationship between pituitary and optic chiasma. Some reports refute any significant field changes as well.
   f. *Visual evoked potential:* Decrease in P100 wave latency is seen during pregnancy.
2. *Pathologic ocular changes:*
   a. *Pregnancy-induced hypertension (PIH):* Preeclampsia is blood pressure of over 140/90 mm Hg, generalized edema, and proteinuria after 20 weeks of pregnancy. If seizures develop, then it is called eclampsia. The most common visual symptom is blurring of vision. Patients may also experience photopsia, scotoma, and diplopia. Visual symptoms may be a precursor of a seizure in preeclamptic patients. The retinal changes resemble hypertensive retinopathy. The most common finding is retinal arteriolar narrowing, usually focal but may also be generalized. Other changes include retinal hemorrhage, retinal edema, hard exudate, nerve fiber layer infarcts, and capillary nonperfusion. There is a positive correlation between the severity of preeclampsia and the degree of retinopathy.

      Most of these findings return to normal following the resolution of preeclampsia. Serous retinal detachment (RD) has been reported in <1% of preeclamptic patients and about 10% of eclamptic patients and usually is bilateral. There is no relation between development of RD and severity of retinopathy. Optic nerve findings that may be seen in preeclampsia include papillary edema, ischemic optic neuropathy, and optic atrophy. Cortical blindness has also been reported rarely in PIH.
   b. *Central serous chorioretinopathy (CSCR):* Pregnancy is a known risk factor for CSCR. Most frequently seen in the third trimester, it tends to resolve spontaneously 1–2 months postpartum. About 90% of pregnant CSCR patients

develop white fibrinous subretinal exudates, compared to only 20% in nonpregnant CSCR. Factors contributing to pathogenesis of CSCR in pregnancy include physiologic changes in hemodynamics, vascular permeability, autonomic nervous function, and hormones.
   c. *Vascular occlusive diseases:* Pregnancy is a hypercoagulable state due to increased platelet adhesiveness, elevated levels of clotting factors, hyperfibrinogenemia, elevated fatty acid levels, and reduced fibrinolytic activity. This may lead to arterial and venous occlusions, disseminated intravascular coagulopathy, thrombotic thrombocytopenic purpura, antiphospholipid antibody syndrome (APS), amniotic fluid embolism, and cerebral venous thrombosis. RVOs are rare as compared to arterial occlusions. Purtscher-like retinopathy may also be seen after delivery due to occlusion of multiple superficial retinal arterioles.
3. *Changes in preexisting diseases:*
   a. *Diabetic retinopathy (DR):* DR may worsen during pregnancy. Progression is seen in both nonproliferative DR (NPDR) and proliferative DR (PDR). With prepregnancy laser treatment, the risk of progression is reduced by 50% and hence it is recommended for patients with severe NPDR and PDR. Diabetic macular edema may develop or worsen during pregnancy, but it often resolves postpartum.
   b. *Tumors:* Asymptomatic pituitary adenoma may enlarge during pregnancy and cause various ophthalmological symptoms. Headache, visual field changes (most frequently bitemporal defect), lowered visual acuity, and rarely diplopia may occur. These tend to resolve postpartum, leaving no visual sequelae. Preexisting meningiomas may vascularize and enlarge causing acute visual loss and is believed to be mediated by estrogen and progesterone. Uveal melanoma is rare, and its incidence and reactivation rate is higher in pregnant women compared to nonpregnant women of same age. Cavernous hemangioma is also noted to have accelerated growth in pregnancy.
   c. *Graves' disease:* It is the most common cause of hyperthyroidism during pregnancy with exacerbation seen in the first trimester. The course follows an improvement in second and third trimester with further worsening postpartum.
   d. *Uveitis:* During pregnancy the increased endogenous steroids along with multifactorial and complex mechanisms cause both ocular and systemic signs of noninfectious uveitis to subside and attack frequency to decrease. Both the ocular and systemic symptoms of sarcoidosis, spondyloarthropathy and rheumatoid arthritis, have been seen to improve in pregnancy. However, frequent relapses may occur after delivery. Toxoplasmosis can result in congenital infection if a primary infection occurs during pregnancy through transplacental transmission from mother to baby. Even though very severe infection occurs in the first trimester, transmission to the fetus is more frequently seen in the third trimester, when maternal and fetal circulations are in greatest contact. Pregnancy may be a triggering factor for ocular recurrence of toxoplasmosis, but recurrent disease has little risk for transmission to the fetus. Vogt–Koyanagi–Harada disease is a bilateral panuveitis which has been seen to regress and in some cases completely resolve during pregnancy and the postpartum period. Some cases of worsening in early pregnancy have also been reported.
   e. *Posterior scleritis:* Posterior scleritis worsens and recurrence increases during pregnancy.
   f. *Multiple sclerosis (MS):* The rate of MS attacks decreases during pregnancy, although it may increase in the first three months postpartum.
   g. *Pituitary apoplexy-Sheehan's syndrome:* It is a pituitary gland enlargement due to sudden infarct or hemorrhage in pituitary adenomas. Pregnancy is one of the risk factors for this condition and occurs as a result of spontaneous postpartum hemorrhage. The condition is vision-threatening and is characterized by sudden headache, vision loss and visual field loss, and/or ophthalmoplegia. Typical vision field loss is bitemporal superior quadrant defect.[1]

 2. Discuss ocular manifestations of dengue fever.

- Ocular involvement in dengue fever is seen in 7–40% of cases. The involvement can be either unilateral or bilateral, and the interval between the onset of the fever and visual symptoms ranges from 2 days to 5 months.
- The usual complaints include redness, blurring of vision, and other infrequent complaints such as scotoma, ocular pain, metamorphopsia, micropsia, and impaired color vision.
- Most frequently reported anterior segment manifestation is subconjunctival hemorrhage. Others include uveitis, angle closure glaucoma, and less common findings such as superficial punctate erosions keratitis and scleritis.
- Posterior segment complications include cotton-wool spots, retinal hemorrhages, foveolitis, macular edema, retinal vascular occlusion, vasculitis, optic neuropathy, chorioretinitis, and/or exudative RD.
- The precise pathophysiologic mechanism of dengue ophthalmic complications is not well understood, the most commonly accepted theory is the possibility of an immune-mediated process leading to deposition of immune complexes rather than a direct viral infection.

3. How will you monitor and manage a case of dengue fever from an ophthalmic standpoint?

Investigations

A complete blood count usually shows thrombocytopenia, and it is one of the most common hematological disorders associated with dengue fever. It is of a transient nature and the platelet count reverts to normal once the infectious process has been successfully controlled. Multimodal ocular investigations are usually indicated for posterior segment pathology.

- Amsler grid test can be used to detect scotomas in patients with dengue-related maculopathy.
- Visual field analysis can be used to record and monitor the scotomas.
- Microperimetry is a beneficial tool to detect a significant reduction of contrast sensitivity related to visual symptoms for quantitative measurements and follow-up of scotomas in dengue foveolitis, even when standard visual field testing is normal.
- Fundus fluorescein angiography (FFA) can be done to aid in diagnosing vascular occlusions, vasculitis, and foveolitis. Findings include blocked fluorescence, leakage from venules, retinal pigment epithelium (RPE) defects, and capillary nonperfusion.
- Optical coherence tomography (OCT) imaging is used to diagnose and monitor the retinal thickness and foveal morphology. Three patterns of dengue maculopathy have been described based on standard OCT: first, retinal thickening of central or paracentral fovea; second, cystoid macular edema (CME); and third, foveolitis. Foveolitis is a unique entity in dengue eye disease, which is characterized by a well-circumscribed yellow-orange lesion at the foveal center corresponding with focal disruption of the outer neurosensory retina and the inner segment/outer segment (IS/OS) junction. Among these patterns, foveolitis tends to have the worst visual outcome.
- Optical coherence tomography angiography (OCTA) findings include capillary flow deficit, enlargement of the foveal avascular zone, and loss of capillaries in the superficial and deep capillary plexus. These features may suggest a retinal vascular micro-occlusion mechanism.

Treatment

- The majority of patients with dengue-related ocular complications have a self-limiting course and hence does not require any treatment.
- Topical corticosteroids can be instilled for anterior segment inflammation. Patients who are persistently symptomatic and have poor vision due to posterior segment ocular complications may be started on oral steroids or intravenous steroids depending on ocular involvement. Oral prednisolone at a dose of 1 mg/kg can be initiated.
- Visual prognosis of dengue ophthalmic complications following treatment with systemic steroids in the form of intravenous or oral prednisolone is favorable. These patients are followed up every 2–4 weeks and steroids are tapered according to clinical response.
- Intravenous immunoglobulin can be administered in patients unresponsive to intravenous methylprednisolone or oral prednisolone.
- Rare cases of nonresolving vitreous hemorrhage may need pars plana vitrectomy.
- Some patients may have persistent scotoma despite clinical resolution of dengue ophthalmic complications. Overall, ophthalmic involvement secondary to dengue fever carries a good visual prognosis.

4. Explain the ocular involvement in systemic lupus erythematosus (SLE).

Ophthalmic manifestations of SLE are not included in the diagnostic scoring system. Even then, ocular involvement may be seen much earlier to definitive establishment of the diagnosis. Ocular involvement can be divided into external, retinal, choroidal, neuro-ophthalmologic, and orbital manifestations.

- *External ocular involvement:* External ocular manifestations may precede the classical diagnostic manifestation of SLE by 1–3 years. Discoid lupus erythematosus (DLE) usually presents similar to chronic blepharitis with erythematous, raised, scaly dermatitis with madarosis and thick lid margins. These lesions usually respond to systemic or topical corticosteroids or both or to systemic hydroxychloroquine. The most common ocular manifestation of SLE is keratoconjunctivitis sicca. Conjunctivitis and interstitial keratitis are rare. DLE patients can rarely have superficial punctate keratitis and recurrent epithelial erosions. SLE may present with diffuse anterior or nodular scleritis and episcleritis as well. These may be presenting clinical manifestations of SLE.

- *Retinal involvement:* Lupus retinopathy is the second most common ocular manifestation of SLE. The most frequent retinal findings include cotton wool spots (CWS), retinal hemorrhages, and vascular tortuosity. Other reported posterior segment changes include retinal hard exudates, retinal vasculitis, retinal artery and/or vein occlusion, arteriolar narrowing, arteriovenous crossing changes, macular pigmentary mottling, retinal scarring, and macular infarction. The underlying pathophysiology in lupus retinopathy is the infiltration of vessel walls with fibrillar material causing vascular constrictions and widespread hyaline thrombus formation. This is not a true vasculitis, as the vessel walls themselves are free of inflammatory cells.
- *Choroidal involvement:* Extensive deposition of immune complexes in choroid is seen due to its profuse blood flow. CSCR-like picture with multifocal serous RD has been observed that resolves with systemic control of the disease. Existence of anti-RPE antibodies is speculated to be the cause of injury.
- *Neuro-ophthalmologic involvement:* Optic nerve involvement in patients with SLE may be in the form of optic neuritis, ischemic optic neuropathy, and disc edema. Central nervous system (CNS) vasculitis affecting the brainstem in patients with SLE may lead to pupillary abnormality, cranial nerve involvement, and diplopia. Other manifestations include ocular motility disorders, internuclear ophthalmoplegia, nystagmus, and homonymous hemianopia.
- *Orbital involvement:* Orbital involvement in SLE resembles orbital pseudotumor with no discrete lesion and a good response to systemic steroids. Orbital myositis with proptosis and pain on external ocular movements may also be seen in SLE.

Ophthalmic manifestations of systemic lupus erythematosus	
External	**Neuro-ophthalmic**
• Keratoconjunctivitis sicca • Conjunctivitis • Superficial punctate keratitis • Recurrent epithelial erosion • Interstitial keratitis • Episcleritis and scleritis • Discoid lupus erythematosus	• Optic neuritis • Ischemic optic neuropathy • Pupillary and oculomotor disturbances • Pseudotumor cerebri • Nystagmus • Homonymous hemianopia • Amaurosis • Internuclear ophthalmoplegia
Retinal	**Choroidal**
• Cotton wool spots • Retinal hemorrhage • Tortuous vessels • Retinal vascular occlusion • Retinal vasculitis • Proliferative retinopathy • Macular infarction	• Ischemic choroidopathy • Multifocal serous retinal detachment • Choroidal vasculitis **Orbital** • Orbital pseudotumor • Orbital myositis

5. What is the ocular involvement in obstructive sleep apnea (OSA) syndrome?

Obstructive sleep apnea syndrome is a sleep disorder with nocturnal pharyngeal collapse leading to partial airway obstruction and hypopneic or apneic events during sleep. Ocular involvement arises due to the mechanical and vascular effects of the syndrome. Appropriate triaging between sleep physicians and ophthalmologists is vital to prevent ocular complications and vision loss in patients with OSA.
- *Floppy eyelid syndrome (FES):* There is a strong association between OSA and FES. Patients may present with foreign body sensation, dryness, redness, eyelid swelling, or papillary conjunctivitis. The tissue damage and eyelid eversion occur at night, and hence symptoms are worse upon waking. Pharyngeal collapse in OSA is due to increased neck thickness which causes connective tissue weakness. Histology of lids in FES reveals decreased elastin content and increased matrix metalloproteinase activity in lid connective tissue, demonstrating a similar connective tissue weakness. There is also a tissue redundancy in lateral canthal tendon. The symptoms are more on the side on which OSA patients sleep, suggesting mechanical stress as well.
- *Nonarteritic anterior ischemic optic neuropathy (NAION):* The majority of NAION patients suffer from vision loss upon waking up, suggesting nocturnal hypotension as a contributing factor. Patients with OSA suffer from defective autoregulation of blood flow, with an imbalance of nitric oxide and endothelin leading to hypoxia and hypoperfusion of tissues. During apneic episodes, intracranial pressure can increase, which limits perfusion to the optic nerve and may lead to NAION.

- *Central serous chorioretinopathy (CSCR):* There is an increase in circulating epinephrine and norepinephrine levels in patients with OSA. This increased sympathetic tone affects the choroidal vasculature and RPE, leading to accumulation of subretinal serous fluid.
- *Retinal vein occlusion (RVO):* The relation between RVO and OSA is attributed to the effect of OSA on blood flow autoregulation and microvasculature. Just like NAION, symptoms of RVO arise upon waking, suggesting relation to nocturnal apnea. Hypercoagulability seen in OSA with further inflammation also contributes to the development of RVO.
- *Glaucoma:* There is an association between OSA and both normal-tension glaucoma and open-angle glaucoma. OSA can contribute to the pathogenesis of glaucoma more through its vascular effects than mechanical process. OSA predisposes the optic nerve head to ischemia and damage through episodes of hypoxia, hemodynamic changes to retinal blood vessels, oxidative stress, mitochondrial dysregulation, and inflammation. Glaucoma patients with OSA tend to have a higher IOP, worse visual field indices, and thinner retinal nerve fiber layer.[2]

6. Describe the ocular features due to deficiency of vitamin A, B1, B2, C, and D.

Vitamin A

Nutritional blindness caused by vitamin A deficiency remains the single leading cause of blindness among children worldwide. Xerophthalmia refers to the irregular, lustreless, and poorly wet surface of conjunctiva and cornea associated with vitamin A deficiency. The World Health Organization has classified xerophthalmia in order of severity from night blindness (XN) to corneal ulceration and keratomalacia along with corneal scar (XS) and xerophthalmic fundus (XF) which is a rare condition.[3]

World Health Organization classification of xerophthalmia	
XN	Night blindness
X1A	Conjunctival xerosis
X1B	Bitot spots
X2	Corneal xerosis
X3A	Corneal ulceration/keratomalacia involving less than one-third of corneal surface
X3B	Corneal ulceration/keratomalacia involving one-third or more of corneal surface
XS	Corneal scar
XF	Xerophthalmic fundus

- *Night blindness (XN):* Earliest manifestation of vitamin A deficiency is night blindness. It occurs due to inadequate or slow recovery of rhodopsin in retina after exposure to bright light. It is reversible with oral replacement, even as fast as 48 hours.
- *Conjunctival xerosis (X1A):* Vitamin A deficiency causes loss of mucin and goblet cells, increased keratinization, and a transition of normal columnar to stratified squamous epithelium of the conjunctiva. The conjunctiva is dry with lack of wettability, loss of transparency, thickening, wrinkling, and pigmentation.
- *Bitot's spot (X1B):* It is pathognomonic of vitamin A deficiency. It is a well-demarcated patch of keratinized, squamous metaplasia of the bulbar conjunctiva usually seen in the temporal conjunctiva. They have a frothy, foamy, cheesy, greasy, or granular appearance. The number of Bitot spots generally correlates with the severity of deficiency and low serum retinol concentrations.
- *Corneal Xerosis (X2):* Cornea undergoes squamous metaplasia with keratinization due to severe vitamin A deficiency. Cornea acquires a lustreless surface with peau d'orange appearance. Superficial punctate keratitis is also seen, mainly in the inferonasal part of cornea, which stains with fluorescein.
- *Corneal ulceration (X3):* It is a round or oval ulcer with a relatively clean and punched-out appearance. These small punched-out ulcers can progress to keratomalacia, a necrotizing condition that affects a large portion or the entire cornea.
- *Xerophthalmic fundus (XF):* It is a rare condition characterized by fine whitish-yellow or grayish dot-like, oval, or linear opacities in the fundus at the RPE level. They appear as window defects on FFA.
- *Corneal scar (XS):* It is not a sign of active vitamin A deficiency. It is a sequela to cornel ulcer and keratomalacia.

Vitamin B1 (Thiamine)

The systemic disease resulting from thiamine deficiency is called beriberi. Ocular features are usually seen in the dry form of beriberi. The main ocular manifestation of thiamine deficiency is optic atrophy. Other features include corneal epithelial changes, rectus muscle palsies leading to unilateral or bilateral ophthalmoplegia, and nystagmus. Dry beriberi also has nervous system involvement such as peripheral neuropathy, Wernicke's encephalopathy, and Korsakoff's syndrome.

Vitamin B2 (Riboflavin)

Ocular manifestation of riboflavin deficiency is likely due to its role in the development and maintenance of the surface structures of epithelial cells. They may manifest with peripheral corneal vascularization and angular blepharoconjunctivitis.

Vitamin B12

Optic neuropathy is rarely seen in vitamin B12 deficiency. Patients typically present with painless, symmetrical, and progressive reduction in visual acuity. It resembles the optic neuropathy seen in Leber's hereditary optic neuropathy as in both there is a typical absence of optic disc leakage on fluorescein angiography. Central scotomas and dyschromatopsia may be present. If severe anemia is present, then flame-shaped and dot-blot retinal hemorrhages may be seen.

Vitamin C (Ascorbic Acid)

Ascorbic acid is about 15–20 times more concentrated in aqueous humor than in plasma. Ocular involvement is primarily due to hemorrhages caused by increased capillary fragility. Proptosis secondary to orbital hemorrhage occurs in cases of infantile scurvy but is rarely seen in adults. Petechiae or larger hemorrhages can occur in the conjunctiva, eyelids, orbit, anterior chamber, vitreous, and retina.

Vitamin D

Deficiency of vitamin D can cause dry eye symptoms and proptosis.

Vitamin deficiency and eye	
Vitamin	Ocular manifestation
B1—thiamine	• Corneal epithelial changes • Ophthalmoplegia • Nystagmus • Optic atrophy
B2—riboflavin	• Peripheral corneal vascularization • Angular blepharoconjunctivitis
B3—niacin	• Optic neuropathy
B6—pyridoxine	• Angular blepharoconjunctivitis • Optic neuritis • Gyrate atrophy (rare)
B12	• Optic neuropathy and • Optic atrophy • Central scotomas • Dyschromatopsia • Flame-shaped and dot-blot hemorrhages
C—ascorbic acid	• Hemorrhage in eyelids, conjunctiva, anterior chamber, retina • Proptosis in infantile scurvy
D	• Dry eye • Proptosis

 7. Discuss eye in epidemic dropsy.

Epidemic dropsy results from ingestion of edible oil adulterated with *Argemone mexicana* (Mexican Poppy) oil. It is a multisystem disease involving the cardiovascular, hepatic, renal, ocular, and other systems. The most striking feature of the disease is the acute onset of edema of the extremities. Other manifestations include cutaneous features such as tenderness, erythema, rash over the edematous parts, gastrointestinal tract symptoms, low-grade fever, and congestive cardiac failure, which can be fatal.

Ocular manifestations occur relatively late in the course of epidemic dropsy.

- The most important ocular manifestation of epidemic dropsy is glaucoma. The incidence of glaucoma in cases of epidemic dropsy is variable. Glaucoma is usually bilateral. Increased activity of aqueous prostaglandin and histamine is hypothesized to cause hypersecretion and increased protein levels in aqueous leads to significant elevation of IOP.
- Patients may develop visual field defects such as nasal defects and enlargement of blind spots. The toxic alkaloid in argemone oil is known to cause a form of leaking microangiopathy. This could have a toxic effect on functional integrity of retina or direct action on ganglion cells leading to visual field defects.
- Anterior segment evaluation characteristically reveals a quite eye with no signs of uveitis, and open angles with normal anterior chamber depth.
- Other ocular manifestations include subconjunctival hemorrhages, retinal venous dilatation with tortuosity, retinal hemorrhages, subhyaloid hemorrhages, disc edema, anemic retinopathy, macular edema, and central RVO.

 8. Discuss lifestyle modification in patients with diabetes.

Lifestyle interventions play a vital role in controlling diabetes and helps in improvement of overall health. Major components of lifestyle modification include dietary modification, exercise, and weight reduction. All these measures aim to improve glycemic control in diabetic patients and thereby increase insulin sensitivity of tissues. Lifestyle interventions also helps to improve the lipid profile in all patients with diabetes, as dyslipidemia has been found to be a risk factor for atherosclerotic cardiovascular disease along with obesity, hypertension, and smoking.

Diabetes Education

This is used to describe a comprehensive diabetes self-management education program that patients with newly diagnosed diabetes should participate in. It includes individualized instruction on nutrition, physical activity, optimizing metabolic control, and preventing complications.

Medical Nutrition Therapy

It is the process of tailoring a dietary plan by taking into account medical, lifestyle, and personal factors. This aims for weight reduction in overweight individuals and weight maintenance in others by monitoring carbohydrate intake and a balanced nutrition.

Weight Reduction

Weight reduction is especially important for diabetics and emphasis should be placed on lowering caloric intake, increasing physical activity, and behavior modification to achieve weight loss. This is more beneficial in type 2 diabetes who are overweight (BMI ≥25–29.9 kg/m^2) or obese (BMI ≥30 kg/m^2). Improved glycemic control induced by weight loss is associated with improvement of insulin resistance and improved insulin secretion, especially in type 2 diabetes.

Exercise

Regular exercise leads to improved glycemic control due to increased responsiveness of body tissues to insulin. It can also delay the progression of impaired glucose tolerance to overt diabetes.

Psychological Interventions

Psychotherapy may reduce psychological distress and improves glycemic control in some diabetics.

Pregnancy Planning

All women of childbearing age with diabetes should be counseled about the potential effects of diabetes, and the potential impact of pregnancy on their diabetes control and any existing complications.

Smoking Cessation

It has been proved that discontinuation of smoking is one of the most important aspects of therapy in patients with diabetes who smoke.

9. Enumerate the various ocular manifestation of Hansen's disease.

Hansen's disease (also known as leprosy) is a systemic disease caused by an acid-fast bacillus, *Mycobacterium leprae*. The majority of the ocular complications of leprosy are sight-threatening and can be avoided if timely treatment is initiated. Ridley and Jopling classified leprosy into five groups with a spectrum of high cellular immunity and low bacterial counts (tuberculoid-TT) at one end to low cellular immunity and high bacterial counts (lepromatous-LL) at the other end. There are three intermediate forms: borderline lepromatous (BL), borderline tuberculoid (BT), and borderline borderline (BB). For therapeutic purposes the smear positive LL, BL, and BB are also called multibacillary disease (MB) and the smear negative TT and BT are termed as paucibacillary disease (PB). Two types of reactions are described in leprosy—erythema nodosum leprosum (ENL) is seen in lepromatous leprosy and reversal reaction (RR) is seen in borderline leprosy.[1,2]

The main potentially sight-threatening ocular manifestations of Hansen's disease include cataract, lagophthalmos, reduced corneal sensation, corneal ulcers, iridocyclitis/uveitis, scleritis, glaucoma, and other ocular complications.

Cataract

Cataract is the most common cause of visual impairment and blindness in leprosy patients. It is usually age-related and less often it may be due to prolonged steroid use in treating inflammation. Rarely, it is due to subclinical chronic iridocyclitis.

Lagophthalmos

The inability to close eyelids is called lagophthalmos. The facial nerve supply to orbicularis oculi through its temporal and zygomatic branches is affected, causing inadequate lid closure. Lower lids are most affected usually. Initially, patients have nocturnal lagophthalmos. These patients also have a decreased blink rate. Lagophthalmos causes cosmetic blemish, but also can lead to corneal ulceration and opacity in the presence of decreased corneal sensation. The amount of lagophthalmos is proportional to the extent of the damage to the facial nerve. Risk factors for lagophthalmos in leprosy include a depigmented, anesthetic, or erythematous skin patch over the zygomatic area, recent commencement of multidrug therapy (MDT), and borderline leprosy.

Reduced Corneal Sensation

The reduced corneal sensation is usually seen in long-standing polar lepromatous leprosy. Sensation may be tested quantitatively by using the Cochet and Bonnet esthesiometer. A cotton wisp is no longer recommended for testing corneal sensation in the field unless it is done in the clinics.

Corneal Ulcers

Corneal ulcers can occur due to an acute microbial infection or as a secondary infection in exposure keratitis. It leads to opacification of cornea. Risk factors for corneal ulcers in these cases include lagophthalmos, impaired corneal sensation, and nasolacrimal infection. Usually, acute corneal ulcers manifest with decreased vision, pain, and red eye. But pain can be absent in insensitive corneas and these patients present late with progressed ulcer and severe diminution of vision. These are medical emergencies and prompt rigorous treatment is needed.

Uveitis/Iridocyclitis

It is one of the most common causes of blindness in MB leprosy patients. Iris and ciliary body being cooler than the core body temperature form a favorable site for growth of *M. leprae*. Acute uveitis typically occurs in borderline lepromatous leprosy while chronicity is seen in lepromatous leprosy. Paucibacillary leprosy rarely account for iridocyclitis. The bacilli can harbor in the eye even after a course of MDT, and a sub-clinical course is commonly seen. Iris pearls (<0.5 mm) are pathognomonic of leprosy. Miosis and iris atrophy may also be seen due to impaired dilator pupillae innervation.

Scleritis

Scleritis is usually seen in lepromatous leprosy patients and requires aggressive treatment with steroid drops and/or usually with oral nonsteroidal anti-inflammatory drug (NSAID) or steroids.

Glaucoma

Glaucoma is secondary to treatment with steroids or due to uveitis. Hence, regular IOP monitoring is warranted in leprosy patients.

Other Ocular Complications

- Thickening and nodules of corneal nerves
- Punctate subepithelial avascular leprous keratitis
- Madarosis
- Band-shaped keratopathy.

Management of Lagophthalmos in Hansen's Disease

Early Lagophthalmos

Eyelids may appear normal in mild weakness of orbicularis oculi. Hence, it is imperative to check voluntary gentle closure of the eyelids, along with forced closure and the measurement of the mid-palpebral height at every visit. Early lagophthalmos can be managed by medical measures such as:

- *Blinking exercises:* Patients have to shut their eyes forcefully for a count of about 10 seconds, 10–20 times a session, for 2–3 sessions a day. This exercise strengthens the orbicularis oculi muscle fibers that have been spared.
- *Tear substitutes:* To keep cornea moist and protected, as exposure can lead to drying. Patients are advised to use topical carboxymethyl cellulose 1%, polyvinyl alcohol 1–3% drops, or other equivalent topical lubricants for at least 6–8 times a day. Long-acting lubricant ointment to be applied at night.
- *Corneal protection:* If cornea is exposed, using protective spectacles or goggles can reduce tear evaporation from ocular surface. At night, cross taping and shield can also be used.

Late Lagophthalmos

Surgery is indicated for lagophthalmos if:

- >6 months duration
- >2 mm gap on forced closure
- Impending corneal damage
- Corneal ulcer development
- Excessive symptoms such as tearing and redness due to dryness.

Surgical options available include lateral tarsorrhaphy, upper lid retractors recession, lower lid tightening and elevation, temporalis muscle transfer, and gold weight implants.

- *Lateral tarsorrhaphy:* It is the most commonly performed surgery for lagophthalmos. It is a simple surgical procedure in which the lateral aspects of the eyelid margins are abraded and sutured together. The palpebral fissure is reduced in size while the lids cover the cornea better and patient can retain useful vision. The surgery can be performed medially as well if the eyelid gap or corneal damage is more medial. The limitation is poor cosmetic appearance.
- *Upper lid retractors recession:* The recession of the upper lid retractors (levator and Muller's muscle) is another useful procedure.
- *Lower lid tightening and elevation:* A tightening procedure such as a lateral tarsal strip procedure will improve apposition of the lower eyelid to the globe. This in turn helps to reduce epiphora or lacrimation as well.
- *Temporalis muscle transfer:* In this procedure, a strip of tendon from the temporalis muscle is undermined and split into two. Then each strip is tunneled subcutaneously along the upper and lower eyelid margins and sutured to the medial canthal tendon. After surgical recovery, the patient is taught to close the eyes by clenching the teeth. Complications of this procedure may include ptosis and ectropion.
- *Gold weight implants:* Gold weights can be implanted into the upper lid to enhance lid closure in a gravity-dependent manner. Gold, being inert, is the ideal material of choice. However, astigmatic shift, migration, and extrusion of the gold weight may occur as a complication.

 10. Discuss ocular effects of systemic medications.

Systemic medications can have adverse ocular effects and can affect the visual function to varying degrees depending on site and extent of involvement.[3] The effects can be seen in eyelids, cornea, uvea, lens, retina, optic nerve, and even the visual cortex.

Adnexa		
Monoclonal antibodies	**Indication**	**Ocular effects**
Epidermal growth factor receptor inhibitors	Treatment of solid tumors	• Trichomegaly—common • Blepharitis—less common • Dry eye syndrome—less common • Cicatricial entropion—rare
Imatinib mesylate- selective inhibitor of tyrosine kinase	Treatment of CML and gastrointestinal stromal tumors	Periorbital edema (after 5–8 weeks of treatment initiation)
Ipilimumab—CTLA-4 antibody	Treatment of metastatic malignant melanoma	Features similar to thyroid eye disease

(CML: chronic myeloid leukemia; CTLA-4: cytotoxic T-lymphocyte-associated protein 4)

Cornea		
Drug	**Indication**	**Ocular effects**
Amiodarone	Cardiac antiarrhythmic agent	• Vortex keratopathy (dose-dependent) • Reversible on cessation • Minimal impairment of visual acuity • No need to discontinue drug
Chloroquine and hydroxychloroquine	Antimalarial agents, treatment of autoimmune connective tissue disorders	• Vortex keratopathy (dose-independent) • Reversible on cessation
Chlorpromazine	• Sedative • Antipsychotic	Diffuse yellowish-brown granular deposits in the endothelium, Descemet membrane, and deep stroma, within the palpebral fissure area
Silver—argyrosis	Iatrogenic or occupational exposure	• Grayish-brown granular deposits in Descemet membrane • Conjunctiva may also be affected
Gold—chrysiasis	Rheumatoid arthritis	• If total dose of gold is >1,500 mg, corneal deposits may occur • Dust-like or glittering purple granules scattered throughout the epithelium and stroma
Amantadine	Parkinson disease	Diffuse white punctate opacities. Epithelial edema +/–

Uvea		
Drug	**Indication**	**Ocular effects**
Rifabutin	Mycobacterial infections	Acute anterior uveitis (AAU) with hypopyon
Cidofovir	CMV retinitis in AIDS	• AAU with few cells and marked fibrinous exudate • Hypopyon • Vitritis
Bisphosphonates	Osteoporosis (to retard bone absorption)	Uveitis and scleritis (by activation of T cell sub-group)
Sulfonamides	Antibiotic	• Uveitis • Ciliary effusion • Steven–Johnson syndrome
Fluoroquinolones	Antibiotic	• Acute extensive anterior segment pigment dispersion • BAIT—bilateral acute iris transillumination • BADI—bilateral acute depigmentation of iris
Etanercept, infliximab, adalimumab (TNF inhibitors)	Immunosuppressants	• Paradoxical uveitis • Induction of sarcoidosis
Topiramate	Anticonvulsant migraine	• Acute angle closure and myopia secondary to ciliochoroidal effusion • Presents with blurred vision, haloes, pain, and redness • Shallow AC • Raised IOP (Also seen with sulfonamide, bupropion, and acetazolamide)

(AC: anterior chamber; AIDS: acquired immune deficiency syndrome; CMV: cytomegalovirus; IOP: intraocular pressure; TNF: tumor necrosis factor)

Lens

Drug	Indication	Ocular effects
Steroids	Systemic and ocular inflammation	• Posterior subcapsular cataract initially • Anterior subcapsular cataract later • Secondary glaucoma (more with topical)
Amiodarone	Cardiac antiarrhythmic agent	Anterior subcapsular lens deposits
Chlorpromazine	• Sedative • Antipsychotic	• Fine, stellate, yellowish-brown granules on anterior lens capsule within pupillary area • Usually if cumulative dose >1000 g
Gold	Rheumatoid arthritis	Anterior capsular deposits
Allopurinol	Gout	Increased risk of cataract formation in elderly

Retina

Drug	Indication	Ocular effects
• Chloroquine • Hydroxychloroquine	• Antimalarial • Autoimmune connective tissue disorders	Bull's eye maculopathy
Phenothiazines		
• Thioridazine	Schizophrenia	• Adverse effect if dose >800 mg/day • Salt and pepper retinopathy—early feature • Progress to plaque-like pigmentation and focal loss of RPE and choriocapillaris • Finally, diffuse loss of RPE and choriocapillaris
• Chlorpromazine	• Sedative • Antipsychotic	Nonspecific pigmentary granularity and clumping
• Digoxin	• Atrial fibrillation • Symptomatic heart failure	• Decreased vision, scotoma, photophobia, and dyschromatopsia (xanthopsia, cyanopsia, chloropsia) • ERG—delayed implicit time and reduced B-wave amplitude
Interferon alfa	• Hepatitis C • Malignancy	• Cotton wool spots and retinal hemorrhages • FA shows focal capillary nonperfusion • Less commonly can cause CME, EOM paresis, Disc edema and RVO
Desferrioxamine	Chelating agent in transfusion	• Rapid visual loss • Initially normal fundus, later mottled pigmentary changes develop • FA shows punctate hyperfluorescence
Nicotinic acid	Cholesterol lowering agent	• If doses >1.5 g/day • Cystoid macular edema without leakage on FA • Mild reduction in VA
Alkyl nitrites ("poppers")	Recreational drugs used before sexual activity	• Bilateral loss of VA and photopsia • Small yellow spot in fovea • Clearly seen in autofluorescence • OCT—defect in foveal ellipsoid band

(CME: cystoid macular edema; EOM: extraocular movement; ERG: electroretinogram; FA: fluorescein angiography; OCT: optical coherence tomography; RPE: retinal pigment epithelium; RVO: retinal vein occlusion, VA: visual acuity)

Drug-induced crystalline maculopathies

Drug	Indication	Ocular effects
Tamoxifen	Antiestrogen drug used in breast carcinoma	• Bilateral fine yellow crystalline deposits in the inner layers of the retina and punctate gray lesions in the outer retina and RPE • OCT—helps in early detection • Rarely optic neuritis
Canthaxanthin	Carotenoid used to simulate sun tanning	Deposition of glistening yellow inner retinal deposits in a doughnut conformation at posterior poles

Contd…

Contd...

Drug	Indication	Ocular effects
Methoxyflurane	Inhalant general anesthetic	• Calcium oxalate crystals deposited in retina • Mild visual impairment, RPE hyperplasia
Nitrofurantoin	Antibiotic used mainly for UTI	• Mild visual impairment • Superficial and deep glistening intraretinal deposits in a circinate pattern at posterior pole.

(OCT: optical coherence tomography; RPE: retinal pigment epithelium; UTI: urinary tract infection)

Optic nerve		
Drug	Indication	Ocular effects
Ethambutol	Tuberculosis	• 18% incidence of neuropathy at a daily dose >35 mg/kg/day • Painless blurring of vision, with reduced VA • Impaired color vision • Swollen disc with splinter hemorrhages • Loss of contrast sensitivity—early sign • Central or peripheral visual field defects
Isoniazid	Tuberculosis	• Toxic optic neuropathy • Risk is higher if given along with ethambutol
Amiodarone	Cardiac antiarrhythmic agent	• Optic neuropathy secondary to demyelination • Unilateral or bilateral disc swelling • Corneal findings • Visual field defects present
Vigabatrin	Antiepileptic	• Bilateral concentric, predominantly nasal visual field constriction • Common if cumulative dose > 3 kg • Other subtle signs include peripheral atrophy, arteriolar narrowing, abnormal macular reflexes, and surface wrinkling • OCT—detects peripapillary retinal nerve fiber layer atrophy even before field defects
Methotrexate	Immunosuppressant	• Rare cause of optic neuropathy • Reduced VA, dyschromatopsia, visual field loss

(OCT: optical coherence tomography; VA: visual acuity)

Visual cortex		
Drug	Indication	Ocular effects
Bevacizumab	Colon and rectal tumors	Cortical blindness

11. Discuss ocular effects of oral contraceptive pills.

Estrogen and progesterone receptors have been observed in many ocular tissues, such as the meibomian gland, conjunctiva, cornea, lens, choroid, and retina. Since oral contraceptive pills (OCPs) usually contain estrogen and progesterone these tissues are at increased risk. OCPs are widely used for contraception, but they are also prescribed in menorrhagia, endometriosis, acne and hirsutism, fibroid uterus, and premenstrual syndrome.

	Symptoms and signs	Mechanisms
Ocular surface		
• Alterations	• Discomfort and reduced tear secretion	• Decreased lipid production and size of sebaceous glands • Alterations in mucus secretion • Alterations in corneal thickness and biomechanics
	• Discomfort and intolerance in contact lens wearers	• Increased vascular permeability and dilatation
• Benefits	• Amelioration of the symptoms in postmenopausal women with keratoconjunctivitis sicca	• Vasodilatory action of estrogens on lacrimal gland • No differences in tear osmolarity

Contd...

Contd...

	Symptoms and signs	Mechanisms
Anterior segment		
• Alterations	• Shape of lens, axis, interpupillary distance, and vision exhibits significant differences	• Modified by serum E2 levels
• Benefits	• Decreases IOP and risk for primary open-angle glaucoma	• Neuroprotective action through the RGCs estrogen receptors • Increase in retinal blood flow
	• Prevention of cataractogenesis	• 17-β-estradiol prevents oxidative stress by neutralizing H_2O_2 and eliminating catalase activity
	• Protection of corneal collagen from degradation	• 17-β-estradiol suspends IL-6, IL-1, TNF-α and metalloproteinases expression
Posterior segment		
Alterations	• Central retinal artery or vein occlusion • Intraocular hemorrhages • Aneurysms • Macular or papillary edema • Acute ischemic optic neuropathy	• Thrombosis of the retinal vessels and angiogenesis • VEGF-D stimulation along with the consequential vascular remodeling and vasodilation • Vascular fragility • Elevated fibrinogen and thromboxane A2 concentrations • Increased PDGF concentrations • NOS and cyclooxygenase endothelial dysfunction • Decreased antithrombin III and HDL cholesterol levels
Benefits	• Age-related macular degeneration • Diabetic retinopathy • Oxygen-induced retinopathy	• Antioxidant activity of estrogens by stimulating SOD2, reducing ROS and DNA replication and diminishing MDA and NADPH oxidase • 17β-estradiol eliminates apoptosis of RGCs, by stabilizing the mitochondrial membrane potential • 17β-estradiol regulates SOD, glutathione peroxidase and catalase • Increase in retinal blood flow
Neuro-ophthalmology		
Alterations	• 6th cranial nerve paralysis • Parietal syndrome • Hemianopsia • Retrobulbar neuritis • Papillary edema • Benign intracranial hypertension	Thrombosis of the cerebral or retinal vessels

(DNA: deoxyribonucleic acid; HDL: high-density lipoprotein; IOP: intraocular pressure; NADPH: nicotinamide adenine dinucleotide phosphate oxidase; NOS: nitric oxide synthase; PDGF: platelet-derived growth factor; RGC: retinal ganglion cells; ROS: reactive oxygen species; SOD: superoxide dismutase)

12. Discuss ocular manifestation of leukemias.

Leukemia is a group of blood neoplasms involving hematopoietic stem cells, which proliferate in bone marrow and lymphoid tissue. These transformed stem cells migrate into peripheral blood and thence other tissues. They are classified into acute or chronic and based on cell type primarily involved into myeloid or lymphoid. The ocular manifestation of leukemia is ubiquitous; it involves almost all ocular structures to varying degrees. The ocular effect can be divided broadly due to those related to direct infiltration of ocular tissues with leukemic cells, changes related to accompanying hematologic abnormalities such as anemia, hyper viscosity, or thrombocytopenia, and the opportunistic infections associated with immunosuppression from disease or its therapy. Posterior segment structures are most frequently affected by leukemias.

Anterior Segment Manifestation

The anterior segment manifestations are rare. They include:
- Conjunctival mass
- Anterior uveitis
- Iris infiltration.

Retinal Manifestation

- *Retinal infiltrates* due to direct infiltration of retina with leukemic cells are seen in leukemic retinopathy and they appear as grayish white nodules associated with local hemorrhage, destruction, and necrosis. They have been associated with fulminant disease and premature mortality.
- *Sheathing* of retinal vessels and intravascular margination of leukemic cells also occur.
- *White centered hemorrhages* are due to accumulations of leukemia cells seen along with cellular debris and capillary emboli.
- *Hard exudates and CWS* are also seen. CWS occur due to actual leukemic infiltration of retina and/or nerve fiber layer infarction.
- *Microaneurysms* are usually seen in chronic leukemias adjacent to areas of ischemia and nonperfusion due to hyper viscosity.
- Other uncommon retinal manifestations include frank sea-fan *neovascularization*, central and branch *RVO*.

Vitreous

Infiltration of vitreous is rare.

Choroid

- Frequent infiltration due with leukemic cells due to high blood flow.
- Choroidal involvement along with overlying retinal pigment epithelial degeneration and clumping is seen commonly in acute leukemias.
- "Leopard-spot" pattern due to involvement of choriocapillaris by leukemic cells.

Optic Nerve

- Direct infiltration of the optic nerve occurs as a prelaminar fluffy, white infiltrate superficial to the lamina cribrosa on the optic nerve head or as a retrolaminar infiltrate visible on neuroimaging.
- Patients can have profound visual loss.
- Leukemic meningitis can cause elevated intracranial pressure which can cause disc edema and hence have to be differentiated from optic nerve infiltration.
- Optic nerve infiltration may mimic optic neuritis as well.

Other Manifestations

- Pseudotumor cerebri
- Leukemic meningitis can cause raised intracranial pressure.
- Multiple cranial nerve palsies have also been reported, with the sixth and seventh cranial nerve palsies being most commonly associated with leukemic meningitis.
- Cytomegalovirus (CMV) is a common opportunistic infection seen in immunocompromised individuals due to chemotherapy for leukemias. Other infections include herpes virus, toxoplasmosis, and fungal infections.

 13. Discuss ocular manifestation of multiple sclerosis.

Multiple sclerosis (MS) is a chronic relapsing and remitting, episodic demyelinating disease of the CNS. It is more common in women than men. There is a wide range of ocular manifestations seen in MS.

Optic Neuritis

- Multiple sclerosis is the most common cause of demyelinating optic neuritis.
- Optic neuritis is the initial presenting feature in 30% of MS patients. It occurs at some point in 50% of established MS.
- After an acute episode of optic neuritis, the overall 15-year risk of developing MS is 50%, if no lesion on magnetic resonance imaging (MRI) then 25% and if at least one lesion risk is >70%.
- In the absence of MRI lesions, lower risk of MS is seen in male gender, absence of a viral syndrome receding the optic neuritis, optic disc swelling, disc/peripapillary hemorrhages or macular exudates, if vision is reduced to no light perception and if there is absence of periocular pain.

Symptoms

- Patients present with subacute monocular visual impairment and can have preceding or accompanying pain on ocular movement.
- Phosphenes (tiny white or colored sparkles), frontal headache, and global tenderness may also be present.
- Bilateral simultaneous presentation is rare, but sequential involvement of the fellow eye is common.

Signs

- Usual visual acuity is 6/18–6/60 (rarely worse).
- Impaired color vision with early red desaturation and contrast sensitivity reduction.
- Relative afferent pupillary defect (RAPD) is usually seen in asymmetric cases.
- In retrobulbar neuritis, the optic disc appears normal while papillitis is seen in the rest.
- The most common visual field defect is diffuse depression of sensitivity in the entire central 30°.
- Other visual field defects include altitudinal/arcuate defects and focal central/centrocecal scotomas.
- Visual field mapping using short-wavelength automated perimetry may provide increased sensitivity.
- Deterioration of vision occurs for about 3 weeks and then improves. More than 90% patients achieve 6/9 or better. Approximately 10% can develop chronic optic neuritis.
- Mild RAPD, residual color vision abnormality may persist.
- Temporal disc pallor or marked optic atrophy may be a consequence.

Ocular Motor Deficits

- Ocular motor disorders range from isolated nuclear or fascicular cranial nerve palsies to bilateral internuclear ophthalmoplegias (INO).
- Most common cranial nerve involved is abducens nerve.
- There may be accompanying deficits in pursuit, saccades, and vestibular eye movements.
- Saccadic abnormalities include square wave jerks, ocular flutter, opsoclonus, or saccadic oscillation.
- Skew deviations and suppression of vestibulo-ocular reflex result in abnormal smooth pursuit.
- Dorsal midbrain syndrome may also be seen with typical convergence retraction nystagmus, decreased vertical saccades, and pupillary light-near dissociation.
- Nystagmus is a frequent ocular motor deficit in MS. INO is the most common, other less common ones being vertical (both upbeat and downbeat), vestibular, pendular, periodic alternating, and gaze-evoked nystagmus.
- INO is characterized by abnormal horizontal ocular movement with lost or limited adduction in the ipsilateral eye and a horizontal abducting nystagmus of the contralateral eye. It is due to lesions involving the medial longitudinal fasciculus and may be either unilateral or bilateral. Bilateral INO is highly in favor of increased risk of MS.
- In INO with a skew deviation, the higher eye is typically on the side of the medial longitudinal fasciculus lesion.

Ocular Inflammation

- Uveitis in MS is 10 times more common than in general population.
- Uveitis can precede or present concomitantly with the diagnosis of MS.
- In MS, intermediate uveitis is characteristically seen with a bilateral presentation in majority.
- There may be associated anterior chamber inflammation in these patients.
- Retinal periphlebitis is also evident and is characterized by perivascular exudation, hemorrhage, and retinal venous sheathing.

 14. Discuss Von Hippel-Lindau disease.

Von Hippel-Lindau (VHL) is a phacomatosis with autosomal dominant inheritance. In this disease, the VHL protein becomes inactivated by germline mutations of the VHL tumor suppressor gene on chromosome 3p25-26. The VHL protein is responsible for the ubiquitination and degradation of hypoxia-inducible factor-1α (HIF-1α), a transcription factor that induces vascular endothelial growth factor (VEGF) expression. Hence, inactivation of the VHL gene leads to overproduction of VEGF in nonhypoxic conditions resulting in the increased angiogenesis seen in VHL. The significant clinical manifestations of VHL are used in the diagnostic criteria of VHL.

Systemic Disorders and Eye

Diagnostic Criteria for Von Hippel-Lindau Disease

Family history	• Required feature • Any one of the following	
Positive	• One or more retinal capillary hemangioma • One or more CNS hemangioma • One or more visceral lesion*	
Negative	• Two or more retinal capillary hemangioma • One retinal hemangioma with a visceral lesion*	• Two or more CNS hemangioma • One CNS hemangioma with a visceral lesion

*Visceral lesions: Renal cysts, renal carcinoma, pheochromocytoma, pancreatic cysts, islet cell tumors, epididymal cystadenoma, endolymphatic sac tumor, adnexal papillary cystadenoma of probable mesonephric origin.
(CNS: central nervous system)

Systemic Findings

- *CNS hemangioma:*
  - Seen in >50% cases of VHL.
  - Most commonly involve the cerebellum (75%) with headache being the most common presenting symptom associated with it.
  - Second most common location is spinal cord (15%), which presents with pain.
  - The tumors are benign but are a major cause of morbidity and mortality due to mass effect on nearby CNS structures.
  - High tumor burden is linked to partial germline mutation and male sex.
- *Renal cell carcinoma (RCC):*
  - Most common cause of mortality in VHL
  - Multiple benign renal cysts can be found on screening in 50–70% VHL patients. They are generally asymptomatic.
  - RCC is usually bilateral and present at a younger age compared to sporadic cases.
  - RCC can have a finding of a renal mass with flank pain or hematuria.
- *Pheochromocytoma:*
  - Occurs in <25% cases.
  - These benign tumors of adrenal gland when associated with VHL are usually multiple and bilateral.
  - It produces elevated serum levels of catecholamines (norepinephrine and epinephrine).
  - This leads to hypertension, tachycardia, palpitations, headaches, sweating, pallor, and nausea.
- *Other features:*
  - Endolymphatic sac tumors are seen in 11% cases of VHL.
  - Pancreatic neuroendocrine tumors and epididymal cystadenomas are rarely seen in VHL.

Ophthalmic Findings

- *Retinal capillary hemangioblastoma (RCH):*
  - Most common tumor seen in VHL
  - They are usually seen in the peripheral but may also occur in the juxtapapillary area.
  - Initially, the RCH may appear as red or gray dot on the retina.
  - As the tumor size increases, tortuous feeder vessels may become visible, and retinal edema and hard exudates may develop around the tumor and in the macula.
  - FFA reveals small vascular lesions located in the superficial retina adjacent to the retinal vein.
- *Other ocular findings:*
  - Other rare associations of VHL include:
    - Exudative RD (secondary to enlarging lesions)
    - Tractional RD
    - Rubeosis iridis.

Treatment

- *Ablative therapy:*
  - Small peripheral RCHs <1.5 mm—observation
  - If progression in size—argon laser photocoagulation or cryotherapy

- Potential complications of treatment are retinal hard exudates and macular edema
- Other ablative therapies include photodynamic therapy, transpupillary thermotherapy (TTT), plaque radiotherapy, external beam radiotherapy, and vitreoretinal surgical ablation.
- Laser photocoagulation or cryotherapy of juxtapapillary RCHs can result in visual loss and scotomas. Observation is the initial management of juxtapapillary RCHs as they can remain relatively static for prolonged periods.
- *Surgical therapy:*
  - Very large tumors are difficult to treat by ablation and carries significant risks, hence surgical resection is warranted.
  - Tractional RD due to contraction of fibrovascular lesions will need surgical interventions.
  - Pars plana vitrectomy with a relaxing retinectomy helps in preserving or improving vision in advanced VHL with tractional RD.
  - Long-term recurrence rate after surgical resection of large RCHs is very high.
- *Pharmacotherapy:*
  - Pharmacotherapy is especially useful in lesions close to macula and optic nerve, which are difficult to treat with ablative therapy.
  - Intravitreal anti-VEGF drugs such as ranibizumab may decrease RCH exudation, especially in small lesions with minimal exudation. It is usually combined with another modality of treatment for superior results.
  - Other treatment options include intravitreal bevacizumab, oral propranolol, and oral sunitinib.
  - Sunitinib is a tyrosine kinase inhibitor that blocks both VEGF and platelet-derived growth factor receptors. Even though it improves retinal edema in some VHL patients, it has multiple adverse effects.

Screening of Von Hippel-Lindau

Von Hippel-Lindau patients have lifelong risk of development of various lesions and hence lifetime screening along with frequent surveillance of existing lesions is needed. The detailed screening guidelines are issued by the VHL Alliance.

	VHL Alliance Active Surveillance Guidelines 2020						
	Age						
Type of surveillance (tumors being screened)	Until age 5 year	Beginning at age 5 year	Beginning at age 11 year	Beginning at age 15 year	Beginning at age 30 year	Beginning at age 65 year	**Pregnancy**
History and physical examination	Yearly from age 1 year	Yearly	Yearly	Yearly	Yearly	Yearly	Prior to conception
Blood pressure and pulse (pheochromocytomas/paragangliomas)	Yearly from age 2 year	Yearly	Yearly	Yearly	Yearly	Yearly	Prior to conception
Dilated eye examination (retinal hemangioblastoma)	Every 6–12 months, beginning before age 1 year	Every 6–12 months	Every 6–12 months	Every 6–12 months	Yearly	Yearly	Prior to conception, then every 6–12 months
Metanephrines (pheochromocytomas/paragangliomas)		Yearly	Yearly	Yearly	Yearly	Stop routine	Prior to conception
MRI brain and spine w/wo contrast (CNS hemangioblastoma)			Every 2 years	Every 2 years	Every 2 years	Stop routine	Prior to conception
Audiogram (endolymphatic sac tumors)			Every 2 years	Every 2 years	Every 2 years	Stop routine	
MRI abdomen w/wo contrast (renal cell carcinoma, pheochromocytoma/paragangliomas, pancreatic neuroendocrine tumors/cysts)				Every 2 years	Every 2 years	Stop routine	Prior to conception
MRI internal auditory canal (endolymphatic sac tumors)				Once			

(CNS: central nervous system; MRI: magnetic resonance imaging; w/wo: with/without)

Q 15. Discuss salient indications and hazards of radiation to the eye.

Indications of Ocular Radiation

- *Conjunctival tumors:*
  - The most common malignant tumors of the bulbar conjunctiva are squamous cell carcinoma and malignant melanoma. The standard treatment for these tumors is excision together with adjunctive therapy consisting of cryotherapy, chemotherapy, or radiotherapy (RT). RT is usually delayed until the conjunctiva has healed.
  - Palpebral conjunctiva and fornix—mucosal-associated lymphoid tissue lymphoma is radiosensitive but requires treatment to the entire conjunctiva.
- *Intraocular tumors:*
  - *Retinoblastoma (RB):* Small localized RBs (i.e., groups A and B) can be treated with TTT or cryotherapy with or without chemotherapy. Plaque brachytherapy is a second-line treatment option for tumors situated anterior to the equator that fails to regress with conservative treatment options such as TTT, cryotherapy, or chemotherapy.
  - *Uveal melanoma:* Uveal melanoma can be treated with plaque, proton therapy, or stereotactic RT.
  - *Choroidal hemangioma:* Local control of the lesion and the secondary RD. It is important that treatment is instituted before visual loss is severe and prolonged.
  - *Choroidal metastases:* The treatment of choroidal metastases depends on the primary site and the extent of metastases. If choroidal metastasis is unresponsive to systemic treatment, then plaque RT for solitary metastasis or external beam RT (EBRT) can be considered.
- *Orbital lesions:*
  - *Vascular tumors:* RT is very useful for adult orbital and intraocular vascular tumors. RT for infantile hemangiomas is kept as a last resort, due to concerns about secondary carcinogenesis and long-term effects of ocular irradiation.
  - *Lymphoid tumors:* Most lymphoid tumors are radio sensitive, with malignant lesions responding better compared to benign lymphoid tumors.
  - *Thyroid eye disease:* Steroid therapy is the first-line treatment for sight threatening disease, followed by RT or surgery as indicated.
  - *Ocular adnexal tumor invasion:* Eyelid, adnexal, and sinus tumors can invade the orbit making complete local resection difficult or incomplete. These situations need EBRT.
  - *Meningioma:* Total surgical excision is recommended when vision is affected or life is at risk. Primary radiation will spare vision in optic nerve sheath meningioma compared to surgical excision.
  - *Optic nerve glioma:* RT is found to be very effective in these conditions. Since optic nerve glioma is seen in children, the risk of collateral damage due to RT is a concern.
  - *Rhabdomyosarcoma:* When it is localized to the orbit, a combination of prompt biopsy, chemotherapy, and RT offers about 90% survival rate.
  - *Orbital metastasis:* RT is being used for treating orbital metastasis for a long time. Prompt RT is advised in cases of orbital metastasis causing optic nerve compression or corneal exposure. Orbital metastasis usually derived from breast cancer in women and from lung cancer in men is typically treated with RT.
  - *Adenoid cystic carcinoma of lacrimal gland:* This is a relatively radio-resistant tumor. RT is administered usually in occult cases after resection of visible tumor or if found to extend outside the capsule.
  - *Orbital pseudotumor:* This condition is usually treated with systemic steroids or immunosuppressive. Radiation is used in this condition to suppress immune reaction and inhibit secondary fibrosis.
  - *Extraocular extension of intraocular lesions:* Usually for extrascleral extension of choroidal melanoma and retinoblastoma.

Hazards of Ocular Radiation

- *Eyelids:*
  - Acute erythema
  - Moist desquamation
  - Depigmentation
  - Skin atrophy
  - Eyelash loss
  - Ectropion or entropion

- *Lacrimal system:*
  - Lacrimal gland atrophy
  - Reduced tear production
- *Cornea:*
  - Dry eye
  - Stem cell dysfunction
- *Lens:* Cataract
- *Sclera:*
  - Scleral thinning
  - Acute scleral necrosis
  - Intense brachytherapy can cause scleral melting
- *Iris:*
  - Iritis
  - Anterior uveitis
  - Neovascularization of iris
  - Neovascular glaucoma
- *Retina:* Radiation retinopathy—arteriolar occlusion, CWS, intraretinal hemorrhage, and neovascularization. If macula is involved, then loss of vision and blindness can also occur.
- *Choroid:* Chorioretinal ischemia
- *Optic nerve:* Radiation optic neuropathy (due to occlusion of vessels within the optic nerve)
- *Orbit:*
  - Improper bone development
  - Hypoplasia of bones
- *Hypothalamus and pituitary dysfunction:* In children, this can occur if irradiated for optic nerve glioma
- *Radiation-induced cancer:*
  - Risk of radiation-induced cancer is greatest in children, less in adolescents, and lowest in adults.
  - Patients with a genetic predisposition to cancer like retinoblastoma are at higher risk for radiation-induced cancer.
  - Certain organs such as thyroid are more susceptible to develop radiation-induced cancers as compared to others.

 16. Describe connective tissue disorders.

Craniofacial Syndromes

Craniosynostosis

The salient features of craniosynostosis include:
- Abnormally shaped skulls as a result of premature closure of one or more cranial sutures.
- Cranial and facial abnormalities, ophthalmic manifestations, and extremity involvement are typical findings.
- Inheritance patterns are largely elucidated although variable expression is the rule.
- Fibroblast growth factor receptor-2 (FGFR-2) mutation-related craniosynostosis disorders include Crouzon, Apert, Pfeiffer, and Jackson–Weiss syndromes.
- The ophthalmic manifestations of FGFR-2 craniosynostosis disorders are:
  - Optic atrophy
  - Exophthalmos and hypertelorism
  - Exposure keratitis
  - Strabismus
  - Amblyopia.

Facial Syndromes

- The unifying characteristic of this group of disorders is that the abnormal facial structures are derived from the first and second branchial arches and the intervening branchial cleft.
- Systemic abnormalities not associated with the branchial arches may occur in these disorders.
- The etiology of many branchial arch syndromes is largely uncertain although patterns of inheritance have been identified in some cases.

Syndrome	Characteristics	Key ocular features	Other features
Syndromes with bilateral, symmetric facial involvement			
Treacher Collins syndrome	• Mandibulofacial dysostosis • Bilateral, symmetric facial involvement • Malformation of structures derived from the first branchial arch, including the zygoma, the ear, the mandible, and the eyelids	• Notching or colobomas of the outer portions of the lower eyelids • Antimongoloid slant of the palpebral fissures • Atresia of the lower lacrimal puncta and canaliculus	• Microtia with conductive hearing loss • Abnormalities of the pinna • Atresia of the auditory canals and middle ear abnormalities • Hypoplasia of the facial bones • Micrognathia • High arched or cleft palate
Hallermann–Streiff syndrome	• Oculomandibulofacial dyscephaly • Cause still remains unclear	• Congenital cataracts • Microphthalmia • Blue sclera • Nystagmus • Strabismus • Down slanting palpebral fissures • Glaucoma • Aniridia • Sclerocornea	• Birdlike facies • Hypoplastic mandible • Beaked nose • Proportionate short stature • Hypotrichosis • Dental anomalies • Cutaneous atrophy • Tracheomalacia
Pierre Robin sequence	• Inheritance can be dominant or recessive • Pathogenesis may be early in utero constraint	• Glaucoma • Myopia • Retinal detachment • Microphthalmia • Cataract	• Neonatal respiratory distress due to micrognathia • Glossoptosis • Cleft palate +/–
Syndromes with asymmetric facial involvement			
Goldenhar syndrome	• Oculo-auriculo-vertebral dysplasia • Defects in structures derived from the first branchial arch	• Dermoid • Lipodermoid • Blepharoptosis • Colobomas of the upper eyelids • Strabismus • Duane retraction syndrome	• Unilateral deformity of the external ear • Unilateral hypoplasia of the mandible • Hemifacial microsomia • Vertebral anomalies
Parry–Romberg syndrome	• Facial hemiatrophy • Onset is in the first two decades of life • Typically occurs in individuals who are morphologically normal at birth	• Progressive enophthalmos • Atrophic changes in the eyelids • Pupillary disturbances • Heterochromia • Uveitis • Cataracts • Strabismus • Fundus depigmentation	• Progressive hemifacial soft tissue atrophy • Localized facial bony depressions • Hyperpigmentation of the skin • Alopecia • Dental abnormalities • Focal or generalized neurologic abnormalities

Disorders of Fibrillin and Elastic Tissue

- A common feature in these syndromes is ectopia lentis, since a major component of the zonular fibrils of the lens is fibrillin, a cysteine-rich glycoprotein.
- Generalized skeletal, ocular, and facial abnormalities are seen usually.
- These disorders include Marfan syndrome, Homocystinuria, and Weil–Marchesani syndrome.

Syndrome	Characteristics	Key ocular features	Other features
Marfan syndrome	• Autosomal dominant • Mutations in the fibrillin gene (*FBN1*) at 15q21.1 • Mental retardation absent	• Ectopia lentis–superotemporal • Myopia • Retinal detachment • Corneal flatness • Stretched zonules	• Very tall • Arachnodactyly • Anterior chest deformity • Joint laxity • Scoliosis • Thoracic lordosis • High arched palate • Dilatation of the aortic root

Contd...

Contd...

Syndrome	Characteristics	Key ocular features	Other features
Homocystinuria	• Autosomal recessive • Deficiency of cystathionine synthase • Leads to accumulation of homocysteine and methionine	• Ectopia lentis–inferonasal • Myopia • Absent and broken zonules	• Tall stature • Kyphoscoliosis • Joint laxity • Osteoporosis with vertebral collapse • Mental retardation • Hypopigmentation • Premature vascular thrombotic disorders
Weil–Marchesani syndrome	• Inheritance can autosomal recessive or dominant mapped onto 19p or 15q21, respectively	• Microspherophakia • Marked myopia • Pupillary block glaucoma	• Short stature • Brachydactyly • Short and stubby hands and feet • Limited joint mobility

Disorders of Collagen

- All disorders in this group have defects in type II collagen which is the major protein of cartilage, the vitreous, and the nucleus pulposus.
- Skeletal abnormalities, ophthalmic manifestations, and cutaneous involvement are typical findings in these disorders of collagen.
- Stickler syndrome, Kniest dysplasia, and spondyloepiphyseal dysplasia congenita are clinically distinct though share significant similarity, especially with regard to ocular manifestations.

Syndrome	Characteristics	Key ocular features	Other features
Stickler syndrome	• Autosomal dominant • Majority have mutations in the structural genes for type II *COL2A1*, which encodes for type II collagen	• Mostly congenital high and nonprogressive myopia • Retinal detachment • Vitreous is mostly liquefied • Wedge shaped and fleck shaped cortical opacities	• Joint hyperextensibility • Muscle hypotonia • Kyphosis • Scoliosis • Arthritis • Pierre Robin sequence • Progressive sensorineural hearing loss • Mitral valve prolapse
Ehlers–Danlos syndromes	• Heterogeneous group of connective tissue disorders with at least 10 subtypes • Significant ocular manifestations are present in EDS types I, VI, and VII	• Looseness of the lids with a reduction in lid folds • Retinal detachment • Ocular fragility with ruptured globe • Myopia • Blue sclera	• Skin fragility • Skin hyperextensibility • Joint hypermobility • Excessive bruising
Osteogenesis imperfecta	• Caused by abnormalities in type I collagen • Different mutations of *COL1A1* on chr 17 and *COL1A2* on chr 7 • They code for the two procollagens that combine to form the mature collagen I	• Blue sclera due to thinning • Posterior embryotoxon • Keratoconus • Zonular cataract • "Saturn ring"—comparative whitening of the sclera near the limbus	• Hearing loss • Dental anomalies • Stature abnormality

Other Connective Tissue Disorders

Disorder	Characteristics	Key ocular features	Other features
Systemic sclerosis	• Rare connective tissue disorder • Abnormal fibroblasts • Female to male ratio is 8:1	• Most common is eye lid stiffness due to deposition of type I collagen in the dermis • Keratoconjunctivitis sicca • Rarely conjunctivitis, episcleritis, anterior uveitis, and hypertensive retinopathy	• Deposition of ECM in skin, blood vessels, and viscera • Characterized by interplay of inflammatory cytokines and antibodies

Contd...

Contd...

Disorder	Characteristics	Key ocular features	Other features
Polymyositis and dermatomyositis	• Autoimmune diseases characterized by inflammation of the skeletal muscles • Skin involvement +/−	• Most common is a heliotrope rash or purplish discoloration of the eyelids • Retinal vasculitis • Internuclear ophthalmoplegia	• HLA-B8, DR3, DR52 • Elevated creatinine kinase and aldolase levels • Histopathology shows deposition of immune complexes in a vascular distribution
ANCA-associated vasculitis	• Antineutrophil cytoplasmic antibody (ANCA) • Three disorders mainly microscopic polyangiitis (MPA), granulomatosis with polyangiitis (GPA) and eosinophilic granulomatosis with polyangiitis (EGPA)	• Conjunctivitis • Episcleritis • Scleritis • Symblepharon in cicatricial disease • Peripheral ulcerative keratitis • Retinal vascular occlusions • Uveitis • Orbital pseudotumor	• Group of small to medium vessel inflammatory diseases • Cause end organ damage from vessel thrombosis that results from inflammation of the vascular endothelial lining

(ECM: extracellular matrix)

 17. Outline important systemic disorders affecting eye and their salient ocular symptoms and signs.

- Many systemic disorders have ocular components that either present simultaneous, earlier or later to the systemic manifestations of the disease.
- Ocular symptoms connected to systemic diseases involve both anterior and posterior eye segments. Hence, there exists a wide variety of ocular symptoms in clinical practice which are crucial in differential diagnosis.

Immunological Disorders

Systemic disease	Systemic features	Ocular symptoms and signs
Rheumatoid disease	Arthritis—hand, wrist and foot, Felty syndrome	Dry eye, episcleritis, scleritis, iridocyclitis, corneal melting, cataract
SLE	Butterfly rash, pleuritis, pericarditis, Raynaud phenomenon	Episcleritis, iritis, lupus retinopathy
Giant cell arteritis	Temporal arteritis, cephalgia, jaw claudication	Extraocular muscle palsies, anterior ischemic optic neuropathy
Sarcoidosis	Granuloma of lymph nodes, lung and CNS, erythema nodosum	Enlargement of lacrimal glands, iridocyclitis, retinal periphlebitis, sarcoid nodule/granuloma
Reiter syndrome	Arthritis, urethritis, plantar rash	Conjunctivitis, uveitis, retinal vasculitis
Poly arteritis nodosa	Pyrexia of unknown origin, myalgia, arthralgia, skin nodules, renal and cardiac failure	Episcleritis, extraocular muscle palsy, uveitis, retinal hemorrhages, papilledema
Vogt–Koyanagi–Harada syndrome	Meningitis, encephalopathy, dysacusis, vitiligo, alopecia	Poliosis, uveitis, choroiditis, exudative retinal detachment
Multiple endocrine neoplasia (MEN 2b)	Medullary carcinoma of thyroid, pheochromocytoma	Mucosal neuromas of lid and conjunctiva, medullated nerve fibers in cornea

(CNS: central nervous system; SLE: systemic lupus erythematosus)

Hematological Disorders

Systemic disease	Systemic features	Ocular symptoms and signs
Lymphocytic leukemia	Lymphadenopathy, hepatosplenomegaly, anemia, leukopenia	Proptosis, iris nodules, retinal edema, hemorrhages, leukemic retinopathy, Roth spots
Myeloid leukemia	Hepatosplenomegaly, bleeding, thrombosis	Orbital chloroma, retinal edema, hemorrhages, peripheral retinal neovascularization

Contd...

Contd...

Systemic disease	Systemic features	Ocular symptoms and signs
Lymphoma	Fever, lymphadenopathy	Lid/orbital deposits, uveitis
Sickle cell anemia	Transient aplastic crisis, stroke, leg ulcers, jaundice, anemia	Dilated conjunctival vessels, retinal capillary occlusion, sea-fan retinal neovascularization, chorioretinal scars

Infectious Diseases

Systemic disease	Systemic features	Ocular symptoms and signs
Viral		
• Herpes simplex	• Blisters and sores around the mouth and genital area	• Vesicles on lid, dendritic keratitis, uveitis, acute retinal necrosis
• Congenital rubella	• Congenital heart disease, sensorineural deafness, mental retardation	• Microphthalmos, cataract, glaucoma, chorioretinitis
• Measles	• Rash, diarrhea, middle ear infection, encephalitis, precipitates malnutrition	• Keratoconjunctivitis, xerophthalmia, optic neuritis
• Infectious mononucleosis	• Fever, malaise, rash, lymphadenopathy, splenomegaly	• Conjunctivitis, uveitis, retinal phlebitis, papillitis
• Cytomegalovirus	• Immunocompromised adults and newborns—fever, hepatitis, pneumonia, encephalitis	• Microphthalmos, necrotizing chorioretinitis, optic atrophy
• AIDS	• Immunocompromised, Kaposi sarcoma	• Kaposi sarcoma, cotton-wool spots, CMV retinitis, HIV vasculopathy
Fungal		
• Candida	• Oral and genital "thrush"	• Conjunctivitis, Keratitis, retinitis, endophthalmitis
• Cryptococcus	• Immunocompromised adults, pneumonia, meningitis	• Papilledema, optic atrophy
Bacterial		
• Tuberculosis	• Fever, malaise, granulomas (lung, lymph node)	• Phlyctenular conjunctivitis, granulomatous uveitis, serpiginoid choroiditis, granuloma, tubercle, tuberculoma, choroidal abscess, vasculitis
• Leprosy	• Thickened peripheral nerves, hypesthetic skin lesions, weakness of peripheral muscles	• Facial palsy, madarosis, iritis, secondary glaucoma, cataract
Parasitic		
• Toxoplasmosis	• Congenital—mental retardation, deafness, encephalitis in immunodeficient persons	• Macular scarring, retinochoroiditis, vitritis
• Toxocariasis	• Visceral larva migrans—liver, lungs, heart, brain	• Vitritis, choroiditis, vitreoretinal granuloma
• Cysticercosis	• Cysticercosis larva—subcutaneous, brain, spine, heart, muscle	• Subconjunctival or EOM cyst, subretinal or vitreous cyst
• Onchocerciasis	• Subcutaneous onchocercoma	• Sclerosing keratitis, uveitis, cataract

(AIDS: acquired immunodeficiency syndrome; CMV: cytomegalovirus; EOM: extraocular muscles; HIV: human immunodeficiency virus)

Endocrine and Metabolic Disorders

Systemic disease	Systemic features	Ocular symptoms and signs
Homocystinuria	Mental retardation, tall, arachnodactyly, thromboembolic episodes	Subluxation of lens
Mucopolysaccharidoses	Dysmorphism, behavioral disorders, cardiac anomalies	Corneal opacification, pigmentary retinopathy, glaucoma, optic atrophy
Wilson disease	Extrapyramidal signs, cirrhosis	Kayser–Fleischer ring, Sunflower cataract
Hyperthyroidism	Tachycardia, tremors of the hand	Exophthalmos, lid retraction, lid lag, superior limbic keratitis, disc edema
Hypoparathyroidism	Tetany, seizures	Fasciculation, cataract, disc edema

Muscular Disorders

Systemic disease	Systemic features	Ocular symptoms and signs
Myasthenia gravis	Fluctuating voluntary muscle weakness affecting speech, swallowing, breathing	Ptosis, diplopia
Muscular dystrophy	Progressive muscle weakness of characteristic muscle groups	Ptosis, ophthalmoplegia, dry eye, cataract, pigmentary retinopathy

Inherited Disorders

Systemic disease	Systemic features	Ocular symptoms and signs
Down syndrome	Mental retardation, muscle hypotonia, congenital heart disease	Mongoloid slant of eyes, epicanthic folds, keratoconus
Sturge–Weber syndrome	Facial port-wine stain, angiomas of occipital meninges	Arteriovenous malformations of episcleral or choroidal (hemangioma), glaucoma
Neurofibromatosis	Café-au-lait spots, subcutaneous neurofibromas	Ptosis, pulsating exophthalmos, optic nerve glioma, neurofibromas of iris, retina and choroid
Albinism	Hypopigmented skin and hair	Nystagmus, translucent iris, albinotic fundus, foveal hypoplasia
Marfan syndrome	Tall, arachnodactyly, aortic aneurysm, cardiac valvular anomalies	Subluxation of the lens, myopia, retinal detachment
Von Hippel-Lindau disease	Angiomatosis of central nervous system and kidneys	Retinal angiomas

Connective Tissue Disorders

Refer earlier Question.

 18. Discuss juvenile systemic disorders affecting the eye.

Ocular manifestations can be the first findings of systemic disease in some pediatric diseases. Recognizing these ocular manifestations is important for the diagnosis and management of pediatric systemic diseases.[1-3]

Juvenile Idiopathic Arthritis (JIA)

- It is an arthritis of unknown etiology that begins before 16 years and persists for at least 6 weeks.
- It is the most common systemic disease associated with childhood anterior uveitis.
- About 50% children with JIA have persistently active disease after 10 years.
- International League of Association of Rheumatology (ILAR) has classified JIA into seven variants depending on joint involvement during the first 6 months.

	Age at onset	Sex	No. of joints	Clinical features	RF	ANA
Oligoarticular	2 years	F > M 5:1	≤4	• Most common form • Most commonly involves knees, then ankles and wrists • 20% have uveitis	Negative	75%
Polyarticular RF negative	3 years	F > M 3:1	≥5	• Both small and large joints • 5–10% have uveitis • Systemic features may include fever and rash	Negative	40%
Polyarticular RF positive	3 years	F > M	≥5	• Resembles adult rheumatoid arthritis • Low risk of uveitis	Positive	Negative
Systemic	5 years	F = M	Variable	• Still's disease • Systemic features precede arthritis • Fever, episodic rash, lymphadenopathy, hepatosplenomegaly • Uveitis rare	Negative	Negative

Contd...

Contd...

	Age at onset	Sex	No. of joints	Clinical features	RF	ANA
Enthesitis related	Late childhood	F > M		• High risk of uveitis		
Psoriatic arthritis	Biphasic 2–4 and 9–11 years	F > M		• High risk of uveitis		
Undifferentiated				• Low risk of uveitis		

(ANA: antinuclear antibodies; RF: rheumatoid factor)

- Anterior uveitis in JIA is usually asymptomatic and is usually detected by screening with slit-lamp examination.
    - There is a characteristic absence of conjunctival injection, even in presence of severe uveitis.
    - Chronic granulomatous inflammation occurs.
    - There is a tendency for symmetrical bilateral involvement.
    - Endothelial dusting during exacerbations may be noted.
    - Posterior synechiae are seen in long-standing cases.
    - Complications in severe cases include cataract and band-shaped keratopathy.
    - Other serious complications include glaucoma, amblyopia, maculopathy, CME, epiretinal membrane, cyclitic membrane, and phthisis.
    - The presence of advanced uveitis and complications at initial presentation is an important risk factor for the development of further complications, regardless of therapy.
- *Screening for JIA:*
    - Initial ophthalmologic examination—within 6 weeks of the first diagnosis of JIA.
    - Newly diagnosed oligoarticular, psoriatic, and enthesitis-related patients, regardless of antinuclear antibodies (ANA) should be evaluated 2 monthly for 6 months, thereafter 3–4 monthly intervals.
    - Polyarticular RF negative JIA—followed up every 3–4 months from the beginning. If any higher risk factor such as ANA positivity, female gender, or onset before 7 years is seen, a modification of frequency of visit might be needed.
    - Initial screening followed by annual follow-up is recommended for systemic onset and polyarticular RF-positive patients.
    - Visual symptoms or ocular signs warrant urgent ophthalmologic evaluation within 1 week.
- *Treatment:*
    - Treatment options are available to control the active inflammation of the disease. They include:
        - Topical corticosteroids
        - Periocular and/or oral corticosteroids
        - Mydriatic cycloplegics—to prevent synechiae formation
        - NSAIDs
        - *Immunomodulatory therapy:*
            - Methotrexate—0.5 mg/kg once a week
            - Mycophenolate mofetil—600 mg/m² body surface area (BSA) twice daily.
            - Cyclosporine—up to 5 mg kg^{-1} day^{-1}
            - Azathioprine—2–3 mg kg^{-1} day^{-1}
            - Chlorambucil—0.1–0.2 mg kg^{-1} day^{-1}
        - *Biologics:*
            - Infliximab
            - Adalimumab
            (Etanercept should be avoided)
        - *Surgical therapy:* For treating refractory glaucoma or cataract.

Hyperthyroidism

- Most common cause of pediatric hyperthyroidism is Grave's disease.
- Uncommon in childhood and occurs mostly in girls.
- *Common ocular features include:*
    - Eyelid edema
    - Lid lag

- Lagophthalmos
- Mild proptosis
- Enlarged extraocular muscles
- Vision-threatening problems are absent and limitation of extraocular movements is rare.
- Has a good prognosis for spontaneous resolution, usually without recurrence or need for major intervention such as intravenous steroids or decompression of orbit.

Hypoparathyroidism

- Hypocalcemia is seen in hypoparathyroidism and is a common metabolic problem in newborns and neonates.
- It presents within 72 hours and is seen in premature infants, in neonates with asphyxiation, and in infants of diabetic mothers.
- Cataract can occur along with other autoimmune manifestations such as keratitis and conjunctivitis.

Diabetes Mellitus

- Both type 1 and increasingly type 2 diabetes are being seen in children and adolescents now.
- Opacities of lens are infrequent and tend to appear in the teenage years. They can start as cortical opacities that rapidly progresses to total lens opacities.
- Prevalence of DR rises consistently following puberty and is generally rare in children.

Porphyria

- Porphyrins accumulate resulting from alteration of the enzymes in the porphyrin pathways.
- Congenital erythropoietic porphyria can have phototoxic changes of the lids, conjunctiva, and sclera.
- Contracture of the lids results in incomplete closure of eyelids, exposure, and keratitis.

Cystinosis

- It is due to failure in the metabolism of cysteine that results in deposition of cystine crystals in the major parts of the body, mainly the kidney, liver, eye, and brain.
- Ocular findings include iridescent elongated crystal deposition in the cornea, uveal tissue and retina, pigmentary retinopathy, and angle closure glaucoma.
- Symptoms include photophobia and visual impairment.

Mucopolysaccharidosis

- It is due to the inability to degrade glycosaminoglycans such as dermatan sulfate, heparan sulfate, and keratan sulfate as a result of mutations of chromosomes coding for lysosomal enzymes needed for their degradation.
- These include—MPS IH (Hurler), MPS IS (Scheie), MPS IH/S (Hurler/Scheie), MPS II (Hunter), MPS III (Sanfilippo), MPS IV (Morquio), MPS VI (Maroteaux-Lamy), and MPS VII (Sly).
- Autosomal recessive inheritance in all except type II (Hunter syndrome) which has X-linked trait.
- Cornea has a "ground glass" appearance except in Hunter syndrome (clear cornea).
- Glaucoma, retinal degeneration, and optic atrophy are seen in most mucopolysaccharidosis.
- Some children may have night-blindness or blurring of vision.

Wilsons Disease

- This occurs due to excess copper deposition in various tissues and presents usually with liver disorder or neurologic symptoms.
- Liver manifestations include chronic active hepatitis, cirrhosis, and fulminant hepatic failure.
- Copper can deposit in peripheral Descemet's membrane and is detected as golden-brown pigmentations—the Kayser-Fleischer ring.
- Yellow–brown opacities in the subcapsular cortex of lens with petal-like spokes are suggestive of sunflower cataract.

Marfan Syndrome

Refer Question on connective tissue disorders.

Weil–Marchesani Syndrome

Refer Question on connective tissue disorders.

Systemic Lupus Erythematosus

Refer Question on SLE.

Q 19. Critically evaluate nutritional factors causing ocular morbidity.

Mineral Disorders

Mineral	Function	Deficiency
Zinc	• Essential trace element • Part of metalloenzymes • Nucleic acid and membrane metabolism • Part of alcohol hydrogenase that converts retinol to retinal and carbonic anhydrase, which is needed for aqueous production	• Distinctive rash develops around the eyes, nose, mouth, anus, and distal extremities • Loss of cilia of brow and lid • Cornea epithelial thinning, loss of polarity and Bowman's layer loss, subepithelial scar forms • Impaired night vision with degeneration of retinal pigment epithelium and photoreceptors • Ciliary body atrophy, optic atrophy, cataract
Copper	• Part of metalloenzymes	• Atrophy of the nerve fiber layer, ganglion cells, and optic nerve and lacy vacuolization of the iris pigment epithelium • Fundus is blond or whitened, but patients do not have nystagmus or photophobia. They are classified as albinoidism
Iron	• Part of hemoglobin, myoglobin, metalloenzymes	• Anemic retinopathy—retinal hemorrhages, tortuous vessels, cotton-wool spots, and central retinal vein occlusion

Vitamin Disorders

Refer to Question about vitamins.

Q 20. Discuss sarcoidosis and eye.

Sarcoidosis is a chronic idiopathic granulomatous inflammatory disease. It is a systemic disorder that affects multiple major organ systems, primarily the lungs in >90% of cases. Extrapulmonary disease frequently involves the lymph nodes, skin, eye, cardiovascular, musculoskeletal, gastrointestinal, renal, and CNSs. The etiology of sarcoidosis is still not clear.

In 2017, the International Workshop on Ocular Sarcoidosis published revised criteria for diagnosing ocular sarcoidosis, identifying seven clinical signs suggestive of ocular sarcoidosis, eight laboratory investigations in suspected ocular sarcoidosis, and three levels of certainty of a sarcoid diagnosis.

Pathogenesis

Histologically, the hallmark of sarcoidosis is a noncaseating granuloma, consisting of epithelioid cells, histiocytes, multinucleated giant cells, $CD4^+$ lymphocytes, and macrophages/monocytes that are surrounded by $CD8^+$ lymphocytes, plasma cells, fibroblasts, and collagen. Granulomas secrete angiotensin-converting enzyme, lysozyme, glucuronidase, collagenase, and calcitriol.

Revised International Workshop on Ocular Sarcoidosis (IWOS) criteria for the diagnosis of ocular sarcoidosis (OS) (2017)

I. Other causes of granulomatous uveitis must be ruled out
II. Intraocular clinical signs suggestive of OS
   – Mutton-fat keratic precipitates and/or iris nodules (Koeppe or Busacca)
   – Trabecular meshwork nodules and/or tent-shaped peripheral anterior synechia
   – Snowballs/string of pearls vitreous opacities
   – Multiple chorioretinal peripheral lesions (active and atrophic)

Contd…

Contd...

- Nodular and/or segmental periphlebitis (+/− candle wax dripping) and/or macroaneurysm in an inflamed eye
- Optic disc nodule(s)/granuloma(s) and/or solitary choroidal nodule
- Bilaterality (assessed by ophthalmologic examination)

III. *Systemic investigations in suspected OS*
- Bilateral hilar lymphadenopathy (BHL) by chest X-ray and/or chest CT scan
- Negative tuberculin test or Interferon-gamma releasing assays
- Elevated serum ACE
- Elevated serum lysozyme
- Elevated CD4/CD8 ratio (>3.5) in bronchoalveolar fluid
- Abnormal 67-gallium scintigraphy or 18F-FDG PET
- Lymphopenia
- Parenchymal lung changes consistent with sarcoidosis, as determined by pulmonologists or radiologists

IV. *Diagnostic criteria*
- *Definite OS:* Diagnosis supported by biopsy with compatible uveitis
- *Presumed OS:* Diagnosis not supported by biopsy, but BHL present with two intraocular signs
- *Probable OS:* Diagnosis not supported by biopsy and BHL absent, but three intraocular signs and two systemic investigations selected from two to eight are present

Ocular Manifestations

Anterior Segment Manifestations

Symptoms

- Redness
- Ocular pain
- Photophobia
- Lacrimation
- Decreased vision.

Signs

- Granulomatous anterior uveitis—most common manifestation
- Mutton-fat keratic precipitates
- Iris nodules (Berlin nodules in the angle)
- Posterior synechiae
- Peripheral anterior synechiae
- Trabecular meshwork obstruction.

Complications

- Ocular hypertension
- Secondary glaucoma
- Corneal band keratopathy
- Cataract formation
- Epiretinal membrane
- CME.

Posterior Segment Manifestations

Symptoms

- Painless decrease in vision
- Floaters.

Signs

- Vitreous opacities
- "Snowball" infiltrates—clumps of cells and proteinaceous debris, located inferiorly in the anterior vitreous

- Snow banking
- String-of-pearls appearance
- Peripheral vasculitis
- Nonobstructive segmental retinal periphlebitis—"candle-wax drippings" or "en taches de bougies"
- Multifocal chorioretinitis with multiple round punched-out lesions
- Retinal macroaneurysm in an inflamed eye
- Choroidal granulomas
- Panuveitis.

Neuro-ophthalmic Manifestation

- Neurosarcoidosis—known as "the great imitator" due to a variety of symptoms and lack of disease-specific clinical signs
- Optic disc nodule/granuloma
- Optic neuropathy
- Cranial neuropathy—most common neuro-ophthalmic presentation
- Papilledema
- Nystagmus
- Pupillary abnormalities
- Visual field defects
- Raised intracranial pressure
- Abnormal eye movement
- Visual hallucinations
- Encephalopathy
- Hydrocephalus
- Seizures
- Aseptic meningitis
- Psychiatric symptoms.

Ocular Surface Manifestation

- Conjunctiva—follicular conjunctivitis, conjunctival nodules, and granulomas
- Cornea—rarely, affected in chronic cases, with keratoconjunctivitis sicca, superficial punctate keratitis, interstitial keratitis and band keratopathy.

Ocular Adnexa and Orbit

- Lacrimal gland infiltration and inflammation—painless enlargement of the palpebral lobes
- Nasolacrimal duct obstruction due to granulomatous inflammation
- Also affects orbital adipose tissue, extraocular muscles and optic nerve sheath, resembling the other inflammatory disorders affecting the orbit.
- The patients can present with watering, pain, proptosis, diplopia, ptosis, and restricted extraocular movements.

Systemic Manifestations

- Usually presents with respiratory symptoms such as cough and dyspnea, also can have constitutional symptoms such as malaise and arthralgia.
- *Skin lesions:*
  - Erythema nodosum—tender erythematous plaques usually of the shins.
  - Lupus pernio—indurated violaceous lesions involving exposed parts of the body such as the nose, cheeks, fingers, and ears.
  - Granulomatous papules or macules
- Lungs show parenchymal infiltration changes which can lead to severe pulmonary fibrosis. Hilar lymphadenopathy is also seen very frequently.
- Cardiological manifestations such as arrhythmia, even though rare could lead to sudden death.
- Lofgren syndrome is an acute presentation carrying a good prognosis, characterized by the triad of erythema nodosum, bilateral hilar lymphadenopathy on chest X-ray, and polyarthralgia, usually seen in women.

Investigations

- IWOS (2017) have suggested carrying out the following investigations:
  - Chest X-ray and/or CT scan to look for bilateral hilar lymphadenopathy
  - Tuberculin test or interferon-gamma release assay
  - Serum ACE levels and/or serum lysozyme
  - Bronchoalveolar lavage fluid (BALF) analysis—shows elevated CD4/CD8 ratio (>3.5)
  - 67Ga scintigraphy or 18F-FDG PET imaging
  - Hemogram—for lymphopenia
- Hypercalciuria is common.
- Histopathological confirmation of sarcoidosis is almost always required before starting treatment and biopsy is done by fiber optic bronchoscopy from the lungs.
- Other biopsy options include thoracic endosonography with needle aspiration and also from superficial lymph nodes or skin lesions, conjunctival nodules, and lacrimal glands.

Treatment

- *Corticosteroids* (topical or periocular) are the mainstay of therapy for ocular sarcoidosis.
- *Cycloplegics* are frequently needed to prevent synechiae.
- *Posterior uveitis* generally requires systemic steroids and occasionally immunosuppressive agents such as methotrexate, azathioprine, ciclosporin, and TNF inhibitors (e.g., adalimumab).
- *CME* may respond to topical NSAIDs.
- *Surgical intervention* for cataract surgery in ocular sarcoidosis should preferably be performed at a quiescent stage after control of aggressive inflammation for at least 3 months.
- *Neovascularization* may regress with systemic anti-inflammatory treatment, though cases with retinal ischemia, persistent neovascularization, or vitreous hemorrhage benefit from laser treatment to ischemic areas demonstrated by angiography.
- *Indication for systemic treatment* in ocular disease includes optic neuritis and severe posterior uveitis.

Key Points

- Systemic diseases can impact the eye in several ways.
- A detailed history including that of nutrition and family history may help in arriving at a diagnosis.
- Management involves a multi-specialty approach.
- The patient may have underlying life threatening conditions. Hence utmost care should be taken while treating such cases.

References

1. Salmon J. Kanski's Clinical Ophthalmology, 9th edition. London: WB. Saunders/Elsevier; 2019.
2. Albert DM, Miller JW. Albert & Jakobiec's Principles and Practice of Ophthalmology, 3rd edition. Philadelphia: WB Saunders/Elsevier; 2008.
3. Tandon R. Parsons' Diseases of the Eye, 23rd edition. India: Elsevier India; 2019.

Question Bank

Deepali Singhal, Pranita Sahay

Anatomy and Physiology

Q1. Development of eye

Orbit

Q2. Anatomy and relation of the medial and lateral orbital wall
Q3. Draw a neat labeled diagram depicting walls of the orbit.
Q4. Discuss the anatomy of superior orbital fissure (with diagram) and associated clinical syndrome.
Q5. Discuss the anatomy of inferior orbital fissure (with diagram).
Q6. Applied anatomy of orbital apex
Q7. Describe the applied anatomy of the optic canal.
Q8. Describe with diagrams the anatomy of orbit and its spaces and their clinical significance.
Q9. Anatomy of cavernous sinus

Orbital Adnexa

Q10. (a) Anatomy and development of upper eyelid. (b) Its blood supply, venous drainage, and lymphatic drainage. (c) Clinical implications of its blood supply.
Q11. Lid margin
Q12. Outline the surgical and functional anatomy of LPS.

Conjunctiva, Lacrimal Apparatus, and Tear Film

Q13. Anatomy of the lacrimal drainage system with the help of a diagram
Q14. Structure of tear film and its changes in iatrogenic situations (medication and disease)
Q15. Methods to evaluate tear film disorders.
Q16. Neural pathway for tear secretion from the lacrimal gland
Q17. (a) Anatomy and development of lacrimal drainage system. (b) Developmental anomalies of lacrimal passages.
Q18. What is physiological lacrimal pump?
Q19. Effects of contact lens on tear film physiology

Cornea, Limbus, and Sclera

Q20. Anatomy and physiology of corneal endothelium. Tests to check the viability of corneal endothelium
Q21. Corneal transparency
Q22. Theories of corneal transparency
Q23. Corneal endothelial pump
Q24. Dua's layer
Q25. Corneal hysteresis
Q26. Surgical anatomy of limbus and relevance to glaucoma surgeries
Q27. Tear film physiology and applied aspects in contact lens

Q28. What are limbal stem cells? Discuss the clinical and applied significance.

Q29. Anatomy and physiology of ocular surface

Q30. Anatomy of limbus and its surgical importance (diagram). Corneal wound healing and the role of limbus and role of limbal stem cells in various ocular conditions

Uvea, Aqueous Humor, and Intraocular Pressure

Q31. Anatomy and embryology of iris and the management of congenital abnormalities of the iris

Q32. (a) Anatomy of ciliary body with the help of diagram(s). (b) Process of aqueous production and various factors that influence it.

Q33. Development of anterior chamber angle

Q34. Ultrastructure of trabecular meshwork and Schlemm's canal/structure, function, and development of the trabecular meshwork with a note on its clinical significance.

Q35. Mechanism of aqueous formation, circulation, and drainage. Physiology of aqueous drainage through trabecular meshwork. Changes with aging.

Q36. How is the IOP maintained?

Q37. Dynamic of aqueous humor synthesis in health and diseases. Mechanism of drugs affecting it

Q38. (a) Production and outflow of aqueous humor. (b) Relationship between central corneal thickness and IOP measurement. (c) The accepted norm for the adjustment of corneal thickness variations to IOP measurement.

Q39. Describe the blood–aqueous barrier and blood–brain barrier.

Q40. Describe the blood–ocular barrier and its clinical importance.

Q41. Blood supply of choroid, ciliary body, and iris

Lens

Q42. Describe the embryology and anatomy of crystalline lens and its structures and applied aspects in cataract surgery.

Q43. Functional and surgical anatomy of lens and maintenance of transparency of lens throughout the life

Q44. Metabolism of lens in the eye. Describe the pathways of glucose metabolism in the lens. What metabolic abnormalities cause cataract in diabetes and galactosemia?

Q45. Metabolism of human crystalline lens. Biomechanical factors responsible for cataract

Q46. Describe the physiology of accommodation, methods of assessment, and disorders of accommodation.

Q47. Theory of accommodation

Q48. Pathway of accommodation

Q49. Ciliary sulcus

Anterior Chamber

Q50. Anatomy and development of anterior chamber. Developmental anomalies of anterior chamber angle

Q51. Describe the stages of development of angle structures and aqueous outflow channels.

Retina and Visual Pathway

Q52. Development of eye. Retinal disorders related to development of eye

Q53. Describe the embryological evolution of the retina.

Q54. Anatomy and blood supply of retina

Q55. Anatomy and histology of macula

Q56. (a) Anatomy and development of the macula. (b) Different zones of macula and their clinical importance. (c) Enumerate the macular function tests.

Q57. Foveal avascular zone

Q58. Anatomical subdivision of optic nerve

Q59. Describe the vascular supply of the optic nerve head and its clinical importance (with a well-labeled diagram).

Q60. Blood supply of retina and ON

Q61. (a) Anatomy and physiology of rods and cones. (b) Their distribution over the retina. (c) Implications in vision quality with rod and cone dysfunction.
Q62. What are the differences between rods and cones? What is the importance of IS-OS junction?
Q63. Factors influencing dark adaptation
Q64. Describe the mechanism of dark adaptation with respect to anatomy and physiology involved.
Q65. Contrast sensitivity
Q66. Anatomy, biochemical composition, and physiological roles of retinal pigment epithelium
Q67. Macular pigments in health and disease
Q68. Phosphenes
Q69. Theories of color vision. Methods of color vision evaluation
Q70. Recent concepts of psychophysiology of color vision. Compare the various modalities available to critically assess color perception.
Q71. Discuss the problems and applied aspects of color vision tests and color visual field examination.
Q72. Describe the physiology and methods of evaluation of the following: (a) Contrast; (b) stereopsis; (c) dark adaptation; (d) color vision.
Q73. Visual cortex
Q74. Anatomy of optic chiasma
Q75. Visual pathway and its blood supply
Q76. Functional anatomy of optic nerve head and its blood supply. Discuss its clinical significance.
Q77. Anatomy of lateral geniculate body and visual cortex
Q78. Supranuclear control of ocular movements
Q79. Describe the anatomy of the visual pathway and lesions affecting it.
Q80. Retinal rivalry

Pupil

Q81. Pupillary reaction pathways with a labeled diagram. Discuss the abnormalities of pupillary reflexes on their basis.
Q82. Causes, grading, and clinical importance of relative afferent pupillary defect

Vitreous

Q83. Development of vitreous and its examination
Q84. Microscopic structure of vitreous and changes with aging

Extraocular Muscle

Q85. Muscle pulley
Q86. Annulus of Zinn
Q87. Discuss the origin, insertion, function, nerve and blood supply of extraocular muscles with a note on their development.
Q88. Describe briefly the origins, insertions, and action of extraocular muscles.
Q89. Anatomy of superior oblique muscle. Mechanism of its muscle action in carious direction of gaze.
Q90. Discuss the various laws governing the ocular movement. Discuss the clinical implication.

Orbital Vasculature and Nerves

Q91. Anatomy, nerve supply, and action of 3rd, 4th, and 6th cranial nerves
Q92. Anatomy of the cavernous sinus and its communications
Q93. Describe the sympathetic nervous system of the eye with the help of a diagram. Describe the various pharmacological tests to diagnose the abnormalities of the sympathetic nervous system.
Q94. Autoregulation of the ocular blood flow

Optics and Refraction

Refraction

Q1. What is Donder's reduced eye? What are the cardinal points?
Q2. (a) What is visual acuity? (b) Principles of Snellen's visual acuity testing. (b) What are the drawbacks of a Snellen chart? (c) Enumerate other charts for testing of visual acuity and give their advantages over Snellen chart.
Q3. Principles, composition, clinical applications, and advantages of an ETDRS visual acuity chart
Q4. Pediatric visual acuity assessment
Q5. Visual milestones and their development
Q6. Etiology and classification of myopia. Indications and techniques of surgical correction of myopia.
Q7. (a) Define hypermetropia and its components. (b) How does it affect accommodation and ocular alignment?
Q8. (a) What is amplitude of accommodation? (b) What is spasm of accommodation? Name two conditions in which this is commonly seen. (c) How do you treat this condition?
Q9. Classification and components of hypermetropia. Approach for subjective verification of refraction
Q10. Classify astigmatisms with example. Methods to treat astigmatism.
Q11. Management of astigmatism in: (a) 20-year-old male and (b) 50-year-old male with cataract
Q12. (a) What are the recent modalities available to treat presbyopia? (b) What are their advantages and limitations?
Q13. Selection of cycloplegic and mydriatic
Q14. Pediatric vision testing
Q15. Visual acuity in children
Q16. Accommodation and its anomalies
Q17. Define retinoscopy. Its principles, types, and techniques. What are the inferences drawn from the retinoscopy of plane and concave mirror?
Q18. Principle and optics of retinoscopy
Q19. What are the problems of retinoscopy?
Q20. Subjective correction (prescription of glasses) in patients aged 15 and 50 years
Q21. Back vertex power
Q22. Cross cylinder
Q23. Guidelines for correction of refractive error with age
Q24. ETDRS
Q25. Selection of contact lenses
Q26. Merits and demerits of modalities of management of myopia
Q27. Management of progressive myopia in a 10-year-old child
Q28. Describe the various aberrations of the optical system of the eye. What are the various corrective mechanisms built in the eye to overcome these?
Q29. (a) What are spherical aberrations? (b) What are negative and positive asphericity of cornea? Give one example of each.
Q30. Streak retinoscopy
Q31. Compound astigmatism
Q32. Anisometropia
Q33. Subjective verification of refraction
Q34. Discuss the basic principles which are applied in Mx and correction of astigmatism
Q35. Presbyopia and its management

Q36. Describe the mechanism of accommodation, and assessment and Mx of presbyopia.
Q37. Detail the selection criteria for your own ophthalmoscopes and the care you should exercise for their maintenance and maximum utilization.
Q38. Discuss subjective verification of refraction and role of autorefractors.
Q39. Principles and problems of retinoscopy
Q40. What is Sturm's conoid? Explain with a labeled diagram.
Q41. What are the surgical options for management of presbyopia?
Q42. Explain the optics of scleral and RGP contact lens. Contact lenses for keratoconus.
Q43. (a) "Progressive glasses" design. (b) When to use it and its advantages over conventional glasses?
Q44. (a) What are the different designs of bifocal spectacle lens? (b) Give two advantages and disadvantages of each type. (c) What is the best design to minimize these pitfalls?
Q45. Types of spectacle lenses

Instruments

Q46. Optics of operating microscope with a labeled diagram
Q47. Discuss with labeled diagrams optical principles of ophthalmic operating microscopes and their various technological advances.
Q48. Principle of Goldmann applanation tonometer
Q49. Principles, techniques, advantages, and possible sources of error in performing Goldmann applanation tonometry.
Q50. Laser interferometry
Q51. Optics of gonioscope
Q52. Gonioscopy
Q53. Optical principles of various means of appreciating angle
Q54. Critically analyze the methodologies available for aiding visualization through gonioscope. Other methods to assess the angle.
Q55. Prisms in ophthalmology—therapeutic and clinical use
Q56. Optical and principle of binocular indirect ophthalmoscope. What are the various lenses used for IDO and what are their advantage and disadvantage?
Q57. Describe the lenses used for examining the central retina on slit lamp biomicroscopy.
Q58. Care of direct ophthalmoscope
Q59. Optical principle of direct ophthalmoscope
Q60. Lensometer
Q61. Critically evaluate the principles, advantages, and limitations of various keratometers. Recent advances in examining and documenting cornea.
Q62. Optics of keratometer
Q63. Details of areas visualized, discuss optics and application of various viewing systems in vitrectomy.
Q64. Specular microscopy
Q65. Use of cross cylinders
Q66. Practical application of ophthalmoscope
Q67. Optical principle of slit lamp biomicroscope and techniques of slit lamp examination
Q68. Specular microscope—types, principle, and interpretation of results
Q69. Confoscan—type, principle, and clinical use
Q70. Optics of 90D lens
Q71. Potential acuity meter

Eyelids

Nonneoplastic Eyelid Lesions

Q1. Capillary hemangioma of the eye
Q2. Chalazion
Q3. Blepharochalasis

Neoplastic Eyelid lesions

Q4. Differential diagnosis of a painless nodular progressively increasing swelling of the lower lid in 60-year-old male.
Q5. Management of a basal cell carcinoma 5 mm in diameter, located in the center of lower lid margin.
Q6. Differential diagnosis and Mx-management of a growth of the lateral part of eyelids
Q7. A 60-year-old patient presents with noduloulcerative lesion involving central lower lid. Discuss differential diagnosis, evaluation, and management of such a case.
Q8. A 65-year-old lady presents with progressively increasing upper lid mass (15 × 10 mm). Discuss differential diagnosis and management.
Q9. (a) Enumerate malignant tumors of eyelid. (b) Clinical presentations and histopathology of sebaceous cell carcinoma. (c) Outline the management strategy for 20 mm-sized sebaceous cell carcinoma of upper eyelid.

Blepharitis

Q10. Demodex infestation
Q11. Etiopathogenesis, clinical features, differential diagnosis, and management of chronic blepharitis

Entropion

Q12. Etiopathogenesis, preoperative assessment, and management modalities of senile entropion
Q13. Entropion correction
Q14. What are the causes of cicatricial entropion?
Q15. Common techniques for correction of trachomatous upper lid entropion
Q16. Classification and management of various subtypes of entropion

Ectropion

Q17. Pathogenesis of senile ectropion. Elucidate tests for assessment and management of senile ectropion.
Q18. Cicatricial ectropion

Ptosis

Q19. Discuss various modalities of Mx in a case of ptosis and their indications. Critically evaluate the operative procedures available and appropriate steps for prevention and treatment of postoperative problems.
Q20. Classification of blepharoptosis and its relevance to management and complication.
Q21. Discuss the management of a case of congenital ptosis.
Q22. Evaluate in detail the surgical Mx and your criteria for decision making in a case of congenital ptosis.
Q23. Complications of LPS resection in ptosis surgery
Q24. Outline your approach for the evaluation and management of a case of failed ptosis surgery.
Q25. Causes, pathophysiology, diagnosis, and management of acquired ptosis
Q26. Senile ptosis
Q27. Outline your approach for evaluation and management of (a) failed ptosis and (b) ptosis in special situations (complicated ptosis).

Q28. A 6-year-old child is brought to the Outpatient Department (OPD) by her parents with complaints of drooping of the left upper lid noticed 3 years ago. How would you evaluate this patient and decide on your course of management?
Q29. Describe the clinical features, evaluation, syndromic association, and management of congenital ptosis.
Q30. Etiopathogenesis, clinical features, and management of unilateral ptosis with Marcus Gunn phenomenon
Q31. Diagnosis and management of a case of unilateral ptosis with jaw-winking phenomenon
Q32. What are the components of blepharophimosis syndrome? Outline various principles in the complete management of this syndrome.

Miscellaneous

Q33. Describe and discuss the principles and techniques of eyelid reconstructions/principles and techniques of lid reconstruction.
Q34. What are the principles of lid reconstruction? Indications, technique, and complications of Cutler–Beard operation.
Q35. Discuss management of lagophthalmos.
Q36. Enumerate four congenital anomalies of eyelids.
Q37. Management of Bell's palsy

Lacrimal Drainage System

Q1. Clinical evaluation in a case of epiphora
Q2. Epiphora
Q3. Lacrimal pump mechanism—structural and functional (dysfunctional) aspects
Q4. Describe tear formation and its drainage mechanism. How would you diagnose and manage different types of lacrimal obstruction?
Q5. Management of epiphora in 30-year-old female
Q6. Etiology, clinical features, and management of a case of pediatric epiphora.

Acquired Obstruction

Q7. Endoscopic lacrimal surgeries
Q8. (a) Anatomy of the lacrimal sac with the help of diagram(s). (b) What are the different types of DCR surgeries and their advantages and disadvantages?
Q9. Management of canalicular obstruction

Congenital Obstruction

Q10. Describe the etiology, clinical feature, differential diagnosis, and management of congenital nasolacrimal duct obstruction.
Q11. Outline the differential diagnosis and management of watering of eye in children.
Q12. Congenital abnormalities of the lacrimal drainage system and their management

Dacryocystitis

Q13. Management of chronic dacryocystitis

Miscellaneous

Q14. Failed DCR—causes and management
Q15. Describe the techniques for repair of a canalicular injury.
Q16. Common causes of severe bleeding during external DCR
Q17. Dacryocystography

Orbit

Proptosis

- Q1. Differential diagnosis of a patient having proptosis
- Q2. Discuss etiology and management of pediatric proptosis.
- Q3. Discuss etiology and Mx of unilateral proptosis in 3-year-old boy.
- Q4. Differential diagnosis and management of unilateral proptosis
- Q5. Discuss the differential diagnosis of bilateral proptosis.
- Q6. Describe the causes, type, investigation, and management of a case of unilateral axial proptosis in adult.
- Q7. A middle-aged female presents with unilateral proptosis of 1 year duration. Discuss differential diagnosis, evaluation, and management.
- Q8. Exophthalmometry
- Q9. Discuss the differential diagnosis of pulsatile proptosis. Outline your approach to their investigation and Mx
- Q10. Acute proptosis in children
- Q11. (a) Causes of bilateral childhood proptosis. (b) How would you investigate such a case?
- Q12. Causes, evaluation, and management of eyelid retraction
- Q13. A 50-year-old female presents with abaxial proptosis. Discuss differential diagnosis, evaluation, and management.
- Q14. Discuss the different approaches of orbitotomy.
- Q15. (a) What is a dermoid cyst? (b) Systemic associations of dermoid cyst. (c) Differential diagnosis of epibulbar swellings.
- Q16. Symptoms, signs, differential diagnosis, and management of lacrimal gland swellings.
- Q17. Describe the clinical feature and management of lacrimal gland tumor.

Thyroid Eye Disease

- Q18. Discuss the etiopathogenesis, clinical features, diagnosis, indication for intervention, and management of thyroid related ophthalmopathy
- Q19. Describe various thyroid function tests, give clinical picture, and management of hyperthyroidism with special regard to ocular involvement/thyroid ophthalmopathy.
- Q20. Orbital decompression techniques in thyroid ophthalmopathy
- Q21. Enumerate the ocular changes in thyroid dysfunction and its Mx.

Orbital Cellulitis

- Q22. Orbital cellulitis grading and management
- Q23. Management of orbital cellulitis in a child
- Q24. Discuss the differential diagnosis and management of unilateral orbital cellulitis
- Q25. Mucormycosis
- Q26. Causes, clinical presentation, and management of infective orbital diseases

Orbital Tumors

- Q27. Lacrimal gland lesions. Differential diagnosis and management
- Q28. Describe in detail the clinical pic, differential diagnosis, Mx of lacrimal gland tumors.
- Q29. Classify extraocular and intraocular tumors with a note on their prognosis.
- Q30. (a) Neurofibromatosis-ocular manifestations. (b) Differential diagnosis of optic nerve glioma.

Q31. Optic nerve glioma
Q32. Rhabdomyosarcoma

Nonneoplastic Vascular Abnormalities

Q33. Differential diagnosis of unilateral axial proptosis. Clinical features, histopathology, and management of cavernous hemangioma
Q34. Carotico cavernous fistula

Miscellaneous

Q35. Indications, techniques, surgical steps, and complications of exenteration. Discuss the methods of rehabilitation.
Q36. Etiology, clinical features, morphologic types, assessment, and management of contracted socket
Q37. Acquired causes and management of different grades of an anophthalmic contracted socket
Q38. What are orbital implants and their indications? Enumerate different materials for orbital implants. What are the advantages and complications of orbital implants?
Q39. Indications of orbital decompression. Importance of medial wall in orbital decompression?
Q40. Discuss the functional and surgical anatomy of orbit along with their development. Their various important disorders and anomalies.
Q41. (a) What are the surgical spaces of the orbit? (b) What are the surgical approaches? (c) Role of MRI and CT in diagnosis of ocular lesions.
Q42. Transfrontal orbitotomy—procedure and indications
Q43. Phakomatoses—definition, types, and ocular manifestations
Q44. (a) Diagnostic criteria for neurofibromatosis. (b) Ocular features of neurofibromatosis types 1 and 2
Q45. Management of ocular manifestation of neurofibromatosis
Q46. Craniosynostosis and eye
Q47. How would you approach and manage a suspected case of blowout fracture?
Q48. (a) Clinical presentation of a case of orbital blowout fracture. (b) How will you investigate such a case? (c) Indications for surgery and the surgical principles.
Q49. Orbital spaces, significance in investigation, and salient disorders
Q50. Describe the spaces of orbit and discuss their surgical importance.
Q51. Describe investigations for intraocular malignancies in an adult and options for their management.
Q52. Orbital fracture in relation to structural anatomy
Q53. What are the surgical options in the management of a blowout fracture of the orbit? Discuss the indications for each.
Q54. Oculo-orbital cysticercosis
Q55. Sclerosing pseudotumor
Q56. Pseudotumor of orbit
Q57. Describe types of orbital implants and their advantages.
Q58. Describe the methods, benefits, and risks of tumor biopsy of extraocular and intraocular tumors.
Q59. How will you evaluate and manage an anophthalmic socket in a 3-year-old child?
Q60. Causes, evaluation, and management of lagophthalmos
Q61. A 27-year-old male presents with acute periorbital swelling, redness, and pain. How will you investigate, diagnose, and treat this case?
Q62. Principles of radio imaging in orbital pathologies
Q63. Discuss indications and techniques of evisceration and enucleation.

Conjunctiva

Conjunctival Degeneration

- Q1. Pterygium
- Q2. Current techniques for management of recurrent pterygium. P.E.R.F.E.C.T. technique for management of pterygium
- Q3. Recent advances in pterygium surgery
- Q4. Recurrent pterygium

Allergic Conjunctivitis

- Q5. Vernal keratoconjunctivitis—clinical features, pathology, and treatment
- Q6. A 25-year-old man complaining of itching and redness of both 5+5 eyes since childhood presents with gradually increasing refractive error and photophobia. Outline the workup and management.
- Q7. Acute hemorrhagic conjunctivitis

Infectious Conjunctivitis

- Q8. Discuss intricacies in diagnosis and management of conjunctivitis.
- Q9. Viral conjunctivitis
- Q10. Clinical features, pathogenesis, differential diagnosis, and management of a case of viral conjunctivitis.
- Q11. Neonatal conjunctivitis/clinical features, differential diagnosis, and management of ophthalmia neonatorum
- Q12. Clinical features and management of adenoviral keratoconjunctivitis
- Q13. Discuss clinical features and lab diagnosis of trachoma. Discuss its management, complications, and prophylaxis. What is SAFE strategy?
- Q14. (a) Etiopathogenesis of lid changes in trachoma. (b) Management outline of stage 2 trachoma.
- Q15. Chlamydia trachomatis

Miscellaneous

- Q16. Phlyctenular conjunctivitis
- Q17. (a) Etiopathogenesis and clinical features of cicatricial conjunctivitis. (b) Complications and management of cicatricial conjunctivitis.
- Q18. A 34-year-old lady presents with chronic inflammation and irritation of superior limbus. What are the most likely diagnosis, pathogenesis, and management of the disease? Superior limbic keratoconjunctivitis

Cornea and External Diseases

Ocular Surface Disease

- Q1. What are the various ocular surface disorders? Discuss the etiopathogenesis, clinical features, and management of ocular surface disorders.
- Q2. (a) Define dry eye as per DEWS 2 report. (b) Role of anti-inflammatory drug for management of dry eye. (c) Diagnosis and management of meibomian gland dysfunction.
- Q3. Describe the etiology, clinical features, diagnosis, and management of dry eye disease.
- Q4. Recent advances in the investigations and management of dry eye disease
- Q5. Clinical features, evaluation, and management of meibomian gland disease
- Q6. Etiopathogenesis, clinical features, diagnosis, and management of Sjögren's syndrome
- Q7. Tear film and its changes in iatrogenic situations

- Q8. Tear film physiology and applied aspects in contact lens wear
- Q9. Discuss etiology, investigations, and treatment with special reference to recent advances in dry eye disease/dry eye syndrome.
- Q10. Ocular surface disorders and their management
- Q11. Classify the various ocular lubricating agents used in the management of dry eye disease.
- Q12. What is the role of preservatives in them? What are the preservatives used in lubricating agents?
- Q13. Tear biological replacement therapy
- Q14. Stem cell deficiencies
- Q15. SJS—etiology, manifestation, and management
- Q16. Describe the clinical features, evaluation, and management of ocular manifestation of Steven Johnson Syndrome (SJS).
- Q17. Management of acute SJS
- Q18. Indications, techniques, and limitations of impression cytology
- Q19. What are cytokines? Enumerate important pro-inflammatory cytokines. What role do they play in ocular inflammation?
- Q20. Write about the secretory immune system of the eye. How does Sjögren's syndrome influence the immunologic architecture of the lacrimal gland?

Corneal Ulcer

- Q21. (a) Clinical and microbiological workup of corneal ulcer patient. (b) Additional workup in suspected acanthamoeba and atypical mycobacterial keratitis.
- Q22. Nonresponding bacterial corneal ulcer
- Q23. Clinical features, diagnosis, and approach in management of fungal keratitis
- Q24. Elaborate the risk factors, clinical presentation, diagnosis, and management of acanthamoeba keratitis.
- Q25. Management of nonhealing corneal ulcer/current concepts in the management of nonhealing corneal ulcer
- Q26. Clinical presentation, differential diagnosis, and management of recurrent herpes simplex keratitis
- Q27. Clinical features and management of corneal epithelial infectious ulcers and immune keratitis in herpes simplex infection
- Q28. What are the ocular manifestations of herpes zoster ophthalmicus in acute and chronic state? How do you manage them? What is the management of postherpetic neuralgia?
- Q29. Management of herpes zoster ophthalmicus
- Q30. Clinical features, complications, and management of a case of herpes zoster ophthalmicus
- Q31. Disciform keratitis
- Q32. Surgical treatment for marginal corneal ulcer
- Q33. Peripheral corneal thinning disorders and their management
- Q34. Role of steroids in keratitis
- Q35. Herpetic stromal keratitis
- Q36. Exposure keratitis
- Q37. Neuroparalytic keratitis
- Q38. Neurotrophic keratopathy
- Q39. Viral keratitis
- Q40. Etiopathogenesis, clinical features, investigation, and management of chronic, nonhealing peripheral corneal ulcer
- Q41. Etiopathogenesis, clinical features, differential diagnosis, investigation, and management of PUK
- Q42. Presentation, pathogenesis, and management of Mooren's ulcer
- Q43. A 30-year-old male reports with acute onset unilateral red eye and diminished vision of 3 days duration with watery discharge, a corneal epithelial lesion, stromal infiltration, and an immune ring on the endothelium. He gives a history of previous episodes of red eye in the same eye and has lesions suggestive of previous corneal disease. Make a flowchart describing how you would arrive at a diagnosis and how you would manage the case.

Q44. Describe the clinical features, evaluation, and management of microsporidial keratitis.
Q45. A 30-year-old female got up at night with severe pain and watering in left eye. She gave history of a nail injury to her eye 1 year back. How would you approach and manage such a case?
Q46. (a) Clinical features and causative organisms of a case of bacterial corneal ulcer. (b) How will you investigate such a case?
Q47. Describe the different types of recurrent corneal erosions. Give an outline of their treatment.

Ectatic Corneal Disorder

Q48. Describe peripheral corneal thinning disorders and their management
Q49. Etiology, pathogenesis, workup, differential diagnosis, and management of keratoconus
Q50. Describe the optical principles and application of corneal topography. Discuss concepts of management of keratoconus.
Q51. Corneal topography changes in keratoconus. How do you grade the severity of keratoconus?
Q52. Posterior keratoconus
Q53. Changes in topography in cases of corneal ectasia
Q54. Corneal crosslinking—principle, indication, technique, and different protocols
Q55. How will you suspect, investigate, and treat a case of preclinical keratoconus?
Q56. A 25-year-old woman presents with inability to correct her vision completely with glasses. Her keratometric values are 48 D@ 95°/52 D@185° (OD), 50 D@65°/55 D@ 155°. What is your plausible diagnosis and discuss important steps in further confirming your diagnosis and factors influencing her management.
Q57. Principles of contact lens fitting in keratoconus
Q58. Prominent corneal nerve and thickened corneal nerve

Corneal Dystrophy

Q59. Highlight the new classification of corneal dystrophy.
Q60. Describe stromal dystrophies with clinical features, histopathological changes, and special stains used for their identification and management.
Q61. TGF-beta-1-related corneal dystrophies
Q62. Describe the inheritance pattern of corneal stromal dystrophies.
Q63. Discuss changing concepts in management of endothelial dysfunction.
Q64. Dystrophies and degenerations in eye

Corneal Degeneration

Q65. Peripheral corneal degeneration
Q66. Spheroidal degeneration

Chemical Injury

Q67. Classify chemical injuries and discuss the prognostic indicators. Outline various management modalities and long-term complications. Role of stem cell transplantation in its management
Q68. (a) Management of unilateral 5-day-old chemical burn. (b) Newer concepts in the management of ocular burns.
Q69. Clinical features, evaluation, and management of alkali ocular injury
Q70. Management of acute chemical burn
Q71. Management of symblepharon following chemical injury
Q72. Discuss the current concepts in the management and prognosis of chemical injury

Degenerative Changes of Cornea

Q73. Peripheral corneal degeneration
Q74. BSK

Q75. Salzmann's nodular degeneration

Q76. Spheroidal degeneration

Congenital Corneal Opacity

Q77. Corneal opacity and its congenital variant

Q78. Staphyloma

Q79. Limbal dermoid

Q80. Sclerocornea

Ocular Surface Surgery

Q81. Limbal stem cell transplant

Q82. SLET

Q83. Describe the use of amniotic membrane in ophthalmology and techniques of amniotic membrane grafting

Q84. Discuss the newly available options for the management of limbal stem cell deficiency.

Q85. Ocular surface surgery

Corneal Transplantation

Q86. High-risk keratoplasty: Risk assessment and management

Q87. Recent advances and concepts in corneal grafting with special reference to high-risk keratoplasty

Q88. Discuss lamellar keratoplasties and their role in corneal disorders

Q89. (a) Enumerate various types of lamellar keratoplasty. (b) How would you decide which lamellar procedure would be appropriate for a patient?

Q90. Indications, techniques, advantages, and disadvantages of deep anterior lamellar keratoplasty (DALK)

Q91. Discuss endothelial keratoplasty.

Q92. Endothelial keratoplasty—indications, surgical techniques, and outcomes

Q93. Indications, advantages, disadvantages, and long-term results of Descemet's stripping endothelial keratoplasty.

Q94. (a) Indications and evaluation of a case for lamellar keratoplasty. (b) What are the causes of failure of a DSAEK procedure? (c) How does DSAEK differ from DMEK surgically?

Q95. Recent advances in the endothelial keratoplasty

Q96. Describe etiology, risk factors, pathogenesis, and management of corneal graft rejection/immunology of graft rejection.

Q97. Corneal graft failure

Q98. Discuss the management of shallow anterior chamber after keratoplasty.

Q99. Eye banking and corneal preservation techniques

Q100. Critically evaluate organization of ideal blood bank with reference to maximize the needs of our region.

Q101. Planning an ideal eye bank at a tertiary ophthalmic hospital.

Q102. Eye banking and legislation

Q103. Corneal preservation

Q104. Disease screening and donor cornea preservation

Q105. (a) Enumerate the various short-term and intermediate-term methods for corneal preservation. (b) What are their main constituents? (c) Advantages and disadvantages of these media.

Q106. Acute ocular graft-versus-host disease

Q107. DSEK

Q108. Keratoprosthesis: (a) Types and (b) indications

Q109. Discuss merits and demerits of endothelial keratoplasty.

Q110. Critically evaluate DSEK/DSAEK and DMEK.

- Q111. A 76-year-old man underwent cataract surgery for grade 4 nuclear sclerosis. There was incomplete recovery followed by diminution of vision 6 weeks after surgery. Discuss the causes for diminution of vision and management in brief.
- Q112. How would you set up an eye bank?

Miscellaneous

- Q113. Clinical features, etiology, and management of corneal edema.
- Q114. What is pseudophakic bullous keratopathy? Causes, clinical presentation, and treatment modalities for pseudophakic bullous keratopathy.
- Q115. Management of Descemet's membrane detachment
- Q116. Collagen shield
- Q117. Discuss corneal wound healing and ways to modulate it.
- Q118. Vital stains in corneal evaluation
- Q119. Cosmetic contact lens
- Q120. Corneal complication of IOLs
- Q121. Management of DMD
- Q122. A 10-year-old child with complaints of blurring of vision and whitish opacities in both eyes is brought to OPD. Discuss differential diagnosis and management of this case.
- Q123. Define and classify xerophthalmia. Give the guidelines of treatment and prophylaxis.
- Q124. Keratomalacia
- Q125. Orthokeratology
- Q126. Origin and genesis of retrocorneal membrane
- Q127. Describe the epidemiology, clinical features, management, and prophylaxis for vitamin A deficiency.

Refractive Surgery

- Q1. Refractive surgeries

Corneal Refractive Surgery

- Q2. (a) How will you workup a case for LASIK surgery? (b) What are the modalities available and which one is preferred and why?
- Q3. LASIK surgery and its complications
- Q4. SMILE refractive surgery—indications, intraoperative and postoperative complications, and their management
- Q5. Customized excimer laser corneal ablation
- Q6. Astigmatic and refractive corneal surgeries
- Q7. Critically discuss recent advances in keratorefractive procedures
- Q8. Discuss the changing scenario in diverse refractive procedures
- Q9. Critical note on selection of patient for refractive surgery
- Q10. Femtosecond laser
- Q11. (a) Enumerate keratorefractive surgeries. (b) Intraoperative and postoperative complications of LASIK and their management.
- Q12. Phakic IOLs—types, indications, intraoperative and postoperative complications, and their management
- Q13. Newer advances in refractive surgery
- Q14. What is conductive keratoplasty? What is the mechanism, indication, advantage, and disadvantage of conductive keratoplasty?
- Q15. What are the causes of dry eye post-LASIK surgery? How will you manage it?

Q16. Corneal ring segments—indications and complications
Q17. SMILE in refractive surgery: Advantages and disadvantages over conventional LASIK surgery
Q18. Recent advances in management of postoperative astigmatism
Q19. Wavefront-guided ablation

Lens-based Refractive Surgery

Q20. What are phakic IOLs? Discuss their indications, techniques, and complications.
Q21. Mention the commonly used phakic IOL. Indications for use. Method for calculation of the power and size of the IOL.
Q22. Refractive surgery for patients not suitable for LASIK

Miscellaneous

Q23. Discuss the surgical procedures to manage corneal astigmatism with or without cataract surgery.

Sclera

Scleritis

Q1. Scleritis
Q2. (a) Etiopathogenesis and clinical features of necrotizing scleritis. (b) Evaluation and management of necrotizing scleritis
Q3. (a) Classification of scleritis. (b) Clinical features, investigation, and management of scleritis
Q4. (a) Clinical features and types of anterior and posterior scleritis. (b) How will you investigate a case of scleritis? (c) Management of necrotizing scleritis

Glaucoma

Q1. Epidemiology of glaucoma in India
Q2. Target IOP
Q3. ONH evaluation
Q4. Ocular blood flow in glaucoma

Ocular Hypertension

Q5. Define ocular hypertension. Investigation and management of a case of ocular hypertension

Normal Tension Glaucoma

Q6. Normal tension glaucoma
Q7. (a) What is normal tension glaucoma? (b) Etiopathogenesis, clinical characteristics, differential diagnosis, and management of a case of normal tension glaucoma

Open-angle Glaucoma

Q8. Visual field defects in open-angle glaucoma
Q9. Medical management of glaucoma
Q10. Discuss preperimetric glaucoma and its diagnosis and factors in progression of field defects.
Q11. Describe the pathogenesis, clinical features, evaluation, differential diagnosis, and management of pigment dispersion syndrome.

Q12. (a) Etiopathogenesis, clinical features, and diagnosis of pseudoexfoliative glaucoma. (b) Give specific features of true exfoliation in eye.
Q13. Criteria for early glaucomatous visual field changes
Q14. Describe the various concepts that explain the pathogenesis of optic nerve damage in glaucoma.
Q15. What is advanced glaucoma? How would you follow up a case of advanced glaucoma? Discuss the various treatment options.

Angle-closure Glaucoma

Q16. Clinical feature and management of ACG
Q17. The EAGLE study

Secondary Glaucoma

Q18. Classify secondary glaucoma. Diagnosis and management of lens-induced glaucomas (make a flowchart).
Q19. Steroid-induced glaucoma
Q20. Drug-induced glaucoma
Q21. Outline the etiopathogenesis clinical features and management of neovascular glaucoma
Q22. Phacolytic glaucoma and Mx
Q23. Discuss the causes of secondary glaucoma. Pattern of rise of IOP in postuveitic glaucoma
Q24. Pathogenesis and management of malignant glaucoma
Q25. Pathogenesis, diagnosis, and management of a case of angle-recession glaucoma.
Q26. Phakomatoses
Q27. Define and enumerate the ICE syndromes. Describe the clinical features and management.
Q28. PEX syndrome
Q29. Aphakic glaucoma
Q30. Causes and management of glaucoma associated with ocular trauma.
Q31. How will you diagnose and classify a case of inflammatory glaucoma? What are the treatment options available?
Q32. What is Sturge–Weber syndrome? Give its classification, clinical signs, investigations, and principles of management of associated glaucoma.
Q33. Epidemic dropsy glaucoma
Q34. Topiramate-induced angle closure

Primary Congenital Glaucoma

Q35. Discuss the genetics, pathophysiology, differential diagnosis, and management of primary congenital glaucoma and its associated syndromes.
Q36. Surgical management of congenital glaucoma
Q37. Briefly discuss disorders exhibiting developmental anomalies of the angle.
Q38. Step ladder classification of anterior cleavage syndrome and its management.
Q39. Axenfeld–Rieger syndrome

Antiglaucoma Drugs

Q40. (a) Classify pharmacological agents available to treat glaucoma. (b) Mechanism of action of topical agents. (c) Adverse effects and contraindications of systemic agents.
Q41. Dynamic of aqueous humor synthesis in health and diseases. Mechanism of drugs affecting it
Q42. Dorzalamide
Q43. Prostaglandins in glaucoma
Q44. Side effects of glaucoma medications
Q45. Neuroprotection and its mechanism of action in glaucoma

Glaucoma Surgery

- Q46. Surgical management options for glaucoma
- Q47. Assessment of glaucoma filtering surgery bleb
- Q48. Releasable sutures
- Q49. Management of refractory glaucoma
- Q50. Discuss wound healing in glaucoma filtration surgery and various methods to modulate it to enhance its surgical success.
- Q51. Augmented trabeculoplasty
- Q52. Diagnosis, management, and prevention of complications of trabeculectomy arising within 6 weeks after surgery
- Q53. Management of postoperative shallow AC following filtering surgery
- Q54. Management of encapsulated bleb following filtering surgery
- Q55. Bleb-associated endophthalmitis
- Q56. Surgical management of failed trabeculectomy
- Q57. Nonpenetrating glaucoma surgery—types, advantages, and limitations
- Q58. Glaucoma drainage devices/newer microsurgical devices for management of glaucoma/indications, procedures, advantages, and complications of glaucoma drainage devices. What is their role in glaucoma management when compared to conventional trabeculectomy?
- Q59. Recent surgical devices in glaucoma surgery
- Q60. Discuss tube versus trabeculectomy study (TUT).
- Q61. A patient with chronic angle closure glaucoma undergoes a trabeculectomy and has a shallow anterior chamber on the first postoperative day. Describe the process by which you would discern the cause of postoperative anterior chamber shallowing and how you would manage this situation.
- Q62. (a) Etiopathogenesis of flat anterior chamber after glaucoma surgery. (b) How would you critically evaluate and manage such a case?
- Q63. Management of intractable glaucoma or multiple failed glaucoma surgeries.
- Q64. (a) Enumerate various implant drainage devices in glaucoma surgery. (b) Indications and adverse effects of Ahmed glaucoma valve surgery
- Q65. Evaluation and management during failure of filtration surgery in glaucoma. What are the indications of antimetabolite in this surgery?
- Q66. Antimetabolites in glaucoma filtration surgery: Agents, doses, and mode of delivery.

Laser Treatment for Glaucoma

- Q67. Describe in brief the indication technique complications of laser peripheral iridoplasty and laser peripheral iridotomy.
- Q68. Selective laser trabeculoplasty
- Q69. Lasers in glaucoma

Miscellaneous

- Q70. The uses and pitfalls of optical coherence tomography in glaucoma
- Q71. Advances in the management of glaucoma and their limitations
- Q72. Nerve fiber layer with reference to glaucoma
- Q73. Management of a painful blind eye with medically uncontrollable intraocular pressure of 50 mm Hg
- Q74. Aniridia
- Q75. Diagnosis of preperimetric glaucoma
- Q76. Short wave automated perimetry

Lens

Acquired Cataract

- Q1. Pathogenesis of senile cataract. IOL power calculation. Newer IOL materials and design.
- Q2. (a) What are the causes of complicated cataract? (b) Principles of management of cataract associated with chronic anterior uveitis
- Q3. Traumatic cataract
- Q4. Evaluation and management of postuveitic cataract
- Q5. Factors contributing to genesis of cataract.
- Q6. Critically evaluate a case of complicated cataract and its management

Posterior Polar Cataract

- Q7. Grading and management of posterior polar cataract

Cataract in Systemic Conditions

- Q8. Risk factors and systemic diseases causing cataract
- Q9. Diabetic cataract

Pediatric Cataract

- Q10. What are the differences in an adult and pediatric eye?
- Q11. Discuss development of lens, with respect to various types of congenital cataract.
- Q12. Discuss the types and management of pediatric cataract.
- Q13. Developmental cataract
- Q14. Management of developmental cataract
- Q15. Types, clinical features, differential diagnosis, and management of PHPV
- Q16. Aphakia in children—management
- Q17. Congenital rubella syndrome
- Q18. Enumerate congenital abnormalities of lens.
- Q19. Management of unilateral cataract in a 2-year-old child
- Q20. Management strategies of bilateral congenital cataract in a 2-year-old child
- Q21. Etiology, inheritance, morphology, and four main systemic metabolic associations of congenital cataract.
- Q22. (a) Calculation of IOL power in children. (b) Selection of IOL in children
- Q23. Pediatric cataract surgery
- Q24. Precautions to be observed during pediatric cataract surgery and why?
- Q25. What is the relationship between pediatric cataract surgery and glaucoma?
- Q26. Infant aphakia treatment study
- Q27. Visual rehabilitation in pediatric cataract surgery

Subluxated Lens

- Q28. Protocols for management of options of subluxated cataract
- Q29. Subluxation of crystalline lens—etiology, clinical features, differential diagnosis, and management (with flowchart)
- Q30. Discuss the clinical examination, investigation, and management of subluxated lens in 6-year-old boy.
- Q31. (a) Systemic associations of ectopia lentis. (b) Management of a case of ectopia lentis.
- Q32. Ten features of Marfan syndrome
- Q33. Causes, clinical features, and management of ectopia lentis

Q34. What is the nature of biochemical abnormality in homocystinuria? Discuss the ocular and systemic manifestations, genetics, and management.

Cataract Surgery

Q35. Parameters involved in fluid dynamics in phacoemulsification

Q36. Differences, advantages, and disadvantages of peristaltic versus venturi pump

Q37. Ophthalmic viscoelastic devices (OVD)

Q38. Techniques of nucleotomy

Q39. Difficulties encountered during phacoemulsification in a small pupil. How will you manage a case of nondilating pupil for phacoemulsification?

Q40. Critically evaluate multifocal IOLs in ophthalmic practice. Mention the types and outcomes of multifocal IOL?

Q41. Pros and cons of accommodative and newer IOLs in ophthalmic practice

Q42. SFIOL. Describe techniques of sutureless SFIOL.

Q43. Enumerate the techniques of secondary IOL implantation in an adult patient with aphakia and discuss the advantage and disadvantage of each technique.

Q44. Newer IOLs

Q45. What is the concept and its applications in various full-range IOLs such as multifocals, accommodative, pseudoaccommodative, and extended-range IOLs?

Q46. Toric IOL

Q47. PCO and its prevention

Q48. CTR

Q49. IOLs to aid near vision

Q50. Aspheric lenses

Q51. Bimanual phacoemulsification

Q52. Newer concepts in phacoemulsification

Q53. Principles of cataract surgery in different ocular situations

Q54. Chop techniques

Q55. Methods of surgical anesthesia in cataract surgery

Q56. SICS

Q57. Procedures to obtain emmetropia in IOL implantation

Q58. Posterior capsulorhexis

Q59. Decentered IOL

Q60. What is the differential diagnosis of postoperative inflammation following cataract surgery with respect to management

Q61. Nd:YAG capsulotomy

Q62. Use of femto laser in cataract surgery

Q63. (a) Principles of Femtosecond laser-assisted cataract surgery (FLACS). (b) Advantages and disadvantages of FLACS over conventional phacoemulsification. Blade-free cataract surgery.

Q64. Management of intraoperative complications of phacoemulsification

Q65. A 70-year-old male with a normal phakic contralateral eye had posterior capsular tear in the center during a phacoemulsification procedure after removal of the cortex. Make a flowchart describing your subsequent actions, explaining why you performed each step.

Q66. An 80-year-old retired school teacher with parkinsonism and modest visual demands was operated for cataract in the right eye and she has a postoperative error of +5 diopter in the first week. Her contralateral eye is pseudophakic and has good uncorrected postoperative vision with which she is satisfied. The current surgery was uncomplicated. (a) Discuss various options for further management of the patient. (b) How would you decide on the best course of action?

Q67. (a) Evaluation of preexisting astigmatism in a patient with cataract. (b) Various surgical methods to manage preoperative astigmatism during cataract surgery.

Q68. Indications, advantages, disadvantages, and complications of a Toric multifocal intraocular lens implantation following cataract extraction.

Q69. How will you diagnose and manage a case of intraoperative zonular dialysis during cataract surgery?

Q70. What are the predisposing factors, preoperative signs, and management of a case of suprachoroidal hemorrhage during an intraocular surgery?

Q71. (a) Types of multifocal IOLs. (b) Case selection and basic principles for premium IOLs.

Q72. How do different types of intraocular lenses influence contrast sensitivity?

Q73. Principle, utility, and advantages of: (a) Square-edged optics, (b) aspheric optics, and (c) heparin-coated optics

Q74. Principles in the management of cataract surgery post vitreoretinal surgery with silicone oil in vitreous.

Q75. A 60-year-old diabetic male presented with sudden onset diminution of vision 1 week after uneventful cataract surgery. Give differential diagnosis and management algorithm.

Q76. IOL power calculation in postrefractive surgery patient

Q77. Advances in biometry, IOL design, and phacoemulsification techniques

Q78. Discuss postoperative shallow anterior chamber after various intraocular surgeries and its management.

Miscellaneous

Q79. Intralenticular foreign body

Q80. Persistent pupillary membrane

Q81. After giving 1 mL of a peribulbar anesthetic, there is sudden proptosis, pain, subconjunctival hemorrhage, severe chemosis, and loss of vision with loss of all ocular movements and inability to close the eyelids. (a) Describe what your further course of action would be. (b) What are the signs of globe perforation during peribulbar block?

Q82. Describe the congenital and developmental anomalies of the lens.

Q83. Describe the techniques of ocular anesthesia with their advantages and disadvantages.

Uveitis

Q1. Classify uveitis, enumerating the role of various investigations with respect to Mx modalities.

Q2. Classification, causes, clinical manifestation, and management of uveitis

Q3. Classify uveitis, describe clinical features of intermediate uveitis, and its management.

Q4. Uveitis—types, etiologies, and recent advances in management.

Q5. Investigative profile in uveitis

Q6. Role of immunosuppressive therapy in uveitis

Anterior Uveitis

Q7. What are the types, ocular clinical features, differential diagnosis, and management of a case of juvenile idiopathic arthritis?

Q8. Still's disease

Q9. Differential diagnosis and management of a 10-year-old boy presenting with bilateral diminution of vision and swelling of the right knee.

Q10. Causes of heterochromia iridocyclitis

Q11. Clinical features and management of Fuchs uveitis syndrome

Q12. (a) Differential diagnosis of heterochromia iridis. (b) Features, complications, and management of a case of Fuchs uveitis syndrome

Q13. Various presentations of uveitis in spondyloarthropathies

Intermediate Uveitis

- Q14. Describe etiopathogenesis, clinical features, and management of intermediate uveitis.
- Q15. What are the indications and modes of application of periocular steroids? What are their advantages and complications and what steps can be taken to prevent them?
- Q16. What are the indications, advantages, and disadvantages of intraocular steroids?
- Q17. Vision loss in intermediate uveitis
- Q18. Pars planitis

Posterior Uveitis

- Q19. Posterior uveitis
- Q20. Vasculitis and describe Wegener's granulomatosis.
- Q21. Chorioretinitis
- Q22. Disseminated choroiditis—causes and management
- Q23. Discuss the differentials and management of posterior parasitic uveitis.

Panuveitis

- Q24. Differential diagnosis and management of bilateral panuveitis
- Q25. Sympathetic ophthalmitis—etiopathogenesis, clinical features, and management
- Q26. VKH

Infectious Uveitis

- Q27. Discuss various ophthalmic manifestations of Hansen's disease
- Q28. Clinical features, diagnostic investigations, and management of ocular tuberculosis.
- Q29. Elaborate ocular manifestation of HIV and its management. What is the impact of HAART on ocular features
- Q30. Diagnostic features of HIV retinopathy and relationship to CD4 counts
- Q31. Ocular toxoplasmosis/toxoplasma retinitis
- Q32. Ocular toxocariasis
- Q33. Clinical feature, evaluation, and management of ocular cysticercosis
- Q34. Clinical features, investigations, treatment, and prognosis in a case of CMV retinitis
- Q35. Acute retinal necrosis

Miscellaneous

- Q36. Clinical presentation, investigation, and management of pediatric uveitis
- Q37. White dot syndrome
- Q38. Differential diagnosis of white dot syndrome
- Q39. Describe the clinical features, evaluation, and management of serpiginous choroidopathy.
- Q40. Describe clinical features, diagnosis, and management of ocular sarcoidosis.
- Q41. Hemorrhagic occlusive retinal vasculitis
- Q42. Heterochromic iridocyclitis
- Q43. Surgical Mx of complications of uveitis
- Q44. Intravitreal implants in uveitis
- Q45. Clinical features, investigations, and management of ocular sarcoidosis
- Q46. Role of biological agents in management of patient with bilateral chronic uveitis
- Q47. A 30-year-old male presented with genital lesions and complained of sudden diminution of vision in one eye followed 6 weeks later by similar diminution in the other eye. What are the possible diagnoses? Give broad guidelines in the management of each situation.

Q48. (a) Indications, routes of administration, dosage schedule, and complication of steroids in uveitis. (b) Role of alternative drugs used in uveitis.

Q49. Sarcoidosis and eye

Retina

Diabetic Retinopathy

Q1. Pathogenesis and sequelae of cotton wool spots and hard exudates on retina in diabetic retinopathy

Q2. Proliferative diabetic retinopathy

Q3. Current concepts in DR and their relevance to Mx

Q4. Discuss the pathogenesis, clinical features, investigation, and management algorithm for diabetic macular edema with reference to recent clinical trials.

Q5. Discuss the role of lasers in management of diabetic macular edema.

Q6. Diagnosis and management of recalcitrant DME/nonresolving DME

Q7. What are the various anti-VEGF drugs available? Mention their pharmacologic features, indications for use, advantages, and disadvantages.

Q8. Bevacizumab—mechanism of action, indications, and differences with other anti-VEGF drugs

Q9. (a) Aflibercept/what is VEGF-Trap? (b) What are its advantages over the current anti-VEGF agents?

Q10. Ocular management of a 50-year-old diabetic patient including medical, surgical, and laser treatment who has 3/60 vision and proliferative diabetic retinopathy in both eyes.

Q11. Vascular endothelial growth factors

Q12. A 65-year-old diabetic man presents with painless diminution of vision with vitreous haze. How will you investigate and treat him?

Q13. (a) Investigations and assessment of a case of long-standing diabetes with moderate nonproliferative diabetic retinopathy with clinically significant macular edema. (b) How will you manage such a case?

Hypertensive retinopathy

Q14. Hypertensive retinopathy

Q15. Hypertension—ocular features with special reference to PIH/Q PIH

Q16. Discuss ocular changes in hypertension and their Mx strategies.

Q17. Pathogenesis, clinical features, diagnosis, and management of different grades of retinopathy in pregnancy-induced hypertension

Vascular Occlusion

Q18. Describe the etiopathogenesis, clinical features, investigations, and current management strategies for CRVO.

Q19. BRVO—etiopathogenesis, clinical features, evaluation, and management

Q20. Clinical features of early and late branch retinal vein occlusion

Q21. Results of important trials in management of BRVO

Q22. Diagnosis and management of ocular ischemic syndrome

Q23. Hemorrhagic occlusive retinal vasculitis

Q24. Etiopathogenesis, clinical features, investigations, and management of central retinal arterial occlusion

Q25. Management of macular edema following retinal vein occlusion

Retinal Vasculitis

Q26. Eales disease

Retinopathy of Prematurity

- Q27. Retinopathy of prematurity staging
- Q28. ROP and plus disease
- Q29. Risk factors, evaluation, classification, and management of ROP
- Q30. Screening guidelines for ROP in India, classification and management of ROP

Other Retinal Vascular Diseases

- Q31. Clinical features, differential diagnosis, and management of a case of Coats disease
- Q32. What is Terson's syndrome? Write its clinical features, differential diagnosis, complications, and management.
- Q33. Retinal artery macroaneurysm
- Q34. Cherry red spot
- Q35. Von Hippel–Lindau disease

Age-related Macular Degeneration

- Q36. Discuss the pathology of dry and wet ARMD and its management.
- Q37. Recent advances in management of ARMD
- Q38. Discuss the ocular and systemic side effects of commercially available anti-VEGF agents. Describe the randomized controlled trial comparing the different anti-VEGFs in AMD.
- Q39. Choroidal neovascular membrane—pathogenesis, differential diagnosis, and management
- Q40. Discuss the pathogenesis, prevention, clinical manifestation, investigations, and treatment of AMD (medical and surgical).
- Q41. Describe management options for a 60-year-old patient suffering from age-related macular degeneration with visual acuity of 3/60 in both eyes. Discuss options for visual rehabilitation of patient.
- Q42. Discuss the CATT 1 and CATT 2 trials. What were the objectives, design, conclusion, and implication of the trial?
- Q43. Pathology of various age-related macular lesions

Polypoidal Choroidal Vasculopathy

- Q44. Clinical features, diagnosis, differential diagnosis, and management of idiopathic polypoidal choroidal vasculopathy

Vitreomacular Traction Syndrome

- Q45. Vitreomacular traction syndrome/VMTS

Macular Hole

- Q46. Etiology, pathogenesis, evaluation, grading, and management of full-thickness macular hole
- Q47. Discuss the OCT features of macular hole in relation to management. Discuss factors prognosticating the treatment outcome.
- Q48. Macular hole management/macular hole surgery
- Q49. Traumatic MH
- Q50. Indications, advantages, and disadvantages of internal limiting membrane (ILM) peeling in vitreoretinal surgery

Epiretinal Membrane

- Q51. Describe the etiopathogenesis, clinical feature, diagnosis, and management of epiretinal membrane.
- Q52. (a) What is an epiretinal membrane (ERM)? (b) Causes of ERM and its management.

Central Serous Chorioretinopathy

- Q53. Pachychoroid
- Q54. Central serous chorioretinopathy—etiology, pathogenesis, clinical features, and management

Q55. Management of central serous choroidopathy
Q56. What are the current management options available for a case of chronic central serous chorioretinopathy?
Q57. FFA findings in CSR

Cystoid Macular Edema

Q58. Pseudophakic CME
Q59. Current trends in the diagnosis and management of macular edema

Degenerative Myopia

Q60. Discuss the changing concepts in Mx of high myopia with a clinical appraisal of the methods available.
Q61. Clinical features of pathological myopia
Q62. Retina and vitreous in myopia

Macular Telangiectasia

Q63. Macular telangiectasia

Hereditary Fundus Dystrophy

Q64. Atypical RP
Q65. Best dystrophy
Q66. Clinical features of Stargardt disease
Q67. Flecked retina syndrome
Q68. Retinoschisis. Differential diagnosis and management
Q69. Heredomacular degeneration

Retinal Detachment

Q70. Physiological basis of retinal detachment
Q71. Lattice degeneration of retina
Q72. Differentiating features between retinoschisis and rhegmatogenous retinal detachment
Q73. Lincoff's rule
Q74. Pneumatic retinopexy
Q75. Intravitreal gases
Q76. RD surgery
Q77. Proliferative vitreoretinopathy—etiopathogenesis, clinical diagnosis, classification, and treatment. Measures to prevent PVR
Q78. Sutureless vitrectomy
Q79. Discuss the changing concepts in Mx of different types of retinal detachment
Q80. Current trends in VRSx and macular procedures
Q81. Management options of PVR
Q82. GRT
Q83. Secondary rhegmatogenous retinal detachment
Q84. (a) Clinical features and differential diagnosis of various types of retinal detachment. (b) Management of giant retinal tear.
Q85. A 21-year-old myopic male presented with a total retinal detachment in the right eye, a single causative break at 11 o'clock anterior to the equator and no PVR. (a) What are the surgical options for management of retinal detachment? (b) Explain clearly why you would recommend your chosen surgical option and outline the surgical steps.

- Q86. (a) Indications and procedure for use of various tamponading agents in retinal surgery. (b) Advantages and disadvantages of tamponading agents used in retinal surgery.
- Q87. Etiopathogenesis and management of exudative retinal detachment.
- Q88. Discuss the role of silicon oil in VR surgery. Describe its complications and method of removal.
- Q89. What are the principles of scleral buckling surgery for retinal detachment? What are its modern day indications and problems?
- Q90. Describe the clinical feature, causes, investigation, and management in a case of tractional retinal detachment.
- Q91. A 21-year-old myope (−2.5 D) presented with sudden onset profound unilateral diminution of vision. Discuss the differential diagnosis, investigation, and management.
- Q92. Highlight the basic principles of vitreoretinal surgery.

Endophthalmitis

- Q93. Endophthalmitis
- Q94. Discuss the investigations and management of a case of postoperative endophthalmitis/postcataract surgery endophthalmitis.
- Q95. Discuss the microbiological profile in infective endophthalmitis with their antibiotic sensitivity profile. Give doses and combination of antibiotics preferred for intravitreal injection. What is the normal ocular flora?
- Q96. Evaluate the rational management of endophthalmitis including a critical note on therapy-induced problems.
- Q97. Pseudophakic endophthalmitis
- Q98. Metastatic endophthalmitis
- Q99. Causes, prevention, investigation, and management of cluster endophthalmitis
- Q100. Toxic anterior segment syndrome
- Q101. Differences between TASS and endophthalmitis
- Q102. Clinical features, causes, evaluation, and management of a case of endophthalmitis, 6 weeks after cataract surgery

Miscellaneous

- Q103. Posterior vitreous detachment
- Q104. Clinical features, diagnostic tests, and management of retained intraocular foreign body
- Q105. Critically evaluate Mx of dropped nucleus.
- Q106. Management of posteriorly dislocated nucleus
- Q107. Management of dislocated nuclear fragments after phacoemulsification in a 65-year-old male presenting 1 month after surgery
- Q108. Retinal artery macroaneurysm
- Q109. Cherry red spot
- Q110. Hematological disorder in retina
- Q111. Types of RIOFB. Evaluation and management of RIOFB
- Q112. Iridofundal coloboma
- Q113. VH
- Q114. Differential diagnosis and management of a 47-year-old female patient presenting with unilateral hazy vitreous
- Q115. Hemorrhagic occlusive retinal vasculitis
- Q116. Discuss the role of anti-VEGF agents in ocular pathologies
- Q117. Wide-angle viewing system
- Q118. Pars plana surgery and its indications
- Q119. ICG dye in ophthalmology
- Q120. Vitreous substitutes
- Q121. PFCL
- Q122. Intravitreal steroids

Q123. 25G vitrectomy
Q124. Terson's syndrome
Q125. Ocular phototoxicity
Q126. ONH drusen
Q127. Verteporfin
Q128. Analyze role of genetics in retinal disorders.
Q129. MIVS
Q130. Evaluation of macular function in opaque media
Q131. MacTel
Q132. Principles, technique, indications, and complications of photodynamic therapy
Q133. What is micropulsed retinal laser? What is the change in concept of application of lasers in a micropulsed design and what are its advantages?
Q134. Approach to a case of amaurosis fugax
Q135. Enumerate macular function test
Q136. Evaluation and management of traumatic subretinal hemorrhage over the macula
Q137. A patient presents with central unilateral metamorphopsia. Discuss differential diagnosis, evaluation, and management of such a case.
Q138. Intravitreal implant and indications for their use. What are their possible side effects?
Q139. What are the recent advances in choroidal assessment on OCT? In which situations has it been applied?
Q140. Discuss the differential diagnosis, investigation, and management in a 22-year male with unilateral, profound, and sudden diminution of vision.
Q141. Classification and diagnosis of choroidal effusions
Q142. Autofluorescence
Q143. Ocular manifestation of leukemia
Q144. Dyes used for ILM peeling

Vitreous

Q1. Asteroid hyalosis and synchysis scintillans
Q2. Aging changes in vitreous
Q3. Vitreous hemorrhage

Ocular Tumors

Epibulbar Tumor

Q1. Management of ocular surface squamous neoplasia
Q2. Histopathology of invasive OSSN
Q3. Clinical presentation, diagnosis, histopathology, and management of two most common premalignant epibulbar ocular tumors
Q4. Clinical features, histopathology, and management of ocular surface squamous neoplasia (OSSN)
Q5. Ocular surface tumors

Choroidal Tumors

Q6. Enumerate the differential diagnosis of pigmented lesion of the iris

Q7. Classification, clinical features, diagnosis, differential diagnosis, histopathology, and management of choroidal melanoma

Q8. Prognostic factors in a case of choroidal melanoma

Q9. (a) Enumerate causes of iris cyst. (b) Discuss briefly the management of different types of iris cysts.

Q10. Pathology, differential diagnosis, adverse prognostic factors, and nonsurgical management of a case of choroidal melanoma

Retinal Tumors

Q11. Histopathological features of retinoblastoma/pathology of round cell tumors

Q12. Give the clinical features, staging, and management of retinoblastoma. Write a note on prognostic factors of retinoblastoma.

Q13. Recent classifications of RB from clinical and pathological viewpoints with special reference to prognosis and Mx.

Q14. Retinoblastoma management protocols

Q15. Role of plaque therapy in RB

Q16. Discuss the various avenues of Mx of bilateral RB in 1-year child

Q17. Critically evaluate treatment strategies for 18-month-old bilateral RB

Q18. Clinical features and genetic screening of primary retinal pigment disorders

Q19. Discuss the role of newer modalities of Mx in RB with their indications and details of the therapies.

Q20. Recent classification of RB

Q21. Indications, procedure, advantages, and disadvantages of chemoreduction for retinoblastoma

Q22. Genetic transmission of RB

Q23. Role of various investigative modalities in retinoblastoma

Q24. Genetics of RB

Q25. Intra-arterial chemotherapy for retinoblastoma.

Q26. Newer advances in the management of 2 DD unilateral retinoblastoma in the presenting eye and when presenting in the fellow eye in bilateral retinoblastoma.

Q27. (a) Recent advances in the management of retinoblastoma. (b) Management of a two-disc diameter raised retinoblastoma in a 3-year-old child.

Q28. Nonsurgical management of retinoblastoma

Q29. A 6-year-old boy presents with unilateral leukocoria. What is the differential diagnosis and describe management of its most common cause.

Q30. What are the various vascular retinal tumors? Briefly discuss presentation, diagnosis, and management of any two of them.

Miscellaneous

Q31. Intraocular metastasis

Q32. Write briefly on metastatic lesions of eye.

Q33. Clinical features (ocular + systemic), investigations, and treatment of a case of primary intraocular lymphoma

Strabismus

Q1. Describe methods of testing visual acuity in children/pediatric vision assessment.

Q2. (a) Various types of eye movements. (b) Various neuroanatomic pathways controlling eye movements.

Binocular Vision

Q3. Binocular vision—evolution, development, grades, and tests for assessment of binocular single vision

Q4. Anatomical and physiological basis of binocular vision

Q5. (a) Sensory adaptation to strabismus. (b) What is fusional vergence?

Q6. Stereopsis

Q7. Define abnormal retinal correspondence. Explain its development and methods of diagnosis.

Q8. What are the methods of measurement of stereopsis? Discuss the sensory and motor adaptations to strabismus.

Q9. What are the sensory adaptations in strabismus and their clinical significance?

Q10. Anomalous retinal correspondence

Q11. Worth four dot test

Q12. Method and significance of Bagolini striated glasses test

Q13. (a) Difference between a Horopter and Panum's area. (b) Sensory and motor adaptations to strabismus.

Esotropia

Q14. Define esotropia. Classification and management of esotropia in children

Q15. Describe investigation and management of esotropia in 1-year child.

Q16. Management of congenital esotropia

Q17. Infantile esotropia—clinical feature, evaluation, indications for intervention, and management. Also write a note on postoperative complications.

Q18. (a) What is AC/A ratio. (b) What are the methods of measuring it? (c) Briefly discuss the disorders resulting from altered AC:A ratio.

Q19. Describe different protocols for management of congenital esotropia.

Q20. Discuss the management of esotropia in a 5 years old child.

Q21. Evaluation and management of accommodative esotropia.

Q22. (a) Classify esotropia. (b) How would you plan the management of convergence excess esotropia in a 5-year-old child? (c) Describe the choice of procedure and surgical planning in detail.

Exotropia

Q23. Discuss IDS management, prognostic factors, and controversies.

Q24. Discuss intermittent divergent squint management, prognostic factors, and controversies.

Q25. Classify exotropia in children. Discuss its management.

Vertical Deviation

Q26. Etiology, diagnosis, and management of superior oblique overaction

Q27. Management of vertical diplopia

Q28. (a) A 45-year-old patient presents with sudden onset vertical diplopia. What is the differential diagnosis? (b) Evaluation and management of acute onset vertical diplopia.

Q29. Dissociated vertical deviation

Q30. What are dissociated vertical deviations (DVD)? How do you differentiate a DVD from an inferior oblique overaction? What is the management of DVDs?

Q31. Double elevator palsy

Q32. Surgical management of monocular elevation deficit

Q33. Management of vertical diplopia

Restrictive Strabismus

Q34. What is congenital cranial dysinnervation disorders? Give classification for CCDS.

Q35. Discuss the etiopathogenesis and clinicoinvestigative approach to restrictive strabismus.

Q36. Brown's syndrome
Q37. (a) What is Duane retraction syndrome? (b) Enumerate the types and describe the clinical features. (c) Management of a case of Duane retraction syndrome with abnormal head posture.
Q38. Classification and principles in the management of Duane retraction syndrome.

Strabismus Surgeries

Q39. Inferior oblique weakening procedures
Q40. Nonsurgical Mx of esotropia
Q41. Faden operation
Q42. Adjustable sutures in squint surgery
Q43. Evaluate various transposition surgeries in strabismus
Q44. IO weakening procedures
Q45. Anterior segment ischemia
Q46. Nonsurgical management of strabismus

Miscellaneous

Q47. Classification of amblyopia/discuss amblyopia and recent trends in management
Q48. Classification and management of amblyopia
Q49. Classification, management, and strategies for prevention of amblyopia
Q50. Microtropia
Q51. Etiology, clinical feature, and management of AV pattern deviations
Q52. A 14-year-old boy is brought by his parents with occasional deviation of the eyes. Discuss differential diagnosis, evaluation, and management of such a case.
Q53. Role of botulinum toxin in strabismus

Neuro-ophthalmology

Optic Nerve

Q1. (a) Signs of optic nerve dysfunction. (b) Various investigations available to assess the optic nerve function.
Q2. How would you evaluate the integrity of visual pathways? Discuss briefly about localization of their lesions in the context of neurological disorder.
Q3. Evaluation and management of disc edema.
Q4. Differential diagnosis, evaluation, and management of unilateral disc edema
Q5. Traumatic optic neuropathy
Q6. Discuss the clinical features, differential diagnosis, and management of optic neuritis.
Q7. Distinguishing glaucomatous from nonglaucomatous optic neuropathy.
Q8. Toxic amblyopia/etiology, clinical feature, and management of toxic optic neuropathy
Q9. Optic disc anomalies
Q10. Orbital apex syndrome
Q11. Cavernous sinus syndrome—clinical presentation and management
Q12. Papilledema and head injury
Q13. Pathogenesis and clinical features of papilledema
Q14. Describe the clinical features, diagnosis, and management of idiopathic intracranial hypertension (IIH)
Q15. Describe etiopathogenesis, clinical features, and management of AION.

- Q16. Describe the typical and atypical clinical features, evaluation, and management of arteritic AION (anterior ischemic optic neuropathy).
- Q17. Describe the approach to a 73-year-old male patient who complains of a profound unilateral loss of vision in one eye, followed by a similar loss on the other after 8 weeks. What are the diagnosis, clinical features, investigations, and management of such a case?
- Q18. Ischemic optic neuropathy—diagnosis and management
- Q19. Optic nerve head drusen
- Q20. Discuss etiopathogenesis, differential diagnosis, and Mx of unilateral swelling of ON head.
- Q21. Multiple sclerosis (ocular aspect)
- Q22. Drug-induced optic neuropathies
- Q23. Congenital optic disc anomalies
- Q24. Describe the clinical features, diagnosis, and Mx of a case of methyl alcohol poisoning.
- Q25. A 45-year-old patient presents with unilateral central scotoma. Discuss differential diagnosis, evaluation, and management of such a case.
- Q26. A 34-year-old pregnant lady presents with sudden bilateral loss of vision. What are the likely causes? How will you treat them?
- Q27. Papilledema and head injury

Pupil

- Q28. Discuss examination of the pupil and its significance.
- Q29. Describe the pupillary pathways in detail and their affections with a diagram. Different tests to elucidate them
- Q30. Types of afferent pupillary defect
- Q31. Physiological basis and causes of light near dissociation
- Q32. Horner's Syndrome. Pharmacological tests for diagnosis/etiology, clinical features, diagnosis, and differential diagnosis of Horner's syndrome.
- Q33. What is anisocoria, indications for its investigation and management.

Chiasmal and Retrochiasmal Lesion

- Q34. Visual pathway and localization of field defects
- Q35. Discuss and compare the type of visual field defects in glaucoma and neuro-ophthalmic conditions.
- Q36. Anatomy of optic chiasma, discuss briefly the various lesions affecting visual fields (role in health and disease).
- Q37. Pituitary lesions for ophthalmologist
- Q38. Chiasmal syndromes
- Q39. Cortical blindness
- Q40. Causes and ocular manifestations of chiasmal lesions

3rd Cranial Nerve Palsy

- Q41. Discuss 3rd cranial nerve palsy—etiology, clinical feature, and management
- Q42. Clinical features and management of 3rd nerve palsy
- Q43. Anatomy of 3rd, 4th, and 6th cranial nerve and enumerate the lesions of each nucleus.
- Q44. Causes, investigations, and management of acute onset 3rd nerve palsy

4th Cranial Nerve Palsy

- Q45. A 27-year-old driver developed left eye hypertropia following an accident. How will you diagnose and manage him?
- Q46. (a) Pathway of 4th cranial nerve. (b) Enumerate the causes of 4th nerve palsy (acquired) with respect to site of affections.
- Q47. Management of unilateral and bilateral 4th nerve palsy

6th Cranial Nerve Palsy

Q48. One and half syndrome
Q49. Describe and discuss investigation and management of a case of ophthalmoplegia.
Q50. Etiology and management of ophthalmoplegias
Q51. Orbital apex syndrome
Q52. Management options in a case of lateral rectus palsy with visually disabling diplopia.

Nystagmus

Q53. (a) Nystagmus—definition and types. (b) Approach and examination of a case of congenital nystagmus. (c) Surgical options for nystagmus and their outcome.
Q54. Clinical conditions in which nystagmus is observed.
Q55. Five features of infantile nystagmus syndrome
Q56. Kestenbaum–Anderson procedure
Q57. Spasmus nutans syndrome
Q58. Upbeat and downbeat nystagmus

Ocular Myopathies

Q59. Myasthenia gravis
Q60. (a) Clinical features and diagnostic tests of ocular myasthenia. (b) Important differential diagnosis and points to differentiate.
Q61. Etiology, types, clinical picture, differential diagnosis, and management of myasthenia gravis

Miscellaneous

Q62. Internuclear ophthalmoplegia
Q63. One and half syndrome—its cause and clinical features
Q64. Superior orbital fissure syndrome—clinical presentation and management
Q65. Tests for malingering
Q66. Describe etiopathogenesis and appearance of visual field changes in neurological disorders.
Q67. Clinical feature and Mx of ocular migraine
Q68. Cerebellopontine angle tumor
Q69. Essential blepharospasm
Q70. (a) Enumerate causes of unilateral profound painless loss of vision. (b) How will you manage such a case in a 65-year-old male patient?
Q71. (a) What are the main types of migraine? (b) Differential diagnoses of the visual phenomena that accompany an attack of migraine.
Q72. Causes of unilateral sudden vision loss in a 16-year-old girl
Q73. Cavernous sinus thrombosis

Investigations

Q1. Describe the electrophysiology and applied aspects of ERG, VER, and EOG.
Q2. Types of ERG and their application
Q3. (a) Genesis of visual evoked potential (VEP). (b) What are the types of VEP and enumerate the conditions for assisting in diagnosis and management of the conditions. (c) Limitation of VEP.
Q4. Discuss the electrophysiological tests and their relevance in ophthalmic disorders.

Q5. OCT angiography—principle and clinical application
Q6. Tests for color vision
Q7. Tests of stereoacuity
Q8. Tests for contrast sensitivity
Q9. Color vision testing
Q10. Tests for malingering
Q11. Corneal topography/describe corneal topography and its documentation and their applied aspects.
Q12. Automated perimetry—indication and utility
Q13. HVF analysis. Interpretation of automated perimetry printout
Q14. ICG angiography
Q15. Multifocal ERG (mfERG) and its clinical importance
Q16. Fundus fluorescein angiography. Causes of hyperfluorescence and blocked fluorescence in fluorescein angiography
Q17. OCT in ophthalmology/principle of optical coherence tomography. Indications of use of above modality in different ocular conditions. Recent advances in OCT.
Q18. Role of OCT in glaucoma and neuro-ophthalmologic disorders
Q19. What is OCT? What are its advantages over conventional imaging? Name the conditions where it helps in precise diagnosis.
Q20. Enumerate the uses of optical coherence principle in ophthalmology. What equipment are based on this principle and their advantages?
Q21. Role of OCT and FFA in retinal disorders
Q22. Ocular USG
Q23. Automated perimetry—indications and utility
Q24. UBM and its role in ophthalmology. (a) Principle and uses of UBM. (b) Its advantages and disadvantages over anterior segment OCT. Enumerate conditions where it is a preferred mode of investigation.
Q25. PENTACAM
Q26. ASOCT
Q27. IOL master
Q28. Pachymetry
Q29. GDx
Q30. HRT
Q31. DCT
Q32. ORBSCAN
Q33. ORA (ocular response analyzer)
Q34. Wavefront imaging
Q35. Laser interferometer
Q36. VER
Q37. Describe newly available modalities for imaging of the anterior segment.
Q38. (a) What is the principle of ophthalmic biometry. (b) Which ophthalmic equipment uses this principle? (c) What are the advantages and disadvantages of this type of biometry?
Q39. Principles of MRI and its role in practice of ophthalmology.

Ocular Trauma

Q1. Discuss the pathophysiology, clinical evaluation, and management of suprachoroidal hemorrhage
Q2. Discuss the classification of blunt ocular trauma and describe the management of case of total hyphema.

Q3. Evaluation and management of near total hyphemia in a 10-year-old boy postinjury with a ball presenting to you on the 2nd day.
Q4. Traumatic hyphema—grading, investigation, complication, and management
Q5. Principle of primary open globe injury repair
Q6. Prognostic significances of various manifestations of ocular trauma on the globe and adnexa as appreciated in your casualty.
Q7. Evaluate vision-threatening injuries and discuss principles for their Mx from the standpoint of best possible outcomes.
Q8. Open globe injury
Q9. Critically analyze the recent advances in orbital and canalicular interventions with special reference to trauma.
Q10. Classification and grading system for mechanical ocular injuries. Discuss medicolegal aspects of ocular trauma.
Q11. Prevention of ocular injuries during Diwali festival.
Q12. Discuss classifications of ocular trauma. Outline the types of IOFBs and their critical Mx
Q13. Ocular manifestations in a case of head injuries vis-a-vis their role in management
Q14. (a) Enumerate the various consequences of a closed globe injury by a blunt object. (b) How would you distinguish between open-globe and closed-globe injury?
Q15. Evaluation and management of a case presenting with iridodialysis.
Q16. Evaluation and management of traumatic subretinal hemorrhage over the macula.
Q17. Siderosis bulbi—clinical features and electrophysiological changes in ERG
Q18. (a) Effect of blunt trauma on normal lens. (b) Management of subluxated lens following trauma
Q19. (a) Posterior segment complications in a case of blunt trauma to the eye. (b) How will you manage them?
Q20. Concussion injuries—classification, management, long-term sequelae, and prognosis
Q21. A patient presented with total loss of vision in one eye, 2 days following trauma to the eye with a cricket ball. Discuss the possible causes.
Q22. Briefly evaluate vision-threatening injuries and discuss the principles of their management from the standpoint of the best possible outcome.
Q23. Discuss ocular manifestations of head injury and its management.

Community Ophthalmology and Biostatistics

Q1. What are the types of prospective studies and their advantages? What are the methods to avoid bias in a study?
Q2. Discuss briefly the causes, magnitude, categories, and preventive strategies for vision impairment.
Q3. Low vision aids
Q4. (a) Categories of low vision and classification of low vision aids (LVA). (b) Evaluation of a patient with low vision.
Q5. Definition of blindness and low vision. What is the recent change in NPCB criteria for blindness and what impact does it have?
Q6. What are the objectives and action plan of "National Programme for Control of Blindness" (NPCB)? Give the definition of blindness as per NPCB and WHO.
Q7. WHO guidelines on visual impairment
Q8. Strategies to decrease morbidity by glaucoma in the country. Ideal model for glaucoma service in a tertiary care center
Q9. Reach in program.
Q10. Strategies to control cataract blindness in India.
Q11. Discuss various LVA available and their clinical applicability.
Q12. What are low vision aids? Discuss their indications and optical principles
Q13. Evaluate strategies to decrease childhood blindness in Vision 2020. Strategies to control cataract blindness in India

Q14. Vision 2020 and India
Q15. Discuss NPCB and Vision 2020 with special reference to combating corneal blindness
Q16. Eye camp approach versus reach in approach
Q17. Discuss briefly the problems in rehabilitation of visually handicapped children. How could you organize an effective eye screening program in a semi-urban school in your community with special reference to refractive errors?
Q18. Discuss strategies to reduce ocular morbidities in diabetics in your country.
Q19. Discuss viable strategies to reduce amblyopia at the community level.
Q20. Discuss in detail about reach in program for management of cataract in community.
Q21. Discuss visual aids and their relevance to our national program for control of blindness and Vision 2020 in India.
Q22. Predominant causes of blindness in India and national initiatives for prevention. Outline the strategies to reduce the incidence of various ocular injuries in the community.
Q23. Diabetic retinopathy and Vision 2020
Q24. Design a suitable screening program for diabetic retinopathy at community level and its importance in light of recent advances in its management.
Q25. Discuss cataract surgical rate in the context of the national program with special reference to the visual outcome of such surgeries.
Q26. Discuss prevention of childhood eye disorders and role of our school health programs.
Q27. Discuss strategies to reduce morbidity caused by preventable ocular trauma in the country.
Q28. Discuss in detail the causes and management of childhood blindness in India.
Q29. Discuss your strategies for tackling major causes of visual impairment in the community with special reference to children under the NPCB and Vision 2020.
Q30. Discuss the various approaches to rehabilitation of visually handicapped.
Q31. Write about the magnitude of blindness in the country and the proportion being contributed by various eye diseases. Discuss the challenges and strategies for elimination of blindness caused by diabetic retinopathy and glaucoma.
Q32. What are the various initiatives under NPCB? Perform a critical analysis of various strategies of the program.
Q33. Evolution, structure, and functioning of eye banks in India
Q34. Childhood blindness
Q35. Role of hospital corneal retrieval program in eye banking
Q36. What are the objectives, strategies, approaches, and organizations of Vision 2020 program? Strategies of Government of India to achieve these targets.
Q37. Types of screening procedures in ophthalmology. Difference between screening and survey procedures. Give an example of screening program in ophthalmic practice
Q38. (a) What is a "randomized control trial"? (b) What is randomization and why is it required? (c) What are confounding factors in a study and how to avoid them?
Q39. (a) Tests of significance. (b) Standard deviation. (c) Confidence interval.
Q40. (a) What are bias and confounding in statistical analysis? (b) A sample of 100 patients was segregated into two groups to check the IOP-lowering effect of two different antiglaucoma medications. Give possible causes of bias and possible confounders.
Q41. (a) Measures of central tendency in a series of observations. (b) Measures of variability of individual observations.
Q42. Enumerate causes of childhood blindness. How will you calculate the sample size and plan a survey for childhood blindness in India.
Q43. How will you calculate the incidence and prevalence of a disease? How will you calculate the sample size and plan a survey for cataract blindness.
Q44. Enumerate two broad headings for study designs and give one example under each category.
Q45. Define specificity and sensitivity in evaluating screening tests. What is their relevance to positive and negative predictive value of the test?
Q46. Guidelines and mandatory requirement for conducting eye camps in India.
Q47. How would you set up a screening camp for glaucoma?

Q48. Describe the magnitude, prevalence, and causes of blindness in India.
Q49. Describe the types and methodology of epidemiologic survey.
Q50. Discuss the cataract surgical rate in context of the national program with special reference to the visual outcome of such surgery.
Q51. Rapid assessment survey

Ophthalmic Microbiology, Pharmacology, and Pathology

Ophthalmic Microbiology

Q1. Laboratory diagnosis of microbial keratitis
Q2. Lab diagnosis of trachoma
Q3. Polymerase chain reaction

Ophthalmic Pharmacology

Q4. Mitomycin C in ophthalmology. Mention its side effects.
Q5. Antiviral agents
Q6. Antifungal drugs/antifungals used in ophthalmology; classification, clinical uses, and adverse effect
Q7. What is the role of anti-VEGF agents in ophthalmic diseases? Discuss the mechanism of action, indication, contraindications, and outcomes of these agents.
Q8. What are the various steroids used in ophthalmology? Discuss common preparation, potency, mode of administration, indication, contraindication, and side effect.
Q9. Classify immunomodulators and discuss their role in various ophthalmic disorders
Q10. (a) Role of immunosuppressive drugs in ophthalmic conditions. (b) Enumerate the commonly used drugs with their dosage and complications.
Q11. Antimetabolites used in ophthalmology
Q12. Enumerate the microbiological techniques available to diagnose and identify the cause of intraocular infection. Discuss the advantages and disadvantages of each technique.
Q13. Botulinum toxin in ophthalmology—mechanism of action, indications, and complications
Q14. Role of antioxidants in ophthalmology
Q15. Indications of pulse steroid therapy in ophthalmology (ON, early rejection PK, VKH, AION)
Q16. (a) Name the commonly used preservatives in ophthalmic medication. (b) What are the advantages and disadvantages of preservatives in ophthalmic medications? (c) What are the various means of preventing these adverse effects?
Q17. Methods to increase the ocular bioavailability and efficacy of drugs used in the treatment of ocular disorders, along with example.
Q18. (a) Role of newer antiviral agents used in ophthalmology. (b) What are the specific advantages of these over available antivirals?
Q19. Describe the barriers to drug penetration in the cornea. What is partition coefficient? Describe the various factors affecting drug penetration with respect to drug formulation and corneal anatomy.
Q20. What is the pharmacological MOA of cyclosporine? What are its clinical uses in ophthalmology?
Q21. What are the various steroids used in ophthalmology? Discuss the preparation, potency, modes of administration, indication, contraindication, and side effects.

Ophthalmic Pathology

Q22. Chemical fixatives for histopathological examination of ophthalmic specimens
Q23. Application of routine and special stains in histopathology

Recent Advances

Q1. Stem cells in ocular conditions
Q2. Immunosuppressives in ophthalmology
Q3. Lasers in ophthalmology
Q4. (a) Classify LASERs used in ophthalmic practice. (b) Uses of LASERs in ocular disorders. (c) Safety precautions in LASER delivery
Q5. Femtosecond laser in ophthalmology
Q6. Drug delivery implants in eye
Q7. Describe briefly recent advances in alleviation of irreversible blindness—LVA, stem cells, and retinal implants.
Q8. Use of nanotechnology in ophthalmic disease
Q9. Role of gene therapy in ophthalmic diseases
Q10. Genetic counseling in ocular disorders
Q11. Drug implant
Q12. Drug delivery system in ophthalmology
Q13. Role and application of telemedicine in ophthalmology
Q14. Write a critical note on role of genetics in important blinding disorders.
Q15. Artificial eye/visual prosthesis/what is a bionic eye? What are the principles of its working and enumerate its indications.
Q16. Enumerate and describe the role of various biomarkers which may be beneficial in diagnosis, pathogenesis, treatment strategies, and prevention of various ocular morbidities
Q17. Indications of fibrin glue in ophthalmology

Systemic Disorders and Eye, Drug Toxicity

Q1. Pregnancy-induced ocular problems
Q2. (a) Ocular manifestations of dengue fever. (b) How will you monitor and manage a case of dengue fever from ophthalmic standpoint?
Q3. Describe the ocular involvement in SLE.
Q4. Describe the ocular involvement in sleep apnea syndrome.
Q5. Describe the ocular features due to deficiency of vitamins A, B1, B2, C, and D.
Q6. Outline important systemic disorders affecting eye and their salient ocular symptoms and signs.
Q7. Juvenile systemic disorders affecting eye
Q8. Eye in epidemic dropsy
Q9. Critically evaluate nutritional factors causing ocular morbidity
Q10. Ocular manifestation of connective disorders
Q11. Lifestyle modification in a diabetic patient
Q12. Enumerate the various ocular manifestations of Hansen's disease. Discuss management of lagophthalmos.
Q13. Common systemic medications and ocular toxicity
Q14. Ocular side effects of oral contraceptive pills
Q15. Sarcoidosis and eye
Q16. Ocular manifestations in collagen disorders
Q17. Ocular manifestation of leukemia
Q18. Discuss juvenile systemic disorders affecting the eye.

Q19. Ocular aspects of multiple sclerosis
Q20. Discuss salient indications and hazards of radiation to the eye.
Q21. Critically evaluate nutritional factors causing ocular morbidity
Q22. Von Hippel–Lindau disease

Miscellaneous

Sterilization and Disinfection

Q1. Describe the various zones in OT. Describe the techniques used for sterilization of the various types of ophthalmic instruments.
Q2. OT disinfection and sterilization
Q3. Discuss various preoperative and perioperative aseptic approaches for prevention of intraocular infection.
Q4. Sterilization techniques—ophthalmic operation theater, surgical instruments, and logistics
Q5. Describe the guidelines for setting up a new ophthalmic operation theater and methods to keep it sterile
Q6. Postoperative infections—prevention and management
Q7. (a) Essential components of modular ophthalmic operating room. (b) Disinfection and sterilization of operating room.

Others

Q8. (a) Define and enumerate vital dyes used in ophthalmology. (b) Clinical applications of vital dyes in diagnosis and treatment of ophthalmic diseases.
Q9. Genetic counseling in ocular disorders
Q10. Vital dyes in ocular surgery
Q11. Various dyes in ophthalmology
Q12. Uniocular diplopia
Q13. How would you approach and manage a case of diplopia?
Q14. Sutures and needles in ophthalmology
Q15. Ocular stem cells
Q16. HLA antigens
Q17. Anterior segment of newborn
Q18. Outline dystrophies and degenerations of eye
Q19. How would you organize an upgraded residency training program in ophthalmology in your institute?
Q20. Hazards of radiation to eye
Q21. Discuss iatrogenic disorders of eye
Q22. A 64-year-old individual presents with sudden profound unilateral loss of vision. Discuss etiology, evaluation, and management.
Q23. Critically evaluate the causes for failing vision in elderly patient.

Index

Page numbers followed by *b* refer to box, *f* refer to figure, *fc* refer to flowchart, and *t* refer to table.

A

Abaxial proptosis 147
   causes of 238*t*
   differential diagnosis of 148*fc*
Abducens
   nerve 128, 353
   nucleus 360*f*
Aberrant regeneration 78
   management of 84
Ablative therapy 892
Ablepharon-macrostomia syndrome 12
Abscess 496
   intracranial 178
   intraorbital 146
   orbital 176*f*, 208
   subperiosteal 146, 176*f*, 179
   subretinal 496
Acanthamoeba
   astronyxis 643
   castellani 643
   culbertsoni 643
   divionensis 643
   keratitis 643, 646*t*, 655, 800
      differential diagnosis of 645*t*
      management of 643
         steroids in 638
   palestinensis 643
   polyphaga 643
   rhysodes 643
Accessory lacrimal gland 240
Accommodative esotropia 369, 375
   evaluation of 375
Acetylcholinesterase
   antibody 32
   inhibitors 291
Achromatopsia 310
   incomplete 450
Acid-fast bacillus 884
Acids 868, 869
Acquired immunodeficiency syndrome 71, 318, 498, 740, 886, 899
Acquired ptosis 22, 23
   causes of 29
   diagnosis of 29
   management of 29
   pathophysiology of 29
Acrocephaly 223*f*
Acrylic prosthesis, spectacle-retained 260
Actinic keratosis 271
Actinomycin D 147
Active force generation test 282, 288
Acute conjunctivitis 613, 615
   clinical features of 613
   etiology of 613
Acute graft rejection, management of 709

Acute graft versus-host disease 728, 730
Acute posterior multifocal placoid pigment epitheliopathy 470, 487, 494, 509
Acyclovir 657
Adalimumab 170, 518, 886, 901, 906
Adenocystic carcinoma 216
Adenoid cystic carcinoma 214, 894
Adenomas
   benign 343
   invasive 343
Adenosine receptor agonist 553, 555
Adenoviral conjunctivitis 616
   treatment of 616
Adhesion bands 246
Adhesive-retained silicone prosthesis 260
Adie's syndrome 341, 641
Adie's tonic pupil 341
Adison's syndrome 327
Adnexa 466, 620, 644
   indication 886
   monoclonal antibodies 886
   ocular effects 886
Adnexal papillary cystadenoma 892
Adrenergic agents 580
Advanced glaucomatous field defect 531
Advantage over laser ablation technique 853
Advantage over laser thermal keratoplasty 853
Age-related macular degeneration 447, 749
Agranulocytosis 162
Agraphia 346
Ahmed glaucoma drainage device 570*f*
Aicardi syndrome 325
Akinetopsia 346
Albinism 411, 900
Alcohol keratoepitheliectomy 201, 275
Alexia 346
Alfa-adrenergic receptor agonists 545, 547
Alkali 868, 869
Alkyl nitrites 887
Allopurinol 887
Alopecia 494
Alumina 263
Aluminum oxide 263
Alzheimer's disease 741
Amantadine 886
Amaurosis fugax 429
Amblyopia 326, 393, 413
   anisometropic 393, 394
   classification of 393 394
   management of 392-394, 789
   prevention of 394
   risk of 233
   therapy 809
      recent advances in 394
Amblyoscopic test 294

Ambrosio-enhanced ectasia display 794
Amebiasis 488
Amelanotic nevi 274
American Joint Committee on Cancer 200, 200*t*, 277
Ametropic amblyopia 393, 394
Aminoglycoside 645, 646
Amiodarone 322, 826, 886, 887, 888
Amitriptyline 350
Ammonia 868
Amniotic band sequence 12
Amniotic membrane
   graft 249, 651, 691, 705, 778
   transplant 515, 705, 771, 872
Amorphous corneal dystrophy, posterior 672, 675
Amorphous stromal dystrophy 675
Amphotericin B 182, 667
Ampulla 303
Amsler grid test 879
Amsler sign 476
Amsler-Krumeich classification 696*t*, 787
Amyloidosis 451, 683
Anaglyph principle 364, 365
Anakinra 170, 518
Ancylostoma caninum 488
Anesthesia, type of 35
Aneurysm 282, 483, 484
   rupture of 240
Angiography 243
Angioid streaks 421
Angioneurotic edema 694
Angioscotomata 531
Angiotensin-converting enzyme 348, 469, 479
Angle
   closure glaucoma 442, 444, 515 549, 583
   developmental anomalies of 522
   kappa 219
Angular blepharitis 14
Angular vein 100
Anidulafungin 668
Aniridia 523, 524*f*, 527, 528, 542
Anisocoria 339
   physiological 339
Ankylosing spondylitis 466, 477
   juvenile 471, 475
Anomaloscope 416
Anomalous dentition 229
Anomalous retinal correspondence 361*f*, 362, 363, 366, 367, 369
Anophthalmia 223, 243, 249, 250
   clinical 223
   congenital 223, 251*f*
   esophageal-genital syndrome 250
   onset of 249

Anophthalmic socket 245
   causes of 249
Anophthalmos 221, 223
   congenital clinical 249
Anterior chamber 425, 426, 466, 566, 566*f*, 624, 632, 644, 709, 710, 723, 725, 774, 864, 869, 886
   depth evaluation 726
   distortion of 749
   gas bubbles 830
   intraocular lens 824
   irregular 824
   paracentesis 625
   phakic intraocular lens 846
   reaction 774
Anterior cleavage syndromes 525
Anterior epithelium layer, cells of 463
Anterior lamellar
   recession 46*f*
   reposition 46
   therapeutic keratoplasty 718, 782
Anterior orbital basal cell carcinoma 260*f*
Anterior segment
   dysgenesis 587, 763
   ischemia 391
   manifestation 889, 904
   optical coherence tomography 230, 471, 543, 563, 564*f*, 629, 631, 677, 678, 691, 698, 778
Anterior stromal puncture 599, 691
Anterior uveitis 481, 498, 505, 513, 519, 690, 889
   cytomegalovirus-associated 505
Anterior visual pathway 322
Anthelminthic therapy 503
Antiapoptosis 725*t*
Antibiotics 640, 871
   preservative-free 769
   therapy 254, 616, 766
   topical 17
Anticholinergic agents 580
Anticoagulants 581
Anticollagenase drugs 650
Antidepressants 581
Antifibrinolytic agents 876
Antifibrotic agents 588
Antifungal drugs 667
Antigen presenting cells 708, 713*f*, 714, 729
Antigenic keratan sulfate 674
Antiglaucoma drugs 627
Antiglaucoma medications 546, 598, 650, 710, 876
   newer 553
Anti-inflammatory drugs 650
Anti-interleukin therapy 518
Antimetabolites 141, 403, 480, 770
Antimicrobial therapy 626
Antimuscle-specific kinase antibody 290
Antineutrophil cytoplasmic antibody 139, 225, 402, 484, 898
Antinuclear antibody 139, 225, 402, 469, 472, 474, 901
Antioxidants 595
Antiphospholipid antibody 225, 484
Antiplatelet agents, role of 333
Antiplatelets 876
Antithrombotic therapy 507
Antithyroglobulin antibodies 160

Antithyroid drugs 161
Antithyroid peroxidase antibodies 160
Anti-toxoplasma antibodies 501
Antitumor necrosis factor-alpha 170
Anti-vascular endothelial growth factor therapy 509, 711
Antiviral therapy 616
Anton syndrome 346
Aortic valvular insufficiency 478
Aphakia 578
Aphakic bullous keratopathy 690
Applanation tonometry 542, 805
Apraclonidine test 33, 339, 340
Aqueous humor replacement 871
Aqueous lacrimal secretion 86
Aqueous misdirection 727
Arcade, peripheral 9
Arcuate keratotomy 843, 855, 857
Arcus
   juvenilis 682
   senilis 682
Arden gratings 311
Argon laser photocoagulation 431
Argyll Robertson pupil 337, 521
Arhinencephaly 243
Arteriovenous malformations 137
   embolization 239
Arteritic anterior ischemic optic neuropathy 330, 334
Artery, frontal 8
Arthralgia 162
Arthritis 474
Artificial tears 850
Ascorbate 872
Ascorbic acid 882
Aspergillus fumigatus 648
Aspheric rigid gas permeable lens 798
Aspiration 819
Asteroid hyalosis 451
Asthma, atopy-bronchial 694
Astigmatic corneal surgeries 843
Astigmatic keratotomy 843, 857
Astigmatism 785, 787
   irregular 835, 838
   management of postoperative 858
Astrocytes, migration of 411
Ataxia telangiectasia 231
Atovaquone 502
Atropine 467
Audiogram 893
Aura, part of 349
Autoimmune diseases 477, 826
Autoimmune disorders 648
Autoimmune pathogenesis 508
Autoimmune thyroid disease 158
Autologous serum eye drops 851, 872
Autosomal dominant
   disorder 464
   inheritance 823
Autosomal recessive disorder 823
Avellino dystrophy 680
Axenfeld-Rieger anomaly 464, 523, 525, 527*f*
Axenfeld-Rieger syndrome 523, 524*f*, 542
Axial system 297
Azathioprine 169, 403, 480, 494, 901, 906
Azelastine 769
Azithromycin 502
Azoles 645, 646, 668

B

Bacillus Calmette-Guérin 402
Bacterial keratitis 648
   clinical features of 622
   differential diagnosis of 623*t*
   etiology of 622
   management of 622, 626*fc*
Bacterial orbital cellulitis 174, 176
Bacterial ulcers, steroids in 636
Bagolini striated glass test 362, 362*f*, 365, 367
Balance technique 52
Balint syndrome 346
Bandage contact lens 631, 634, 640, 660, 673, 691, 866
   use of 649
Bartonella infection 479
Basal cell
   carcinoma 112*f*, 116, 257*f*
      management of 118
   nevi syndrome 327
Base cryotherapy 275
Basiliximab 712
B-carotene 766
Behçet's disease 466, 472, 484, 489, 516, 520
Bell's palsy 4
Bell's phenomenon 36, 67, 75
Benedikt's syndrome 281*f*
Benzalkonium chloride 792
Berlin nodules 904
Best fit
   sphere 698
   toric ellipsoid 698
Best-corrected visual acuity 427, 696, 721, 832
Beta-adrenergic
   blockers 547
   receptor antagonists 545
Beta-irradiation therapy 570
Bevacizumab 888
   topical 711
Bick's procedure 49
Bielschowsky's theory 380
Biguanides 645, 646
Bilobed flap 57, 58
Bimanual microincision phacoemulsification 816
Binocular function 281
Binocular stimulation imbalance 380
Binocular vision 360
   anatomical basis of 363
   assessment of 360
   development of 360
   evolution of 360
   physiological basis of 363
   tests for 361
Bio-hazardous waste disposal 740
Biometry 808, 827
Biopsy 514
Biplanar incision 603*f*
Birdshot
   chorioretinopathy 508
   uveitis 507
Birmingham eye trauma terminology 862
Bisphosphonates 886
Bitot's spot 763, 763*f*, 881
Bjerrum scotoma 530
Blau syndrome 474, 475, 507

Bleb 560
    assessment of 561
    classification 563
Bleeding 847
Bleomycin 239
Blepharitis 14
    acute 14
    anterior 14
    categorization of 16*t*
    chronic 14
    classification of 14
    clinical features of 14
    management of 14
    marginal 14
    pathogenesis of 14
    posterior 14, 15, 17
    presentation, differential diagnosis of 16
    risk factors of 14
    types of 14
Blepharophimosis 23, 28, 29
    syndrome 21, 29*f*
        components of 28
Blepharoptosis 19
Blepharospasm 295, 702
    benign essential 60, 61*f*, 350
    management of essential 350
Blind eye 294
Blind spot
    enlargement of 531
    mechanism 367, 369
Blindness 293
    nutritional 881
    partial 294
Blinking exercises 885
Blood
    agar, fresh 402
    borne growth 662
    investigations 282, 320, 430
    pressure 893
    sugars, fasting 802
    thinners 802
    urea nitrogen 469
    vessels 460
Blue cone monochromatism 450
Blue dot cataract 808
Blue rubber bleb nevus syndrome 238, 239
Blue-field entoptic phenomenon 458
Blue-yellow color vision 310
Blunt trauma 859
Blurred vision 508, 653, 780
B-lymphocyte inhibitor 141
Body tissues 205
Boeck candy test 370, 397
Bone
    autogenous 136
    bleeding 100
    defect, repair of 244
    flaps replaced 235
    fossa formation 210*f*
    lytic lesions 209
    marrow 215, 518
        biopsy 229, 348
    removal 235
Bony abnormalities 225
Bosma arhinia microphthalmia syndrome 250
Botulinum toxin 47*f*, 60, 68, 282, 351
    cosmetic indications of 62

    injection 61*f*, 392
        complications of 62*t*
    role of 396
Botulism 289
Bourneville disease 231
Bowel disease, inflammatory 471, 477, 478
Bowman's layer 678, 779, 788
    micro-distortions 838
    transplant 717
Bowman's membrane 515, 677, 682, 683
    transplant 717
Brachycephaly 223*f*
Bradycardia 291
Brain 315, 327
    parenchyma 207*f*
    stem, tumors of 304
    tributaries from 307
Branch retinal vein occlusion 451
Brimonidine 595
Brodsky's theory 381
Broken zonules, signs of 824
Bromophenol blue 433
Bronchoalveolar lavage 514
Brow complex 76, 76*fc*
    examination of 75
Brow ptosis, management of 83
Brown's pigmentation 274
Brown's syndrome 383, 385
    acquired 384
    grades of 385
Bruch's membrane 326, 413, 463
    synthesis 413
Brücke's muscle 461
Brugia malayi 488
B-scan ultrasonography 335, 491
Buccal mucosa transplantation 873
Buckling theory 129
Bullous serous retinal detachments 493
Burkitt's lymphoma 347
Burning sensation 15
Burnt out open-angle glaucoma 585
Busacca's nodules 466

C

C chart 398
Café au lait spots 144, 209*f*
Calcineurin inhibitor 141, 710, 770
Calcitonin gene-related peptide 713
Calcium
    channel blockers 595
    hydroxide 869
Caldwell projection 204
Calhoun staging 378
Cam vision stimulator 393
Canalicular agenesis 92
Canalicular injury, repair of 105
Canalicular laceration, repair of 861
Canalicular obstruction 105
    management of 103
Canalicular trephination 103, 104
Canalicular wall dysgenesis 92
Canaliculitis, etiological factors for 101
Canaliculoplasty 104
Canaliculops 93
Canaliculus 87
    lower 87
Canaloplasty 556, 558

Cancer, radiation-induced 895
Candida 499, 899
Candidial endophthalmitis 499
Candidiasis 512
Candle wax dripping 484, 513
Cannulation technique 110
Canthal fixation, adequate 52
Canthal injury, repair of lateral 861
Canthal laxity, lateral 42*f*
Canthal tendon 5
    lateral 5, 82, 84
Canthaxanthin 887
Canthi 2
Cantholysis, lateral 54
Canthopexy, lateral 234
Canthoplasty 234
Canthotomy, lateral 54, 164
Capillary plexuses 411
Capsular contraction syndrome 754
Capsular opacification, posterior 749, 820
Capsular tear, early posterior 454
Capsulopalpebral fascia 6
Capsulorhexis
    continuous circular 819
    incomplete 819
Carbamazepine 351
Carbonic anhydrase inhibitors 329, 545, 547
Cardiorespiratory anomalies 229
Cardiovascular disease 478
Carotid artery 298
    external 8, 125
    internal 8, 240, 305*f*
Carotid bruits 330
Carotid cavernous fistula 147, 240
Carotid Doppler 430
Caruncle 277
Caspofungin 668
Cataract 400, 454, 473, 476, 771, 801, 884
    bilateral 806, 806*t*
    congenital 806
    development, mechanism for 811
    extraction, intracapsular 824
    late rosette 811
    management 515
    membranous 811
    morphology of 807*t*, 812
    partially absorbed 811
    posterior subcapsular 467
    postsurgery for congenital 577
    removal 818
    screening for 807
    surgery 601, 748, 749, 801, 817, 856, 857
        indications for 817
        preoperative testing for 801
        small pupil during 813
        surgical intervention for 906
    traumatic 810, 813
    unilateral 806, 806*t*
    visually significant 515
Cataractogenesis 848
Catarrhal marginal ulcer 777
Catford drum test 370, 397
Cat-scratch disease 639
Cavernous hemangioma 139, 237, 238, 342
    management of 237
    pathology of 238
Cavernous sinus 240, 306, 340
    anatomy of 306, 306*f*

communication of 306, 307f
    drains 307
    thrombosis 146, 173, 176f, 178, 307
Ceftazidime 753
Cefuroxime 753
Cells 864
    density 745
    simple 300
Cellular mechanisms 151
Cellulitis, fungal orbital 180, 182f
Cenegermin, role of 642
Central corneal
    edema 566f
    guttae 688
    thickness 700, 795
Central nervous system 178, 194, 222, 479, 493, 880, 892, 893, 898
    lymphoma, primary 194
Central retinal artery 124, 408
    occlusion 421
Central retinal vein occlusion 125, 421, 451
Central vision, loss of 568
Cephalocele 243
Cerebellar artery, inferior 306
Cerebellar peduncle, inferior 303
Cerebellum 303
Cerebral achromatopsia 345
Cerebral artery 298
    posterior 313
Cerebral vasculitis 509
Cerebral vision loss, acute-onset 345
Cerebrospinal fluid 100, 131, 167, 191, 215, 235, 318, 469, 492, 509, 532
    diversion procedures 329
    leak 134, 259
    pleocytosis 494
Certolizumab 518
Cervical lymph node examination 75
Chamber intraocular lens decentration, posterior 754
Chamber-associated immune deviation 713
Charge syndrome 12, 325
Charleux sign 694
Chemical
    chelation 515
    injury 248, 649
        acute 868
        Dua's classification of 870
Chemoreduction 275
Chemosis 185f, 622
    conjunctival 730
Chemotherapeutic agents, topical 275
Chemotherapy 191, 229, 234, 279
    adjuvant 227, 229
    intravenous 191
    role of 227
Cherry red spot 423, 424
    causes of 423, 424
Chest X-ray 225, 469, 514
Chiasm, arterial supply of 298
Chiasma 297
    anatomy of 342
    prefixed 297
Chiasmal diseases 344
Chiasmal lesion 342
    ocular manifestation of 342
Chiasmal syndromes 342

Chlamydia 478
    trachomatis 45, 617, 618
Chlorambucil 403, 494, 901
Chloroquine 886, 887
Chlorpromazine 887
Choanal atresia 464
Chocolate agar 402
Cholesterol plaques 430
Cholinergic crisis 291
Chondroitin sulfate enriched optisol media 747
Chordoma 342
Choriocapillaris 510
    basement membrane of 463
    layer of 463
Chorioretinal atrophic scars 477
Chorioretinal atrophy 488, 509
Chorioretinal scar 504
Chorioretinitis 486, 521
Chorioretinopathy
    heterogeneous group of inflammatory 507
    central serous 447, 520, 877, 881
Choristoma 229
Choroid 425, 426, 462, 499, 890, 895
    coloboma of 418
    inflammation of 441
    stroma of 461
Choroidal detachment 400, 428, 565, 726, 727
Choroidal fluorescence, blockage of 491
Choroidal melanomas, small 189
Choroidal neovascular membrane 467
Choroidal neovascularization 441, 470, 491, 509
Choroiditis 467
    ampiginous 510
    punctate inner 507
Choroidopathy
    geographical 510
    punctate inner 487, 512
Chromic acid 868
Chromophores 436
Chromosomal disorders 576
Chromosome 675, 823
Chromovitrectomy 432
Chronic angle-closure glaucoma 571
Chronic obstructive pulmonary disease 803
Churg-Strauss syndrome 483, 485
Ciancia syndrome 372
Cicatricial ectropion 49, 50, 77fc
Cicatricial entropion 45
    etiology of 45b
    management of 45f
Cicatricial lagophthalmos 70, 72
Ciclosporin 906
Cidofovir 886
Ciliary artery
    anterior 463
    posterior 124, 408, 463
Ciliary body 459, 461, 495
    excision of 570
    extension of 461
    layer of 461
    nonpigmented epithelium of 461
    parts of 461
    pigmented epithelium of 461
Ciliary epithelium 461, 462
Ciliary membrane formation 820

Ciliary muscle spasm 467
Ciliary nerves, trauma to 647
Ciliary process 462
    blood supply of 463
    microscopic structure of 462
Ciliary stroma 461
    muscle in 461
Ciliochoroidal detachment 428
Circinate balanitis 478
Citicoline 394, 596
Citrate 872
Classical teardrop sign 132f
Clear corneal tunnel incision 603t, 856
Climatic proteoglycan stromal keratopathy 685
Clindamycin 502
Clinical activity score 154, 154t
Clostridium botulinum 60, 351
Clotrimazole 668
Canalicular mucosa 106f
Coats disease 503, 504
Cobalt 215
Cocaine test 339, 340
Cogan's lid 32
Co-glycolic acid 483
Cohen and Osher's technique 573, 574f
Coin test 397
Collagen
    abnormal 684
    connective tissue fibrils 462
    cross-linking 627
    disorders of 897
    fibrils, secret 463
    shrinkage 852
Collier's sign 66
Colloidal iron 676
Coloboma
    posterior segment 418
    simple 12
Color Doppler ultrasound 219
Color vision 307, 314, 316, 323, 333
    anomalies of 309, 310fc
    defects, congenital 309
    methods to check 416
    physiology of 308
    tests for 308
    theories of 307, 416
Color-opponent ganglion cells, types of 308
Common contrast sensitivity tests 412
Common lacrimal gland lesions, radiological features of 226t
Complete blood count 139, 146, 402, 484, 501
Complex cells 300
Computed tomography 32, 132, 139, 153, 175, 189, 193, 202, 203, 225, 228, 230, 238, 240-243, 252f, 253, 479, 485, 865
    high-resolution 402, 469, 514
    orbit 207f-213f, 221f
    scan 132, 205, 242
Conductive keratoplasty 852, 853f
    advantages of 852
    disadvantages of 852
    indication of 852
Cone 449
    dysfunction syndromes 450
    types of 416

Confocal microscopy 625, 629, 645, 664, 686, 845
Confocal scanning laser
  polarimetry 534
  tomography 534
Congenital anophthalmia 223
  evaluation of 250
  management of 250
Congenital hereditary endothelial dystrophy 687, 690, 763
Congenital ptosis 19f, 20, 23
  clinical features of 22
  evaluation of 22
Congestion 240
  conjunctival 185f
Conjunctiva 2, 268, 424, 425, 466, 486, 495, 498, 569f, 600, 620, 624, 628, 632 639, 644, 697, 703, 864
  bulbar 870
  epithelial tumors of 268
  inferior forniceal 196f
  normal 570
  palpebral 763f
Conjunctival defect, closure of 275
Conjunctival disease, cicatrizing 245
Conjunctival epithelial
  cells 851
  cyst 270
  tumors 267
Conjunctival flap 627, 652, 872
Conjunctival fornices 870
Conjunctival hyperemia, mild 730
Conjunctival inflammation 246, 647
Conjunctival injection 731
Conjunctival intraepithelial neoplasia 273, 703
Conjunctival lesions 829
  pigmented 195
  surgical removal of 275
Conjunctival limbal allograft 706
Conjunctival mass 889
Conjunctival melanoma 195, 201, 257
  classification of 199
  clinical features of 199
Conjunctival nevus 195, 196f
  clinical features of 196
  excision of 197b
  management of 196
Conjunctival papillae 622
Conjunctival peritomy, types of 604fc
Conjunctival pigmented tumors 195
Conjunctival pseudoepitheliomatous hyperplasia 270
Conjunctival resection 634
Conjunctival retention cyst, right 266f
Conjunctival swab 650
Conjunctival transplantation 873
Conjunctival vessels, cork screwing of 240
Conjunctival-limbal autograft 705, 705
Conjunctiva-Muller muscle flap 403
Conjunctivitis
  acute 613, 615
  adenoviral 616
  allergic 615t
  bacterial 617, 621
  causes of 614t
  chemical 618
  chlamydial 619, 621
  classification of 731t
  fungal 621
  giant papillary 15
  gonococcal 619, 621
  herpes 617
  infective 615t
  management of acute 613
  microbial 618
  pseudomembranous 730
Conjunctivodacryocystorhinostomy 84, 91
Conjunctivoplasty 48f
Connective tissue 462
  disorders 401, 576, 895, 897, 900
Consensual reflex 336
Contact lens 599, 643, 699, 700, 781, 797, 826
  fitting
    principles of 797
    types of 797
  use 623
  wear 647, 696
Contrast sensitivity 310, 311, 316, 323, 328, 333, 412
Convergence excess esotropia 375
  management of 375
Conversion reaction 293
Cordarone 826
Corectopia 464
Cornea 425, 426, 435, 453, 486, 495, 498, 600, 620, 624, 628, 632, 635, 639, 644, 695, 697, 703, 863, 864, 877, 895
  allocation criteria 743t
  anatomy of 600
  central flattening of 851
  conjunctivalization of 703
  ectatic disorders of 777
  indication 886
  ocular effects 886
  physiology of 600
Corneal abrasion 38, 56
Corneal allograft rejection 708
  differential diagnosis of 710t
  immunology of 712
  management of high-risk 717
  mechanism of 713
  prevention of high-risk 716
  risk factors for 707t
  signs of 709f
Corneal amyloid degeneration 685
Corneal astigmatism, manage 856
Corneal biomechanics 698, 795, 827
Corneal biopsy 625
Corneal blood staining 875
Corneal breakdown 153
Corneal button, excision of 255f
Corneal cellular factors 607
Corneal cross-linking 700, 701, 791, 792, 841
  indications for 791
  plus refractive procedures 841
Corneal decompensation 749, 750
Corneal degeneration 681
  types of 682fc
Corneal dehydration 607f
Corneal dystrophy 609, 641, 671, 677, 681, 687
  classification of 671
Corneal ectasia 694, 695f, 789, 791
  types of 789
Corneal edema 505, 691
  diffuse 774
  severe 774
Corneal endothelial
  cells, loss of 848
  pumps, mechanism of action of 608f
  reflex 694
Corneal endothelium 608t, 612, 692
  anatomy of 600
  embryology of 600
Corneal epithelial
  abnormalities 644
  cells 702
  dendrites 833
  edema, stage of 686, 689
Corneal epithelium 605
  pathological responses on 609
Corneal erosions, management of recurrent 630
Corneal excision set 739
Corneal exposure, management of 79
Corneal fluorescein staining 731
Corneal gluing 650
Corneal graft
  failure 800
  rejection 706, 711t
    management of 706
    signs of 709t
  survival 724t
Corneal guttae, stage of 686
Corneal haze 841
Corneal hydrops 695, 780
Corneal hypoesthesia 33
Corneal implants 854
Corneal incision
  internal 602
  paired opposite 856
  types of clear 604fc
Corneal infection 622
Corneal injury, management of 865
Corneal inlays 842
Corneal lacerations 866
Corneal melt 703
  postsurgical peripheral 777
Corneal nerve 799
  enlarged 800
  grading of 799
  prominent 694, 695f, 799
  thickened 799
Corneal opacity 788
  bilateral healed 764f
Corneal pachymetry 691
Corneal pam, recurrent 199
Corneal perforation 771, 831
  size of 649
Corneal preservation
  methods for 744, 746
  techniques 744
Corneal protection 885
Corneal refractive surgery 825
Corneal ring segments 851
Corneal scarring 694, 763, 771, 838, 881
  stage of 686
Corneal scleral segment 742
Corneal scraping 625, 650, 778
Corneal sensation 624, 884
Corneal shrinkage procedures 854
Corneal stroma 679, 684, 869
  pathological responses of 610

Corneal stromal edema, stage of 686, 689
Corneal surgery 422
Corneal suturing 866
Corneal thickness 696f, 849
Corneal thinning 694, 790
Corneal tissue
  harvesting 738
  modeling 854
Corneal topography 629, 778, 780, 783, 789, 826, 849
  application of 783
Corneal transparency 605, 605fc, 606f,
Corneal transplantation 652, 700, 706, 873
  high-risk 715, 716
  immunological rejection of 714t
Corneal tumors 267
Corneal ulcer 442, 444, 637t, 647, 649, 881, 884
  management of nonhealing 647
  perforated 648
  risk factors for nonhealing 647t
  trial, steroids for 636, 637
Corneal vascularization, theories of 606
Corneal wound
  closure of 866
  full-thickness nonself-sealing 866
  healing 608, 826
Corneal xerosis 763, 881
Corneopalpebral adhesion 12
Corneoscleral wounds, closure of 867
Cornisol 747
Corona ciliaris 461
Coronal cut, posterior 207, 207f
Coronal incision 166, 167
Cortical blindness 344
  etiology of 345
  features of 345
Corticosteroids 292, 331, 403, 468t, 482, 480, 482, 507, 509, 514, 716, 770, 876, 906
  indications of 638t
  intravenous 403
  therapy 480
  topical 468, 519, 616, 627, 709, 871, 901
  use of topical 649
Corynebacterium diphtheria 648
Cosmesis 52
Cotton wool spots 484, 498, 880
Cough 905
Counter coup injury 811
Coup injury 811
Cover test 284
Cramps, abdominal 291
Cranial dysinnervation disorders, congenital 383
Cranial nerve 27, 126, 287, 304, 360f
  function 285
Craniofacial syndromes 895
Craniopharyngioma 342, 343
Craniosynostosis 142, 221, 327, 895
  manifestations of 221t
C-reactive protein 282, 485
Creutzfeldt-Jakob disease 740, 741
Cribriform plate 164, 204
Criterion-free procedure 412
Crocodile forceps 848
Crocodile tears 78, 84
Crohn's disease 478, 483
Crouzon syndrome 168
Crow's feet 63

Crutch glasses 292
Cryotherapy 191, 279, 480, 515
Cryptophthalmos 12, 13, 221, 223
  complete 13
  incomplete 13
Crystalline lens 436, 459, 865
  dislocated 455
Crystalline maculopathies, drug-induced 887
Cultivated oral mucosal epithelial transplantation 706
Cultured limbal epithelial transplantation 705, 706
Cupula 303
Curly collagen fibers 678
Curry-Jones syndrome 250
Curvularia keratitis 666f
Cushing's syndrome 473
Custom ocular prosthesis 245f
Custom-designed plaque radiotherapy 277
Customized corneal cross-linking 793
Cutler beard bridge technique 55, 56f, 861
Cyanoacrylate glue 650, 670, 866
Cyanolabe 416
Cyclitic membrane 820
Cyclocryotherapy technique 570, 571f
Cyclodestruction 598
Cyclodestructive procedures 588, 592, 597
Cycloelectrolysis 570
Cycloheximide 664
Cyclopentolate 473
Cyclophosphamide 147, 403, 494
Cycloplegia test 294
Cycloplegics 710, 906
  agents 467, 627
Cyclosporine 169, 403, 480, 494, 710, 711, 716, 717, 770, 901
Cyclovergence 363
Cyproheptadine 351
Cystadenoma, epididymal 892
Cystathionine B-synthase deficiency 823
Cystic eye, congenital 221, 224
Cystic fibrosis 242
Cystic lesions 241
Cysticercosis 488, 899
Cysticercus cellulosae 503
Cystinosis 902
Cystoid macular edema 454, 467, 473, 481, 485, 516, 820, 901
Cysts 609, 612
  conjunctival 373, 422
  epidermoid 241
  formation of 134, 134f
  hinders conformer placement 253
  large 224
  orbital 225
  orbitopalpebral 248f, 252
  pancreatic 892
  renal 892
  translucent 241
Cytomegalovirus 426, 476, 484-487, 500, 504, 506, 711, 886, 899
  retinitis 497, 498, 504-506
Cytoplasmic antineutrophil cytoplasmic antibody 402
Cytoskeleton 413
Cytotoxic T-lymphocyte
  antigen 518
  associated protein 4 886

D

Daclizumab 518
Dacryoadenitis, first episode of 226
Dacryoadenoma 270
Dacryocele, congenital 95
Dacryocystitis 619
  management of chronic 96
Dacryocystography 104, 110
  digitally subtracted 104
Dacryocystorhinostomy 93, 95, 98, 110
  types of 96
Dacryoendoscopy 104
Dacryops 240
  etiopathogenesis of 241fc
Dacryoscintigraphy 111
Dalen-Fuchs nodules 491
Dalrymple's sign 66
Dark adaptation
  curve 417
  mechanism of 417
  values of 418
Darkfield microscopy 521
De novo melanoma 201
Decompression retinopathy 568
Decorin gene 675
Deep anterior lamellar keratoplasty 674, 700, 718, 719f, 796
Deep capillary plexus 411
Deep lamellar endothelial keratoplasty 422
Deep temporal fascia 36
Dehydration 609f
  relative state of 607
Delleman syndrome 12
Dementia 741
Dendritic ulcer 654
Dengue fever, ocular manifestation of 878
Dentate processes 407
Deorsumvergences 363
Deoxyribonucleic acid 276f, 659, 889
  epitheliums synthesis of 426
Dermal fillers 62
Dermatitis 50f, 479
Dermatomyositis 898
Dermoid 210f
  adnexal 230t
  cyst 229, 241
  systemic associations of 229
Descemet's membrane 662, 695, 723, 745, 778
  endothelial keratoplasty 706, 722, 723t, 724
  folds, grading of 745f
  forms 406
Descemet's stripping
  automated endothelial keratoplasty 720, 724
  endothelial keratoplasty 706
Descemetorhexis 721, 724
Desferrioxamine 887
Deuteranopia 310
Dexamethasone 438, 480, 519, 753
  intravitreal implants 483
  sodium succinate 770
Dexsol 747
Diabetes mellitus 156, 332, 337, 344, 802, 902
  history of 287
Diamidines 645, 646

Diarrhea 291
Dichromacy 310
Diffuse lamellar keratitis 833
    grading of 833*t*
Diffuse unilateral subacute neuroretinitis 487, 488
    management of 488
Digital bleb massage 570
Digital massage 569*f*
Digital rasterstereography-based topography system 783
Digoxin 887
Dihydrofolate reductase 518
Dilator muscles 460, 463
Dimethyl fumarate 321
Diode laser cyclophotocoagulation 822
Dioptric power 783
Diplopia 134, 280, 290
    charting 133, 281, 288
    management of vertical 379, 380, 383
Diquafosol ophthalmic solution 851
Direct capsular rupture 811
Direct lacrimal gland stimulation 108
Disc 400
    drusen 334
    edema 315*fc*, 880
        bilateral 314
        management of 314, 316
        true 314
        unilateral 314
    neovascularization of 470, 484
    pole, rotation of 326
    stereo-photography 543
Distraction test 42, 43*f*
Diuretics 428
Diurnal variation 32, 542
Dominant modulator theory 308
Donder's law 358
Donnenfeld proposed classification 832
Donor
    cornea
        evaluation 744
        preservation 744
    eyes, grading of 746, 746*t*
    sclera 403
    screening 740
    serologic testing 740
    tissue 722
        antigenic load of 712
Dorsal midbrain syndrome 66, 891
Dorzolamide 549, 749
Dot visual acuity test 397
Double elevator palsy 382
    management of 382*fc*
Double Maddox rod test 285
Double prism test 294
Double vision 38
Down's syndrome 327, 694, 807, 900
Doxycycline 17, 239, 521
Drop method 110
Drugs
    therapy, targeted 669
    topical 647
Dry age-related macular degeneration 410
Dry eye 62, 731
    disease 684, 730, 824
    post-laser-assisted in situ keratomileusis 8850*fc*

management of 850
surgery, causes of 850
postoperative 839
refractory 851
testing 826
treatment 851
Dua's layer 604
Duane's retraction syndrome 229, 359, 371, 383, 385
    esotropic 386, 387*fc*
    management of 386
Dyschromatopsia 309
Dysphagia 290
Dyspnea 905
Dysthyroid
    ophthalmopathy 379
    optic neuropathy 156, 163
Dystrophy 681, 681*t*
    lateral 677

E

E chart 398, 864
Eales disease 516
Ear
    anomalies 464
    infirmary keratoconus classification 786
    nose, and throat 73
Eccentric fixation 366, 367, 369
Ecchymoses 863
Echinocandins 668
Echocardiogram 803
Echography, quantitative 219
Econazole 668
Ectasia 838
    anterior 695*f*
    posterior 695*f*
Ectoderm, surface 464
Ectopia et pupillae 823
Ectopia lentis 584, 821
    causes of 822*t*
Ectopic caruncle 91
Ectopic lacrimal gland 90
    cysts 241
Ectropion 38, 40, 47, 77*fc*
    classification of 47, 48*t*
    correction of 50*f*
    management of 49
    preoperative assessment of 47
    uvea, congenital 542
Edema 609, 612
    periorbital 863
Edinger-Westphal nuclei 337
Edridge-green lantern test 309
Edrophonium test 32, 291
Ehlers-Danlos syndrome 240, 897
Elastic tissue 896
    layer 463
Electrocardiogram 803
Electrode 311
Electrolyte imbalance 547
Electromyography 291
Electron microscopy 674
Electro-oculogram 488
Electrophysiological test 323, 535
Electroretinogram 457, 469, 488, 535, 901
    focal 457
Elliot and Nankin method 388

Embryotoxon, posterior 523, 523*f*, 525
Emedastine 769
Encephalitis 337
Encephalocele 224, 243
    types of 243*t*
Encephalocraniocutaneous lipomatosis 12
Endocrine
    disorders 899
    neoplasia, multiple 898
Endodermal sinus tumor 342
Endolymphatic sac tumors 892, 893
Endophthalmitis 253, 453, 454, 466, 496, 737, 752, 775*t*, 867
    bacterial 505
    chronic 503
    clinical signs of 867
    fungal 505
    postoperative 435, 491
    post-traumatic 867
    vitrectomy study 753
Endothelial cell 711
    health 805
    indices 601*t*
    loss 719, 720
Endothelial corneal dystrophy 689*t*
Endothelial dysfunction, causes of 690
Endothelial graft rejection rates 721
Endothelial keratoplasty 691, 692, 720, 724
    recent advances in 724
Endothelial rejection 709
    treatment of 711
Endotheliitis 656
    spectrum of 655
Endothelium 456, 612, 745
    active pump of 607
    function of 607
Enophthalmos 859, 863
    absence of 863
    minimal 245*f*
Entopic phenomena 457, 458
Entoptic phenomenon 458
Entropion 40, 44*f*
    classification of 40*t*
    clinical tests for 43*f*
    congenital 46
    correction of 44*f*, 46*f*
    grading of 41*t*
    signs of 41*t*
    symptoms of 41*t*
Enucleation 254, 257, 275, 599, 873
    techniques of 253
Enyedi's postoperative target refraction 808
Enzyme 672
    linked immunosorbent assay 402, 469, 501, 656
Epiblepharon 13, 63
    bilateral 47*f*
    correction 47*f*
Epibulbar choristoma 229, 274
Epibulbar dermoid 229
Epibulbar swellings, differential diagnosis of 229, 230*t*
Epicanthus 29
    inversus syndrome 13, 28, 29*f*
    palpebralis 13
    superciliaris 13
    tarsalis 13

Epidemic dropsy 882
  glaucoma 536
Epidermal growth factor 872
  receptor inhibitors 886
Epilepsy 327
Epinastine 769
Epinephrine 773
Epiphora 590
  clinical evaluation of 108
  evaluation of 108
  management of 83
  true 108
Epiretinal membrane 453, 480, 516, 749
  formation 481
Episcleral venous pressure 577
Episcleral vessels, superficial 400
Episcleritis 399, 401t
  features of 401
Epithelial adhesion 643
Epithelial basement membrane dystrophy 628
Epithelial defect 622, 831, 838
  recurrent 703
Epithelial haze 644
Epithelial ingrowth 834, 838
  classification of 834t
Epithelial keratitis, management of 656
Epithelial rejection 709, 720
  treatment of 710
Epithelial thickness mapping 795
Epitheliopathy, dendritic 655
Epithelium 745
  and stroma, replacement of 717
  anterior pigment 400
  function of 607
  removal of 792
Erythema nodosum 513
Erythrocyte sedimentation rate 139, 146, 282, 402, 472, 485
Erythrolabe 416
Erythropoietin 321
Escherichia coli 402, 619, 645
Esotropia 361f, 369, 375
  accommodative 389
  classification of 369
  congenital 371, 374
  incomitant 370
  infantile 372
  investigation of 370
  management of 369-372, 374, 375
Etanercept 170, 480, 518, 886
Ethambutol 322, 888
Ethanol 324
Ethmoid
  mucosa 100
  neurovascular bundles 259
  sinuses 173
  sinusitis 182f
Ethylenediaminetetraacetic acid 515, 683
Evisceration 253, 257, 599, 873
  techniques of 253
Exaggerated donor-derived lymphocytic reaction 728
Excimer laser
  corneal ablation 839
  stromal photoablation 855
Excision biopsy 238
  principles 117, 119

Exenteration
  complications of 257
  indications of 257
  surgical steps of 257
  types of 258
Exercise 883
Exophthalmometry 133, 149, 150
  absolute 150
  classification of 149
  importance of 149
  types of 149
Exotropia 376, 378
  classification of 378
  management of 378
Ex-press glaucoma filtration device 556
External beam radiation therapy 192, 227
Extracellular matrix 463, 898
Extraconal space 172, 216
Extraocular extension 193, 894
Extraocular movements 281, 284, 287, 314, 328, 901
Extraocular muscles 89, 150, 207f, 216, 290, 352, 353, 424
  action of 356, 357t
  attachments 253
  congenital fibrosis of 23, 384
  development of 355
  paralysis of 489
  pulley system 353f
Extraorbital space 217
Exudative retinal detachment 400, 504, 521
Eye 221, 790t, 877, 882, 894, 900, 903
  absence of 223
  adduction of 281
  bank 738, 744
    laboratory 740
    system, composition of 738f
    training center 738
  chronic redness of 702
  contralateral 245, 793
  development of 221, 405
  diseases 474
  donation 739
  dryness of 649
  end-stage 873
  fetal development of 406t
  lid tissue, origin of 10
  loss
    chronic infection-related 245
    trauma-related 245
  margin 259f
  movements 301, 359
    pathways for 302
    slow 359
    types of 359
  normal development of 221
  outward bulge of 185f
  painful blind 253, 596, 598
  rubbing 697
  warming devices 851
  watering of 90, 653
  whitish patch in 702
Eyeballs 220
  contour, loss of 257f
Eyebrow
  asymmetry 24
  hair loss 495
Eyelash, loss of 56

Eyelid 51, 234, 406, 424, 425, 498, 624, 632, 635, 639, 644, 697, 703, 859, 894
  anatomy 1
  anomalies, congenital 10
  blepharoptosis, right upper 266f
  capillary hemangioma of 114
  closure 640
    adequate 52
  contour defects 37
  crease approach 69
  defect 860, 861
  developmental anomalies of 12
  ectropion, bilateral severe lower 49f
  edema 162
  embryological development of 10
  eversion 34
  examination 859
  formation 11
  glands of 7
  hygiene 17
  involvement 486
  laceration 859
    management of 860
    repair of 860
  lamellae 277
  lateral aspect of 118
  laxity
    horizontal 42
    vertical 42
  lesions
    common benign 112f
    treatment of 498
  lower 41f, 76, 77
  lymphatic drainage of 7
  malignant tumors of 119
  malposition 134
  margin 53, 55f, 860
    reconstruction of 53, 53
    sutures 861
  mass 228
  mobility, normal 52
  multiple upper 30f
  neurofibroma 232
    management of 232
  position 295
    anomalies of 70
  protractor muscles of 65f, 65t
  reconstruction 51
    techniques of 52
  retraction 56, 62, 65
    causes of 66
    central neurogenic causes of 66
    classification of 66t
    left lower 266f
    management of 65
  structure 2
    development of 10t
    maturation of 11
  surgery 158
  swinging 237f
  tension 52
  trauma 859
    management of 859
  tumors 111, 208
    benign 111, 113t, 114f
    malignant 112f, 113t
  vascular supply to 8

F

Face, development of 121*f*
Facial
 artery, transverse 8
 asymmetry 284
 functional units 76*t*
 movements, lower 84
 nerve
  anatomy of 70, 72
  branches of 73*fc*, 74*fc*
  intracranial course of 73*fc*
  palsy 71*f*, 76*fc*, 77*fc*
  terminal branches 74*f*
 palsy 77*fc*
  reflex lacrimation in 76*fc*
 syndromes 895
 synkinesis 62
Faden operation 389
Famciclovir 657
Farnsworth Munsell D-15 test 416
Fascia lata 36
Fascicular lesions 280
Fasciculus, median longitudinal 287, 302*f*
Fat
 adherence syndrome 388
 decompression 165
 predominant, development of 152*f*
Fatigue test 32, 291
Fecal-oral route 503
Feeder vessels 279
Fellow eye 625, 703
 axial length of 261
Femtosecond laser 854, 855
 application 836
 assisted dissection 852
 disadvantages of 856
 flaps 855
 refractive platforms 854
Femtosecond lenticule extraction 855
Femtosecond over microkeratome flaps, advantages of 828
Ferrara ring segment 851
Fiber electromyography, single 291
Fiberoptic bronchoscopy 906
Fibrillin, disorders of 896
Fibrin glue 651
 application 325
Fibrinous reaction 774
Fibroblasts 460, 684
 abnormal 897
Fibrocytes 462
Fibromuscular dysplasia 240
Fibronectin 872
Fibrosis 609, 610, 612
Fibrous lamina cribrosa forms 406
Fibrovascular ingrowth 263
Filament, debridement of 661
Filamentary keratitis 659, 660*t*
 management of 659
Fine needle aspiration
 biopsy 190
 cytology 228
Fingolimod-macular edema 749
Fink's method 388
Fixation disparity method 373
Flap striae 832
 classification of 832*t*

Flare 864
Flashes 440
Flatter corneas 823
Fleck corneal dystrophy 672, 675
Fleischer's ring 694, 695*f*
Flexible nylon iris hooks 814*f*
Floppy eyelid syndrome 880
Flucinolone acetonide 514
Fluconazole 668
Fluid, abnormal accumulation of 428
Fluidics, role of 815
Fluocinolone 480
 acetonide 437, 483
 acetonide intravitreal implants 482
Fluorescein
 angiography 193, 469, 470, 470*fc*, 488, 491, 496, 506, 508, 509, 510, 511, 512, 887
 dye disappearance test 75, 110
 endoscopic dye test 101, 110
 fundus angiography 333
 treponemal antibody absorption test 402, 521
Fluorine isotope 214
Fluoro-2-deoxy-D-glucose 213
Fluoroquinolone 769, 886
 topical fourth-generation 833
Fluorouracil 249, 275, 588
Flying spot 458
F-M 100 hue test 416
Forced duction test 133, 281, 285, 288, 387
Forced upward traction test 67
Forehead flap, median 58
Forme fruste keratoconus 698, 793
Fornices adequate depth 245
Fornix 201
 contracture 246
 formation suture 249
Fossa formation 209
Four intravitreal corticosteroid implants 437
Fourth cranial nerve
 anatomy of 283, 305, 305*f*
 palsy 283, 305, 348
 etiology of 283
Fovea centralis 407
Foveal avascular zone 410, 411
Foveal hypoplasia 411
Foveola 407
Foville syndrome 287, 287*f*
Fracture 130*f*
Fragments, loss of 866
Francis Felix rundle 153
Francois central cloudy dystrophy 672, 676
Fraser and Manitoba syndrome 223
Free tarsoconjunctival graft 57
Free thyroxine 160
 index 160
Frequency doubling technology 534
Fricke flap 57, 58
Friend test 294
Frisby-Davis test 364, 366
Frizzled-related protein gene 334
Frontoethmoidal encephaloceles 243
Frontoethmoidal lynch incision 217*f*
Frosted branch angiitis 484
Fuchs endothelial corneal dystrophy 688, 689*t*, 800
 differential diagnosis of 690*t*
 management of 688

Fuchs heterochromic
 iridocyclitis 466, 476
 uveitis 472
Fuchs uveitis syndrome 475-477
 complications of 476
 features of 476
 management of 476
Functional acuity contrast test 311
Functional endoscopic sinus surgery 146, 177
Fundoscopy 330
Fundus 316, 332, 632
 autofluorescence 327, 335, 469, 471, 508, 509, 511, 512
 classic orange-red discoloration of 493
 evaluation 780
 examination 287, 314, 328, 697, 826, 865
 fluorescein angiography 315, 331, 452, 484, 485, 493, 496, 879
 mass 400
 photography 285
Fungal keratitis 648, 663, 663*f*, 665*f*, 666*f*
 clinical features of 664*b*
 development of 662*b*
 diagnosis of 661, 664
 incidence of 662
 medical therapy of 667*t*
 steroids in 637
Fungi, dematiaceous 663
Fusarium solani 648
Fusion 361, 366, 369
 Horopter and Panum's area of 368*f*

G

Gabapentin 350
Gadolinium 215
Gallium scanning 514
Ganciclovir 499
Ganglion
 cells 406, 407, 416
 ciliary 127, 341
Garcia's sign 488
Gastrointestinal tract disturbances 291, 547
Gaucher's disease 424
Gene therapy 712, 724*t*, 725*t*
Genetics 589, 806
Germinoma 342
Gerontoxon 682
Giant cell arteritis 330, 442, 898
Giant retinal tears 436
Giardiasis 488
Giemsa stain 642
 methods 402
Glabellar flap 57, 58
Glands 406
Glaucoma 400, 413, 453, 454, 476, 481, 520, 522, 531, 539, 540, 542, 548, 555, 577-579, 593, 593*fc*, 771, 823, 881, 884, 885
 acute congestive 615
 adult refractory 587
 advanced 596
 childhood 529
 classification of secondary 576
 congenital 542, 591, 591*fc*, 619, 763, 800
 drainage device 570, 588, 592
  implantation 428
 drug-induced 580
 epidemiology of 528

family history of 542
filtering surgery 514
following cataract surgery 809
high pressure 585
lens
　induced 582, 812
　　particle 583
management of 546, 554, 567f
normal-tension 585
open-angle 529, 545, 582
optical coherence tomography in 539
pathogenesis 593
phacoantigenic 583
phacolytic 582
phacomorphic 583
preperimetric 532
primary congenital 522, 587, 589
pupillary block 515, 848
refractory 515, 586, 588fc
secondary 473, 515, 529, 542, 774
　adult 577
　angle-closure 578
　childhood 576
　open-angle 577
steroid induced 577
surgery 428, 515, 873
　complications of 565
　nonpenetrating 557
traumatic 577
uses of 539
Glaucomatocyclitic crisis 477, 504
Glaucomatous visual field changes, criteria of 535
Glaukos IStent 556
Glioma 342
Globe dystopia 183f, 228, 238, 242, 243
　inferior 243
　inferotemporal 184f
Glucocorticoids 156, 169
　receptor agonists, selective 712
Glucose-6-phosphate dehydrogenase 502
Glutamate, role of 532
Glycerine 748
Glycosaminoglycan 151
Gnathostoma 488
Gnathostomiasis 488, 489
Goblet cells 7
　conjunctival 851
Goldenhar syndrome 12, 229, 325, 386, 896
Goldmann perimetry 312
Goldmann visual fields 509
Golimumab 518
Goniotomy 591, 592f
Gopal Krishna classification 248
Gorlin syndrome 229, 327
Gorlin-Chaudhry-Moss syndrome 250
Gormaz 150
Graether ring 815f
Graft lenticule, insertion of 721
Graft rejection
　differential diagnosis of 709
　treatment of 709
Graft-versus-host disease 728, 730t, 731
　chronic 729, 730, 731t
　ocular 728, 729
　pathophysiology of
　　acute 729, 729f
　　chronic 729
　prevention of 732

treatment of 732
　acute 732
　chronic 732
　ocular 732, 733t
Gram's stain 642
Granit's dominator 416
Granular corneal dystrophy 677, 679, 680
Granulomas 246
　peripheral 503
Granulomatosis 486
Graves' disease 158, 159, 878, 901
　systemic manifestations of 159t
Graves' hyperthyroidism 162
Graves' ophthalmopathy 150, 153f, 154
Graves' orbitopathy 140
　classification 154
Graves' thyrotoxicosis 158
Grocott's methenamine silver stain 642
Ground-glass appearance 678
Growth, management of 118
Guillain-Barré syndrome 66
Gunderson flap 599
Gustatory lacrimation 78, 84

H

Haemophilus influenzae 174, 613, 625
Haidinger's brushes 458
Hallermann-Streiff syndrome 896
Halo sign 331
Hansen's disease 884, 885
　ocular manifestation of 884
　ophthalmic manifestations of 494
Haploscopic method 373
Haploscopic principle 364, 365
Harada disease 509, 878
Harmonious arc 362f
Hartmann-Shack sensor 840
Hassall-Henle bodies 683, 686, 690
Headache 62, 280, 349
　causes of primary 349
Hearing loss 330
Heart defects 464
Heavy eye syndrome 379
Heerfordt syndrome 513
Heidelberg retinal tomography 543, 557
Helicoid peripapillary chorioretinal degeneration 510
Helium-neon laser 457
Helper T-cells 714
Hemangioma
　acquired capillary 115
　benign cavernous 210f
　capillary 114, 144, 145, 237
　choroidal 189, 894, 880
　congenital 239
　　capillary 115
　partially involuting congenital 239
Hemangiomatosis 115
Hematological disorders 898
Hematoma 216
Hemianopic offset 530
Hemicoronal incision 218
Hemifacial spasm 4, 60, 61f
Hemifield slide phenomenon 344
Hemodilution 740
Hemorrhage 38, 133, 388, 749, 890
　choroidal 727
　intragel 451

intraretinal 498
macular 424, 836
retinal 425, 489, 500
retrobulbar 802
subarachnoid 431
suprachoroidal 437, 567
Hemosiderosis bulbi 453
Hemostatic multiple figure-of-eight sutures 233
Hemostatic sutures 235
Hepatotoxicity 162
Hereditary benign intraepithelial dyskeratosis 271
Hering's law 162, 358
Herpes infection 426
Herpes simplex 426, 899
　keratoconjunctivitis 619
　virus 486, 487, 653, 654, 657, 707
　　conjunctivitis 621
　　keratitis 498, 628, 653, 654, 655, 657, 690
Herpes zoster
　keratitis 655
　ophthalmicus 466, 498
　virus 639
Herpetiform keratitis, central 687
Herring's law 67
Herring's opponent theory 308, 416
Hess chart 281, 284, 288
Heterochromia 475
　iridis, differential diagnosis of 475
　iridocyclitis, causes of 475t, 477
Heterophoria method 373
Hexagonal cells, percentage of 746
High-efficiency particulate air 739
High-energy photons pass 213
Highly active antiretroviral therapy 497
High-pass resolution perimetry 535
Hilar lymphadenopathy, bilateral 402, 514
Hinge location 850
Hirschberg test 371
Histamine H1 and H2 receptor antagonists 581
Histoplasmosis 512
Hoddap-Parrish-Anderson classification system 535, 535t
Hodgkin's lymphoma 342
Holland-Mannis classification 703
Hollenhorst plaques 430
Holmgren's wool test 309, 416
Homatropine, topical 667
Homocystinuria 542, 823, 897, 899
Hormone, adrenocorticotropic 321, 344
Horner's muscle 4, 88
Horner's syndrome 7, 338f, 339, 342
　central 339
　congenital 340
　ipsilateral 287
　postganglionic 340
　preganglionic 340
Horner-Duverney's muscle 88
Host antigens 728
Hounsfield units 205
House-Brackmann scoring system 78t
Huber's classification 386
Hughes tarsoconjunctival flap 54
　technique 861

Human immunodeficiency virus 194, 272, 483, 486, 497, 500, 639, 803, 899
　associated retinal vascular endothelial infection 500
　infection status 279
　paraviral syndrome 483
　retinopathy 498, 500
　　etiology of 500
　　features of 500
Human leukocyte
　antigen 469, 472, 485
　　matching, role of 716
　cell 714
Human lymphocyte antigen 508
Human papillomavirus 272
Human T-lymphotropic virus 484
Hummelsheim procedure 390
Humphrey's visual field 312, 313, 805
Huntington's chorea 741
Hyaline degeneration 683
Hyaloid system 406
Hyaluronic acid 63, 68
　gel filler 68*f*
Hydraulic theory 129, 130*f*
Hydrocephalus 244
Hydrocortisone sodium succinate 770
Hydrofluoric acid 868
Hydrogel conformers 250
Hydrogel lens, conventional 782
Hydrogen atom, nucleus of 214
Hydrophobic acrylic lens 808
Hydroxyamphetamine
　mechanism of action of 339, 340
　test 339, 340
Hydroxyapatite 254, 263
Hydroxychloroquine 826, 886, 887
Hyperacuity 458
Hyperautofluorescent 511
Hypercalcemia 683
Hypercalciuria 906
Hypercholesterolemia 332
Hyperemia 424
Hyperfluorescence 491
Hyperhomocystinemia 332
Hyperintense 228
Hyperlacrimation 62, 108
Hyperosmotic agents 546, 548
Hyperostosis, localized 209
Hyperphosphatemia 683
Hypertelorism 220, 221
　grading of 220*t*
　management of 221*fc*
Hypertension 332, 344, 802
　history of 287
　pregnancy-induced 877
　severe 428
Hyperthyroidism 158, 161*fc*, 899, 901
　management of 158
Hypertonic saline 599
Hypertrophy, benign prostatic 802
Hypertropia, right 286
Hyphema 466, 568, 864
　grading of 875
　traumatic 874
Hypoautofluorescence, central 512
Hypocalcemia 902
Hypoesthesia, infraorbital 133, 864
Hypofluorescence 491
Hypoparathyroidism 899, 902
Hypoplasia 90, 464
Hypopyon 481, 774, 864
　uveitis, causes of 466
Hypothalamus 895
Hypotony 454, 467, 473, 516, 565, 566, 820
Hysteria 293

I

Iatrogenic iris damage 815
Ice pack test 32, 291
Ideal anophthalmic socket 245*f*
Ideal bleb 560, 561*f*
Idiopathic intracranial hypertension 327
　management of 327
　treatment in 328
Idiopathic orbital inflammatory disease 137, 138, 140
Ifosfamide 147
Illiterate charts 864
Imatinib mesylate 886
Imbibition pressure 607
Immersion scan 219, 803
Immune
　recovery uveitis 499
　rejection 706
　responses 609 612
　　modulation 725*t*
　stromal keratitis 655, 656
　system, restored 499
Immunization, history of 287
Immunoglobulin
　G 402
　intravenous 292, 320
Immunological disorders 898
Immunomodulation 226
Immunomodulator therapy 485
Immunosuppressants 292
Immunosuppression 226
Immunotherapy 279
Implant
　complications 265, 265*f*
　exposure 246
　types of 262, 264*t*
Implantable collamer lens 782
Implantable phakic contact lens 782
In vitro confocal microscopy 274, 564, 691
In vivo laser scanning confocal microscopy 704
Incision 35
Incisional refractive procedures 843, 854, 857
Indiana Bleb Appearance Grading Scale 562*f*
Indocyanine green
　angiography 193, 433, 452, 469, 470, 488, 491, 496, 508-512
　dye, uses of 422
　role of 421
Indoleamine dioxygenase 713
Infantile esotropia 372
　nonsurgical management in 389
Infections 373, 401, 660, 832, 838
　chronic bacterial 520
　fungal 426
　postoperative 259
　risk factors for 867
Infectious epithelial keratitis 654, 658
　sequelae of 655

Infectious keratitis 619, 791
　sequelae 688
Infectious retinal vasculitis 485
Infective keratitis 648
　treatment of 650
Inferior oblique tendon, insertion of 357*f*
Inferior orbital
　fissure 132*f*, 166*f*
　wall fracture 209*f*
Inferior rectus 354
　muscle, entrapment of 132*f*
Inflammation 151, 343, 599, 609-612
　chronic 473, 848
　　low-grade 820
　granulomatous 491
　mild 468, 519
　paucity of 503
　preoperative control of 818
　primary site of 464
Inflammatory disease, recurrent bilateral 510
Inflammatory disorders 622
Infliximab 480, 494, 518, 886, 901
Infracyanine green 433
Infraorbital foramen 204
Injury
　prognostication of 863
　type of 859
Inner choroidal
　ischemia, multifocal areas of 511
　vessels 510
Inosine monophosphate 711
Insulin-like growth factor 1 151
Interface vascularization 720
Interferon 152
　alfa 887
　gamma release assay 402, 497
Interleukin 152, 479, 518, 627, 713*f*
Intermittent divergent squint 376-378
　management of 376, 377
Internal transconjunctival incision 133*f*
International Classification of Retinoblastoma 191*t*
International League of Associations of Rheumatology 471
International Society for Study of Vascular Anomalies 239, 239*fc*
International Uveitis Study Group 478
Interpupillary distance 164, 221
Intra-arterial chemotherapy 191
Intrabubble technique 719
Intracameral therapy 669
Intraconal space 172, 216
Intracorneal ring segments 700, 782, 851, 855
Intracranial extension 234
Intracranial tension, signs of raised 234
Intraocular drugs 773
Intraocular foreign body 453, 867
　removal 437
Intraocular hemorrhage, treatment of 432
Intraocular inflammatory disease 521
Intraocular lens 436, 473, 578, 801, 812, 815*f*, 824
　choice of 808
　decentration of 754, 847
　dislocated 453
　implantation 819
　multifocal 842
　power calculation 808, 846

Intraocular lesions, extraocular extension of 894
Intraocular lymphoma 508
    management of primary 194
Intraocular malignancy 186
Intraocular neoplasm, secondary to 577
Intraocular pressure 188, 467, 483, 506, 598, 599, 606*f*, 607*f*, 625, 647, 703, 710, 775, 848, 864, 870, 877, 886, 889
    elevated 566, 567, 710, 726
    low 727
    uncontrolled 598
Intraocular steroids 482
Intraocular surgery, complications of 441
Intraocular tumors 185*f*, 186, 188*fc*, 189*t*, 193, 579, 894
    biopsy for 190
    classification of 187*fc*
    risk of dissemination of 257
Intraoperative floppy iris syndrome 802, 814
Intraorbital pressure 130*f*
Intraorbital trigeminal nerve 127*f*
Intrastromal ablation 854
Intrastromal corneal ring segment 700
Intrastromal therapy 669
Intratumoral calcification 209
Intravenous pulsed corticosteroid therapy 710
Intravitreal gas 431
Intravitreal implants 437, 480
Intravitreal injections 511, 602, 818
Intravitreal triamcinolone acetonide 438
    ideal dose of 439
    uses of 438
Intrinsic eye disease 741
Invaginated scolex 504
Iridocorneal angle 425
Iridocorneal endothelial syndrome 690
    Chandler variant of 687
Iridocorneal touch, peripheral 566*f*
Iridocyclitis 884
    acute 495, 615
    chronic 495
    risk of acute 495
Iridodonesis 824
Iridofundal coloboma 418
Iridotomy lens 550
Iris 459, 495, 466, 624 632, 644, 865, 895
    absence of 464
    anatomy 812
    atrophy 464
    chromicity of 476*t*
    coloboma 419, 464
    congenital anomalies of 464
    depigmentation 493
    dilator, pharmacologic stimulation of 341
    embryology of 463, 464*t*
    forms, dilator muscle of 406
    infiltration 889
    management of 814
    muscles of 460*t*
    nodules 493, 904
    posterior pigment epithelium of 460
    prolapse 649, 819
    retraction 848
    root 341, 461
    sphincter 340, 406
        pharmacologic stimulation of 340
    stroma 406, 460
        muscles of 460
    surgery 816*t*

Iron 215
Irregular corneal surface 655
Irrigation 819
Irvine-Gass syndrome 750
Ischemic optic neuropathy 313, 332, 880
Ishihara's pseudo-isochromatic plate 346
Islet cell tumors 892
Isodense homogeneous lesion 228
Isointense 228
Isoniazid 322, 888
    toxicity 324
Isopter contraction 531
Itraconazole 668

J

Jackson's convex and concave cylinder test 294
Jaw wink
    gradation of 27
    mild-to-moderate 28
    phenomenon 27, 84, 78
    severe 28
Jensen's procedure 390
Johnstone's technique 574, 575*f*
Jones procedure 43
Juvenile idiopathic arthritis 471, 472, 474, 818, 900
    clinical features of 472*t*

K

Kaltreider formula 261
Kaplan regimen, traditional 480
Kaposi's sarcoma 466, 498
Kasabach-Merritt syndrome 144
Kemp's and Collin's grading of entropion 41*f*
Keratectasia
    iatrogenic 841
    postoperative 834
Keratectomy
    photorefractive 631, 653
    phototherapeutic 515, 673
Keratic precipitates 465, 466, 655, 709, 710
Keratitis 400, 636
    chronic 703
    endothelial 658
    exposure 638
    fungal 648, 663, 663*f*, 665*f*, 666*f*
    healed infective 763
    human 662*b*
    infectious 619, 791
    infective 648
    interstitial 686, 690
    management of microsporidial 634
    microbial 153, 771
    noninfective 648
Keratoacanthoma 270
Keratoconjunctivitis, adenoviral 636*t*
Keratoconus 693, 695, 695*f*, 696*f*, 696*t*, 697, 698, 786, 790, 793, 797
    arresting progression of 781
    classification of 699*t*, 787*t*
    diagnosis of 785*t*
    differential diagnosis of 697*t*, 781*t*
    grading severity of 785
    management of 700*fc*, 779, 783, 784, 795, 796
    ocular associations of 779*t*
    posterior 787, 788

    preclinical 793, 796
    progression of 795*t*
    severity index 785
    severity of 784
    signs of 780
    stable 845
    subclinical 793
    treatment of 699
Keratoderma blennorrhagicum 478
Keratoepithelin 677
Keratoepithelioplasty 634
Keratoglobus 790
Keratolenticular contract 524*f*
Keratolimbal allograft 705
Keratomalacia 761-763, 765*fc*, 881
    healed 764*f*
    treatment of 765
Keratometry 697, 780, 784, 804, 808, 849
Keratopathy
    band-shaped 466, 473, 515, 683, 685
    bullous 599, 791
    exposure 38, 649
Keratoplasty 422, 670
    endothelial 691, 692, 720, 724
    full-thickness 642
    high-risk 713, 715*f*
    large-diameter 779
    management of high-risk 715
    penetrating 647, 674, 692, 700, 707, 796, 855
    therapeutic 627, 666*f*, 670
Keratoprosthesis 706, 735, 873
    indications of 733
    procedures 735*t*
    types of 733, 734
Keratorefractive procedures 841
    recent advances in 841
Keratorefractive surgeries 854
Keratotic plaque 271
Keratotomy, transverse 843, 857
Keratouveitis, herpetic 658
Ketoconazole 668
Ketotifen 769
Kidney function test 385
Kinetic B-scan ultrasonography 452
Kinetic echography 219
Klippel-Feil syndrome 229, 386
Klippel-Trénaunay syndrome 239
Knapp's palsy, inverse 391
Knapp's procedure 391, 383
    augmented 383
    modified 383
Koeppe nodules 466
Kolker's technique 573, 574*f*
Krachmer grading scale 689*b*
Krause accessory lacrimal gland cysts 241
Krause gland 86
Krimsky's method 371
Kyrieleis arteriolitis 501

L

Lacerations 863
Lacrimal anlage duct 93
Lacrimal disorders 62
    acquired 96
Lacrimal drainage system
    congenital abnormalities of 90
    patency of 247

Lacrimal ductal cysts 240
Lacrimal excretory system 87
 developmental disorders of 91
Lacrimal fistula 93
Lacrimal gland 7, 85, 103*f*, 216, 227*t*, 238, 425
 adenoid cystic carcinoma 227, 258, 894
 agenesis 90
 anatomy 123*f*
 aplasia 90
 based therapies 103
 boundaries of 124*t*
 lesions 225, 226*fc*, 237
  clinical features of 225*t*
 swellings, management of 225
Lacrimal irrigation 109
Lacrimal nerve 353
Lacrimal papilla 2, 87
Lacrimal pump 64
 mechanism 88, 89*f*
Lacrimal sac 88, 96, 624
 compressions 94
 diverticula 93
Lacrimal secretory system 85
 developmental disorders of 90
Lacrimal system 122, 895
 anatomy of 85
 congenital disorders of 90
Lacrimal valves, congenital absence of 96
Lactosylceramidosis 424
Lacus lacrimalis 2
Lagophthalmos 38, 64, 67, 73, 164, 638, 884, 885
 causes of 70
 early 885
 management of 78, 84, 84*t*, 885
 mechanical 70
 pathophysiology of 70*fc*
Lambert-Eaton syndrome 289, 292, 293*t*
Lamellar corneal transplantation 723
Lamellar keratectomy 634
 evolution of 717*f*
Lamellar keratoplasty 634, 647, 675, 700, 717, 855
 peripheral 779
 superficial anterior 718
Lamellar procedure 717
Lamellar reconstruction, posterior 55*f*
Lamellar sclerectomy 275
Lamellar treatment technique 858
Lamina fusca 462
Lamina papyracea 130
Laminar airflow hood 739
Landolt C chart 864
Lang's microtropia 395
Lang's syndrome 373
Lang's two-pencil test 365, 366
Langer's lines 50
Larger self-sealed lacerations 866
Laser 551
 ablation corneal refractive procedures 844, 857
 delivery 456
 holographic interferometry 784
 hyaloidotomy 453
 interaction 426
 interferometry 457, 805
 peripheral iridoplasty 551, 549
 photocoagulation 189, 191, 325, 426, 427
  indirect 480

 platform 855
 power
  settings 427
  titration 427
 trabeculoplasty, selective 559
 treatment 597
 wavelength 426
Laser-assisted in situ keratomileusis 653, 665*f*, 826*fc*, 827, 831, 848, 855
 complications of 829, 829*fc*
 evolution of 827
 presbyopic 842
 surgery 825, 827
  conventional 827, 838
 work-up 828
Lash
 loss of 495
 ptosis 38
Lateral canthal resuspension procedure 43, 82, 82*f*
Lateral canthotomy 54, 164
 incision 217*f*
Lateral distraction test 42
Lateral geniculate body 299
 anatomy of 299, 300*f*
Lateral rectus 302*f*, 303, 354, 360*f*, 387
 palsy 287
Lateral semicircular skin flap 54
Lateral tarsal strip 43, 49*f*, 82, 82*f*
Lateral traction test 43*f*
Lattice corneal dystrophy 678
Lazy-T procedure 49
Le Fort's theory 129
Lee's chart 288, 398
Lee's medial canthoplasty 81
Lee's screen 362
Leflunomide 331
Lens 435, 632, 644, 877
 capsule, posterior 473
 Clarke classification of congenital dislocation of 822
 dislocation, anterior 578
 exfoliation of 824
 fitting 797
 fragments
  removal of 455
  retained 820
 hardness of 812
 indication 887
 ocular effects 887
 partial displacement of 821
 placode 405
 status of 445
 subluxation 464
 suspensory ligaments of 462
 vesicle, formation of 405
 zonules of 462
Lenticular refractive surgery 700
Lenticule
 extraction 836
 extraction of 838
 tearing of 837
 tissue 837
Leprosy 639, 899
 lepromatous 495
 reactions 495
Lerdelimumab 170

Lesion
 asymptomatic 238
 detection, screening for 219
 extraorbital 237
 inflammatory 227*t*
 intraconal 237
 localization of 339, 340
 orbital extension of 257*f*
 posterior segment 495
 size determination 456
 space-occupying 143, 237
 well-circumscribed 229
Letter test 311, 807
Leukemia 342, 347, 424
 chronic myeloid 886
 lymphocytic 898
 ocular manifestation of 889
Leukemic cells 424
Leukocoria 185*f*
Leukocytes, role of 607
Levator aponeurosis 19*f*
 recession 81
 repair 35
Levator disinsertion 30
Levator function technique 26
Levator muscle resection 35
Levator palpebrae superioris 6, 20, 24, 25, 65, 68, 84
 muscle 19*f*
Levator recession 69, 158
Levocabastine 769
Levodopa 394
Lhermitte's sign 319
Lid 466, 495, 620
 coloboma of 12
 crease 1
 crutches 33
 drop 31
 edema 863
 fissure, contralateral widening of 20
 lag 38
 lower 8
 margin 2
  abnormalities of 639, 703
  irregularity 56
 opening, apraxia of 61
 peaking of 38
 position of 2
 reconstruction
  principles of 51
  techniques of 51
 retractors, inferior 6
Light
 absorption 413
 adjustable lens calhoun vision 843
 flashes of 400
 intensity of 435
 microscopy 674, 686
 more anisocoria in 340
 near dissociation 337
  causes of 337
 wavelength of 435
Limbal corneal tunnel incision 603*t*
Limbal epithelial transplantation, simple 705, 706
Limbal ischemia 869
Limbal relaxing incisions 843, 857

Limbal stem cell
  deficiency 702, 705, 771, 870
    causes of 702*t*
    management of 702, 705*fc*
    unilateral partial 705
  transplant 873
Limbal transition zone theory 272
Limbus 644, 703, 863
  anatomy of 601, 602*f*
Linear nevus sebaceous syndrome 12
Linear skin defects syndrome 250
Linezolid 322
Lipid keratopathy 683
Lipoidal degeneration, primary 685
Lipopolysaccharide 729
Lipoprotein, high-density 889
Lippman's HOTV test 398, 807
Listing's law 358
Liver function test 385, 402
Local invasion, assessment of 116
Locoregional metastasis, assessment of 116
Lodoxamide 769
Lofgren syndrome 513
Loose zonules, signs of 824
Loteprednol 403
Louis-Bar syndrome 231
Low contrast optotype tests 412
Lowe syndrome 542
Lower eyelid 41*f*, 76, 77
  island flap 57, 58
  margins 19*f*
  medial ectropion, bilateral 48*f*
  retraction 158
    and ectropion, management of 82
    mechanism of 77*fc*
  spacer grafts 83
Lower lid 8
  anterior lamella of 67
  central 117
  lateral canthus 112*f*
  malignant melanoma of 112*f*
  near lateral canthus 112*f*
  seborrheic keratosis over 112*f*
  swelling of 117
  tightening 885
  transconjunctival incision 217*f*
  transcutaneous incision 217*f*
Lower motor neuron 287, 301
Low-molecular-weight heparin 803
Lubricants 770
Lumbar puncture 328
Lutein 414
Lyme disease 479, 639
Lymph node 8, 229, 278
  peripheral 514
Lymphangioma 142, 146, 184*f*, 224
Lymphatic channels, proximity of 201
Lymphatic malformations 239
Lymphedema distichiasis syndrome 23
Lymphoma 194, 211*f*, 214, 227, 899
  disorder of malignant 210*f*
Lymphoproliferative lesions, diagnostic workup of 225
Lynch incision 218

M

MAB21l2 variants 250
Mackie classification 642*t*
Macrolides 17
Macrophage 460
  migration inhibitory factor 713
Macula
  anatomical terminology of 409*t*
  anatomy of 409, 410
  assessment of 805
  development of 410
  different zones of 410
  histology of 409
  lutea 407
Macular buckling 325
Macular coloboma 419
Macular corneal dystrophy 672, 674, 674*t*
  types of 673
Macular dystrophy 686
Macular edema 400, 438, 481, 509, 749
  diabetic 410, 438
Macular function
  crude assessment of 457
  tests 456
Macular granuloma 503
Macular pigments 414
Maculopathy 481
  hypotonic 726
Maddox rod 285, 457
  test 457
Maffucci syndrome 238
Magnesium hydroxide 868
Magnetic implants 260
Magnetic resonance venography 315
Malar sulci 1
Malaria 488
Malignant tumor 225
  management for 119
Malingering, tests for 293, 294
Malyugin ring 815*f*
Manganese 215
Manitoba oculotrichoanal syndrome 12
Mantoux 225
Marcus Gunn jaw-winking
  phenomenon 28
  syndrome 27
  ptosis 20, 21
Marcus Gunn phenomenon 27
Marfan syndrome 694, 822, 896, 900, 902
Margin reflex distance 19*f*, 24, 26, 164
  technique 26
Marginal rotation procedure 45*f*
Marionette lines 63
Martsolf syndrome 250
Masquerade syndromes 507
Mass
  choroidal 448
  painless 241
Massachusetts eye 786
Masson's trichrome 677, 679, 680
Mast cell 460
  stabilizers 769
Match tissue 52
Maternal infection 806
Matrix metalloproteinase-9 629
Matthew-Wood syndrome 250
Maudgal theory 659
Maurice theory 606*f*
Maxillary sinus 132*f*, 173
McDonald's criteria 318*t*
McDonald's diagnostic criteria 318
Measles 639, 899

Mechanical theory, depiction of 532*fc*
Medial canthal
  laxity 42*f*
  plication 83
  tendon 3, 5, 42, 48*f*, 83, 84, 259*f*
Medial distraction test 42
Medial forehead flap 57
Medial orbitotomy approaches 218
Medial rectus 302*f*, 303, 354, 360*f*, 387
  pulleys of 352*f*
Medial spindle 49
  procedure 83
Medial traction test 43*f*
Medial transnasal canthopexy 234
Medial wall decompression 168
Medical nutrition therapy 883
Medicamentosa keratitis 655
Medulloepithelioma
  clinical features of 192
  clinical implications of 192*t*
  differential diagnosis of 192
  management of 192
Megalocornea 823
Meibomian gland 7
  dysfunction 14
Meige syndrome 350
Melanocytes 462
Melanoma
  choroidal 219
  malignant 118
  management of conjunctival 199
Melanosis
  acquired 198
  complexion-associated 195, 196*f*, 197
Melanotic nevi 274
Memantine 596
Membranes, premature rupture of 618
Menace reflex 295
Meninges, tributaries from 307
Meningioma 234, 342, 343, 894
Meningocele 147
Meningoencephalocele 243
Meniscus sign 838
Mental retardation 464
Mersilene mesh 36
Mesenchymal dysgenesis 788
Mesenchyme 405
Meso-zeaxanthin 414
Metabolic diseases 806
Metabolic disorders 304, 576, 899
Metabolically active tissues 213
Metallic artifacts 212
Metamorphopsia 510, 749
Metastasis, choroidal 189, 894
Metastatic endophthalmitis 512
Metastatic lesions 216
Metastatic tumors 189, 509
Methicillin-resistant Staphylococcus aureus 617, 621
Methotrexate 170, 189, 403, 888, 901, 906
Methoxyflurane 888
Methyl alcohol 322
  poisoning 335
  toxicity 323
Methyl methacrylate 473
Methylprednisolone 320, 403, 494
  intravenous 156, 480
Micafungin 668
Miconazole 668

Microaneurysm 500, 890
Microbial keratitis, superadded 686
Microcoria 464
Microcysts 644
Micro-incision vitrectomy surgery 434
Microinvasive glaucoma surgery 556
Microkeratome heads 833
Microphthalmia 224
    lie 223
Microphthalmos 28, 221, 223, 224, 254
Micropulse
    laser therapy 426
    retinal laser 426
Microspherophakia 823
Microsporidia 636t
    species 635t
Microsporidial keratitis
    clinical features of 634
    evaluation of 634
Microtrauma 779
Microtropia 369, 394
    classification of 395
    management of 395
Microvitreoretinal entry 809
Midface complex 75, 77
Midface ptosis, management of 83
Mid-pupil lid distance 67f
Migraine 62, 415
    acute 350
    aura 349
    basilar 349
    hemiplegic 350
    management of 349
    prophylaxis of 350
    with aura 349
    without aura 349
Miliary iris lepromas 495
Millard-Gubler syndrome 287, 287f
Miltefosine 646
Mimicking glaucomatous optic neuropathy 585
Mineral disorders 903
Miniature toy test 397
Minimum inhibitory concentration 668
Mini-scleral lens 798
Minocycline 17
Miosis 400
Miotic agents 548
Mitochondrial deoxyribonucleic acid 32
Mitochondrial respiratory complex 250
Mitomycin C 275, 276f, 588
    use of 770
Mobius syndrome 287
Moist chamber method 746
Molecular mechanisms 151
Moll gland 7
Molluscum contagiosum 112f, 498
Monitor disease activity 509
Monoclonal antibodies 712, 716
Monocular elevation deficit 20, 21
    surgical management of 383
    types of 382
Monocular metamorphopsia 442
Monocular vision loss, sudden 430
Monofocal intraocular lens 843
Mononucleosis, infectious 899
Monovision 843
    testing 827

Mooren's ulcer 632t, 633 634, 777
    classification of 632
    differential diagnosis of 633
    management of 631
Moorfields bleb grading system 562, 563f
Moraxella 648
    catarrhalis 614
Morgagnian, congenital 807
Morning glory syndrome 325
Motility 864
Motion artifact 212
Moutsouris sign 722
Moxifloxacin 753
Moyamoya disease 234
Mucin
    peripheral 659
    secretion 851
Mucocele 242
    clinical features of 242t
    commonly occurs 242
    etiopathogenesis of 242, 242fc
    management of 242, 243fc
    treatment of 242
Mucopolysaccharidoses 462, 899, 902
Mucor, features of 181
Mucous membrane graft 249
Müller cells inhibit 411
Muller's muscle 6, 7, 34, 65, 68, 162, 462
    conjunctival complex 34
    excision 68, 69f
    resection 25, 34
Müller's smooth muscle fibers 162
Müllerectomy 81, 158
Multi-drug therapy 494
Multifocal choroidal tubercles 496
Multifocal choroiditis 470, 487, 507, 512
Multifocal discrete yellowish lesion 496
Multifocal panuveitis 487
Multilayered amniotic membrane graft 627
Multiple basal-cell carcinomas 229
Multiple canalicular wall
    aplasia 92
    dysgenesis 92
    hypoplasia 92
Multiple myeloma 225
Multiple sclerosis 304, 313, 318t, 335, 337, 413, 478, 479, 483, 517, 741, 890
    ocular manifestation of 890
Mumps 426
Munson sign 695
Muscle
    contraction of 290
    cut 256f
    entrapment 384
    fibrosis 384
    peripheral 301
    predominant disease 151, 152f
    pulley 352
        heterotopia of 352, 395
    tendon, slippage of 373
    twitching 291
Muscular branches 100
Muscular disorders 900
Muscular dystrophy 900
Musculoaponeurotic system, superficial 50
Mustarde's double Z-plasty 29
Myasthenia gravis 22, 31, 289, 290, 293t, 379, 741, 900

    management of 289
    therapies for 291
Mycobacteria 322
Mycobacterium
    leprae 495, 884
    tuberculosis antigen 497
Mycophenolate mofetil 169, 403, 480, 494, 716, 717, 901
Mycotic keratitis 661
Mydriasis, congenital 464
Mydriatic cycloplegics 901
Myectomy 388
Myelin coating 296
Myelinated nerve fibers 326
Myelinated retinal fibers 327
Myeloid leukemia 424, 898
Myoconjunctival sutures 256f
Myoconjunctival technique 256
Myocutaneous flaps 57
Myocysticercosis 211f, 384, 504
Myokymia 4
Myopia 439, 787
    correction of 845
    high 326
    pathological 448, 804
    severe 415
    transient 400
Myopic astigmatism 845

N

N-acetylcysteine 660
Nafziger's sign 149
Nagel's anomaloscope 309
Nail injury 628
Nanophthalmos 542
Nasal cavity 103f
Nasal mucosa transplantation 873
Nasal visual field 337
Nasociliary nerve 348, 353
Nasojugal flap 57, 58
Nasolabial folds 63
Nasolacrimal duct 88, 89, 259f
    obstruction 96, 647
        congenital 91, 93, 619
Nasopalpebral lipoma-coloboma syndrome 12
Nasopharyngeal carcinoma 342
Natamycin 667
Necrotizing retinitis 521
Necrotizing scleritis 272, 399, 404
    management of 403
Necrotizing stromal keratitis 655, 657
Nedocromil 769
Neisseria 648
    gonorrhoeae 617 618
Neoadjuvant chemotherapy 227
Neodymium-doped yttrium aluminum garnet 631
Neoplasia 272
Neoplasms 347
Neovascular age-related macular degeneration 410
Neovascular bleeding 831
Nerve
    course of 304
    fibers 462
    intracranial portion of 296, 297

peripheral 126
stimulation test, repetitive 291
stretching of 164
superior division of 305
Nerve palsy 281
management of
fourth 286
third 283
sixth 288f
Nervous system, peripheral 242
Neural crest cell 464
Neuritis 643
Neurocutaneous syndromes 12
Neurocysticercosis 504
Neuroectoderm, layer of 463
Neuroectodermal cells 407
Neurofibromatosis 144, 147, 209f, 231, 232fc, 542, 900
diagnostic criteria of 231
ocular features of 231
ocular manifestation of 231, 233fc
Neurogenic innervations, abnormal 20
Neurologic examination 243
Neurological disorder, context of 307
Neuromuscular junction 289, 289f, 290
abnormality 289
physiology of 289
Neuron, first-order 338
Neuro-ophthalmic manifestation 905
Neuropathic pain 836
Neuropathic tonic pupil 341
Neuroprotective agents 594, 594f
Neuroretinitis 318, 483, 485, 496, 521
Neurotoxins 741
Neurotrophic epithelial keratopathy 655
Neurotrophic factors 594
Neurotrophic keratitis 641, 642t, 658
management of 656
treatment of moderate-severe 642
Neurotrophic keratopathy 640
Nevoid basal cell carcinoma syndrome 229
Newer drug delivery system 555
Newer modern techniques 625
Newer technology 421
Newer treatment modalities 18
Niacin 749
Nicotinamide 595
adenine dinucleotide phosphate oxidase 889
Nicotinic acid 887
Niemann-Pick disease 424
Night blindness 763, 881
Night vision disturbances 835
Nishida's procedure 390
Nitric acid 868
Nitric oxide synthase 889
Nitrofurantoin 888
Nocturnal lagophthalmos 70, 72
Nodular iris lepromas 495
Nodular scleritis 399
Noduloulcerative lesion 117
Noise artifact 212
Nonaccommodative esotropia 369
Nonarteritic anterior ischemic optic neuropathy 322, 332, 880
management of 331
Noncontact specular microscopy 690
Noncontiguous areas 511

Noncorticosteroid immunomodulatory therapy 468, 517
Nonendoscopic endonasal 100
Non-Hodgkin's lymphoma 342
Noninfectious causes 486
Noninfective causes 499
Noninvoluting congenital hemangioma 239
Nonmarginal eyelid laceration, repair of 860
Nonmelanocytic benign epithelial tumors 268
Nonneoplastic vascular abnormalities 239
Non-nutrient agar 402
Nonpigmented epithelium 460
Nonporous implants 262
advantages of 263
Nonproliferative diabetic retinopathy, severe 427
Nonspecific orbital inflammatory disease 225, 226
Nonsteroidal anti-inflammatory drugs 226, 329, 403t, 473, 660, 871
Norepinephrine transporter inhibition 553
Nothnagel syndrome 281f
Nuclear lesions 280
Nucleus management 819
Numerous radial contraction folds 459
Nummular chorioretinal depigmented scars 494
Nummular corneal endotheliitis 505
Nutritional supplements 851
Nystagmus 62, 326, 807, 891

O

Objective prism test 294
Obstructive sleep apnea syndrome 880
Occipital cortex
layer of 300
types of cells in 300
Occipital encephaloceles 243
Occipital lobe 300
Occlusive retinal vasculitis 484, 516
Occlusive vasculitis 181f
Occult choroidal
lesions 470
neovascularization 456
Ocular adnexa 62, 905
tumor invasion 894
Ocular albinism 406
Ocular anomalies 386, 806
Ocular biometry 811, 812
Ocular blood flow 593
role of
Ocular causes 647
Ocular changes 495
Ocular chemical injuries 868
Ocular cicatricial pemphigoid 647, 703
Ocular clinical features 436, 471
Ocular coloboma 464
Ocular colobomata 418
Ocular conditions 800
Ocular cysticercosis 504
management of 503
Ocular developmental anomalies 542
Ocular dimension, anomalies of 822
Ocular discomfort 246
Ocular disease 413, 906
isolated 494

Ocular disorders 424, 428
Ocular examination 281, 284, 500, 512, 764, 807, 824, 859
Ocular features 343, 472, 486
Ocular herpes simplex virus 825
Ocular histoplasmosis syndrome 508
Ocular history 23
Ocular hypertension 153, 413, 481
Ocular immune privilege, breach of 713
Ocular inflammation 428, 683, 891
Ocular injury 810
classification of 862
Ocular investigations 778
Ocular lesions 494
Ocular lubricants 640
Ocular lymphoma 451
Ocular manifestation 511, 512, 762, 823
management of 231
Ocular melanocytosis 195, 198
Ocular motility, laws of 358
Ocular motor
deficits 891
nerve palsies 521
Ocular movements, supranuclear control of 301
Ocular mucous membrane pemphigoid 16
Ocular myasthenia
diagnostic tests of 289
gravis, signs for 290t
Ocular myopathy 289
Ocular pain 653
Ocular perfusion pressure 593t
role of 593f
Ocular phototoxicity 435
Ocular prosthesis 245, 599
Ocular radiation
hazards of 894
indications of 894
Ocular sarcoidosis 513, 903, 906
diagnosis of 903
Ocular screening criteria 474t
Ocular side-effects 520, 546, 547, 548
Ocular signs 290
Ocular structure, anomalies of 822
Ocular surface 76, 208, 272
disease 660
index 731
disorder 623, 648, 705
epithelium 869
manifestation 905
system 86
treatment of 230t
tumors of 267
Ocular surface squamous neoplasia 272, 275, 276, 278
diagnosis of 274
management for 274
microscopic appearance of 273
Ocular surgery 649, 697
Ocular torticollis 20
Ocular toxocara 502
Ocular toxocariasis 503
Ocular toxoplasmosis 500
Ocular trauma 428, 649, 859, 862, 868, 874
management of penetrating 862
penetrating 253, 862, 865, 867
score 863, 863t
Ocular tuberculosis 496
Oculocerebrocutaneous syndrome 12

Oculoectodermal syndrome 12
Oculomotor nerve 126
   fascicle 341
   palsy 379
Oculomotor nucleus 360, 360*f*
Oculoplasty 1
Ointments 691
Oligoarticular arthritis type 472
Olopatadine 769
Omega-3 essential fatty acids 851
Onchocerciasis 899
One-and-a-half syndrome 302*f*, 304
Opaque bubble layer 830, 838
Opaque dark green solution 456
Opaque media 456
Open door fractures 129
Open-angle glaucoma, juvenile 541
Ophthalmia neonatorum 618
   clinical features of 618
   etiology of 618
   management of 618
Ophthalmic artery 408, 463
   branch of 124*f*, 353
Ophthalmic complications 62
Ophthalmic signs 424
Ophthalmic solution 642
Ophthalmic viscoelastic device 773
Ophthalmic work-up 802
Ophthalmologic evaluation 863
Ophthalmoplegia 207
   bilateral internuclear 891
   chronic progressive external 22, 24, 32, 289*f*
   external 32
   internuclear 302, 304
Ophthalmoscopy
   direct 780
   indirect 285
Optic atrophy 312, 494, 501, 875
Optic canal 296
Optic chiasma 296, 336
   anatomy of 297, 342
   formation of 298
Optic cup
   formation of 405
   neuroectoderm of 463
Optic disc 317, 323, 407
   anomalies 324
   coloboma 325
   edema 481, 509
      and atrophy 234
   hyperemia 493
   pit 324
   swelling 332
   tilted 326
Optic glioma 343
Optic nerve 126, 137, 138, 146, 164, 107*f*, 209*f*, 217*f*, 297, 307, 327, 336, 413, 425, 426, 888, 890, 895
   anatomical subdivision of 295
   coloboma of 419
   cut 256*f*
   cut section, length of 256*f*
   damage, pathogenesis of 531
   develops 407
   diseases 443
   drusen 334
   dysfunction, signs of 307
   function tests 307
   glioma 209*f*, 234, 894
   hypoplasia 503
   indication 888
   intraocular portion of 296*f*
   intraorbital portion of 296*f*
   lesions 237
   ocular effects 888
   position related to 217
   tumors 234
      lateral to 217
      medial to 217
Optic nerve head 297, 317
   damage 529
   drusen 334, 420
      complications of 421
      treatment of 421
   vascular supply of 297
Optic nerve sheath 334
   decompression 329
   meningioma 140
Optic neuritis 321*t*, 415, 442, 890
   atypical 319*t*
   management of 317
   steroids in 320
   treatment 320
      of demyelinating 320
   typical 319*t*
Optic neuropathy 240, 454, 882
   anterior ischemic 330, 421
   drug-induced 335
   traumatic 316, 317
Optic pathways, myelination of 326
Optic tract 336
Optic vesicle 405
   formation of 405
Optical biometry 805
Optical coherence tomography 189, 196, 312, 315, 319, 323, 328, 335, 410, 446, 470, 485, 491, 493, 496, 501, 509, 510, 534, 540, 699*f*, 784, 879, 887, 888
   angiography 319, 333, 335, 411, 471, 508-512, 879
Optical iridectomy 766
Optical penetrating keratoplasty 766
Optical property 415
Optical quality 848
Optical shadowing, posterior 501
Optical therapy 392
Optokinetic nystagmus test 295
Ora serrata 407, 461
Oral antiviral drugs 657
Oral carbonic anhydrase inhibitors 545
Oral contraceptive pills 888
   ocular effects of 888
Oral corticosteroids 403, 901
Oral maintenance therapy 498
Oral medications 351
Oral mucosal epithelial cell transplantation 872
Oral steroids 638, 646
Oral valacyclovir, use of 499
Oral vitamin A 765*t*
Orbicularis muscle 53*f*
   ciliaris 461
   oculi 2, 3
   weakness of 33
Orbit 212, 217*f*, 424, 425, 905
   applied anatomy of 172
   blowout fracture of 129
   bony walls of 121*f*
   congenital lesions of 220
   contents of 122
   cystic lesions of 219
   development of 121
   functional anatomy of 120
   pathology 204
   pseudotumor of 384
   surgical anatomy of 120
   surgical approaches to 217
   surgical spaces of 173*f*, 216, 216*f*
   temporal extraconal space of 176*f*
   vascular lesions of 239
   venous drainage of 125
Orbital adnexa 253
Orbital anatomy 120
Orbital apex 220
   syndrome 347
Orbital bones 163
Orbital canal and fissures 128
Orbital cavity
   postoperative rehabilitation of 260
   reduces 207*f*
Orbital cellulitis 146, 171, 172, 175, 176*f*, 180*f*, 182*f*
   clinical features of 174 185*f*
   complications of 178
   differential diagnosis of 182
   treatment of 146*fc*
Orbital computed tomography 335
Orbital cysticercosis 184
Orbital decompression 157, 165*f*, 167, 168
   bilateral 234
   indications of 168
   techniques 164
Orbital dermoids 142, 230*t*
Orbital disease 193, 202
Orbital exenteration 275
   anterior 257*f*, 258*f*
Orbital fascia 122, 123*f*
Orbital fat 163
Orbital fibroblast 151
   two subgroups of 152*f*
Orbital floor 130, 164
   defect 136*f*
   fracture 379, 384, 859
   titanium implant 136*f*
Orbital fracture 129, 132*t*, 133*f*
   reconstruction of 134
   repair 218
      indications for 131
Orbital hematoma 859
Orbital hypertelorism 220
Orbital imaging 202, 214, 228
   modalities 145*t*
Orbital implants 134, 261
   complications of 261
Orbital inflammation 185*f*
Orbital lesions 139*t*, 145*t*, 202, 894
Orbital lobe cysts 241
Orbital lymphangioma 184
Orbital lymphatic drainage 125
Orbital mass, anterior 228
Orbital metastasis 894
Orbital mucormycosis 258*f*
Orbital myositis 384

Orbital neurofibroma 234
Orbital pathology 202, 205, 217
Orbital pseudotumor 894
Orbital pyramid, bones forming walls of 120t
Orbital radiotherapy 157
Orbital retinoblastoma 184
Orbital roof 131
Orbital septa 2
Orbital septum 4
Orbital spread, suspected 208
Orbital structural factors 395
Orbital trauma 208, 262
    clinical evaluation of 131
Orbital tumor 168
    lateral posterior 234
Orbital venous drainage 126f
Orbital wall 130f
    blowout fractures 863
Orbitopalpebral cysts, management of 252f
Orbito-palpebral plexiform neurofibroma 232
Orbitopathy, inflammatory 168
Orbitotomy 217, 218, 236
    anterior 217, 217f
    incisions for 237f
    lateral 217
    surgical incisions for 217f
Oréfice's sign 488
Organ transplant 505
Organic amblyopia 393
Organoid nevus syndrome 229
Organophosphate toxicity 299
Oropharynx, examination of 75
Ortho Duane's retraction syndrome, management of 387
Orthophoria 362f
Orthoptic treatment 392
Oscillopsia 62
Osler-Weber-Rendu disease 239
Osseo-integrated orbital prosthesis 260, 261f
Osteogenesis imperfecta 897
Osteo-keratoprosthesis 737
Osteoma 211f
Osteomeshó orbital implant 136f
Osteo-odonto-keratoprosthesis, modified 736, 736f
Otolith organs 303
Otorhinolaryngological evaluation 75
OTX2 variants 250
Oxycephaly 223f
Oxygen
    radicals 456
    tension 435
Oxymetazoline 33
Ozurdex 438, 483

P

P16 gene 272
Pachymetry 542, 697, 785, 789, 826
    map 834
Pagetoid sebaceous gland carcinoma 274
Pagetoid spread 119
Pain 246, 622 628
    facial 330
    severe 628
Painless lower eyelid nodules, differential diagnosis of 117t

Palinopsia 347
Palmaris longus tendon 36
Palpable orbital mass 207
Palpation 863
Palpebral fissure
    horizontal 250, 251f
    narrowing of 84
Palpebral lobe cysts 241
Pancreatic neuroendocrine tumors 892
Panophthalmitis 496
Panretinal photocoagulation 598
Panum's area 368
Panuveitis 512
    bilateral 489
Papilla 295
Papilledema 314, 328
    Frisen's grading of 314
    optical coherence tomography in 313
    pathogenesis of 314
Papillitis 318
    isolated 521
Para sellar tumors 344
Paracentral scotoma 530
Paragangliomas 893
Paralysis
    accommodation 295
    lingual 330
Paralytic lagophthalmos 70, 71, 75, 80f
Paramedian pontine reticular formation 360f
Paranasal sinus 132, 173, 216, 257
    disease, orbital signs of 208
Paraproteinemia, suspected 225
Parasitic uveitis, posterior 488
Parasympathetic innervation 124
Parasympathetic outflow 340
Parietal lobe lesions 347
Parinaud's syndrome 66, 337
Park's method 388
Park's monofixation syndrome 395
Park's three-step test 284
Parkinson's disease 66, 741
Parkinson's syndrome 741
Parotid gland, palpation of 75
Parry-Romberg syndrome 896
Pars ciliaris 2
Pars lacrimalis 2
Pars plana 461
    incision 567f
    surgery 453
    vitrectomy 325, 453, 477, 480, 504
        surgery 602
Pars planitis 479, 481
Pars plicata 461
Partial density averaging 212
Partial levator myectomy 28
Patch graft 627, 670, 766
Patellar fossa 821
Patent fistula beneath sclera 564f
PAX gene 464
PAX6 genes 464
Pediatric cataract
    aspects of 806
    morphology 807
Pediatric hyperthyroidism, causes of 901
Pediatric orbital
    cellulitis 179fc
    fractures 131

Pediatric proptosis
    causes of 141f
    etiology of 141
    management of 141, 142
Pediatric retinal detachment 437
Pediatric uveitis 507
Pediatric vision assessment 397
Pegging system 264
Pelli-Robson contrast sensitivity chart 311
Pellucid marginal degeneration 700, 777
Pen torch method 726
Penicillin
    allergic patients 521
    desensitization 521
    intravenous 499, 521
Pentacam parameters 698t
Perfluorocarbon liquid 436
Perfluorocarbon perfused vitrectomy 437
Perfluorodecalin 436
Perfluorooctane 436
Perfluoro-octyl bromide 436
Perfluoroperhydrophenanthrene 436
Perfluoropropane 442
Perfluorotributylamine 436
Peribulbar block 865
Pericentral scotomas 511
Perilesional edema 504
Perinuclear antineutrophil cytoplasmic antibody 402
Periocular adjunctive procedures 83
Periocular steroids 481, 485, 519
    indications for 519
Perioral complex 75, 78
Perioral lines 63
Periorbital complex 76
    examination of 75
Periorbital lines 63
Periosteal flaps 59
Peripapillary retinal fiber 313
Peripheral corneal thinning 404
    disorders 777
        differential diagnosis of 777t
Peritomy 255f, 256f
Peroxisome proliferator-activated receptor 170
Persistent corneal epitheliopathy 730
Persistent fetal vasculature 407, 504
Persistent infection 647
Persistent pupillary membrane 464
Persistent vitreous opacities 501
Peters' anomaly 524, 524f, 526, 527f, 542
Phace syndrome 144
Phacodonesis 824
Phacoemulsification 602, 602fc, 818
Phakic intraocular lens 844, 848
    indications of 845
    posterior chamber 846
    rotation 848
    types of 845, 845t
Phakic toric intraocular lens 782
Phakomatosis 230, 231t, 576
    pigmentovascularis 231
Phenothiazines 887
Phenylephrine 33
    test 34
Phenytoin 351
Pheochromocytoma 892, 893
Phosphenes 415

Phosphocholines 646
Photodocumentation 865
Photodynamic therapy 189, 455
Photophobia 590, 622, 653, 669, 702, 875
Photopsia 400
   central 508
   peripheral 508
Photoreceptor dysfunction 450*t*
Photoreceptors develop inner segments 406
Phthalmic surgery 801
Phthisis bulbi 245*f*
Pierre-Robin sequence 896
Piezoelectric crystals 219
Pigment epithelium, posterior 460
Pigmentary retinopathy 24
Pigmented epibulbar lesions, differential diagnosis of 195*t*
Pigmented epithelium 460
Pigmented filamentary fungi 662
Pilocarpine 773
Pilocytic astrocytomas 343
Pimaricin 667
Pinch technique 233
Pinhole test 294
Pituitary abnormalities 250
Pituitary adenoma 342
Pituitary apoplexy 342, 343, 878
Pituitary carcinomas 343
Pituitary dysfunction 895
Pituitary tumors 343
Placido disc principle 783
Placido-based videokeratography 794
Placoid chorioretinitis, relentless 509, 511
Plagiocephaly 223*f*
Plana surgery 453
Plaque brachytherapy 192, 277
Plasma
   dilution 740
   exchange 320
   proteins, accumulation of 684
   regain, rapid 402, 479, 521
Plasmapheresis 292
Plasmodium falciparum infection 488
Platelet-derived growth factor 889
Pleomorphic adenoma 216
Pleomorphism 601
Pleoptics 394
Plica semilunaris 2, 70*f*, 277
Plus 10 reading test 294
Pneumatic displacement 442
Pneumatic retinopexy 752
Pneumocystis carinii 499
Polar cataract, small posterior 808
Polaroid scotometer 362
Polio 639
Poliosis 494
Polyangiitis 486
Polyarteritis nodosa 483, 486, 484, 487, 898
Polycaprolactone 135, 136*f*
Polycoria 464
Polyenes 667
Polyglactin 263
Polyglycolic acid 135
Polylactic acid 483
Polymegathism 601
Polymerase chain reaction 469, 521, 620, 656, 664

Polymethyl methacrylate implant, insertion of 255*f*
Polymethylmethacrylate 254, 814, 845
Polymyositis 898
Polyneuropathy, chronic idiopathic demyelinating 741
Polytetrafluoroethylene 482
Polytrauma 862
Pontine reticular formation, posterior 287, 302, 302*f*
Porous implants 263
   advantages of 263
Porous polyethylene 135, 263
Porphyria 902
Porphyrins accumulate 902
Posaconazole 669
Posner-Schlossman syndrome 477, 504
Postenucleation socket syndrome 246
Posterior polymorphous
   corneal dystrophy 690
   dystrophy 690
Posterior uveal melanoma
   clinical features of 193
   clinical manifestations of 193*t*
   differential diagnosis of 193
Posterior vitreous detachment 439, 836
   classification of 440
   clinical implications of 440
   effects of 439
Postfixed chiasma 297
Post-Hotz procedure 47*f*
Post-Jones procedure 44*f*
Postkerato-refractive surgery ectasia 790
Post-laser therapy 551
Post-LASIK 851
   dry eyes 836
   fungal keratitis 665*f*
   ocular dryness 851
Postlateral tarsorrhaphy 80*f*
Postpars plana vitrectomy surgery glaucoma 587
Postrefractive ectasias 791
Postseptal tissues 9
Postsynaptic acetylcholine 289
Potassium hydroxide 402, 868
Preauricular skin appendages 229
Preaxial system 297
Pre-descemet
   corneal dystrophy 672, 676
   endothelial keratoplasty 722, 723*t*
   membrane 604
      microscopic anatomy of 604*fc*
Prednisolone acetate 468, 519, 809
Prednisone 502
Preloaded graft 724
Presbyopia 826
Presbyopic refractive surgery 856
Preseptal cellulitis 146, 174, 176*f*, 183, 183*f*, 208
Preseptal tissues 9
Presumed ocular histoplasmosis syndrome 512
Pretectal nucleus 336
Previous socket surgery 245
Primary acquired melanosis 195, 196*f*
   clinical features of 198
   histopathology of 198

Primary acquired nasolacrimal duct obstruction 96
Primary intraocular lymphoma 494
   clinical features of 194
   clinical manifestations of 194*t*
   differential diagnosis of 194
Primitive neuroectodermal tumor 187
Prism 392
   bars 364
   dioptre 286, 387
   test 295
Progestational steroids 871
Progression, assessment of 543
Propamidine isethionate 645
Prophylactic laser photocoagulation 485, 507
Propionibacterium 15
Propranolol 350
Proptosis 136, 136*fc*, 137*t*, 140*f*, 142, 143*fc*, 144*fc*, 185*f*, 212*f*, 228, 234, 242, 639
   acute 184*f*
   bilateral 136
   differential diagnosis of 142*t*
   intermittent 138
   management of unilateral axial 137, 139
   measurement of 210
   painful 138
   unexplained 207
Propylthiouracil 161
Prosopagnosia 346
Prostaglandin 475
   analogs 544-546
Prostanoid receptor agonist 554, 555
Prosthesis 246*f*
   examination of 247*f*
   thickness of 247*f*
   volume of 247*f*
   weight of 247*f*
Protanopia 310
Protein
   kinase, rho-associated 692
   water-soluble 607
Proteinaceous fluid 215
Protein-energy malnutrition 767
Pseudo-argyll robertson pupil 281
Pseudo-cherry red spot 424
Pseudodendrites 644
Pseudo-glaucoma 585
Pseudoguttae 687
Pseudoisochromatic chart test 308
Pseudomembrane, conjunctival 622
Pseudomonas 174
Pseudopapilledema 314
Pseudophakic bullous keratopathy 690
Pseudophakic cystoid macular edema 750
Pseudoproptosis 136*fc*
Pseudoptosis 20
Pseudo-von Graefe's sign 281
Pseudoxanthoma elasticum 421
Psoriatic arthritis 478, 901
   juvenile 471
Ptosis 23, 28, 281, 290, 295, 863
   acquired 22, 23
   aponeurotic 30*f*
   congenital 19*f*, 20, 23, 23*t*
      aponeurotic 21
      dysgenetic 20
   correction 29
   crutch 33

evaluation 24t
examination 19f
management of 33
    congenital 22, 23, 25fc
    unilateral 27
mechanical 241
mild 25
moderate 26
severe 26
simple congenital 20
surgery 36
true 20
Pulfrich's phenomenon 319
Pulsatile proptosis 138, 148fc, 149fc
    differential diagnosis of 147
Pulse
    duration 426
    echo technology 219
    therapy 403
Puncta 87
Punctal agenesis 91
Punctal apposition 52
Punctal canalization, incomplete 91
Punctal occlusion 79, 640, 661
Punctal plugs 851
Punctate epithelial keratitis 654
Punctate erosions 644
Pupil 281, 314, 323, 332, 335, 624, 863
    dilatation 815f
    dilation 388
    enlargement 819
    examination of 295, 335, 826
    nondilating 515, 813
    normal 337
    ovalization 848
Pupillary dysfunction, unexplained
    efferent 208
Pupillary examination 875
Pupillary fibers 337
Pupillary margin plastered 466
Pupillary membrane 463
    begins 464
    formation 820
    peeling 816
    removal of 819
Pupillary pathway 336, 337f
    defect 336
Pupillary reaction 164, 864
Pupillary reflex 294
    assessment 859
Pupillary zone 459
Pupillomotor fibers 341
Pure blowout fracture 129
Purified protein derivative 402, 469, 485, 497
Purkinje vascular entopic phenomenon 458
Pursuit originates, neural pathway for 302
Pursuit pathway 303f
Putaminal hemorrhage 351
Pyrex Lester-Jones tubes 103f
Pyrimethamine 502

Q

Quadrilateral bone flap 235
Quantiferon gold 225
Quenching singlet oxygen 414
Quickert procedure 45

R

Rab18 deficiency 250
Rabinowits–McDonnel grading 786
Racial melanosis 195, 197
Radiation necrosis 234
Radioactive iodine therapy 162
Radioactive tracer accumulation 213
Radiotherapy
    forms of 277
    role of 227
Rainbow glare 834
Ramsay Hunt syndrome 639
Randot test 364, 366
Rapamycin 716, 717
Rapid eye movements 359
Rare syndromes 12
Rathke's pouch 343
RBP4 gene 250
Reactive arthritis 474, 478
    syndrome 477, 478
Recombinant human interferon alpha-2b 275
Recovery instruments 739
Recti muscles, insertion of 356f
Recurrent corneal erosion syndrome 628, 631t, 686
    differential diagnosis of 628
    etiology of 629t
    management of 630t
Red blood cell 500, 864
Red eye 653
    causes of 615t
Redundant skin 20
Re-epithelialization, rapid 769
Reflection aberrometry 840
Reflex 397
    lacrimation 108
Refraction 371, 374
Refractive corneal surgery 843
Refractive correction 789
Refractive error 28, 807, 832, 849
Refractive lens exchange 701, 842, 848
Refractive lenticular extraction 829, 854
Refractive procedures 841
Refractive surgery 801, 825, 848, 849t, 855
    newer advances in 841
    prior 825
Refractory macular edema 453
Regional lymph node examination 229
Rehabilitation, methods of 257
Reid's baseline 206f, 207f
Reis–Bückler's corneal dystrophy 677, 800
Reiter's disease 520
Reiter's syndrome 520, 898
Relapsing polychondritis 484, 517
Relative afferent pupillary defect 164, 228, 335, 863
    quantification of 336
Renal carcinoma 892
Renal cell carcinoma 892
Renal failure, chronic 683
Restrictive strabismus 383, 384
    etiology of 383
    pathogenesis of 383
Retina 405, 425, 426, 435, 441, 453, 498, 503, 895
    anatomy of 407
    blood supply of 407, 408
    cryopexy of peripheral 480
    embryological evolution of 406
    inflammation of 441
    lesions 510
    neurosensory 407
    outer 507
Retinal arterial microaneurysm 430
Retinal blood vessels 531
Retinal break 504
Retinal capillary hemangioblastoma 892
Retinal coloboma 405
Retinal detachment 400, 436, 454, 481, 504, 516, 749, 751, 810, 823, 865
    detection of 219
    surgery 507
Retinal diseases 443
Retinal disorders 405
Retinal ganglion cells 889
Retinal hemangioblastoma 189, 893
Retinal infections 498
Retinal infiltrates 890
Retinal ischemia 430
Retinal lesions, active 511
Retinal manifestation 890
Retinal necrosis 484
    acute 484, 487, 505, 506
    progressive outer 483, 506
    treatment of acute 506
Retinal nerve fiber layer 488
Retinal pigment epitheliitis, acute 487
Retinal pigment epithelium 187, 189, 193, 407, 413, 414, 461, 470, 494, 887, 888
    functions of 413
Retinal tear 454
Retinal toxicity, dye-induced 422
Retinal toxoplasmosis, punctate outer 501
Retinal vascular
    attenuation 509
    endothelium 498
Retinal vasculitis 483, 496, 497, 521
    idiopathic 483, 485
    stages of 484
Retinal vein occlusion 240, 509, 881, 887
    secondary to 427
Retinal vessels 407, 451
    normal 451
    reach periphery 406
    sheathing of 890
Retinal-neuro-cutaneous cavernous hemangioma syndrome 231
Retinitis 467
    focal 521
    peripheral 506
    pigmentosa 421, 448
Retinoblastoma 258, 272, 504, 894
    classification of 191
    clinical features of 190t
    diagnosis of 191
    differential diagnosis of 190, 190t
    treatment modalities for 191
Retinochoroidal coloboma 419
    classification of 420
Retinochoroiditis 501
Retinochoroidopathy 508
Retinoic acid 872
    synthesis pathway members 250
Retinol-binding protein, role of 250

Retinopathy
    acute zonal occult outer 507
    diabetic 436, 448, 878
    leukemic 425
    of prematurity 437, 504
Retrabeculectomy 570
Retraction, mild-to-moderate 69
Retractor reinsertion 49
Retrobulbar bilobed cystic lesion 185*f*
Retrobulbar injection 598
Retrobulbar neuritis 318
Retrochiasmal lesion 342
Retro-illumination mode 681*f*
Retrolaminar region 297
Retrolental cells 865
Retroprosthetic membrane 736, 737
Rhabdomyosarcoma 146, 183, 224, 227, 228, 228*fc*, 229*t*, 347, 894
    clinical features of 228
Rhegmatogenous
    complications 503
    retinal detachment 419, 453, 504
Rhese position 205
Rheumatoid arthritis 402
Rheumatoid disease 898
Rheumatoid factor 901
Rhizomelic skeletal dysplasia 250
Rhizopus-induced orbital cellulitis 182*f*
Rho kinase inhibitors 725
Rhokinase inhibitors 553
Rhomboid flap 57, 58
Riboflavin 779, 882
    deficiency, ocular manifestation of 882
Ribonucleic acid 276, 724
Riddoch phenomenon 346
Rieger anomaly 523, 525
Rieger syndrome 525
Rifabutin 886
Rigid gas permeable 700, 796
    keratoconic design 798
    lens 798
Rim deformities 864
Ring of Zinn 347
Rituximab 170, 189, 518
Rizzuti phenomenon 694
Rochon-Duvigneaud syndrome 128
Rod dysfunction syndromes 450
Rods and cones
    anatomy of 448
    dysfunction 448, 449
    physiology of 448
    spatial distribution of 449
Rome-Vienna protocol 736
Rosette cataract, early 811
Rosiglitazone 749
Rowsey–Hay's technique 866
Rubella syndrome, congenital 687, 899
Rundle's curve 153, 153*f*
Ruptured capsule 812
Rural injury setting 867

S

Sabin's tetrad occurring 501
Sabouraud dextrose agar 402, 664
Saccades 359
Saccadic abnormalities 891
Salmonella 478, 648

Salzmann nodular degeneration 683, 685
Salzmann's nodules 610
Sands of Sahara 833
Sarcoidosis 337, 448, 474, 475, 479, 508, 513, 898, 903, 906
    early-onset 507
    test for 402
Satellite lesions 644
Sattler's layer 462
Scaphocephaly 223*f*
Scarring, stage of 689
Scheimpflug imaging 698
    principle 783
Schirmer's test 68, 75, 826, 850
    score 731
Schlemm canal appears 406
Schnyder corneal dystrophy 672, 674
Sclera 399, 424, 426, 486, 624, 632, 864, 895
    condenses 406
Scleral buckling 752
    surgery 602
Scleral flap 569*f*
Scleral incisions, type of external 602*f*
Scleral inflammation 399, 403*t*
    classification of 399*fc*
Scleral injury, management of 865
Scleral lens 798
Scleral perforation 864
Scleral show 67
Scleral wounds, closure of 866
Sclerectomy, deep 557
Scleritis 399, 401*t*, 402, 404, 884
    anterior 399, 400, 403
    classification of 399
    diffuse 399
    features of 401
    grading of 400, 400*t*
    infectious 402
    medical management of 402
    posterior 399, 400, 403, 494, 878
    surgical management of 403
    treatment of 402
    types of 404
Sclerocorneal tunnel 602
    incision 603*t*
Scleromalacia perforans 399, 403, 404
Sclerosant therapy 146, 239
Sclerosing panencephalitis, subacute 487
Sclerosis, amyotrophic lateral 741
Sclerotomy, posterior 567*f*
Scotoma
    absolute 511
    central suppression 362*f*
    suppression 362
Sea blue histiocyte syndrome 424
Sebaceous cell carcinoma, histopathology of 119
Sebaceous gland carcinoma 55*f*, 112*f*, 116
Sebaceous nevus, cutaneous 229
Seborrheic blepharitis 14, 17
Second-order neuron 338
Seidel scotoma 530
Seidel's test 864, 866
    positive 649
    pressure 649*p*, 650
Seizures 504
Self-sealed corneal wounds 866

Sella
    anatomy of 298*f*
    turcica 204
Semicircular canals 303
Semicooked fish 489
Senile furrow degeneration 777
Senile ptosis
    causes of 29
    diagnosis of 29
    management of 29
    pathophysiology of 29
Sensation, foreign body 241
Sensory root, smaller lateral 72
Sentinel lymph node biopsy 201
Septic choroiditis 512
Sequential ray tracing aberrometry 840
Seronegative spondyloarthropathy 472
    treatment of 478
Serotonin
    antagonist 351
    reuptake inhibitor, selective 428
Serous 429
    choroidal effusions 429
Serpiginous choroiditis 467, 496, 509, 510
Serpiginous choroidopathy, management of 513
Serum
    angiotensin-converting enzyme 139, 225, 402, 514
    calcium 225
    thyroid-stimulating hormone 159
Sheehan's syndrome 878
Sheridan's ball test 371, 397
Sheridan's letter chart 398
Sherrington's law 358, 359
Shield ulcer 768, 771
    treatment for 770*fc*
Shigella 478, 648
Shimmer sign 838
Shin's technique 573, 573*f*
Short-wavelength automated perimetry 535, 537, 538*f*
    advantages of 539*t*
    disadvantages of 539*t*
Sickle cell anemia 899
Siedel's test 561
Silicone 36, 135, 262
    elastomers 260
    hydrogels 782, 798
    oil-filled eyes 804
Simultanagnosia 346
Simultaneous macular perception 360
Sine wave gratings 412
Single canalicular wall
    aplasia 92
    dysgenesis 92
    hypoplasia 92
Sino-orbital mucormycosis 181*f*
Sinskey hook 725
Sinus
    frontal 173
    ostium, obstruction of 242
Sixth cranial nerve
    anatomy of 283, 305
    palsy 287
Sjögren hand 398
Sjögren's syndrome 659
Skeletal anomalies 229

Skewed radial axis 698
Skin
    closure of 244
    crease
        defects 37
        high 31
    flaps 50
    graft 56
        full-thickness 56, 56
    ichthyosis of 48f
    incision 234, 259f
        line of 235f
Skull, fontanelles of 222f
Sleep apnea 332
Sleep test 32, 291
Slice thickness 206
Sliding tarsoconjunctival flap 58
Slit-lamp 624, 739
    biomicroscopy 440, 455, 763, 780
        bleb grading systems 561
    examination 92, 663, 675, 679f, 695, 742, 862, 864
Slit-scanning corneal tomography system 783
Small incision cataract surgery 601
Small-incision lenticule extraction 829, 841, 855
    complications of 837t
Smile refractive surgery 836, 838
Smooth eyelid margin 52
Smooth mucosal lining of eyelid 52
Smooth muscle fibers 400
Smooth pursuit 359
Snake bites 741
Snap-back test 42, 43f
Snellen's visual activity 310, 412
Snowballs 479, 513
Socket surgery complications 266f
Sodium
    chloride, topical 660
    cromoglycate 769
    hyaluronate 819
    hydroxide 868
    tetradecyl sulfate 239
Soft hydrogel lenses 798
Soft keratoconic designs 782, 798
Soft tissue 225, 424
    contracture 248
    moderate 204
    structures 105f
    window 209f-211f
Solid tissue biopsy 402
Solid tumors, treatment of 886
Solitary choroidal tuberculoma 496
Solitary fibrous tumor 137, 141
Somatostatin 713
Soutter scalp incision 234
SOX2
    anophthalmia syndrome 249
    genes 249, 250
    protein 250
Spastic entropion 46, 61
Spatial contrast sensitivity 412
Special surgical instruments 814t
Spectacles 699
Spectral domain optical coherence tomography 431, 508, 511, 512
Specular examination 742

Specular microscopy 686, 739, 745, 845
Sphenoid door jamb 166f
Sphenoid sinus 173
    mucocele 342
Spheroidal degeneration 684
Sphincter pupillae 460, 463
Spielmann's theory 380
Spin-spin relaxation 215
Spiramycin 502
Spirochete treponema pallidum 520
Split thickness dermis 403
Spondyloarthropathies 477
    juvenile-onset 474, 507
Squamous cell carcinoma 112f, 116, 271
    demonstrate intense 214
    invasive 273
Squamous papilloma 269
Squint surgery 390
Squint, evaluation of 371, 374
Staining antineutrophil cytoplasmic antibody 486
Stallard–Wright lateral orbitotomy incisions 217f
Staphylococcal blepharitis 14, 15
Staphylococcal marginal keratitis 654
Staphylococcus
    aureus 15, 174, 613, 619
    epidermidis 15, 174
Staphylomas 404
Static procedures 79
Stellate wounds 866
Stem cell transplantation, types of 728
Stepladder classification 525, 526f
Stereoacuity 458
Stereopsis 361, 364, 365, 378
    development of 364
    physiological basis of 364
    tests for 294
Stereostatic dissociation 346
Sterile keratitis 838
Sterile melts 737
Steroid 17, 333, 650, 887
    advantages of 637t
    after keratoplasty 638
    appropriate use of 809
    complications of 519
    disadvantages of 637, 637t
    effects of 637
    intravitreal 438, 473
    role of 636, 646
    sparing agent 331, 770
    supplemented 520
    therapy 468
    use of 317
Steven's scissors 253
Stevens–Johnson syndrome 245, 703
Stickler syndrome 897
Still's disease 474
Stimulus 311, 416
    deprivation amblyopia 394
Strabismic amblyopia 393, 394
Strabismus 28, 326, 352, 365, 396, 788, 823-825
    acquired restrictive 384
    congenital restrictive 383
    fixus 352
    motor adaptations of 366-368
    nonsurgical management of 392

sensory adaptation to 363, 367, 366
surgery 157, 292, 387
transposition surgeries in 390
Streptococcus pneumoniae 174, 613, 619, 648
Stroma 462, 678, 745
    choroidal 462
    superficial 677
Stromal anatomy 855
Stromal atrophy 493
Stromal corneal dystrophy
    congenital 672, 675
    types of 672, 673t
Stromal disease 655
Stromal dystrophies 672
Stromal fibrosis 611
Stromal invasion 643
Stromal keratitis 655, 658
    management of 656
    pressure-induced 834
Stromal lamellae, peculiar arrangement of 605
Stromal rejection 709
    treatment of 710
Stromal scarring 655
Stromal swelling pressure 607
Stromal thinning 644
Stromal ulceration 644
Stromal vascularization 611
Sturge–Weber syndrome 231, 239, 428, 542, 900
Subciliary incision 218
Subconjunctival betamethasone sodium phosphate solution 482, 519
Subconjunctival fibrosis 703
Subcutaneous areolar tissue 2, 3
Subdural hematoma 304
Subepithelial fibrillary lines 694
Subepithelial scar 695f
Subepithelial zone, pathological responses of 610
Subhyaloid hemorrhage 450
Submacular hemorrhage, classification of 441
Submandibular lymph nodes 201
Submuscular areolar tissue 2
Suborbicularis dissection 258
Suborbicularis oculi fat 83, 84
Subperiosteal space 172, 216
Subretinal cysticercosis 504
Subretinal neovascularization 470
Subsequent neovascularization 483
Subtarsal incision 218
Sub-Tenon's
    injection, posterior 818
    space 172
    triamcinolone 482, 519
Sugiura's sign 466, 493
Sulfa-based drugs 581
Sulfadiazine 502
Sulfamethoxazole 502
Sulfonamides 428, 886
Sulfuric acid 868
Sun classification 464
Sunglasses 685
    protective 836
Superior oblique muscle, anatomy of 357
Superior oblique overaction
    diagnosis of 378, 379

etiology of 378
management of 378, 379
Superior oblique palsy 379, 380
management of 285, 286*fc*
Superior oblique tendon
insertion of 356*f*
transfer 391
Superior ophthalmic vein 240, 306, 353
Superior orbital fissure 234, 287, 348*f*, 353*f*
syndrome 128, 347
Superior rectus
contralateral 305
transposition 387
Superior sulcus deformity 246*f*
Superomedial neurovascular bundles 258
Superotemporal homogenous mass 209*f*
Superotemporal hypodense lesion 210*f*
Superoxide dismutase 889
Suppression, extent of 362
Suprachoroidal effusion 454
Suprachoroidal lamina 462
Suprachoroidal space 428
Supraciliary lamina 462
Supranuclear lesions 280
Supranuclear pathways 301
Surgery
basic principles of 243
goals of 217, 233
principle of 220
timing of 808
Surgical debulking 146
Surgical excision 146, 275
Surgical limbus, application of 601, 602
Surgical management 68, 133, 766
principles of 227
Surgical procedure, basic selection criteria for 849
Surgical technique 253, 255, 651, 735
and principles 233
Surgical treatment 79
Surgical viewing systems 454
Surgicel 259
Susac syndrome 484, 517
Suspensory materials 36
Suture
granuloma 373
lid margin 53
lines 229
material 715
removal, technique of 575
tarsal plate 53
tarsorrhaphy, temporary 80
Sutureless micro-incision vitrectomy 434
Sutureless surgery 434
Suturing technique 715
Swan syndrome 749
Swinging flashlight test 336
Switch flap 59
Swollen lens 578
Symblepharon
congenital 13, 223
lysis 872
Sympathetic fibers 340
Sympathetic hyperactivity 342
Sympathetic nervous system 338
diagnose abnormalities of 338
Sympathetic ophthalmia 254, 508
risk of 257
Sympathetic ophthalmitis 487, 489, 490

Symptomatic band keratopathy 473
Syndromic craniosynostosis 222*t*
Syndromic variants 12
Synechiae, posterior 467, 493, 515, 820
Synechiolysis 819
Synoptophore 361, 361*f*, 365-366
test 294
Syphilis 402, 499, 520
acquired 521
neuro-ophthalmic manifestations of 521
primary 521
secondary 521
tertiary 521
Systemic agents, mechanism of action of 545
Systemic anomalies 224, 243
Systemic antibiotics 627
Systemic anticoagulants 876
Systemic antifungal therapy 669
Systemic connective tissue disorders 485
Systemic disease 227, 413, 421, 503, 641, 660, 898-900
Systemic disorders 542, 877, 898
Systemic evaluation 193, 229
Systemic immunosuppression 517
Systemic immunosuppressive therapy 474
Systemic inflammatory disorders 226, 337
Systemic lupus erythematosus 402, 479, 484-486, 490, 516, 879, 898, 903
ophthalmic manifestations of 880
tests for 402
Systemic lymphoma 451
Systemic metastasis 278
Systemic nonsteroidal anti-inflammatory drugs 403
Systemic sclerosis 897
Systemic steroids 485, 499, 505, 710
role of 515
Systemic therapy 473, 519, 715
Systemic thyroid status 164

T

T cell
activation 7813*f*
differentiation 714*f*
inhibitors 403, 480
receptor 708, 713*f*
regulatory 714*f*
T helper cells, role of 152*f*
T2-weighted image 215, 216
Taches de Bougie 513
Tachyzoite 500
eventually ceases 500
Tacrolimus 403, 716, 717
Taenia solium 184, 503
Tamoxifen 887
Tangent screening 294
Tardive dyskinesia 350
Tarsal plate 2, 5
Tarsal surface, anterior 19*f*
Tarsoconjunctival flaps 58
Tarsorrhaphy 80, 157, 885
lateral 80
temporary 254
Taurine deficiency 322
Taxonomy 459
Tear
breakup time 24, 75, 642
drop sign 132

drop supplements 627
film 24, 605
evaporation 609*f*
meniscus height 75
secretion 86
basics of 86
substitutes 885
preservative-free 872
supplements 660
Tectonic keratoplasty 766
Tectonic patch graft 627
Telangiectasia
focal 332
hereditary hemorrhagic 239
Telecanthus 28, 29, 220, 221
Teller acuity
card 397, 807
chart 370
Template technique 233
Temporal artery biopsy 331
Temporal contrast sensitivity 412
Temporal retinal fibers 337
Temporalis muscle transfer 885
Tenectomy, posterior 379
Tenon's advancement 872
Tenon's capsule 253, 399
anterior 256*f*
dissection 255*f*, 256*f*
fibrous 217
posterior 256*f*
Tenon's patch graft 627, 651
Tenon's prolapse 373
Tenon's space 217
Tenoplasty flaps 872
Tenotomy 379
Tenzel flap 54, 57
Teprotumumab 170
Teriflunomide 321
Terrien's marginal degeneration 777
Terson syndrome 431, 432, 445
Tetracycline 17, 428, 872
hydrochloride 521
Thalamic infarct 351
Therapeutic indications 60
Therapeutic vitrectomy 516
Thiamazole dosage 161
Thiamine 882
Thiel-Behnke corneal dystrophy 677
Thinner slices 206
Thioridazine 887
Third cranial nerve
anatomy of 283
palsy 280
congenital 21
Third nerve palsy 280, 283*fc*
management of acute onset 283
procedures for 391
Third-order neuron 338, 340
Thoracic endosonography 906
Thygeson's superficial punctate keratitis 636*t*
Thymectomy 292
Thymic hyperplasia 289
Thyroglobulin 160
Thyroid
associated ophthalmopathy 150
dysfunction 162
ophthalmopathy 158, 164, 384
stimulating immunoglobulins 161
tests 160

Thyroid eye disease 62, 66, 67f, 137, 140, 150, 157, 170, 211f, 894
   orbital decompression for 218
   pathogenesis of 152f
   pathophysiology of 151f
Thyroid function test 155, 158, 159, 291
   interpretation of 160, 160t
Thyroidectomy 162
Thyroid-related ophthalmopathy
   clinical features of 150
   diagnosis of 150
   etiopathogenesis of 150
   management of 150
Thyroid-stimulating hormone 151, 159, 161
   receptor 151
      antibodies 160, 161
Thyroid-stimulating immunoglobulin 160
Thyrotropin-releasing hormone 159
Tissue 35
   acoustic impedance 219
   adhesives 627, 634, 670, 778
   autogenous 263
   biopsy 514
   cyst 500
      infraorbital 500
   defects, large 860
   donors 740
   engineered endothelial keratoplasty 725
   high-density 203
   intermediate-density 203
   labelling 743
   low-density 203
   origin 113t
   processing 742
   removal 839
   storage of 742
Titanium mesh 136f
Titmus stereo test 364, 366
TNM classification, drawbacks of 278
Tobacco 322, 324
Tocilizumab 170, 331, 518
Toluidine blue 274
Tonic convergence 363
Tonic pupil, etiology of 341
Tonometry 826
Topical agents, classes of 545
Topical steroid 634, 638, 646, 660, 809, 833
   sparing agents 616
Topiramate 329, 350, 886
Topographic echography 219
Topography systems, application of 784
Topography-guided
   laser treatment 840
   photorefractive keratectomy 782, 796
   procedure 839
Toric intraocular lens implantation 857
Torsion, evaluation of 285
Torsional kestenbaum 388
Toxic amblyopia 321
Toxic anterior segment syndrome 772, 775t
   etiology of 773b
Toxic optic neuropathy 313, 321-323
   differential diagnosis of 323
   ethyl alcohol-induced 324
   management of 321
   neuroimaging in 323
Toxin 342, 343
   theory 768

Toxocara
   canis 488, 503
   cati 503
   larvae 503
Toxocariasis 488, 504, 899
Toxoplasma 506
   gondii 500
   retinitis 500, 505
   retinochoroiditis 448, 499
Toxoplasmosis 488, 499, 500, 512, 899
   acquired 501
   congenital 501, 502
Trabectome 556
Trabecular meshwork fibers, inflammation of 467
Trabeculectomy 570, 571, 591
   complications of 565
   releasable sutures in 572
Trabeculitis 476
Trabeculotome 591, 592f
Tractional retinal detachment 453, 485
Transconjunctival anterior retinal cryotherapy 598
Transconjunctival medial
   orbital approach 218
   orbitotomy incision 217f
Transcranial orbitotomy 218
Transforming growth factor 152, 713f, 714
Transfrontal orbitotomy 234, 235
Transient disc ischemia 334
Transient ischemic attacks, episodes of 429
Transient light sensitivity syndrome 834
Translaminar pressure 532
Transplantation of Human Organs Act 740
Transpupillary thermotherapy 189, 191
Transscleral cyclophotocoagulation 515, 570
Transscleral diode cyclophotocoagulation 515
Transscleral microwave cyclodestruction 570
Trapdoor fracture 129
Trapezoid incision 602
Trauma 342, 347, 444
   penetrating 437, 859
   signs of 132f
Traumatic chiasmal syndrome 343
Traumatic subluxation 822
Traumatic subretinal hemorrhage, management of 441
Treacher Collins syndrome 896
Treponema pallidum 402, 521
Tretinoin 826
Triamcinolone acetonide 433, 770, 818
Tricarbocyanine anionic dye 433
Trichromacy, anomalous 309
Trichromatic theory 308, 416
   extension of 416
Trigeminal nerve 126, 495
Trigonocephaly 223f
Trimethoprim 502
Triplanar incision 603f
Trocar placement 604t
Trochlear nerve 353
Tropicamide 467, 473
Trypan blue 432, 773
Tscherning aberroscope 840
Tubercles, choroidal 496
Tuberculin sensitivity test 497
Tuberculin skin test 402, 497

Tuberculoma, choroidal 496
Tuberculosis 137, 138, 143, 226, 479, 496, 500, 639, 899
   tests for 402
Tuberous sclerosis 231
Tubulointerstitial nephritis 507
Tuck-in lamellar keratoplasty 779
Tumor 1, 193, 225, 274, 878
   adnexal 257
   conjunctival 267, 894
   diagnosis of 219
   epithelial 268
   extraocular 186
   growth of 233
   larger size 193
   lymphoid 894
   measurement of 219
   medium-size 193
   necrosis factor 152, 518, 713, 714, 729, 886
      alpha 141, 473, 770
   primary 277
   secondary 234
   small-size 193
   vascular 894
Tunnel creation, manual technique of 852
Turner syndrome 327, 464

U

Ulcer
   geographic 654
   heals 771
   marginal 624, 654
Ulcerative colitis 478
Ulcerative keratitis, peripheral 777
Ultrasonic endoscopic dacryocystorhinostomy 99
Ultrasonography 139, 153, 202, 238
   B scan 193
Ultrasound biomicroscopy 189, 507, 778, 808
Ultra-wide-field fluorescein angiography 471
Unilateral axial proptosis
   causes of 137, 138b, 237t
   differential diagnosis of 237
   etiology of 138b
   investigation of 137
Unilateral proptosis 136, 147
   differential diagnosis of 147b
Unilateral ptosis
   clinical features of 27
   diagnosis of 27
   etiopathogenesis of 27
Unilateral wipe-out syndrome 488
Upper canaliculus 87
Upper eyelid 24, 29f, 41f, 42f, 76, 119, 176f
   cicatricial entropion 46f
   crease incision 218
   defect, full-thickness 56f
   entropion 46f, 56
   loading 81, 81f
   margins 19f
   nevus 112f
   retraction 67f, 158
      management of 81
   skin 217
Upper lid 8, 112f
   capillary hemangioma of 112f
   mass 118

retractors recession 885
skin 217*f*
squamous papilloma of 112*f*
Upper motor neuron 301
Upper respiratory tract infection 143, 184
Urinary tract infection 888
Urrets-Zavalia syndrome 719
Uthoff's phenomenon 319
Uvea 435, 459, 886
    effusion syndrome 448, 494
    indication 886
    lymphoid infiltration 494
    lymphoma 189, 194
    ocular effects 886
    tissue, anatomy of 459
    tract, blood supply of 463
Uveal melanoma 214, 258, 894
    management of posterior 193
Uveitic cataract 809, 816*f*
Uveitic glaucoma 577, 579
Uveitic stage, acute 492, 493
Uveitis 400, 451, 459, 465*t*, 466, 468, 468*t*, 470, 471, 473, 486, 507, 517, 519, 568, 817, 848, 878, 884
    acute anterior 467
    bilateral chronic 517
    cataract surgery 817
    chronic 817
        anterior 467
    classification of 464
    complications of 514
    glaucoma hyphema syndrome 749
    granulomatous 465*t*
    infectious 818
    infective 499
    intermediate 477, 478, 481, 508
    lens associated 491
    management of intermediate 478
    moderate-to-severe 468, 519
    nongranulomatous 465*t*, 476
    noninfectious 482
    periocular steroids for 481
    posterior 486, 505, 906
    recurrence of 516, 820
    requires intensive treatment 495
    severe unilateral anterior 481, 519
    steroid treatment trial, multicenter 483
    subretinal fibrosis with 512
    syndrome 507
    traumatic 507
    type of posterior 486
    unilateral intermediated 481, 519
    unilateral posterior 481, 519
    vitrectomy in 516
Uveitis nomenclature 465*t*, 467*t*
    classification 465*t*
        standardization of 464, 465*t*
Uveoparotid fever 513

V

Valacyclovir 657
Valleys of Kuhnt 461, 462
Valve of Rosenmüller 88, 96
van Herrick's technique 726*t*
Vancomycin 753, 833
Vancomycin-resistant S. aureus 177
Varicella zoster 426

uveitis 516
virus 486, 487, 499
Vascular endothelial growth factor 724, 871, 891
Vascular occlusive diseases 878
Vasculitic diseases 401
Vasculitides 226
Vasointestinal peptide 713
Vasostimulatory factor, mechanism of action of 607*fc*
Venereal disease research laboratory 402, 479, 485, 521
Venous dilatation and tortuosity 425
Venous drainage 9
Venous lymphatic malformation 143
Venous malformations 239
Ventral pontine syndrome 287
Ventriculocele 243
Vernal keratoconjunctivitis 700, 702, 768
Vernier acuity 458
Verteporfin 455
Vertical diplopia, evaluation of 379
Vertical lid split incision 217*f*, 218
Vertical muscle palsy, procedures for 391
Vertical saccades 302
Vertical steps 530
Vertigo 330
Vessels, choroidal 406
Vestibular nuclei 303
Vestibular reflex 359
Vestibulo-ocular
    pathway 303*f*
    reflex 302
Vicryl interrupted sutures 256*f*
Vicryl suture 256
Victus femtosecond laser platform 855
Videokeratography 698
Vigabatrin 322, 888
Vigorous therapy 499
Vincristine 147, 191
Viral conjunctivitis 616
Viral culture 656
Viral endotheliitis 655
Viral hepatitis, active 740
Viral infections, history of 287
Viral keratitis 638*t*, 648
    steroids in 637
Viral uveitis 466
Visa classification 154
Visa system 155*t*
Visceral larvae migrans 503
Visceral lesions 892
Visceral mesoderm 405
Viscocanalostomy 557
Viscoelastic technique mimicking 719
Vision 677, 678, 680
    awareness, disorders of 346
    bilateral diminution of 474
    decrease of 702
    diminution of 788
    poor gain of 749
    quality 448
    threatening necrotizing process 399
    unilateral sudden diminution of 442
Vision loss 348, 708
    acute 345
    chronic 345
    moderate-to-severe 675

nonorganic 312
permanent 509
prevention of irreversible 467
Visual acuity 281, 284, 312, 314, 316, 323, 328, 410, 624, 697, 703, 726, 780, 824, 826, 833, 834, 859, 864, 887, 888
    assessment of 397, 807
    diminution of 674
    functional 311
    meter test, potential 457
    methods of testing 397
    mild reduction of 774
    reduced 400
    uncorrected 832
Visual agnosia 345
Visual allesthesia 346
Visual assessment 397, 398
Visual axis 684
    opacification formation 809
Visual complaints, nonorganic 295
Visual compromise 874
Visual cortex 299, 300, 888
    anatomy of 301*f*
    electric stimulation of 415
Visual decrease 678
Visual development, abnormalities of 20
Visual evoked 807
    potential 224, 311, 457, 535, 765, 877
    response 317, 319, 333, 370, 805, 811
Visual fibers' representation 299
Visual field 312, 315, 317, 319, 322, 327, 333, 342, 508, 511, 512, 537*f*, 877
    analysis 879
    central depression of 531
    changes 529, 536
    defect 313, 313*t*, 335, 420
        types of 529, 530*f*
    evaluation of 312
    examination 323, 331
    loss, peripheral 530
    testing 344
Visual hallucinations 347
Visual impairment 345, 868
Visual loss 441
Visual outcome 334
    postoperatively 515
Visual pathway 299*f*
    anatomy of 299
    diseases 413
    integrity of 307
Visual prognosis 818, 879
Visual rehabilitation 514, 598, 781, 809
Visual status assessment 374
Visualizing vascular lesions 216
Visually evoked response 397
Visual-spatial relation, disorders of 346
Vital structures 130, 131
Vitamin 882
    A 881
        deficiency 415, 762, 766, 881
    B_1 882
        deficiency of 881
    B_{12} 882
    B_2 882
        deficiency of 881
    B_3 595
    C 882
        deficiency of 881

Index

D 882
    deficiency of 881
  deficiency 882
  disorders 903
Vitiliginous chorioretinitis 508
Vitiligo 494
Vitreal inflammation 499
Vitrectomy 507, 752, 809
  cutter 453
  diagnostic 516
  setup, basic components of 453
  surgery, evolution of 434
  timing of 455
Vitreomacular traction 453, 480, 749
Vitreoretinal complication 836, 848
Vitreoretinal lymphoma, primary 189
Vitreoretinal surgery 436, 490, 516
Vitreoretinopathy
  familial exudative 503
  proliferative 422
Vitreous 454, 471, 498, 503, 824, 865
  amyloidosis of 451
  biopsy 453
  cavity 436
  inflammatory reaction 493
  opacification, progressive 490
  opacities 477
  procedures 579
  syneresis 453
Vitreous detachment
  management of posterior 440
  partial posterior 440
  stages of posterior 440
Vitreous hemorrhage 150, 451, 453, 465, 490
  causes of 451
  complications of 453
  diagnosis of 452
  etiology of 451t
  fate of 451
  pathogenesis of 432
  recurrent 516
  treatment of 452
  types of 450
Vitritis 451
Vogt's limbal girdle 682
Vogt's striae 694, 695f

Vogt-Koyanagi-Harada disease 492
Vogt-Koyanagi-Harada syndrome 447, 487, 489, 491, 494, 498, 508
  diagnostic criteria of 493
Voltage-gated sodium channels 290
Vomiting 373
von Hippel-Lindau disease 231, 891, 900
von Recklinghausen disease 231
Voriconazole 645

Waardenburg anophthalmia syndrome 250
Walker-Warberg syndrome 325
Warburg micro syndrome 250
Watson's classification 632t
Wave theory 600, 600fc
Wavefront testing 827
  methods of 840
Wavefront-guided
  ablation 840
  procedure 839
Weber syndrome 281f
Wedge-resection procedure 46f
Wegener's granulomatosis 483, 485, 486, 648
Weil-Marchesani syndrome 897, 903
Weis procedure 43
Weskamp-Cotlier syndrome 231
White dot syndrome 507
  multiple evanescent 470, 487
White eye blowout fracture 131
Whitnall's ligament 10f, 86
Wildervanck syndrome 386
Willis circle 298, 298f, 342
Wilson's disease 899, 902
Wilson's technique 572, 573f
Wolfring accessory lacrimal gland cysts 241
Wolfring gland 86
Woods classification 464
Worth four dot test 361, 362f, 367
Worth's ivory ball test 371, 397
Wound
  closure 860
  construction, types of 602fc
  exploration 860
  leaks 435, 727

repair 860
tension, assessment of 53
Wyburn-Mason syndrome 231, 239

Xanthelasma over upper lid and lower lid 112f
Xerophthalmia 762, 765t, 881
  classification of 762t
  ocular manifestation of 763
Xerophthalmic fundus 763, 881
Xerosis, conjunctival 763, 881
X-linked recessive 450
X-ray
  clinical applications of 204
  orbit 132, 865
  principle of 203, 203f

Yellow lid sign 486
Yellow-white
  lesions 507
  nodule 334
Yersinia
  enterocolitica 159
  species 478
Yttrium aluminum garnet laser hyaloidotomy 431

Z

Zaidman theory 659
Zeaxanthin 414
Zehenders 150
Zeis gland 7
Zinn annulus 353, 353f
Zonular dehiscence 454
Zonular weakness 754
Zonulolysis 819, 820
Z-plasty 50
Zygomatic artery 8
Zygomatic bone 204
  lysis 210f
Zygomycetes 181

EU GSPR Authorised Reprsentative
Logos Europe, 9 rue Nicolas Poussin
1700, La Rochelle, France
Phone: +33 (0) 6 67 93 73 78
E-mail: contact@logoseurope.eu